# Handbook of Radiation Oncology

## Basic Principles and Clinical Protocols

Edited by

**Bruce G. Haffty, MD**
*Professor and Chairman*
*Department of Radiation Oncology*
*University of Medicine and Dentistry of New Jersey*
*Robert Wood Johnson Medical Center*
*and*
*Associate Director*
*Cancer Institute of New Jersey*
*New Brunswick, NJ*

**Lynn D. Wilson, MD, MPH**
*Professor*
*Clinical Director and Vice Chairman*
*Residency Training Program Director*
*Department of Therapeutic Radiology*
*Yale University School of Medicine*
*New Haven, CT*

JONES AND BARTLETT PUBLISHERS
*Sudbury, Massachusetts*
BOSTON    TORONTO    LONDON    SINGAPORE

*World Headquarters*
Jones and Bartlett Publishers
40 Tall Pine Drive
Sudbury, MA 01776
978-443-5000
info@jbpub.com
www.jbpub.com

Jones and Bartlett Publishers
Canada
6339 Ormindale Way
Mississauga, Ontario L5V 1J2
Canada

Jones and Bartlett Publishers
International
Barb House, Barb Mews
London W6 7PA
United Kingdom

Jones and Bartlett's books and products are available through most bookstores and online booksellers. To contact Jones and Bartlett Publishers directly, call 800-832-0034, fax 978-443-8000, or visit our website, www.jbpub.com.

Substantial discounts on bulk quantities of Jones and Bartlett's publications are available to corporations, professional associations, and other qualified organizations. For details and specific discount information, contact the special sales department at Jones and Bartlett via the above contact information or send an email to specialsales@jbpub.com.

The authors, editor, and publisher have made every effort to provide accurate information. However, they are not responsible for errors, omissions, or for any outcomes related to the use of the contents of this book and take no responsibility for the use of the products and procedures described. Treatments and side effects described in this book may not be applicable to all people; likewise, some people may require a dose or experience a side effect that is not described herein. Drugs and medical devices are discussed that may have limited availability controlled by the Food and Drug Administration (FDA) for use only in a research study or clinical trial. Research, clinical practice, and government regulations often change the accepted standard in this field. When consideration is being given to use of any drug in the clinical setting, the health care provider or reader is responsible for determining FDA status of the drug, reading the package insert, and reviewing prescribing information for the most up-to-date recommendations on dose, precautions, and contraindications, and determining the appropriate usage for the product. This is especially important in the case of drugs that are new or seldom used.

**Production Credits**
Executive Publisher: Christopher Davis
Associate Editor: Kathy Richardson
Editorial Assistant: Jessica Acox
Production Director: Amy Rose
Production Editor: Daniel Stone
Associate Marketing Manager: Ilana Goddess
Manufacturing Buyer: Therese Connell
Composition: Auburn Associates, Inc.
Cover Design: Kate Ternullo
Printing and Binding: Malloy, Inc.
Cover Printing: Malloy, Inc.

**Library of Congress Cataloging-in-Publication Data**
Haffty, Bruce G., 1950-
    Handbook of radiation oncology : basic principles and clinical protocols / Bruce G. Haffty, Lynn D. Wilson.
        p. ; cm.
    Includes bibliographical references and index.
    ISBN-13: 978-0-7637-3143-4
    ISBN-10: 0-7637-3143-9
    1. Cancer—Radiotherapy—Handbooks, manuals, etc.    I. Wilson, Lynn D. II. Title.
    [DNLM: 1. Neoplasms—radiotherapy—Handbooks. 2. Radiation Oncology—methods—Handbooks.
QZ 39 H138h 2009]
    RC271.R3H33 2009
    616.99'40642—dc22
                                                                                    2008007269

6048

Printed in the United States of America
14  13  12  11  10      10  9  8  7  6  5  4  3

## Dedication

We dedicate this book to our families.

### The Hafftys
To my wife Kathy and children Lauren, Sarah, and Brian.


### The Wilsons
To my wife Nancy and children Hunter and Victoria.
Also to my parents who taught me the value of hard work, discipline,
and integrity.

# Contents

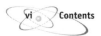

# Foreword

We hope that this book will be a valuable resource to those caring for patients undergoing radiation therapy. It is our intent that this handbook can be used by a broad range of professionals, including radiation and medical oncologists, residents and fellows, medical students, physicists, dosimetrists, therapists, and nurses, as a brief, but thorough reference. Although all of the chapters cover general oncologic principles, workup, staging, and multidisciplinary aspects of treatment, the book is focused on those issues most pertinent to patients undergoing radiation therapy.

The first 9 chapters of the book are devoted to the basic principles of physics and radiobiology, specific technologies including brachytherapy, radiosurgery, unsealed sources, as well as some general oncologic principles. These are followed by disease site-specific chapters that cover the majority of malignancies treated with radiation therapy.

It is difficult, in the context of a relatively limited pocket-size handbook, to completely cover all of the issues related to radiation treatment. In our original concept and design of the book, we decided to reach out to experts, who would contribute what they felt to be the most pertinent, relevant and practical information. In this regard, we are pleased that we have been able to include many of the leading experts throughout the fields of radiation oncology, biology, and physics in this effort.

Throughout the book, brief text boxes are inserted, which highlight specific points and studies. The intent of these text boxes is to highlight critical issues or landmark studies that are felt to be essential to our understanding or management of the disease.

Whether you are a practicing radiation oncologist looking for a brief reference for patient management; a student of medicine, nursing, physics, dosimetry, or therapy orienting yourself to the field; or a resident, fellow, or practicing radiation oncologist looking for a general review, we hope you will find this book a practical and useful resource.

**Bruce G. Haffty, MD**
**Lynn D. Wilson, MD, MPH**

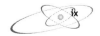

# Contributing Authors

**Kaled M. Alektiar, MD**
Department of Radiation Oncology
Memorial Sloan-Kettering Cancer Center
New York, NY

**Penny Anderson, MD**
Department of Radiation Oncology
Fox Chase Cancer Center
Philadelphia, PA

**Johanna Bendell, MD**
Division of Medical Oncology
Duke University Medical Center
Durham, NC

**James D. Brierley, MB**
Professor
Department of Radiation Oncology
University of Toronto
Princess Margaret Hospital
Toronto, ON, Canada

**Thomas A. Buchholz, MD**
Professor and Chairman
Department of Radiation Oncology
The University of Texas
M.D. Anderson Cancer Center
Houston, TX

**Paul M. Busse, MD, PhD**
Clinical Director
Department of Radiation Oncology
Massachusetts General Hospital
Associate Professor
Department of Radiation Oncology
Harvard Medical School
Boston, MA

**Mark K. Buyyounouski, MD, MS**
Associate Member
Department of Radiation Oncology
Fox Chase Cancer Center
Philadelphia, PA

**Ömür Karakoyun Çelik, MD**
Assistant Professor of Radiation Oncology
Department of Radiation Oncology
Celal Bayar University Faculty of Medicine
Turkey

**Brian Chang, MD**
Radiation Oncologist
Radiation Oncology Associates, P.C.
Fort Wayne, IN

**Daniel T. Chang, MD**
Assistant Professor
Department of Radiation Oncology
Stanford University
Stanford, CA

**Michael G. Chang, MD**
Assistant Professor
Director Residency Program
Department of Radiation Oncology
Virginia Commonwealth University
Richmond, VA

**Seungtaek Choi, MD**
Department of Radiation Oncology
The University of Texas
M.D. Anderson Cancer Center
Houston, TX

**Peter W.M. Chung, MD**
Department of Radiation Oncology
Princess Margaret Hospital
University of Toronto
Toronto, ON, Canada

**Joseph Colasanto, MD**
Radiation Oncologist
Department of Radiation Oncology
St. Francis Hospital
Hartford, CT

**Brian G. Czito, MD**
Assistant Professor
Department of Radiation Oncology
Duke University Medical Center
Durham, NC

**Bouthaina Dabaja, MD**
Assistant Professor
Section Chief Lymphoma
Radiation Oncology Department
The University of Texas
M.D. Anderson Cancer Center
Houston, TX

**Roy H. Decker, MD, PhD**
Assistant Professor
Department of Therapeutic Radiology
Yale University School of Medicine
New Haven, CT

**Patricia J. Eifel, MD**
Professor of Radiation Oncology
Department of Radiation Oncology
The University of Texas
M.D. Anderson Cancer Center
Houston, TX

**Deborah Frassica, MD**
Associate Professor
Residency Program Director
Department of Radiation Oncology and
    Molecular Radiation Sciences
Johns Hopkins University
Baltimore, MD

**Molly Gabel, MD**
Associate Professor and Director of
    Clinical Services
Department of Radiation Oncology
The Cancer Institute of New Jersey
Robert Wood Johnson Medical School
New Brunswick, NJ

**Daniel R. Gomez, MD**
Resident
Department of Radiation Oncology
Memorial Sloan-Kettering Cancer Center
New York, NY

**Sharad Goyal, MD**
Instructor
Department of Radiation Oncology
Cancer Institute of New Jersey
University of Medicine and Dentistry of
    New Jersey
Robert Wood Johnson Medical School
New Brunswick, NJ

**Chul Soo Ha, MD**
Professor and Chair
Department of Radiation Oncology
University of Texas Health Science Center
San Antonio, TX

**Bruce G. Haffty, MD**
Professor and Chairman
Department of Radiation Oncology
University of Medicine and Dentistry of
    New Jersey
Robert Wood Johnson Medical School
The Cancer Institute of New Jersey
New Brunswick, NJ

**Michael P. Hagan, MD, PhD**
Professor
Department of Radiation Oncology
Virginia Commonwealth University
Richmond, VA

**Stephen M. Hahn, MD**
Henry K. Pancoast Professor and Chairman
Department of Radiation Oncology
University of Pennsylvania Medical Center
Philadelphia, PA

**Peter Han, MD**
Radiation Oncology
SUNY Downstate Medical Center
Brooklyn, NY

**Louis B. Harrison, MD**
Clinical Director
Department of Radiation Oncology
Continuum Cancer Centers of New York
Chairman of Radiation Oncology
Beth Israel Medical Center and St. Luke's and
    Roosevelt Hospitals
Professor of Radiation Oncology
Albert Einstein College of Medicine
New York, NY

**Jeffrey C. Haynes, MD**
Resident
Department of Radiation Oncology
University of Pennsylvania Medical Center
Philadelphia, PA

**Russell W. Hinerman, MD**
Assistant Professor
Department of Radiation Oncology
University of Florida/Shands Cancer Center
Gainseville, FL

**Eric M. Horwitz, MD**
Associate Professor
Chairman and Clinical Director
Department of Radiation Oncology
Fox Chase Cancer Center
Philadelphia, PA

**Janet K. Horton, MD**
Assistant Professor
Department of Radiation Oncology
Wake Forest University Baptist Medical Center
Winston-Salem, NC

**Kenneth Hu, MD**
Assistant Professor
Department of Radiation Oncology
Continuum Cancer Centers of New York
Beth Israel Medical Center and St. Luke's and
    Roosevelt Hospitals
Albert Einstein College of Medicine
New York, NY

**Geoffrey S. Ibbott, PhD**
Professor and Chief, Section of Outreach
    Physics
Department of Radiation Physics
The University of Texas
M.D. Anderson Cancer Center
Houston, TX

**Salma K. Jabbour, MD**
Assistant Professor
Department of Radiation Oncology
The Cancer Institute of New Jersey
University of Medicine and Dentistry
    of New Jersey
Robert Wood Johnson Medical School
New Brunswick, NJ

**Anwar Khan, MD**
Department of Therapeutic Radiology
Yale University School of Medicine
New Haven, CT

**Sung Kim, MD**
Assistant Professor
Department of Radiation Oncology
The Cancer Institute of New Jersey
University of Medicine and Dentistry
    of New Jersey
Robert Wood Johnson Medical School
New Brunswick, NJ

**Christopher R. King, MD, PhD**
Associate Professor
Department of Radiation Oncology
Stanford Cancer Center
Stanford, CA

**Jonathan P.S. Knisely, MD, FRCP**
Associate Professor
Therapeutic Radiology
Co-Director
Yale-New Haven Gamma Knife Center
Yale University School of Medicine
New Haven, CT

**Andre Konski, MD, MBA, MA, FACR**
Member
Department of Radiation Oncology
Fox Chase Cancer Center
Chief Medical Officer
Fox Chase Cancer Center Partners
Philadelphia, PA

**Nancy Lee, MD**
Associate Attending
Department of Radiation Oncology
Memorial Sloan-Kettering Cancer Center
New York, NY

**Roger M. Macklis, MD**
Professor of Medicine
Department of Radiation Oncology
Cleveland Clinic Lerner College of Medicine
Cleveland, OH

**Ronald McGarry, MD, PhD**
Clinical Associate Professor
Department of Radiation Medicine
University of Kentucky
Lexington, KY

**William M. Mendenhall, MD**
Department of Radiation Oncology
University of Florida/Shands Cancer Center
Gainesville, FL

**James M. Metz, MD**
Assitant Professor and Chief of Clinical
    Operations
Department of Radiation Oncology
Editor-in-Chief, OncoLink
Hospital of the University of Pennsylvania
Philadelphia, PA

**William P. O'Meara, MD**
Department of Radiation Oncology
Memorial Sloan-Kettering Cancer Center
New York, NY

**Brian O'Sullivan, MD**
Department of Radiation Oncology
Princess Margaret Hospital
University of Toronto
Toronto, ON, Canada

**Alan Pollack, MD, PhD**
Professor and Chair
Department of Radiation Oncology
University of Miami Miller School of Medicine,
Miami, FL

**Barry S. Rosenstein, PhD**
Department of Radiation Oncology
Mount Sanai School of Medicine
New York University School of Medicine
New York, NY

**Benjamin D. Smith, MD**
Adjunct Assistant Professor
Department of Radiation Oncology
The University of Texas
M.D. Anderson Cancer Center
Houston, TX

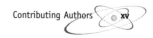

**John H. Suh, MD**
Chairman
Department of Radiation Oncology
Cleveland Clinic
Cleveland, OH

**Joel E. Tepper, MD**
Hector MacLean Distinguished Professor
    of Cancer Research
Department of Radiation Oncology
University of North Carolina School of
    Medicine
Chapel Hill, NC

**Vipul V. Thakkar, MD**
Radiation Oncologist
Southeast Radiation Oncology
Charlotte, NC

**Robert D. Timmerman, MD**
Professor and Vice Chairman
Department of Radiation Oncology
University of Texas Southwestern
Dallas, TX

**Prabhakar Tripuraneni, MD**
Scripps Clinic
La Jolla, CA

**Richard Tsang, MD**
Professor
Department of Radiation Oncology
University of Toronto
Princess Margaret Hospital
Toronto, ON, Canada

**Christina Tsien, MD**
Assistant Professor
Department of Radiation Oncology
University of Michigan Medical Center
Ann Arbor, MI

**Andrew T. Turrisi, III, MD**
Radiation Oncologist-in-Chief
Detroit Medical Center
Professor
Department of Radiation Oncology
Wayne State University School of Medicine
Detroit, MI

**Christopher G. Willett, MD**
Professor and Chairman
Department of Radiation Oncology
Duke University Medical Center
Durham, NC

**Lynn D. Wilson, MD, MPH**
Professor
Vice Chairman and Clinical Director
Department of Therapeutic Radiology
Yale University School of Medicine
New Haven, CT

**Charles G. Wood, MD**
Department of Radiation Oncology
Mary Bird Perkins Cancer Center
Baton Rouge, LA

**Joachim Yahalom, MD**
Attending and Member
Memorial Sloan-Kettering Cancer Center
Professor of Radiation Oncology
Weill Medical College of Cornell University
New York, NY

**Torunn I. Yock, MD, MCH**
Assistant Professor
Harvard Medical School
Department of Radiation Oncology
Massachusetts General Hospital
Boston, MA

**Michael J. Zelefsky, MD**
Professor of Radiation Oncology
Chief, Brachytherapy Service
Memorial Sloan-Kettering Cancer Center
New York, NY

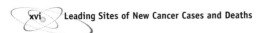
## Leading Sites of New Cancer Cases and Deaths—2008 Estimates

| Estimated New Cases* | | Estimated Deaths | |
|---|---|---|---|
| **Male** | **Female** | **Male** | **Female** |
| Prostate 186,320 (25%) | Breast 182,460 (26%) | Lung & bronchus 90,810 (31%) | Lung & bronchus 71,030 (26%) |
| Lung & bronchus 114,690 (15%) | Lung & bronchus 100,330 (14%) | Prostate 28,660 (10%) | Breast 40,480 (15%) |
| Colon & rectum 77,250 (10%) | Colon & rectum 71,560 (10%) | Colon & rectum 24,260 (8%) | Colon & rectum 25,700 (9%) |
| Urinary bladder 51,230 (7%) | Uterine corpus 40,100 (6%) | Pancreas 17,500 (6%) | Pancreas 16,790 (6%) |
| Non-Hodgkin lymphoma 35,450 (5%) | Non-Hodgkin lymphoma 30,670 (4%) | Liver & intrahepatic bile duct 12,570 (4%) | Ovary 15,520 (6%) |
| Melanoma of the skin 34,950 (5%) | Thyroid 28,410 (4%) | Leukemia 12,460 (4%) | Non-Hodgkin lymphoma 9,370 (3%) |
| Kidney & renal pelvis 33,130 (4%) | Melanoma of the skin 27,530 (4%) | Esophagus 11,250 (4%) | Leukemia 9,250 (3%) |
| Oral cavity & pharynx 25,310 (3%) | Ovary 21,650 (3%) | Urinary bladder 9,950 (3%) | Uterine corpus 7,470 (3%) |
| Leukemia 25,180 (3%) | Kidney & renal pelvis 21,260 (3%) | Non-Hodgkin lymphoma 9,790 (3%) | Liver & intrahepatic bile duct 5,840 (2%) |
| Pancreas 18,770 (3%) | Leukemia 19,090 (3%) | Kidney & renal pelvis 8,100 (3%) | Brain & other nervous systems 5,650 (2%) |
| All sites 745,180 (100%) | All sites 692,000 (100%) | All sites 294,120 (100%) | All sites 271,530 (100%) |

*Excludes basal and squamous cell skin cancers and in situ carcinoma except urinary bladder.

©2008, American Cancer Society, Inc., Surveillance Research

# 1

# Radiation Physics

*Geoffrey S. Ibbott, Ph.D.*

## ATOMIC STRUCTURE

Our understanding of atomic structure continues to evolve, but we have for many decades understood the atom to be the smallest unit of matter that possesses the physical and chemical properties characteristic of each of the 106 known elements. An atom consists of a central nucleus surrounded by a cloud of electrons moving in orbits around the nucleus. The nucleus contains protons and neutrons, and in a neutral atom, the number of negatively charged electrons balances the number of positively charged protons in the nucleus. We use the terminology $^{A}_{Z}X$ to characterize an atom, where A is the number of nucleons (protons + neutrons) in the nucleus, Z is the number of protons (or electrons in a neutral atom), and X represents the chemical symbol for the element. The symbol A is known as the mass number while Z is known as the atomic number of the atom. The element is defined by the atomic number, but an element can have several mass numbers depending on the number of neutrons in the nucleus. Atoms with the same Z but different values of A are known as *isotopes* of the element X.

The nucleus is held together by nuclear binding energy; an energy deficit represented by the observation that the mass of an atom weighs less than the combined mass of its constituents. For example, one gram-atomic mass of $^{12}C$ is exactly 12 grams. However, the combined mass of protons, neutrons, and electrons to make up this amount of carbon is 12.09888 grams. The mass deficit is the mass equivalent of the energy that must be supplied to overcome the nuclear binding energy and separate a carbon atom into its constituents.

### Electron Energy Levels

The Bohr model of the atom describes the electrons in an atom as occupying orbits or shells around the nucleus.[1,2] Each shell can hold a maximum number of electrons described by $2n^2$, where n is the number of the electron shell. The first shell (n = 1 or K) can hold up to two electrons, the second shell (n = 2 or L) can contain up to eight electrons and so on.

Electrons are held in their orbits by their electron binding energy, a concept similar to nuclear binding energy, in that energy must be supplied to remove an electron from its shell. An electron can be elevated from, say, the K shell to the L shell if it is provided with an amount of energy exactly equal to the difference in the binding energies of these two orbits. Table 1-1

TABLE 1-1  Binding Energies (electron volts) for Electrons in Hydrogen and Tungsten
Atoms. Binding Energies are Shown as Negative Values Because They Represent
Energy That Must be Supplied.

| | | Binding Energy | |
| n | Shell | Hydrogen | Tungsten |
|---|---|---|---|
| 1 | K | −13.50 | −69,500 |
| 2 | L | −3.40 | −11,280 |
| 3 | M | −1.50 | −2,810 |
| 4 | N | −0.90 | −588 |
| 5 | O | −0.54 | −73 |

shows the binding energies for electrons in the hydrogen and tungsten atoms. The table indicates that to move an electron from the K shell to the L shell of hydrogen requires –3.4 eV – (−13.5 eV) = 10.1 eV.

> A unit of energy, the electron volt (eV), describes the energy gained by an electron as it is accelerated by a potential difference of 1 volt. Larger amounts of energy can be expressed in kilo electron volts (keV) or million electron volts (MeV).

If the amount of energy provided to the electron is greater than or equal to its binding energy, the electron can be removed completely from the atom.

If an electron falls from its orbital to an orbital closer to the nucleus, energy is emitted. This can happen only if a vacancy exists in the inner orbital. If an electron was to fall from the M shell of tungsten to the K shell, the energy emitted would be 69,500 eV − 2,810 eV = 66,690 eV or 66.7 keV.

Energy released as a result of the transition of an electron from an outer to an inner orbital, or by an electron falling from outside the atom into an inner orbital, is called *characteristic radiation*. When amounts of energy greater than a few keV are emitted, the radiation appears as X-rays.

When a vacancy occurs in an atom of high atomic number, a cascade of transitions is likely to occur, as electrons fall from ever more distant orbitals to fill the vacancies being created in the inner orbitals. This may result in a series of characteristic X-rays being emitted.

## RADIOACTIVITY AND RADIOACTIVE DECAY

Many atoms are stable, but in some the ratio of the number of neutrons to protons leads to instability and these nuclei frequently undergo changes that lead to a more stable configuration. These changes are accompanied by the emission of particles and electromagnetic radiation as the nucleus releases energy corresponding to the increase in binding energy of the nucleons as they arrive at their final configuration. These changes are referred to as *radioactive decay*, and the process of emission of radiation is described as *radioactivity*. In some cases, the number of protons in the final configuration differs from the number in the original nucleus, and the nucleus is said to have been *transmuted* from one chemical element to another. The processes of radioactive decay most important to radiation therapy are:

- **Beta-minus decay.** An electron is emitted from the nucleus when, in effect, a neutron is converted to a proton and an electron. The emitted electron is called a beta-minus particle or *negatron*. An antineutrino carries away some of the energy but is otherwise irrelevant in medicine. One or more gamma rays may be emitted.

$$\;_0^1 n \rightarrow\;_1^1 p +\;_{-1}^0 e + \tilde{\nu}$$

$$\;_Z^A X \rightarrow\;_{Z+1}^A Y + \beta^{-1} + \tilde{\nu} + \gamma$$

- **Beta-plus decay.** Within the nucleus, a proton and an electron can combine to form a neutron. This requires creating an electron (and a positively charged electron called a *positron*, to maintain the balance of charge) from available energy. The positron is emitted as well as a neutrino and possibly one or more gamma rays.

$$_1^1p + \left( _{-1}^0e + _{+1}^0e \right) \rightarrow _0^1n + _{+1}^0e + \nu$$

$$_Z^AX \rightarrow _{Z-1}^AY + \beta^+ + \nu + \gamma$$

- **Electron capture.** A nucleus without sufficient energy to create a negatron—positron pair may capture an inner-orbital electron, which combines with a proton to produce a neutron. This process achieves the transition to a more stable nucleus without the emission of a particle. Generally, one or more gamma rays is emitted, as well as characteristic X-rays which are produced as electrons fall to fill the inner-orbital vacancy.

$$_Z^AX + _{-1}^0e \rightarrow +_{Z-1}^AY + \nu + \gamma$$

## Radioactive Decay

The rate of decay of a radionuclide is directly proportional to the number of atoms of a radionuclide present in a given sample. As the number of atoms of the radionuclide decreases (as they change into the progeny nuclide) the rate of decay, or *radioactivity,* of the sample decreases. This relationship is expressed as:

$$N = N_0 e^{-\lambda t}$$

where $N_0$ is the number of atoms present at time $t = 0$. The decay constant $\lambda$ is determined as:

$$\lambda = \frac{(\ln 2)}{T_{1/2}}$$

where ln 2 is the natural logarithm of 2 and has the value 0.693. $T_{1/2}$ is the physical *half life,* which is the time required for the number of radioactive atoms in the sample to decrease to 1/2 of the initial value. This means that the activity of a radioactive sample decreases exponentially; the same amount of decrease occurs during each equal time interval. For example, during one half life, the activity decreases to 1/2 of its original value. During a second half life, the activity decreases by half again or to one quarter of its original value.

The *average life* $T_{avg}$ of a radioactive sample, also known as the *mean life*, is the average time for decay of atoms in the sample. The average life is:

$$T_{avg} = \frac{1}{\lambda} = 1.44 \left( T_{1/2} \right)$$

Cobalt-60 decays by beta minus emission. During the decay of $^{60}$Co to $^{60}$Ni, a negatron and an anti-neutrino are emitted, and gamma rays having energies of 1.17 MeV and 1.33 MeV are released.

Carbon-11 decays by beta plus emission. During decay to $^{11}$O, a positron and a neutrino are ejected, and a gamma ray is emitted.

Palladium-103 is an example of a radionuclide that decays by electron capture. During the decay of $^{103}$Pd to $^{103}$Rh, gamma rays are emitted from the nucleus, and characteristic X-rays are emitted as the K-shell vacancy is filled.

The activity of a sample of a radionuclide is the number of atoms decaying per second. The SI unit of activity is the becquerel [Bq], and an activity of 1 Bq corresponds to a rate of decay of 1 atom per second. The historical unit of activity, the curie [Ci], represents a rate of decay of 3.7 3 $10^{10}$ atoms per second.

Iodine-131, a radionuclide used for unsealed source brachytherapy, has a half life of 8.0 days. A sample having an activity of 15 millicuries [mCi] decays to 3.75 mCi over the course of 16 days.

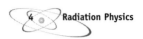 

**4**

The average life is sometimes used in calculations of dose delivery from permanent brachytherapy implants.

## Decay Schemes

A decay scheme is often a convenient way to describe the transitions that take place during decay of a radioactive nuclide. The decay scheme of $^{137}$Cs is shown in Figure 1-1A, and indicates that this nuclide decays by two primary competing pathways; most often a negatron or negative beta particle is emitted, followed by a gamma ray of 0.662 MeV. About 6.5% of the time, however, a single beta particle which carries away all of the decay energy is emitted. In contrast, the decay scheme for $^{125}$I is shown in Figure 1-1B. This nuclide decays by electron capture. The electron capture event is followed by the emission of a gamma ray having 35 keV of energy. The resulting tellurium atom, $^{125}$Te, has a vacancy in the k electron orbital, and a cascade of electrons follows with the emission of characteristic tellurium X-rays. The gamma ray, as well as several of these X-rays, are useful in cancer treatment with sealed sources of $^{125}$I.

---

**FIGURE 1-1** **(A) Decay scheme of cesium-137. (B) Decay scheme of iodine-125. (C) Decay scheme of fluorine-18.**

---

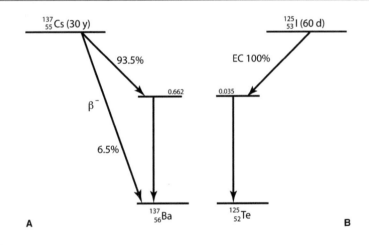

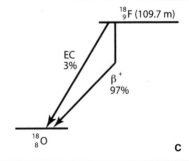

On the other hand, Figure 1-1C depicts the decay of $^{18}$F, a nuclide used for positron emission tomography (PET) imaging. $^{18}$F emits a positron which carries all of the decay energy and therefore is not followed by a gamma ray. The arrow representing the positron emission is drawn vertically downward for a short distance to indicate that energy must be provided by the nucleus before the positive beta particle is emitted. The energy requirement is 1.02 MeV; this amount is sufficient to create the positron and electron pair that are needed.

## Electromagnetic Radiation

X-rays and gamma rays occupy part of a continuous spectrum of radiation known as electromagnetic radiation. EM radiation is characterized by sinusoidally varying electric and magnetic fields which carry energy and travel through space at the speed of light. X-rays and gamma rays, having high energy, are at the upper end of the EM spectrum; EM radiation with moderate energy may be manifested as visible light, while low-energy EM radiation appears as microwaves and radiowaves. We tend to think of EM radiation as particles or "packets" of energy; a concept that is permitted by quantum physics. The relationship between the energy of a photon and its wavelength is given by $E = h\nu$ where $h$ is Planck's constant and has a value $h = 6.62 \times 10^{-34}$ J·sec. The frequency $\nu$ and wavelength $\lambda$ of EM radiation are related by the expression $\nu = c/\lambda$ where $c$ is the speed of light in a vacuum.

X-rays and gamma rays differ only in their origin: gamma rays are emitted during transitions between isomeric energy states of a nucleus, while X-rays are emitted during electron transitions between energy shells.

## Production of X-Rays

As described earlier, the movement of electrons between energy shells in an atom can result in the emission of characteristic radiation. A vacancy can occur in the K shell if an energetic electron from outside the atom collides with a K-shell tungsten electron, transferring sufficient energy to the orbital electron to remove it from the atom. Ionization of the tungsten atom then leaves a vacancy which can be filled by an electron from outside the atom, or by a cascade of electrons falling from one shell to another within the tungsten atom.

X-rays can also be produced when electrons lose energy as a result of passing close to an atomic nucleus. The attractive force between a positively charged nucleus and a negatively charged electron can slow the electron and change its path, resulting in the emission of energy, known as *Bremsstrahlung*, or "braking radiation." The atomic nucleus must be large, and atoms such as tungsten serve this purpose well.

Figure 1-2 is a simplified diagram of a modern diagnostic X-ray tube. The principal elements of the X-ray tube are a filament which releases electrons by thermionic emission, and a target made of tungsten embedded in a large anode. A high voltage is placed across the filament (or cathode) and the anode, to accelerate electrons from the filament and slam them into the target. The focal spot is the region on the target where the electrons strike. Modern X-ray tubes are often provided with two filaments, one large and one small. The size of the filament determines the size of the focal spot on the target, and consequently the size of the region from which X-rays are emitted. A smaller focal spot produces more detailed images but limits the electron flow (*tube current*) and the production of X-rays to lower levels.

X-ray tubes of similar design are used for CT scanners, radiographic and fluoroscopic simulators, kV imaging systems used for image-guided radiation therapy and orthovoltage X-ray equipment. Linear accelerators also produce X-rays by directing high-energy electrons into a target, but the means of accelerating the electrons is different and will be addressed later.

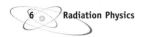 

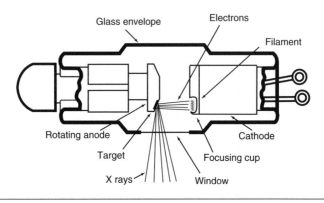

**FIGURE 1-2** Diagram of an X-ray tube showing the cathode, filament, rotating anode, and target.

## INTERACTIONS OF X-RAYS AND GAMMA RAYS

When an X-ray or gamma ray enters a material, one of three outcomes is possible: the photon may be scattered in a different direction during one or more interactions, it may be absorbed during an interaction, or it may be transmitted through the material without interaction. Photons that traverse a material without interaction are called primary radiation, while photons that interact through processes that change their direction are called scattered radiation. A photon that is absorbed or scattered is described as having been *attenuated*, and the amount by which a beam of photons is attenuated is a characteristic of the attenuating material and the photon beam spectrum.

Measurements of the attenuation of a beam of photons leads to the determination of a characteristic called *half value layer* (HVL). The HVL is the thickness of that material that reduces the intensity of a radiation beam to $1/2$ of its original value. Under conditions of "good geometry," in which the radiation beam is fairly small and the measuring device is located at some distance beyond the attenuating material, a monoenergetic beam will be attenuated exponentially with increasing thickness of absorber. A polyenergetic beam, such as the X-ray beam from a linear accelerator, is not attenuated exponentially because the absorber preferentially removes low energy photons. As a result the second HVL (the thickness of material required to reduce the beam intensity from $1/2$ to $1/4$ of its original value) might be larger than the first HVL.

Measurements of the HVL of a photon beam allow estimation of the linear attenuation coefficient $\mu = 0.693/\text{HVL}$. When the HVL is expressed in cm, $\mu$ is expressed in $\text{cm}^{-1}$. The linear attenuation coefficient can then be used to estimate the transmitted beam intensity for any thickness of absorbing material from $I = I_0 e^{-\mu x}$, where $I$ is the transmitted intensity, $I_0$ is the initial intensity, and $x$ is the thickness of absorbing material. The exponential in this equation must be dimensionless, so the units of $\mu$ must be the reciprocal of the units of $x$.

The HVL of a 6 MV photon beam from a linear accelerator might be 1.5 cm of a field-shaping alloy such as Cerrobend. Field-shaping blocks generally are designed to attenuate the radiation beam to <5% of its original intensity. This requires a thickness of at least 5 HVLs leading to a transmitted primary beam of $(1/2)^5$ or $1/32 = 3.1\%$. Therefore, a thickness of $5 \cdot 1.5 \text{ cm} = 7.5 \text{ cm}$ would be necessary.

For example, a Cerrobend block having a thickness of 5 cm would attenuate the 6 MV beam described earlier to:

$$\frac{I}{I_0} = e^{-\left(\frac{0.693}{1.5} \cdot 5\right)}$$

$$\frac{I}{I_0} = 0.099 \approx 10\%$$

Photons can interact with matter through a number of possible interactions, but in radiation therapy three are of greatest importance. These are photoelectric absorption, Compton scattering, and pair production.

## Photoelectric Absorption

Photoelectric absorption occurs when the energy of an x or gamma ray is transferred entirely to an inner orbital electron in an absorber atom. This interaction results in the complete absorption of the photon and its energy is used by the electron to escape from the atom. See Figure 1-3. The *photoelectron* is ejected from the atom with kinetic energy KE = energy of the incoming photon—binding energy of the electron orbital from which it was ejected. The photoelectron can interact with other atomic electrons and atomic nuclei. The vacancy created in the absorber atom is filled by an electron from an outer orbital or one from outside the atom leading to emission of characteristic radiation.

The probability that a photon will interact through photoelectric absorption is a function of both the photon's energy and the atomic number of the target atom. For the process to occur at all, the incident photon must have energy greater than the binding energy of the involved orbital electron. In general, the probability that a photon will undergo photoelectric absorption decreases with the cube of the photon energy and increases with the cube of the atomic number of the target atom.

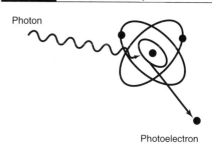

**FIGURE 1-3** Photoelectric absorption.

Photon

Photoelectron

## Compton Scattering

Photons with therapeutic energies are most likely to interact in biologic materials through Compton scattering. See Figure 1-4. The photon loses a portion of its energy to a loosely-bound outer-orbital electron. The Compton electron easily escapes as its binding energy is negligible; the photon may be scattered through any angle up to 180°, in which case it is called "backscatter."

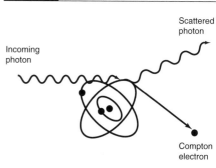

**FIGURE 1-4** Compton scattering.

Scattered photon

Incoming photon

Compton electron

The probability of Compton interactions is independent of the atomic number of the absorber but increases with the electron density ($e/cm^3$).

The maximum energy carried by a photon scattered through 90° is 511 keV, and a photon scattered through 180° can have a maximum energy of 255 keV. These relationships are important when designing room shielding to protect against scattered radiation.

## Pair Production

High energy photons can interact in materials through a process known as pair production. The name is an accurate description of the event in which the incoming photon disappears and its energy is converted to the mass of two particles. See Figure 1-5. The two particles are an electron and a positron (a positively charged electron). The energy equivalent of the mass of an electron is 0.51 MeV. Therefore, pair production cannot occur unless the incoming photon has an energy of at least double this amount, or 1.02 MeV. Photons with energies greater than 1.02 MeV are increasingly likely to undergo pair production as their energy increases and as the atomic number of the absorber increases. Energy carried by the incoming photon in excess of 1.02 MeV is divided equally between the pair of particles in the form of kinetic energy. Pair production occurs in the vicinity of the nucleus of an absorber atom. After losing its kinetic energy, the positron will combine with a free electron. The two particles will disappear and their mass will be converted to two annihilation photons having 0.51 MeV each and traveling in opposite directions.

## RADIATION THERAPY TREATMENT UNITS

### Low Energy X-ray Units

The practice of radiation therapy began very soon after Roentgen's discovery of X-rays. Until the development of $^{60}$Co units in the 1950s, most radiation therapy was delivered with X-rays generated at potentials below about 300 kV. Today, many departments retain low energy X-ray units for use with occasional patients, but they have largely been replaced by megavoltage linear accelerators. Low energy X-ray units fall into the following classifications:

- **Contact therapy units.** These operate at potentials of 40–50 kV and produce X-rays with HVLs of 1 or 2 mm Al. The X-ray tube is designed to be placed in contact with the surface to be irra-

---

**FIGURE 1-5** Pair production. Annihilation radiation is produced when the positron combines with an electron.

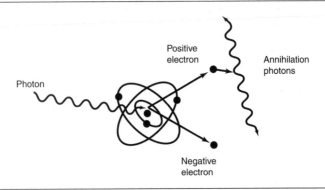

diated, at approximately 2 cm from the X-ray target. These beams are suitable only for the treatment of surface lesions.

- **Superficial therapy units.** This classification refers to units operating in the range of 50–150 kV and producing HVLs in the range of 1–8 mm Al. The field is limited and defined by a glass or stainless steel cone, and the surface to be treated is placed in contact with the end of the cone.
- **Orthovoltage therapy units.** These units operate in the range 200–350 kV. For many years, these units provided the most penetrating X-ray beam available in radiation therapy, and were therefore known as "deep therapy" machines. Orthovoltage machines typically used adjustable collimators, rather than fixed cones.

## Isotope Teletherapy Units

Teletherapy units based on sources of radioactive material were developed during the early years of radiation therapy, but it was not until 1951 and the availability of high activity sources of $^{60}$Co that these units came into widespread use. At this point, it is estimated that there are about 50 cobalt units in active clinical use in North America, but throughout the rest of the world there may be more than 2,000. In developing countries, where service capabilities for complex equipment may be limited, a cobalt unit is a relatively trouble free and lower cost option.

Cobalt units contain a source of $^{60}$Co with an activity in the range of 10,000 Ci. The specific activity of cobalt, about 1,100 Ci/g, means that a clinical cobalt source may be 2 cm in diameter. This large size means that the *penumbra* (the "fuzzy" edge of the radiation beam) may be as much as 2 cm at normal treat-ment distances.

Because of the size of the source, the collimator of a cobalt unit is more complex than the simple diaphragm used in a low energy X-ray unit. See Figure 1-6. The radiation beam is turned on and off by moving the source from a shielded position to an exposed position. The mechanism used for moving the source is frequently mechanical but might also be pneumatic.

> Because the source of a cobalt unit must be moved mechanically from the shielded position, the source is partially exposed briefly before arriving at the exposed position. This leads to exposure that is not reflected by the timer setting and is described by a correction for timer error.

---

**FIGURE 1-6** Two types of multivaned collimators used with cobalt units.

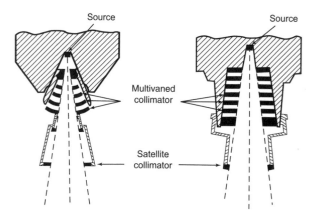

Source

Source

Multivaned collimator

Satellite collimator

---

Hendee, WR, Ibbott GS. Radiation Therapy Physics, 2nd ed Philadelphia (PA), Mosby-Year Book: 1996.[3]

Unlike early low energy X-ray units, some cobalt units were manufactured with isocentric gantries. The gantry of an isocentric unit rotates about a horizontal axis, so that the source remains in a plane perpendicular to this axis, and the radiation beam always passes through a single point in space, known as the *isocenter*.

## Linear Accelerators

Modern linear accelerators (also known as *linacs*) are now found in virtually all radiation therapy departments and have replaced most low energy X-ray units and isotope teletherapy units. See Figure 1-7. Most medical linacs accelerate electrons, and the resulting electron beam can be directed through a scattering foil and then to the patient for electron beam therapy. Alternatively, the electron beam can be caused to strike a target, producing X-rays that are collimated and directed to the patient. Most electron accelerators consist of the following components:

- **Microwave power source.** The source of microwave power is a tube, either a *magnetron* or a *klystron*. The magnetron or klystron converts electrical power to microwaves and the resulting pulse of microwaves is directed to the linear accelerator guide to accelerate electrons.
- **Linear accelerator guide.** In the linear accelerator guide, electrons are accelerated to nearly the speed of light.
- **Bending magnet.** Accelerator guides designed for energies greater than 6 MeV must be mounted horizontally in the upper part of the gantry and the electrons must be bent toward the patient. A 270° bending magnet is generally used as this type of magnet can be made *achromatic*. See Figure 1-8. Electrons whose energy varies from the intended energy by more than a small amount are stopped. When the energy of the beam is changed intentionally, as in multimodality accelerators, the strength of the bending magnet has to be adjusted.

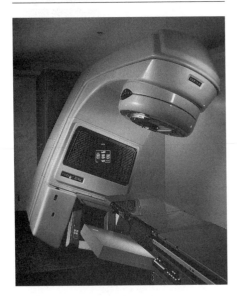

**FIGURE 1-7** A representative modern medical linear accelerator.

- **X-ray target and flattening filter.** To produce an X-ray beam in a linear accelerator, the accelerated electron beam must be directed into an X-ray target. The target in an accelerator is a *transmission* target, meaning that the X-rays continue in the forward direction toward the patient. In an accelerator with an achromatic bending magnet, the target is placed at the focus of the magnet. The X-ray beam may be strongly *forward peaked*. A *flattening filter* is necessary to create a beam of sufficient area and uniformity for clinical use.
- **Scattering foil.** Dual modality linear accelerators allow the X-ray target and flattening filter to be removed from the beam, so that the accelerated electron beam can be directed toward the patient. The accelerated beam is a narrow pencil beam and must be broadened and made uniform for patient treat-

ment. This is generally accomplished through the use of a scattering foil; a thin foil (or multiple foils) of intermediate- or high-Z material.

- **Monitor ionization chamber.** The dose rate of an accelerator beam may vary unpredictably or by design. It is not possible to rely on the elapsed time to control the dose delivered to a patient. Instead, the radiation leaving the target or the scattering foil passes through a monitor ionization chamber where it produces an ionization current that is proportional to the beam intensity. The ionization current is conducted to the accelerator control panel, where it is converted to a digital display of *monitor units*. The dose delivered to the patient is controlled by programming the accelerator to deliver a prescribed number of monitor units, often referred to as the "meter setting." Monitor chambers contain multiple segments and are able to monitor the flatness and symmetry of the radiation beam, as well as the machine output.

- **Collimator.** Shaping of the beam is handled by the collimator. Because the source of radiation in an accelerator is nearly a point source, the collimator can be of simpler design than in a $^{60}$Co teletherapy unit. For X-ray beams, the collimator often consists of jaws made of a high atomic number material such as lead or tungsten. In most cases, the jaws are adjusted under motor control to create rectangular beams of any size and shape up to 40 cm × 40 cm.

**FIGURE 1-8** A modern 270 achromatic bending magnet.

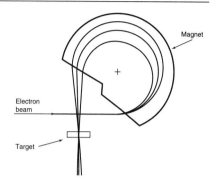

It is customary to calibrate a linear accelerator monitor ionization chamber so that the meter setting corresponds to the dose to a patient under standard conditions of field size, distance, and depth in tissue.

Because electrons can be easily scattered by the intervening air between the scattering foil and the patient, the final stage of collimation of an electron beam must be close to the skin surface. A cone or "electron applicator" is used to shape electron beams.

Most modern linear accelerators incorporate a multileaf collimator (MLC), either as a replacement for one pair of accelerator jaws, or as a tertiary device mounted below conventional collimator jaws. For many treatment applications MLCs replace customized cerrobend blocking and are able to conform to relatively complex shapes. (See Figure 1-9).

MLCs were originally envisioned as a field shaping device to eliminate the hazards and tedious work of creating custom cerrobend blocks. With the advent of intensity-modulated radiation therapy, MLCs have become a key element in treatment delivery, and their characteristics must be precisely known for treatment planning. A comprehensive quality assurance program addressing the MLC is essential.[4]

## MEASUREMENT OF IONIZING RADIATION

A number of different parameters are used to describe radiation quantity. Each of these parameters is useful for different purposes; some are more easily measured than others, but some enable us to

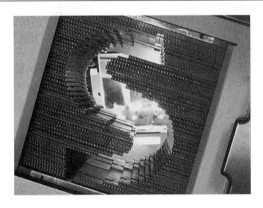

Courtesy of Siemens Medical Solutions USA, Inc.

relate measurable quantities to patient doses. In general, these quantities express the intensity of a beam of radiation, the exposure or energy transferred from the beam to a material, or the dose absorbed by a material from the beam of radiation.

## Radiation Exposure

Radiation exposure is defined as the ability of the radiation to produce ionization in air. The measurement of radiation exposure is a key factor in radiation dosimetry, and is relatively straightforward to measure. A historical unit of radiation exposure is the Roentgen, where $1R = 2.58 \times 10^{-4}$ coulombs of charge produced per kilogram of air. However, the Roentgen has virtually disappeared from use as the SI unit of coulombs/kg has become accepted.

## KERMA

Kerma is an acronym for kinetic energy released in matter. It is a measure of the amount of energy transferred from an ionizing radiation beam but does not consider what happens to the energy after it is lost by the beam. It applies only to "indirectly ionizing" radiation such as photons and neutrons. In the radiation therapy context, kerma describes the mean energy transferred from a beam of photons to charged particles (electrons) in the medium per unit mass. If the medium of interest is air, as is the case inside an air-filled ionization chamber, the quantity is referred to as air kerma. The unit of kerma is the joule per kilogram (J/kg). However, kerma is expressed in units of gray (Gy), where 1 Gy = 1 J/kg.

## Stopping Power

Stopping power is a measure of the loss of energy by directly ionizing radiation, such as the electrons set in motion by a beam of photons. Stopping power is not generally measured but is calculated from theory. The linear stopping power describes the energy lost per unit path length of a charged particle. The mass stopping power is defined as the linear stopping power divided by the density of the absorbing medium. Dividing by the density of the medium eliminates dependence of the mass stopping power on the density of the medium. This facilitates the comparison of energy lost from charged particles in media of widely differing densities such as air, tissue, and lead. Linear stopping power is generally expressed in MeV/cm while mass stopping power is typically expressed in MeV cm$^2$/g.

## Free-Air Ionization Chamber

Fundamental measurements of radiation exposure are accomplished in standards laboratories using an instrument known as a free-air ionization chamber. The simpler instruments commonly used in a clinic are compared with standards established by free-air ionization chambers to yield calibration coefficients for the simpler instruments. Free-air chambers, as will be seen below, are bulky and impractical for use in a clinic, but their design eliminates the correction factors and assumptions needed for simpler instruments.

A free-air chamber is shown schematically in Figure 1-10. It consists essentially of a box with an aperture on one side to define a radiation beam. The radiation beam passes through the box, in this case from left to right, and passes between two electrodes. The dimensions of the radiation beam are defined by the aperture and are known with great precision. Similarly, the length of the region in which ionization is collected is defined by the length of the collecting electrode. The electrodes are designed to ensure that the dimensions of the collection region can be known to high precision. Therefore, ionizations in the air inside the chamber that are produced by the radiation passing through the chamber can be collected and the total number of coulombs of charge per unit mass of air in the collection region (C/kg) can be determined very accurately.

The dimensions of the free-air chamber must be sufficiently large to allow for *electronic equilibrium*. That is, ionizations that are produced within the collection region but escape from it must be compensated for by ionizations that are produced upstream from the collection region but travel into it and therefore are collected by the collecting electrode. The range of electrons set in motion by high energy photons increases as the photon energy increases. Therefore, free-air chambers are effectively limited to orthovoltage X-ray and $^{60}$Co beams.

## Thimble Ionization Chamber

As previously mentioned, a free-air chamber is not a practical instrument for routine clinical use. Instead, thimble ionization chambers are used, which function in much the same way. A thimble ionization chamber is shown in Figure 1-11. Thimble chambers for calibration of megavoltage photon beams often have an air volume of approximately 0.6 cm$^3$. By itself, this volume is not suffi-

cient to establish electronic equilibrium but equilibrium can be maintained if the wall of the ionization chamber is made of air-equivalent material of greater density, whose thickness is equivalent to the thickness of air that would be required.

Under some circumstances, a parallel plate chamber might be used rather than a thimble chamber. A parallel plate chamber is designed somewhat like a very small free-air chamber, in that it consists of two parallel electrodes. The electrodes are generally close together, often 1 mm apart. The electrode diameters are also small, frequently less than 1 cm. A parallel plate chamber is most often irradiated with the beam perpendicular to the electrodes. The electrode facing the source is ordinarily made of very thin plastic or foil, with a conductive coating on the

**FIGURE 1-10** A free-air ionization chamber. The collecting volume is defined by the area of the beam and the length L.

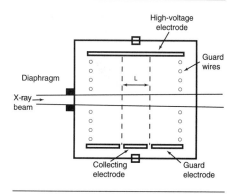

## FIGURE 1-11  A typical thimble ionization chamber.

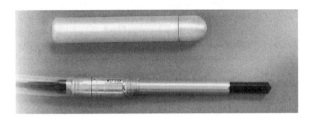

Courtesy of Scanditronix-Wellhofer.

inner surface. This design allows the measurement of ionizing radiation at very shallow depths, as is often necessary in low energy electron beams. See Figure 1-12.

## RADIATION DOSE

In radiation oncology, we are concerned about the chemical and biological changes in tissue as a result of exposure to ionizing radiation. These changes are caused by the deposition of energy from the radiation into the tissue. As stated earlier, the *kerma* is the amount of energy transferred from a photon beam to the ion pairs produced in the absorbing medium. The *absorbed dose* is the energy actually absorbed per unit mass of the irradiated volume. If ion pairs escape the region under consideration without depositing all of their energy, and if they are not compensated by ion pairs originating outside the volume under consideration (electronic equilibrium), the kerma exceeds the absorbed dose. Under conditions in which electronic equilibrium is achieved and the radiative energy loss is negligible, the kerma and absorbed dose are identical. The unit of absorbed dose is the gray (Gy) defined as one joule per kilogram of irradiated medium. The relationship between kerma and absorbed dose is shown in Figure 1-13. The figure shows that the kerma is greater than the absorbed dose in the buildup region, where electronic equilibrium has not been established. At the depth of maximum dose, kerma and dose are equal. At greater depths, because the photon beam is attenuated a small amount over the range of the electrons set in motion by photon interactions, the absorbed dose is slightly greater than the kerma.

## FIGURE 1-12  A representative parallel-plate ionization chamber.

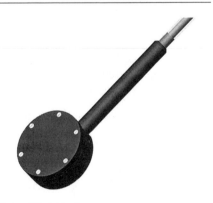

Courtesy of Standard Imaging.

## MEASUREMENT OF RADIATION DOSE

Ionization chambers do not measure radiation dose directly. Instead, they measure the energy transferred to a small volume of air (kerma or exposure) by ionizing radiation. Because the air is contained in a small cavity (an ionization chamber) that is displacing the medium of interest (tissue or tissue-equivalent material), a number of corrections are required to determine the absorbed dose in the medium of interest. These corrections will be discussed in a later section.

However, several devices exist for measuring radiation dose directly. Such a device would be most useful if its characteristics (density, effective atomic number) matched those of the medium of interest (tissue). This is rarely the case, and even with devices that measure dose directly, corrections are often required. Some of these devices are:

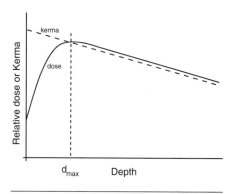

**FIGURE 1-13** The relationship between kerma and absorbed dose in water.

- **Calorimeter.** Almost all of the energy absorbed by a medium from a beam of ionizing radiation is converted ultimately to heat. A calorimeter is a device, usually manufactured from water or graphite, whose temperature can be measured extremely accurately. The measurement volume must be surrounded by a mass of similar tissue-equivalent material that also insulates the measurement volume from its surroundings. When it is irradiated, the increase in temperature of the calorimeter is measured. The absorbed dose is determined from the specific heat of the medium.

- **Film dosimetry.** The emulsion of a photographic film contains crystals of a silver halide embedded in a gelatin matrix. Exposure to radiation causes the formation of a latent image, which is manifested by the deposition of silver when the film is subsequently processed. The amount of silver deposited is proportional to the radiation dose. The darkening of the developed film is expressed as the optical density OD, where $OD = \log(1/T)$. The transmittance T is the reduction in light intensity when the film is placed between a light source and a detector. *Photographic* film dosimetry is subject to error, largely because the presence of silver in the emulsion causes the effective atomic number of film to be considerably higher than that of tissue. In contrast, *Radiochromic* film contains no high Z elements. Instead, it consists of a plastic film to which is attached a radiation sensitive dye. When exposed to radiation, the dye changes color, producing a visible image. No processing is required. The color change can be detected by a densitometer.

- **Thermoluminescence dosimetry.** A thermoluminescence dosimeter (TLD) releases light when it is heated following exposure to ionizing radiation. Materials such as lithium fluoride (LiF) store some of the energy deposited by ionizing radiation by elevating electrons into the crystal matrix into "traps." When LiF is subsequently heated, the electrons are lifted from the traps, and allowed to fall down to the ground state. As they fall, light is emitted, and the amount of light is proportional to the radiation dose absorbed by the dosimeter. The effective atomic number of LiF is 8.18, sufficiently close to that of soft tissue (7.4) that these dosimeters exhibit only a small amount of energy dependence. Because of its low cost and relatively easy handling, LiF is widely used as a mailed dosimetry system for conducting dosimetry audits.[5]

- **Optically-Stimulated Luminescence (OSL).** OSL detectors perform in a similar fashion to TLD, except that the energy stored in the dosimeter material by the absorption of ionizing radiation is released not by heat but by the application of light from a laser. OSL dosimeters have been widely used for personnel monitors and are now being investigated for clinical dosimetry uses.

• **Other solid state detectors.** Electronic diodes, MOSFETs, diamonds, and certain organic scintillators have been used as radiation dose detectors. The response of these systems is generally proportional to dose, although some of these devices show a dependence on the energy or dose rate of the radiation.

## CALIBRATION OF MEGAVOLTAGE BEAMS OF X-RAYS AND ELECTRONS

The preferred instrument for calibrating a therapeutic beam of X-rays or electrons is a thimble ionization chamber. Ionization chambers do not measure dose directly, so it is necessary to relate absorbed dose to the ionization measured by the chamber. This is done at a calibration laboratory and in the United States, the AAPM-Accredited Dosimetry Calibration Laboratories (ADCLs) provide this service.[6] At an ADCL, an ionization chamber is compared with an ADCL instrument that is traceable to the National Institute of Standards and Technology (NIST) in a water phantom in a beam of $^{60}$Co gamma rays. The ratio of absorbed dose to chamber signal is the *dose to water calibration coefficient*, $N_{D,w}$. A calibration protocol published by the AAPM describes a recommended technique for using an ionization chamber and an ADCL-provided calibration coefficient to determine the dose to water.[7] The protocol specifies that, for photon beams, an ionization chamber should be placed at 10 cm depth in water, in a $10 \times 10$ cm field at the standard treatment distance, and a measurement of ionization made for a set number of monitor units. This reading, designated $M_{raw}$, must be corrected for environmental conditions as well as some aspects of operation of the instrument as indicated in the equation below.

$$M = M_{raw} \cdot P_{TP} \cdot P_{ion} \cdot P_{pol} \cdot P_{elec}$$

where $P_{TP}$ is a correction for the temperature (T) and pressure (P) at the time of measurement, compared with the conditions to which the chamber response has been normalized. In the US, ion chamber calibration coefficients are referred to a temperature of 22°C (72°F) and a pressure of 760 mm Hg. Consequently, the temperature-pressure correction is:

$$P_{TP} = \left( \frac{273 + T}{295} \right) \cdot \left( \frac{760}{P} \right)$$

At high elevations, such as in Denver (elevation 5,280 ft), the pressure correction to an ionization chamber reading is approximately 1.2. In other words, the reading must be increased by 20% to correct for the reduced air density.

$P_{ion}$ is a correction for the incomplete collection of ions in the ion chamber. $P_{ion}$ is always greater than unity, but values larger than 1.05 are an indication that the ion chamber is not suitable for the measurement conditions.

$P_{pol}$ is a correction for differences in the sensitivity of the ionization chamber when the collection voltage is reversed. Particularly for electron beams, it is advisable to average the measurements made with the collection voltage set to first one, then the other polarity.

$P_{elec}$ is a correction factor for the response of the electrometer to which the ionization chamber is connected. This correction factor is provided by the ADCL.

Once the corrected ionization reading, M, is determined, the dose to water at the depth of measurement is calculated as follows:

$$D_w = M \cdot N_{D,w} \cdot k_Q$$

To account for changes in the response of the instrument at other megavoltage energies, a quality conversion factor, $k_Q$, is applied. $k_Q$ is determined from a table or graph published in the protocol for the specific ionization chamber and the energy of radiation. The energy of a photon beam is characterized by the percent depth dose at 10 cm, measured under well-defined conditions.

$D_W$ determined this way is usually divided by the *clinical percent depth dose* value at 10 cm depth, to arrive at the dose at $d_{max}$.

For calibration of electron beams, the AAPM protocol recommends determination of the quality conversion factor as follows:

$$k_Q = P_{gr} \cdot k_{ecal} \cdot k'_{R_{50}},$$

where $P_{gr}$ is a gradient correction and is necessary because, in an electron beam, the percent depth dose may change over the dimensions of the chamber.

$k_{ecal}$ is termed the "photon-electron conversion factor," and converts $k_Q$ into the appropriate correction for an electron beam having an energy of approximately 15 MeV.

$k'_{R_{50}}$ is an energy-dependent correction that accounts for differences in the chamber response at different electron beam energies. The electron beam energy is characterized by $R_{50}$, the depth at which the dose in the electron beam falls to 50% of the maximum dose.

## Dosimetry of Radiation Fields

The radiation dose delivered to a point of interest in a patient can rarely be measured directly. Instead, it is customary to estimate the dose in a patient from doses measured in a phantom. Measurements are usually made with a small ionization chamber, although other detectors can be used. Most often, the measurements are obtained at depths along the central axis of the radiation beam and expressed as fractions of the amount of radiation measured at a reference location. These fractions are most commonly described as percent depth doses, tissue-air ratios, tissue-phantom ratios, or tissue-maximum ratios.

### Percent Depth Dose

The percent depth dose (%dd) is the ratio of absorbed dose at depth along the central axis of the radiation beam divided by the dose at the depth of dose maximum ($d_{max}$). For X-rays generated at voltages below 400 kVp, the maximum dose occurs at the surface of the phantom, and the reference dose is measured on the central axis at the phantom surface. For higher energy photons, the reference dose is determined on the central axis at $d_{max}$. A graph showing the change in $d_{max}$ with beam energy appears in Figure 1-14.

Percent depth dose is influenced by several parameters:

- **Depth.** Beyond the depth of maximum dose, the percent depth dose decreases nearly exponentially. For a beam of 6 MeV X-rays, the decrease is approximately 4% per centimeter of depth. For 18 MV photons, the decrease is roughly 3% per centimeter.
- **Field size and shape.** As the dimensions of a megavoltage radiation beam increase, the amount of scatter generated in the field increases, and the slope of the percent depth dose curve decreases. Figure 1-15 shows the change in percent depth dose for 6 MV X-ray beams of different dimensions.
- **Source to surface distance (SSD).** The percent depth dose decreases with depth in a phantom or patient for two reasons: the radiation is attenuated (absorbed and scattered) by the medium, and because the beam is diverging from the source. If a phantom is moved from the standard treatment distance to a greater distance, the change in percent depth dose will be less rapid, because the beam diverges a smaller amount over a given depth when the surface is at a larger distance. This change is expressed by the *Mayneord F factor*[8] where,

$$\left(\%dd\right)_{SSD_2} = \left(\%dd\right)_{SSD_1} \cdot F^2$$

**FIGURE 1-14** The percent depth dose for 10 cm × 10 cm beams of photons of several energies.

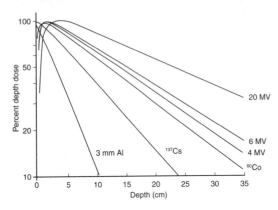

From Johns, HE and Cunningham, JR (B). Used with permission.

$$F^2 = \left( \frac{\dfrac{SSD_2 + d_{max}}{SSD_2 + d}}{\dfrac{SSD_1 + d_{max}}{SSD_1 + d}} \right)^2$$

## Tissue-Air Ratio

The tissue-air ratio (TAR) is the dose at depth in a phantom divided by the dose in air, or:

$$TAR = \frac{D_d}{D_{air}}$$

where $D_{air}$ is the dose to a small mass of tissue (just enough to provide electronic equilibrium, or $d_{max}$) and is measured at the same distance from the source as $D_d$. Because both measurements for TAR are made at the same distance from the source, the distance itself is not important. However, measurements of TAR are frequently made at the isocenter of the treatment machine. For megavoltage machines, TAR has reduced usefulness, because measurements in air become increasingly difficult at higher beam energies. The TAR at a depth of $d_{max}$ is also known as the backscatter factor (BSF), or peakscatter factor (PSF).

## Tissue-Phantom Ratio

The tissue-phantom ratio (TPR) is conceptually very similar to the TAR, except that the reference measurement is made at a reference depth in a phantom. Therefore,

$$TPR = \frac{D_d}{D_{ref}}$$

Again, both $D_d$ and $D_{ref}$ must be measured at the same distance from the source of radiation, meaning that a different thickness of phantom material must be placed over the ionization chamber for each measurement.

**FIGURE 1-15** The change in percent depth dose for 6 MV X-ray beams of several field sizes.

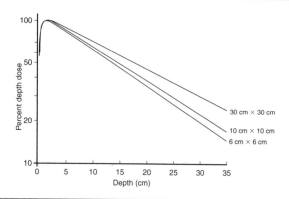

The value of the TPR in calculating doses for isocentric treatments should be clear; if the reference dose rate is known at the isocenter of the machine, under a depth $d_{ref}$, it is a straightforward matter to calculate the dose rate at any other depth as,

$$Dose\ rate\ at\ d_{tumor} = Dose\ rate\ at\ d_{ref} \cdot TPR\ at\ d_{tumor}$$

Very often, the reference depth is chosen to be the depth of maximum dose, $d_{max}$. When this is done, the TPR is known as the tissue-maximum ratio, TMR.

## Isodose Curves

Figure 1-15 shows the variation in dose along the central axis of a radiation beam (the depth dose curve). However, the dose to tissue away from the central axis cannot be determined from these data. To estimate the absorbed dose to off-axis points, isodose curves for the X-ray beam can be consulted.

Figure 1-16 shows the isodose curves for a 10 × 10 cm beam of 10 MV photon at 100 cm SSD. Each isodose curve defines points in a homogeneous tissue-equivalent medium at which the absorbed dose is a specific percentage of the dose on the central axis at $d_{max}$.

## Wedged Isodose Curves

Radiation beams are sometimes modified by inserting a wedge filter, a wedge-shaped metal filter that differentially attenuates the radiation beam from one side of the beam to the other. A typical wedge filter is shown in Figure 1-17, and the corresponding isodose distribution is shown in Figure 1-18.

The wedge angle is defined as the angle between an isodose curve near 10 cm depth and a line perpendicular to the central axis. In other words, it is the angle through which the isodose curve has been tilted. Wedged isodose curves also can be produced by moving one collimator jaw across the field while the beam is on, thus changing the radiation intensity in a more or less linear fashion from one side of the beam to the other. A general term for such a technique is *programmed wedge filter,* but more common terms are "dynamic" or "virtual" wedge.

**FIGURE 1-16** Isodose curves from a 10 MV X-ray beam.

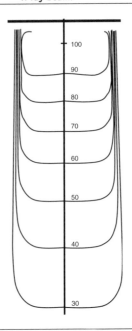

## Electron Depth Dose and Isodose Curves

The percent depth dose along the central axes of electron beams of several energies is compared in Figure 1-19. Electron beam depth dose curves are characterized by a relatively high surface dose and rapid fall-off beyond a certain depth. Consequently, the dose from an electron beam is fairly uniform up to approximately the depth of the 90% dose, after which the dose falls rapidly.

Representative isodose curves are shown in Figure 1-20. Electron beams typically show a constriction of the higher isodose curves and a bulging of the lower isodose curves. Attention must be paid to this characteristic when prescribing electron beam field sizes. This broadening of the penumbra also can lead to difficulties when beams of radiation are to be matched.

## Scatter-Air Ratio (SAR) and Scatter-Phantom Ratio (SPR)

Scattered radiation contributes significantly to the dose at points in an irradiated patient. It is often of interest to estimate the contributions to dose at a point from primary and scattered radiation. This is particularly useful, for example, to calculate the dose under a block or to an organ just outside a radiation field. Although more sophisticated algorithms are available today, for many years the

**FIGURE 1-17** A 45° wedge filter.

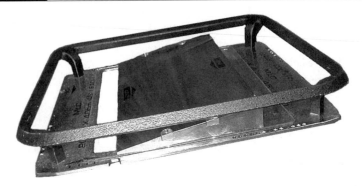

concept of the scatter-air ratio (SAR) facilitated these calculations.

For a beam of zero field size, no scattered radiation is produced in the medium, and the value of $TAR_0$ at any depth is solely a measure of the primary radiation reaching that depth.[9] The difference between the TAR for a field of finite size $fs$ compared with the $TAR_0$ reflects the contribution of scattered radiation at that depth. The difference is the SAR:

$$SAR_d = TAR_{fs,d} - TAR_{0,d}$$

The value of SAR varies with the depth of overlying tissue, the beam energy, and the field size and shape.

Scatter-phantom ratio (SPR) bears the same relationship to TPR and is calculated in a similar fashion. The SPR is more useful for high energy megavoltage radiation, when measurements in air are impractical.

SAR or SPR can be used to calculate the dose caused by scattered radiation in a patient. The technique is especially useful when calculating

**FIGURE 1-18** Isodose curves for a 6 MV X-ray beam with a 45° wedge filter.

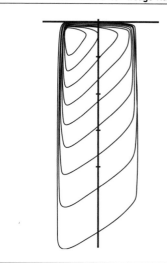

doses in irregularly shaped fields. The effective SAR can be computed for an irregular field by breaking the field into smaller segments and summing the fractional SAR for each segment. The effective SAR is then added to the $TAR_0$ to produce the effective TAR for the irregular field:

$$TAR_{eff,d} = TAR_{0,d} + SAR_{eff,d}$$

**FIGURE 1-19** Central axis depth dose curves for several electron beam energies.

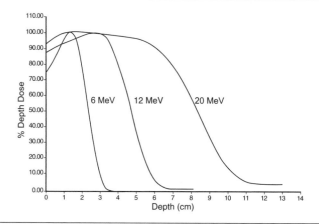

**22** Radiation Physics


**FIGURE 1-20** Isodose curves for a 16 MeV electron beam from a linear accelerator.

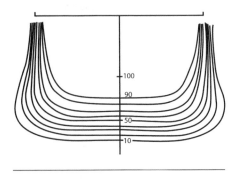

A similar procedure can be followed using TPR and SPR values.

## TREATMENT PLANNING

Treatment planning is defined here as the process of estimating the dose at a point in a patient, or the relative dose distribution throughout the irradiated volume, as well as the process of determining the optimum field arrangement to most effectively treat the patient's condition. Today, it is rare for relative dose distributions to be determined using manual methods, as sophisticated computer algorithms are widely available for this purpose. However, it is more common for the dose at a point, or inversely, the *treatment time* (or *meter setting*) required to deliver the prescribed dose at a point to be determined using manual techniques.

## POINT DOSE CALCULATIONS

Calculations of dose at a point are performed for two purposes: to determine the meter setting to carry out a prescription and to determine the dose at points other than the prescription point. The calculations may consider irregularities in the field shape or tissue composition, although such corrections are often complex and time consuming when performed manually. The method for calculating the dose at a point depends on the complexity of the treatment situation and the manner in which the treatment unit was calibrated. Figure 1-21 illustrates the relationship between calibration conditions and several treatment conditions.

## METER SETTING CALCULATIONS

Determining the meter setting requires first that the prescribed dose be related to the dose per monitor unit at the calibration point. As illustrated in Figure 1-21, this requires the use of parameters that relate the dose at the prescription point depth to the depth of $d_{max}$, adjust for differences between the prescribed field size and 10 × 10 cm² field, differences in the distance from the source to the prescription point and to the reference point, and corrections for attenuation by materials placed in the beam to modify its shape or beam intensity.

The meter setting can be calculated as follows:

- SSD technique:

$$\text{Meter setting} = \frac{\text{prescribed dose @ depth}}{\dfrac{\%dd}{100} \cdot D_{ref} \cdot S_c \cdot S_p \cdot ISR \cdot T}$$

- SAD technique:

$$\text{Meter setting} = \frac{\text{prescribed dose @ depth}}{TMR \cdot D_{ref} \cdot S_c \cdot S_p \cdot ISR \cdot T}$$

Each of these parameters will be addressed in turn.

**FIGURE 1-21** Comparison between calibration conditions and treatment conditions.

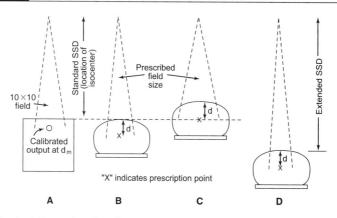

"X" indicates prescription point

    **A**        **B**        **C**        **D**

**(A)** Calibration is frequently performed to provide the machine output in terms of dose rate at $d_{max}$ in water for a $10 \times 10$ cm$^2$ field at the standard *SSD*. **(B)** Treatment at the same SSD as the calibration. The depth of the prescription point is usually greater than $d_{max}$. The prescribed field size is defined at the patient's surface. **(C)** Treatment using isocentric positioning. The prescribed field size is defined at the isocenter. **(D)** Treatment at an extended *SSD*. The prescribed field size may be defined at the patient's surface or at the depth of the prescription point.

## Reference Dose Rate $D_{ref}$

This is generally 1 cGy/MU at $d_{max}$ in a $10 \times 10$ cm field at 100 cm SSD. To simplify calculation procedures, the calibration may be performed at the isocenter, or a $d_{ref}$ other than $d_{max}$ may be used.

## Depth

To relate the dose or dose rate at the prescription point to that at $d_{max}$, a percent depth dose or TMR (TPR) must be used. The choice of which parameter to use is generally made as follows:

- **SSD technique.** For patients treated with the skin surface at a standard SSD (for example, 100 cm) it is most convenient to use %dd to relate the dose at the prescription depth to dose at $d_{max}$.
- **Isocentric technique.** When patients are treated isocentrically, the prescription point is placed at the isocenter, and the TMR can be used to determine the corresponding dose at isocenter with an overlying thickness of $d_{max}$. It is then straightforward to relate the calibration dose rate to the dose at isocenter at a depth of $d_{max}$. Note that if the treatment unit is calibrated at a reference depth that is not equal to $d_{max}$, it is necessary to use a tissue-phantom ratio (TPR) whose reference depth is equal to the depth used for calibration.

## Field Size and Shape

When field sizes and shapes other than a 10 cm $\times$ 10 cm square are used to treat patients, the output of the treatment unit may be different from the calibration output, and the dose rate in the patient may change due to the presence of more or less scatter. Although more sophisticated computer-based techniques are available, a straightforward method suitable for manual calculations is as follows:

- **Collimator scatter factor (S$_c$).** S$_c$ is a measure of the treatment unit output as a function of collimator setting, relative to a 10 cm × 10 cm field. S$_c$ considers only the effects of changing the collimator setting.
- **Phantom scatter factor (S$_p$).** S$_p$ describes the change in dose rate at d$_{max}$ with changes in field size relative to 10 cm × 10 cm, independent of the collimator setting. S$_p$ can be based on the effective field size, which is most often determined as follows:

$$\text{effective FS} = 4 \cdot \frac{\text{field area}}{\text{field perimeter}}$$

The effective or *equivalent square field* method is suitable when fields are only moderately irregular. When extremely irregular fields are used, a method such as the SAR technique of scatter summation should be used, or more sophisticated computer-based techniques should be used.

A graph representing the variation in S$_c$ and S$_p$ is shown in Figure 1-22. The output (dose rate at d$_{max}$) for any field size and shape, and any collimator setting, is the product of S$_c$ and S$_p$:

$$\text{Output at d}_{max} = S_c \cdot S_p$$

**FIGURE 1-22** Collimator and phantom scatter factors.

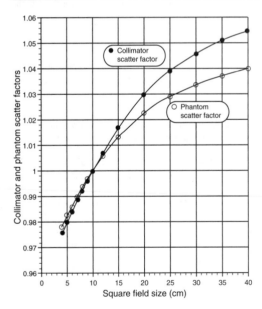

Representative normalized collimator scatter factors (Sc) and normalized phantom scatter factors (Sp) plotted as a function of field edge for square fields. Data for a 6 MV linac, measured by the author.

### Treatment Distance

If the patient is treated at a distance different from that used for calibration, a correction must be applied. As a correction has already been applied to relate the dose at the prescription depth to the dose at a reference depth (either the %dd, TMR or TPR) the purpose of a distance correction is to adjust for any difference between the distance from the source to the reference point in the patient and the distance from the source to the calibration point:

- **Treatment at standard SSD.** If the patient is treated at the standard SSD used for calibration, no distance correction is required. See Figure 1-21A and Figure 1-21B.
- **Treatment at non-standard SSD.** Treatment at extended SSD is sometimes necessary to obtain unusually large field sizes, such as for treatment of the

*cranio-spinal axis*. For example, a patient may be treated at 150 cm SSD to obtain a field of 60 cm length. In this case, the reference point in the patient is at 150 cm + $d_{max}$, while the calibration reference point is most likely at 100 cm + $d_{max}$. The dose rate at the patient's reference point is reduced by the square of the inverse ratio of the distances (inverse-square ratio or ISR). In this case, the ISR is:

$$ISR = \left( \frac{100 + d_{max}}{150 + d_{max}} \right)^2$$

For a 6 MV X-ray beam with $d_{max}$ = 1.5 cm, the ISR = $\left( \frac{101.5}{151.5} \right)^2$ or 0.449, indicating that the dose rate at the patient's reference point is less than ½ the dose rate at the calibration point. See Figure 1-21A and Figure 1-21D.

- **Isocentric treatment.** Refer to Figure 1-21A and Figure 1-21C. For isocentric treatment, the reference point in the patient is actually slightly closer to the source than the distance to the calibration reference point. Most commonly, the patient will be positioned with the center of the target at 100 cm from the source, while the calibration reference point is at 100 cm + $d_{max}$. Therefore, the ISR is calculated as:

For isocentric treatment using a 6 MV beam with $d_{max}$ = 1.5 cm, the ISR = $\left( \frac{101.5}{100} \right)^2 = 1.030$.

$$ISR = \left( \frac{100 + d_{max}}{100} \right)^2$$

## Transmission Factors

Any material placed in the beam between the source and patient has the potential to attenuate the beam, reducing the dose rate to the patient. Examples of such devices include plastic trays used to support beam shaping blocks, and wedge filters. The transmission factor (T) for any such device is the ratio of the dose rate at the calibration reference point with the device present divided by the dose rate with the device removed. Typical values of T are 0.97 for plastic beam shaping trays and 0.50 for a 45° wedge filter. It is essential that transmission factors be determined on-site for each device used on each treatment unit.

## EFFECTS OF TISSUE INHOMOGENEITIES

Measurements of radiation beam characteristics made in a water phantom do not indicate the effects of patient tissues that are dissimilar to water. *Inhomogeneities* for which corrections might be necessary include bone, lung and air, and fat. The correction to be applied depends on the type and energy of the radiation, the size of the radiation field, and the size and composition of the *inhomogeneity*. Several manual calculation techniques may be used to account for the presence of inhomogeneous tissue:

- **Ratio of tissue air ratios method.** A correction factor is calculated from the ratio of TARs determined for the effective depth of the point of calculation divided by the TAR for the physical depth of the point of calculation:

$$CF = \frac{TAR_{d_{eff},fs}}{TAR_{d,fs}}$$

**FIGURE 1-23** Terminology and schematic representation of inhomogeneous tissues, for use with the ratio of *TAR*s method, and the Power-Law method.

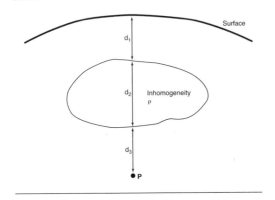

$d_{eff}$ is the water-equivalent depth of the point of calculation. The water-equivalent depth is determined by summing the products of the thickness of each tissue layer and its electron density as shown in Figure 1-23. The relative electron density $\rho_e$ has units of electrons/ cm$^3$ of the heterogeneity relative to that of water. The distances $d_2$ and $d_3$ are explained in Figure 1-23. The electron density $\rho_e$ of lung tissue is generally taken to be 0.3 while a representative value for bone is 1.2. Air is considered to have a density of 0. The ratio of TARs technique can also be used to correct for obliquity of the skin surface. The corrected dose at the point of interest is the product of the dose calculated ignoring the inhomogeneity multiplied by the correction factor.

- **Power law TAR method.** The ratio of TARs method described above is considered an "effective pathlength" method. In other words, it is a one-dimensional correction that ignores inhomogeneous tissues other than those on a line between the point of calculation and the source, nor does it consider the location of the point of the interest relative to the heterogeneity. The power law TAR method is an attempt to consider the distance from the heterogeneity to the point of interest.[10] A correction factor is calculated based on the thickness of the heterogeneity, its density, and the distance from the heterogeneity to the point of interest:

$$CF = \left( \frac{TAR_{d_2+d_3,fs}}{TAR_{d_3,fs}} \right)^{\rho_e - 1}$$

- **Equivalent TAR method.** Neither of the correction techniques described previously consider the lateral extent of the heterogeneity. Many heterogeneities of significance in radiation therapy are small in size or are located so that they intercept only a portion of the beam. Frequently, the heterogeneity does not intersect the central axis of the radiation beam. The equivalent TAR method was developed to consider the effects on scattered radiation of inhomogeneous regions of defined extent and location.[11] It is not easily calculated manually.

- **Coefficient of equivalent thickness (CET) method for electron beams.** A correction for the transmission of electron beams through inhomogeneous tissues has been developed using a coefficient of equivalent thickness (CET).[12] The effective thickness of inhomogeneous tissue is determined by multiplying the physical thickness by the CET.

$$d_{eff} = d - z(1 - CET)$$

where d is the physical depth of the point of interest and z is the thickness of inhomogeneous tissue overlying the point of interest. Recommended values of CET are 1.65 for compact bone and 0.5 for lung.

## Separation of Adjacent Fields

To treat large volumes of tissue, it is often necessary to abut two or more radiation fields. When this is done, the divergence of the fields must be considered, and regions of overlap or low dose must be avoided. With photon beams, it is often necessary to calculate a gap or separation on the patient surface to avoid regions of excessively high dose at shallow depths below the surface. See Figure 1-24. The separation between the two fields is determined by calculating the gap width required for each field:

$$G_1 = \left(\frac{fs_1}{2}\right)\left(\frac{d}{SAD}\right)$$

where $fs_1$ is the field length at the SAD and d is the depth at which the fields are to abut. For SSD treatments, the SSD is used in place of the SAD and the field length is determined at the surface. The gap $G_2$ is determined in the same way, and the total gap G is determined by adding the two gaps together:

$$G = G_1 + G_2$$

> Care must be taken when opposing pairs of fields are abutted, such as might be used when treating superior and inferior AP-PA fields. If the superior and inferior pairs have different lengths, it is possible for overlap regions to occur between the abutment depth (often the patient's midline) and the surface. This can create a hot spot at the level of the spinal cord.

## VOLUME SPECIFICATION

Comparing patient treatments delivered at multiple centers, as is done in cooperative group trials, requires that the treatments be described in a consistent fashion. One important aspect of this is in the definition of target volumes. Many institutions and several cooperative groups now routinely use the volume definitions published by the International Commission on Radiation Units and Measurements (ICRU) for a generalized dose-specification system.[13,14] The ICRU has defined the following volumes:

- **Gross Tumor Volume (GTV).** The GTV is the demonstrable extent and location of malignant tissue, determined by palpation, direct visualization, or imaging techniques.
- **Clinical Target Volume (CTV).** The tissue surrounding the GTV may be invaded by subclinical microscopic extensions of the tumor. Consequently, a margin is often added around the GTV.
- **Planning Target Volume (PTV).** The CTV is likely to change in size, shape, and location during a course of treatment, as a result of movements of the patient and the tissues containing or adjacent to the CTV. A margin is drawn around the CTV to accommodate these variations and is identified as the PTV.
- **Treated volume.** The treated volume is the region of tissue enclosed by a selected isodose surface, often 95% of the prescription isodose, and identifies tissues receiving doses at or near the prescribed dose.

**FIGURE 1-24** An illustration of the procedure for calculating the gap between adjacent X-ray beams.

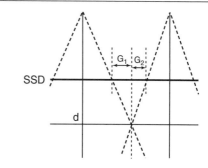

- **Irradiated volume.** The irradiated volume is that tissue receiving a significant dose, perhaps $\geq$ 20% of the prescribed dose.
- **Organ at Risk (OAR).** OARs are normal tissues whose radiation sensitivity may influence the treatment planning process.
- **Planning Risk Volume (PRV).** The PRV is a geometric concept that takes into account the possible geometric variations in organs at risk.

The ICRU has also made recommendations regarding specification of target dose. In general, the ICRU recommends that the dose be specified at or near the center of the PTV, although the maximum and minimum dose to the PTV should also be reported. However, many clinical trials today require that the volume of the PTV receiving the prescribed dose be specified. Frequently, the goal of treatment planning is to ensure that, say, 95% of the PTV receives the prescribed dose, and 99% of the PTV receives at least 90% of the prescribed dose. Of course, the parameters offered here are for illustration only.

## COMPUTERIZED TREATMENT PLANNING

Treatment planning by computer has undergone a significant evolution in recent years. As computer hardware and software have increased in sophistication and complexity, treatment planning capabilities have seemingly been limited only by the imagination of radiation oncologists and physicists. Treatment planning and delivery techniques such as intensity-modulated radiation therapy (IMRT) and image-guided radiation therapy (IGRT) will not be discussed explicitly here, as the details are beyond the scope of this chapter. However, some of the basic principles of image handling and dose calculation will be described.

The steps associated with treatment planning are as follows:

### Beam Data Entry

As part of commissioning a treatment planning system, data characterizing the institution's radiation beams must be entered. The amount of data required depends on the calculation algorithm; for some systems, a complete map of dose measurements in a water phantom is required, while for other systems, only a few depth doses and off-axis measurements are needed. Of course, even systems that require only a small amount of data to be entered still require validation; a process that often involves a comparison between calculations and very detailed and comprehensive measurements.

- **Data-based systems.** These planning systems require the measurement and entry into the computer of comprehensive matrices of data for a variety of field sizes. These data generally consist of central axis depth dose curves and beam profiles for square fields of ten or more different sizes. Similar data sets are required for each of the different beam energies in use at the institution.
- **Model-based systems.** These systems function by constructing a mathematical model from which the dose at any point in a medium irradiated by a beam of any size can be calculated. These systems generally require prior knowledge of the treatment machine characteristics, and then are fine tuned through the use of measurements made at the clinic.

### Patient Data Entry

To generate the treatment plan for a specific patient, certain information regarding the patient is required. This generally consists of the following steps:

- **CT imaging.** Images of the patient are obtained with the patient in the treatment position, and on a surface that mimics the linear accelerator treatment couch. This ensures that the target volume within the patient will be in the same relationship to other structures as at the time of treatment.
- **Image transfer.** The CT images must be transferred from the CT scanner, generally across a network, to the treatment planning system. Some processing is often required before the images are available for treatment planning. In particular, the CT data (CT number or Hounsfield units) must be converted to relative electron densities. See Figure 1-25, for a representative CT number to density curve.[15]
- **Image segmentation or contouring.** A key step in preparing CT images for treatment planning is identifying the target volume. Generally, a physician identifies the GTV or CTV, depending on the type of tumor and previous treatment such as surgery. The CTV is then expanded by a margin to produce the PTV. It is also important to identify other issues of interest, particularly organs at risk. The primary purpose for doing this is to facilitate the calculation of dose to these volumes, although it also facilitates the clear identification of OARs so they can be avoided.

## Energy and Field Selection

At this point, some basic choices are made regarding the beam energy to be used and the field size and shape needed to cover the target volume without encroaching on organs at risk. Modern planning systems include tools to assist in the field shaping process, including a *beams-eye view* (BEV). The BEV illustrates the projection of the PTV on a surface perpendicular to the beam, and allows the operator, or automated software, to determine the positions of multileaf collimator leaves or the shape of customized shielding to match the PTV. Often, the BEV is superimposed upon a digitally reconstructed radiograph (DRR) that is produced by tracing ray lines from the effective position of the radiation source through the CT data set.

---

**FIGURE 1-25** Relationship between CT number and electron density. The relationship is not necessarily a smooth function, and it may be different from one CT scanner to another.

---

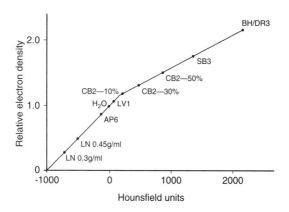

From Constantinou, C., Harrington, J.C., and DeWerd, L.A. An electron density calibration phantom for CT-based treatment planning computers. *Med. Phys.* 1992; 19:325–327. Used with permission.

## Forward Planning

Most treatment plans throughout the history of treatment planning computers have been generated using so-called *forward planning*. This process requires that an operator position radiation beams at appropriate angles and with appropriate weighting to yield the desired dose distribution. Even with the benefit of years of experience, this is often a trial and error process, requiring that the operator make fine adjustments and gradually iterate toward an ideal or optimal solution.

## Inverse Planning

Automatic optimization techniques have been investigated for several decades, but it has only been in recent years that true *inverse planning* has become available. Inverse planning is extremely demanding of computer resources, and requires that the target volumes and organs at risk, as well as their dose constraints, be defined explicitly. In effect, the operator must identify the desired *dose volume histogram* for each tissue of importance, and instruct the computer to search for a beam arrangement that most nearly meets the desired goals. Inverse planning is most often used when IMRT techniques are employed, because the minute adjustments required in MLC leaf position and beamlet weights exceed the capabilities of a human planner.

## Dose Volume Histograms

A dose volume histogram (DVH) is a graphical representation of the dose received by the patient, and the volume of tissue receiving the dose. Figure 1-26 illustrates the comparison between two competing dose volume histograms for a particular patient and organ. At any point along the curves, the DVH indicates the volume of tissue (generally expressed as a percentage of total organ or target volume), that is receiving at least the indicated dose. For example, Figure 1-26 illustrates that with plan 2, 30% of the volume of the OAR is receiving 55 Gy or more.

## Calculation Algorithm

Intensity-modulated radiation therapy (IMRT) permits the design of highly conformal dose distributions that can deliver high doses to a target volume while sparing nearby sensitive normal structures. This is done through a sophisticated process of dividing each field into beamlets, and assigning unique intensities to each beamlet. IMRT can provide improved dose distributions over conventional techniques in the prostate, head and neck, and other clinical sites.

Most treatment planning systems use one of several broad classes of calculation algorithm. In general, the simpler the algorithm, the more rapidly results can be obtained, but also the less accurate the results can be expected to be.

- **Clarkson scatter summation.** The scatter summation technique described earlier has been implemented in treatment planning computers.[16] The use of a computer generally allows for more precise interrogation of the scattered radiation, and under conditions of uniform patient density and little surface obliquity, the technique can accommodate well for irregularly shaped fields. However, when tissue inhomogeneities are encountered or large variations in surface obliquities exist, the Clarkson calculation generally relies on simple heterogeneity correction algorithms such as the ratio of TARs technique. As this technique ignores the extent of heterogeneities other than along the ray line between the source and point of calculation, this form of heterogeneity correction is likely to be fairly inaccurate. In particular, when the point of calculation is near an interface between tissues of two different densities, such as at the surface of the lung, the correction technique is unable to consider the transport of energy by electrons set in motion by photon interactions, and the resulting loss of electronic equilibrium.

- **Pencil beam method.** The pencil beam technique was developed in the 1960s, and allows the rapid calculation of dose distributions by simulating large radiation fields as a number of small (1 cm × 1 cm) pencil-like beams. Each pencil beam can be corrected independently for changes in surface obliquity and for the presence of tissue inhomogeneities (generally using the ratios of TARs technique) and the results are summed.
- **Three-dimensional integration methods.** These techniques generally rely at least in part on Monte Carlo calculations. The Monte Carlo simulation is a computational technique in which statistical methods

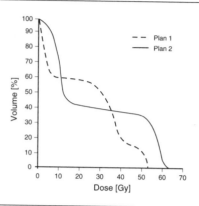

**FIGURE 1-26** Dose-volume histogram for an organ at risk.

are used to simulate a large number of radiation interactions.[17] Individual photons are simulated, and the sequence of likely interactions is traced from their production until their eventual absorption or escape from the volume of interest. These so called *histories* are summed, generally for many millions of particles, to produce the resulting dose distribution. Monte Carlo simulations are generally extremely time consuming and impractical for routine clinical treatment planning. However, the use of Monte Carlo techniques to simulate the dose distribution from a pencil beam can be used in the superposition/convolution technique described next.
- **Superposition/convolution technique.** The Monte Carlo simulation process can be used to generate a dose kernel: the dose distribution resulting from interactions of a pencil beam of radiation in a medium, considering the scattering of photons and the generation and transport of secondary electrons. Dose kernels must be computed for a variety of energies. These kernels can than be *convolved* with the spectrum of the radiation beam from a linear accelerator. The resulting dose distributions are then summed to produce the final dose distribution. In the process, adjustments are made for the shape of the patient and for variations in tissue densities.

## BRACHYTHERAPY

The placement of sealed radioactive sources in or near a tumor is one of the earliest techniques for treating cancer with ionizing radiation. For many years, radium ($^{226}$Ra) was used, but this source has more recently been replaced with nuclei such as cesium ($^{17}$Cs, $^{131}$Cs), iridium ($^{192}$Ir), iodine ($^{125}$I), and palladium ($^{103}$Pd). Techniques for implant therapy can be divided into four categories:

- **Molds or plaques.** Radioactive sources can be placed a short distance above the skin or mucosa in the region of a superficial lesion. The distance between the sources and the lesion is seldom greater than 1 or 2 cm. The intervening space is generally filled with material such as wax or plastic.
- **Interstitial implant.** Radioactive needles, wires, or small encapsulated sources called seeds can be inserted directly into a lesion or the adjacent tissue.
- **Intracavitary implant.** Radioactive sources can be placed in a body cavity adjacent to the target tissue.

- **Intraluminal implant.** Radioactive sources can be introduced into the lumen of a blood vessel, duct, or airway.

Brachytherapy procedures can be further broken down into *temporary* or *permanent* implants. Temporary implants can be delivered on an outpatient basis or can require that the patient be hospitalized for the duration of the treatment, which generally lasts no more than a few days. Permanent implants, which are practical only for interstitial treatments, require that the sources remain in the tissue permanently. For these treatments, sources with relatively short half-lives are used, so that the majority of the dose is delivered within a few weeks or months. Permanent implants must employ sources with low energy emissions, so that the dose rate at the patient's external surface does not present a significant risk of radiation exposure to others. These patients frequently can be released from the hospital as soon as their medical condition permits.

## Specification of Brachytherapy Sources

The specification of brachytherapy sources is undergoing an evolution. Radium sources were specified in terms of the mass of radium in milligrams incorporated into the source. To facilitate the introduction of radium substitutes, newer sources have been specified in terms of milligram equivalents of radium (mg-Ra-eq). This figure is the mass of radium required to produce the same exposure rate at 1 cm as from the substitute source. For radium substitutes, the relationship between mCi and mg-Ra-eq is determined from the ratio of the exposure rate constants for the two nuclei.

A $^{137}$Cs source is described by the manufacturer as having an activity of 20 mg-Ra-eq. How many mCi of cesium are contained in the source?

The exposure rate constants for radium and cesium are shown in Table 1-2. The activity of cesium is determined as follows:

$$\text{mCi of } ^{137}\text{Cs} = \text{mg Ra eq of } ^{137}\text{Cs}\left(\frac{\Gamma_{Ra}}{\Gamma_{Cs}}\right)$$

$$\text{mCi of } ^{137}\text{Cs} = 20 \text{ mg Ra eq } \frac{8.25 \text{ R} \cdot \text{cm}^2/\text{hr} \cdot \text{mg}}{3.28 \text{ R} \cdot \text{cm}^2/\text{hr} \cdot \text{mCi}}$$

Activity = 50.3 mCi

In 1987, the AAPM recommended specification of brachytherapy sources in terms of the air-kerma strength.[18] The air-kerma strength ($S_K$) is the air-kerma rate specified at a standard distance, usually 1m. $S_K$ is expressed in units of $\mu$Gy m$^2$/hr, and is determined by measurement at a standards laboratory, or with an ADCL-calibrated well ionization chamber.

## BRACHYTHERAPY SOURCES

### $^{137}$Cs

The most common radium substitute is $^{137}$Cs. Sources of $^{137}$Cs are constructed as tubes containing radioactive microspheres embedded in a ceramic matrix. A representative $^{137}$Cs source is shown in Figure 1-27. The tubes are typically 2.65 mm external diameter, 20 mm long and active length of 14 mm. The encapsulation must be thick enough to absorb energetic beta particles emitted as $^{137}$Cs decays, because these would deliver a high dose to tissues very close to the surface. These sources are safer to use than radium because the radioactive material is a solid rather than a powder, and because no gaseous radioactive decay products are produced.

TABLE 1-2 Physical Properties of Several Radioactive Nuclides Used in Radiation Therapy

| Element | Isotope | Beta Particle Energy (MeV)* | Gamma Ray Energy (MeV)† | Exposure Rate Constant (R · cm²/ h · mCi) | Half life | HVL in water (cm)‡ | HVL in lead (mm)‡ | Clinical Uses | Source Form |
|---|---|---|---|---|---|---|---|---|---|
| Cesium | $^{137}$Cs | 0.514–1.17 | 0.662 | 3.28 | 30 yr | 8.2 | 6.5 | Temporary intracavitary and interstitial implants | Tubes, needles |
| Cobalt | $^{60}$Co | 0.313 | 1.17–1.33 | 13.07 | 5.26 yr | 10.8 | 11 | Temporary implants | Plaques, tubes, needles |
| Gold | $^{198}$Au | 0.96 | 0.412–1.088 | 2.327 | 2.7 days | 7.0 | 3.3 | Permanent implants of prostate and other sites | Seeds |
| Iodine | $^{125}$I | None | 0.0355 | 1.45# | 59.6 days | 2.0 | 0.02 | Permanent interstitial implants of prostate, lung, and other sites, temporary implants of eye | Seeds |
| Iodine | $^{131}$I | 0.25–0.61 | 0.08–0.637 | 2.2 | 8.06 days | 5.8 | 3.0 | "Cocktail" for thyroid therapy | Liquid, capsules wires, seeds |
| Iridium | $^{192}$Ir | 0.24–0.67 | 0.136–1.062 | 4.62‖ | 74.2 days | 6.3 | 3.0 | Temporary interstitial implants of head, neck, breast, and other sites | Seeds |
| Palladium | $^{103}$Pd | — | 0.020–0.0227 | 1.48 | 17 days | — | 0.01 | Permanent implants of prostate | Seeds |

(continues)

## TABLE 1-2 (continued)

| Element | Isotope | Beta Particle Energy (MeV)* | Gamma Ray Energy (MeV)† | Exposure Rate Constant (R cm²/h · mCi) | Half life | HVL in water (cm)‡ | HVL in lead (mm)‡ | Clinical Uses | Source Form |
|---|---|---|---|---|---|---|---|---|---|
| Phosphorus | $^{32}$P | 1.71 | None | — | 14.3 days | 0.1 | 0.1 | Sodium phosphate injection, for bone and blood diseases; chromicphosphate pleural and intraperitoneal effusions | Liquid |
| Ruthenium | $^{106}$Ru, $^{106}$Rh | 3.5 MeV max. | — | — | 366 days | — | — | Temporary implants of eye | Plaques |
| Strontium | $^{89}$Sr | 1.46 | None | — | 50 days | — | — | Injection for widespread bone metastases | Liquid |
| Strontium | $^{90}$Sr, $^{90}$Y | 0.54–2.27 | None | — | 28.9 yr. 64 hr | 0.15 | 0.14 | Temporary application for shallow lesions (outpatient treatments) | Applicator |
| Ytterbium | $^{169}$Yb | — | 0.060–0.100 | 1.58‖ | 32.0 days | — | — | Temporary & permanent implants | Seeds |

*A dash separates the minimum and maximum energies of the β particles in the spectra. All energies listed are the maximum energy of each particle.
†A dash separates the minimum and maximum energies of the γ rays in the spectra.
‡Assumes narrow beam geometry, a condition usually not found in practical brachytherapy applications.
§For an encapsulated source with a wall thickness equivalent to 0.5 mm Pt-Ir alloy. For radium and radon, the exposure rate constant is expressed in R · cm²/h · mg.
‖For an unfiltered point source with δ ≥ 11.3 keV.[40,41]
¶Neutrons/fission
#This value is reduced to 1.208 by the attenuation of the filtration incorporated into commercially available seeds, together with a correction for anisotropy.

$^{137}$Cs is used almost exclusively for low dose rate temporary implants of the cervix or uterine canal. Treatment involves the placement of an applicator designed to hold the sources in a fixed position against the cervix and in the uterus. A representative Fletcher-Williamson applicator consisting of a tandem and ovoids is shown in Figure 1-28. The applicator is placed while the patient is anesthetized in an operating room. Sources are not introduced into the applicator until the patient has returned to a specially designed hospital room. The hospital room may be equipped with shielded walls, and is situated to minimize the risk of exposure of other patients and staff. This procedure eliminates risk of exposure to operating room personnel, and allows treatment planning calculations to be performed after the applicator is placed but before active sources are introduced into the applicator. This technique is referred to as "afterloading." The sources can be introduced manually, but automatic remote afterloading devices have been manufactured that can introduce the sources from within a shielded container under remote control.

## $^{192}$Ir

Radioactive iridium has been used for both low dose rate (LDR) and high dose rate (HDR) applications and recently for a hybrid technique called pulsed dose rate (PDR) treatment.

- **LDR $^{192}$Ir.** Low dose rate applications of $^{192}$Ir are temporary interstitial placements, in which catheters are placed in an array into the tissue to be treated, and ribbons of iridium seeds are introduced into the catheters. The catheters are placed in an array consisting of one or several planes, depending on the volume of tissue to be treated. After treatment generally lasting a few hours to a few days, the seeds and the catheters are removed.

- **HDR $^{192}$Ir.** Sources of $^{192}$Ir have been produced with activities as high as 10 Ci ($S_K = 4 \times 10^4$ μGy m$^2$/hr) for treatment at high dose rate. The hazards of such high activity sources require that they be transferred from a shielded safe into an applicator or implant catheters using an automatic remote afterloader. See Figure 1-29. $^{192}$Ir has a half life of 74 days. Consequently, the source in an HDR remote afterloader must be replaced approximately every 3 months. This source emits gamma rays with an average energy of 0.38 MeV.

- **PDR $^{192}$Ir.** A remote afterloader containing a source of $^{192}$Ir of approximately 1 Ci has been developed for PDR therapy. In this procedure, conventional LDR brachytherapy is simulated by delivering the source to the applicator for brief, regularly spaced intervals, of approximately

**FIGURE 1-27** A representative $^{137}$Cs source.

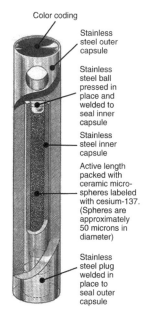

Color coding

Stainless steel outer capsule

Stainless steel ball pressed in place and welded to seal inner capsule

Stainless steel inner capsule

Active length packed with ceramic micro-spheres labeled with cesium-137. (Spheres are approximately 50 microns in diameter)

Stainless steel plug welded in place to seal outer capsule

Courtesy of 3M.

**FIGURE 1-28** Fletcher-Williamson applicator for $^{137}$Cs intracavitary brachytherapy.

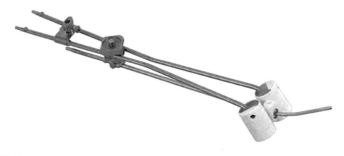

Courtesy of Nucletron.

10 minutes per hour. This regimen is believed to confer the same radiobiological advantages as LDR treatment, while permitting unrestricted access to the patient for much of the time.

## $^{198}$Au

On rare occasions, radioactive gold is used as a substitute for radon seeds which have been abandoned due to the hazard associated with the escape of radioactive gas. $^{198}$Au has a 2.7 day half life and emits gamma rays of 0.412 meV.

**FIGURE 1-29** An automatic remote afterloader for PDR brachytherapy treatments.

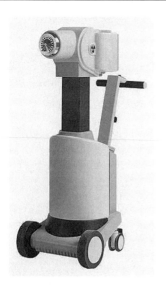

Courtesy of Nucletron.

## $^{125}$I

Many permanent interstitial brachytherapy procedures, especially those of the prostate, are performed with radioactive iodine seeds. Representative sources of $^{125}$I are shown in Figure 1-30. This nuclide has a half life of 59.6 days and decays by electron capture. This decay process presents a significant advantage in that it has no particulate emissions that must be filtered. As a result, the encapsulation of the source can be made thinner and sources can be made extremely small. The gamma rays and X-rays emitted from this source have energies in the range of 28 to 35 keV. With such a low photon energy, the radiation can be shielded easily with lead, for which $^{125}$I has an HVL of 0.02 mm.

## $^{103}$Pd

Sources of radioactive palladium are used as an alternative to $^{125}$I and again are largely used for permanent implants of the prostate. $^{103}$Pd decays by electron capture and emits characteristic X-rays in the range of 20–23 KeV. The half life is approximately 17 days.

## $^{131}$Cs

This isotope of cesium has a half life of 9.7 days and decays by electron capture producing gamma and X-rays in the range of 30 keV. As such, the dose distributions are comparable to those produced by $^{125}$I and $^{103}$Pd.

## Ophthalmic Irradiators

Certain ophthalmic conditions such as pterygium of the cornea as well as certain intraorbital malignancies such as melanomas, can be treated effectively with small radioactive applicators positioned on or near the sclera for a short time. Applicators for the treatment of pterygium contain radioactive strontium ($^{90}$Sr) in secular equilibrium with yttrium ($^{90}$Y). The low energy beta particles from $^{90}$Sr are absorbed by the encapsulation of the applicator, but the higher energy betas from $^{90}$Y (2.27 MeV maximum) are useful for treatment of the sclera. The dose rate from a strontium applicator may be as high as 100 cGy/s, but may vary greatly across the surface of the applicator.

Eye plaques are sometimes used to

**FIGURE 1-30** Several models of $^{125}$I and $^{103}$Pd brachytherapy seeds.

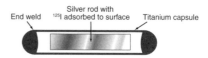

Amersham Health model 6711 source

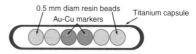

NASI model MED3631-A/M or MED3633 source

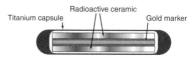

Bebig model I25.S06 source

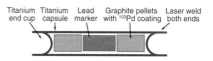

Theragenics model 200 source

treat malignancies of the eye such as choroidal melanoma. A gold shield is constructed to match the curvature of the globe of the eye, and sources of $^{125}$I, $^{103}$Pd, or beta emitters such as ruthenium ($^{106}$Ru) in equilibrium with rhodium ($^{106}$Rh) are placed on the concave surface. The applicator is then attached to the globe for a treatment duration on the order of 3 or 4 days.

## Brachytherapy Dose Calculations

Calculation of the dose distribution around single implanted brachytherapy sources can be complicated by a number of factors. Many sources produce anisotropic dose distributions. Gynecological implant applicators frequently incorporate shielding to protect the rectum and bladder, and the use of correction factors to account for this shielding exceeds the ability of most treatment planning methods. Consequently, a number of approximation techniques are used for the calculation of brachytherapy doses.

## $^{137}$Cs Dose Calculations

Dose distributions around $^{137}$Cs tube sources are most often determined from *along and away tables*. These tables provide dose rates at points defined by their distance along the source axis, measured from the center of the source, and perpendicularly away from the source axis. See Table 1-3. The dose rate at a point in a patient is determined by first finding the *along and away* distances to the point from the source, then multiplying the dose rate at that point (from Table 1-3) by the activity of the source. When multiple sources are used, the dose rates from the sources are summed.

Treatment planning computers for brachytherapy applications can be programmed with data corresponding to that in Table 1-3.

## Radiographic Localization of Implants

The calculation of dose distribution from a brachytherapy implant must be based on the actual location of the sources within the patient because these locations may differ from the original intended locations. Consequently, the source location is determined either from CT images or from pairs of radiographic images. When afterloading techniques are used, the location of the sources must be simulated through the use of *dummy sources*; inert metal rods designed to mimic the sources being used for the procedure. In the case of HDR implants, in which the source will be stepped from one location to another to simulate the use of multiple low dose rate sources, dummy sources that either indicate each dwell position or represent the extremes of a series of equally spaced dwell positions are used.

## Sources Other Than $^{137}$Cs Tubes

Calculations of dose rate around sources of $^{192}$Ir, $^{125}$I, $^{103}$Pd, and $^{131}$Cs are generally performed following a protocol published by the AAPM and known as the TG-43 formalism.[20,21] This formalism uses the air-kerma strength specification of source strength, and provides for the calculation of dose as follows:

$$\dot{D}(r,\theta) = S_K \cdot \Lambda \cdot \frac{G_L(r,\theta)}{G_L(r_0,\theta_0)} \cdot g_l(r) \cdot F(r,\theta)$$

where $\dot{D}(r,\theta)$ is the dose rate at a specific location defined by its distance r from the center of the source, and its angle $\theta$ from the longitudinal axis of the source.

$\Lambda$ is the dose rate constant, expressed in units of cGy/hr per unit air-kerma strength, at 1 cm from the source along its perpendicular bisector ($\theta = 90°$).

$G(r,\theta)$ is the geometry function. This parameter describes the change in dose rate as a function of distance and angle from the source and considers the distribution of activity within the source.

$g(r)$ is the radial dose function. This accounts for absorption and scatter along the transverse axis of the source normalized to the value at the reference point $r_0 = 1$ cm.

$F(r, \theta)$ is the anisotropy function. This function accounts for absorption and scatter in the medium and in the source encapsulation. It is obtained from relative dose measurements and is normalized to the measurement at $\theta_0 = 90°$ for each value of r.

The preceding equation allows a determination of dose rate at any point in a medium near a brachytherapy source, by explicitly separating all of the contributing effects. However, it also requires knowledge of the exact orientation of the source, so that the angle $\theta$ can be determined. It is impractical to determine the orientation of each source in a seed implant. Therefore, it is customary to approximate the TG-43 method by considering each source to be a point source. Thus:

$$\dot{D}(r) = S_K \cdot \Lambda \cdot \left(\frac{r_0}{r}\right)^2 \cdot g_P(r) \cdot \phi_{an}(r)$$

where only the distance from the source is considered, an inverse square calculation is used in place of the geometry function, and an averaged one-dimensional anisotropy function is used

**TABLE 1-3 Dose Rate per Unit Air-Kerma Strength for the Amersham CDCS, J-type Intracavitary Tube**

| Distance along (cm) | Distance away (cm) | | | | | | | | | | | | | |
|---|---|---|---|---|---|---|---|---|---|---|---|---|---|---|
| | 0.00 | 0.25 | 0.50 | 0.75 | 1.00 | 1.5 | 2.00 | 2.5 | 3.00 | 3.50 | 4.00 | 5.00 | 6.00 | 7.00 |
| 7.00 | 0.0186 | 0.0186 | 0.0183 | 0.0182 | 0.0183 | 0.0183 | 0.0180 | 0.0175 | 0.0167 | 0.0159 | 0.0149 | 0.0130 | 0.0111 | 0.00945 |
| 6.00 | 0.0259 | 0.0258 | 0.0254 | 0.0254 | 0.0255 | 0.0254 | 0.0247 | 0.0236 | 0.0222 | 0.0207 | 0.0192 | 0.0161 | 0.0134 | 0.0111 |
| 5.00 | 0.0380 | 0.0379 | 0.0372 | 0.0374 | 0.0376 | 0.0370 | 0.0352 | 0.0329 | 0.0302 | 0.0275 | 0.0249 | 0.0201 | 0.0162 | 0.0130 |
| 4.00 | 0.0608 | 0.0604 | 0.0595 | 0.0602 | 0.0600 | 0.0573 | 0.0527 | 0.0474 | 0.0420 | 0.0370 | 0.0325 | 0.0249 | 0.0193 | 0.0151 |
| 3.50 | 0.0806 | 0.0798 | 0.0791 | 0.0798 | 0.0789 | 0.0735 | 0.0658 | 0.0577 | 0.0499 | 0.0430 | 0.0370 | 0.0276 | 0.0209 | 0.0161 |
| 3.00 | 0.112 | 0.110 | 0.110 | 0.110 | 0.107 | 0.0966 | 0.0834 | 0.0707 | 0.0594 | 0.0499 | 0.0421 | 0.0304 | 0.0225 | 0.0171 |
| 2.50 | 0.165 | 0.162 | 0.163 | 0.161 | 0.153 | 0.130 | 0.107 | 0.0868 | 0.0705 | 0.0576 | 0.0475 | 0.0332 | 0.0241 | 0.0181 |
| 2.00 | 0.271 | 0.264 | 0.266 | 0.252 | 0.229 | 0.180 | 0.138 | 0.106 | 0.0829 | 0.0657 | 0.0530 | 0.0359 | 0.0256 | 0.0189 |
| 1.50 | 0.539 | 0.522 | 0.500 | 0.434 | 0.363 | 0.250 | 0.176 | 0.128 | 0.0958 | 0.0737 | 0.0581 | 0.0383 | 0.0268 | 0.0196 |
| 1.00 | — | 1.589 | 1.141 | 0.805 | 0.585 | 0.341 | 0.218 | 0.149 | 0.108 | 0.0807 | 0.0625 | 0.0403 | 0.0278 | 0.020l |
| 0.50 | — | 6.577 | 2.484 | 1.350 | 0.854 | 0.426 | 0.252 | 0.165 | 0.116 | 0.0854 | 0.0654 | 0.0415 | 0.0284 | 0.0205 |
| 0.00 | — | 8.084 | 3.087 | 1.612 | 0.979 | 0.463 | 0.266 | 0.171 | 0.119 | 0.0872 | 0.0664 | 0.0419 | 0.0286 | 0.0206 |

To obtain cGy/mgRaEq·h, multiply table entries by 7.227. From Williamson[19] with permission.

rather than the two dimensional form. Recommended values for the various parameters used and this formalism are available in publications prepared by the AAPM.[21]

## REFERENCES

1. Bohr N. On the constitution of atoms and molecules. *Philos. Mag.* 1913; 26:476, 875.
2. Hendee WR, Ibbott, GS, and Hendee, EG. Radiation Therapy Physics. 3rd ed. Hoboken, NJ: John Wiley & Sons, Inc. Publications; 2005.
3. Hendee WR, Ibbott, GS. Radiation Therapy Physics, 2nd ed. Philadelphia, (PA), Mosby-Year Book: 1996.
4. LoSasso T, Chui CS, and Ling CC. Comprehensive quality assurance for the delivery of intensity modulated radiotherapy with a multileaf collimator used in the dynamic mode. *Med Phys* 2001; 28:2209–2219.
5. Kirby TH, Hanson WF, Gastorf RJ, Chu CH, Shalek RJ. Mailable TLD System for Photon and Electron Therapy Beams. *Int J Radiat Oncol Biol Phys.* 1986; 12:261–265.
6. Ibbott GS, Attix FH, Slowey TW, Fontenla DP, Rozenfeld ML. Uncertainty of calibrations at the accredited dosimetry calibration laboratories. *Med Phys.* 1997; 24:1249–1254.
7. Almond PR, et al. AAPM's TG-51 protocol for clinical reference dosimetry of high-energy photon and electron beams. *Med. Phys.* 1999; 26:1847–1870.
8. Mayneord W and Lamerton L. A survey of depth dose data. *Br J Radiol.* 1941; 14:255–264.
9. Johns HE and Cunningham, JR. The Physics of Radiology. 4th ed. Springfield, IL: Charles C Thomas Publisher; 1983.
10. Batho HF. Lung corrections in $^{60}$Co beam therapy. *J Can Assoc Radiol* 1964; 15:79.
11. Sontag MR and Cunningham JR. The equivalent tissue/air ratio method for making absorbed dose calculations in a heterogeneous medium. *Radiology.* 1978; 129:787.
12. Laughlin JS et al. Electron-beam treatment planning in inhomogeneous tissue. *Radiology.* 1965; 85:524.
13. International Commission on Radiation Units and Measurements, Report 50. *Prescribing, recording and reporting photon beam therapy.* 1993.
14. International Commission on Radiation Units and Measurements, Report 62. *Prescribing, recording and reporting photon beam therapy.* (Supplement to ICRU Report 50). 1999.
15. Constantinou C, Harrington JC, DeWerd LA. An electron density calibration phantom for CT-based treatment planning computers. *Med. Phys.* 1992; 19:325–327.
16. Cunningham JR. Keynote Address: Development of computer algorithms for radiation treatment planning. *Int J Radiat Oncol Biol Phys.* 1989; 16:1367–1376.
17. Mackie TR et al. Generation of photon energy deposition kernels using EGS Monte Carlo code. *Phys Med Biol.* 1988; 33:1–20.
18. AAPM Task Group No. 32. *Specification of brachytherapy source strength.* Report No. 21. June 1987.
19. Williamson JF. Monte Carlo-Based Dose-Rate Tables for the Amersham CDCS.J and 3M Model 6500 $^{137}$Cs Tubes. *Int J Radiat Oncol Biol Phys.* 1998; 41: 4, 959–970.
20. Nath R, Anderson LL, Luxton G, Weaver KA, Williamson WF, Meigooni AS. Dosimetry of interstitial brachytherapy sources: Recommendations of the AAPM Radiation Therapy Committee Task Group No. 42. *Med Phys.* 1995; 22, 209–234.
21. Rivard MJ, Coursey BM, DeWerd LA, Hanson WF, Huq MS, Ibbott GS, Mitch MG, Nath R, Williamson JF. Update of AAPM Task Group No. 43 Report: A revised AAPM Protocol for brachytherapy dose calculations. *Med Phys.* 2004; 31: 3, 633–642.

# 2

# The Biologic Basis of Radiotherapy

*Barry S. Rosenstein, PhD*

## INTRODUCTION

Radiobiology is the scientific field dedicated to investigating the effects of ionizing radiations on biologic systems. For the purpose of this chapter, the material presented focuses upon those forms of radiation which are used for the treatment of cancer and benign diseases that are amenable to therapy with radiation. Hence, attention is concentrated primarily upon X- and γ-rays, which are used for the vast majority of treatments. What distinguishes X- and γ-ray photons from other forms of electromagnetic radiation is their ability to eject electrons from atoms. Hence, these are ionizing forms of radiation. Also discussed are particulate types of radiation that are employed in radiotherapy, including protons, neutrons, and carbon ions.

## INTERACTION OF RADIATION WITH MATTER

The initial interaction of radiation with matter is to deposit energy by ejecting electrons from atoms. These fast electrons continue on to produce additional ionizations, thereby magnifying the effect of the initial photon interactions. The deposition of energy is random and discrete with spurs (<100 eV), blobs (100–500 eV), and short tracks (500–5000 eV) producing ionizations. Since the majority of the cell consists of water, an important interaction of X-rays is with water molecules, resulting in creation of ion pairs that lead to the formation of free radicals, particularly hydroxyl radicals, which may react with cellular constituents. This process represents the indirect action of radiation and is the mechanism through which the majority of damage in irradiated cells is created. It is in contrast to direct action in which modifications form directly in a target molecule as a result of ionizations produced within that cellular constituent.

Although radiation induces damage to a variety of cellular components, much attention has focused upon DNA as a critical molecule whose alteration by radiation plays a significant role in the events that take place following irradiation. There is substantial evidence to suggest that the DNA double strand break represents the most important lesion whose lack of repair or misrepair can result in cell killing and other biologic effects of radiation.[1] However, double strand breaks are often located in a site where there are several areas of damages, referred to as a local multiply damaged site or clustered lesion, which may represent the critical form of damage.[2,3]

## Linear Energy Transfer

When ionizing radiations traverse biological material, the ionizations are not produced in a random manner but along tracks whose pattern is dependent upon the particular type of radiation[4] (Figure 2-1). In order to quantitate the density of ionizations along a radiation track, the linear energy transfer (LET) is calculated. The LET is equal to the energy transferred per unit track length expressed in units of keV/$\mu$m and depends upon certain characteristics of the radiation:

- **Energy.** For a given particle, the higher the energy and therefore the greater the velocity, the lower is the LET.
- **Mass.** For a given energy, LET increases with particle mass.
- **Charge.** LET increases with particle charge.

---

**FIGURE 2-1** Low LET and high LET radiation tracks.

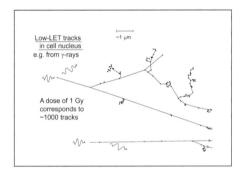

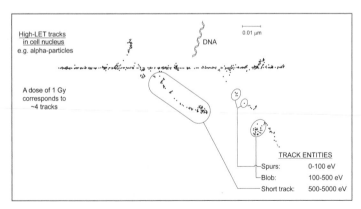

Schematic representation of tracks from low LET $\gamma$-rays (upper panel) or high LET $\alpha$-particles (lower panel). Note that the scale for the $\alpha$-particle track is magnified 100-fold compared with the scale used for the $\gamma$-rays to show the fine structure of this track more distinctly.

Adapted from Goodhead DT: The initial physical damage produced by ionizing radiations. *Int J Radiat Biol* 56:623–634, 1989, with permission.

X- and γ-rays are sparsely ionizing and are characterized by a low LET, whereas particulate forms of radiation such as neutrons and carbon ions are densely ionizing and have a high LET. The importance of direct compared with indirect action increases with LET.

## RELATIVE BIOLOGIC EFFECTIVENESS

The relative biologic effectiveness (RBE) is a parameter used to quantify differences in the biologic impact of a given dose for diverse forms of radiation. It is equal to:[5]

$$RBE = \frac{\text{X-ray dose to produce biologic effect}}{\text{Dose of test radiation to produce effect}}$$

It is important to note that there is not a set RBE for a particular type of radiation since RBE depends on:

- LET
- Biologic end point
- Biologic system
- Fractionation
- Dose rate

For a given end point and mode of radiation delivery, the RBEs for a series of radiations increase with LET up to about 100 keV/μm and then decrease for radiations with greater LET values (Figure 2-2).

## CHROMOSOMAL ABERRATIONS

Radiation damage to DNA often results in breakage of the phophodiester chain. These breaks may either restitute, fail to rejoin and result in deletion of a portion of the chromosome, or the broken ends may reassort and give rise to a chromosomal aberration whose presence could prove lethal to a cell (Box 2-1).[6] The phase of the cell cycle in which the cell is located at the time of irradiation is critical to the type of aberration produced. Chromosome-type aberrations result if the cell is irradiated prior to DNA replication, whereas chromatid-type aberrations are produced by irradiation of cells which have completed DNA synthesis[7] (Box 2-1 and Figure 2-3).

The dose response for the induction of chromosomal aberrations depends on various factors:

- For low LET radiations, the relationship between the number of chromosomal aberrations (E) and dose (D) is linear-quadratic, where $E = \alpha D + \beta D^2$, for exchange-type aberrations which result from the interaction between two chromosomal damages. α and β are parameters specific to the particular chromosomal aberration, radiation, and cell type.
- The dose response is linear for chromosome or chromatid deletions that arise from only one break.
- The yield of aberrations decreases when the dose rate or fraction size is reduced for low LET radiations.

**FIGURE 2-2** LET, RBE, and OER.

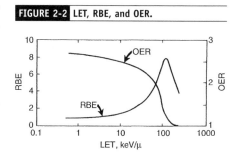

Variation of the RBE and OER as a function of the LET of the radiation used.

Adapted from Hall EJ, Giaccia AJ, *Radiobiology for the Radiologist*, Lippincott Williams and Wilkins, Philadelphia, 2006, with permission.

**BOX 2-1 CLASSES OF CHROMOSOMAL ABERRATIONS**

**Chromosome-Type Aberrations**

- Intra-arm exchanges: An interaction between damages on the same arm of a single chromosome (interstitial deletion, acentric ring, and inversion).
- Inter-arm exchanges: An interaction between damages on opposite sides of the centromere on the same chromosome (centric ring).
- Interchanges: An interaction between damages on different chromosomes (dicentric and translocation).
- Discontinuity: Single chromosome break (terminal deletion).

**Chromatid-Type Aberrations**

- Intra-chromatid exchanges: Alteration of only one chromatid, often together with centric structures
- Inter-chromatid exchanges: Results in a sister chromatid exchange when exchange occurs between homologous chromatids
- Discontinuity: Single chromatid break results in loss of a fragment in one chromatid and the appearance of an acentric fragment in anaphase. Breaks at homologous sites in both chromatids are termed "isochromatid" breaks. Usually join, distinguishing them from chromosome breaks. Lead to the formation of an anaphase bridge.

- The dose response tends towards linearity, regardless of aberration-type, for cells irradiated with high LET forms of radiation.

## Biologic Dosimetry Using Chromosomal Aberrations

The measurement of chromosomal aberrations in peripheral blood lymphocytes represents a useful system to estimate dose for individuals not wearing a radiation monitoring device as may occur during an accident involving exposure to radiation.[8,9] One approach has been to measure dicentric chromosomes in peripheral blood lymphocytes. However, since mature lymphocytes are gradually lost and the presence of chromosome aberrations in lymphocyte progenitor cells may result in their

**FIGURE 2-3 Chromosome-type aberrations.**

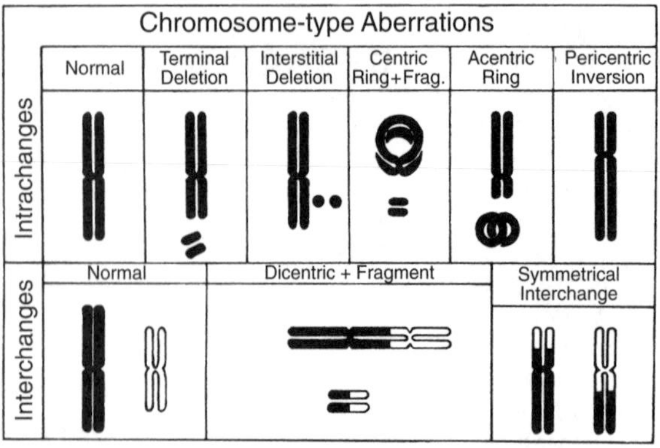


Major classes of chromosome-type aberrations induced by radiation as they would be visualized at mitosis.

Adapted from Evans HJ: Actions of radiations on human chromosomes. *Phys in Med and Biol* 17:1–13, 1972, with permission.

death, the yield of this type of "unstable" aberration diminishes over time. An alternative is the use of chromosomal probes and either fluorescent in situ hybridization (FISH) or genome-wide screening techniques such as spectral karyotyping (SKY), through which it is possible to detect stable aberrations such as traslocations, even decades following irradiation.[10]

### Radiation-Induced Bystander Effects

It has been demonstrated that cells not directly exposed to radiation may nevertheless exhibit effects resulting from the irradiation in the form of genomic instability and cellular lethality. The mechanism for this bystander effect appears to be mediated by a signal received from the irradiated cells.[11] It has also been suggested that bystander effects may be associated with low-dose hypersensitivity in which cells exhibit greater sensitivity to a low dose compared with a higher dose, as well as the adaptive response in which a low dose can provide protection against a subsequent high dose irradiation.[12,13]

## MODELS OF CELL SURVIVAL

The determination of a radiation cell survival curve is useful for many reasons, including measurement of the radiation sensitivity for a particular cell type, the effectiveness of a radiosensitzer/protector, and the modification to cell survival associated with a fractionated or low dose-rate protocol. Examples of survival curves for sparsely and densely ionizing radiations[14] are shown in Figure 2-4. There are two popular approaches to modeling the radiation survival curve (Box 2-2).

---

**FIGURE 2-4** Radiation cell survival curves

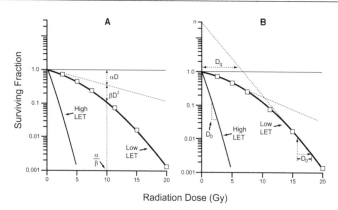

Radiation Dose (Gy)

The fraction of cells surviving a series of doses from either a low or high LET radiation plotted on a logarithmic scale. **(A)** Linear quadratic model. The survival curve used to fit the data is $S = e^{-(\alpha D + \beta D^2)}$. At the dose equal to $\alpha/\beta$, the portion of cell killing due to the $\alpha D$ or linear component of irreparable lesions is equal to the portion of cell killing due to the $\beta D^2$ or quadratic component resulting from the accumulation of sublethal lesions. **(B)** Target model. $D_0$ is the inverse of the final slope of the survival curve and represents a parameter of radiosensitivity. The Dq and n provide an indication as to the extent of the "shoulder" of the survival curve. Increasing values for these parameters are predictive of greater sparing resulting from either dose fractionation or irradiation at a low dose-rate.

---

**BOX 2-2** RADIATION CELL SURVIVAL CURVE MODELS

**Target Models**
- Single-hit, single-target model: Cell killing results from a single lethal damage to one target. The equation describing this model is $S = e^{-D/D_0}$ where D is the dose and $D_0$ is the inverse of the final slope of the survival curve and represents a parameter of radiosensitivity. This model usually provides an acceptable fit for data obtained from cells exposed to high LET radiations, but generally not low LET radiations.
- Single-hit, multi-target model: Cell death results from inactivation of n targets each by a single lethal event. The equation describing this model is $S = 1-(1-e^{-D/D_0})^n$ where n is the number of sublethal targets.
- Two component model: Cell killing results from either a single lethal event or by the accumulation of sublethal damages. The equation describing this model is $S = (e^{-D/_1D_0})[1-(1-e^{-D/_nD_0})]^n$ where $_1D_0$ and $_nD_0$ are the coefficients for the production of either lethal or sublethal events, respectively. Although data obtained for X-irradiated cells can be fit reasonably well to this equation, it is difficult to manipulate mathematically.

**Linear Quadratic Model**
- Origins of this model are in target theory and the shape of the dicentric chromosome induction curve.
- Widely used primarily because it represents a good fit for most survival data and is relatively simple mathematically.
- The equation to represent the survival curve is $S = e^{-(\alpha D+\beta D^2)}$ where $\alpha$ is in units of $Gy^{-1}$ and $\beta$ is in units of $Gy^{-2}$.
- Model describes the nature of the survival response which is thought to have a linear component indicative of cell death due to the induction of "non-reparable" damage and a quadratic component for cell kill resulting from the accumulation of "sublethal" damage.
- $\alpha$ and $\beta$ are parameters of sensitivity and therefore provide a measure of either inherent cellular radiosensitivity, the radiation effectiveness, or the impact of a radiosensitizer/radioprotector.
- $\alpha/\beta$ ratio (in units of Gy) is indicative of the radiobiological response of a particular cell population to a radiation dose delivered over a series of fractions as opposed to a single exposure.

It is important to note that the $\alpha D$ component of the cell killing depends primarily on the total dose and not how it is delivered. In contrast, the $\beta D^2$ component is sensitive to both fraction size and dose rate for a continuous irradiation. Fractionation will have relatively little impact on the survival of cells whose dose response curve is characterized with a large $\alpha/\beta$ ratio whereas there will be a substantial sparing for cells that display a survival curve with a small $\alpha/\beta$. An important observation is that the $\alpha/\beta$ values for tumors and early responding tissues are often high ($\sim 10$ Gy), whereas they tend to be small for late-responding tissues ($\sim 3$ Gy).[15] Hence, use of small fraction sizes or exposure at a low dose rate will generally have a greater sparing effect upon late responding tissues compared with early responding tissues and tumors (Figure 2-5). This represents a fundamental basis for fractionated radiotherapy. However, it should be noted that there may be instances when the $\alpha/\beta$ ratio for a particular type of cancer is comparable to the $\alpha/\beta$ ratio for the critical dose-limiting late effect in the normal tissue/organ irradiated.[16,17] In such cases, it might be feasible to design a radiotherapy protocol that utilizes a large dose per fraction since the impact of fraction size should be comparable in the tumor and normal tissue.

## CELLULAR REPAIR OF RADIATION DAMAGE

It is useful to describe two operational definitions of radiation induced cell damage; potentially lethal damage[18] (Box 2-3) and sublethal damage.[19]

**FIGURE 2-5** Effect of fraction size on early and late radiation effects.

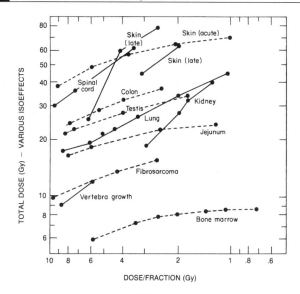

The total dose necessary to produce a series of either early or late radiation effects as well as tumor control plotted as a function of the dose per fraction used to produce the effect. The dashed lines represent early effects, whereas the solid lines used are late effects. As can be observed, the slopes of the late isoeffect curves are generally steeper than the slopes of the early isoeffect curves indicating that fraction size has a greater impact upon late effects compared with early effects.

Adapted from Withers HR: Biologic basis for altered fractionation schemes, *Cancer* 55:2086–2095, with permission.

## TUMOR CONTROL PROBABILITY

If a dose is delivered in a series of fractions, as is nearly always the case in radiotherapy, rather than in a single exposure, then the resulting effective survival curve will be exponential and the effective $D_{10}$ ($_eD_{10}$), the dose required to result in a surviving fraction of 0.1, will be equal to the $_eD_0$ multiplied by 2.3. When the dose response for a large number of identical tumors is plotted, the shape of the tumor control probability (TCP) curve above a certain threshold is sigmoidal because killing is assumed to be a random process and the probability of tumor cure provided by the following equation:

$$P_{cure} = e^{-(M)(SF)}$$

where SF is the clonogen surviving fraction and M is the initial number of clonogens.

Hence, a tumor with $10^9$ clonogens will require a dose that produces a surviving fraction of $10^{-10}$ to result in a 90% probability of cure. However, because of tumor and treatment variability, the clinical data yield TCP curves with shallower slopes than predicted by this equation. It is useful to remember for calculations of TCP that the volume of a sphere is equal to $\pi d^3/6$. Thus, a doubling of the tumor diameter results in an eight-fold increase in volume and, in principle, a similar increase in cell number, representing three cell doublings. Therefore, an increase from a 1 cm

---

**BOX 2-3** OPERATIONAL DEFINITIONS OF CELLULAR DAMAGE

**Potentially Lethal Damage (PLD)**

- Damage that can be modified by postirradiation environmental conditions.
- PLD is considered to have been repaired (PLDR) if survival increases due to alteration of the postirradiation environment such as maintaining cells under conditions that do not permit cell growth.
- PLD is expressed if survival decreases due to the manipulation of the postirradiation environment such as forcing cells to divide shortly after they are irradiated.

**Sublethal Damage (SLD)**

- Damage which, under normal circumstances, can be repaired in hours unless additional sublethal damage is added that interacts to form lethal damage.
- Sublethal damage repair (SLDR) is manifested as the increase in survival when a dose of radiation is split into two or more parts separated by a time interval.
- The smaller the $\alpha/\beta$ ratio, the greater will be the extent of SLDR exhibited by these cells.
- SLDR may result in a therapeutic advantage since late responding normal tissues often exhibit smaller $\alpha/\beta$ values than tumors.
- Little or no SLDR occurs following exposure to high LET radiations.
- For continuous irradiations, as dose-rate decreases, the toxicity of the treatment diminishes due to the repair of sublethal damage during the course of the irradiation.[23] Effect most apparent for dose rates between 0.01 and 1 Gy/min.
- For some cell types over certain dose-rate ranges, dose rate lowering may result in increased cell killing, a phenomenon termed the inverse dose rate effect.[24] One explanation for this effect is that during irradiation at these dose-rates, cells may still be able to progress through the cell cycle but are blocked in $G_2$, a cell cycle phase when cells are particularly sensitive to radiation. It has also been suggested that the inverse dose-rate effect may have as its basis events that are in common with low dose hypersensitivity.[12]

---

to a 2 cm diameter tumor may require nearly an additional $_eD_{10}$ to maintain the same level of tumor control. Dose response curves for the incidence of a particular effect or complication in normal tissues are also sigmoidal above a threshold but tend to be steeper than those for tumor control due to the relative homogeneity of normal tissue radiation responses.

## Radiosensitivity and Cell Cycle Phase

Sensitivity of cells to radiation differs depending upon their position in the cell cycle at the time of irradiation.[20]

- Cells are generally most sensitive during $G_2$ and in M.
- Resistance is usually greatest in the latter part of S.
- Early S and $G_1$ cells exhibit intermediate radiosensitivity, although a resistant period may be evident early in $G_1$.

This differential cell cycle phase radiosensitivity represents an important factor in radiotherapy since surviving cells that were in a resistant phase at the time of an initial irradiation may continue through the cell cycle. Therefore, at the time of a second irradiation, a cell which may have been in a relatively resistant portion of the cell cycle could have progressed into a more sensitive phase and sustain radiation damage which will result in lethality. Reassortment sensitization occurs primarily in more actively dividing cell populations, which may be found in certain types of cancers, and is largely absent in late-responding normal tissue. This represents an important basis for fractionated radiotherapy since, without cell cycle reassortment, a substantially higher radiation dose may be necessary to eradicate a tumor with a single irradiation due to the presence of cells in radiore-sistant portions of the cell cycle (Figure 2-6).

## THE OXYGEN EFFECT

Exposure of biologic systems to low LET forms of radiation in the presence of oxygen results in greater lethality than irradiation under conditions of diminished oxygen.[21] Oxygen sensitizes cells to radiation as its presence increases the yield, variety, and lifetime of the radicals formed upon

**FIGURE 2-6**  Repair, reassortment, and repopulation.

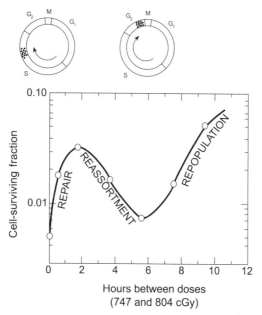

Hours between doses
(747 and 804 cGy)

Chinese hamster cells were irradiated with two doses separated by different time intervals. When the cells were allowed to incubate at 37°C for 1 to 2 hours following the first dose, the surviving fraction was greater than when both fractions were delivered without incubation. This increase in survival was due to repair of sublethal damage between fractions. However, if the cells were incubated 4 to 6 hours following the first dose, the surviving fraction increased, but not with the same magnitude associated with the shorter incubations. This result was obtained since the cells surviving the first radiation expo-sure were primarily S phase cells. Although these cells had repaired much of the sublethal damage induced by the first dose, the resulting diminished radiation toxicity was counterbalanced by the re-assortment of these cells into the more radiation sensitive G$_2$ phase of the cell cycle. Permitting the cells to incubate longer than approximately 6 hours once again resulted in an increased surviving frac-tion since the cells which were not killed due to the first irradiation were able to divide and increase the total number of cells irradiated with the second fraction, thereby resulting in a greater cell-surviving fraction due to repopulation.

Adapted from Hall EJ, Giaccia AJ, *Radiobiology for the Radiologist*, Lippincott Williams and Wilkins, Philadelphia, 2006, with permission.

irradiation. The parameter used to measure the radiation sensitization produced by oxygen is the oxygen enhancement factor (OER), which is generally in the range of 2.5–3.5 for sparsely ionizing radiations and is defined as:

$$\text{OER} = \frac{\text{dose to produce biologic effect under hypoxic conditions}}{\text{dose to produce biologic effect under aerated conditions}}$$

There are a number of points important to consider for the role of oxygen in radiotherapy:

1. OER is inversely proportional to LET of the radiation. This may represent a reason for use of a high LET radiation in radiotherapy.[22] If hypoxic cells are present in a tumor, particularly if they do not reoxygenate well, then use of a high LET radiation could be therapeutically advantageous since a potential survival advantage conferred to hypoxic tumor cells would be eliminated.

2. As the oxygen concentration decreases from fully aerated to hypoxic conditions, survival increases, with the large change in radiobiolgic effectiveness taking place in the range of 0–30 mmHg. This is of significance because oxygen tension in most normal tissues is similar to the 20–40 mmHg characteristic of venous blood. Therefore, a small drop in the normal oxygen level can result in radiation resistance.

3. Chronic hypoxia results from the limited diffusion distance of oxygen through tissue[25] whereas acute hypoxia[26] is a result of the temporary closing of a tumor blood vessel and is therefore transient.

4. Initially following irradiation of a tumor, a large portion of the aerated cells may be killed and the percentage of viable tumor cells that are hypoxic rises dramatically, but does not remain high since tumor cells reoxygenate.[27] Reoxygenation is thought to be essential since in its absence relatively few tumors possessing hypoxic cells would in theory be curable.

5. Tumor hypoxia, independent of considerations of radioresistance, is a marker of tumor aggressiveness as hypoxic conditions cause an increase in genomic instability and malignancy.[28]

## RADIOSENSITIZERS, BIOREDUCTIVE DRUGS, AND RADIOPROTECTORS

There are many chemicals capable of rendering cells or tissues more sensitive to radiation, but it is only those drugs for which there is a differential response between the tumor and dose-limiting normal tissues, that may be of benefit in radiotherapy. In addition to molecular approaches involving the use of targeted therapies, which are discussed separately, drugs that enhance the effects of a radiation treatment are outlined in Table 2-1.

## RADIOPROTECTORS

The goal of a radioprotector is to reduce the radiation response of normal tissues while not affecting the cytotoxicity of radiation against tumor cells. Most attention has focused upon the development of sulfhydryl compounds that protect through a mechanism of free-radical scavenging against oxygen-based free-radical production by radiation. Sulfhydryl compounds are most effective against low LET radiations.[34] The lead compound being tested in clinical trails is amifostine (WR2721, Ethyol), which is a prodrug and does not readily permeate cells because of its terminal phosphorothioic group that reduces the toxicity of the drug. When dephosphorylated by alkaline phosphatase, it is converted to the active metabolite which readily enters cells and scavenges free radicals. Amifostine has a potential use in radiotherapy based upon data suggesting its more rapid uptake by normal tissues compared with tumors.[35]

**TABLE 2-1 Radiosensitizers**

| Drug | Mode of Action |
|---|---|
| Halogenated pyrimidines | • DNA polymerase incorporates halogenated pyrimidines such as 5-bromo- or iodo-deoxyuridine in place of thymidine.<br>• Incorporation of analog in DNA enhances radiation sensitivity.<br>• Therapeutic gain expected for tumors possessing rapidly proliferating clonogens with slowly growing surrounding normal tissues.[29] |
| Hypoxic cell radiosensitizers | • Enhance radiosensitivity of cells deficient in molecular oxygen.[30]<br>• Improvement in the therapeutic index based on the premise that hypoxic cells occur primarily in tumors and not in normal tissues.<br>• Main drugs investigated have been misonidazole, etanidazole, and nimorazole. |
| 5-fluorouracil (5-FU) | • Converted to FdUMP which forms a stable covalent compound with thymidylate synthase leading to its inhibition.<br>• Radiosensitization may result from either dTMP depletion resulting in defective DNA synthesis and DNA repair or abrogating radiation-induced $G_2$ arrest.[31] |
| Gemcitabine (difluorodeoxy-cytidine) | • Causes depletion of deoxynucleotide pools and incorporation into DNA inhibits DNA synthesis.<br>• Deoxynucleotide depletion could lead to misrepair in irradiated cells.[31] |
| Cisplatin | • May radiosensitize cells either through enhanced formation of toxic platinum intermediates in the presence of radiation-induced free radicals and/or inhibition of DNA repair and cell cycle arrest.[31] |
| Taxanes | • Paclitaxel (Taxol) and docetaxel (Taxotere) are mitotic inhibitors that stabilize microtubules by promoting their assembly and preventing depolymerization.<br>• Cells are arrested in $G_2/M$, a radiosensitive portion of the cell cycle.[32] |
| Hypoxic cell cytotoxins | • Selectively kill hypoxic cells.[33]<br>• Require bioreductive activation by nitroreductase enzymes resulting in their conversion to a cytotoxic intermediate which is oxidized back to the parent compound in the presence of oxygen.<br>• Three categories; (1) quinone antibiotics (mitomycin C), (2) nitroheterocyclic compounds (misonidazole and etanidazole), (3) benzotriazine di-N-oxides (tirapazamine). |

## CELL, TISSUE, AND TUMOR KINETICS

Several parameters (Table 2-2) are useful to describe cell, tissue, and tumor kinetics.[36]

## TIME, DOSE, AND FRACTIONATION

Although it is anticipated that molecularly based basic and translational radiobiologic research will play a key role to enhance the effectiveness of radiotherapy, it is arguable that the area of radiation biology with the greatest clinical impact has been the development of altered radiotherapy protocols based upon radiobiologic considerations of time, dose, and fractionation.

---

**TABLE 2-2  Cell Kinetic Parameters**

| Parameter | Description | Formula |
|---|---|---|
| Mitotix index (MI) | Fraction of cells exhibiting mitoric figures | $MI = \dfrac{\lambda T_M}{T_C}$<br><br>where $T_M$ is the length of mitosis, Tc is the length of the cell cycle and $\lambda$ is a correction factor to account for the non-linear distribution of cells through the cell cycle (usually 0.7–1.0) |
| Labeling index (LI) | Fraction of cells that incorporate a DNA label | $LI = \dfrac{\lambda T_S}{T_C}$<br><br>where $T_S$ is the length of S phase |
| Growth fraction (GF) | Fraction of viable cells in a population that are cycling | $GF = \dfrac{\text{proliferating cells}}{\text{proliferating + quiescent cells}}$ |
| Potential doubling time ($T_{pot}$) | Time required for a cell population to double in number allowing for growth fraction | $T_{pot} = \dfrac{\lambda T_S}{LI}$ |
| Cell loss factor ($\phi$) | The rate of cell loss as a fraction of the rate cells are added through division | $\phi = 1 - \dfrac{T_{pot}}{T_d}$<br><br>where $T_d$ is the tumor volume doubling time |

## Time and Fraction Size

Extending the time over which a specific radiation dose is delivered lessens its toxicity because tissues and tumors have a means of counteracting the lethal effects of radiation by either stimulating cells to proceed through the cell cycle, triggering molecular events that diminish radiation-induced cell death, recruiting a larger portion of cells into the cell cycle or decreasing the rate of normal cell loss. The resulting enhanced rate of cell production is referred to as compensatory proliferation or accelerated repopulation and is often observed in early responding tissues and many tumors.[37] Hence, if the time to deliver a series of radiation doses is extended, a higher total dose will be necessary either to provide a particular level of tumor control or will be tolerated by an acutely-responding tissue[38] (Figure 2-7). Thus, even though treatment prolongation may diminish the severity of acute radiation toxicity, this modification could also lead to a loss of tumor control. In contrast, varying the length of a radiotherapy protocol does not generally affect radiation tolerance for late radiation responses. In addition to the impact of time upon treatment dose, fraction size also plays a critical role in radiation response. The dose to achieve a particular level of tumor control or the tolerance dose for normal tissues, particularly late-responding organs, generally decreases with increasing fraction size.[15]

**FIGURE 2-7** | **Tumor control and treatment time.**

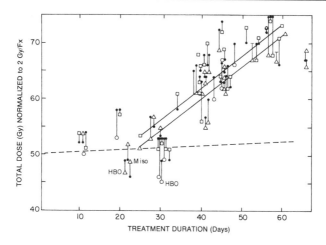

The $TCD_{50}$ (dose to control tumors in 50% of patients) values are plotted as a function of overall time to treat a series of head and neck cancers. Data are provided for T2($\bigcirc$), T3($\square$) or a combination of more than two stages ($\triangle$). For treatments not using 2 Gy fractions, the dose was normalized to the 2 Gy equivalent dose using an $\alpha/\beta$ of 25 Gy. The dose and control rate from which the $TCD_{50}$ was calculated is presented ($\bullet$) to indicate the extent of the extrapolation. The rate of increase in $TCD_{50}$ predicted from a two month clonogen doubling rate(-----). Increase in $TCD_{50}$ (—) with time for T3 ($\square$) and mixed T stages ($\triangle$). HBO designates the use of hyperbaric oxygen and Miso indicates treatment with misonidazole.

Adapted from Withers HR, Taylor JMG, Maciejewski B: The hazard of accelerated tumor clonogen repopulation during radiotherapy, *Acta Oncologica* 27:131–146, 1988, with permission.

## Non-Standard Radiotherapy

Radiotherapy protocols have been developed employing either hyperfractionation or accelerated treatment which involve the use of multiple fractions per day for at least a portion of the treatment. These non-conventional regimens attempt to either take advantage of the greater sparing of late-responding tissues with fractionation or address the problem of tumor repopulation during treatment.[39] In addition, hypofractionation may be used in certain circumstances (Table 2-3).

There is generally little or no impact upon late effects associated with an accelerated treatment since the total dose and fraction size may be only slightly altered. However, a complication of accelerated treatment may be an increase in the level of acute normal tissue toxicity. An important requirement associated with multiple treatments per day protocols is that the minimum time between fractions should be no shorter than 6 hours so as to permit full repair of sublethal damage in normal tissues. This is a particular concern for late radiation effects, especially those that arise in the CNS, which may have a relatively slow rate of repair.[41,42]

## CALCULATION OF BIOLOGICALLY EFFECTIVE DOSES

It is often useful to have a means to compare with a numerical score the theoretical biologic impact of different treatment regimens. This can be accomplished using the linear-quadratic

TABLE 2-3 **Altered Radiotherapy Schedules**

| | Hypo-fractionation | Hyper-fractionation | Accelerated Treatment |
|---|---|---|---|
| Fraction size compared with a conventional protocol[a] | Larger | Smaller (~1.1–1.3 Gy) | May be smaller (~1.4–1.6 Gy), the same or larger |
| Total treatment time compared with conventional protocol | Either unchanged or shorter | Generally unchanged | Shorter |
| Purpose | Complete radiotherapy in fewer treatments | Reduce incidence of late effects while maintaining the same level of tumor control or accept a constant level of late effects, but increase probability of tumor control | Limit the extent of tumor repopulation during treatment |
| Situation when most beneficial | Tumor has either a similar or lower $\alpha/\beta$ ratio than the normal tissues in the radiation field[40] | Tumor exhibits a relatively high $\alpha/\beta$ ratio compared with the dose-limiting normal tissue in the radiation field | Rapidly growing tumors |

[a]Conventional protocol defined as use of 1.8–2.0 Gy fraction sizes delivered daily Monday–Friday to a total dose at which the incidence of adverse effects for critical normal tissues in the radiation field is acceptable.

model to calculate the biologically effective dose (BED)[43–45] which is used to compare different fractionation regimens employing the equations that follow.[46–48] It is assumed that two protocols yielding identical BED values will result in either a similar probability of tumor control or normal tissue effect, depending upon whether the BED was calculated using the $\alpha/\beta$ characteristic of the irradiated tumor or normal tissue. However, in view of the sigmoidal responses for both the tumor control probability and normal tissue adverse effect curves, it must be recognized that a change in the BED for an altered protocol compared with a standard treatment may have little or no clinical impact if the BED for the standard regimen produces either a relatively high or low level of control and/or effects. It is also important to note BED values may not be accurate for protocols involving only one or a few fractions and that BEDs can only be compared when computed using the same $\alpha/\beta$ ratio. In addition, it is possible to add BED values when more than one treatment is used as long as the same $\alpha/\beta$ ratio is employed to calculate the BED. This is helpful when either a change is made in fraction size during the course of treatment or use of a protocol involving both fractionated external beam radiotherapy plus brachytherapy. It should be acknowledged that the equations outlined below do not take dosimetric considerations into account. However, models which enable calculation of normal tissue complication probability (NTCP) curves to reflect partial organ irradiations have been formulated.[49,50]

## (1) Basic Equation

The basic equation that can be used to calculate the BED for a protocol when, (1) the radiation is delivered over a series of fractions at a high dose rate, (2) there is a time period of at least 24 hours between fractions to permit complete repair of sublethal damage, and (3) repopulation does not need to be taken into account either because the lengths of treatment for the protocols being compared are the same or the irradiated tumor/normal tissue is slowly proliferating, is:

$$BED = nd\left[1 + \frac{d}{\alpha/\beta}\right]$$

where n is the number of fractions, d is the dose per fraction and the $\alpha/\beta$ ratio is characteristic of the irradiated tumor or normal tissue.

## (2) Proliferation During Treatment

The basic BED equation can be modified to take into account cellular proliferation during treatment by adding a proliferation term:

$$BED = nd\left[1 + \frac{d}{\alpha/\beta}\right] - \left[\frac{0.693T}{\alpha T_{pot}}\right]$$

where $T_{pot}$ is the potential doubling time, T is the treatment time during which cellular proliferation occurs after any initial lag period and $\alpha$ is a radiosensitivity parameter specific for the irradiated tissue.

## (3) Incomplete Repair

When using a schedule involving multiple fractions per day, there is the possibility that repair may not be complete between fractions. This is not a concern for a conventional treatment when there is generally a 24-hour period between fractions, but for regimens involving two or three fractions per day for which there may be only 4 to 6 hours between fractions, there is the possibility that this time interval may not be adequate for complete repair. Hence, an incomplete repair factor, $h_M$, which can either be calculated from the equation below[51] or obtained from published tables,[52] should be included in the BED calculation[53] to account for either a relatively long repair half-time or a short interval between fractions:

$$BED = nd\left[1 + \frac{d(1 + h_M)}{\alpha/\beta}\right]$$

and

$$h_M = \left[\frac{2}{M}\right]\left[\left(\frac{\phi}{1-\phi}\right)\right]\left[M - \frac{1 - \phi^M}{1 - \phi}\right]$$

where M is the number of fractions delivered per day, $\phi$ is equal to $e^{-\mu(t+\Delta T)}$, t is the exposure duration, $\Delta T$ is the interval between fractions and $\mu$ is the repair rate constant which is equal to $0.693/t_{1/2}$, with $t_{1/2}$ the tissue repair half-time.

## (4) Constant Continuous Low Dose-Rate Irradiations

The BED for a continuous low dose rate treatment at a constant dose rate can be calculated from the equation:

$$BED = RT\left\{1+\left[\frac{2R}{\mu(\alpha/\beta)}\right]\left[1-\frac{1-e^{-\mu T}}{\mu T}\right]\right\}$$

where R is the dose rate, T is the length of the irradiation, and $\mu$ is the repair rate constant.

## (5) Permanent Implant With a Decaying Source

The BED for a continuous low dose-rate treatment delivered by a permanent implant with a decaying source can be calculated as follows:

$$BED = \frac{R_0}{\lambda}\left\{1+\left[\frac{R_0}{(\mu+\lambda)(\alpha/\beta)}\right]\right\}$$

where $R_0$ is initial dose rate of implant, $\lambda$ is the radioactive decay constant of the radioisotope used and is equal to $0.693/T_{1/2}$, $T_{1/2}$ is the radioactive half-life of the isotope and $\mu$ is the repair rate constant.

## PARTICULATE FORMS OF RADIATION

Although the vast majority of radiotherapy is performed using photons, there is increasing interest in the use of particulate forms of radiation (Box 2-4).

---

**BOX 2-4** PARTICULATE FORMS OF RADIATION

**Neutrons**

- High LET and low OER; may be advantageous in treatment of tumors possessing radioresistant hypoxic regions, although reoxygenation generally reduces tumor hypoxia in a conventional fractionated protocol.[54]
- May be useful for the treatment of a limited number of slow-growing tumors.
- Limited clinical potential because of relatively poor ability to deliver a high dose of radiation to a tumor while sparing normal tissues compared with contemporary methods for delivery of X-rays.

**Boron Neutron Capture Therapy (BNCT)**

- Administration of a boron-containing drug that is taken up preferentially by tumor cells.[55]
- Patient exposed to a low energy beam of neutrons that interact with boron to produce short range, densely ionizing $\alpha$-particles and Li ions which irradiate the tumor.

**Protons**

- Dose deposited reaches a sharp maximum near the end of the particle's range that is termed the Bragg peak.[56]
- Main advantage is the ability to confine the high-dose region to the tumor while minimizing irradiation of surrounding normal tissue.
- Radiobiologic properties of the high energy protons used in radiotherapy similar to photons due to their low LET.

**Carbon Ions**

- Excellent dose distribution due to Bragg peak.[57]
- High RBE and low OER, particularly in region of Bragg peak.

## Predictive Assays

As we are entering an era of personalized medicine, it is of increasing interest to determine the optimal treatment plan for each patient individually, rather than using a single standard protocol. The interest in the development of a predictive assay for normal tissue responses is based upon the concept that there are differences between people in their radiation sensitivity. It would therefore be helpful to predict whether a specific patient may be either particularly sensitive or resistant to radiation. Sensitive patients could be encouraged to seek a method of treatment such as surgery or chemotherapy, not involving the use of radiation if these present acceptable options. Alternatively, it is possible that radiosensitive patients could still be suitable candidates for radiotherapy, but a standard dose may be inappropriately high for such patients who might be treated successfully with a lower total dose, assuming that their cancers are also radiosensitive.

In contrast, it may be feasible to treat patients more aggressively who are predicted to be relatively radioresistant and possibly increase the probability of tumor control, which could be of particular importance for more radioresistant forms of cancer. Similarly, it would be of value if it was possible to predict prior to the initiation of radiotherapy whether the cancer being treated in a specific patient would likely either respond well or be resistant to a standard treatment for a particular tumor type. Some of the predictive assays that have been developed are listed in Table 2-4.[58]

## Hyperthermia

The use of heat in combination with radiation has long been of interest in the treatment of cancer.[59] Among the main radiobiologic findings associated with hyperthermia are:

1. The slope of an Arrhenius plot, the inverse of the $D_0$ plotted as a function of the inverse of the temperature, suggests that protein represents the target for heat-induced cell killing.
2. The cell cycle response for heat complements that for X rays in that S phase, the portion of the cell cycle with greatest resistance to X rays, is sensitive to hyperthermia[60] (Figure 2-8).
3. Cells held at acid pH or deficient in nutrients are heat sensitive. Therefore, chronically hypoxic cells that are radioresistant may be sensitive to heat.
4. Heat treatment causes thermotolerance, which is the development of a transient resistance to subsequent heating by an initial heat treatment. The level of heat-shock proteins appears to correlate with the onset and loss of thermotolerance.
5. The biological impact of a combined treatment with heat and radiation may be a consequence of the independent but additive cytotoxic effects of the heat and radiation with their complementary patterns of cell cycle sensitivity and the greater sensitivity to heat of cells at low pH. In addition, the enhancement of radiation cytotoxicity resulting from inhibition of the repair of radiation-induced damage by heat may be of importance.

## Normal Tissue Radiation Response

The purpose of this section is to discuss general principles associated with the response of normal tissues to radiation. The specific histopathologic effects in each tissue/organ system and a detailed description of clinically relevant normal tissue reactions are, however, beyond the scope of this chapter and the reader is referred to a text devoted to this subject.[76]

Radiation responses are commonly divided into early/acute effects and late/chronic effects. Early effects occur within days to weeks after the start of radiotherapy in tissues with a rapid turnover rate. The time of onset for early reactions correlates with the relatively short lifespan of the mature functional cells that comprise these tissues. In contrast, late effects appear after a delay of months or years and occur predominantly in slowly proliferating tissues. An important difference between the two classes of damage lies in their progression. Acute injury is usually repaired

**TABLE 2-4 Predictive Assays**

| Assay | Outcome |
|---|---|
| | *Normal Tissue* |
| Skin fibroblast radiosensitivity | Although there is some evidence indicating an association between skin fibroblast radiosensitivity and the severity of early and late skin effects, this correlation has generally not been observed. |
| Lymphocyte assays | The results of initial lymphocyte radiosensitivity studies were disappointing due to experimental variation, but it may be possible to discriminate differences in radiation-induced cytotoxicity between individuals by taking into account cell-type specific radiosensitivities. |
| Micronuclei formation | Well-established role as a biologic indicator of radiation damage, but efforts to predict radiosensitivity have been inconclusive. |
| Circulating factors | Results have been reported linking a susceptibility for the development of radiation injury in patients undergoing radiotherapy with levels of circulating cytokines, including TGF-$\beta$1, IL-1$\alpha$, IL-6 and KL-6 as well as angiotensin-converting enzyme. However, conflicting results have been reported as to a consistent correlation between these biomarkers with adverse effects.[61–62] |
| Expression arrays | Alterations in gene expression in irradiated normal tissue have been reported to correlate with the development of radiation-induced fibrosis.[63–64] |
| Radiogenomics | Gene-PARE (Genetic Predictors of Adverse Radiotherapy Effects) and GENEPI (GENEtic pathways for the Prediction of the effects of Irradiation) represent two major consortia. Goal is to identify single nucleotide polymorphisms (SNPs) that are predictive for the development of adverse normal tissue effects. Reflective of the HapMap project[65] and the development of high-density SNP arrays which have facilitated the performance of genome-wide studies reporting associations between specific SNPs with either disease susceptibility or treatment responses.[66] |
| | *Tumor* |
| Intrinsic cellular radiosensitivity | A correlation between $SF_2$ (surviving fraction after a dose of 2 Gy) and tumor control has been reported[67] although this assay has not proven useful to predict the response of individual patients to radiotherapy. |
| Proliferative potential | $T_{pot}$ can be estimated through flow cytometric analysis of cells derived from a biopsy obtained from patients who had been administered a halogenated pyrimidine. However, results of a multicenter trial did not support the hypothesis that $T_{pot}$ can be used to predict which patients are the best candidates for an accelerated treatment.[68] |
| Microarray analysis | Several studies have demonstrated the predictive power of pretreatment expression profiling for human tumors treated with chemotherapy.[69] Studies are in progress to identify genes whose expression may correlate with radiotherapy response.[70–71] |
| Oxygen status | Among the approaches that have been developed to identify hypoxic cells[72–75] are labeled nitroimidazoles compounds such as [18]F-misonidazole for PET studies, pimonidazole in immunohistochemical studies, use of Eppendrof polarographic electrodes, and endogenous markers including HIF1-$\alpha$, GLUT-1 and CA9. |

**FIGURE 2-8** Variation in sensitivity to heat and radiation with cell cycle phase.

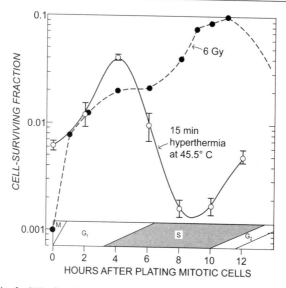

Surviving fraction for CHO cells either heated for 15 min at 45.5°C or irradiated with 6 Gy of X-rays. The position of the cell in the cycle at the time of treatment was determined from uptake of $^3$H-thymidine.

Adapted from Dewey WC, Hopwood LE, Sapareto SA, Gerweck LE: Cellular responses to combinations of hyperthermia and radiation, *Radiology* 123:463–474, 1977, with permission.

because of stem cell proliferation and may be completely reversible. In contrast, late damage could improve, but may never be completely reversed. If the radiation protocol is so severe that it depletes the stem cell population below levels needed for tissue restoration, an early reaction may persist as a chronic injury. Such a response is termed a consequential late effect, as it is a late effect that is a consequence of a persistent severe early effect. Renewal systems may be broadly classified into two categories, hierarchical and flexible (Box 2-5).[77]

## Radiation Late Effects and Cytokine Cascades

It is important to note that the hierarchical and flexible tissue models proposed for the development of early and late radiation effects that are based upon a target cell hypothesis are appropriate only for those organs in which radiation-induced cell depletion plays the major role leading to organ dysfunction. In fact, cell killing alone may play only a modest role in the development of most late effects, such as fibrosis, which are triggered by a radiation-induced cascade of cytokines, particularly involving the vasculature and connective tissue.[78–82] Although radiation-induced late effects are generally defined as responses to radiation that are manifested no earlier than 3 months following the completion of therapy, the events leading to the development of chronic effects likely begin immediately upon exposure to the first dose of radiation. Thus, these events can be viewed as a continuum with progression resulting from an early activation of an inflammatory reaction leading to

---

**BOX 2-5** **NORMAL TISSUE MODELS**

**Hierarchical (Type H) Tissues**

- Rapid turnover rate.
- Suppression of stem cell proliferation by irradiation results in reduced influx of mature cells that continue to be lost at the pre-irradiation rate thereby resulting in depletion of the mature cell compartment.
- Life-span of mature cells is generally limited in type-H tissues, therefore depletion becomes evident shortly after irradiation and is expressed as an early (acute) clinical response.
- The latent period before manifestation of a radiation effect is a reflection of the life-span of the mature functioning cells.

**Flexible (Type F) Tissues**

- Slow turnover rate.
- Because of the long life span of mature cells, suppression of proliferative activity does not result in a rapid decrease in the mature cell population and these tissues exhibit late (chronic) reactions.
- Under normal conditions most cells exist in a differentiated $G_0$ state, but proliferative activity is resumed if cell loss occurs, such as after irradiation.
- If recruited cells were damaged by radiation, they may die upon attempting division.
- The interval between irradiation and manifestation of a radiation effect tends to shorten as the dose increases.

---

the expression and maintenance of a cytokine cascade. Hence, there may be no latent period in a biologic sense, although clinical effects might not be observable for weeks to months post-irradiation. There are immediate and persistent intercellular communications between cells, which lead to the release of autocrine and paracrine messages that determine the course of events once a radiation dose has been delivered. Evidence has been obtained that the inflammatory cytokines, including interleukin (Il)-1, 4, and 6 and TNF$\alpha$ and the fibrotic cytokines TGF$\beta$1, PDGF, and bFGF play important roles in this process. This sequential progression of pro-inflammatory gene expression followed by fibrotic messages and changes is also typical of most wound healing processes. Cytokines and growth factors have been identified as having a wide range of activities and are expressed following a variety of injurious events. Their induction following irradiation is similar to those expressed after other types of injury, such as surgery and chemotherapy, suggesting there are shared pathways of induction or expression of cytotoxic damage. These common events include immunomodulation, angiogenesis, tissue necrosis, and fibrogenic activities.

## ACUTE EFFECTS OF TOTAL BODY IRRADIATION

Early radiation lethality resulting from whole body irradiation is death occurring within approximately 1 to 2 months which can be ascribed to a specific high intensity whole body irradiation.[83,84] The acute radiation syndrome is characterized by four distinct periods:

- Prodromal
- Latent
- Illness
- Recovery or death

During the prodromal period, gastrointestinal and neuromuscular symptoms appear within minutes to hours following irradiation, depending upon the dose received, and generally last several days. Several key symptoms suggestive of a lethal radiation dose are diarrhea, hypotension, and fever. The three major radiation syndromes are described in Table 2-5.

During the hematopoietic syndrome, blood counts show characteristic changes with a relatively rapid onset of lymphocyte depression and a more gradual decrease in neutrophil and platelet counts (Figure 2-9). An important parameter within the dose range that induces bone marrow syndrome is the $LD_{50/60}$, estimated at 3.5 Gy, representing the dose that results in lethality to 50% of an irradiated population within 60 days following irradiation. The $LD_{50/60}$ can be doubled with good medical care. However, above 10–12 Gy, death from GI syndrome is inevitable. In the region of approximately 8–10 Gy, a bone marrow transplant may enhance survival.

## Management of Acute Radiation Syndrome

For doses less than 2 Gy, close observation and management of symptoms, which may be appropriate on an outpatient basis, is recommended. The medical management for people who receive a dose greater than 2 Gy would include treatment of any physical trauma, supportive care in a clean environment (reverse isolation), prevention/treatment of infections using antibiotics, tissue typing for a possible stem-cell transplant, platelet transfusion, and stimulation of hematopoiesis using G-CSF and GM-CSF and psychological support.

## Low Dose Radiation Effects

Although high doses of radiation are used in an effort to eradicate or control the growth of cancer in a patient, concerns associated with exposure to low radiation doses may arise for both radiotherapy personnel and patients, resulting from scattered radiation (both external and internal) and exposure to radioisotopes. The three principal areas of concern are carcinogenesis, hereditary

### TABLE 2-5  Acute Radiation Syndromes

| Syndrome | Cerebrovascular (central nervous system) | Gastrointestinal (GI) | Hematopoietic (bone marrow) |
|---|---|---|---|
| Latent period | Minutes–hours | 3–5 days | 2–3 weeks |
| Dose to induce | >20–50 Gy | >5–8 Gy | >1–3 Gy |
| Period before death | 1–2 days | 3–10 days | 3 weeks–2 months |
| Cause of syndrome | Not certain, but likely due to a cerebral edema, increased intracranial pressure, and cerebral anoxia | Loss of intestinal crypts and breakdown of the GI mucosa | Killing of bone marrow stem and progenitor cells |
| Cause of death | | Infections and marked dehydration as the GI mucosa becomes increasingly atrophic and large amounts of plasma are lost | Infection and hemorrhage may result in death if platelet and white cell counts fall to critically low levels |

---

**FIGURE 2-9** Hematologic response to whole body irradiation.

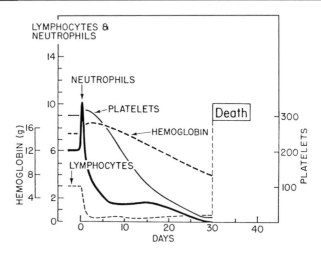

Levels of different blood constituents following a whole body dose of 4.5 Gy. Cell numbers are indicated in units of 10⁹/liter. Hemoglobin values are in gm/100 ml.

Adapted from Andrews GA: Radiation accidents and their management, *Radiat Res Suppl* 7:390–397, 1967, with permission.

effects and fetal effects. In a discussion of low dose radiation effects, it is helpful to define the terms stochastic and deterministic effects (Box 2-6).

## RADIATION CARCINOGENESIS

There is generally a period of years following irradiation before the appearance of a radiation-induced cancer. The average latent period for leukemia is approximately 5 years whereas solid tumors show a much longer latency and may arise decades following irradiation. Although epidemiologic studies for many irradiated populations have been performed to estimate risk for radiation-induced cancer,[85] the Japanese survivors of the atomic bomb attacks on Hiroshima and Nagasaki represent the most important single group that have been followed because they represent a large general population exposed to a wide range of doses.[86,87] An important observation for this population is that the excess relative risk decreased for radiation-induced cancer with both increasing age at time of exposure and attained age. In contrast, although the absolute excess risk also decreased with increasing age at exposure, it increased with attained age[88] (Figure 2-10).

The data obtained for the Japanese atomic bomb survivors and other irradiated populations are consistent with the conclusion that the excess relative risk exhibits a linear increase with dose for solid cancers. It had been suggested that the risk reaches a peak and then decreases with increasing dose due to cell killing, but this concept has been challenged with data indicating that the risk for radiation-induced cancer may plateau or even continue to increase at high doses.[91] The response for leukemia displays a better fit with a linear-quadratic dose response. An association between cancer induction and exposure *in utero* to X rays has been controversial, but it appears

---

**BOX 2-6** **STOCHASTIC AND DETERMINISTIC EFFECTS**

**Stochastic Effects**

• Any dose, however small, may cause the effect, although the probability for induction of the effect is related to the dose received.
• A threshold does not exist for induction of the effect and the severity of the effect is not related to dose.
• Genetic effects and carcinogenesis[89] are examples, although there is controversy as to the existence of a dose threshold for cancer induction by radiation.[90]
• Genetic effects and cancer are considered to be the principal health risks associated with exposure to low radiation doses.[85]

**Deterministic Effects**

• A minimum or threshold dose exists below which induction of the effect cannot be detected.
• The severity of the effect is related to dose.
• Examples are organ/tissue damage and fetal effects.

---

that even a small radiation dose to the developing fetus may increase the cancer risk.[92] In addition, there was a significant dose-response for the development of fatal cancers observed for Japanese atomic-bomb survivors irradiated *in utero*.[93] Although it is difficult to determine the precise role of radiation in the development of second malignancies, data have been obtained suggesting that radiotherapy may induce second cancers.[94–101]

## HERITABLE EFFECTS OF RADIATION

In the absence of data clearly demonstrating statistically significant radiation-induced heritable effects in humans, the risk estimates are based primarily upon animal data.[102] The doubling dose,

---

**FIGURE 2-10** **Excess risk of radiation-induced solid cancers.**

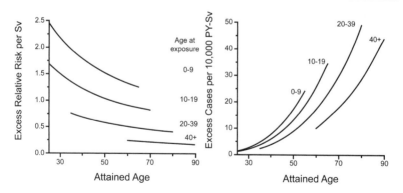

Cohort of Japanese atomic bomb survivors followed by the Radiation Effects Research Foundation. The sex-averaged excess relative risk and excess absolute risk estimates are provided in the left and right panels, respectively, for age-at-exposure groups 0–9, 10–19, 20–39, and 40+ years.

Adapted from Preston DL, Shimizu Y, Pierce DA, Suyama A, Mabuchi K: Studies of mortality of atomic bomb survivors. Report 13: Solid cancer and noncancer disease mortality: 1950–1997, *Radiat Res* 160:381–407, 2003, with permission.

TABLE 2-6  Radiation-Induced Fetal Effects

| Type of effect | Time of gestation when produced |
| --- | --- |
| Prenatal death | Before or immediately after implantation of the embryo into the uterine wall or produced by relatively high doses at later stages of gestation. |
| Congenital malformations | Characteristic of the organ system undergoing active development at the time of irradiation. May result in neonatal death. |
| Growth disturbances | Organogeneis and fetal period. |

which represents a measure of radiation effectiveness to produce hereditary effects, is the dose required to double the spontaneous mutation rate. It has been estimated at approximately 1–2 Sv for humans.[103] Two important findings of animal experiments[104] are that there is a substantial dose rate effect and the genetic consequences of a given dose can be reduced if a time interval is allowed between irradiation and conception.

## RADIATION EFFECTS IN THE DEVELOPING EMBRYO AND FETUS

The major effects of radiation on the embryo and fetus can be classified as outlined in Table 2-6. In terms of human experience,[105,106] information comes primarily from studies of the Japanese atomic bomb survivors. A variety of abnormalities have been reported after *in utero* irradiation, but the most common ones are microcephaly and mental retardation. Severe mental retardation was not observed in this population if the fetus was irradiated earlier than 8 weeks or after 25 weeks of gestation. The relationship between the incidence of mental retardation and dose appears linear and suggests a 40% probability of mental retardation at a dose of 1 Gy received during the most sensitive 8- to 15-week period.

## RADIATION PROTECTION

The objectives of radiation protection are to prevent clinically significant radiation-induced deterministic effects by adhering to dose limits that are below a practical threshold and to limit the risk of stochastic effects (cancer and heritable effects) to a reasonable level . Generally, radiation doses resulting from medical procedures are not included in radiation protection guidelines as these are considered to be of direct benefit to patients in terms of diagnosis or treatment of disease. For the purpose of radiation protection, it is assumed that the risk of stochastic effects is proportional to dose without threshold, throughout the dose range of importance in radiation protection. Given the above assumptions, any selected dose limit will have an associated level of risk. The dose units used in radiation protection are outlined in Table 2-7.

The National Council on Radiation Protection (NCRP) has recommended maximum permissible dose limits for occupational exposure to members of the public which apply to the sum of the effective doses from external radiation and the committed effective doses from internal exposures (Box 2-7).[107] The recommended maximum permissible doses represent upper limits and are subject to the concept of as low as reasonably achievable (ALARA).[108] Hence, exposure of both personnel and patients should be kept as low as possible by either improving shielding, minimizing time spent exposed, increasing the distance from a radiation source, or decreasing the amount of a radioisotope. Implementation of these factors should take into account both economic and radiation risk considerations.

**TABLE 2-7 Radiation Units**

| Unit | Definition | Purpose | SI[1] Units | Conv.[2] Units |
|------|-----------|---------|-------------|----------------|
| Absorbed dose | Energy absorbed per unit mass | Provides a measure of the amount of radiation absorbed by a certain tissue mass | gray (Gy) = 1 J/kg | rad = 100 erg/g<br>1 Gy = 100 rads |
| Equivalent dose | Absorbed dose multiplied by a quality (Q) or radiation weighting factor ($W_R$) | Places biologic effects from exposure to different types of radiations on a common scale based upon RBE values | sievert (Sv) | rem<br>1 Sv = 100 rem |
| Effective dose | Sum of equivalent doses to different organs multiplied by specific tissue weighting factors ($W_T$) for all tissues irradiated | Addresses differential radiation sensitivity among organs to radiation-induced cancers and genetic effects as well as irradiations not resulting in uniform whole body exposure | sievert | rem |
| Committed dose | Integral over 50 years of the equivalent or effective dose after intake of a radionuclide | Accounts for dose resulting from internally deposited radionuclides | sievert | rem |
| Collective dose | Product of the average dose and the number of people exposed | Provides population-based measure of radiation effect | person-sievert | man-rem |
| Genetically significant dose (GSD) | Average equivalent dose to the gonads weighted for the age and sex distribution of the irradiated population to account for expected number of offspring | Provides a dose that can be used to estimate the number of children who will possess radiation-induced mutations due to parental irradiation | sievert | rem |
| Radioactivity | Number of atoms that disintegrate per unit time | Measure of radionuclide's activity | becquerel (Bq)<br>1 Bq = 1 disintegration/sec | curie (Ci)<br>1 Ci = $3.7\times10^{10}$ disintegrations/sec<br>1 Ci = $3.7\times10^{10}$ Bq |

[1]International system of units based upon the metric system which should be used in all scientific communications.
[2]Units commonly used in non-scientific publications.

---

**BOX 2-7 RECOMMENDED DOSE LIMITS**

**Occupational Exposure**

- The individual worker's lifetime effective dose should not exceed age in years X 10 mSv.
- An annual effective dose limit of 50 mSv.
- An annual dose limit of 150 mSv for the lens of the eye.
- An annual dose limit of 500 mSv for localized areas of the skin and the hands and feet.
- A monthly dose limit of 0.5 mSv to the fetus once a pregnancy is declared.
- No occupational exposure should be permitted until age 18 years.

**Public Exposure**

- An annual effective dose limit of 1 mSv for continuous exposure and 5 mSv for infrequent exposure.
- An annual dose limit of 50 mSv for the hands and feet, localized areas of the skin and 15 mSv for the lens of the eye.
- For educational and training purposes involving people younger than age 18 years, an annual effective dose limit of 1 mSv.

---

## References

1. Nunez MI, McMillan TJ, Valenzuela MT, et al. Relationship between DNA damage, rejoining and cell killing by radiation in mammalian cells. *Radiother Oncol* 39: 155–65, 1996.
2. Ward JF. Complexity of damage produced by ionizing radiation. *Cold Spring Harb Symp Quant Biol* 65: 377–382, 2000.
3. Dianov GL, O'Neill P, Goodhead DT. Securing genome stability by orchestrating DNA repair: removal of radiation-induced clustered lesions in DNA. *Bioessays* 23: 745–9, 2001.
4. Goodhead DT. The initial physical damage produced by ionizing radiations. *Int J Radiat Biol* 56: 623–634, 1989.
5. Barendsen G. Responses of cultured cells, tumours and normal tissues to radiation of different linear energy transfer. *Current Topics in Radiation Research* 4: 293–356, 1968.
6. Bender MA. Cytogenetics research in radiation biology. *Stem Cells* 13 Suppl 1: 172–81, 1995.
7. Evans HJ. Actions of radiations on human chromosomes. *Phys Med Biol* 17: 1–13, 1972.
8. Leonard A, Rueff J, Gerber GB, et al. Usefulness and limits of biological dosimetry based on cytogenetic methods. *Radiat Prot Dosimetry* 115: 448–454, 2005.
9. Rodrigues AS, Oliveira NG, Gil OM, et al. Use of cytogenetic indicators in radiobiology. *Radiat Prot Dosimetry* 115: 455–460, 2005.
10. Braselmann H, Kulka U, Baumgartner A, et al. SKY and FISH analysis of radiation-induced chromosome aberrations: a comparison of whole and partial genome analysis. *Mutat Res* 578: 124–133, 2005.
11. Morgan WF. Is there a common mechanism underlying genomic instability, bystander effects and other nontargeted effects of exposure to ionizing radiation? *Oncogene* 22: 7094–7099, 2003.
12. Prise KM, Schettino G, Folkard M, et al. New insights on cell death from radiation exposure. *Lancet Oncol* 6: 520–528, 2005.
13. Mothersill C, Seymour CB. Radiation-induced bystander effects and the DNA paradigm: An "out of field" perspective. *Mutat Res* 597: 5–10, 2006.
14. Hall EJ, Giaccia AJ. *Radiobiology for the Radiologist.* Lippincott Williams & Wilkins, Philadelphia. 6th ed. 2006.
15. Withers HR. Biologic basis for altered fractionation schemes. *Cancer* 55: 2086–2095, 1985.

16. Dasu A. Is the alpha/beta value for prostate tumours low enough to be safely used in clinical trials? *Clin Oncol (R Coll Radiol)* 19: 289–301, 2007.
17. Owen JR, Ashton A, Bliss JM, et al. Effect of radiotherapy fraction size on tumour control in patients with early-stage breast cancer after local tumour excision: long-term results of a randomised trial. *Lancet Oncol* 7: 467–471, 2006.
18. Belli JA, Shelton M. Potentially lethal radiation damage: repair by mammalian cells in culture. *Science* 165: 490–492, 1969.
19. Elkind MM, Sutton H. Radiation response of mammalian cells grown in culture. 1. Repair of X-ray damage in surviving Chinese hamster cells. *Radiat Res* 13: 556–593, 1960.
20. Bernhard EJ, McKenna WG, Muschel RJ. Radiosensitivity and the cell cycle. *Cancer J Sci Am* 5: 194–204, 1999.
21. Barendsen GW, Koot CJ, Van Kersen GR, et al. The effect of oxygen on impairment of the proliferative capacity of human cells in culture by ionizing radiations of different LET. *Int J Radiat Biol Relat Stud Phys Chem Med* 10: 317–327, 1966.
22. Broerse JJ, Barendsen GW, van Kersen GR. Survival of cultured human cells after irradiation with fast neutrons of different energies in hypoxic and oxygenated conditions. *Int J Radiat Biol Relat Stud Phys Chem Med* 13: 559–572, 1968.
23. Hall EJ. Radiation dose-rate: a factor of importance in radiobiology and radiotherapy. *Br J Radiol* 45: 81–97, 1972.
24. Mitchell JB, Bedord JS, Bailey SM. Dose-rate effects on the cell cycle and survival of S3 HeLa and V79 cells. *Radiat Res* 79: 520–536, 1979.
25. Groebe K, Vaupel P. Evaluation of oxygen diffusion distances in human breast cancer xenografts using tumor-specific in vivo data: role of various mechanisms in the development of tumor hypoxia. *Int J Radiat Oncol Biol Phys* 15: 691–697, 1988.
26. Brown JM. Evidence for acutely hypoxic cells in mouse tumours, and a possible mechanism of reoxygenation. *Br J Radiol* 52: 650–656, 1979.
27. Kallman RF. The phenomenon of reoxygenation and its implications for fractionated radiotherapy. *Radiology* 105: 135–142, 1972.
28. Brizel DM, Scully SP, Harrelson JM, et al. Tumor oxygenation predicts for the likelihood of distant metastases in human soft tissue sarcoma. *Cancer Res* 56: 941–943, 1996.
29. McGinn CJ, Kinsella TJ. The clinical rationale for S-phase radiosensitization in human tumors. *Curr Probl Cancer* 17: 273–321, 1993.
30. Saunders M, Dische S. Clinical results of hypoxic cell radiosensitisation from hyperbaric oxygen to accelerated radiotherapy, carbogen and nicotinamide. *Br J Cancer Suppl* 27: S271–8, 1996.
31. Wilson GD, Bentzen SM, Harari PM. Biologic basis for combining drugs with radiation. *Semin Radiat Oncol* 16: 2–9, 2006.
32. Milas L, Milas MM, Mason KA. Combination of taxanes with radiation: preclinical studies. *Semin Radiat Oncol* 9: 12–26, 1999.
33. Brown JM, Wilson WR. Exploiting tumour hypoxia in cancer treatment. *Nat Rev Cancer* 4: 437–447, 2004.
34. Grdina DJ, Kataoka Y, Murley JS. Amifostine: mechanisms of action underlying cytoprotection and chemoprevention. *Drug Metabol Drug Interact* 16: 237–279, 2000.
35. Yuhas JM. Active versus passive absorption kinetics as the basis for selective protection of normal tissues by S-2-(3-aminopropylamino)-ethylphosphorothioic acid. *Cancer Res* 40: 1519–1524, 1980.
36. Tubiana M. Tumor cell proliferation kinetics and tumor growth rate. *Acta Oncol* 28: 113–121, 1989.

37. Thames HD, Bentzen SM, Turesson I, et al. Time-dose factors in radiotherapy: a review of the human data. *Radiother Oncol* 19: 219–35, 1990.

38. Withers HR, Taylor JM, Maciejewski B. The hazard of accelerated tumor clonogen repopulation during radiotherapy. *Acta Oncol* 27: 131–146, 1988.

39. Nguyen LN, Ang KK. Radiotherapy for cancer of the head and neck: altered fractionation regimens. *Lancet Oncol* 3: 693–701, 2002.

40. Brenner DJ, Martinez AA, Edmundson GK, et al. Direct evidence that prostate tumors show high sensitivity to fractionation (low alpha/beta ratio), similar to late-responding normal tissue. *Int J Radiat Oncol Biol Phys* 52: 6–13, 2002.

41. Landuyt W, Fowler J, Ruifrok A, et al. Kinetics of repair in the spinal cord of the rat. *Radiother Oncol* 45: 55–62, 1997.

42. Bentzen SM, Saunders MI, Dische S, et al. Radiotherapy-related early morbidity in head and neck cancer: Quantitative clinical radiobiology as deduced from the CHART trial. *Radiother Oncol* 60: 123–135, 2001.

43. Fowler JF. The linear-quadratic formula and progress in fractionated radiotherapy. *Br J Radiol* 62: 679–694, 1989.

44. Barendsen GW. Dose fractionation, dose rate and iso-effect relationships for normal tissue responses. *Int J Radiat Oncol Biol Phys* 8: 1981–1997, 1982.

45. Thames HD, Jr., Withers HR, Peters LJ, et al. Changes in early and late radiation responses with altered dose fractionation: implications for dose-survival relationships. *Int J Radiat Oncol Biol Phys* 8: 219–226, 1982.

46. Dale RG. The application of the linear-quadratic dose-effect equation to fractionated and protracted radiotherapy. *Br J Radiol* 58: 515–258, 1985.

47. Jones B, Dale RG, Deehan C, et al. The role of biologically effective dose (BED) in clinical oncology. Clin Oncol (R Coll Radiol) 13: 71–81, 2001.

48. Dale RG, Jones B. The clinical radiobiology of brachytherapy. *Br J Radiol* 71: 465–483, 1998.

49. Lyman JT. Complication probability as assessed from dose-volume histograms. *Radiat Res Suppl* 8:S13–9, 1985.

50. Niemierko A. A generalized concept of equivalent uniform dose (EUD). *Med Phys* 26: 1100, 1999.

51. Nilsson P, Thames HD, Joiner MC. A Generalized Formulation of the 'Incomplete-repair' Model for Cell Survival and Tissue Response to Fractionated Low Dose-rate Irradiation. *Int J Radiat Biol* 57: 127–142, 1990.

52. Thames HD, Hendry JH. *Fractionation in Radiotherapy*. Taylor & Francis, London, 1987.

53. Thames HD. An 'incomplete-repair' model for survival after fractionated and continuous irradiations. *Int J Radiat Biol Relat Stud Phys Chem Med* 47: 319–339, 1985.

54. Britten RA, Peters LJ, Murray D. Biological factors influencing the RBE of neutrons: implications for their past, present and future use in radiotherapy. *Radiat Res* 156: 125–135, 2001.

55. Barth RF, Coderre JA, Vicente MG, et al. Boron neutron capture therapy of cancer: current status and future prospects. *Clin Cancer Res* 11: 3987–4002, 2005.

56. Levin WP, Kooy H, Loeffler JS, et al. Proton beam therapy. *Br J Cancer* 93: 849–854, 2005.

57. Jakel O, Schulz-Ertner D, Karger CP, et al. Heavy ion therapy: status and perspectives. *Technol Cancer Res Treat* 2: 377–387, 2003.

58. Ho AY, Atencio DP, Peters S, et al. Genetic Predictors of Adverse Radiotherapy Effects: the Gene-PARE Project. *Int J Radiat Oncol Biol Phys* 65: 646–655, 2006.

59. Dewhirst MW, Vujaskovic Z, Jones E, et al. Re-setting the biologic rationale for thermal therapy. *Int J Hyperthermia* 21: 779–790, 2005.

60. Dewey WC, Hopwood LE, Sapareto SA, et al. Cellular responses to combinations of hyperthermia and radiation. *Radiology* 123: 463–474, 1977.
61. Fleckenstein, K, Gauter-Fleckenstein, B, Jackson, IL, et al. Using biological markers to predict risk of radiation injury. *Semin Radiat Oncol* 17: 89–98, 2007.
62. Zhao L, Wang L, Ji W, et al. Association between plasma angiotensin-converting enzyme level and radiation pneumonitis. *Cytokine* 37: 71–75, 2007.
63. Alsner J, Rodningen OK, and Overgaard J. Differential gene expression before and after ionizing radiation of subcutaneous fibroblasts identifies breast cancer patients resistant to radiation-induced fibrosis. *Radiother Oncol* 83: 261–266, 2007.
64. Rodningen OK, Borresen-Dale AL, Alsner J, et al. Radiation-induced gene expression in human subcutaneous fibroblasts is predictive of radiation-induced fibrosis. *Radiother Oncol*, 2007.
65. International HapMap Consortium: A second generation human haplotype map of over 3.1 million SNPs. *Nature* 449: 851–861, 2007.
66. Christensen K, Murray JC. What genome-wide association studies can do for medicine. *N Engl J Med* 356: 1094–1097, 2007.
67. West CM. Invited review: intrinsic radiosensitivity as a predictor of patient response to radiotherapy. *Br J Radiol* 68: 827–837, 1995.
68. Begg AC, Haustermans K, Hart AA, et al. The value of pretreatment cell kinetic parameters as predictors for radiotherapy outcome in head and neck cancer: a multicenter analysis. *Radiother Oncol* 50: 13–23, 1999.
69. Lonning PE, Sorlie T, Borresen-Dale AL. Genomics in breast cancer-therapeutic implications. *Nat Clin Pract Oncol* 2: 26–33, 2005.
70. Ogawa K, Murayama S, Mori M. Predicting the tumor response to radiotherapy using microarray analysis. *Oncol Rep* 18: 1243–1248, 2007.
71. Ojima E, Inoue Y, Miki C et al. Effectiveness of gene expression profiling for response prediction of rectal cancer to preoperative radiotherapy. *J Gastroenterol* 42: 730–736, 2007.
72. Vordermark D, Brown JM. Endogenous markers of tumor hypoxia predictors of clinical radiation resistance? *Strahlenther Onkol* 179: 801–811, 2003.
73. Rajendran JG, Krohn KA. Imaging hypoxia and angiogenesis in tumors. *Radiol Clin North Am* 43: 169–187, 2005.
74. Vaupel P. Tumor microenvironmental physiology and its implications for radiation oncology. *Semin Radiat Oncol* 14: 198–206, 2004.
75. Olive PL, Aquino-Parsons C. Measurement of tumor hypoxia using single-cell methods. *Semin Radiat Oncol* 14: 241–248, 2004.
76. Fajardo LF, Berthrong M, Anderson RE. *Radiation Pathology*. Oxford University Press, New York, 2001.
77. Wheldon TE, Michalowski AS, Kirk J. The effect of irradiation on function in self-renewing normal tissues with differing proliferative organisation. *Br J Radiol* 55: 759–766, 1982.
78. Denham JW, Hauer-Jensen M. The radiotherapeutic injury—a complex 'wound'. *Radiother Oncol* 63: 129–145, 2002.
79. Williams J, Chen Y, Rubin P, et al. The biological basis of a comprehensive grading system for the adverse effects of cancer treatment. *Semin Radiat Oncol* 13: 182–188, 2003.
80. McBride WH, Chiang CS, Olson JL, et al. A sense of danger from radiation. *Radiat Res* 162: 1–19, 2004.
81. Anscher MS, Vujaskovic Z. Mechanisms and potential targets for prevention and treatment of normal tissue injury after radiation therapy. *Semin Oncol* 32: S86–91, 2005.

82. Bentzen SM. Preventing or reducing late side effects of radiation therapy: radiobiology meets molecular pathology. *Nat Rev Cancer* 6: 702–713, 2006.

83. Waselenko JK, MacVittie TJ, Blakely WF, et al. Medical management of the acute radiation syndrome: recommendations of the Strategic National Stockpile Radiation Working Group. *Ann Intern Med* 140: 1037–1051, 2004.

84. Turai I, Veress K, Gunalp B, et al. Medical response to radiation incidents and radionuclear threats. *Bmj* 328: 568–572, 2004.

85. National Research Council, Health Risks from Exposure to Low Levels of Ionizing Radiation: BEIR VII Phase 2 (2006). National Academies Press, Washington, DC, 2006.

86. Ron E. Cancer risks from medical radiation. *Health Phys* 85: 47–59, 2003.

87. Preston DL, Shimizu Y, Pierce DA, et al. Studies of mortality of atomic bomb survivors. Report 13: solid cancer and noncancer disease mortality: 1950–1997. *Radiat Res* 160: 381–407, 2003.

88. Preston DL, Ron E, Tokuoka S, Funamoto S, et al. Solid cancer incidence in atomic bomb survivors: 1958-1998. *Radiat Res* 168: 1–64, 2007.

89. Brenner DJ, Doll R, Goodhead DT, et al. Cancer risks attributable to low doses of ionizing radiation: assessing what we really know. *Proc Natl Acad Sci USA* 100: 13761–13766, 2003.

90. Tubiana M, Aurengo A, Averbeck D, et al. Recent reports on the effect of low doses of ionizing radiation and its dose-effect relationship. *Radiat Environ Biophys* 44: 245–251, 2006.

91. Sachs RK, Brenner DJ. Solid tumor risks after high doses of ionizing radiation. *Proc Natl Acad Sci U S A* 102: 13040–13045, 2005.

92. Wakeford R, Little MP. Risk coefficients for childhood cancer after intrauterine irradiation: a review. *Int J Radiat Biol* 79: 293–309, 2003.

93. Delongchamp RR, Mabuchi K, Yoshimoto Y, et al. Cancer mortality among atomic bomb survivors exposed in utero or as young children, October 1950-May 1992. *Radiat Res* 147: 385–395, 1997.

94. Brenner DJ, Curtis RE, Hall EJ, et al. Second malignancies in prostate carcinoma patients after radiotherapy compared with surgery. *Cancer* 88: 398–406, 2000.

95. Boice JD, Jr., Engholm G, Kleinerman RA, et al. Radiation dose and second cancer risk in patients treated for cancer of the cervix. *Radiat Res* 116: 3–55, 1988.

96. Horwich A, Swerdlow AJ. Second primary breast cancer after Hodgkin's disease. *Br J Cancer* 90: 294–208, 2004.

97. Neglia JP, Robison LL, Stovall M, et al. New primary neoplasms of the central nervous system in survivors of childhood cancer: a report from the Childhood Cancer Survivor Study. *J Natl Cancer Inst* 98: 1528–1537, 2006.

98. Bassal M, Mertens AC, Taylor L, et al. Risk of selected subsequent carcinomas in survivors of childhood cancer: a report from the Childhood Cancer Survivor Study. *J Clin Oncol* 24: 476–483, 2006.

99. Sigurdson AJ, Ronckers CM, Mertens AC, et al. Primary thyroid cancer after a first tumour in childhood (the Childhood Cancer Survivor Study): a nested case-control study. *Lancet* 365: 2014–2023, 2005.

100. Perkins JL, Liu Y, Mitby PA, et al. Nonmelanoma skin cancer in survivors of childhood and adolescent cancer: a report from the childhood cancer survivor study. *J Clin Oncol* 23: 3733–3741, 2005.

101. Henderson TO, Whitton J, Stovall M, et al. Secondary sarcomas in childhood cancer survivors: a report from the Childhood Cancer Survivor Study. *J Natl Cancer Inst* 99: 300–308, 2007.

102. Neel JV. Reappraisal of studies concerning the genetic effects of the radiation of humans, mice, and Drosophila. *Environ Mol Mutagen* 31: 4–10, 1998.

103. Schull WJ. The children of atomic bomb survivors: a synopsis. *J Radiol Prot* 23: 369–384, 2003.
104. Russell LB, Russell WL. Frequency and nature of specific-locus mutations induced in female mice by radiations and chemicals: a review. *Mutat Res* 296: 107–127, 1992.
105. Streffer C, Shore R, Konermann G, et al. Biological effects after prenatal irradiation (embryo and fetus). A report of the International Commission on Radiological Protection. *Ann ICRP* 33: 5–206, 2003.
106. International Commission on Radiological Protection, ICRP Publication 90: Biological Effects after Prenatal Irradiation (Embryo and Fetus). Elsevier, New York, 2004.
107. National Council on Radiation Protection and Measurements, NCRP Report No. 116— Limitation of Exposure to Ionizing Radiation. Bethesda, 1993.
108. National Council on Radiation Protection and Measurements, NCRP Report No. 107, Implementation of the Principle of As Low As Reasonably Achievable (ALARA) for Medical and Dental Personnel. Bethesda, 1990.

# 3

# Molecular Radiobiology

*Barry S. Rosenstein, PhD*

## INTRODUCTION

Although the principal impact of radiobiology upon the clinical practice of radiation oncology has come primarily from cellular studies and radiobiologic modeling of clinical effects, a major emphasis of current research efforts involves the elucidation on a molecular scale of the events taking place in cells, tissues, and tumors following irradiation. It is anticipated that many of the future research advances that will translate into the clinical practice of radiation oncology will have as their basis an understanding of the events that occur on a molecular level after exposure to radiation.

## ONCOGENES, TUMOR SUPPRESSOR GENES, AND GENOME STABILITY GENES

Cancer is fundamentally a genetic disease in that neoplastic transformation of normal cells results from a series of genetic alterations including point mutations, deletions, amplifications, chromosomal translocations, and inversions.[1] These modifications result in a cell that has escaped normal growth control and displays aberrant proliferative activity. Thus, cancers arise through a multistage process in which both germline and somatic mutations lead to waves of clonal expansion resulting in selection of cells with the greatest growth potential. The genes that are affected in cancer can be broadly classified into three types, oncogenes, tumor suppressor genes, and genome stability genes, whose products generally play important roles in the regulation of cell growth, division, and maintenance of genome integrity.

### Oncogenes

Gain-of-function mutations occur in normal cellular genes termed proto-oncogenes causing them to be converted to active oncogenes,[2] which permit enhanced cellular proliferation (Table 3-1). Therefore, an activated oncogene is dominant in action over a proto-oncogene since only a single copy of an activated oncogene will have an impact upon the neoplastic potential of a cell. Many oncogenes encode growth factors and their receptors which play a central role in the regulation of cell proliferation. Growth factors represent high affinity ligands for transmembrane receptor tyrosine kinases (RTKs). The process through which growth factors and RTKs mediate signal transduction involves ligand binding, receptor dimerization, phosphorylation of the intracellular domain, and

**TABLE 3-1 Oncogenes**

| Oncogene | Neoplasm | Mechanism of Activation | Protein Function |
|---|---|---|---|
| *Growth factors* | | | |
| v-sis | Glioma/fibrosarcoma | Constitutive production | B-chain PDGF |
| int2 | Mammary carcinoma | Constitutive production | Member of FGF family |
| KS3 | Kaposi sarcoma | Constitutive production | Member of FGF family |
| HST | Stomach carcinoma | Constitutive production | Member of FGF family |
| *Growth factor receptors* | | | |
| *Tyrosine kinases: integral membrane proteins* | | | |
| EGFR | Squamous cell carcinoma | Gene amplification/increased protein | EGF receptor |
| v-fms | Sarcoma | Constitutive activation | CSF1 receptor |
| v-kit | Sarcoma/GIST | Constitutive activation/point mutation | Stem-cell factor receptor |
| v-ros | Sarcoma | Constitutive activation | ? |
| MET | MNNG-treated human osteo-carcinoma cell line | DNA rearrangement/ligand-independent constitutive activation (fusion proteins) | HGF/SF receptor |
| TRK | Colon/thyroid carcinomas | DNA rearrangement/ligand-independent constitutive activation (fusion proteins) | NGF receptor |
| NEU | Neuroblastoma/breast carcinoma/NSCLC | Gene amplification/point mutation | ? |
| RET | Carcinomas of thyroid; MEN2A, MEN2B | DNA rearrangement/point mutation (ligand-independent constitutive activation/fusion proteins) | GDNF/NTT/ART/PSP receptor |
| *Receptors lacking protein kinase activity* | | | |
| mas | Epidermoid carcinoma | Rearrangement of 5' non-coding region | Angiotensin receptor |
| *Signal transducers* | | | |
| *Cytoplasmic tyrosine kinases* | | | |
| SRC | Colon carcinoma | Constitutive activation | Protein tyrosine kinase |
| v-yes | Sarcoma | Constitutive activation | Protein tyrosine kinase |
| v-fgr | Sarcoma | Constitutive activation | Protein tyrosine kinase |
| v-fes | Sarcoma | Constitutive activation | Protein tyrosine kinase |
| ABL | CML | DNA rearrangement translocation (constitutive activation/fusion proteins) | Protein tyrosine kinase |
| *Membrane-associated G proteins* | | | |
| H-RAS | Colon, lung, pancreas carcinomas | Point mutation | GTPase |
| K-RAS | AML, thyroid carcinoma, melanoma | Point mutation | GTPase |

| Gene | Tumor | Mechanism | Function |
|---|---|---|---|
| N-RAS | Carcinoma, melanoma | Point mutation | GTPase |
| BRAF | Melanoma, thyroid, colon, ovary | Point mutation | Ser/Thr kinase |
| gsp | Adenomas of thyroid | Point mutation | Gs alpha |
| gip | Ovary, adrenal carcinoma | Point mutation | Gi alpha |
| **GTPase exchange factor (GEF)** | | | |
| Dbl | Diffuse B-cell lymphoma | DNA rearrangement | GEF for Rho and Cdc42Hs |
| Vav | Hematopoietic cells | DNA rearrangement | GEF for Ras? |
| **Serine/threonine kinases: cytoplasmic** | | | |
| v-mos | Sarcoma | Constitutive activation | Protein kinase (ser/thr) |
| v-raf | Sarcoma | Constitutive activation | Protein kinase (ser/thr) |
| pim-1 | T-cell lymphoma | Constitutive activation | Protein kinase (ser/thr) |
| **Cytoplasmic regulators** | | | |
| v-crk | | Constitutive tyrosine phosphorylation of cellular substrates (eg, paxillin) | SH-2/SH-3 adaptor |
| **Trancription Factors** | | | |
| v-myc | Carcinoma, myelocytomatosis | Deregulated activity | Transcription factor |
| N-MYC | Neuroblastoma; lung carcinoma | Deregulated activity | Transcription factor |
| L-MYC | Carcinoma of lung | Deregulated activity | Transcription factor |
| v-myb | Myeloblastosis | Deregulated activity | Transcription factor |
| v-fos | Osteosarcoma | Deregulated activity | Transcription factor API |
| v-jun | Sarcoma | Deregulated activity | Transcription factor API |
| v-ski | Carcinoma | Deregulated activity | Transcription factor |
| v-rel | Lymphatic leukemia | Deregulated activity | Mutant NF-kappa B |
| v-ets-1 | Erythroblastosis | Deregulated activity | Transcription factor |
| v-ets-2 | Erythroblastosis | Deregulated activity | Transcription factor |
| v-eRbA1 | Erythroblastosis | Deregulated activity | T3 Transcription factor |
| v-eRbA2 | Erythroblastosis | Deregulated activity | T3 Transcription factor |
| **Others** | | | |
| BCL2 | B-cell lymphomas | Constitutive activity | Antiapoptotic protein |
| MDM2 | Sarcomas | Gene amplification/increased protein | Complexes with p53 |

AML = acute myeloid leukemia; CML = chronic myelogenous leukemia; CSF = colony stimulating factor; EGF = epidermal growth factor; FGF = fibroblast growth factor; GTPase = guanosine triphosphatase; HGF = hepatocyte growth factor; NGF = nerve growth factor; PDGF = platelet-derived growth factor.

Adapted from MA, Frattini M, Sozzi G, Croce CM, Oncogenes, pp 68-85 In *Cancer Medicine 7*, Kufe DW, Bast RC, Hait W et al, Eds, BC Decker, Hamilton, 2006.

activation of cytoplasmic signaling molecules that transmit signals to the nucleus. In addition, onco-genes may encode signal transducers, transcription factors, and regulators of apoptosis.

## Tumor Suppressor Genes

Tumor suppressor genes[3] act in a recessive fashion since the genetic alterations associated with these genes in carcinogenesis are loss of function mutations, and both copies of the gene must be inactivated for transformation to occur (Table 3-2). However, it should be noted that cancer predis-position resulting from a mutation in a tumor suppressor gene is inherited in a dominant fashion. Therefore, it is only necessary for an individual to inherit just one copy of a mutated tumor suppres-sor gene to render that person susceptible to cancer development since the other copy of the gene is likely to be lost or inactivated in a cell which will then undergo clonal expansion to become a tumor. Thus, a hallmark of tumor suppressor genes is loss of heterozygosity (LOH) in the region of the chromosome where the tumor suppressor gene resides.[4] LOH may occur through a variety of mechanisms including localized deletion, mitotic recombination, gene conversion, translocation, chromosomal nondysjunction, and chromosome breakage.

One of the most extensively studied tumor suppressors is the retinoblastoma tumor suppressor protein (Rb).[5] In a hypo-phosphorylated state, Rb suppresses cell growth through binding E2F transcription factors. This block is relieved through the action of cyclinD-CDK4/CD6 which phos-phorylates Rb causing release of E2F resulting in transcription of genes necessary for cell cycle pro-gression. p53 also represents an important tumor suppressor protein as mutations in the gene which encodes this protein are found in more than 50% of all cancers, making this the most com-monly altered gene in human cancer.[6] p53 plays a critical role in cell cycle regulation delay induced by DNA damage and modulates apoptosis. An important regulator of p53 is MDM2 which possesses E3 ubiquitin ligase activity toward p53.[7] Because of its ability to ubiquitinate p53 and target it for proteasomal degradation, MDM2 generally maintains p53 at low levels. However, p53 phosphoryla-tion caused by ATM activation following DNA damage induction by radiation inhibits the associa-tion of p53 with MDM2 and thus reduces p53 degradation. One of the main transcriptional targets for p53 is p21, which inhibits cyclin dependent kinoses (CDKs) responsible for the Rb phosphoryla-tion that are necessary for the G1-S transition. p53 also plays an important role in apoptosis follow-ing the induction of radiation damage in many cell types through activation of pro-apoptotic proteins including BAX, NOXA and PUMA. Alterations in p53 and Rb and/or their pathways likely occur in the vast majority of all human cancers.

## DNA REPAIR PATHWAYS

Because of the detrimental effects of unrepaired or misrepaired DNA damages, the cell devotes sig-nificant resources to the removal of these lesions. DNA double strand breaks (DSBs) are of partic-ular importance because they can result in chromosomal aberrations that may lead to cell death. The two main pathways for repair of DSBs (Box 3-1) are homologous recombination (HR) (Figure 3-1) and non-homologous end joining (NHEJ) (Figure 3-2).[8]

In addition to repair of DSBs, radiation induces base damages, whose removal via base excision repair may be of importance to cell survival.[9] A battery of glycosylases, each recognizing a relatively narrow spectrum of lesions, removes the damaged base through its cleavage from the sugar-phosphate backbone. An AP endonuclease produces a nick in the DNA at the site where the base was removed fol-lowing which a DNA polymerase restores the missing base and DNA ligase III seals the break.

## MECHANISMS OF CELL DEATH

The goal of radiotherapy is to cause reproductive death of all malignant cells in a tumor in order to prevent the cancer from regrowing, but with an acceptable level of damage to normal tissues and

**TABLE 3-2 Tumor Suppressor and Stability Genes Associated with Inherited Cancer Predisposition Syndromes**

| Gene (synonym)* | Syndrome | Pathway** | Major heredity tumor types*** |
|---|---|---|---|
| **Tumor-suppressor genes** | | | |
| APC | FAP | APC | Colon, thyroid, stomach, intestine |
| AXIN2 | Attenuated polyposis | APC | Colon |
| CDH1 (E-cadherin) | Familial gastric carcinoma | APC | Stomach |
| GPC3 | Simpson-Golabi-Behmel syndrome | APOP | Embryonal |
| CYLD | Familial cylindromatosis | GLI | Pilotrichomas |
| EXT1,EXT2 | Hereditary multiple exostoses | GLI | Bone |
| PTCH | Gorlin syndrome | GLI | Skin, medulloblastoma |
| SUFU | Medulloblastoma predisposition | GLI | Skin, medulloblastoma |
| FH | Hereditary leiomyomatosis | HIF1 | Leiomyomas |
| SDHB, C, D | Familial paraganglioma | HIF1 | Paragangliomas, pheochromocytomas |
| VHL | Von Hippel–Lindau | HIF1 | Kidney |
| TP53 (p53) | Li-Fraumeni | P53 | Breast, sarcoma, adrenal, brain . . . |
| WT1 | Familial Wilms tumor | P53 | Wilms |
| STK11 (LKB1) | Peutz-Jeghers | PI3K | Intestinal, ovarian, pancreatic |
| PTEN | Cowden syndrome | PI3K | Hamartoma, glioma, uterus |
| TSC1, TSC2 | Tuberous sclerosis | PI3K | Hamartoma, kidney |
| CDKN2A (p16INK4A, P14ARF) | Familial malignant melanoma | RB | Melanoma, pancreas |
| CDK4 | Familial malignant melanoma | RB | Melanoma |
| RB1 | Hereditary retinoblastoma | RB | Eye |
| NF1 | Neurofibromatosis | RTK | Neurofibroma |
| BMPR1A | Juvenile polyposis | SMAD | Gastrointestinal |
| MEN1 | Multiple endocrine neoplasia type I | SMAD | Parathyroid, pituitary, islet cell, carcinoid |
| SMAD4 (DPC4) | Juvenile polyposis | SMAD | Gastrointestinal |
| BHD | Birt-Hogg-Dube | – | Renal, hair follicle |
| HRPT2 | Hyperparathyroidism jaw-tumor | – | Parathyroid, jaw fibroma |
| NF2 | Neurofibromatosis type 2 | – | Meningioma, acoustic neuroma |

(continues)

## TABLE 3-2 (continued)

| Gene (synonym)[*] | Syndrome | Pathway[**] | Major heredity tumor types[***] |
|---|---|---|---|
| **Stability genes** | | | |
| MUTYH | Attenuated polyposis | BER | Colon |
| ATM | Ataxia telangiectasia | CIN | Leukemias, lymphomas, brain |
| BLM | Bloom | CIN | Leukemias, lymphomas, skin |
| BRCA1, BRCA2 | Hereditary breast cancer | CIN | Breast, ovary |
| FANCA, C, D2, E, F, G | Fanconi anemia | CIN | Leukemias |
| NBS1 | Nijmegen breakage syndrome | CIN | Lymphomas, brain |
| RECQL4 | Rothmund-Thomson syndrome | CIN | Bone, skin |
| WRN | Werner | CIN | Bone, brain |
| MSH2, MLH1, MSH6, PMS2 | HNPCC | MMR | Colon, uterus |
| XPA, C; ERCC2–5; DDB2 | Xeroderma pigmentosum | NER | Skin |

[*]Representative genes of all the major pathways and hereditary cancer predisposition types are listed. Approved gene symbols are provided for each entry. Alternative names appear in parentheses.

[**]In many cases, the gene has been implicated in many pathways. The single pathway that is listed for each gene represents a "best guess" (when one can be made) and should not be regarded as conclusive.

[***]In most cases, the non-familial tumor spectrum caused by somatic mutations of the gene includes those occurring in familial cases but also additional tumor types. For example, mutations of p53 and CDKN2A are found in many more tumor types than those to which the Li-Fraumeni and familial malignant melanoma patients, respectively, are predisposed.

APC=adenomatous polyposis coli; APOP=apoptotic pathway; BER=base excision repair; CIN=chromosomal instability; FAP=familial adenomatous polyposis; GLI=glioma associated oncogene; HIF1=hypoxia inducing factor 1; MMR=mismatch repair; NER=nucleotide excision repair; PI3K=phosphatidylinositol 3-kinase; RB=retinoblastoma; RTK=receptor tyrosine kinase pathway; SMAD=SMA and MAD related protein 4; wt=wild type.

Adapted from Park BH, Vogelstein B, Tumor suppressor genes, pp 85–103 In Cancer Medicine 7, Kufe DW, Bast RC, Hait W et al, Eds, BC Decker, Hamilton, 2006.

## BOX 3-1   REPAIR OF DNA DOUBLE STRAND BREAKS

### Homologous Recombinational Repair (HR)

- Accurate repair through use of the undamaged sister chromatid as a template.[10,11]
- Most efficient in the S and $G_2$ phases of the cell cycle when there is the availability of sister chromatids as repair templates.

### Non-Homologous End-Joining (NHEJ)

- Does not make use of a template for repair and is therefore intrinsically error prone.
- Uses little or no homology to couple DNA ends.[12,13]
- Predominant process for repair of DSB, particularly during the $G_1$ phase of the cell cycle.
- Required to process the DSB intermediates generated during V(D)J recombination.

## FIGURE 3-1   Homologous recombinational repair of DSBs.

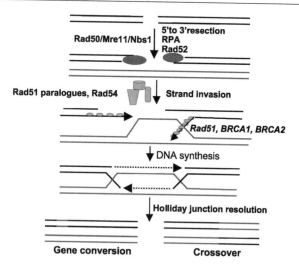

Irradiation of cells stimulates the autophosphorylation of the ATM protein converting it from an inactive dimer to the active monomer form which has kinase activity.[14] This dissociation may be accomplished through recruitment of ATM to damaged DNA and facilitated by the MRE11-RAD50-NBS1 complex (MRN) by tethering DNA.[15] In addition, phosphorylation of histone H2AX occurs which appears to play a role in the formation of repair foci.[16] To promote strand invasion into homologous sequences, there is nucleolytic resection of the flush ends to expose 3′ overhanging single stranded DNA. The 3′ tail is coated with RPA protein to protect it from degradation. RAD51 polymerizes onto the single-stranded DNA to form a nucleoprotein filament and searches for the homologous duplex DNA (strand invasion). DNA strand exchange then generates a joint molecule (Holliday junction) between the homologous damaged and undamaged duplex DNAs in a reaction that is stimulated by the RAD52 and RAD54 proteins. Other proteins implicated in the coordination of a proper RAD51 response include BRCA1, BRCA2, and RAD51 paralogues. The Holliday junction formed is then resolved thereby permitting separation of the repaired duplexes and resulting in either a nonreciprocal or reciprocal exchange.

Adapted from Zhang J, Powell SN: The role of the BRCA1 tumor suppressor in DNA double-strand break repair. *Molecular Cancer Research* 3: 531–539, 2005, with permission.

---

**FIGURE 3-2** Non-homologous end joining repair of DSBs.

---

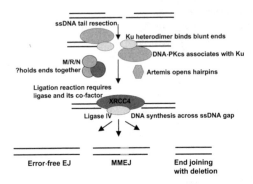

The KU heterodimer, which consists of a tight complex of KU70 and KU80, and has a high affinity for DNA ends, forms a close-fitting asymmetrical ring which threads onto a free end of DNA. KU then recruits DNA-PKcs to a DNA end. This results in formation of the DNA-protein kinase holoenzyme complex and permits activation of its kinase activity. Artemis cleaves any residual loops or hairpins that are formed in this process. DNA ligase IV is present in a tight complex with XRCC4 which ligates the broken DNA ends.[12]

Adapted from Zhang J, Powell SN: The role of the BRCA1 tumor suppressor in DNA double-strand break repair. *Molecular Cancer Research* 3: 531–539, 2005, with permission.

---

organs. Radiation can cause the loss of reproductive integrity either through cell death processes or the induction of senescence/differentiation.[17]

1. Senescence: DNA damage caused by radiation can induce a cell to undergo replicative senescence. A senescent cell typically exhibits morphological changes, such as flattened cytoplasm and increased granularity.
2. Mitotic/post-mitotic death: Following irradiation, cells may die during or subsequent to division, often due to the presence of radiation-induced chromosomal aberrations. This may involve mitotic catastrophe in which an aberrant mitosis results in the formation of multinucleate, giant cells with uncondensed chromatin.
3. Interphase cell death: Some cells die within hours after irradiation by death in the absence of division, often through apoptosis. This is most prominent in lymphocytes, spermatogonia, intestinal crypt cells and salivary gland serous cells, but also occurs in many normal tissues and tumors.

In addition to mitotic catastrophe, the three major mechanisms of cell death following irradiation are apoptosis, autophagy, and necrosis (Box 3-2). Table 3-3 lists some of the commonly employed assays used for detection of apoptosis.[18]

## Caspases

The morphological and biochemical characteristics of apoptosis[19,20] generally result from activation of caspases which are cysteine aspartyl-specific proteases. Initiator caspases are activated by death signals whereas effector caspases are activated by initiator caspases and act upon a number of substrates to cause the morphological features associated with apoptotic cell death. Apoptosis can occur by either an extrinsic or intrinsic pathway (Figure 3-3 and Box 3-2).

BOX 3-2 MECHANISMS OF CELL DEATH

**Apoptosis**

- Cell shrinkage accompanied by an increase in cell density.
- Nuclear fragmentation (pyknosis).
- Convolution and blebbing of the cell membrane.
- Chromatin condensation.
- Non-random degradation of nuclear DNA into oligonucleosome-sized fragments.
- Separation of the cell into a cluster of membrane-bound apoptotic bodies which are cleared by phagocytosis.
- Deletion of single cells in isolation.
- Lack of an inflammatory response.

**Autophagy**

- Mechanism to eliminate damaged proteins or organelles, but cells that undergo excessive autophagy may die.
- Organelles and other cell components are encased in autophagosomes that fuse with lysosomes causing degradation of the autophagosomal contents.
- Increased endocytosis, vacuolation, membrane blebbing, and nuclear condensation.

**Necrosis**

- Loss of osmotic stability.
- Irreversible cell swelling and plasma membrane rupture.
- Groups of cells affected.
- Random DNA fragmentation manifested as a smear on a gel.
- Lysosomes disrupted and release proteolytic enzymes.
- Generation of an inflammatory response in the area of tissue affected.
- May also be a form of programmed cell death.

## CELL CYCLE REGULATION

The progression of cells through the cell cycle is a highly ordered process which is regulated primarily through CDKs, cyclins, and CDK inhibitors.[21,22] CDK levels tend to remain relatively constant

TABLE 3-3 **Assays for Detection of Cells Undergoing Apoptosis**

| Assay | Description |
|---|---|
| DNA ladder formation | Presence of oligonucleosomal fragments manifested as distinct bands on a DNA agarose gel resulting from DNA cleavage in linker-regions |
| TUNEL (TdT-mediated dUTP nick end labeling) | Visualization of DNA breaks using terminal deoxynucleotidyl transferase (TdT) to catalyze the polymerization of fluorescein-labeled nucleotides (dUTP) onto 3'-OH ends |
| Annexin-V binding | High affinity probe for phosphotidylserine exposed on the outer cell membrane leaflet |
| Bisbenzimide (Hoechst 33342 and 33258) | Cell-permeable DNA dye |
| DAPI (4', 6-Diamidine 2'-phenylindole dihydrochloride) | Blue fluorescent DNA stain |

**FIGURE 3-3** Intrinsic and extrinsic apoptosis pathways.

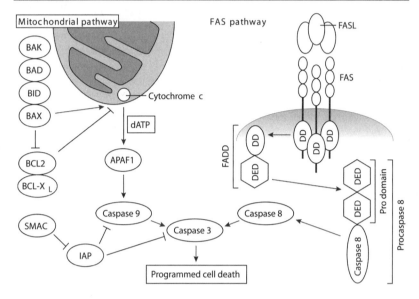

The intrinsic pathway (left) takes place through the mitochondria via release of cytochrome c which interacts with a multi-protein caspase activating complex, termed the apoptosome, a central component of which is APAF1 and together with ATP/dATP causes activation of pro-caspase 9. Regulatory control over release of cytochrome c is exerted through members of the BCL-2 family which includes both anti-apoptotic (BCL-2, BCL-xL) and pro-apoptotic BAX, BAK, BID, BAD) members. Stimulation of p53 following irradiation activates molecules such as BAX that act upon the mitochondria to cause release of cytochrome c. In addition, irradiation on the cell membrane activates acid sphingomyelinase resulting in the production of ceramide which serves as a second messenger to stimulate the mitochondrial pathway.[23] The extrinsic pathway (right) involves signals from the microenvironment which can be induced by radiation. Ligands including FAS ligand (FASL), tumor necrosis factor (TNF), and TNF-related apoptosis-inducing ligand (TRAIL) bind to FAS receptor, TNF receptor or death receptor 4 (DR4/TRAIL-R1), respectively, which causes recruitment of FAS-associated death domain (FADD) protein. The death effector domain (DED) of FADD then binds to the DED of procaspase 8 causing activation of caspase 8, caspase 3, and the pro-caspase activation cascade that results in the apoptotic response. Inhibitor of apoptosis proteins (IAPs) are important regulators of apoptosis through binding and inhibition of caspase activity. SMAC/DIABLO promotes apoptosis by binding to IAPs and preventing them from sequestering caspases.

Adapted from Fesik SW: Promoting apoptosis as a strategy for cancer drug discovery, *Nat Rev Cancer* 5:876–85, 2005, with permission.

through the cell cycle, but synthesis of cyclins fluctuates. The restriction point is the stage in $G_1$, past which, cells are committed to enter into S phase. The main elements associated with progression through the restriction point are Rb, cyclin D, CDK4, CDK6, and CDK inhibitors. Cyclins E and then A form complexes with CDK2 initiating entry and progression through S phase. Cyclin A and then cyclin B associate with CDK1 to promote movement through $G_2$ into M. ATM also plays a critical role in regulation of the cell cycle[24] (Figure 3-4).

**FIGURE 3-4** Mammalian cell cycle checkpoints.

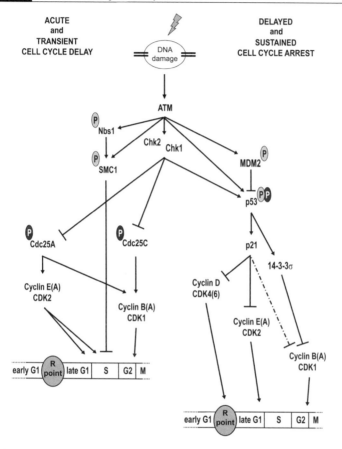

Following irradiation, ATM phosphorylates p53, resulting in stimulation of p21 transcription which delays progression of cells from G1 into S through inhibition of cyclin D/CDK4(6) and cyclinE(A)/CDK2. ATM also phosphorylates and activates CHK2 kinase, which in turn phosphorylates p53, thereby interfering with its binding to MDM2 and preventing targeting of p53 for degradation via ubiquitination. In addition, ATM phosphorylates MDM2 which inhibits the nuclear export of the p53-MDM2 complex, a prerequisite for p53 degradation. ATM plays a role in S phase arrest after irradiation both through involvement of the MRN complex and SMC1 as well as through phosphorylation of CDC25A by activated CHK1/CHK2 resulting in CDC25A inhibition. This prevents CDC25A phosphatase from activating CDK2, which is necessary for replicon initiation. The regulation of the $G_2$ checkpoint by ATM is thought to occur through activation of CHK1/CHK2 which phosphorylates CDC25C phosphatase thereby preventing it from dephosphorylating CDK1, a step necessary for progression from $G_2$ into M. The 14-3-3$\sigma$ protein inhibits $G_2$/M progression by cytoplasmatic sequestration of cyclin B/CDK1 complexes.

Adapted from Lukas J, Lukas C, Bartek J: Mammalian cell cycle checkpoints: signaling pathways and their organization in space and time. *J DNA Repair* 3:997–1007, 2004, with permission.

## TELOMERES AND TELOMERASE

Ends of chromosomes, telomeres, are protected by a nucleoprotein complex preventing them from being perceived by the cell as DNA double-strand breaks.[25] The DNA component of telomeres consists of short repetitive G-rich sequence ending in a 3′ single-stranded overhang that bends back on itself creating a "t-loop". However, because DNA polymerases responsible for DNA replication synthesize DNA in the 5′→3′ direction and require a primer and template, there is loss of genetic information from the 5′ end of DNA during each round of replication associated with synthesis of the lagging DNA strand. The loss of telomeric DNA appears to signal a DNA damage response that leads to cellular senescence. To address this limit upon continued cell division, many cancer cells activate telomerase, which possesses a reverse transcriptase activity capable of restoring telomeric sequences thereby maintaining telomere length. It is interesting to note that the telomere binding protein TRF2, which is involved in preserving telomere stability, is associated with a variety of proteins involved with recognition and repair of DNA double-strand breaks, thereby linking DNA repair and maintenance of telomere integrity.

## TUMOR MICROENVIRONMENT

It is important to recognize that tumors are not simply clonal populations of cells, but exist within a stroma in which the microenvironment plays a role. Hypoxia in particular plays a critical role in this environment as it stimulates signaling pathways, especially through activation of hypoxia-inducible factor 1 (HIF-1), a transcription factor that binds to hypoxia regulatory elements in the nucleus to stimulate the expression of multiple genes involved in tumor metabolism, growth, and angiogenesis.[26] In addition, radiation causes HIF-1 levels to increase, resulting in upregulation of proteins such as VEGF. Evidence has been obtained suggesting that the tumor reoxygenation which occurs following irradiation of solid tumors plays an important role stimulating the increase in HIF-1.[27] Thus, HIF-1 affects tumor radiosensitivity through its impact upon angiogenesis, apoptosis, metabolism, and proliferation.

## SIGNAL TRANSDUCTION PATHWAYS

Exposure of cells to radiation causes the activation of signal transduction pathways that regulate both enhanced cellular proliferation as well as stimulation of cell death processes[28] (Figure 3-5). These events are mediated primarily through the action of either protein kinases that phosphorylate substrate molecules or phosphatases that remove phosphate groups, resulting in regulation of cytoprotective and cytotoxic responses. The epidermal growth factor (ERBB) receptor family plays a particularly important role and consists of four transmembrane receptor tyrosine kinases whose function it is to transmit extracellular signals directing proliferation, differentiation, and survival responses.[29] The receptors are activated by ligand binding to the extracellular domain of a receptor monomer that leads to dimerization. Once the receptors have dimerized, the cytoplasmic domains, which possess tyrosine kinase activity, are activated thereby inducing recruitment of proteins that stimulate signaling cascades. Epithelial tumors frequently dysregulate receptor signaling by escaping regulatory control.[30,31] The responses that enhance survival are initiated by receptors in the cell membrane and are transmitted primarily via the RAS/MAPK[32] pathway which is activated by ERBB family members such as EGFR or through the PI3K/AKT pathway that increases survival either by stimulating proliferation or inhibiting apoptosis. In particular, radiation-induced activation of EGFR may represent a principal molecular mechanism underlying the accelerated repopulation that is observed during radiotherapy. The cytotoxic responses can be stimulated directly through induction of apoptosis or transmitted through the SAPK/JNK path-

**FIGURE 3-5** RAS signal transduction pathway.

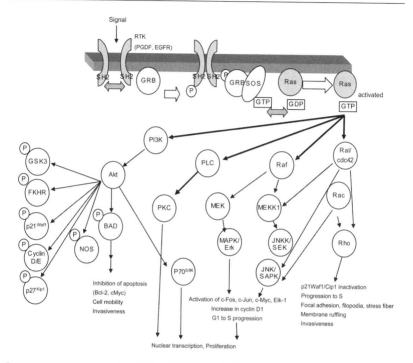

Receptor tyrosine kinases such as EGFR and PDGFR are stimulated by an extracellular signal resulting in dimerization and autophosphorylation of SH2 domains on the intracellular surface of the protein. The adapter protein GRB then binds via its SH2 domains, associates with SOS, and attaches it to the cell membrane surface where it is able to interact with RAS. This stimulates GTP–GDP exchange. Activated GTP-RAS stimulates cellular proliferation through activation of multiple pathways including the RAF, MEK, JNK, RAC/RHO, PLC, and PI3K/AKT pathways. AKT has multiple downstream targets (GSK3; FKHR; p21; cyclin D/E; P27Kip1, NOS; BAD; P70S6K; mTOR).

Adapted from Brunner TB, Hahn SM, McKenna WG, Bernhard EJ: Radiation sensitization by inhibition of activated Ras. *Strahlentherapie und Onkologie* 11:731–740, 2004, with permission.

way which in certain cells promotes apoptosis whereas in other cell types this signal transduction cascade may result in a cytoprotective effect following irradiation.

## MOLECULAR APPROACHES TO RADIOSENSITIZATION

An important focus of current radiobiologic research is the development of drugs that specifically sensitize cancer cells to the lethal effects of radiation. Many of these approaches use "targeted therapy" in which an agent specifically affects a particular molecular target in the tumor cells, typically using small molecule inhibitors and monoclonal antibodies.

TABLE 3-4 Targeted Radiosensitizers

| Drug | Target | Basis of Action | Possible Mechanism of Radiosensitization |
|---|---|---|---|
| cetuximab (Erbitux) | EGFR | Monoclonal antibody | Disruption of signal transduction pathways that promote cellular survival following irradiation[33] |
| trastuzumab (Herceptin) | ERBB2 | Monoclonal antibody | Disruption of signal transduction pathways that promote cellular survival following irradiation |
| gefitinib (Iressa) | EGFR | Small molecule tyrosine | Disruption of signal transduction pathways that promote cellular survival following irradiation |
| erlotinib (Tarceva) | EGFR | TKI | Disruption of signal transduction pathways that promote cellular survival following irradiation |
| imatinib (Gleevec) | ABL, KIT, PDGFR | TKI | Disruption of signal transduction pathways that promote cellular survival following irradiation |
| bevacizumab (Avastin) | VEGF | Monoclonal antibody | Inhibition of angiogenesis[34] |
| sunitinib (Sutent) | VEGFR, KIT, PDGFR, FLT3 | Small molecule TKI | Inhibition of angiogenesis and tumor cell proliferation[35] |
| tipifarnib (Zarnestra) | RAS | Farnesyl transferase inhibitor | Inhibition of RAS activation which is associated with radiation resistance[36,37] |
| sorafenib (Nexavar) | RAF, KIT, FLT3, VEGFR, PDGFR | Small molecule multi-kinase inhibitor | Inhibition of angiogenesis and tumor cell proliferation[38] |
| bortezomib (Velcade) | Proteasome | Inhibition of the chymotrypsin-like activity of the 26S proteasome | Interaction to produce radiosensitization[39] |
| histone deacetylase inhibitors | Histone deacetylases | Hydroxamic acid derivatives, carboxylates, benzamides, electrophilic ketones and cyclic peptides | Inhibition of pro-mitogenic and DNA repair processes[40,41] |
| sirolimus (Rapamune, rapamycin) | mTOR/FRAP (mammalian target of rapamycin) | Binds to the FKBP12 complex and inhibits in TROR/FRAP | Inhibition of the PI3K/AKT pro-survival pathway[42] that is activated by radiation. mTOR/FRAP is a downstream target of AKT (temsirolimus and everolimus are also mTOR/FRAP inhibitors) |
| irinotecan (Camptosar) | Topoisomerase I | Topoisomerase I cleavable complex poison | Inhibition of repair processes[43] |
| celecoxib (Celebrex) | Cyclooxygenase(COX)-2 | Diarylheterocyclic that inhibits COX-2 through interaction with specific amino acids | Inhibition of the production of radioprotective prostaglandins through COX.[44] Radiation activates cytoplasmic phospholipase A2 which triggers release of arachidonic acid from membrane phospholipids and production of prostaglandins. COX-2 is over-expressed in a variety of tumors. |

# REFERENCES

1. Vogelstein B, Kinzler KW. Cancer genes and the pathways they control. *Nat Med* 10: 789–799, 2004.

2. Pierotti MA, Frattini M, Sozzi G, et al. Oncogenes pp 68–84 In *Cancer Medicine 7,* Kufe DW, Bast RC, Hait W, et al, Eds., B.C. Decker, Hamilton, 2006.

3. Park BH, Vogelstein B. Tumor suppressor genes pp 85–103 In *Cancer Medicine 7,* Kufe DW, Bast RC, Hait W, et al, Eds., B.C. Decker, Hamilton, 2006.

4. Thiagalingam S, Foy RL, Cheng KH, et al. Loss of heterozygosity as a predictor to map tumor suppressor genes in cancer: molecular basis of its occurrence. *Curr Opin Oncol* 14: 65–72, 2002.

5. Mittnacht S. The retinoblastoma protein—from bench to bedside. *Eur J Cell Biol* 84: 97–107, 2005.

6. Sengupta S, Harris CC. Traffic cop at the crossroads of DNA repair and recombination. *Nat Rev Mol Cell Biol* 6: 44–55, 2005.

7. Chene P. Inhibiting the p53-MDM2 interaction: an important target for cancer therapy. *Nat Rev Cancer* 3: 102–109, 2003.

8. O'Driscoll M, Jeggo PA. The role of double-strand break repair—insights from human genetics. *Nat Rev Genet* 7: 45–54, 2006.

9. Fortini P, Pascucci B, Parlanti E, et al. The base excision repair: mechanisms and its relevance for cancer susceptibility. *Biochimie* 85: 1053–1071, 2003.

10. Zhang J, Powell SN. The role of the BRCA1 tumor suppressor in DNA double-strand break repair. *Mol Cancer Res* 3: 531–539, 2005.

11. West SC. Molecular views of recombination proteins and their control. *Nat Rev Mol Cell Biol* 4: 435–445, 2003.

12. Lieber MR, Ma Y, Pannicke U, et al. Mechanism and regulation of human non-homologous DNA end-joining. *Nat Rev Mol Cell Biol* 4: 712–720, 2003.

13. Collis SJ, DeWeese TL, Jeggo PA, et al. The life and death of DNA-PK. *Oncogene* 24: 949–961, 2005.

14. Bakkenist CJ, Kastan MB. DNA damage activates ATM through intermolecular autophosphorylation and dimer dissociation. *Nature* 421: 499–506, 2003.

15. Dupre A, Boyer-Chatenet L, Gautier J. Two-step activation of ATM by DNA and the Mre11-Rad50-Nbs1 complex. *Nat Struct Mol Biol,* 2006.

16. Thiriet C, Hayes JJ. Chromatin in need of a fix: phosphorylation of H2AX connects chromatin to DNA repair. *Mol Cell* 18: 617–622, 2005.

17. Okada H, Mak TW. Pathways of apoptotic and non-apoptotic death in tumour cells. *Nat Rev Cancer* 4: 592–603, 2004.

18. Watanabe M, Hitomi M, van der Wee K, et al. The pros and cons of apoptosis assays for use in the study of cells, tissues, and organs. *Microsc Microanal* 8: 375–391, 2002.

19. Danial NN, Korsmeyer SJ. Cell death: critical control points. *Cell* 116: 205–219, 2004.

20. Fesik SW. Promoting apoptosis as a strategy for cancer drug discovery. *Nat Rev Cancer* 5: 876–885, 2005.

21. Kastan MB, Bartek J. Cell-cycle checkpoints and cancer. *Nature* 432: 316–323, 2004.

22. Lukas J, Lukas C, Bartek J. Mammalian cell cycle checkpoints: signalling pathways and their organization in space and time. *DNA Repair (Amst)* 3: 997–1007, 2004.

23. Kolesnick R, Fuks Z. Radiation and ceramide-induced apoptosis. *Oncogene* 22: 5897–5906, 2003.

24. Lobrich M, Jeggo PA. The two edges of the ATM sword: co-operation between repair and checkpoint functions. *Radiother Oncol* 76: 112–118, 2005.

25. Bailey SM, Murnane JP. Telomeres, chromosome instability and cancer. *Nucleic Acids Res* 34: 2408–2017, 2006.

26. Semenza GL. Targeting HIF-1 for cancer therapy. *Nat Rev Cancer* 3: 721–732, 2003.

27. Moeller BJ, Dewhirst MW. HIF-1 and tumour radiosensitivity. *Br J Cancer* 2006.
28. Dent P, Yacoub A, Contessa J, et al. Stress and radiation-induced activation of multiple intracellular signaling pathways. *Radiat Res* 159: 283–300, 2003.
29. Marmor MD, Skaria KB, Yarden Y. Signal transduction and oncogenesis by ErbB/HER receptors. *Int J Radiat Oncol Biol Phys* 58: 903–13, 2004.
30. Hynes NE, Lane HA. ERBB receptors and cancer: the complexity of targeted inhibitors. *Nat Rev Cancer* 5: 341–54, 2005.
31. Krause DS, Van Etten RA. Tyrosine kinases as targets for cancer therapy. *N Engl J Med* 353: 172–87, 2005.
32. Coleman ML, Marshall CJ, Olson MF. RAS and RHO GTPases in G1-phase cell-cycle regulation. *Nat Rev Mol Cell Biol* 5: 355–366, 2004.
33. Schmidt-Ullrich RK, Contessa JN, Lammering G, et al. ERBB receptor tyrosine kinases and cellular radiation responses. *Oncogene* 22: 5855–5865, 2003.
34. Jain RK, Duda DG, Clark JW, et al. Lessons from phase III clinical trials on anti-VEGF therapy for cancer. *Nat Clin Pract Oncol* 3: 24–40, 2006.
35. Atkins M, Jones CA, Kirkpatrick P. Sunitinib maleate. *Nat Rev Drug Discov* 5: 279–280, 2006.
36. Brunner TB, Hahn SM, McKenna WG, et al. Radiation sensitization by inhibition of activated *Ras*. *Strahlenther Onkol* 180: 731–740, 2004.
37. Mesa RA. Tipifarnib: farnesyl transferase inhibition at a crossroads. *Expert Rev Anticancer Ther* 6: 313–319, 2006.
38. Sridhar SS, Hedley D, Siu LL. Raf kinase as a target for anticancer therapeutics. *Mol Cancer Ther* 4: 677–685, 2005.
39. Richardson PG, Mitsiades C, Hideshima T, et al. Bortezomib: proteasome inhibition as an effective anticancer therapy. *Annu Rev Med* 57: 33–47, 2006.
40. Minucci S, Pelicci PG. Histone deacetylase inhibitors and the promise of epigenetic (and more) treatments for cancer. *Nat Rev Cancer* 6: 38–51, 2006.
41. Chinnaiyan P, Allen GW, Harari PM. Radiation and new molecular agents, part II: targeting HDAC, HSP90, IGF-1R, PI3K, and Ras. *Semin Radiat Oncol* 16: 59–64, 2006.
42. Shinohara ET, Cao C, Niermann K, et al. Enhanced radiation damage of tumor vasculature by mTOR inhibitors. *Oncogene* 24: 5414–5422, 2005.
43. Wu HG, Choy H. Irinotecan in combination with radiation therapy for small-cell and non-small-cell lung cancer. *Oncology* (Williston Park) 16: 13–8, 2002.
44. Choy H, Milas L. Enhancing radiotherapy with cyclooxygenase-2 enzyme inhibitors: a rational advance? *J Natl Cancer Inst* 95: 1440–1452, 2003.

# 4

# Combined Modality

*Charles G. Wood, MD*
*Stephen M. Hahn, MD*

## OVERVIEW

Combining different treatment modalities to improve outcome is by no means a recent trend in oncology. Historical data have demonstrated gains in survival, locoregional control, and functional results when local, locoregional, and systemic treatments have been used in concert, particularly in such sites as head and neck,[1–6] lung,[7–10] breast,[11–13] gastrointestinal tract,[14–16] bladder,[17] and cervix.[18–21] Contemporary clinical approaches to many solid tumors have placed an increasing emphasis on combined therapy, as the biology of both radiation and systemic treatment continues to be better understood, the efficacy and toxicity of concomitant treatments better described, and the interactions between different treatments better defined. This chapter is designed to explore the rationale behind the use of multiple therapies in definitive treatment regimens and to briefly summarize treatment evolution for several disease sites in which combination modality approaches have yielded improved outcomes.

## CHEMOTHERAPY

The term chemotherapy classically encompasses those systemic agents that exert cytotoxic or cytostatic effects on neoplastic cells. Multiple classes of chemotherapeutic compounds such as antimetabolites, vinca alkaloids, epipodophyllotoxins, and taxanes induce cell damage during specific phases of the cell cycle.[22] Others, such as platinum and alkylators, are cell cycle-nonspecific. This portends important consequences for anti-cancer therapy: cell cycle-specific drugs generally plateau in concentration-dependent effects, as only a proportion of tumor cells are actively dividing at a specific point in time; cell cycle-nonspecific compounds may display linear dose-response curves, as increasing drug concentration increases cell kill. Additionally, because cell cycle-specific agents plateau as concentration increases, further cytotoxicity must be achieved through increased duration of response, and so those drugs are often schedule-dependent.[23]

The limitations of single-agent therapy have been somewhat addressed by multi-agent regimens.[22] Cell kill may be increased with multi-agent chemotherapy regimens by overcoming drug-specific resistance of heterogeneous tumor cells. The use of multiple agents with different mechanisms of action may result in additive or synergistic effects. Conversely, toxicity may be reduced by using lower doses of drugs versus those necessary with single agent use, and by using compounds with non-overlapping toxicity profiles.

Human tumors are heterogeneous and are not thought to demonstrate constant logarithmic growth patterns. Smaller tumors may display more rapid growth; however, as tumor size increases, cells may outgrow their blood supply and become quiescent or undergo necrosis, resulting in slower growth rates. This can cause the tumors to become less sensitive to cytotoxic agents, both because of a greater percentage of nonproliferating cells and the issue of drug distribution disruption due to a compromised blood supply.

Chemotherapy alone, however, rarely produces tumor eradication or "cure" in the most common solid malignancies; consequently, there has been a strong rationale to combining chemotherapy with other treatment modalities such as radiation and/or surgery with such efforts beginning in earnest in the 1980s.

## RADIATION

Radiation, like surgery, is a locoregional treatment for conditions both malignant and benign. It utilizes high energy photons or particles such as electrons, and to a lesser extent, protons and neutrons. Photon radiation is most commonly used in the clinical setting, and usually interacts with tissue via Compton effects, in which the incoming high energy photon possesses energy sufficient to remove an orbital electron.[24] The unbound electron may then react directly with DNA (termed direct action), or react with water to form a hydroxyl radical which then reacts with DNA (termed indirect action). Radiation causes cellular demise by inducing DNA double-strand breaks which lead to cell death when replication is attempted. It is often delivered in small daily doses, or fractions, to take advantage of such biologic factors as repair, cell cycle redistribution, repopulation, and reoxygenation. It has potential for use in the definitive treatment of many solid malignancies, and also has a role in curative and palliative treatment of several hematologic malignancies.

## COMBINED MODALITY THERAPY

Nearly all chemotherapy drugs have been combined in clinical trials with radiation treatment for improvement of outcome via increased local control, decreased distant metastases, or both.[25] Combining the two modalities represents an attempt to exploit the mechanisms of spatial cooperation, independent cell kill, debulking, and enhanced tumor response through interactive means. Spatial cooperation refers to a situation in which one modality, usually radiation, is used to address the primary tumor, while another, usually chemotherapy, is delivered to prevent systemic spread. Independent cell kill refers simply to the use of two effective therapies at full dose, though not necessarily simultaneously, to achieve a greater tumor response versus that demonstrated with either agent alone. A third non-interactive model, debulking, describes the use of chemotherapy prior to radiation to shrink tumors, increasing the effectiveness of radiotherapy due to decreased cell number, and potentially decreasing toxicity by allowing smaller radiotherapy portals.

Enhanced tumor response may also be achieved by interactive mechanisms, including the inhibition by chemotherapy of radiation damage repair and the killing by one modality of subpopulations of cells resistant to the other modality. When such interactive mechanisms are thought to occur for a specific drug, that agent is often said to be "radiosensitizing." The degree to which a chemotherapy agent is a radiosensitizer is often described in preclinical studies by the use of the term "sensitizer enhancement ratio" or "SER." The SER refers to the ratio of cell or tumor kill from radiation in combination with a chemotherapy agent to radiation alone.

### Therapeutic Gain

The concept of therapeutic gain must be considered when assessing perceived benefits with combined modality regimens. Therapeutic gain describes the ratio of tumor response to toxicity, and is realized when the addition of a second modality increases tumor response with respect to either modality alone, at comparable levels of toxicity. In other words, an enhanced therapeutic gain refers to a better effect of chemoradiotherapy on tumor compared to normal tissues. Essentially, the added "good" of a combination treatment regimen must significantly outweigh the added "bad", with the "bad" being increased normal tissue toxicity. Unfortunately, comparison of treatment toxicities is largely based on acute morbidities, as late toxicity is less often reported and less well understood.

Concurrent administration of multiple modalities has been found to be associated with the greatest increase in side effects, particularly when chemotherapy agents with specific toxicities for organs within the radiation field are given in a concomitant fashion. For this reason, concurrent chemoradiation regimens are generally composed of agents that demonstrate non-overlapping toxicity profiles (avoiding bleomycin in lung cancer or doxorubicin with concurrent radiation in breast cancer).

The key to effective clinical radiosensitization is the therapeutic gain that one achieves with the use of the concurrent use of chemotherapy and radiation. The ideal situation is one in which radiation is combined with an agent that enhances the effect on tumor but not normal tissues, thereby increasing therapeutic gain. This selective radiosensitization is not completely achieved with conventional chemotherapy agents because of the increased normal tissue toxicity described in prior paragraphs. However, with the advent of molecularly targeted therapies and the recent report of the use of cetuximab, an inhibitor of epidermal growth factor receptor (EGFR), in combination with radiation for locally advanced head and neck cancer[3] the promise of selective radiosensitization may be realized.

## Chemotherapy

Cisplatinum is the classic example of a radiosensitizing chemotherapeutic, and pre-clinical evidence of its sensitizing properties, initially against leukemic cells, was reported in the 1970s.[26,27] A second early pre-clinical study, this in the setting of bladder cancer, is summarized as follows.

---

**BOX 4-1**

An animal tumor model was utilized by Soloway *et al.* to compare the cytotoxicity of radiation alone, cisplatinum or cyclophosphamide alone, and radiation with either concurrent cisplatinum or cyclophosphamide in mice with transplanted transitional cell carcinoma. Mice receiving radiation and concurrent cisplatinum achieved the highest number of cures, mice receiving radiation alone achieved approximately half as many cures, and mice receiving cisplatinum alone had no discernable benefit compared to mice receiving no treatment. The authors concluded that the data suggested "cooperation" between cisplatinum and radiation.

Soloway MS, Morris CR, Sudderth B. Radiation Therapy and cis-diammine-dichloroplatinum (II). In Transplantable and primary murine bladder cancer. *Int J Radiat Oncol Biol Phys* 1979;5:1355–1360.

---

Cisplatinum forms intrastrand and interstrand crosslinks with DNA that lead to DNA strand breaks and miscoding.[28] When combined with radiation, an increased number of radiation-induced strand breaks are noted to occur, perhaps by the conversion of easily repaired single-strand breaks to potentially lethal double-strand breaks during repair of DNA-platinum adducts.[29] This inhibition of radiation-induced damage repair is currently the most widely accepted explanation for the supra-additive effects of cisplatinum and radiotherapy. Other proposed mechanisms of interaction include a radiation-induced increase in cellular uptake of cisplatinum, a radiation-induced amplification of toxic platinum intermediates, and cytokinetic cooperation between the two.[29] Cisplatinum and its derivatives carboplatin and oxaliplatin are commonly used in the clinic as radiosensitizers.

5-FU is another drug thought to modulate radiation effects on tissue. It produces cytotoxicity through several mechanisms, with both DNA and RNA as targets. Its interaction with radiation is not fully understood, though it appears to involve inappropriate cell cycle progression.[30] Because laboratory and clinical data have suggested that extended infusions of 5-FU are required to maximize radiation interaction,[31,32] patients are often placed on protracted or continuous infusion courses requiring prolonged vascular access, and increasing morbidity secondary to thrombosis and infection. This prompted the development of capecitabine, an oral 5-FU pro-drug that is converted to the active metabolite by thymidine phosphorylase, which has been shown to selectively reside at increased concentrations in several tumor types.[33,34] Enthusiasm for capecitabine has been prompted further by recent data suggesting that radiation is capable of inducing an upsurge in thymidine phosphorylase levels.[35]

Gemcitabine, a pyrimidine analogue, has demonstrated potent radiosensitization in both normal tissue and tumor cells.[36] The interaction of gemcitabine and radiation is maximal when cells are exposed to the drug for at least 24 hours prior to radiation, and sensitization may still occur for several or more days after a brief exposure to the compound. Gemcitabine appears to inhibit DNA repair, though elucidation of its mechanisms of interaction with radiation is ongoing. Gemcitabine is such a potent and non-selective radiosensitizer that it is not commonly used in the United States in combined modality regimens. Significant morbidity and mortality have been reported when gemcitabine is used with radiation,[37] and it is common in clinical practice to wait three to four weeks between the use of radiation and gemcitabine.

Temozolomide is an alkylating agent that is metabolized to its active form, methyltriazeno-imidazole-arboxamide (MTIC). It is taken orally, is readily absorbed, and can rapidly cross the blood-brain barrier. The primary antitumor activity is via methylation of DNA, and cytotoxicity involves at least three DNA repair activities.[38] Pre-clinical data has suggested at least an additive effect when combined with radiation, and a recent large phase III randomized trial in patients with newly-diagnosed glioblastoma multiforme demonstrated a survival advantage for combined therapy followed by adjuvant temozolomide as discussed here.

Paclitaxel and docetaxel are derivatives of the yew tree and possess a 14-member ring, the taxane, for which the class is named.[22] Taxanes are microtubule stabilizing agents and promoters of microtubule assembly (in contrast to another class of plant-derived agents, the vinca alkaloids, that inhibit microtubule assembly).[39] These drugs block or prolong passage through the G2/M cell

---

**BOX 4-2**

Stupp and colleagues randomized patients with newly-diagnosed glioblastoma multiforme to radiation (60 Gy in 30 fractions) with or without concurrent daily temozolomide followed by adjuvant temozolomide for an additional 6 cycles. When compared with the radiation alone arm at a median follow-up of 28 months, patients in the combined treatment arm demonstrated improved overall survival (OS) (median OS 14.6 versus 12.1 months and 2-year OS 26.5% vs. 10.4%, $p < 0.001$) and improved progression free survival (PFS) (median PFS 6.9 vs. 5.0 months, $p < 0.001$).

A follow-up study performed to determine which patients received the most benefit from concomitant treatment found a correlation between those patients with promoter methylation "silencing" of the MGMT ($O^6$-alkylguanine-DNA alkyltransferase) DNA repair gene and improved OS. When all patients for whom MGMT status could be determined were considered, patients with MGMT promoter methylation were shown to have increased OS. When both treatment group and MGMT status were considered, those with MGMT promoter methylation in the combined modality arm demonstrated the

*(continues)*

**BOX 4-2** (CONTINUED)

greatest benefit. Conversely, those without MGMT promoter methylation in the combined modality arm received only a marginal benefit with the addition of temozolomide to radiation.

Stupp R, Mason WP, van den Bent MJ, et al. Radiotherapy plus concomitant and adjuvant temozolomide for glioblastoma. *N Engl J Med* 2005;352:987–996. Hegi ME, Diserens AC, Gorlia T, et al. MGMT gene silencing and benefit from temozolomide in glioblastoma. *N Engl J Med* 2005;352:997–1003.

cycle checkpoint secondary to the inability of cells to achieve or dissociate from a microtubule spindle, and are cytotoxic at sufficient concentrations. Surviving cells accumulate in the radiosensitive G2/M phase, creating a potential for synergism radiation and taxane agents.[40–42] These compounds demonstrate significant antineoplastic activity across a broad range of solid tumors and are included as part of combined modality therapy for such sites as head, neck, and lung.

## Hypoxic Cell Cytotoxins

Because ionizing radiation has been shown in mammalian cells to be dependent upon the presence of oxygen, efforts have been made to target the resistant fraction of hypoxic cells present in human tumors.[43] Most animal studies have shown tumors to contain hypoxic fractions of 10%–20%, and comparable proportions are estimated in human tumors.[44] Hypoxic cell targeting has the added benefit of intrinsic selectivity, as hypoxia is much less prevalent in normal tissues versus tumors, creating a potential for therapeutic gain with radiation.

Tirapazamine is one of several bioreductive drugs that selectively eradicates hypoxic cells, killing hypoxic cells at drug concentrations 50–300 times lower than that needed for oxic cells.[45] The compound is reduced under hypoxic conditions to a highly reactive free radical, producing cell kill via DNA strand disruption. It is converted back into the non-toxic parent compound under toxic conditions.[25] Tirapazamine has been shown to increase response to radiation in mouse models, and produces enhanced responses to cisplatinum as well.[46] Multiple phase III trials that include tirapazamine as part of the investigational arm are pending in such sites as advanced NSCLC, head and neck cancer, and cervical cancer.

Mitomycin is another example of a directly cytotoxic agent that preferentially targets hypoxic cells, and could be considered the prototype bioreductive drug.[47] It, like tirapazamine, is reduced under conditions of low oxygen tension, and the resulting multifunctional alkylating products lead to DNA cross-linking and cell demise.[43] Several prospective randomized trials employing mitomycin and radiotherapy in head and neck cancer have demonstrated increased locoregional control and/or survival versus radiation alone, in the setting of an acceptable toxicity profile.[48–50] Investigation of mitomycin in altered radiation schedules and in combination with other systemic agents in head and neck, gynecologic, and gastrointestinal cancers is ongoing.

## Hypoxic Cell Radiosensitizers

Other attempts to overcome the radioresistance of hypoxic cells have made use of agents able to mimic the sensitizing effects of oxygen. These drugs are less subject to rapid metabolic breakdown and can diffuse adequate distances from perfusing vessels to reach the more hypoxic cells situated away from the blood supply.[51] The nitroimidazoles, the third-generation of such sensitizers, were found to have radiation dose-modifying effects in animal studies, though this effect was reduced with fractionated treatment, possibly due to reoxygenation of tumor cells.[43] Misonidazole, the most potent of the nitroimidazoles, has shown generally disappointing results in clinical trials, probably due to dose-limiting neurotoxicity. Alternatively, nimorazole, a much less active agent but with a more attractive toxicity profile, has produced significant gains in locoregional control and disease-free survival (DFS) in a large Danish head and neck cancer study,[52] and is currently included as part of the standard of care in Denmark for patients with head and neck cancer.

## Targeted Agents

A variety of different molecular-signaling pathways are involved in the response to radiation and chemotherapy,[53,54] and strategies to target these tumor-specific defects are currently being studied in the clinic. A major potential advantage of these targeted therapies over conventional chemotherapy is a significantly decreased side effect profile, as the target of many of these agents is often exclusive to or upregulated in neoplastic cells. The demonstration of an increased therapeutic gain from the addition of cetuximab with radiation as described in following paragraphs is an important advance in combined modality therapy because it shows that selective radiosensitization is feasible. The challenge, however, is to understand how to integrate targeted therapies with conventional chemotherapy and radiotherapy while still maintaining the benefit of tumor selectivity.

The ErbB receptor tyrosine kinase family is a logical target for combined modality therapy, as these receptors are known to be overexpressed in a variety of epithelial tumors[55] and have been correlated with adverse outcomes and radioresistance.[56,57] Pre-clinical evidence has demonstrated interaction between radiation and ErbB-1 (EGFR) targeting, with enhanced radiation effects considered secondary to induction of apoptosis and hindrance of proliferation.[58]

Cetuximab, an EGFR inhibitor, was found to confer a survival advantage when added to conventional radiation versus radiation alone in locally advanced head and neck cancer patients and is discussed further in the head and neck section. EGFR inhibitors have also been evaluated in non-small cell lung cancer (NSCLC), and gefitinib has now been replaced by erlotinib owing to the survival benefit shown by erlotinib versus best supportive care in patients with relapsing or persistent disease following first- or second-line chemotherapy.[59] It has been approved by the FDA for use as second-line systemic treatment in patients with locally advanced or metastatic lung cancer, and in combination with gemcitabine as first-line treatment for advanced pancreatic cancer.

Trastuzumab targets the ErbB-2 receptor (HER-2/neu), found to be overexpressed in 25%–30% of all breast cancers and associated with an increased rate of relapse and a worse prognosis. The drug has produced survival benefits in both the metastatic and non-metastatic setting in patients whose tumor cells strongly express the HER-2/neu protein. It has been linked to increased cardiotoxicity when given with doxorubicin as well as when given alone, particularly in patients with extensive past exposure to doxorubicin. Preliminary data has suggested an acceptable acute toxicity profile when delivered concurrently with radiotherapy, including those patients with left-sided lesions in which the heart may be subjected to moderate radiation doses.[60]

Other molecular agents are currently being evaluated, including angiogenesis inhibitors, apoptotic inducers, and farnesyl transferase inhibitors. Pre-clinical and clinical work is ongoing to assess the effects of these targeted drugs on malignant and normal tissues.

## LUNG CANCER

### Non-small Cell Lung Cancer

Until recently, radiation therapy alone functioned as the standard of care for patients with locally advanced or medically inoperable non-small cell lung cancer (NSCLC). Long-term survival, however, was uncommon with this approach, no better than 5% at 5 years in locally advanced disease, with poor control of both local and distant disease.[61] These suboptimal results led to the investigation of adding chemotherapy to definitive radiotherapy. Initially, studies focused on the sequential use of chemotherapy and radiation.[7,62–64] More recently, combined, concurrent chemotherapy and radiation regimens have been utilized.[65–67] Strategies utilizing more frequent chemotherapy administration at lower doses, as well as higher dose chemotherapy at less frequent intervals, has been employed. More frequent drug dosing is aimed at increasing local control (LC) and theoretically takes advantage of radiosensitization properties believed to be associated with cisplatinum. Higher dose systemic treatment, alternatively, may impart advantages in controlling metastatic spread.

Early cooperative group trials demonstrated improvements in overall survival (OS) when chemotherapy was delivered prior to radiation in patients with locally advanced NSCLC. The CALGB conducted a trial in the mid-1980s that randomized patients with stage III NSCLC to cisplatinum/vinblastine followed by radiation treatment versus radiation treatment alone.[62,63] With a median follow-up of more than 8 years, the chemoradiation group displayed superior survival compared to those treated without induction chemotherapy (median OS 13.7 vs. 9.6 months and 7-year OS 13% vs. 6%, p = 0.012), with a 1% frequency of life-threatening pneumonitis or esophagitis.

A follow-up intergroup trial within the RTOG, ECOG, and SWOG randomized patients with unresectable stage II or III NSCLC to one of three treatment arms: induction cisplatinum and vinblastine followed by conventional radiation, conventional radiation alone, and hyperfractionated radiation alone (twice-daily to a dose of 69.6 Gy).[7,64] OS was found to be statistically improved for the chemoradiation group versus the other two arms (p = 0.04), although long-term survival was still poor, no better than 8% in any arm.

Chemoradiation delivered concurrently has also been shown to improve outcome versus radiation alone in NSCLC patients. The EORTC 08844 study compared split-course radiation with or without daily or weekly cisplatinum.[68] The daily chemotherapy arm demonstrated significantly improved OS versus the radiation alone arm at 3 years (16% vs. 2%, p = 0.009), though no survival difference was seen at 3 years between the daily and weekly chemotherapy groups (16% vs. 13%, p = 0.36).

A phase III trial out of Yugoslavia compared hyperfractionated radiation (twice-daily to 64.8 Gy) with or without weekly or every other week carboplatin and etoposide.[69] Three-year survival was found to be significantly different between the three groups (p = 0.003), with the weekly chemotherapy arm demonstrating the best results.

A second phase III trial from Yugoslavia compared hyperfractionated radiation (twice-daily to 69.6 Gy) with or without daily carboplatin and etoposide therapy.[70] Jeremic and colleagues reported superior 4-year OS (23% vs. 9%, p=0.021) and 4-year local relapse-free survival (42% vs. 19%, p = 0.015) in the combined modality arm. In all three trials, the survival benefit was thought due to improved LC, lending support to the principle of frequent, low-dose administration of radiosensitizing chemotherapy for purposes of increasing local eradication of tumor.

Concurrent versus sequential chemotherapy has likewise been evaluated in a phase III setting. Furuse *et al.* of the West Japan Lung Cancer Group compared mitomycin-C, vindesine, and cisplatinum (MVP) administered prior to or with radiation in unresectable stage III NSCLC patients.[65] The concurrent arm demonstrated a modest but statistically significant median and 5-year survival advantage (16.5 vs. 13.3 months and 15.8% vs. 8.9%, p = 0.04). A patterns of failure analysis suggested that the survival benefit was, again, due to LC.

A second trial, RTOG 94-10, reported and updated in abstract form only, also compared sequential versus concomitant cisplatinum and vinblastine with conventional radiation.[66,67] A third arm employed hyperfractionated radiotherapy with concurrent cisplatinum and oral etoposide. The concurrent cisplatinum/vinblastine arm displayed significantly improved 4-year overall survival versus the sequential arm (21% vs. 12%, p = 0.04), with the concurrent hyperfractionated group producing intermediate results (17% alive at 4 years).

Despite the results reported across multiple randomized trials for concurrent versus sequential chemoradiation, concurrent treatment has by no means been a "home run" in lung cancer, yielding improved but still modest long-term survival. A common feature of combined, concurrent chemoradiotherapy is an increase in moderate and severe esophagitis compared to radiation alone. Because of the modest benefits and increased risks of toxicity, the concurrent approach should be offered only to patients with good performance status with the reserve necessary to tolerate this rigorous regimen. Sequential chemoradiation remains an acceptable definitive treatment for locally advanced disease in those patients who present with multiple or significant co-morbidities or disease-related sequelae.

## Small Cell Lung Cancer

Small cell lung cancer (SCLC) is treated primarily with chemotherapy with or without radiation, except in those uncommon cases in which surgical resection is performed for both treatment and diagnostic purposes in patients who are assumed to have NSCLC. Local therapy, either surgery or radiation, was originally the mainstay of treatment for patients with SCLC. Long-term survival rates with this approach, however, were anecdotal at best. In the 1970s, the disease was noted to be highly responsive to chemotherapy, and various drug combinations were utilized. Though complete responses were not uncommon with chemotherapy alone, the cancer almost invariably relapsed, with local failure on the order of 80%. Early attempts to combine radiation with chemotherapy produced a finite number of long-term remissions, a major paradigm shift for the disease. This was reflected in separate meta-analyses published in the early 1990s reporting absolute benefits in both OS and LC for patients receiving chemotherapy and radiation versus chemotherapy alone.[71,72]

Although extensive stage disease patients still fare exceedingly poorly with current treatment, the approximate one-third of SCLC patients who demonstrate limited stage disease (disease confined to one hemithorax and able to be reasonably encompassed within a single radiation portal) at diagnosis are potentially curable and best managed with concurrent chemoradiation.

This was most clearly demonstrated in an intergroup study by Turrisi *et al.* shown here.

---

**BOX 4-3**

The Intergroup 0096 trial randomized patients to cisplatinum and etoposide chemotherapy with concurrent radiation beginning with the first chemotherapy cycle and delivered either twice-daily to a dose of 45 Gy over 3 weeks or once-daily to a dose of 45 Gy over 5 weeks. Prophylactic cranial radiation was offered to those patients in both groups with a complete response. At a median follow-up approaching 8 years, a statistically significant survival advantage was seen in the twice-daily radiation group versus the once-daily radiation group (median OS 23 vs. 19 months and 5-year OS 26% vs. 16%, p = 0.04). Grade 3 esophagitis was significantly increased in the twice-daily radiation arm (27% vs. 11%, p < 0.001), though hematologic and pulmonary toxicity were similar between the arms.

Turrisi AT, 3rd, Kim K, Blum R, et al. Twice-daily compared with once-daily thoracic radiotherapy in limited small-cell lung cancer treated concurrently with cisplatin and etoposide. *N Engl J Med* 1999;340:265–271.

---

A subsequent Japan Clinical Oncology Group trial by Takada *et al.* reported a trend toward improved survival in limited stage SCLC patients treated with cisplatinum/etoposide chemotherapy concurrent with twice-daily thoracic radiation begun with the first cycle of chemotherapy versus once-daily thoracic radiation begun after the fourth cycle of chemotherapy (median OS 27.2 months vs. 19.7 months and 5-year OS 23.7% vs. 18.3%, p = 0.097), followed by prophylactic cranial radiation in those with a complete or near-complete response.[73]

## HEAD AND NECK CANCER

Carcinoma of the head and neck has long been treated with surgery, radiation, or a combination of the two modalities. Recently, chemotherapy has been selectively included in the management of high-risk head and neck cancer, determined by such variables as primary site location, number of involved nodes, presence of extranodal extension, and surgical margin status. Though the roles of neoadjuvant and adjuvant chemotherapy remain controversial, concurrent use of chemotherapy and radiation has been shown to confer a survival benefit across several randomized trials and meta-analyses.

Two meta-analyses of early trials employing radiation with or without chemotherapy for head and neck cancer reported a modest improvement in survival for patients treated with concomitant therapy.[74,75] A more recent meta-analysis, MACH-NC, analyzed over 16,000 patients in 87 randomized-controlled studies between 1965 and 2000 comparing radiation with or without chemotherapy, 50 of which employed concurrent chemoradiation schedules.[76,77] The authors reported a 5-year OS advantage of 5% for patients treated with both chemotherapy and radiation and 8% for patients treated with concurrent chemoradiation, with the greatest benefit seen in platinum-based drug regimens.

In locally advanced head and neck cancer, multiple phase III trials have supported the use of concurrent chemoradiation, a particularly attractive option for technically unresectable patients and those in whom appropriate surgical resection might result in suboptimal functional and/or cosmetic outcome.

The feasibility of chemoradiation as an alternative to surgery in locally advanced laryngeal cancer was demonstrated by The Department of Veterans Affairs Laryngeal Cancer Study Group in the early 1990s.[78] Up until this time, the standard treatment for high-risk laryngeal cancer was total laryngectomy, with a resulting loss of normal speech and the placement of a permanent tracheostomy. The VA larynx study randomized patients to induction cisplatinum/5-FU followed by radiation in those patients with a good response to chemotherapy, or to surgery and adjuvant radiotherapy. Laryngeal preservation was possible in 64% of patients in the chemoradiation arm, and no survival difference was evident after more than 10 years of follow-up.[79] The increased locoregional recurrence in the chemoradiation arm was offset by decreased distant metastases, and T stage was prognostic for local failure, with 56% of T4 laryngeal cancers undergoing salvage total laryngectomy.

These results were built upon by RTOG 91-11 which enrolled patients with locally advanced resectable laryngeal carcinoma,[80] though this cohort included only 10% of patients with T4 tumors as opposed to 25% in the VA larynx study. Participants were treated with induction cisplatinum/5-FU followed by radiation, concurrent cisplatinum and radiation, or radiation alone. The concurrent chemoradiation arm demonstrated increased LC and an increased laryngeal preservation rate compared to the other arms and chemotherapy was found to suppress distant metastases in the induction and concurrent arms, OS was equivalent between the three groups. The authors concluded that the majority of locally advanced laryngeal cancer patients (T2, T3, and low-volume T4 disease) could be managed adequately with a non-surgical approach, and that concurrent chemoradiation represented the best non-surgical treatment option.

The addition of chemotherapy to radiation has also been shown to confer a survival benefit in those patients with unresectable disease. A head and neck Intergroup study compared radiation alone, radiation with concurrent cisplatinum, and split-course radiation with cisplatinum/5-FU in patients with locally advanced squamous cell carcinoma of the head and neck, excluding primaries of the nasopharynx, paranasal sinuses, and parotid glands.[6] Concurrent chemoradiation was shown to provide a median survival advantage over radiation alone (37% vs. 23%, p = 0.014), and the split-course combined modality arm produced intermediate results not significantly different from either of the other two arms.

Renewed interest in the addition of induction chemotherapy to concurrent chemoradiation schedules has come about due to recent outcome data presented by Posner et al.[81] The authors reported on the preliminary results of the TAX 324 study in abstract form, comparing induction cis-platinum/5-FU with or without docetaxel and followed by radiation (median dose of 70 Gy in 7.1 weeks) with concurrent carboplatin. Patients with stage III or IV squamous cell carcinoma of the oral cavity, oropharynx, larynx, or hypopharynx were randomized between the two induction chemotherapy regimens, and surgery was performed following chemoradiation in patients with residual or initially bulky disease. Patients in the cisplatinum/5-FU/docetaxel induction group were found to have an improved median OS (70.6 months vs. 30.1 months, p = 0.0058) and DFS (3-year DFS 49% vs. 37%, p = 0.004) versus those in the cisplatinum/5-FU induction group, with similar acute toxicity profiles. Data on local and distant control and late toxicity were not yet available at the time of the report; nevertheless, the authors argued that the cisplatinum/5-FU/docetaxel arm represented the new standard of care in locally advanced head and neck cancer.

In patients treated primarily by surgery, postoperative radiotherapy (PORT) has been found to increase LC, though it has not been proven to extend survival.

---

**BOX 4-4**

The RTOG 95-01/Intergroup trial randomized patients to conventional radiation (60–66 Gy in 30–33 fractions) with or without concurrent bolus cisplatinum (100 mg/m2) delivered every 3 weeks for a total of three cycles (days 1, 22, 43). Compared to the PORT alone arm, the postoperative chemoradiation group demonstrated significantly improved locoregional control (82% vs. 72% at 2 years, p=0.01) and DFS at a median follow-up of 46 months, though OS was not statistically different.

The EORTC 22931 trial randomized patients to conventional radiation (66 Gy in 33 fractions) with identical cisplatinum dosing and scheduling. Compared to the PORT alone arm, the postoperative chemoradiation group demonstrated significantly decreased locoregional relapse (18% vs. 31%, p = 0.007), improved PFS (47% vs. 36%, p = 0.04), and improved OS (53% vs. 40%, p = 0.02) at a median follow-up of 60 months.

Cooper JS, Pajak TF, Forastiere AA, et al. Postoperative concurrent radiotherapy and chemotherapy for high-risk squamous-cell carcinoma of the head and neck. *N Engl J Med* 2004;350:1937–1944.

Bernier J, Domenge C, Ozsahin M, et al. Postoperative irradiation with or without concomitant chemotherapy for locally advanced head and neck cancer. *N Engl J Med* 2004;350:1945–1952.

---

Similar trials from the RTOG and EORTC, mentioned previously, evaluated the role of PORT with or without concurrent chemotherapy following surgical resection for squamous cell carcinoma of the oral cavity, oropharynx, larynx, or hypopharynx with high-risk pathologic features. Pathologic features defining eligibility for the RTOG 95-01/Intergroup trial included involvement of two or more nodes, extranodal extension, and microscopically positive margins of resection. The EORTC 22931 study included these patients, as well as those with pT3 or pT4 primaries and any nodal stage except T3N0 of the larynx; perineural involvement; vascular tumor embolism; and oral cavity or oropharyngeal tumors with involved level IV or V nodes. Both studies demonstrated improved locoregional control and DFS in the chemoradiation arm, and an OS advantage for combined therapy was seen in the EORTC study.

Among head and neck subsites, nasopharyngeal carcinoma is rather unique in that surgery rarely plays a role in treatment due to the restrictive nature of the anatomy and the functional deficits that would result, a high propensity for cervical and retropharyngeal nodal metastases, and a high responsiveness to radiotherapy. The Intergroup 0099 trial randomized patients with nasopharyngeal carcinoma to radiation with or without chemotherapy consisting of concurrent cisplatinum delivered every 3 weeks followed by adjuvant cisplatinum and 5-FU for an additional three courses [4,82]. Patients in the chemoradiation arm demonstrated superior 5-year OS (67% vs. 37%, p = 0.001) and 5-year DFS (74% vs. 46%, p < 0.001) at a minimum follow-up of five years.

Similar results were reported by Lin et al., who randomized patients to radiation with or without cisplatinum and 5-FU during weeks one and five of radiation treatment.[5] At a median follow-up of 65 months, patients in the combined treatment arm displayed improved 5-year OS (72.3% vs. 54.2%, p = 0.0022) and 5-year progression-free survival (PFS) (71.6% vs. 53.6%, p = 0.0012). It was the first trial to demonstrate a survival advantage with combined modality therapy for nasopharyngeal carcinoma patients in an endemic area.

The benefit of systemic therapy in combination with radiation is not limited to conventional chemotherapy alone in head and neck cancer. As shown in the following box, Bonner et al. recently reported on radiation with or without cetuximab, a monoclonal antibody against the EGFR receptor, in patients with locoregionally advanced squamous cell carcinoma of the head and neck.

---

**BOX 4-5**

A phase III, multicenter study randomized 424 patients with non-metastatic stage III or IV squamous cell carcinoma of the oropharynx, hypopharynx, or larynx to once-daily, twice-daily, or concomitant boost radiotherapy with or without cetuximab. In the combined treatment group, intravenous cetuximab was begun 1 week prior to radiation at a loading dose of 400 mg/m2, followed by weekly infusions of 250 mg/m2 throughout the duration of radiotherapy. At a median follow-up of 54 months, patients in the concurrent arm displayed a longer duration of locoregional control (24.4 months vs. 14.9 months, p=0.005), improved PFS (17.1 vs. 12.4 months, p = 0.006), and superior OS (49.0 months vs. 29.3 months, p = 0.03). With the exception of infusion reactions and acneiform rash, the incidence of grade 3 or greater toxicity was similar between the two arms.

Bonner JA, Harari PM, Giralt J, et al. Radiotherapy plus cetuximab for squamous-cell carcinoma of the head and neck. *N Engl J Med* 2006;354:567–578.

---

The benefits in locoregional control, PFS, and OS were encouraging, especially with the superior toxicity profile of cetuximab. Current trials are underway comparing concurrent chemoradiation with and without cetuximab in head and neck cancer patients.

## GASTROINTESTINAL CANCER

Though surgery remains the basis of curative treatment in gastric, pancreatic, and large bowel cancers, chemoradiation continues to be more extensively integrated into the treatment of gastrointestinal (GI) malignancies. Chemoradiotherapy now functions as the standard of care in anal cancer,[83] and when added to surgery may offer benefits in a variety of GI tract subsites.[25] 5-FU represents the cornerstone to which other agents have been added in combination, and protracted or continuous infusion is often favored over bolus administration. Oxaliplatin is emerging as another useful agent for GI malignancies, and is often delivered with 5-FU and folinic acid (leucovorin) in a combination known as FOLFOX for treatment of colorectal cancer.[84,85]

## Esophageal Cancer

Surgical resection remains part of the standard treatment for patients with stage I and II disease, and also in selected cases of stage III tumors. However, the proportion of patients alive at 5 years is low, with significant failure both locoregionally and distantly. The addition of neoadjuvant chemoradiation to esophagectomy offers theoretical benefits both locally and systemically, and has been shown in multiple randomized trials to yield a survival benefit. Walsh and colleagues randomized patients with resectable esophageal adenocarcinoma to esophagectomy with or without preoperative chemoradiation consisting of two courses of cisplatinum and 5-FU and concurrent radiation (40 Gy in 15 fractions).[86] Patients in the combined treatment arm demonstrated improved survival versus the surgery alone arm (median OS 16 vs. 11 months and 3-year survival 32% vs. 6%, p = 0.01), though the surgery alone group was noted to have fared worse than expected.

The CALGB 9781 trial, recently presented in abstract format, included patients with either adenocarcinoma or squamous cell carcinoma of the esophagus.[14] Treatment arms consisted of neoadjuvant chemoradiation followed by esophagectomy versus esophagectomy alone. Patients with stages I-III disease and tumors ≥ 2 cm from the gastroesophageal junction were eligible. At a median follow-up of 6 years, a survival advantage was demonstrated by the trimodality group versus the surgery alone group (median OS 4.5 vs. 1.8 years, 5-year OS 39% vs. 16%, p = 0.005). The authors concluded that neoadjuvant chemoradiation followed by esophagectomy represented the new standard of care in resectable esophageal cancer.

The addition of chemotherapy to radiation in patients with locally advanced disease has also been shown to yield improvements in survival. Although at least six phase III randomized trials have compared chemoradiation with radiation alone, only the RTOG 85-01 study, as discussed in this section, is considered to have utilized adequate doses of chemotherapy and radiation.

Despite the encouraging results of RTOG 85-01, locoregional control was less than 50%, and the Intergroup 0123 trial attempted to improve upon this via radiation dose escalation.[87] Patients were treated with cisplatinum/5-FU chemotherapy and concurrent radiation to doses of either 50.4 Gy in 28 fractions or 64.8 Gy in 36 fractions. No difference was seen between the two groups with

---

**BOX 4-6**

The RTOG 85-01 trial included patients with adenocarcinoma or squamous cell carcinoma of the esophagus. Treatment arms consisted of either radiation alone (64 Gy in 32 fractions) or radiation (50 Gy in 25 fractions) with concomitant cisplatinum and 5-FU chemotherapy. Combination chemotherapy was begun on day 1 of radiation and continued for a total of 4 cycles (weeks 1, 5, 8, 11). Patients on the chemoradiation arm demonstrated improved OS versus those treated with radiation alone (median OS 14.1 vs. 9.3 months and 5-year OS 27% vs. 0%, p < 0.001), with 22% alive at 8 years of follow-up and a projected 10-year OS of 20%. Patients treated with chemoradiation were less likely to have persistent disease and demonstrated greater locoregional and distant control.

Herskovic A, Martz K, al-Sarraf M, et al. Combined chemotherapy and radiotherapy compared with radiotherapy alone in patients with cancer of the esophagus. N Engl J Med 1992;326:1593–1598.

Al-Sarraf M, Martz K, Herskovic A, et al. Progress report of combined chemoradiotherapy versus radiotherapy alone in patients with esophageal cancer: an intergroup study. J Clin Oncol 1997;15:277-284.

Cooper JS, Guo MD, Herskovic A, et al. Chemoradiotherapy of locally advanced esophageal cancer: long-term follow-up of a prospective randomized trial (RTOG 85-01). Radiation Therapy Oncology Group. JAMA 1999;281:1623–1627.

respect to survival or locoregional control, and greater toxicity was reported in the higher dose arm, though it did not appear to be related to the increased radiation dose. The authors concluded that the standard dose of radiation when delivered with cisplatinum/5-FU remained 50.4 Gy.

## Rectal Cancer

Management of rectal cancer relies primarily on resection of bowel and neighboring lymph nodes. Implementation of advanced surgical techniques such as total mesorectal excision (TME), in which the node-bearing mesorectum is included in the resection specimen, have been associated with a reduction in local relapse rates by as much as 20%.[88] However, pelvic failure can have devastating effects on quality of life and remains a significant concern in patients with deep bowel wall penetration or nodal metastasis, regardless of the surgical technique employed.

Adjuvant chemoradiation following resection in locally advanced disease has proven superior to either radiation or chemotherapy alone in the postoperative setting. This was demonstrated early on by the 4-arm GITSG 7175 trial, in which patients with T3/4 disease or node positivity and without gross residual tumor following surgery were randomized to radiation, chemotherapy, chemoradiation, or no further treatment.[89] Patients in the chemotherapy-alone arm received bolus 5-FU and MeCCNU, and those in the chemoradiation group received only bolus 5-FU. Participants receiving radiation achieved improved locoregional control versus those who did not (84% vs. 75%, p = 0.06), and chemoradiation arm demonstrated the highest OS and DFS rates among all arms, with statistically significant outcomes versus the surgery alone group (7-year OS 57% vs. 32%, p = 0.005, and 5-year DFS 67% vs. 45%, p = 0.009).

The NCCTG undertook a study comparing postoperative radiation with or without chemotherapy in patients with locally advanced disease.[90] Patients in the chemoradiation arm displayed significant improvements versus those treated with postoperative radiation alone with respect to OS, DFS, LC, and distant metastasis (DM).

A subsequent Intergroup trial evaluated different combinations of chemotherapy in a similar population of patients receiving chemoradiotherapy following surgical resection.[91] The four drug regimens tested included bolus 5-FU and protracted venous infusion (PVI) 5-FU, each with or without MeCCNU. Patients receiving radiation and PVI-5FU demonstrated superior 4-year DFS and OS rates versus those treated with radiation and bolus 5-FU, and no benefit was seen when MeCCNU was added to either regimen. Interestingly, no differences in LC were observed between patients treated with PVI and bolus 5-FU.

The necessity of the inclusion of radiation with chemotherapy in adjuvant treatment was addressed by the 4-arm NSABP R-02 trial, in which T3/4 or node-positive rectal cancer patients were treated postoperatively with MeCCNU/vincristine/5-FU (MOF) or 5-FU/leucovorin, each with or without radiation.[92] Only male patients were eligible for randomization to MOF. Females received postoperative 5-FU/leucovorin with or without radiation, and were not included in the chemotherapy comparison analysis. No difference was noted between patients receiving chemotherapy versus chemoradiation with respect to 5-year DFS (50% vs. 51%, p = 0.90) or 5-year OS (58% vs. 59%, p = 0.89). The benefit of radiation was limited to improvements in 5-year LC for patients in the chemoradiation arm (92% vs. 87%, p = 0.02). Additionally, men treated with MOF displayed decreased 5-year DFS versus men treated with 5-FU/leucovorin (47% vs. 55%, p = 0.009), providing further support for inclusion of 5-FU and elimination of MeCCNU in combined modality rectal cancer regimens.

Efforts to improve upon results with surgery alone have not been confined to the postoperative setting. The EORTC 40971 trial randomized patients with resectable tumors to TME with or without preoperative radiation.[93] Patients in the combined treatment arm received 25 Gy in 5 Gy fractions via a 3- or 4-field arrangement and underwent TME within 1 week. Those patients in the surgery alone arm received postoperative radiotherapy in cases of close surgical margins or intra-operative tumor spillage. At a median follow-up of 2 years, the preoperative radiation group demonstrated superior LC versus the TME alone arm (97.5% vs. 91.8%, $p < 0.001$).

A similar preoperative radiation scheme was utilized in the Swedish Rectal Cancer Trial, which randomized patients with resectable tumors to surgery with or without neoadjuvant radiotherapy.[16,94] Unlike in the EORTC study, a TME technique was not required, and postoperative radiotherapy was not delivered to selected patients in the surgery alone arm. The addition of radiation was observed to confer significant improvements versus surgery alone with respect to 5-year OS (58% vs. 48%, $p = 0.004$), 5-year DFS (74% vs. 65%, $p = 0.002$), and 5-year LC (89% vs. 73%, $p < 0.001$). Additionally, the authors reported similar postoperative mortality and quality of life between the two groups.

The issue of optimal timing of preoperative treatment was addressed by Francois *et al.* in the Lyon R90-01 trial comparing long and short intervals between neoadjuvant radiation and surgery.[95] Patients with resectable disease were treated with preoperative radiation to a dose of 39 Gy in 3 Gy fractions via a 3-field technique. They were then randomized to surgery either 2 weeks following radiotherapy or 6 to 8 weeks following radiotherapy. The long-interval arm displayed improved pathologic downstaging (26% vs. 10.3%, $p = 0.007$) versus the short-interval arm, but no significant differences were noted in sphincter preservation rates (76% vs. 68%, $p = 0.27$).

Preoperative treatment has also been compared with postoperative treatment. In a recent trial conducted by the German Rectal Cancer Study Group, patients with T3/T4 nodal involvement or T3/T4 disease per ultrasonagraphy were randomized to one of two arms.[96–98] Patients in the preoperative group received two cycles PVI 5-FU with concurrent radiotherapy (50.4 Gy), TME within 4 to 6 weeks, and four cycles of bolus 5-FU. Patients in the postoperative group underwent TME followed within 4 weeks by six cycles of 5-FU, and concurrent radiotherapy (50.4 Gy and 5.4 Gy boost) was begun with the first or second cycle of 5-FU with PVI. The preoperative arm compared to the postoperative arm achieved an increased rate of sphincter preservation in low-lying tumors (39% vs. 19%, $p < 0.004$) and a decreased rate of 5-year local relapse (7% vs. 11%, $p = 0.02$) and chronic anastomotic recurrence (2.7% vs. 8.5%, $p = 0.001$). OS, DFS, and DM at 5 years were similar between the two groups, and both acute toxicity (diarrhea and any grade 3–4) and late toxicity (strictures and any grade 3–4) were significantly increased in the postoperative arm.

## Anal Cancer

Prior to the advent of combined modality approaches, invasive squamous cell carcinoma of the anus was treated by abdominoperineal resection (APR), leaving the patient with a permanent colostomy. Even with such extensive treatment, however, local relapse was frequent. Primary external beam radiotherapy was found to produce results similar to surgery, although OS at 5 years was no better than 50%–70%. Attempts to combine concurrent multi-agent chemotherapy with radiation began to be reported in the 1970s, with APR reserved for relapsing or persistent disease.

Two phase III randomized trials performed by the UKCCCR[99] and the EORTC[100] compared concurrent chemoradiation with radiation alone in patients with non-metastatic anal carcinoma. Both trials utilized concomitant 5-FU and mitomycin in the experimental arm, and initial radiation doses of 45 Gy were employed, with a 15–25 Gy boost in patients with at least a partial response to treatment. Patients with stable or progressing disease underwent salvage surgical resection. Though neither trial was able to show a benefit in OS, the clear improvements in LC and colostomy-free survival led to the institution of chemoradiation as the standard of care.

A phase III intergroup trial conducted by the RTOG and ECOG randomized patients with non-metastatic anal carcinoma to radiation and concurrent 5-FU with or without mitomycin.[101] As with the European studies, no benefit in OS was achieved, although the addition of mitomycin translated to decreased 4-year local failure (16% vs. 34%, p < 0.01) and increased 4-year DFS (73% vs. 51%, p = 0.003) and 4-year colostomy-free survival (71% vs. 59%, p = 0.014). Based on these results, and despite the increased early grade 4+ toxicity in the mitomycin-containing arm (23% vs. 7%, p < 0.001), the use of mitomycin was considered justified.

Interestingly, patients not achieving a complete pathologic response in the intergroup trial were initially salvaged not with APR, but with additional chemoradiation. More than half of the patients (12/22) with persistent disease demonstrated a pathologic complete response following pelvic radiation (9 Gy in five fractions) and concurrent cisplatinum/5-FU. Of those 12 patients, four remained disease- and colostomy-free at 4 years, and an additional four underwent successful salvage APR and remained free of disease at 4 years. These results have contributed to the increasing acceptance of attempting salvage with chemoradiation before resorting to radical surgery.

## CONCLUSION

Contemporary cancer therapy is undergoing a paradigm shift in which single-modality treatment is becoming more an exception than a rule. Combined chemoradiotherapy regimens are already in common use in a variety of other solid tumors including some not focused upon in this chapter, including CNS malignancies, pancreatic cancer, and even prostate cancer. The key to the use of chemoradiotherapy is developing regimens that improve the therapeutic index (improving tumor control and patient outcome without a significant increase in early or late toxicities). A new era of targeted therapy is being defined by this concept of therapeutic gain and its emphasis on tumor specificity. As advances in molecular biology continue to accelerate the development of clinically relevant targeted anticancer agents, the challenge of integrating multiple treatment modalities in an optimal manner will likewise increase.

## REFERENCES

1. Cooper JS, Pajak TF, Forastiere AA, *et al.* Postoperative concurrent radiotherapy and chemotherapy for high-risk squamous-cell carcinoma of the head and neck. *N Engl J Med* 2004;350:1937–1944.
2. Bernier J, Domenge C, Ozsahin M, *et al.* Postoperative irradiation with or without concomitant chemotherapy for locally advanced head and neck cancer. *N Engl J Med* 2004; 350: 1945–1952.
3. Bonner JA, Harari PM, Giralt J, *et al.* Radiotherapy plus cetuximab for squamous-cell carcinoma of the head and neck. *N Engl J Med* 2006;354:567–578.
4. Al-Sarraf M, LeBlanc M, Giri PGS, *et al.* Superiority of five year survival with chemradiotherapy (CT-RT) vs radiotherapy in patients (Pts) with locally advanced nasopharyngeal carcinoma (NPC). Intergroup (0099) (SWOG 8892, RTOG 8817, ECOG 2388) Phase III Study: Final Report. American Society of Clinical Oncology. San Francisco, CA; 2001.
5. Lin JC, Jan JS, Hsu CY, *et al.* Phase III study of concurrent chemoradiotherapy versus radiotherapy alone for advanced nasopharyngeal carcinoma: positive effect on overall and progression-free survival. *J Clin Oncol* 2003;21:631–637.
6. Adelstein DJ, Li Y, Adams GL, *et al.* An intergroup phase III comparison of standard radiation therapy and two schedules of concurrent chemoradiotherapy in patients with unresectable squamous cell head and neck cancer. *J Clin Oncol* 2003;21:92–98.
7. Sause W, Kolesar P, Taylor SI, *et al.* Final results of phase III trial in regionally advanced unresectable non-small cell lung cancer: Radiation Therapy Oncology Group, Eastern Cooperative Oncology Group, and Southwest Oncology Group. *Chest* 2000;117:358–364.
8. Arriagada R, Bergman B, Dunant A, *et al.* Cisplatin-based adjuvant chemotherapy in patients with completely resected non-small-cell lung cancer. *N Engl J Med* 2004;350:351–360.

9. Douillard JY, Rosell R, De Lena M, *et al.* Adjuvant vinorelbine plus cisplatin versus observation in patients with completely resected stage IB-IIIA non-small-cell lung cancer (Adjuvant Navelbine International Trialist Association [ANITA]): a randomised controlled trial. *Lancet Oncol* 2006;7:719–727.

10. Winton T, Livingston R, Johnson D, *et al.* Vinorelbine plus cisplatin vs. observation in resected non-small-cell lung cancer. *N Engl J Med* 2005;352:2589–2597.

11. Clarke M, Collins R, Darby S, *et al.* Effects of radiotherapy and of differences in the extent of surgery for early breast cancer on local recurrence and 15-year survival: an overview of the randomised trials. *Lancet* 2005;366:2087–2106.

12. Effects of chemotherapy and hormonal therapy for early breast cancer on recurrence and 15-year survival: an overview of the randomised trials. *Lancet* 2005;365:1687–1717.

13. Romond EH, Perez EA, Bryant J, *et al.* Trastuzumab plus adjuvant chemotherapy for operable HER2-positive breast cancer. *N Engl J Med* 2005;353:1673–1684.

14. Tepper JE, Krasna M, Niedzwiecki D, *et al.* Superiority of trimodality therapy to surgery alone in esophageal cancer: Results of CALGB 9781. American Society of Clinical Oncology. Atlanta, GA; 2006.

15. Macdonald JS, Smalley S, Benedetti J, *et al.* Postoperative combined radiation and chemotherapy improves disease-free survival (DFS) and overall survival (OS) in resected adenocarcinoma of the stomach and gastroesophageal junction: update of the results of the Intergroup Study INT-0116 (SWOG 9008). ASCO Gastrointestinal Cancers Symposium. San Francisco, CA; 2004.

16. Improved survival with preoperative radiotherapy in resectable rectal cancer. Swedish Rectal Cancer Trial. *N Engl J Med* 1997;336:980–987.

17. Grossman HB, Natale RB, Tangen CM, *et al.* Neoadjuvant chemotherapy plus cystectomy compared with cystectomy alone for locally advanced bladder cancer. *N Engl J Med* 2003; 349:859–866.

18. Whitney CW, Sause W, Bundy BN, *et al.* Randomized comparison of fluorouracil plus cisplatin versus hydroxyurea as an adjunct to radiation therapy in stage IIB-IVA carcinoma of the cervix with negative para-aortic lymph nodes: a gynecologic oncology group and southwest oncology group study. *J Clin Oncol* 1999;17:1339–1348.

19. Keys HM, Bundy BN, Stehman FB, *et al.* Cisplatin, radiation, and adjuvant hysterectomy compared with radiation and adjuvant hysterectomy for bulky stage IB cervical carcinoma. *N Engl J Med* 1999;340:1154–1161.

20. Eifel PJ, Winter K, Morris M, *et al.* Pelvic irradiation with concurrent chemotherapy versus pelvic and para-aortic irradiation for high-risk cervical cancer: an update of radiation therapy oncology group trial (RTOG) 90-01. *J Clin Oncol* 2004;22:872–880.

21. Peters WA, 3rd, Liu PY, Barrett RJ, 2nd, *et al.* Concurrent chemotherapy and pelvic radiation therapy compared with pelvic radiation therapy alone as adjuvant therapy after radical surgery in high-risk early-stage cancer of the cervix. *J Clin Oncol* 2000;18:1606–1613.

22. Takimoto CH, Calvo E. Principles of oncologic pharmacotherapy. In: Pazdur R, Coia LR, Hoskins WJ, *et al.*, editors. *Cancer Management: A Multidisciplinary Approach.* Ninth ed. Lawrence, KS: CMP Healthcare Media; 2005. pp. 23–42.

23. Ratain MJ. Pharmacology of cancer chemotherapy: pharmacokinetics and pharmacodynamics. In: Devita VT, Hellman S, Rosenberg SA, editors. *Cancer Principles & Practice of Oncology.* 6th ed. Philadelphia: Lippincott Williams & Wilkins; 2001. pp. 335–344.

24. Gazda M, Coia L. Principles of radiation therapy. In: Pazdur R, Coia L, Hoskins WJ, *et al.*, editors. *Cancer Management: A Multidisciplinary Approach.* 9th ed. Lawrence, KS: CMP Healthcare Media; 2005. pp. 11–22.

25. Stewart FA, Bartelink H. The combination of radiotherapy and chemotherapy. In: Steel GG, editor. *Basic Clinical Radiobiology*. 3rd ed. New York, NY: Arnold; 2002. pp. 217–230.

26. Morris CR, Blackwell LH, Loveless VS. Antileukemic properties of combinations of radiation and malonato(1,2-diaminocyclohexane) platinum(ii) (NSC-224964). *J Med* 1977;8:253–259.

27. Wodinsky I, Swiniarski J, Kensler CJ, *et al.* Combination radiotherapy and chemotherapy for P388 lymphocytic leukemia in vivo. *Cancer Chemother Rep 2* 1974;4:73–97.

28. Wilson GD, Bentzen SM, Harari PM. Biologic basis for combining drugs with radiation. *Semin Radiat Oncol* 2006;16:2–9.

29. Hennequin C, Favaudon V. Biological basis for chemo-radiotherapy interactions. *Eur J Cancer* 2002;38:223–230.

30. Davis MA, Tang HY, Maybaum J, *et al.* Dependence of fluorodeoxyuridine-mediated radiosensitization on S phase progression. *Int J Radiat Biol* 1995;67:509–517.

31. Byfield JE, Calabro-Jones P, Klisak I, *et al.* Pharmacologic requirements for obtaining sensitization of human tumor cells in vitro to combined 5-Fluorouracil or ftorafur and X rays. *Int J Radiat Oncol Biol Phys* 1982;8:1923–1933.

32. Rich TA, Lokich JJ, Chaffey JT. A pilot study of protracted venous infusion of 5-fluorouracil and concomitant radiation therapy. *J Clin Oncol* 1985;3:402–406.

33. Nishimura G, Terada I, Kobayashi T, *et al.* Thymidine phosphorylase and dihydropyrimidine dehydrogenase levels in primary colorectal cancer show a relationship to clinical effects of 5'-deoxy-5-fluorouridine as adjuvant chemotherapy. *Oncol Rep* 2002;9:479–482.

34. Hotta T, Taniguchi K, Kobayashi Y, *et al.* Increased expression of thymidine phosphorylase in tumor tissue in proportion to TP-expression in primary normal tissue. *Oncol Rep* 2004;12:539–541.

35. Sawada N, Ishikawa T, Sekiguchi F, *et al.* X-ray irradiation induces thymidine phosphorylase and enhances the efficacy of capecitabine (Xeloda) in human cancer xenografts. *Clin Cancer Res* 1999;5:2948–2953.

36. Shewach DS, Lawrence TS. Gemcitabine and radiosensitization in human tumor cells. *Invest New Drugs* 1996;14:257–263.

37. Talamonti MS, Catalano PJ, Vaughn DJ, *et al.* Eastern Cooperative Oncology Group Phase I trial of protracted venous infusion fluorouracil plus weekly gemcitabine with concurrent radiation therapy in patients with locally advanced pancreas cancer: a regimen with unexpected early toxicity. *J Clin Oncol* 2000;18:3384–3389.

38. Newlands ES, Stevens MF, Wedge SR, *et al.* Temozolomide: a review of its discovery, chemical properties, pre-clinical development and clinical trials. *Cancer Treat Rev* 1997;23:35–61.

39. Hall EJ. Chemotherapeutic Agents from the perspective of the radiobiologist. In: *Radiobiology for the Radiologist*. 5th ed. Philadelphia: Lippincott Williams & Wilkins; 2000. pp. 470–494.

40. Tishler RB, Geard CR, Hall EJ, *et al.* Taxol sensitizes human astrocytoma cells to radiation. *Cancer Res* 1992;52:3495–3497.

41. Liebmann J, Cook JA, Fisher J, *et al.* In vitro studies of Taxol as a radi-ation sensitizer in human tumor cells. *J Natl Cancer Inst* 1994;86:441–446.

42. Leonard CE, Chan DC, Chou TC, *et al.* Paclitaxel enhances in vitro radiosensitivity of squamous carcinoma cell lines of the head and neck. *Cancer Res* 1996;56:5198–5204.

43. Horsman MR, Overgaard J. Overcoming tumour radioresistance resulting from hypoxia. In: Steel GG, editor. *Basic Clinical Radiobiology*. 3rd ed. London: Arnold; 2002. pp. 169–181.

44. Horsman MR. The oxygen effect and tumour microenvironment. In: Steel GG, editor. *Basic Clinical Radiobiology*. 3rd ed. New York: Arnold; 2002. pp. 158–168.

45. Brown JM. SR 4233 (tirapazamine): a new anticancer drug exploiting hypoxia in solid tumours. *Br J Cancer* 1993;67:1163–1170.

46. Kovacs MS, Hocking DJ, Evans JW, *et al.* Cisplatin anti-tumour potentiation by tirapazamine results from a hypoxia-dependent cellular sensitization to cisplatin. *Br J Cancer* 1999; 80:1245–1251.

47. Sartorelli AC, Hodnick WF, Belcourt MF, *et al.* Mitomycin C: a prototype bioreductive agent. *Oncol Res* 1994;6:501–508.

48. Haffty BG, Son YH, Papac R, *et al.* Chemotherapy as an adjunct to radiation in the treatment of squamous cell carcinoma of the head and neck: results of the Yale Mitomycin Randomized Trials. *J Clin Oncol* 1997;15:268–276.

49. Dobrowsky W, Naude J. Continuous hyperfractionated accelerated radiotherapy with/ without mitomycin C in head and neck cancers. *Radiother Oncol* 2000;57:119–124.

50. Zakotnik B, Smid L, Budihna M, *et al.* Concomitant radiotherapy with mitomycin C and bleomycin compared with radiotherapy alone in inoperable head and neck cancer: final report. *Int J Radiat Oncol Biol Phys* 1998;41:1121–1127.

51. Adams GE. Hypoxic cell sensitizers for radiotherapy. In: Becker FF, editor. *Cancer.* Vol 6. New York: Plenum Press; 1977.

52. Overgaard J, Hansen HS, Overgaard M, *et al.* A randomized double-blind phase III study of nimorazole as a hypoxic radiosensitizer of primary radiotherapy in supraglottic larynx and pharynx carcinoma. Results of the Danish Head and Neck Cancer Study (DAHANCA) Protocol 5-85. *Radiother Oncol* 1998;46:135–146.

53. Bernhard EJ, Maity A, Muschel RJ, *et al.* Effects of ionizing radiation on cell cycle progression. A review. *Radiat Environ Biophys* 1995;34:79–83.

54. Maity A, Kao GD, Muschel RJ, *et al.* Potential molecular targets for manipulating the radiation response. *Int J Radiat Oncol Biol Phys* 1997;37:639–653.

55. Mendelsohn J, Baselga J. The EGF receptor family as targets for cancer therapy. *Oncogene* 2000;19:6550–6565.

56. Haffty BG. Molecular and genetic markers in the local-regional management of breast cancer. *Semin Radiat Oncol* 2002;12:329–340.

57. Chakravarti A, Dicker A, Mehta M. The contribution of epidermal growth factor receptor (EGFR) signaling pathway to radioresistance in human gliomas: a review of preclinical and correlative clinical data. *Int J Radiat Oncol Biol Phys* 2004;58:927–931.

58. Huang SM, Bock JM, Harari PM. Epidermal growth factor receptor blockade with C225 modulates proliferation, apoptosis, and radiosensitivity in squamous cell carcinomas of the head and neck. *Cancer Res* 1999;59:1935–1940.

59. Shepherd FA, Rodrigues Pereira J, Ciuleanu T, *et al.* Erlotinib in previously treated non-small-cell lung cancer. *N Engl J Med* 2005;353:123–132.

60. Tan-Chiu E, Yothers G, Romond E, *et al.* Assessment of cardiac dysfunction in a randomized trial comparing doxorubicin and cyclophosphamide followed by paclitaxel, with or without trastuzumab as adjuvant therapy in node-positive, human epidermal growth factor receptor 2-overexpressing breast cancer: NSABP B-31. *J Clin Oncol* 2005;23:7811–7819.

61. Perez CA, Stanley K, Rubin P, *et al.* A prospective randomized study of various irradiation doses and fractionation schedules in the treatment of inoperable non-oat-cell carcinoma of the lung. Preliminary report by the Radiation Therapy Oncology Group. *Cancer* 1980;45: 2744–2753.

62. Dillman RO, Seagren SL, Propert KJ, *et al.* A randomized trial of induction chemotherapy plus high-dose radiation versus radiation alone in stage III non-small-cell lung cancer. *N Engl J Med* 1990;323:940–945.

63. Dillman RO, Herndon J, Seagren SL, *et al.* Improved survival in stage III non-small-cell lung cancer: seven-year follow-up of cancer and leukemia group B (CALGB) 8433 trial. *J Natl Cancer Inst* 1996;88:1210–1215.

64. Sause WT, Scott C, Taylor S, *et al.* Radiation Therapy Oncology Group (RTOG) 88-08 and Eastern Cooperative Oncology Group (ECOG) 4588: preliminary results of a phase III trial in regionally advanced, unresectable non-small-cell lung cancer. *J Natl Cancer Inst* 1995;87:198–205.

65. Furuse K, Fukuoka M, Kawahara M, *et al.* Phase III study of concurrent versus sequential thoracic radiotherapy in combination with mitomycin, vindesine, and cisplatin in unresectable stage III non-small-cell lung cancer. *J Clin Oncol* 1999;17:2692–2699.

66. Curran WJ, Scott C, Langer C, *et al.* Phase III comparison of sequential vs concurrent chemoradiation for patients (Pts) with unresected stage III non-small cell lung cancer (NSCLC): initial report of radiation therapy oncology group (RTOG) 9410. American Society of Clinical Oncology; 2000.

67. Curran WJ, Scott CB, Langer CJ, *et al.* Long-term benefit is observed in a phase III comparison of sequential vs concurrent chemo-radiation for patients with unresected stage III nsclc: RTOG 9410. American Society of Clinical Oncology; 2003.

68. Schaake-Koning C, van den Bogaert W, Dalesio O, *et al.* Effects of concomitant cisplatin and radiotherapy on inoperable non-small-cell lung cancer. *N Engl J Med* 1992;326:524–530.

69. Jeremic B, Shibamoto Y, Acimovic L, *et al.* Randomized trial of hyperfractionated radiation therapy with or without concurrent chemotherapy for stage III non-small-cell lung cancer. *J Clin Oncol* 1995;13:452–458.

70. Jeremic B, Shibamoto Y, Acimovic L, *et al.* Hyperfractionated radiation therapy with or without concurrent low-dose daily carboplatin/etoposide for stage III non-small-cell lung cancer: a randomized study. *J Clin Oncol* 1996;14:1065–1070.

71. Warde P, Payne D. Does thoracic irradiation improve survival and local control in limited-stage small-cell carcinoma of the lung? A meta-analysis. *J Clin Oncol* 1992;10:890–895.

72. Pignon JP, Arriagada R, Ihde DC, *et al.* A meta-analysis of thoracic radiotherapy for small-cell lung cancer. *N Engl J Med* 1992;327:1618–1624.

73. Takada M, Fukuoka M, Kawahara M, *et al.* Phase III study of concurrent versus sequential thoracic radiotherapy in combination with cisplatin and etoposide for limited-stage small-cell lung cancer: results of the Japan Clinical Oncology Group Study 9104. *J Clin Oncol* 2002;20:3054–3060.

74. Munro AJ. An overview of randomised controlled trials of adjuvant chemotherapy in head and neck cancer. *Br J Cancer* 1995;71:83–91.

75. El-Sayed S, Nelson N. Adjuvant and adjunctive chemotherapy in the management of squamous cell carcinoma of the head and neck region. A meta-analysis of prospective and randomized trials. *J Clin Oncol* 1996;14:838–847.

76. Pignon JP, Bourhis J, Domenge C, *et al.* Chemotherapy added to locoregional treatment for head and neck squamous-cell carcinoma: three meta-analyses of updated individual data. MACH-NC Collaborative Group. Meta-Analysis of Chemotherapy on Head and Neck Cancer. *Lancet* 2000;355:949–955.

77. Bourhis J, Amand C, Pignon JP. Update of MACH-NC (meta-analysis of chemotherapy in head & neck cancer) database focused on concomitant chemoradiotherapy. American Society of Clinical Oncology; 2004.

78. Induction chemotherapy plus radiation compared with surgery plus radiation in patients with advanced laryngeal cancer. The Department of Veterans Affairs Laryngeal Cancer Study Group. *N Engl J Med* 1991;324:1685–1690.

79. Hong WK, Lippman SM, Wolf GT. Recent advances in head and neck cancer—larynx preservation and cancer chemoprevention: the Seventeenth Annual Richard and Hinda Rosenthal Foundation Award Lecture. *Cancer Res* 1993;53:5113–5120.

80. Forastiere AA, Goepfert H, Maor M, *et al.* Concurrent chemotherapy and radiotherapy for organ preservation in advanced laryngeal cancer. *N Engl J Med* 2003;349:2091–2098.

81. Posner MR, al. e. Induction carboplatin (P) and fluorouracil (F) with or without docetaxel (T) followed by chemoradiation (CTRT) and surgical resection as indicated for locally advanced squamous cell carcinoma (LASCC) of the head and neck: preliminary results of the TAX 324 study. American Society of Clinical Oncology. Atlanta, GA; 2006.

82. Al-Sarraf M, LeBlanc M, Giri PG, *et al.* Chemoradiotherapy versus radiotherapy in patients with advanced nasopharyngeal cancer: phase III randomized Intergroup study 0099. *J Clin Oncol* 1998;16:1310–1317.

83. Rousseau DL, Jr., Thomas CR, Jr., Petrelli NJ, *et al.* Squamous cell carcinoma of the anal canal. *Surg Oncol* 2005;14:121–132.

84. Andre T, Boni C, Mounedji-Boudiaf L, *et al.* Oxaliplatin, fluorouracil, and leucovorin as adjuvant treatment for colon cancer. *N Engl J Med* 2004;350:2343–2351.

85. Sun W, Haller DG. Adjuvant therapy for colon cancer. *Curr Oncol Rep* 2005;7:181–185.

86. Walsh TN, Noonan N, Hollywood D, *et al.* A comparison of multimodal therapy and surgery for esophageal adenocarcinoma. *N Engl J Med* 1996;335:462–467.

87. Minsky BD, Pajak TF, Ginsberg RJ, *et al.* INT 0123 (Radiation Therapy Oncology Group 94-05) phase III trial of combined-modality therapy for esophageal cancer: high-dose versus standard-dose radiation therapy. *J Clin Oncol* 2002;20:1167–1174.

88. Ellenhorn JDI, Cullinane CA, Coia LR, *et al.* Colon, rectal, and anal cancers. In: Pazdur R, Coia LR, Hoskins WJ, *et al.*, editors. *Cancer Management: A Multidisciplinary Approach.* 9th ed. Lawrence, KS: CMP Healthcare Media; 2005. pp. 343–376.

89. Prolongation of the disease-free interval in surgically treated rectal carcinoma. Gastrointestinal Tumor Study Group. *N Engl J Med* 1985;312:1465–1472.

90. Krook JE, Moertel CG, Gunderson LL, *et al.* Effective surgical adjuvant therapy for high-risk rectal carcinoma. *N Engl J Med* 1991;324:709–715.

91. O'Connell MJ, Martenson JA, Wieand HS, *et al.* Improving adjuvant therapy for rectal cancer by combining protracted-infusion fluorouracil with radiation therapy after curative surgery. *N Engl J Med* 1994;331:502–507.

92. Wolmark N, Wieand HS, Hyams DM, *et al.* Randomized trial of postoperative adjuvant chemotherapy with or without radiotherapy for carcinoma of the rectum: national surgical adjuvant breast and bowel project protocol R-02. *J Natl Cancer Inst* 2000;92:388–396.

93. Kapiteijn E, Marijnen CA, Nagtegaal ID, *et al.* Preoperative radiotherapy combined with total mesorectal excision for resectable rectal cancer. *N Engl J Med* 2001;345:638–646.

94. Local recurrence rate in a randomised multicentre trial of preoperative radiotherapy compared with operation alone in resectable rectal carcinoma. Swedish Rectal Cancer Trial. *Eur J Surg* 1996;162:397–402.

95. Francois Y, Nemoz CJ, Baulieux J, *et al.* Influence of the interval between preoperative radiation therapy and surgery on downstaging and on the rate of sphincter-sparing surgery for rectal cancer: the Lyon R90-01 randomized trial. *J Clin Oncol* 1999;17:2396.

96. Sauer R, Fietkau R, Wittekind C, *et al.* Adjuvant versus neoadjuvant radiochemotherapy for locally advanced rectal cancer. A progress report of a phase-III randomized trial (protocol CAO/ARO/AIO-94). *Strahlenther Onkol* 2001;177:173–181.

97. Sauer R, Fietkau R, Wittekind C, *et al.* Adjuvant vs. neoadjuvant radiochemotherapy for locally advanced rectal cancer: the German trial CAO/ARO/AIO-94. *Colorectal Dis* 2003;5:406–415.
98. Sauer R, Becker H, Hohenberger W, *et al.* Preoperative versus postoperative chemoradiotherapy for rectal cancer. *N Engl J Med* 2004;351:1731–1740.
99. Epidermoid anal cancer: results from the UKCCCR randomised trial of radiotherapy alone versus radiotherapy, 5-fluorouracil, and mitomycin. UKCCCR Anal Cancer Trial Working Party. UK Co-ordinating Committee on Cancer Research. *Lancet* 1996;348:1049–1054.
100. Bartelink H, Roelofsen F, Eschwege F, *et al.* Concomitant radiotherapy and chemotherapy is superior to radiotherapy alone in the treatment of locally advanced anal cancer: results of a phase III randomized trial of the European Organization for Research and Treatment of Cancer Radiotherapy and Gastrointestinal Cooperative Groups. *J Clin Oncol* 1997;15:2040–2049.
101. Flam M, John M, Pajak TF, *et al.* Role of mitomycin in combination with fluorouracil and radiotherapy, and of salvage chemoradiation in the definitive nonsurgical treatment of epidermoid carcinoma of the anal canal: results of a phase III randomized intergroup study. *J Clin Oncol* 1996;14:2527–2539.

# 5

# Brachytherapy

Daniel R. Gomez, MD
Kaled M. Alektiar, MD
Michael J. Zelefsky, MD

## OVERVIEW

Brachytherapy is derived from the Greek word *brachios*, meaning short distance, and has been in practice since the early twentieth century. It has remained a common treatment modality in multiple tumor sites, most commonly for prostate and gynecological tumors but also less frequently in breast, head and neck, eye, central nervous system tumors, lung cancers, and sarcomas. Apart from an oncologic setting, brachytherapy has been used to prevent restenosis of coronary arteries in the technique of endovascular brachytherapy, though treatment of this nature is now less often used secondary to the advent of drug-eluting stents.

| BOX 5-1 | KEY DEFINITIONS |
|---|---|
| Brachytherapy | Radiation treatment given by placing radioactive material directly in or near the target, most often a tumor. |
| Interstitial Brachytherapy | Radioactive material placed within the interstices or spaces within an organ. |
| Intracavitary Brachytherapy | Radioactive material placed within a pre-existing body cavity. |
| Permanent Brachytherapy | An implant that remains in place indefinitely and is not removed. |
| Temporary Brachytherapy | Implants that are left within an organ or cavity for a specified period of time and are then removed after delivering the desired dose. |
| High Dose Rate Brachytherapy | The delivery of temporary radioactive sources that utilize dose rates in excess of 0.2 Gy/min. |
| Low Dose Rate Brachytherapy | Brachytherapy in which the radioactive sources are left in place for the duration of treatment, usually utilizing doses at the rate of 40 to 200 cGy/hour. Note that low dose rate brachytherapy can be either temporary, and removed after several days, or permanent. |

## PHYSICS AND BIOLOGY OF BRACHYTHERAPY

### Commonly Used Sources and the Concepts of Activity and Radioactive Decay

This section is a brief overview of key concepts and equations pertinent to brachytherapy. Table 5-1 is derived from Perez et al[1] and describes the physical characteristics of commonly used sources.

Note that the first isotope used in brachytherapy was Radium 226, which is a decay product of the element $^{238}$U. However, it is essentially obsolete, mainly because of the risk of radon gas emission into bone from its sources and its high cost of extraction.[1,2] It has been replaced by a number of other radioactive nuclides. Iodine and palladium will be discussed in detail with regard to their use in prostate brachytherapy and relevant studies comparing the two isotopes. Iridium-192 is a common isotope used in HDR brachytherapy. Cesium-137 and Ytterbium-169 have more recently come into clinical use, particularly in prostate brachytherapy.

## Important Concepts in the Physics of Brachytherapy

### Total Activity and Dose Rate

In order to understand the physics underlying brachytherapy, it is essential to comprehend the concept of radioactive decay. The relationship between the total activity of a source and the activity at any given time can be summarized by the following equation:

$$A(t) = A(0) \times e^{-t \times 0.693/T_{1/2}}$$

Where $A(0)$ is the initial activity of the source (at the time of placement), $t$ is time, and $T_{1/2}$ is the half life of the radionuclide, as given in the table below. It can be shown that dose *rate* is proportional to activity, and thus the equation above can be rewritten using initial dose rate and current dose rate in place of $A(0)$ and $A(t)$, respectively. Thus, the dose rate of a radionuclide has a reciprocal relationship with its half-life.[1] This is reasonable considering that the faster an isotope decays, or deposits dose, the shorter the half life that is expected. Therefore, radon, which has an initial dose rate that is over 10 times greater than iodine (75 cGy · hr$^{-1}$ versus 7.0 cGy · hr,$^{-1}$ respectively), has a half life that is 15 times shorter (3.83 days versus 59.6 days, respectively).

### Specific Activity

While the initial dose rate of a source is a straightforward method of categorizing a specific radionuclide into LDR or HDR therapeutic modalities (with LDR sources being those with a lower initial dose rate, such as iodine or palladium), a related component is that of *specific activity*, or activity per unit mass (usually measured in Curies/gram). For instance, consider a radionuclide that has a high initial dose rate but low specific activity. Although theoretically this nuclide could be used for HDR brachytherapy, the amount of isotope required would preclude any practical use in this regard. When

**TABLE 5-1 Common Isotopes Used in Brachytherapy**

| Element | Isotope | Energy (MeV) | Half Life | Clinical Application |
|---------|---------|--------------|-----------|----------------------|
| Radium | $^{226}$Ra | 0.83 (average) | 1,626 years | LDR intracavitary and interstitial |
| Radon | $^{222}$Rn | 0.83 (average) | 3.83 days | Permanent interstitial |
| Cesium | $^{137}$Cs | 0.662 | 30 years | LDR intracavitary and intersitial |
| Iridium | $^{192}$Ir | 0.397 (average) | 73.8 days | LDR and HDR, interstitial and intracavitary |
| Cobalt | $^{60}$Co | 1.25 | 5.26 years | HDR intracavitary |
| Iodine | $^{125}$I | 0.028 | 59.6 days | LDR permanent interstitial |
| Palladium | $^{103}$Pd | 0.020 | 17 days | LDR permanent intersitial |
| Cesium | $^{131}$Cs | 0.030 | 9.69 days | LDR permanent |
| Ytterbium | $^{169}$Yb | 0.093 | 32 days | LDR temporary intersitial |

examining common isotopes, for example, [137]Cs and [103]Pd have specific activities that are much too low for use in HDR brachytherapy (87 Ci/g and 60 Ci/g, respectively), while isotopes such as [192]Ir and [169]Yb are much more ideal in this respect (7760 Ci/g and 33,700 Ci/g, respectively). Note that [125]I has a high specific activity (17,400 Ci/g), but as its initial dose rate is classified in the "ultra-low" category, it is not of practical clinical use in HDR, highlighting the importance of both factors.

### Exposure and Delivered Dose

In order to calculate the exposure from a single radionuclide source, it can be assumed that the source is a point in space emitting radiation in all directions (an *isotropic* point source). This assumption can be made if the diameter of the source is much less than the distance to which it is emitting radiation. Since this is often the case (the diameter of most radionuclide sources is approximately 0.5 cm, emitting radiation to a target centimeters away), the following equation relates exposure rate and distance:

$$X(d) = (\Gamma \cdot A) / d^2,$$

where $X(d)$ is the exposure rate at a given distance, $\Gamma$ is the exposure at 1 cm from a mCi point source, A is the activity, and d is the distance from the source.

However, it is clear that the actual dose received by a tumor cannot be calculated in such a straightforward manner. Many other factors play a role in dose distribution from a radionuclide source. Specifically, radioactivity from the source is attenuated as it traverses the tissue, through interactions such as Compton scattering and the photoelectric effect. Second, as a result of these interactions, secondary photons are emitted which increase the theoretical dose at any given point, an effect known as *scattered-photon buildup*. Indeed, this effect is much more pronounced than what is observed for external beam radiation.

In addition, brachytherapy sources exhibit the property of anisotropy, which means that the amount of radiation emitted varies along axes in different directions, such that the dose emitted along one axis does not match the dose in a different direction. There are multiple etiologies of anisotropy, such as distribution of radioactivity within the source, source self-absorption, the shape of the source being used, and a high source-length to treatment distance ratio.

Today, computer programs are used to account for these confounding interactions and to determine an accurate dose deposited in tissue. However, before these programs were commonplace, various pre-calculated systems were in place to optimize the therapeutic ratio from various collections of sources. The two systems used before the popularity of computer programs were the Manchester, or Paterson-Parker, and the Quimby system. The details of each of these systems are beyond the scope of this chapter, but in essence they provide tables to estimate dose based on the distribution of sources and volume of the target tissue. In addition, they provide rules as to how to distribute radioactive sources as well as dose-specification criteria to calculate factors such as strand length and strand arrangement. The Paris system was devised to determine distribution and dosing guidelines for removable implants such as [192]Ir.

### Air-Kerma Strength (Absorbed Dose)

No overview of brachytherapy physics would be complete without a discussion of air-kerma strength. Kerma is an acronym for *kinetic energy released in materials*, and thus is an alternative term for absorbed dose (measured in the unit gray). Air-kerma strength is defined as the product of air-kerma rate at a point along the transverse axis of the source in free space. Mathematically, it is defined as

$$S_{k} = K_{air}(d) \cdot d^2,$$

where $S_K$ is air kerma-strength, measured in U, d is the distance from the source, and $K_{air}$ (d) is the kerma in air, or the kerma as if the source were in a vacuum.

In addition to providing standardization among various sources, air-kerma strength provides a type of quality assurance process for radionuclide sources. As the number of patients treated with brachytherapy has increased in recent years, so have the number of commercially available manufacturers. The AAPM task force recommended that calibrations of all brachytherapy sources be directly traceable to the National Institutes of Standards and Technology (NIST), meaning that the source must be calibrated against a national standard at an accredited dosimetry laboratory.[3]

## CLINICAL APPLICATIONS OF BRACHYTHERAPY

### Prostate Brachytherapy—Low Dose Rate

#### Indications

In terms of treating patients based on clinical stage, Gleason score, and PSA level, the majority of patients with *localized* disease are potential candidates for LDR brachytherapy, either as monotherapy or when used in combination with external beam radiotherapy (EBRT). However, other factors must also be taken into account. Table 5-2 lists relative and absolute contraindications to brachytherapy as practiced at MSKCC.

Note that patients with prostate glands >60 cc are candidates for cytoreductive hormonal therapy. The size criteria is present to avoid pubic arch interference as well as the high number of seeds that would be required for large glands, which in turn is associated with increased urinary related morbidity.

Table 5-3 outlines criteria for monotherapy and combination therapy (with EBRT). Thus far no prospective, randomized trials have been completed comparing the clinical outcomes of patients who have received LDR monotherapy versus combination therapy with EBRT. RTOG 0232 is currently in the accrual phases and is examining that question (Figure 5-1).[4] The study is expected to accrue 1520 total patients.

#### Technique

Prostate brachytherapy can be performed with either a preplanning or intraoperative technique. In the preplanning technique, the patient visits the hospital prior to the day of his implant and images

---

**TABLE 5-2  Relative and Absolute Contraindications to Prostate Brachytherapy**

| | |
|---|---|
| **Absolute Contraindications** | History of severe urinary symptoms in the past, such as recurrent urethral strictures/TURP procedures or an international prostate symptom score (IPSS) ≥ 16 |
| | Medically poor surgical candidate |
| | Overt seminal vesicle invasion |
| **Relative Contraindications** | Prior history of transurethral resection of the prostate (TURP) or transurethral needle ablation of the prostate (TUNA) |
| | IPSS less than 15 but patient requiring continuous use of alpha blockers |
| | Prostate gland > 60 cc (unless androgen deprivation given for volume reduction) |

**TABLE 5-3  Clinical Criteria for LDR Monotherapy and Combination Therapy with EBRT**

| | |
|---|---|
| Monotherapy (must meet all criteria) | Clinical stage T1–T2b |
| | Gleason score 6 or selected low-volume Gleason 3+4 |
| | PSA <10 |
| | < 50% of biopsy cores involved |
| Combination therapy (any one of criteria) | Clinical stage T2c or higher |
| | Gleason score 4+3 or higher |
| | PSA >10 |
| | ≥ 50% of biopsy cores involved |

**FIGURE 5-1** RTOG 0232.

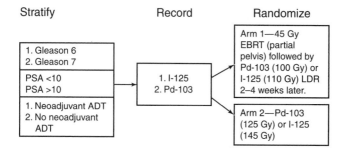

of his prostate are taken (either with ultrasound or a CT scan). The physician and physicists then contour the prostate and devise a plan for seed implantation that is replicated during the LDR procedure. In intraoperative planning, an ultrasound is performed during the implant procedure and the planning is done at that time. Table 5-4 highlights advantages and disadvantages of each technique.

**TABLE 5-4  Preplanning versus Intraoperative Prostate Brachytherapy**

| | Advantages | Disadvantages |
|---|---|---|
| Preplanning Technique | • Decreases OR time and anesthesia risk<br>• Number of seeds can be accurately ordered in advance | • Does not account for intraoperative changes due to needle placement<br>• Necessitates recreating seed placement from the preplan in the OR |
| Intraoperative Technique (real-time planning) | • Accounts for intraoperative prostatic edema related to needle placement<br>• Doses to normal tissues (rectum, urethra) estimated real-time<br>• Optimization takes into account intraoperative geometry of target and normal tissues | • Slightly greater anesthesia risk with increased operating time<br>• Must estimate prostate size based on prior imaging, which may require more or less seeds than anticipated |

The following is the step by step technique used at MSKCC for an intraoperative planning procedure. A preplanning system would use a similar technique but with steps 8 and 9 completed prior to the patient's visit.

---

**BOX 5-2 SUMMARY OF PLANNING TECHNIQUE**

1. Patient placed under general anesthesia.
2. Preoperative antibiotics and Decadron (to reduce prostatic edema) delivered.
3. Patient placed in dorsal lithotomy position.
4. Rectum cleared by irrigation.
5. Foley catheter inserted into bladder.
6. Transrectal ultrasound probe secured to operative bed and then placed into rectum. Template secured onto probe.
7. Prostate visualized on ultrasound and applicator needles placed within prostate gland.
*8. Images at 5 mm intervals captured onto treatment planning computer system.
*9. Prostate and normal tissue strictures (rectum and uretha) contoured on computer system and plan generated using inverse planning optimization to adhere to predetermined dose constraints to normal tissues and target.
10. Seeds placed into prostate in accordance with the plan.

*denotes steps that pertain only to intraoperative treatment planning

---

It is notable that in a study by Zelefsky et al[5] comparing patients treated with the a preplanning CT-based technique versus two different intraoperative techniques (ultrasound-guided and 3D-conformal optimization), the patients treated with the intraoperative 3D technique had superior target coverage for all evaluated dosimetric variables (V100, V90, D90).

After seed placement is performed, it is standard practice to obtain a post-implant CT scan to assess the final positions of the seeds and to ensure that the planned dose is similar to the administered dose. Table 5-5 delineates the constraints that are used to define an adequate implant when assessing the final dosimetry.

### Outcomes

Many centers have reported PSA relapse-free survival rates in patients who have undergone brachytherapy monotherapy to the prostate. The results of selected major studies are summarized in Table 5-6.

**TABLE 5-5 Constraints for Post-Implant Dosimetry of the Prostate**

| Constraint | Definition | Acceptable Threshold |
|---|---|---|
| D90 | The dose delivered to 90% of the prostate | Minimum of 95% of prescribed dose |
| V100 | The volume of the prostate receiving at least 100% of the prescribed dose | Minimum of 90% of prostate volume |
| V150 | The volume of the prostate receiving at least 150% of the prescribed dose | Less than or equal to 70% of the prostate volume |
| Urethral Dose | Percent of prescription dose to urethra | Maximal dose less than 150% of prescription dose |
| Rectal Dose | Percent of prescription dose to rectum | Less than or equal to 100% to <2.5 cc of rectal wall |

TABLE 5-6 Studies Examining LDR Brachytherapy as Monotherapy for Prostate Cancer

| Study | Number of Patients | Median follow-up | PSA-free survival |
|---|---|---|---|
| Zelefsky et al[6] | 367 | 63 months | 96% favorable |
| Kollmeier et al[7] | 243 | 75 months | 89% intermediate at 5 years<br>88% favorable |
| Grimm et al[8] | 125 | 81 months | 81% intermediate<br>65% unfavorable at 8 years<br>87% favorable at 10 years |
| Potters et al[9] | 1,449 (1,148 with PPI alone) | 82 months | 91% favorable<br>80% intermediate<br>66% unfavorable at 10 years |
| Ragde et al[10] | 140 | 93 months | 66% favorable at 10 years |
| Zelefsky et al[11] | 2,693 | 63 months | 82% favorable<br>70% intermediate<br>48% unfavorable at 10 years |

Several authors have also observed the dose response relationship for LDR prostate brachytherapy. See Table 5-7.

In addition to the randomized trial comparing monotherapy with combination therapy previously described (RTOG 0232), multiple single-arm and retrospective studies have examined the efficacy of combination therapy in controlling disease for higher risk patients. These are summarized in Table 5-8.

## Toxicity

The common toxicities arising from brachytherapy implants can be generally divided into three categories—rectal, urinary, and erectile. Table 5-9 cites the incidences of these side effects as well as general management strategies.

## Iodine versus Palladium

A long-standing question in prostate brachytherapy has been whether or not the implant type, Iodine-125 or Palladium-103, makes a difference in regard to outcome. A randomized study by Wallner et al is attempting to answer this question.

TABLE 5-7 Dose Response Studies for LDR Prostate Brachytherapy

| Study | Number of Patients | Median follow-up | PSA-free survival |
|---|---|---|---|
| Stock et al[12,13] | 181 | 44 months | 68% for D90 <140 Gy<br>96% ≥ 140 Gy at 5 years |
| Potters et al[14] | 520 | 30 months | 80% D90 < 90%<br>92% ≥ 90% at 4 years<br>V100 and D90 ≥ 100% with no effect |
| Zelefsky et al[11] | 2,693 | 63 months | 93% for D90 ≥ 130 Gy<br>76% for D90 < 130 Gy at 8 years |

**BOX 5-3**

This randomized control trial of 600 patients with stage T1c-T2a prostate carcinoma (Gleason score 5-6, PSA 4-10) is currently under accrual. Preliminary results from 126 patients randomized to either [125]I or [103]Pd demonstrated at 3 years, the freedom-from-failure rate was 89% for [125]I and 91% for [103]Pd (p=NS).

Wallner et al. [125]I versus [103]Pd for low-risk prostate cancer: preliminary PSA outcomes from a prospective randomized multicenter trial.[28] *Int J Radiat Oncol Biol Phys* 2003 Dec 1; 57(5).

TABLE 5-8 **Summary of Studies Utilizing Combination Therapy**

| Study | Number of Patients | Median follow-up | PSA-free survival |
|---|---|---|---|
| Singh et al[15] | 65 | 36 months | 85% intermediate<br>85% unfavorable at 3 years |
| Critz et al[16,17] | 1,469 | 72 months | 93% favorable<br>80% intermediate<br>61% unfavorable at 10 years |
| Sylvester et al[18] | 232 | 63 months(mean) | 85% favorable<br>77% intermediate<br>47% unfavorable at 10 years |

TABLE 5-9 **Side Effects for LDR Prostate Brachytherapy**

| Side Effect | Incidence | Management Strategy |
|---|---|---|
| Urinary | 80–90% acute grade 1 nocturia/ irritative symptoms (IPSS peaks at 2 weeks)<br>40–50% acute dysuria<br>1–2% with urethral stricture<br>Incontinence 1% or less[19–22] | 1. Alpha-blockers<br>2. Urinalysis and potential treatment with antibiotics<br>3. Referral to urologist for possible cystoscopy (if symptoms nonresponsive to above) |
| Rectal | 15–30% with acute grade 1 or 2 rectal symptoms<br>2–10% acute rectal proctopathy/ rectal bleeding<br>1% grade 3 rectal bleeding or higher[23–25] | 1. Stool softeners to minimize constipation<br>2. Cortisone suppositories and oral mesalamine to minimize inflammation<br>3. Referral to GI for possible colonoscopy *Note:* Invasive procedures such as laser coagulation should be used very cautiously due to risk of fistula formation |
| Erectile | 15–50% potency loss[26,27] | 1. Phosphodiesterase inhibitors such as Sildenafil, if no contraindication with other medications<br>2. Intracavernosal prostaglandin injections<br>3. Penile implant, referral to sexual dysfunction specialist |

Although these results are still early, over the next several years these data should be able to answer whether higher failure rates are seen in one isotope over the other. In regard to toxicity, theoretically [103]Pd may have a radiobiologic advantage due to a half life of 17 days, versus 60 days for [125]I. However, a recent retrospective study of 976 patients demonstrated that when patients were stratified by prostate size, there was no difference in time to IPSS peak, prolonged catheter dependency, IPSS resolution, or postimplant surgical intervention.[29]

## Prostate Brachytherapy—High Dose Rate

### Indications

While HDR brachytherapy is often utilized in patients with higher risk disease, as indicated by higher Gleason score or PSA levels, or for those with extracapsular extension or seminal vesicle invasion, it is also employed in patients without these high-risk features as well. It is suitable for patients with extracapsular disease because HDR catheters can be inserted into the interstitium of the gland as well as into regions surrounding the prostate. This is in contrast to LDR brachytherapy, in which it is relatively difficult to provide an adequate dose to regions outside of the prostate capsule due to the requirement that the seed is "anchored" in the gland. A drawback, however, to HDR brachytherapy is the inconvenience of an inpatient hospital stay and bed rest over a period of 2 days so that the catheters remain intact and in place. The technique of HDR is described in the following paragraphs.

### Technique

In contrast to LDR prostate brachytherapy, during which all of the operative planning and radiation delivery are done during a single operative session, HDR brachytherapy involves placement of catheters into the prostate gland under anesthesia followed by delivery of fractionated treatments over the next 1 to 2 days, as described here.

---

**BOX 5-4  SUMMARY OF PLANNING TECHNIQUE**

1. Patient brought to the operating room and placed under general anesthesia, foley catheter placed, patient immobilized in dorsal lithotomy position.
2. High dose rate catheters placed into prostate gland, template sutured into place.
3. Cystoscopy performed to ensure that catheters do not penetrate bladder mucosa.
4. Patient transferred to recovery suite in a modified supine position with legs elevated on a ramp.
5. After recovery, patient undergoes CT simulation.
6. Treatment plan designed to deliver multiple fractions to the target at risk.
7. Patient brought to the radiation suite for each treatment, with inter-fraction intervals of at least 4–6 hours.
8. After the final treatment, template and Foley catheter removed and patient discharged back to hospital room. After ambulation and sufficient recovery, the patient is discharged home (usually the same night).

---

### Results

There has been a significant amount of experience in treating prostate cancer with combination HDR brachytherapy and external beam radiation. General treatment regimens have consisted of HDR brachytherapy, 5.5 to 7 Gy for 3–4 fractions, delivered as an inpatient, followed by external beam radiation therapy to a dose of 45–50.4 Gy beginning 3 weeks after the HDR procedure. Table 5-10 demonstrates three trials utilizing combination HDR brachytherapy. All three studies included patients of all three risk groups using the various risk classification schemes. The results are analogous to LDR for patients with low- or intermediate-risk disease and improved in patients with high-risk disease.

TABLE 5-10 Studies Examining the Effect of Combination HDR and EBRT

| Study | Number of Patients | Median Follow-Up | PSA-Free Survival |
|-------|-------------------|------------------|-------------------|
| Demanes et al[30] | 209 | 87 months | 90% favorable<br>87% intermediate<br>69% unfavorable at 10 years |
| Galalae et al[31] | 611 | 60 months | 96% favorable<br>88% intermediate<br>69% unfavorable at 5 years |
| Yamada et al[32] | 105 | 44 months | 100% favorable<br>98% intermediate<br>92% unfavorable at 5 years |

---

**BOX 5-5**

In this retrospective trial, 149 patients with early-stage prostate cancer were treated with either $^{103}$Pd to 120 Gy (84 patients) or HDR brachytherapy using $^{192}$Ir to a dose of 38 Gy, delivered in four fractions. At a median follow-up of 35 months, biochemical control was essentially the same (97% for LDR versus 98% for HDR), but there were decreased rates of acute dysuria, urinary frequency/urgency, and rectal pain with HDR.

Grills et al. High dose rate brachytherapy as monotherapy reduces toxicity compared to low dose rate palladium seeds.[33] *Journal of Urology* 2004 Mar 171(3)

---

High dose rate monotherapy is a more novel technique. However, much work has been done at William Beaumont Hospital in this regard, as illustrated in the following study.

## Dose Escalation

The following is a dose escalation study utilizing HDR brachytherapy at doses of 5.5–11.5 Gy per fraction.

**BOX 5-6**

Between 1991 and 2000, 207 patients were treated with combination external beam radiation therapy and HDR brachytherapy. In regards to the HDR treatment, patients were either treated with 3 fractions if they were in the low dose group (5.50–6.50 Gy) or 2 fractions in the high dose group (8.25–11.5 Gy). The 5-year biochemical control rate was significantly higher in the high dose group than in the low-dose group (87% vs. 52%, $p = 0.014$).

Martinez et al. Dose escalation using conformal high dose rate brachytherapy improves outcome in unfavorable prostate cancer.[34] *Int J Radiat Oncol Biol Phys*; 2002 Jun 1; 53(2).

---

## Toxicity

As with LDR, side effects from HDR brachytherapy can be grouped into the categories of urinary, rectal, and erectile dysfunction. Up to 40% of patients report no urinary symptoms, while grade 3 urinary toxicity has been cited as 3%–7%.[30,31] Rectal toxicity is rare, with 2%–7% of patients experiencing symptoms, the most common being self-limiting rectal bleeding. Erectile dysfunction has been reported to be 33%–50%, with up to 80% of patients achieving erections with the aid of a potency medication.[30,31,34]

# Brachytherapy for Cervical Cancer

## Indications

The American Brachytherapy Society recommends that brachytherapy should be a component of treatment in all patients receiving definitive irradiation for cervical carcinoma.[36,37] The treatment algorithm for cervical cancer is complex and depends on stage, bulk of disease, and whether the patient is an operative candidate. In general, patients with early stage disease who are not operative candidates receive a combination of external beam radiation and brachytherapy. Patients with locally advanced disease generally receive a combination of external beam radiation, brachytherapy, and chemotherapy. For further discussion in this regard, we refer the reader to the cervical cancer chapter of this textbook.

Standard brachytherapy for cervical cancer generally refers to intracavitary brachytherapy, which uses a tandem and ovoids technique for LDR and either a tandem and ovoids or ring and tandem technique for HDR, outlined later in this section. However, there are certain instances during interstitial implantation when needles are implanted directly into the cervix. These situations include patients with: 1) extensive parametrial involvement, 2) narrow or distorted vagina, 3) inability to insert a tandem into the endocervical canal, 4) local/vaginal recurrences after a hysterectomy, and 5) distal vaginal involvement.[36]

## Technique, Low Dose Rate Cervical Intracavitary Brachytherapy

Historically, low-dose-rate brachytherapy has been an essential component of managing cervical cancer, and it is still commonly used at many institutions. However, as outlined later in this section, several studies have demonstrated similar results when comparing LDR and HDR techniques. For this reason, HDR has supplanted LDR at a large percentage of institutions. Following is an outline of the technique as performed at our institution.

---

**BOX 5-7  SUMMARY OF RING AND TANDEM TECHNIQUE**

1. Anesthesia given (general, spinal, or local).
2. Patient placed in dorsal lithotomy position. Foley catheter and rectal tube inserted.
3. Pelvic examination performed to assess extent of tumor and position of uterus (including bimanual examination).
4. Gold seeds placed into anterior and posterior lips of cervix, to be used as a reference point for treatment planning.
5. Cervix grasped with tenaculum and metallic probe placed into os.
6. Os progressively dilated using progressive dilators with increasing diameters.
7. Tandem placed into cervix, equidistant from the pubis, sacral promontory, and the lateral pelvic wall (position verified with fluoroscopy).
8. Applicator inserted over the tandem and placed into the vaginal fornices, tenaculum removed.
9. Vagina packed with gauze to displace the bladder and rectum and secure applicator into position.
10. Correct positioning of applicator and tandem confirmed by fluoroscopic imaging.
11. Treatment planning films taken in radiation oncology suite; bladder and rectal contrast given to improve visualization of these structures.
12. Patient transferred back to room and treatment plan generated to deliver prescription dose, usually over a period of 2 to 3 days.
13. Patient brought back to radiation oncology suite and radioactive sources placed into tandem and ovoids; patient on strict bedrest and radiation precautions over this time period.
14. After dose is delivered, radioactive sources removed and patient discharged home.

### Dose Points to Target and Critical Normal Tissue Structures:

To calculate the dose delivered to several critical structures, it is customary to use several hypothetical dose points, as defined by the International Commission of Radiological Units (ICRU). These points are as follows:

- **Point A:** 2 cm cephalad to the cervical os along the tandem and 2 cm perpendicular to the plane of the tandem (visualized by a radiopaque ring in a keel affixed to the tandem)
- **Point B:** 2 cm cephalad to the os and 5 cm lateral to the patient's midline (3 cm lateral to point A), represents parametrial tissue
- **Point C:** 1 cm lateral to point B, represents pelvic sidewall
- **Bladder point:** Most posterior point in the bulb of the Foley catheter on the lateral film and in the center of the film on the AP film
- **Rectal point:** 0.5 cm posterior to the vaginal mucosa on the lateral film at the mid-ovoid level
- **Point $V_S$:** Vaginal point, lateral edge of ovoid on AP film and middle of the ovoid on the lateral film

These points were selected because they represent a true three-dimensional volume that can then be correlated with the tumor geometry as visualized on imaging such as a CT or MRI scan. They also allow for calculation of normal tissue irradiation (that of the bladder, rectum, vagina, and pelvic wall). In patients receiving LDR brachytherapy alone (IA patients), the ABS recommended dose is 60–70 Gy to point A. When given in combination with external beam radiation (45 Gy), the recommended total dose is 85 Gy to point A (on the right and the left, with the LDR brachytherapy component contributing 40 Gy to the total dose). The total bladder dose (from external beam radiation and brachytherapy) should be below 80 Gy, and the rectal dose below 75 Gy. The total dose to $V_S$ should be 150% of the Point A dose.[36]

### Technique, Low Dose Rate Cervical Interstitial Brachytherapy

In contrast to the tandem-ovoid technique, interstitial cervical brachytherapy is delivered through a template applicator that is analogous to the template used for prostate brachytherapy. There are several different commercial applicators in use, but two of the most common are the Syed-Neblett applicator and the Martinez applicator.

---

**BOX 5-8 SUMMARY OF TECHNIQUE**

1. Patient placed under anesthesia (local, spinal, or general).
2. Pelvic examination performed.
3. Radiopaque markers placed in the cervix at the superior/inferior borders of the lesion of interest.
4. Tandem placed into cervical os.
5. Template sutured into place.
6. Needles placed into template, both laterally and in a cephalocaudal direction to adequately cover the tumor volume.
7. Patient allowed to recover from anesthesia.
8. Treatment planning films taken. Dummy ribbons, with unique sequences of dummy seeds of different sizes, loaded into various needles to assist in source position reconstruction.
9. Treatment plan generated, usually to deliver the desired dose in 2 to 3 days.
10. Patient brought back down to radiation suite and sources loaded.
11. After desired dose delivered, sources and template removed.

The use of a tandem in interstitial cervical brachytherapy is controversial, because it can create hot spots. To avoid these hot spots the obturator surface of the needles should not be loaded.[36,38]

It is recommended that the physician prescribe at the minimum target dose, rates of 0.5–0.7 Gy/hour. Dose homogeneity is also very important because serious complications have occurred with dose inhomogeneity. Finally, the source strength of interior needles should be twice that of peripheral needles.[39] The total dose of LDR Syed implant at MSKCC is 30–35 Gy.

### Technique, High Dose Rate Intracavitary Brachytherapy for Cervical Carcinoma

In general, the operative technique used in HDR intracavitary brachytherapy is similar to that described for LDR brachytherapy. Indeed, the use of anesthesia, tandem placement, and vaginal packing, are all the same, and either the ring and tandem or tandem and ovoids technique can be used.

The main difference between LDR and HDR is that rather than the sources being inserted over a period of 2 to 3 days, the treatment plan is generated on the day of the procedure and the patient is treated in a matter of minutes. Patients thus do not require an inpatient hospital stay or the inconvenience of the radiation precautions and bed rest that accompany LDR brachytherapy. However, patients generally receive several treatments. As a result, a Smit sleeve is often placed on the cervix during the first treatment to facilitate applicator placement while decreasing the risk of uterine perforation. The level of anesthesia varies with institution and physician preference, ranging from local anesthesia delivered in the physician's office to conscious sedation.

Regarding dosing for HDR cervical intracavitary brachytherapy, the dose can be alternatively prescribed to Point H rather than Point A. Point H is found by drawing a line connecting the mid-dwell positions of the ring or ovoids (depending on which delivery system is used).[37] From the intersection of this line with the tandem, the point is 2 cm superiorly, plus the thickness of the ring/ovoid, and then 2 cm perpendicular to the tandem in the lateral direction.

Dosing regimens vary significantly among institutions. External beam radiation doses range between 20–50.4 Gy. The brachytherapy component begins after 20–45 Gy of external beam radiation therapy, to allow for some reduction in the size of the tumor, and thus to facilitate tandem placement, but with the overall treatment time being less than 8 weeks. As will be explained later in this section, multiple studies have demonstrated decreased control rates if treatment time is prolonged.

Fractionation schemes vary between institutions from 5.3–7.5 Gy per fraction × 4–8 fractions.[37] At MSKCC, we employ a dose of 30 Gy in 5 fractions, plus 50.4 Gy of external beam radiation with a midline block (4 cm transverse × 10–12 cm longitudinal dimensions) placed after 45 Gy to reduce the dose to the bladder and rectum.

### Technique, Interstitial High Dose Rate Cervical Brachytherapy

The operative technique of high dose rate interstitial brachytherapy, including anesthesia, vaginal packing, use of bladder and rectal contrast, and placement of the template and needles, is similar to that described for LDR interstitial brachytherapy and thus will not be reviewed in detail again. In contrast to HDR intracavitary brachytherapy, however, patients are admitted to the hospital, usually 1 week after the completion of their external beam radiation (generally 45 Gy), and the template is left in place over a period of 2 to 3 days. The patient is then brought to the radiation oncology suite and treatments are delivered at time periods of greater than or equal to 6 hours, for a total of five fractions. The total dose delivered is generally 20–25 Gy given at 4.5–5 Gy per fraction. After the final treatment, the patient is discharged home. Note that little data have been published on interstitial HDR brachytherapy of the cervix, and thus total doses and fraction sizes have not been standardized.

TABLE 5-11  Acute Toxicity of Cervical Brachytherapy[40–45]

| Toxicity/Complication | Management |
| --- | --- |
| Pulmonary Embolus (0.3%) | *Prophylaxis* for all LDR cases with venocompression devices and heparin or low molecular weight heparin |
| Fever/Infection (15–20%) | Cultures and directed antibiotic regimen |
| GI (diarrhea, cramping, rectal discomfort) | Imodium or Lomotil for diarrhea, hydrocortisone enemas or anti-inflammatory suppositories (Anusol) for rectal discomfort |
| GU (dysuria, frequency) | Pyridium for pain, Detrol for urgency, antibiotics for UTI |
| Vaginal discomfort and vaginitis | Aquaphor for skin irritation, daily douching with hydrogen peroxide and water |

## Toxicity of Brachytherapy for Cervical Cancer

Table 5-11 illustrates some common acute toxicities and their general management. Pulmonary embolus, while very rare, can be fatal, and thus prophylaxis is a must.[40] Severe late toxicity to the vagina or bladder is relatively rare with intracavitary cervical cancer. These toxicities include vaginal stenosis, rectal fistulas, bowel obstruction, and fracture of the femoral head, and Grade 3 or higher complications have generally been reported to be less than 5%.[41–44] The use of vaginal dilators after treatment should be used to prevent the late complications of vaginal shortening and stenosis.[45] Toxicity comparisons between the LDR and HDR techniques are illustrated further in the Results section following.

## Outcomes, Low Dose Rate Brachytherapy of the Cervix

Several Patterns of Care studies have demonstrated improvement in local control when LDR brachytherapy is added to external beam radiation. A representative study is listed here and forms the basis for the ABS' "strong" recommendation that definitive irradiation for cervical carcinoma include brachytherapy as a component.

---

**BOX 5-9**

In 1973 and 1978, the Patterns of Care Study conducted two national surveys of patients for squamous cell carcinoma of the cervix. In addition, a survey of patients treated in 1973 was used to establish outcome of treatment (where patients were assumed to have received optimal treatment). The only treatment factor associated with improved pelvic control in multivariate analysis was the use of intracavitary irradiation. There was also a statistically significant relationship between the dose delivered to point A and complications, with the highest amount of complications occurring when the total dose to point A exceeded 85 Gy.

Lanciano RM et al Pretreatment and treatment factors associated with improved outcome in squamous cell carcinoma of the uterine cervix: a final report of the 1973 and 1978 patterns of care studies.[46] *Int J Radiat Oncol Biol Phys* 1991 Apr; 20(4):667–676

---

There have also been several studies demonstrating decreased tumor control and overall survival rates when the overall time of treatment is prolonged.[47–49] One pertinent study is listed here.

Studies such as these provide the rationale for performing brachytherapy during the delivery of external beam radiation, as tumor repopulation in cervical cancer is relatively rapid.

---

**BOX 5-10**

Between 1973 and 1983, 386 patients with stage IIB and stage III cervical cancer were treated with external beam radiation and LDR intracavitary brachytherapy. There was a loss of local control and overall survival of approximately 1% per day when treatment exceeded 52 days.

Girinsky T, Rey A. et. al. Overall treatment time in advanced cervical carcinomas: a critical parameter in treatment outcomes.[48] *Int J Radiation Oncol Biol Phys* 1993 Dec; 27:1051–1056.

---

Regarding correlation of dose to local control, a large study was performed by Fyles et al, which identified dose as a significant prognostic factor.

---

**BOX 5-11**

In this retrospective analysis of 965 patients with cervical cancer treated at Princess Margaret Hospital between 1976 and 1981, on multivariate analysis FIGO stage was the most significant factor affecting disease free survival, followed by radiation dose and treatment duration. If the analysis was limited to patients who received 75 Gy or more, radiation dose was no longer a significant factor.

Fyles AW et al. Prognostic factors in patients with cervix cancer treated by radiation therapy: results of a multiple regression analysis.[50] *Radiother Oncol* 1995 May; 35(2): 107–17.

---

### Outcomes, High Dose Rate Cervical Brachytherapy

There have been several randomized studies comparing LDR to HDR brachytherapy for cervical cancer. Table 5-12 outlines three of the largest and most recent studies. In summary, local control and survival have been found to be approximately equal. In regard to toxicity, some studies have found higher rectal toxicity with the HDR technique, and others with LDR. However, the absolute rate of complications, particularly the rate of grade III-IV complications, has been acceptable with either method. It is often stated that the most significant theoretical disadvantage to HDR brachytherapy is an increased propensity for late reactions due to the high doses per fraction. However, in randomized trials this has not been shown to be significant.

---

**TABLE 5-12  Selected Randomized Studies Comparing HDR and LDR Brachytherapy**

| Study | N | Local Control/OS | Toxicity |
|---|---|---|---|
| Lertsanguansinchai et al[42] | 237 | Local Control: 86% HDR, 89% LDR at 3 years (p=0.51) OS: 68.4% HDR, 71% LDR at 3 years (p=0.75) | Grade 3 and 4 complications 2.8% in LDR group, 7.1% in HDR group (p=0.23) |
| Patel et al[43] | 482 | Local Control: 80% LDR, 76% HDR OS: 73% for LDR, 78% for HDR at 5 years (p=NS) | Higher rectal complication rate in LDR group (20 vs. 6%), 2.4% vs. 0.4% severe complications (p=NS) |
| Hareyama et al[44] | 132 | Local Control (Stage II/III): 100/70% LDR, 89/69% HDR at 5 years (p=NS) | Overall complication rate 13% in LDR group, 10% in HDR group (p=NS) |

Of note, many nonrandomized and retrospective trials have supported the findings of randomized trials. In general, HDR and LDR are thought to be similar in regard to control and toxicity, but because HDR offers the advantages of less radiation exposure for providers and caregivers, as well as the fact that it is done on an outpatient basis and does not require multiple days of bed rest (which reduces patient discomfort and the medical risks associated with the lack of ambulation), many centers have made the transition from LDR to HDR in the past several years, a trend that is likely to continue as HDR becomes more widely available.

## Brachytherapy for Endometrial Cancer

### Indications

At MSKCC, most early stage endometrial cancer patients with stage IA Grade 3–stage IIB, superficial stromal invasion and comprehensive surgical staging are candidates for intravaginal brachytherapy. In patients without comprehensive nodal staging, postoperative intravaginal treatment is usually reserved for stages IA-IB Grade 2, with stages IB Grade 3–stage IIB receiving pelvic radiation.

Patients with recurrences at the vaginal cuff, or with inoperable disease, receive either intravaginal brachytherapy or interstitial Syed implantation, depending on the extent of disease.[51] For a more detailed discussion in this regard, the reader is referred to the review by Alektiar[52] and the endometrial cancer section of this textbook.

### Technique

For HDR intravaginal brachytherapy at MSKCC a cylinder is used, the diameter of which ranges from 2–3 cm. The dose per fraction is generally 6–7 Gy given in three fractions with 1 to 2 week intervals. It is an outpatient treatment and requires no sedation. The dose is prescribed to a depth of 0.5 cm from the vaginal surface. If the diameter of the cylinder is less than 3 cm the dose per fraction is 6 Gy instead of 7 Gy to decrease the dose to the vaginal mucosal surface. If external beam radiation is used in addition to intravaginal HDR, the dose per fraction is usually 4–5 Gy. The length of the vagina treated ranges from 4–7 cm depending on the stage and grade of tumor. Patients with grade 3 are generally treated to 7 cm length while those with I-B grade 1,2 are treated to 4 cm length. If LDR intravaginal brachytherapy is used, it is given as an inpatient treatment, generally with a cylinder or ovoids. The dose is usually 60 Gy prescribed to the vaginal surface.

For patients with vaginal recurrence from endometrial cancer the treatment generally consists of pelvic radiation to 45 Gy followed by intravaginal brachytherapy for nonbulky disease that responds well to external beam radiation. For these patients, the dose is prescribed to one centimeter from the vaginal mucosa for the first two fractions and to 0.5 cm for fractions three to five. For patients with bulky disease, or tumors that do not respond to external beam radiation, a Syed implant is often recommended. A dose of 18 Gy is given in four fractions of 4.5 Gy with HDR or 25–30 Gy with LDR. For patients with medically inoperable disease the treatment guidelines are similar to those for definitive radiation in cervical cancer.

### Toxicity

Acute complications with HDR intravaginal brachytherapy are minimal and usually consist of bladder and intestinal irritation or vaginal discharge. The risk of Grade 3 or higher complications is approximately 1%. The risk of late complications is also low (1%–2%).[53–56] As is the case with brachytherapy for cervical cancer, patients should receive instruction on dilator use to prevent vaginal stenosis.

## Outcomes

The rate of vaginal recurrence after intravaginal HDR is low, at approximately 1%–2%.[53–55] The risk of pelvic recurrence is also low (1%–2%) as long as the patients with high risk of pelvic lymph nodes metastasis (IB grade 3–IC) had a negative lymph node dissection.[53,56–57] Two randomized trials have shown a benefit to postoperative pelvic irradiation when compared to surgery alone.[58,59] In addition, a prospective study by Aalders et al[60] has shown an advantage in local recurrence with the addition of pelvic radiation to intravaginal brachytherapy (versus intravaginal brachytherapy alone) in patients with stage IB to IC disease after TAH/BSO without lymph node sampling. However, no randomized trials have been done comparing surgery alone versus surgery with intravaginal brachytherapy. Postoperative HDR intravaginal brachytherapy after hysterectomy in stage I-II patients has been studied in multiple single institution trials with excellent levels of locoregional control and acceptable morbidity. The results of selected larger and more recent trials are outlined in Table 5-13. Of these trials, three examined HDR brachytherapy alone after surgery, and the final study, by Knocke et al[61], is the largest series examining HDR intravaginal brachytherapy alone (256 of the 280 included patients) in nonoperable patients.

# Brachytherapy for Carcinoma of the Vagina and Urethra

## Indications

Patients with vaginal carcinoma in situ can be treated with intravaginal brachytherapy alone. Patients with more infiltrative tumors are generally treated with a combination of external beam radiation, intravaginal and interstitial brachytherapy. External beam radiation can only be omitted in the subset of patients with stage I disease in whom there is superficial invasion. Brachytherapy is used as an alternative to surgery for early stage tumors of the distal urethra. In more bulky tumors (T3/T4 or node positive tumors) it is used as part of a combined modality regimen with external beam radiation ± surgery.

## Techniques

Intracavitary brachytherapy of the vagina utilizes a technique similar to that described for endometrial cancer, with a vaginal cylinder. Interstitial brachytherapy of the vagina, as well as that of the urethra or vulva, utilizes a technique similar to that previously described for interstitial brachytherapy of the cervix.

**TABLE 5-13  Selected Studies in HDR Brachytherapy for Endometrial Cancer**

| Study | N | Median Follow-Up | Local Control | Toxicity |
|---|---|---|---|---|
| Anderson et al[53] | 102 | 49 months | 97% at 5 years | 0% grade 3 or 4 acute GI/GU toxicity, 0% late toxicity |
| Alektiar et al[54] | 382 | 48 months | 95% vaginal/pelvic control at 5 years | 0.8% of patients with grade 3 or worse toxicity |
| Horowitz et al[56] | 164 | 65 months | 95% at 5 years | 0% grade 3 or 4 toxicity |
| Knocke et al[61] (no surgery) | 280 (24 with EBRT) | 58 months | 75% at 5 years | 0% grade 3 or 4 acute toxicity 5% grade 3 or higher late toxicity at 5 and 10 years |

## Outcomes

Regarding definitive irradiation of the vagina, Samant et al[62] recently published a report of primary vaginal cancer treated with definitive chemoradiation.

The success of brachytherapy for urethral cancer is largely dependent on the stage of disease, because proximal urethral cancers are considered a higher stage than distal tumors. For early-stage tumors of the distal urethra, 5-year local control rates have been reported to be up to 80%–90% with radiation alone (often brachytherapy with external beam radiation).[63,64] However, for tumors of the proximal urethra, or those that encompass a large portion of the urethral canal, control rates are generally in the 20%–50% range.[63,65]

## Carcinoma of the Lip

### Indications

Brachytherapy or external beam radiation therapy can be effectively used alone for early-stage tumors of the lip, and particularly those near the commissure where the risk of cosmetic deformity with surgical resection is greatest. Brachytherapy can also be used as an alternative to external beam radiation therapy postoperatively for selected patients with advanced tumors who have residual disease or adverse pathologic features such as perineural invasion.

### Technique

The technique for brachytherapy in the head and neck involves the interstitial placement of multiple source applicators into the tumor bed and surrounding areas of risk. It will therefore be briefly outlined here and can be extrapolated to each site in the head and neck. Note that before any head and neck brachytherapy procedure, a pretreatment dental evaluation is mandatory. All tooth extractions or other major dental procedures should be considered prior to the brachytherapy procedure.[66]

In general, patients are placed under either local or general anesthesia for the placement of source applicators. A guide needle is typically placed into the region of the tumor (or surgical bed), followed by the source applicator. When all of the applicators have been placed into the desired treatment region, a treatment plan with a 0.5–1 cm tumor margin is generated. If LDR brachytherapy is being performed, the source is then placed into the applicator and remains there for 3 to 5 days to deliver the intended prescription dose, during which time the patient is placed into radiation isolation. After the treatment is finished, the applicators are removed and the patient is discharged shortly thereafter.

If the patient is being treated with HDR brachytherapy, the applicators are often placed in the operating room (or a procedure room) and a CT simulation is subsequently performed. A plan is generated and the patient is taken to a hospital bed, returning for BID treatments, at least 4 to 6 hours apart, until the desired dose is given. The total treatment time also ranges from 3 to 5 days.

### Results

Table 5-14 includes a series examining the efficacy and toxicity of brachytherapy in carcinoma of the lip.

## Carcinoma of the Oral Cavity (excluding lip)

### Indications

For most early stage cancers of the oral tongue (stage T1 or T2), brachytherapy can be used as an alternative to surgery or external beam radiation. However, tumors that are in close proximity to the mandible, such as anterior floor of mouth tumors, are often managed with other modalities due to the increased dose that the mandible will receive and the resultant risk for osteonecrosis.[70,71] For more advanced lesions, brachytherapy can be used in the postoperative setting in conjunction with external beam radiation. It can also be used as an alternative to external beam radiation therapy with early-stage lesions that have adverse pathologic findings during surgery such as close margins or perineural invasion.

### Results

One of the largest studies of brachytherapy of the oral cavity is from France by Decroix and Ghossein.

There have also been multiple retrospective trials comparing HDR brachytherapy to LDR brachytherapy, and these are summarized in the Table 5-15.

---

**BOX 5-13**

Six-hundred-two patients with stages T1-T3 carcinoma of the oral tongue were treated between 1959 and 1972. Three-hundred-twelve of these patients were treated with brachytherapy alone, mostly in T1/T2 lesions; 148 patients received combination external beam radiation therapy and brachytherapy, 69 patients had brachytherapy and surgery, and the rest of the patients (73) received either surgery alone (6 patients) or external beam radiation therapy alone (67 patients). Five-year locoregional control (either in the primary site or in the neck) was achieved in 76% of T1 lesions, 69% of T2 lesions, and 60% of T3 lesions.

Decroix Y, Ghossein NA. Experience of the Curie Institute in treatment of cancer of the mobile tongue: Treatment policies and result.[72] *Cancer* 1981 Feb 1;47(3):496–502.

---

**TABLE 5-14  Outcome with Brachytherapy for Carcinoma of the Lip**

| Study | Patients Included | N | Control | Toxicity |
|---|---|---|---|---|
| Beauvois et al[67] | 89% T1/T2, all with LDR alone | 247 | 95% at 5 years | 11% ulceration, 0.5% tissue necrosis |
| Petrovich et al[68] | T1-T3, LDR | 91 | 96% at 5 years | 4% tissue necrosis, 11% changes in skin pigmentation |
| Guinot et al[69] | T1-T4, HDR | 39 | 91% at 3 years | Toxicity similar to LDR (percentages not given) |

**TABLE 5-15 Series Comparing HDR and LDR Brachytherapy for Oral Cavity Cancer**

| Series | Patients Included | N | Local Control | Toxicity |
|---|---|---|---|---|
| Kakimoto et al[73] | T3 oral tongue cancer | 75 (61 LDR, 14 HDR) | 85% LDR, 84% HDR at 3 years | Soft tissue ulcer: LDR 3/61, HDR 3/14 Bone exposure; LDR 12/61, HDR 0/14 |
| Inoue et al[74] | T1/T2 oral tongue cancer | 29 (15 LDR, 14 HDR) | 86% LDR, 100% HDR at 2 years (p=0.157) | Soft tissue ulcer: 0/15 LDR, 1/14 HDR Bone exposure: 0/15 LDR, 1/14 HDR |
| Inoue et al[75] | T1/T2 floor of mouth cancer | 57 (41 HDR, 16 LDR) | 69% LDR, 94% HDR at 5 years (p=0.113) | Bone exposure and/or soft tissue ulcer: 13/41 LDR, 6/16 HDR |

Thus, the trials up to now, although small in size and with short follow-up, have shown HDR and LDR brachytherapy to be essentially equivalent in regard to local tumor control and late complications.

## Base of Tongue Cancer

### Indications

Due to the high risk of lymph node involvement in oropharyngeal cancers, brachytherapy is almost always used in combination with external beam radiation to treat the cervical lymph nodes (rather than as monotherapy).[71] Often, the external beam component is given prior to brachytherapy (to a dose of 5000–5400 cGy), with the latter being performed approximately 3 weeks after the final external beam treatment. For more advanced disease (stage III and IV), concurrent chemotherapy is also administered, which can be expected to increase toxicity.

### Results

Multiple retrospective studies have demonstrated high rates of local control using brachytherapy implants alone for T1/T2 base of tongue tumors, as well as in combination with external beam radiation for larger tumors. Four of the most significant studies are outlined in Table 5-16. All of these studies utilized a combined modality approach of external beam radiation and implants. Only the Karakoyun-Celik et al[79] study utilized chemotherapy as part of the treatment regimen in a significant proportion of patients, likely because this study is the most recent.

Therefore, brachytherapy plus external beam radiation offers similar control rates to high dose external beam radiation alone. With the advent of intensity modulated radiotherapy, there is some controversy in the radiation oncology community as to the utility of brachytherapy for base of tongue lesions. With IMRT, which has been shown to reduce treatment-related toxicity, and the now proven benefit of chemotherapy in locally advanced disease, high dose external beam radiation may supplant brachytherapy in this regard.[80] However, it has been argued that the data for IMRT in this setting is still short-term in scope, and that the high conformality of this technique increases the chance for geographic misses.[81] More follow-up is needed in this regard, but as of now brachytherapy continues to be used for this disease.

**TABLE 5-16  Efficacy of Brachytherapy Implants for Base of Tongue Tumors**

| Study | Patients Included | N | Local Control | Toxicity |
|---|---|---|---|---|
| Harrison et al[76] | T1–T4 | 17 | T1- 4/4, T2-5/6, T3–5/6, T4–1/1 at 2 years | Soft tissue ulcers: 5/16 Osteoradionecrosis: 1/16 More complications in patients receiving implant first (4/7 vs. 2/10) |
| Puthawala et al[77] | T3, T4, N2, N3 | 70 | 83% at 2 years | Soft tissue ulcers/ osteora-dionecrosis: 8/70 (11.4%) |
| Gibbs et al[78] | T1–T4 | 41 | 82% at 5 years | Soft tissue ulceration: 7% Osteoradionecrosis: 5% |
| Karakoyun-Celik et al[79] | T1–T4 (60% received chemotherapy) | 40 | 78% at 5 years, 70% at 10 years | Osteoradionecrosis: 2/40 (5%) Trismus: 2/40 (5%) |

## Brachytherapy as Salvage for Recurrent Head and Neck Tumors

Patients with recurrent tumors of the head and neck generally have limited therapeutic options. Because re-irradiation of this region is often associated with significant morbidity,[82] brachyther-apy has been used in conjunction with surgery and chemotherapy to improve local control with the advantage of a rapid dose fall off. Studies utilizing this technique are limited, but the retrospec-tive analysis by Narayana et al[83] is one of the largest in this regard.

---

**BOX 5-14**

Thirty patients with recurrent head and neck cancers received brachytherapy as part of a salvage reg-imen between September 2003 and October 2005. Eighteen patients were treated with postoperative brachytherapy to a dose of 3.4 Gy BID × 10 fractions, nine patients were treated with 4 Gy BID × 10 fractions for definitive treatment, and three patients were treated with 4 Gy BID × 5 fractions in con-junction with EBRT to 39.6 Gy. Local control was 71% at 2 years and overall survival was 63%. At a median follow-up of 12 months, those patients that underwent surgery had an improved rate of local control (88% vs. 40%, p = 0.05). There were six Grade II and four Grade III complications, all in the postoperative group.

Narayana A, Cohen GN et al. HDR interstitial brachytherapy in recurrent and previously irradiated head and neck cancers: preliminary results.[83] *Brachytherapy*. 2007 Apr-Jun; 6(2): 157–63.

---

The authors concluded that brachytherapy was feasible in terms of local control and with no reported grade IV/V delayed toxicity, likely secondary to the fractionation regimen and the lack of chemotherapy.

## Endobronchial Brachytherapy

### Indications

As the name implies, endobronchial brachytherapy is used for tumors situated in the bronchus. While in the past endobronchial brachytherapy has been used alone for curative intent, more common uses of this modality are in combination with external beam radiation, in patients who have had prior radiation therapy and then experienced a recurrence of their disease, and for patients who require palliation of symptoms such as dyspnea or hemoptysis.

## Technique

Typically, the patient is placed under general anesthesia for the procedure, which is often done with a thoracic surgical team present. A bronchoscope is placed through the mouth into the airway. Next, a guidewire is placed through the bronchoscope into the region of the tumor. Dummy seeds are then placed over the guidewire into the affected region. A 1–2 cm margin is typically given both proximal and distal to the tumor. After the region of interest is identified and agreed upon by the radiation oncologist and the surgical team (as visualized through bronchoscopic images), the radioactive source is placed into the catheter. Traditionally, LDR brachytherapy with iridium has been used, but in recent years HDR brachytherapy has supplanted LDR therapy in most large centers. A plan is generated and the source is applied for several minutes while the dose is delivered.[84]

Note that endobronchial brachytherapy is often used for patients with significant bronchial involvement that obstructs the lumen. In these cases, laser resection is sometimes used to create a lumen and thus provide a passageway for the bronchoscope. In order to limit toxicity, some clinicians advocate waiting 2 to 3 days after this procedure prior to performing endobronchial brachytherapy.

## Results

There have been multiple retrospective studies examining brachytherapy as definitive therapy, as a boost with external beam radiation, and for palliation. The data on endobronchial brachytherapy for curative intent as monotherapy has been limited, generally being reserved for patients with early-stage disease who are medically inoperable.[1] Indeed, when used as part of a definitive treatment regimen the brachytherapy component would be used as a boost to external beam therapy. Following is a table of the largest, representative studies in this regard. As can be seen in Table 5-17, serious toxicities that can result from the procedure include hemoptysis and a tracheo-esophageal fistula.

**TABLE 5-17 Studies Utilizing Brachytherapy in Combination with External Beam Radiation for Treatment of Lung Cancer**

| Study | Patients Included | N | Overall Survival | Toxicity |
|---|---|---|---|---|
| Chang et al[85] | Symptomatic malignant airway obstruction | 59 | Maximum survival 18 months from first treatment | Hemoptysis–four patients Radiation pneumonitis–three patients |
| Agyun et al[86] | Medically inoperable | 62 | Median survival 13 months Stage I–20 mos Stage IIIA-B–10 mos | Fatal hemoptysis–nine patients |
| Cotter et al[87] | Medically inoperable | 65 | 38% at 1 year, median survival 8 mos | Hemoptysis–one patient Fistula Formation–three patients |
| Mantz et al[88] | Early stage medically inoperable | 39 | 15% with combo EBRT, 9% with monotherapy at 3 years | Benign bronchial stricture–one patient Hemoptysis–no patients |

Multiple studies have also been performed on endobronchial brachytherapy for symptom palliation. One of the most pertinent studies in this regard is that by Speiser and Spratling described as follows.

---

**BOX 5-15**

The study was designed to standardize endobronchial brachytherapy and to assess the efficacy of palliation of symptoms. Patients received either medium dose rate or high dose rate brachytherapy at doses ranging from 750-1000 cGy. Overall, hemoptysis was palliated in 99% of patients, obstructive pneumonia 99%, cough 85%, and dyspnea 86%. The authors concluded that endobronchial brachytherapy provides significant improvement of symptoms relating to bronchial obstruction.

Speiser BL, Spratling L. Remote afterloading brachytherapy for local control of endobronchial carcinoma.89 *Int J Radiat Oncol Biol Phys* 1993 Mar 15; 25(4): 579–87.

---

## Episcleral Brachytherapy

### Indications

Table 5-18 lists criteria for episcleral plaque brachytherapy, as derived from the recommendations for uveal melanoma from the American Brachytherapy Society.[90]

Note that these are general guidelines for selecting patients with plaque brachytherapy versus enucleation. Indeed, some large tumors or tumors situated close to the macula can be treated successfully with episcleral plaques. The preceding indications are thus at the discretion of the treating ophthalmologist and radiation oncologist.

### Technique

The episcleral eye plaque is made prior to the operative procedure, with the desired dose prescriptions as determined by the height and basal diameter of the tumor. After a diagram of the exact location and size of the tumor is generated, this is transferred to a treatment planning system. The margin placed around the tumor varies somewhat among institutions, but is typically in the range of 1–3 mm. At most institutions, $^{125}$I is the isotope used, but $^{60}$Co, $^{222}$Rn, $^{106}$Ru, $^{192}$Ir, $^{103}$Pd have all been used at various institutions.[85] For ocular melanomas, at our institution the dose is typically 8500 cGy, while for retinoblastoma the dose at our institution is approximately 4000 cGy.

During delivery of the eye plaque, the patient is placed under general anesthesia. The skin around the eye is prepped by the ophthalmologic team and a corneal protector is placed. The conjunctiva is dissected and a dummy plaque is first inserted to ensure an appropriate fit prior to insertion of the radioactive plaque. If possible, the lateral rectus muscle is preserved, but in the event

---

TABLE 5-18 **Patient Selection for Episcleral Plaque Placement**

| Enucleation | Plaque Brachytherapy |
|---|---|
| Blind, painful eye | Asymptomatic patients desiring visual preservation |
| Tumor involving >40% of the intraocular volume | Small to medium size tumors that have demonstrated growth |
| Tumors located close to the macula/peripapillary tumors in which vision would be difficult to preserve | Tumors situated relatively far from the macula |

that this muscle is ligated, it will be resutured during removal of the plaque and the patient can expect to have full function of this muscle. The active plaque is then placed around the tumor and the conjunctiva is closed. The patient then recovers and returns to the hospital room. After the desired dose is delivered (usually in the range of 2 to 3 days), the patient returns to the operating room and the plaque is removed.

### Results

The most important study in the area of episcleral plaque brachytherapy has been the Collaboratoive Ocular Melanoma Study (COMS) randomized trial of [125]I brachytherapy for choroidal melanoma. In this study, 1,317 patients with tumors from 2.50–10.0 mm in height and 16.0 mm in basal diameter were randomized to either enucleation or episcleral plaque brachytherapy to a dose of 8,500 cGy. This study produced a series of papers based on the results, which included visual acuity, local control, and overall survival. These are summarized in Table 5-19.

The COMS studies demonstrated that episcleral plaque brachytherapy for melanoma was equivalent to enucleation in terms of overall survival, with a small proportion of patients requiring enucleation. In regard to visual toxicity, this was found to be mainly size and location dependent.

## Endovascular Brachytherapy

### Indications

Endovascular brachytherapy is an example of a non-oncologic use of therapeutic radiation. The utility of this modality arises because after stent placement in the coronary arteries for atherosclerotic disease, 20%–30% of patients experience restenosis of the vessel.[94] Although endovascular brachytherapy has been utilized with peripheral vessels, such as the femoropopliteal artery and the renal artery, this discussion will focus on coronary artery brachytherapy. For a further review of endovascular brachytherapy in peripheral arteries, the reader is referred to the reviews by Schillinger et al[95] and Reilly et al.[96]

Virtually any patient who requires stent placement is a candidate for coronary artery brachytherapy (CAB). However, some factors, such as diabetes, unstable angina, prior episodes of restenosis, longer lesions, and vein-graft lesions place patients at higher risk for restenosis. These patients would thus theoretically have the most benefit with a more aggressive approach following balloon angioplasty.

TABLE 5-19　Results of COMS Study for Episcleral Plaque Brachytherapy in Ocular Melanoma

| Local Control[91] | Overall Survival[92] | Visual Acuity[93] |
|---|---|---|
| 12.5% of patients receiving brachytherapy undergoing enucleation by 5 years, 10.3% treatment failure | 5-year OS 81% in enucleated arm, 82% in brachytherapy arm ($p = 0.48$) | 43–49% of eyes had substantial impairment in visual acuity at 3 years, more common in large tumors and shorter distance between tumor and foveal avascular zone |
| **Conclusion:** Local treatment failure and enucleation infrequent, typically occurred early | **Conclusion:** Mortality rates do not differ between enucleation and episcleral plaque brachytherapy | **Conclusion:** Episcleral plaque brachytherapy can decrease visual acuity in a significant proportion of patients and is tumor size and location dependent |

## Technique

Coronary artery brachytherapy can be delivered using either β radiation in the form of electrons ($^{32}$P, $^{90}$Sr/Y, $^{188}$Re), or γ radiation in the form of photons ($^{192}$Ir). The choice of isotope, like other areas of brachytherapy, is largely institution dependent, but in general γ radiation, being more highly penetrating, requires additional shielding.[94] In addition, the radiation can be delivered either with permanent radioactive stents or, similar to other forms of HDR, with individual seeds that are exposed to the area at risk for several minutes. The latter form of delivery is much more commonly used and is the method utilized in the following pertinent clinical trials.

## Results

Several published randomized trials regarding CAB are summarized in Table 5-20.

These studies have demonstrated that CAB is effective in reducing the rates of restenosis, myocardial infarction, and survival. However, there have been two concerns with coronary artery brachytherapy. The first is the rate of late thrombosis, as was demonstrated in the PREVENT and GAMMA-1 studies in Table 5-20. The second is known as the "candy wrapper" or "edge" effect, in which there are increased rates of thrombosis in the region adjacent to the stent (so named due to the resemblance of the partial blockages to the shape of a candy wrapper on angiogram). Both of these effects decrease the overall efficacy of CAB.

**TABLE 5-20 Randomized Studies of Coronary Artery Brachytherapy**

| Study | Isotope | N | Results | Conclusion |
|---|---|---|---|---|
| Teirstein et al[97] (Scripps Study) | $^{192}$Ir | 55 | 17% restenosis with radiation, 54% with placebo | Decreased restenosis, increased lumina diameter with radiation |
| Leon et al[98] (GAMMA-1 Study) | $^{192}$Ir | 131 | Early stenosis: 43% with radiation, 29% with placebo (p=0.02) Late thrombosis: 5.3% with radiation, 0.8% with placebo (p=0.09) | Lower rates of restenosis but higher rates of late thrombosis |
| Raizner et al[99] (PREVENT study) | $^{32}$P | 105 | Restenosis: 8% with radiation, 39% with placebo (p=0.012); increased stenosis adjacent to target site, increased late thrombosis with radiation | Lower rates of restenosis but higher rates of stenosis adjacent to target site and more late thrombotic events |
| Waksman et al[100] (INHIBIT study) | $^{32}$P | 332 | Myocardial infarction/ revascularization 15% with radiation, 31% with placebo | Decreased rate of myocardial infarction and revascularization with radiation |
| Popma et al[101] (START study) | $^{90}$Sr | 47 | Death/MI/revascularization 28% with radiation, 44% with placebo | Decreased death, revascularization, MI with radiation |

With the noted concerns about CAB, along with the requirement for special equipment and the advent of drug eluting stents, it is unclear what future role for the prevention of restenosis brachytherapy will play. However, it is still practiced in several institutions and does indeed occupy a niche for the prevention of restenosis in this prevalent disease.

## RADIATION SAFETY

The American Brachytherapy Society (ABS), The American College of Medical Physics (ACMP), and the American College of Radiation Oncology (ACRO) have recently developed consensus guidelines for performance standards of brachytherapy.[102]

Many of these regulations are institutional standards and include such key points as properly shielded rooms, pretreatment reviews, device preparation, and quality assurance for both the sources and brachytherapy equipment.

However, for the practicing physician, the following key points can assist in maintaining a high level of radiation safety during brachytherapy procedures (taken from the preceding consensus guidelines[102]).

1) A comprehensive brachytherapy team should include a radiation oncologist, medical physicist, radiation therapist, medical dosimetrist, patient support staff, and a radiation safety officer, or RSO. The RSO should be contacted for any concerns regarding safety of the patient or staff.
2) The radiation oncologist and medical physicist should be present during all source loading. Any other participating caregivers should also have training in stopping the remote afterloader and managing medical and technical emergencies.
3) Patient safety is optimized when all source placement is verified, either by imaging or by intraoperative findings. Inadequate verification of applicator placement can lead to misplaced sources and catastrophic consequences.
4) The delivered dose should be verified on all patients, particularly the correlation between calculated dose and dose actually administered. If, during the procedure, it is found that the dose cannot be delivered with less than 20% deviation from the prescribed dose, after adjusting for patient position, then the physician should consider aborting the procedure.
5) All individuals approved to handle radioactive materials are under the control of a radiation safety committee. These individuals must adhere to a program that, among other components, instructs each individual on the proper way to "receive, transport, and dispose of radioactive materials." In addition, written emergency procedures should be well-defined and readily available for all appropriate staff.

For more information in this regard, the interested reader is advised to read the consensus guidelines[102] and to contact their institutional radiation safety officer with any questions or concerns.

## REFERENCES

1. Perez CA, Halperin EC. *Principles and Practice of Radiation Oncology*. Lippincott Williams and Wilkins; Philadelphia, Pennsylvania, 2004.
2. Stanton R, Stinson S. *Applied Physics for Radiation Oncology*, Medical Physics Publishing; Madison, Wisconsin, 1996.
3. Nath R, Anderson LL et al. Dosimetry of brachytherapy sources: Recommendations of the AAPM Brachytherapy Task Force No. 43, *Medical Physics*; 22(2): 209–234.
4. Radiation Therapy Oncology Group, RTOG 0232; A phase 3 study comparing combined external beam radiation and transperineal interstitial permanent brachytherapy with brachy-

therapy alone for selected patients with intermediate risk prostatic carcinoma. http://www.rtog.org/members/protocols/0232.

5. Zelefsky MJ, Yamada Y et al. Postimplantation dosimetric analysis of permanent transperineal prostate implantation: improved dose distributions with an intraoperative computer-optimized conformal planning technique. *IJROBP* 200;48(2): 601–608.

6. Zelefsky MJ, Yamada Y et al. Five-year outcome of intraoperative conformal permanent I-125 interstitial implantation for patients with clinically localized prostate cancer. *IJROBP* 2007; 67(1): 65–70.

7. Kollmeier MA, Stock RG, Stone N. Biochemical outcomes after prostate brachytherapy with 5–year minimal follow-up: importance of patient selection and implant quality. *IJROBP* 2003; 57(3): 645–653.

8. Grimm PD, Blasko JC et al. 10–year biochemical (prostate-specific antigen) control of prostate cancer with (125)I brachytherapy. *IJROBP* 2001; 51(1): 31–40.

9. Potters L, Morgenstern C et al. 12–year outcomes following permanent prostate brachytherapy in patients with clinically localized prostate cancer. *J Urol* 2005; 173(5): 1562–1566.

10. Ragde H, Korb LJ et al. Modern prostate brachytherapy prostate specific antigen results with up to 12 years of observed follow-up. *Cancer* Nov 2000; 89(1): 135–141.

11. Zelefsky MJ, Kuban DA. Multi-institutional analysis of long-term outcome for stages T1–T2 prostate cancer treated with permanent seed implantation. *IJROBP* 2007; 67(2): 327–333.

12. Stock RG, Stone NN et al. What is the optimal dose for $^{125}$I prostate implants? A dose response analysis of biochemical control posttreatment biopsies and long-term urinary symptoms. *Brachytherapy* 2002; 1: 83–89.

13. Stock RG, Stone NN et al. A dose-response study for $^{125}$I prostate implants: definitions and factors affecting outcome. *IJROBP* 1998; 41: 101–108.

14. Potters L, Cao Y et al. A comprehensive review of CT-based dosimetry parameters and biochemical control in patients treated with permanent prostate brachytherapy. *IJROBP* 2001; 50: 605–614.

15. Singh A, Zelefsky MJ et al. Combined 3–dimensional conformal radiotherapy and transperineal Pd-103 permanent implantation for patients with intermediate and unfavorable risk prostate cancer. *Int J Cancer* 2000; 90: 275–280.

16. Critz FA, Williams WH et al. Simultaneous irradiation for prostate cancer: intermediate results with modern techniques. *J Urol* 2000; 164: 738–741.

17. Critz FA, Levinson K. Ten-year disease free survival rates after simultaneous irradiation for prostate cancer with a focus on calculation methodology. *J Urol* 2004 Dec; 172 (6 Pt 1): 2232–2238.

18. Sylvester JE, Blasko JC et al. Ten-year biochemical relapse-free survival after external beam radiation and brachytherapy for localized prostate cancer: the Seattle experience. *IJROBP* Nov 2003; 57(4): 944–952.

19. Kleinberg L, Wallner K et al. Treatment-related symptoms during the first year following transperineal 125I prostate implantation. *IJROBP* Mar 1994; 28(4): 985–990.

20. Brown D, Colonias A et al. Urinary morbidity with a modified peripheral loading technique of transperineal $^{125}$I prostate implantation. *IJROBP* May 2000; 47(2): 353–360.

21. Gelblum DY, Potters L et al. Urinary morbidity following ultrasound-guided transperineal prostate implantation *IJROBP* Aug 1999; 45(1): 59–67.

22. Merrick GS, Butler WM et al. Temporal resolution of urinary morbidity following prostate brachytherapy. *IJROBP* Apr 2000; 47(1): 121–129.

23. Kang SK, Chou RH et al. Gastrointestinal toxicity of transperineal interstitial prostate brachytherapy. *IJROBP* May 2002; 53(1): 99–103.

24. Gelblum DY, Potters L. Rectal complications associated with transperineal interstitial brachytherapy for prostate cancer. *IJROBP* Aug 2000; 48(1): 119–124.

25. Tran A, Wallner K et al. Rectal fistular after prostate brachytherapy. *IJROBP* Sep 2005; 63(1): 150–154.

26. Zelefsky MJ, Wallner KE et al. Comparison of the 5–year outcome of three-dimensional conformal radiotherapy versus transperineal permanent I-125 implantation for early-stage prostatic cancer. *J Clin Onc* 1999 Feb; 17(2): 517–522.

27. Bhatnagar V, Stewart ST et al. Estimating the risk of long-term erectile, urinary and bowel symptoms resulting from prostate cancer treatment. *Prostate Cancer Prostatic Dis* 2006; 9(2):136–146.

28. Wallner K, Merrick S et al. 125I versus 103Pd for low-risk prostate cancer: preliminary PSA outcomes from a prospective randomized multicenter trial. *IJROBP* Dec 2003 1; 57(5): 1297–1303.

29. Niehaus A, Merrick GS et al. The influence of isotope and prostate volume on urinary morbidity after prostate brachytherapy. *IJROBP* Sep 2006; 64(1): 136–143.

30. Demanes DJ, Rodriguez RR et al. High-dose-rate intensity-modulated brachytherapy with external beam radiotherapy for prostate cancer: California endocurietherapy's 10–year results. *IJROBP* Apr 2005; 61(5): 1306–1316.

31. Galalae RM, Martinez A et al. Long-term outcome by risk factors using conformal high-dose-rate brachytherapy (HDR-BT) boost with or without neoadjuvant androgen suppression for localized prostate cancer. *IJROBP* 2004; 58: 1048–1055.

32. Yamada Y, Bhatia S et al. Favorable clinical outcomes of three-dimensional computer-optimized high-dose-rate prostate brachytherapy in the management of localized prostate cancer. *Brachytherapy* 2006; 5:157–164.

33. Grills IS, Martinez AA et al. High dose rate brachytherapy as prostate monotherapy reduces toxicity compared to low dose rate palladium seeds. *J Urol* Mar 2004; 171(3): 1098–1104.

34. Martinez AA, Gustafson G et al. Dose escalation using conformal high-dose-rate brachytherapy improves outcomes in unfavorable prostate cancer. *IJROBP* Jun 2002; 53(2): 316–327.

35. Thin T, Phan A. High-dose rate brachytherapy as a boost for the treatment of localized prostate cancer. *J Urol* 2007; 177(1); 123–127.

36. Nag S, Chao C et al. The American Brachytherapy Society recommendations for low-dose-rate brachytherapy for carcinoma of the cervix. *Int J Radiat Onc Biol Phys* Jan 2002; 52(1): 33–48.

37. Nag S, Erickson B et al. The American Brachytherapy Society recommendations for high-dose-rate brachytherapy for carcinoma of the cervix. *Int J Radiat Onc Biol Phys* Aug 2000; 48(1): 201–211.

38. Aristizabal SA, Surwit EA et al. Treatment of advanced cancer of the cervix with transperineal interstitial irradiation. *Int J Radiat Onc Biol Phys* July 1983; 9(7): 819–827.

39. International Commission on Radiation Units and Measurements. ICRU Report 58: Dose and volume specification for reporting interstitial therapy. Bethesda, MD. International Commission on Radiation Units and Measurements, 1997.

40. Kuske RR, Perez CA et al. Phase I/II study of definitive radiotherapy and chemotherapy (cis-plating and 5–fluorouracil) for advanced for recurrent gynecologic malignancies. Preliminary report. *Am J Clinic Oncol* Dec 1989; 12(6): 467–473.

41. Okkan S, Atkovar G et al. Results and complications of high dose rate and low dose rate brachytherapy in carcinoma of the cervix: Cerrahpasa experience. *Radiother Oncol* 2003; 67: 97–105.

42. Lertsanguansinchai P, Lertbutsayanukul et al. Phase III randomized trial comparing LDR and HDR brachytherapy in treatment of cervical carcinoma. *IJROBP* 2004; 59(5): 1424–1431.

43. Patel FD, Sharma SC et al. Low dose rate vs. high dose rate brachytherapy in the treatment of carcinoma of the uterine cervix: a clinical trial. *Int J Radiat Oncol Biol Phys* Jan 1994; 28(2):335–341.

44. Hareyama M, Sakata K et al. High-dose-rate versus low-dose rate intracavitary therapy for carcinoma of the uterine cervix. *Cancer* 2002; 94(1): 117–124.

45. Bruner DW, Lanciano R et al. Vaginal stenosis and sexual function following intracavitary radiation for the treatment of cervical and endometrial carcinoma. *Int J Radiat Oncol Biol Phys* Nov 1993; 27(4): 825–830.

46. Lanciano RM et al. Pretreatment and treatment factors associated with improved outcome in squamous cell carcinoma of the uterine cervix: A final report of the 1973 and 1978 patterns of care studies, *Int J Radiat Oncol Biol Phys* Apr 1991; 20(4):667–676.

47. Fyles A, Keane TJ et al. The effect of treatment duration in the local control of cervical cancer. *Radiother Oncol* 1992:25:273–279.

48. Girinsky T, Rey A. et al. Overall treatment time in advanced cervical carcinomas: a critical parameter in treatment outcomes. *Int J Radiation Oncol Biol Phys* 1993; 27:1051–1056.

49. Lanciano RM, Pajak TF et al. The influence of treatment time on outcome for squamous cell carcinoma of the uterine cervix treated with radiation: a patterns of care study. *Int J Radiat Oncol Biol Phys* 1993; 25:391–406.

50. Fyles AW, Milosevic M et al. Prognostic factors in patients with cervix cancer treated by radiation therapy: results of a multiple regression analysis. *Radiother Oncol* 1995; 35(2): 107–117.

51. Nag S, Erickson B et al. The American Brachytherapy Society recommendations for high-dose-rate brachytherapy for carcinoma of the endometrium. *Int J Radiat Oncol Biol Phys* 2000; 48(3): 779–790.

52. Alektiar KM. When and how should adjuvant radiation be used in early stage endometrial cancer? *Semin Radiat Oncol* Jul 2006; 16(3): 158–163.

53. Anderson JM, Stea B et al. High-dose-rate postoperative vaginal cuff irradiation alone for stage IB and IC endometrial cancer. *IJROBP* 2000; 46(2): 417–425.

54. Alektiar KM, Venkatraman E et al. Intravaginal brachytherapy alone for intermediate-risk endometrial cancer. *IJROBP* 2005; 62(1): 111–117.

55. MacLeod C, Fowler A et al. High-dose-rate brachytherapy alone post-hysterectomy for endometrial cancer. *Int J Radiat Oncol Biol Phys* Dec 1998; 42(5): 1033–1039.

56. Horowitz NS, Peters WA et al. Adjuvant high dose rate vaginal brachytherapy as treatment of stage I and II endometrial carcinoma. *Obstet Gynecol* 2002; 99(2): 235–240.

57. Chadha M, Nanavati PJ et al. Patterns of failure in endometrial carcinoma stage IB grade 3 and IC patients treated with postoperative vaginal vault brachytherapy. *Gynecol Oncol* Oct 1999; 75(1): 103–107.

58. Creutzberg CL, van Putten WL et al. Surgery and postoperative radiotherapy versus surgery alone for patients with stage-1 endometrial carcinoma: multicentre randomised trial. *Lancet* 2000; 355(9213): 1404–1411.

59. Keys HM, Roberts JA et al. A phase III trial of surgery with or without adjunctive external pelvic radiation therapy in intermediate risk endometrial adenocarcinoma: a Gynecologic Oncology Group Study. *Gynecol Oncol* Mar 2004; 92(3): 744–751.

60. Aalders JG, Abeler V et al. Postoperative external irradiation and prognostic parameters in stage I endometrial carcinoma: clinical and histopathologic study of 540 patients. *Gynecol Oncol* 1980; 56(4): 419–427.

61. Knocke TH, Kucera H et al. Primary treatment of endometrial carcinoma with high-dose-rate brachytherapy: results of 12 years of experience with 280 patients. *Int J Radiat Oncol Biol Phys* 1997; 37(2): 359–365.

62. Samant R, Lau B et al. Primary vaginal cancer treated with concurrent chemoradiation using cis-platinum. *Int J Radiat Oncol Biol Phys* Nov 2007; 69(3): 746–50.

63. Milosevic M, Padraig RW et al. Urethral carcinoma in women: results of treatment with primary radiotherapy. *Radiother Oncol* 2000; 56: 29–35.

64. Prempree T, Amornmarn R, Patanphan V. Radiation therapy in primary carcinoma of the female urethra. II. An update on results. *Cancer* 1984; 54: 729–733.

65. Weghaupt K, Gerstner GJ et al. Radiation therapy for primary carcinoma of the female urethra: a survey over 25 years. *Gynecol Oncol* 1984; 17: 58–63.

66. Casino AR, Toledano IP et al. Brachytherapy in lip cancer. *Oral Medicine and Pathology* 2006; 11:E223–229.

67. Beauvois S, Hoffstetter S et al. Brachytherapy for lower lip epidermoid cancer: tumoral and treatment factors influencing recurrences and complications. *Radiother Oncol* 1996; 55:69.

68. Petrovich Z, Kuisk H et al. Carcinoma of the lip. *Arch Otolaryngol* 1979; 105: 187–191.

69. Guinot JL, Arribas L et al. Lip cancer treatment with high dose rate therapy. *Radiother Oncol* 2003; 69:113–115.

70. Harrison, LB. Applications of brachytherapy in head and neck cancer. *Sem Surg Onc* 1997; 13:177–184.

71. Nag S, Cano ER et al. The American Brachytherapy Society recommendations for high-dose-rate brachytherapy for head-and-neck carcinoma. *Int J Radiat Oncol Biol Phys*. Aug 2001; 50(5): 1190–1198.

72. Decroix Y, Ghossein NA. Experience of the Curie Institute in treatment of cancer of the mobile tongue: treatment policies and result. *Cancer* 1981; 47(3): 496–502.

73. Kakimoto N, Inoue T et al. Results of low- and high-dose rate interstitial brachytherapy for T3 mobile tongue cancer. *Radiother Oncol* 2003; 68(2): 123–128.

74. Inoue T, Inoue T et al. Phase III trial of high and low dose rate interstitial radiotherapy for early oral tongue cancer. *Int J Radiat Oncol Biol Phys* 1996; 36(5): 1201–1204.

75. Inoue T, Inoue T et al. High dose rate versus low dose rate interstitial radiotherapy for carcinoma of the floor of mouth. *Int J Radiat Oncol Biol Phys* 1998; 41(1): 53–58.

76. Harrison, LB, Sessions RB et al. Brachytherapy as part of the definitive management of squamous cancer of the base of tongue. *Int J Radiat Onc Biol Phys* Dec 1989; 17(6): 1309–1312.

77. Puthwala AA, Syed AM et al. Limited external beam and interstitial 192iridium irradiation in the treatment in carcinoma of the base of tongue: a ten year experience. *Int J Radiat Onc Biol Phys* May 1988; 14(5): 839–848.

78. Gibbs IC, Le QT et al. Long-term outcomes of after external beam irradiation and brachytherapy boost for base-of-tongue cancers. Oct 2003; 57(2): 489–494.

79. Karakoyn-Celik O, Norris CM et Al. Definitive radiotherapy with interstitial implant boost for squamous cell carcinoma of the tongue base. *Head & Neck*. Feb 2005; 27(5): 353–361.

80. Lee N, Point/Counterpoint: Brachytherapy versus intensity-modulated radiation therapy in the management of base-of-tongue cancers. *Brachytherapy* 2005; 4(1): 5–7.

81. Hu K, Harrison LB. Point/Counterpoint: Brachytherapy versus intensity-modulated radiation therapy in the management of tongue cancers. *Brachytherapy* 2005; 4(1): 1–4.

82. Haraf D, Weischelbaum R et al. Re-irradiation with concurrent hydroxyurea and 5–fluorouracil in patients with squamous cell cancer of the head and neck. Ann Oncol 1996; 7: 913–918.

83. Narayana A, Cohen GN et al. HDR interstitial brachytherapy in recurrent and previously irradiated head and neck cancers—Preliminary result. *Brachytherapy* Apr-Jun 2007; 6(2): 157–163.

84. Gaspar LE, Brachytherapy in lung cancer. *J of Surgical Oncology* 1998; 67:60–70.

85. Chang LF, Horvath J et al. High dose rate afterloading intraluminal brachytherapy in malignant airway obstruction of lung cancer. *Int J Radiat Oncol Biol Phys* Feb 1994; 28(3): 589–596.

86. Aygun C, Weiner S et al. Treatment of non-small cell lung cancer with external beam radiotherapy and high dose rate brachytherapy. *Int J Radiat Oncol Biol Phys* 1992; 23(1): 127–132.

87. Cotter GW, Lariscy Y et al. Inoperable endobronchial obstructing lung cancer treated with combined endobronchial and external beam irradiation: a dosimetric analysis. *Int J Radiat Oncol Biol Phys* Oct 1993 20; 27(3): 531–55.
88. Mantz CA, Dosoretz DE et al. Endobronchial brachytherapy and optimization of local disease control in medically inoperable non-small cell lung carcinoma: a matched pair analysis. *Brachytherapy* 2004; 3(4): 183–190.
89. Speiser BL, Spratling L. Remote afterloading brachytherapy for the local control of endo-bronchial carcinoma. *Int J Radiat Oncol Biol Phys* Mar 1993; 25(4): 579–587.
90. Nag S, Quivey JM et al. The American Brachytherapy Society recommendations for brachy-therapy of uveal melanomas. *Int J Radiat Oncol Biol Phys* 2003; 56(2): 544–555.
91. Jampol LM, Moy CS et al. The COMS randomized trial of iodine 125 brachytherapy for choroidal melanoma: IV. Local treatment failure and enucleation in the first 5 years after brachytherapy. COMS report no. 19. *Ophthalmology* Dec 2002; 109(12): 2197–2206.
92. The Collaborative Ocular Melanoma Study Group. The COMS randomized trial of Iodine 125 brachytherapy for choroidal melanoma, III: Initial mortality findings. COMS report no. 18. *Arch Ophthalmol* July 2001; 119: 969–982.
93. Melia BM, Abramson DH et al. Collaborative ocular melanoma study (COMS) randomized tial of I-125 brachytherapy for medium choroidal melanoma. I. Visual acuity after 3 years. COMS report no. 16. *Ophthalmology* Feb 2001; 108(2): 348–366.
94. Sheppard R, Eisenberg MJ et Al. Intracoronary brachytherapy for the prevention of resteno-sis after percutaneous coronary revascularization. *American Heart Journal* Nov 2003; 146(5): 775–786.
95. Schillinger M, Minar E. Advances in vascular brachytherapy over the past 10 years. Focus on femoropopliteal applications. *J Endovasc Ther* Dec 2004; 11 Suppl 2 II180–191.
96. Reilly JP, Ramee SR. Vascular brachytherapy in renal artery restenosis. *Curr Opin Cardiol* Jul 2004; 19(4): 332–335.
97. Teirstein PS, Masullo V et al. Catheter-based radiotherapy to inhibit restenosis after coronary stenting. *N Engl J Med* 1997; 336: 1697–1703.
98. Leon MB, Teirstein PS et al. Localized intracoronary gamma-radiation therapy to inhibit the recurrence of restenosis after stenting. *New Eng J Med* Jan 2001; 344(4): 250–256.
99. Raizner AE, Oesterle SN et al. Inhibition of restenosis with beta-emitting radiotherapy: Report of the Proliferation Reduction with Vascular Energy Trial (PREVENT). *Circulation* Aug 2000; 102(9): 951–958.
100. Waksman R, Raizner AE et al. Use of localized intracoronary β radiation in treatment of in-stent restenosis: the INHIBIT randomized controlled trial. *Lancet* 2002; 359: 551–557.
101. Popma JJ, Suntharalingham M et al. Randomized trial of $^{90}Sr/^{90}Y$ β-radiation versus placebo control for treatment of in-stent restenosis. *Circulation* 2002; 106: 1090–1096.
102. Nag S, Dobelhower R et al. Inter-society standards for the performance of brachytherapy: a joint report from the ABS, ACMP and ACRO. *Crit Rev Onc Hematol* Oct 2003; 48(1): 1–17.

# 6

# Stereotactic Radiosurgery/ Stereotactic Body Radiation Therapy

*Brian Chang, MD*
*Robert D. Timmerman, MD*

## OVERVIEW

**Stereotactic radiosurgery (SRS)**—a specialized radiation technique, delivering a large single dose of highly collimated radiation to one or more intracranial targets, with submillimeter precision.

**Fractionated Stereotactic Radiotherapy (FSR)**—an extension of SRS, delivered via a fractionated schedule (2 to 30 fractions) utilizing nonrigid immobilization, thereby providing the precision of stereotaxy while allowing adjacent normal structures to repair sublethal damage.

**Stereotactic body radiation therapy (SBRT)**—the precise delivery of large fraction sizes (8–30 Gy) delivered over 1 to 5 fractions to an extracranial site, by either taking inherent organ/target motion into account (gating) or limiting it (abdominal compression).

Both SRS and SBRT utilize external three-dimensional reference systems (stereotaxy) for accurate target localization and treatment delivery. These techniques utilize multiple beams spread in a large solid angle to minimize entrance dose and, ultimately, volume of normal tissue irradiated. Thus the therapeutic window using a stereotactic approach is related primarily to geographic accuracy and rapid dose fall-off outside the tumor volume rather than exploiting the differential ability of normal and tumor tissue to repair DNA damage as seen with large field, conventionally fractionated radiotherapy (CFR) which includes normal tissue within its target volume.

In this chapter we will discuss the clinical applications of these technologies with an emphasis on topics not presented elsewhere in this text.

## CENTRAL NERVOUS SYSTEM (CNS)

### PRIMARY PARENCHYMAL

#### Malignant Glioma

GBM is a notoriously radioresistant malignancy that inevitably recurs, usually within 2 cm of the original tumor. SRS has been evaluated in one randomized controlled trial in an effort to improve survival.

**BOX 6-1**

Randomized trial of 203 patients with supratentorial GBM ≤4 cm were randomized to postoperative SRS followed by EBRT (60Gy) plus BCNU or EBRT with BCNU alone. There was no significant difference in median, 2-year, or 3-year survival. Likewise, SRS did not impact the pattern of failure, quality of life or cognitive decline.

Souhami et al. Randomized Comparison of Stereotactic Radiosurgery Followed by Conventional Radiotherapy with Carmustine to Conventional Radiotherapy with Carmustine for Patients with Glioblastoma Multiforme: Report of Radiation *Therapy Oncology Group* 93-05 Protocol. IJROBP. 2004 Nov 1; 60(3):853–860.

Unless part of a clinical trial, based on the negative results of this study, SRS should not be used as a boost in the primary management of patients with GBM.

SRS continues to be used in selected patients with recurrent malignant glioma (small, well demarcated, enhancing lesions), although it is unclear if this approach offers any additional benefit.

## Ependymoma

Intracranial ependymoma is a rare entity, and the literature describing the use of an SRS boost in the primary management of this neoplasm is limited, with only a few single institutional series reported in the literature. The available data appears to suggest an improved local control rate and survival with this aggressive approach, although further study in clinical trials is needed.[1]

## SECONDARY PARENCHYMAL

### Brain Metastases

Stereotactic radiosurgery in the setting of brain metastases is a noninvasive local modality meant to eradicate gross tumor that is poorly controlled with conventional doses of whole brain radiation therapy (WBRT).[2,3] The initial use of SRS in the setting of brain metastases was based on surgical data that noted a significant benefit in survival, local recurrence, time to recurrence, time to neurologic death, and quality of life when given in conjunction with WBRT in a favorable subset of patients with a single brain metastasis.[2] SRS appears to offer similar local control rates to surgery, although no prospective randomized trials have compared the two modalities.

### Dose

The doses utilized for SRS are based on the results of the RTOG 90-05 dose escalation trial which treated patients with prior gliomas (median prior dose 60 Gy) and prior brain metastases (median prior dose 30 Gy). The recommended single doses are listed in Table 6-1.

TABLE 6-1 **RTOG 90-05 Dose Escalation Trial Recommendations**

| Tumor Size | Dose |
|---|---|
| ≤2 cm | 24 Gy* |
| >2–3 cm | 18 Gy |
| ≥3–4 cm | 15 Gy |

*Dose did not reach MTD.

*Whole brain radiation therapy with or without stereotactic radiosurgery as a boost*

Two prospective randomized trials investigating the benefit of SRS with whole brain radiation versus whole brain radiation alone have been reported in the peer-reviewed literature.[4] Both trials report a significant benefit in local control with addition of a radiosurgery boost following WBRT. The results of both trials are depicted in Table 6-2.

*SRS with or without WBRT*

The argument for withholding WBRT is based on the perception of late neurotoxicity associated with global therapy. The data to support this conclusion in the adult population is founded on retrospective data utilizing unconventional fractionation schemes without validated neurocognitive testing.[5] Given the consistent evidence derived from the surgical and SRS literature supporting a clear increase in the rate of intracranial recurrences when whole brain radiation therapy is withheld,[6,7] and the strong association of intracranial recurrences with a detriment in neurocognitive function,[8] the authors would not recommend the routine use of SRS alone.

## VASCULAR

### Arteriovenous Malformation (AVM)

An AVM is a congenital disorder of the vascular system resulting from an abnormal communication (shunt) between a high pressure artery and low pressure vein that bypasses the capillary bed. Numerous shunts form the AVM nidus, which can be extremely fragile, posing a risk for bleeding which can lead to significant morbidity and potential mortality. Because there is little to no functional brain tissue within the lesion, the nidus can be a reasonable target for SRS. Furthermore, a zone of gliosis surrounds the nidus, constituting a buffer zone in many patients. Obliteration of an AVM nidus may take up to 3 years, making it a second-line therapy to surgical resection in most patients. Often AVMs in deep or more eloquent locations are treated with SRS.

### Epidemiology/Presentation

AVMs occur in 0.14% of the general population in the United States of whom 50% present with hemorrhage and 50% present with nonfocal symptoms (headache, seizure) or focal neurological deficit, as an incidental finding. The annual rate of spontaneous hemorrhage is between 2%–4%.

**TABLE 6-2  Randomized Trials of Whole Brain Radiation Therapy With or Without a Stereotactic Radiosurgical Boost**

| Study | n | Median Survival | | 1-Year Local Relapse | |
|---|---|---|---|---|---|
| | | SRS | No SRS | SRS | No SRS |
| RTOG 9508 | 331 | 6.5 months | 5.7 months | 18% | 29% |
| Univ. of Pitt | 27 | 11 months | 7.5 months | 8% | 100% |

**BOX 6-2**

Randomized trial of 331 patients with 1–3 brain metastases treated with either whole brain radiation therapy with or without a stereotactic radiosurgery boost. Overall there was a significant improvement in local control with the addition of radiosurgery which translated into a significant improvement in performance status and steroid use but not overall survival. However, radiosurgery did confer a statistically significant survival benefit to the subset of patients with a single brain metastasis over whole brain radiation therapy alone.

Andrews et al. Whole brain radiation therapy with or without stereotactic radiosurgery boost for patients with one to three brain metastases; phase III results of the RTOG 9508 randomised trial. *Lancet.* 2004 May 22;363(2):1665–72.

*Workup*

### TABLE 6-3 AVM Diagnostic Testing

| Diagnostic Test | Description |
|---|---|
| Laboratory Studies | CBC, PT/PTT, Type and Screen |
| MRI | First choice in the nonemergent setting. Identifies location, size, and relationship to surrounding intracranial structures. Hemosiderin can be detected indicating a previous hemorrhage. |
| MRA | Noninvasive view of AVM anatomy with lower resolution than conventional angiography. |
| Digital-subtraction Angiography | Invasive test that provides definitive diagnosis. Allows grading of AVM via Spetzler and Martin criteria. |

### TABLE 6-4 AVM Treatment

| Treatment | Pros | Cons |
|---|---|---|
| Surgery | Immediate Cure | Intraoperative bleeding, infection, edema, damage to adjacent neural tissue, ischemic CVA, death* |
| Endovascular Therapy | Significant decrease in blood flow through the lesion. Adjunct to surgery to decrease risk of intraoperative bleeding or decrease target size for SRS | Several procedures usually needed, rarely achieves complete eradication of lesion and nidus usually recanalizes over time, risks similar to surgery, |
| SRS | Can treat deep-seated tumors | Time to obliteration 2-4 years, size limitations (<3 cm) |

*Increasing operative risk with increasing score on the Spetzler-Martin scale. Grade 1–3 operated upon, sometimes grade 4, and never grade 5.

### Treatment

The goal of therapy is total obliteration of the AVM because any residual could lead to hemorrhage.

### Dose

Successful obliteration after SRS correlates with the minimum dose delivered but not the volume or maximum dose.[9] The optimal SRS dose requires balancing the expected obliteration rate and toxicity to normal tissue.

### TABLE 6-5 Dose/In-field Obliteration

| Dose | In-Field Obliteration |
|---|---|
| 26.9Gy | 99% |
| 24.8Gy | 98% |
| 22.0Gy | 95% |
| 19.8Gy | 90% |
| 17.4Gy | 80% |
| 15.8Gy | 70% |
| 13.3Gy | 50% |

Flickinger et al.[9]

## Cavernous Hemangioma (also known as cavernous angioma or cavernoma)

This is a vascular disorder characterized by grossly dilated blood vessels with a thin wall composed of a single layer of endothelium. The walls of this lesion are leaky due to the absence of the other layers that constitute a normal vessel wall. Up to 40% of the

TABLE 6-6  Spetzler-Martin Scale*

| Characteristic of Lesion | Number of Points |
|---|---|
| **Size** | |
| Small (diameter <3 cm) | 1 |
| Medium (diameter 3–6 cm) | 2 |
| Large (diameter >6 cm) | 3 |
| **Location** | |
| Non-eloquent site | 0 |
| Eloquent site (sensorimotor, language, or visual cortex; hypothalamus or thalamus; internal capsule; brainstem; cerebellar peduncles, or cerebellar nuclei) | 1 |
| **Pattern of Venous Drainage** | |
| Superficial only | 0 |
| Any deep | 1 |

Total scores range from 0–5; high scores are associated with high risk of permanent neurological deficit after surgery.
*Spetzler, RF and NA Martin, A proposed grading system for arteriovenous malformations. J Neurosurg, 1986. 65(4): p. 476–483.

time an associated venous angioma occurs with this lesion and this can complicate surgical intervention.

### Epidemiology/Presentation

Cavernous hemangiomas occur in 0.5%–1% of the general population in the United States. Over 30% develop symptoms related to local mass effect and hemorrhage in the third to fourth decade of life. At least 20% of cases are inherited in an autosomal dominant fashion with a higher occurrence in patients of Mexican-American heritage.

### Workup

MRI with T2 weighted sequences—diagnostic test of choice
*Angiogram—does not visualize these lesions because of their low blood flow.

### Treatment

Surgery is the treatment of choice. However, for lesions located in eloquent regions of the brain where the risks of an invasive procedure are felt to be unacceptable, SRS has been offered as an alternative, based on the AVM experience. Multiple single institutional studies report conflicting results regarding the rebleed rate following SRS. This may be partially due to differences in patient selection, definition of bleeding episodes, follow-up time, mode of lesion diagnosis, and variation in frequency of follow-up imaging. The optimal dose is unknown, and the prescribed dose is driven primarily by the perceived risk of toxicity to the surrounding normal tissue. Similar to the AVM literature, the bulk of the rebleeding risk reduction is seen 2 years after treatment.

## SKULL BASE

### Meningioma

SRS is an excellent, noninvasive approach for small skull base meningiomas (<3 cm in diameter) with a reported local control rate of ≥89% and minimal late toxicity (2.5%–5.5%) with a median follow-up of 7 to 8 years.[10–12] These results compare favorably with modern series of microsurgical resection given the high risk of recurrence (10%–33% for completely resected tumors and 55%–75%

for partially resected tumors at 10 years), permanent neurologic complications (16%–56%), and potential operative mortality (3.6%) associated with this invasive approach. Based on these data the authors recommend radiosurgery when technically feasible, reserving microsurgery for patients in need of immediate decompression in the setting of progressive neurologic deficits.

### Dose

The local control and complication rates quoted in the previous paragraph were attained with median doses of 12–14.5 Gy prescribed to the tumor margin. A tumor size greater than 10cc is associated with a significantly lower 5-year local control rate of 68% vs. 91.9% with 14 Gy prescribed to the tumor margin.[13] However, the potential benefit of dose escalation is unclear, and would certainly increase the risk of late term complications. Thus for larger tumors conventionally fractionated radiotherapy may be the preferred treatment under those conditions.

### Volume

The gross disease defined on gadolinium enhanced MRI scan is treated without inclusion of the dural tail, given the increased morbidity associated with larger treatment volumes and lack of data to support an elevated marginal recurrence rate by omitting the dural tail from the treatment volume.

## Acoustic Neuroma (vestibular schwannoma)

Acoustic neuroma is a benign tumor originating from the Schwann cells surrounding the 8th cranial nerve (95% vestibular, 5% cochlear) at Hensen's node, the point where the peripheral and central portions of the nerve meet as it exits the brainstem at the cerebellopontine angle.

### Epidemiology

Acoustic neuromas are clinically diagnosed in 1/100,000 population, with 2,500 new cases per year. Most occur sporadically; however, roughly 10% of cases are attributable to familial neurofibromatosis type II. Patients with this disorder classically have bilateral involvement and often involve the whole nerve rather than a discrete area.

### Presentation

Presenting symptoms are related to direct compression of the acoustic nerve or adjacent structures. Typical presentation involves unilateral sensorineural hearing loss (80%), vertigo (<10%), headaches (<10%) and/or tinnitus. Brainstem compression can lead to hydrocephalus, and facial nerve (CN VII) compression can lead to weakness of the facial muscles (10%), or decreased salivation, tearing, and taste. Trigeminal nerve compression can lead to loss of the corneal reflex and facial anesthesia (25%).

### Workup

Gadolinium-enhanced MRI—diagnostic test of choice. Appearance may be pathognomonic.

### Treatment

Treatment options include microsurgery, SRS, FSR, or observation.

### Dose

The optimal SRS dose is unclear, although with a short median follow up of 24 months, median doses of 12–13 Gy appear to provide excellent local control (98.6%) with no incidence of facial nerve dysfunction and a low 4.4% rate of trigeminal neuropathy.[14] Hearing preservation was seen in 70.3%. This appears to be comparable to the surgical outcome of 0.7% local recurrence, 6% incidence of facial nerve dysfunction, no risk of trigeminal neuropathy, and a 47% hearing preservation rate. Given the apparent absence of late recurrences between years 4 and 10 status post-SRS,

TABLE 6-7  **Acoustic Neuroma Treatment**

| Treatment | Pros | Cons |
|---|---|---|
| Microsurgery | Complete removal of tumor. Less frequent radiographic follow-up necessary. | Increased risk of cranial nerve deficits (VII, VIII), longer postoperative recovery, risk of CSF leakage, HA, meningitis, mortality. |
| SRS | Noninvasive, outpatient procedure with excellent local control and very low morbidity. | Risk of cranial nerve deficits: CN VIII (30%), CN VII (2–5%). |
| FSR | Noninvasive, outpatient procedure with a lower risk of toxicity than SRS (CN VIII toxicity in <5%). | Inconvenience of several weeks of daily treatments. No long term data. |
| Observation | No intervention. | Follow-up MRIs for several years at 6 month intervals to determine tumor progression. |

the previously reported local control rate at a median dose of 13 Gy is likely to remain durable, although further follow-up to confirm these results is needed.[15]

## Pituitary Adenoma

The aim of radiotherapy in the case of pituitary adenomas is to address one or both of the following processes:

- Function—oversecretion of hormones naturally produced in the pituitary gland (GH, ACTH, prolactin, TSH, LH, FSH) resulting in well defined clinical syndromes.
- Clonogenic proliferation—associated mass effect, leading to visual field deficits and/or hypopituitarism.

### Outcome

Radiobiological studies demonstrate that high doses per fraction are required to obliterate cell function in nonproliferating systems, whereas conventional fractionation schemes are sufficient to remove the proliferative capacity of the tumor. Although there have been no randomized trials comparing SRS and CFR or FSR, SRS doses of 15–30 Gy to the tumor margin appear to provide comparable clonogenic control of 85%–95%, and a shorter latency period to functional obliteration than CFR or FSR. Ultimately, 50%–70% of patients appear to achieve functional control with SRS, usually within the first 2 years after treatment, although these rates vary dramatically from series to series based on the definition of functional control and length of follow-up.[16]

### Toxicity

Another added benefit of SRS appears to be its toxicity profile with an apparent lower reported risk of hypopituitarism, visual deterioration, and radiation-induced neoplasms.

Optic neuropathy—affects 1% of patients, and is not typically seen at doses below 8–9 Gy.[17] Tolerance of the optic apparatus may be reduced by nerve compression by the adenoma, ischemic changes, previous interventions, age, and other comorbidities.

Hypopituitarism—the true incidence of radiation-induced hypopituitarism is difficult to determine because most patients have previously undergone resection and/or received conventionally fractionated radiotherapy.

Memory—both SRS and FSR allow less of the dose to spill into the hypothalamus and medial temporal lobes compared to CFR.

## Paraganglioma

Paragangliomas are benign tumors that rarely lead to death. Therefore, the goal of therapy is to preserve neurologic function and quality of life, while providing durable local control. Radiotherapy is an attractive treatment option because one can avoid the morbidity (new cranial nerve palsies, CSF leaks, etc.) and mortality associated with surgery. Conventionally fractionated radiotherapy, at modest doses, has shown excellent local control rates of 86%–97% with ≥10 year follow-up. Radiosurgery appears to provide an excellent local control rate of 100% with minimal risk of complications, while offering the convenience of a single treatment.[18] Although promising, given the relatively short follow-up with SRS, further long term follow-up is needed to characterize the efficacy and complication rate associated with this modality.

## Trigeminal Neuralgia (Tic Douloureux)

Trigeminal Neuralgia is a debilitating neuropathic disorder causing severe pain in the distribution of the trigeminal nerve (CNV). Although this is not a fatal disease, it has been labeled the "suicide disease" as a result of patients taking their lives because of refractory pain.

### Epidemiology

Roughly 1:50,000 incidence in the United States, although this may be higher due to the frequent misdiagnosis of this disorder. This disorder typically develops after the fifth decade of life and is seen more commonly in women than men, with a 2:1 ratio.

### Presentation

Episodic pain in the trigeminal distribution is described as electric shocks. The pain is typically unilateral, lasting several seconds to minutes at a time. These episodes can be triggered by light touch, exposure to cold, and daily activities (shaving, brushing teeth).

### Workup

MRI scan to rule out a mass or aberrant vessel that may be compressing the trigeminal nerve.

### Treatment

Medical management with anticonvulsants (carbamazepine) remains the primary treatment of choice. A number of other options remain for patients refractory to medical therapy, including: alcohol injection, glycerol injection, balloon compression, electric current, microvascular decompression, sensory rhizotomy, and SRS. All of these therapies are successful in the majority of patients, although each carries its own unique side effect profile.

A subset of patients who remain refractory to these invasive second line therapies, refuse invasive procedures, or are elderly with multiple comorbidities warrant a noninvasive approach. For these patients, SRS remains an excellent option, providing complete pain relief in 60%–80% (requiring no medical therapy), 50%–90% pain reduction (severity/frequency) in 16%–20%, and <50% pain improvement in ≤10%, with a latency period of 3 months.[19] Among those who fail, the median time to failure is 3 years, and thus long term follow-up is needed.

### Dose

Based on the results of one multi-institutional retrospective review it appears that maximum doses ≥70 Gy improved complete pain relief rates over lower doses of 72% vs. 9%, respectively.[20]

**TABLE 6-8 Trigeminal Neuralgia Treatment**

| Treatment | Description | Side Effects |
|---|---|---|
| Anticonvulsants | Carbamazepine (treatment of choice). | Drowsiness, decreased alertness, dizziness, blurred vision. |
| Microvascular decompression | Displaces blood vessels in contact with the trigeminal root with a small pad. High success rate (>75%). | Risk of hearing loss, facial weakness/anesthesia, diplopia, CVA, mortality. |
| Partial sensory rhizotomy | Transects a part of the trigeminal nerve. Usually successful. | 100% facial anesthesia. |
| Percutaneous stereotactic radiofrequency thermal rhizotomy | Utilizes electric current to heat and thereby damage the nerve root fibers associated with pain. Successfully controls pain in most. | Facial anesthesia is common. |
| Alcohol injection | Injections of alcohol into the branches of the trigeminal nerve. Pain relief. | Pain relief is only temporary. |
| Percutaneous glycerol injection | Glycerol is injected into the trigeminal cistern. Pain relief in most. | Facial anesthesia/paresthesias common. |
| Percutaneous balloon compression | Balloon is inflated causing a pressure effect on the nerve and ultimately nerve damage. Successful pain relief in most. | Most experience facial numbness, and more than half have nerve damage resulting in temporary or permanent weakness of the muscles of mastication. |

However, the optimal dose remains to be defined in a prospective fashion. Based on the reported literature, 70–90 Gy prescribed to the maximum dose using a 4 mm isocenter focused on the proximal trigeminal nerve just anterior to the pons seems to be a reasonable approach.

*Toxicity*

Facial anesthesia occurs in 20% with a median follow-up of 5 years.[19]

## FUNCTIONAL

Leksell and Larsson developed SRS as a method for cerebral lesion generation without opening the skin and skull for the management of functional brain disorders (Parkinson's, epilepsy). Using high single doses of 50–200 Gy to produce tissue necrosis, they were able to produce a similar effect to surgical transection.

## Parkinson's

Parkinson's disease is a chronic, progressive, neurodegenerative, movement disorder, resulting from insufficient formation and action of dopamine in the brain.

*Epidemiology*

Approximately 1 million people, or 0.3% of the United States population, are affected. The incidence is between 50,000 to 60,000 cases per year with a median age of onset of 55 to 60 years. There is a slight male predominance with a male to female ratio of 1.5:1.

**TABLE 6-9 Parkinson's Target Localization**

| SRS | Target | Localization |
|---|---|---|
| Thalamotomy | Ventralis intermedius nucleus (VIM)—measures 3–4 mm in the anteroposterior dimension | 7–8 mm anterior, 11–13 mm lateral, 2 mm superior to the posterior commissure along the intercommissural line. |
| Pallidotomy | Globus pallidus interna (Gpi) | Immediately lateral to the internal capsule, just superior to the optic tract, and immediately posterior to the mammillary bodies. 2–3 mm anterior to the midcommissural point, and 18–23 mm lateral and 4–6 mm inferior to the intercommissural line. |

### Presentation

Characterized by muscle rigidity, tremor, bradykinesia, and akinesia.

### Treatment

Medical therapy is the primary treatment of choice. Patients refractory to medical management are candidates for surgical interventions that either ablate (thalamotomy or pallidotomy) or stimulate (deep brain stimulation—DBS) overactive brain nuclei. These invasive interventions are highly accurate, utilizing both stereotactic guidance and electrophysio-logic confirmation for target localization. The results are immediate and durable in 90% of patients. However, these invasive procedures carry the inherent surgical risks of death, hemorrhage, and infection.

SRS is a noninvasive alternative for producing ablative lesions that is reserved for those patients who are deemed poor neurosurgical candidates as a result of advanced age or comor-bid conditions. The disadvantages of SRS include delayed therapeutic effect of 4 to 8 weeks, and lack of electrophysiologic confirmation for target localization. One large series with long term follow-up reported a roughly 90% near complete/complete response rate that appears comparable to the results seen with radiofrequency thalamotomy and pallidotomy.[21] In addition, no late term side effects were seen in this study which appears to be superior to the reported surgical literature.

SRS treatment planning is conducted with an MRI scan using stereotactic coordinates calculated relative to a line connecting, but not including, the anterior and posterior commissures (intercommissural line) that typically measures 2.4–3.2 cm in length. Table 6-9 describes the details of SRS targeting, and the figure depicts the anatomic relationship of the two anatomic targets.

### Dose

Based on the reported literature, 120–140 Gy prescribed to the maximum dose using a 4 mm isocenter appears effective and well tolerated.[21]

**TABLE 6-10 Epilepsy SRS Target Volume**

| SRS | Target Volume |
|---|---|
| Mesial temporal lobe epileptogenic zone | The anterior part of the parahippocampal region, the entorhinal area adjacent to the collateral sulcus, and the rhinal sulcus; the head of the hippocampus; the anterior part of the hippocampal body; and the amygdalofugal part of the amygdaloid complex. |

# Epilepsy

Epilepsy is a chronic neurologic disorder characterized by recurring, unprovoked seizures.

## Epidemiology

There is a 1% incidence in the general population, predominantly affecting patients in the pediatric and elderly age groups.

## Presentation

The presenting symptoms can vary depending on the function of the areas of brain involved. In general, seizures are classified as partial (simple/complex) or generalized depending on whether there is localized or generalized involvement of the cortex, respectively. The presence of an altered consciousness differentiates complex partial from simple partial seizures.

## Treatment

The primary treatment of choice is medical therapy. For the 20% of patients who remain refractory to medical intervention, surgery is an effective second-line therapy, with an associated 68% success rate. The role of SRS, as a noninvasive alternative to surgery, is an area of active investigation. One small prospective trial evaluated the role of SRS (24 $\pm$ 1 Gy prescribed to the margin) in 21 patients with mesial temporal lobe epilepsy. At 2 years post-SRS, 65% were rendered seizure-free, with a significant reduction in seizure frequency, and an improvement in quality of life measures of mental health and role functioning. However, there was a delay between treatment and the reduction of seizure activity, and a transient increase in seizure activity was seen in all patients during the interim. Visual field deficits were present in fewer than half of these patients, which appears comparable to the complication rate seen with surgery.[22] Otherwise, no permanent neurologic deficits were noted.

SRS appears to be promising as a safe and effective noninvasive therapy for medically refractory epilepsy. However, further study is necessary to establish its long term safety and efficacy.

For epileptogenic foci located elsewhere in the brain, MRI is frequently utilized to identify areas of atrophy associated with the epileptogenic focus. Noninvasive functional imaging studies such as FDG-PET, single-photon-emission tomography (SPECT), and magnetoencephalography (MEG) act in a complementary fashion and can aid in target delineation when the MRI appears normal.

# STEREOTACTIC BODY RADIOTHERAPY (SBRT)

## Lung

Approximately 20% of patients with non-small cell lung cancer (NSCLC) present with early, localized disease. Surgery is the treatment of choice for operable patients with a 65% 5-year survival rate reported for stage I patients. Conventionally fractionated radiotherapy (CFR) offers an inferior outcome for those patients who are medically inoperable (50% local control, 15% 5–year overall survival). Dose escalation in an attempt to improve local control and survival is hampered by accelerated tumor repopulation, increased risks of toxicity, and logistical difficulties associated with extending treatment for a population burdened by multiple comorbidities. SBRT theoretically provides the biologic advantages of dose escalation while avoiding the disadvantages of the previously outlined CFR dose escalation.

One phase I dose escalation trial of 47 patients (T1-2 N0) revealed a total of 10 local failures, with 9/10 occurring at doses $\leq$ 16 Gy.[23,24] The MTD was 22 Gy $\times$ 3 for T2 tumors larger than 5 cm, and was not reached at 20 Gy $\times$ 3 for T1 tumors or at 22 Gy $\times$ 3 for T2 tumors smaller than 5 cm. A phase II trial based on these results has reached its accrual goal of 70 patients with stage I NSCLC. The results of other studies utilizing SBRT for early lung cancer with differing dose fractionation and prescription schemes appear promising (80%–100% local control, 40%–100% 2 to 3 year survival, 0%–4% grade 3 toxicity), although the median follow-up for these studies is short. The RTOG is currently accruing patients with T1–2 and T3 (chest wall only) N0 NSCLC to a multi-institutional phase I/II trial.

### Treatment Planning

Respiratory motion must be accounted for either by limiting diaphragmatic movement with abdominal compression, breath hold devices, gating, or by incorporating tumor motion into the PTV. The GTV should be contoured on CT pulmonary windows. Bronchial injury with collapse of the distal lung tissue is a toxicity unique to SBRT. Thus treatment of tumors in close proximity to the proximal bronchial tree depicted in Figure 6-1 is not recommended outside of a clinical trial. Patients with tumors located in this zone are currently excluded from the RTOG 0236 protocol.

Table 6-11 lists maximum dose limits based on radiobiologic conversion models and reported clinical experience using large doses per fraction. Although the risks of symptomatic pneumonitis are not well defined with SBRT, it appears that a V13 ≤10% and mean lung dose ≤7–8 Gy should result in acceptable toxicity.

## Liver

The liver is a common site of metastasis. Surgical resection of liver metastases in carefully selected patients is associated with a 30%–40% 5-year survival. A number of other invasive therapies including laser-induced thermo-therapy, cryosurgery, ethanol injection, intra-arterial chemotherapy, and radiofrequency ablation have been studied with varying results. Unfortunately, however, many patients are not candidates for these invasive approaches. SBRT is a noninvasive alternative that could potentially offer survival benefits similar to those seen with SRS in the setting of a single brain metastasis, while avoiding the inherent risks associated with an invasive procedure.[4]

There have been two SBRT phase I dose escalation trials published in the literature reaching 26 Gy in a single fraction and 60 Gy in three fractions without any reported dose limiting toxicities.[25,26] A phase II trial is underway to evaluate the local control rate associated with the three

---

**FIGURE 6-1** *RTOG 0236 protocol.

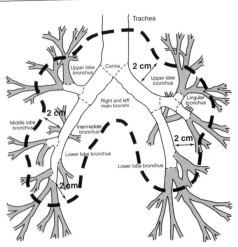

TABLE 6-11  RTOG 0236: Organ, Volume, Dose

| Organ | Volume | Dose |
|---|---|---|
| Spinal cord | Any point | 18 Gy (6 Gy per fraction) |
| Esophagus | Any point | 27 Gy (9 Gy per fraction) |
| Ipsilateral brachial plexus | Any point | 24 Gy (8 Gy per fraction) |
| Heart | Any point | 30 Gy (10 Gy per fraction) |
| Trachea and ipsilateral bronchus | Any point | 30 Gy (10 Gy per fraction) |

*RTOG 0236 protocol (*Note:* these tolerance figures have not been validated with long term follow-up).

fraction regimen. The results of other studies utilizing SBRT for liver metastases with differing dose fractionation and prescription schemes show promising results (65%–81% local control), although the median follow-up for these studies is short.

### Treatment Planning

Similar to SBRT treatments for the lung, diaphragmatic motion of the tumor must be accounted for. A CT simulation is performed with IV contrast, and the images are obtained during the arterial phase to optimize the differential between tumor and normal liver parenchyma enhancement. The authors also recommend obtaining T2-weighted fat suppressed MRI images with the patient in the treatment planning position. These images can be fused with the planning CT to help define the GTV.

Table 6-12 lists the maximum dose limits based on known tolerance data, radiobiologic conversion models, and reported clinical experience using large doses per fraction.

## SPINAL/PARASPINAL

Metastases involving the spinal and paraspinal regions are a common problem, with an incidence of 18,000 new cases per year. These tumors are frequently symptomatic, with associated pain or neurologic dysfunction. CFR is an effective therapeutic option offering palliation to the majority of patients; however, the ability to deliver doses that can effectively control gross tumor with this approach is limited by spinal cord tolerance. As a result, those patients who go on to develop symptomatic progression within their previous radiation field are offered surgery to avoid the potential complications associated with re-irradiation. SBRT can potentially offer a noninvasive alternative to surgery in this setting by providing adequate palliation while minimizing the cumulative dose to the spinal cord.

No dose escalation trials have been performed to date due to concerns of irreversible spinal cord myelopathy. Thus, SBRT doses delivered to the tumor (10–16 Gy in one fraction, 20–30 Gy in five fractions) are conservative, keeping the dose to the cord within conventional fraction sizes. This approach appears to offer durable palliation in the majority of patients (85%–90%) without any apparent neurologic toxicity.[27–29] SBRT appears to be a safe and effective palliative treatment for

TABLE 6-12  Liver: Organ, Volume, Dose Constraints

| Organ | Volume | Dose |
|---|---|---|
| Liver | 700 cc or 35% | 15 Gy (5 Gy per fraction) |
| Right kidney | 67% | 15 Gy (5 Gy per fraction) |
| Total kidney | <35% | 15 Gy (5 Gy per fraction) |
| Spinal cord | Any point | 18 Gy (6 Gy per fraction) |
| Stomach | Any point | 0 Gy (10 Gy per fraction) |

*Note:* these tolerance figures have not been validated with long term follow-up.

spinal and paraspinal metastases, although further study is necessary to establish the long term safety and efficacy of this approach, as well as to better define the dose constraints to the cord.

### Treatment Planning

Given the proximity of the spinal cord to the treated volume, one must ensure an accurate, reproducible treatment setup via patient immobilization with an invasive or noninvasive stereotactic body frame and image guidance at the time of treatment to minimize setup error.

## RETROPERITONEUM

### Renal Cell Carcinoma (RCC)

In the United States, 31,000 new cases of renal cell carcinoma are diagnosed each year. Nephrectomy is the primary treatment option with curative outcome in 90% of patients with tumor confined to the kidney (40%). Nephron-sparing surgery (NSS) allows preservation of the uninvolved kidney while providing comparable outcome to patients with a solitary lesion, reduced renal function, and medical conditions that place the patient at risk of developing reduced renal function in the future. In an effort to minimize the inherent risks associated with open surgery, minimally invasive procedures have been developed (laparoscopic partial nephrectomy, cryoablation, radiofrequency ablation), although the long term efficacy of these approaches is unknown. Although RCC is considered to be radioresistant to CFR, it appears to be radiosensitive to large doses per fraction. Based on the encouraging response to large doses per fraction, SBRT is a logical noninvasive alternative to NSS. Reported SBRT experience, though limited, appears to corroborate the apparent sensitivity of RCC to large doses per fraction. Two small retrospective series found a roughly 90% local control rate with a total dose of 40 Gy in 5 fractions, although the follow-up was short.[30,31] The use of SBRT in this setting is currently being investigated in prospective phase I trials.

### Pancreatic Cancer

The standard of care for unresectable pancreatic cancer is chemoradiation, which has a generally poor outcome. SBRT as the sole local modality may offer improved local control over CFR while allowing systemic doses of chemotherapy to be initiated without delay. One prospective phase I trial of 18 patients reached a dose of 25 Gy in one fraction without any reported grade 3 GI toxicities or local failures at this dose level over a median follow-up of 9 months.[32] A phase II trial by the same group utilized the 25 Gy in one fraction schema following a course of CFR with concurrent 5-FU in 16 patients.[33] Only two grade 3 toxicities were reported with 94% local control, although the natural history of the disease was not altered by this aggressive approach. Another phase II trial utilizing a different fractionation scheme (15 Gy × 3) found unacceptable toxicity with poor local control.[34] Further study is needed. However, given the absence of chemotherapeutic regimens capable of providing successful systemic control, the potential benefit with SBRT in this setting may be limited to patient convenience and the earlier initiation of systemic doses of chemotherapy.

## PELVIS

### Prostate

CFR is a definitive modality that appears to offer a comparable outcome to radical prostatectomy for low to intermediate risk prostate cancer. Although well tolerated, CFR requires 7 to 10 weeks of daily therapy which is not only inconvenient to the patient, but may not offer a differential benefit in tumor control over normal tissue toxicity implicit in protracted fractionated schedules, given the low $\alpha/\beta$ ratio associated with prostate cancer (1.5–3). Several investigators have shown comparable tumor control and toxicity outcomes utilizing hypofractionated schedules with fraction sizes ranging from 2.5–3.13 Gy. SBRT would provide an even shorter course of therapy with the potential for both improved disease control and acute/late toxicity.[35] Several phase I trials are currently underway. Long term follow-up will be necessary to establish the safety and efficacy of this approach.

## CONCLUSION

SRS and SBRT are precise methods of delivering high doses of radiation to a well defined target volume that were previously unattainable with conventional techniques. The radiobiologic implications of delivering these large doses promise improved tumor control outcomes. The literature reviewed in this chapter appears to support the utility of SRS and SBRT as effective treatment modalities with acceptable morbidity. Further scientific study is necessary in the form of carefully constructed prospective trials to further our understanding of these powerful tools.

## REFERENCES

1. Lo, SS, et al. The role of gamma knife radiosurgery in the management of unresectable gross disease or gross residual disease after surgery in ependymoma. *J Neurooncol,* 2006.
2. Patchell, RA, et al. A randomized trial of surgery in the treatment of single metastases to the brain. *N Engl J Med,* 1990. 322(8): p. 494–500.
3. Noordijk, EM, et al. The choice of treatment of single brain metastasis should be based on extracranial tumor activity and age. *Int J Radiat Oncol Biol Phys,* 1994. 29(4): p. 711–717.
4. Kondziolka, D., et al. Stereotactic radiosurgery plus whole brain radiotherapy versus radiotherapy alone for patients with multiple brain metastases. *Int J Radiat Oncol Biol Phys,* 1999. 45(2): p. 427–434.
5. DeAngelis, LM, JY Delattre, and JB Posner. Radiation-induced dementia in patients cured of brain metastases. *Neurology,* 1989. 39(6): p. 789–796.
6. Patchell, RA, et al. Postoperative radiotherapy in the treatment of single metastases to the brain: a randomized trial. *Jama,* 1998. 280(17): p. 1485–1489.
7. Sneed, PK, et al. A multi-institutional review of radiosurgery alone vs. radiosurgery with whole brain radiotherapy as the initial management of brain metastases. *Int J Radiat Oncol Biol Phys,* 2002. 53(3): p. 519–526.
8. Meyers, CA, et al. Neurocognitive function and progression in patients with brain metastases treated with whole-brain radiation and motexafin gadolinium: results of a randomized phase III trial. *J Clin Oncol,* 2004. 22(1): p. 157–165.
9. Flickinger, JC, et al. A dose-response analysis of arteriovenous malformation obliteration after radiosurgery. *Int J Radiat Oncol Biol Phys,* 1996. 36(4): p. 873–879.
10. Eustacchio, S, et al. Preservation of cranial nerve function following gamma knife radiosurgery for benign skull base meningiomas: experience in 121 patients with follow-up of 5 to 9.8 years. *Acta Neurochir Suppl,* 2002. 84: p. 71–76.
11. Kobayashi, T, Y Kida, and Y Mori. Long-term results of stereotactic gamma radiosurgery of meningiomas. *Surg Neurol,* 2001. 55(6): p. 325–331.
12. Kreil, W., et al. Long term experience of gamma knife radiosurgery for benign skull base meningiomas. *J Neurol Neurosurg Psychiatry,* 2005. 76(10): p. 1425–1430.
13. DiBiase, SJ, et al. Factors predicting local tumor control after gamma knife stereotactic radiosurgery for benign intracranial meningiomas. *Int J Radiat Oncol Biol Phys,* 2004. 60(5): p. 1515–1519.
14. Flickinger, JC, et al. Acoustic neuroma radiosurgery with marginal tumor doses of 12 to 13 Gy. *Int J Radiat Oncol Biol Phys,* 2004. 60(1): p. 225–230.

15. Kondziolka, D, et al. Long-term outcomes after radiosurgery for acoustic neuromas. *N Engl J Med,* 1998. 339(20): p. 1426–1433.

16. Witt, TC. Stereotactic radiosurgery for pituitary tumors. *Neurosurg Focus,* 2003. 14(5): p. e10.

17. Losa, M., et al. Gamma knife surgery for treatment of residual nonfunctioning pituitary adenomas after surgical debulking. *J Neurosurg,* 2004. 1000(3): p. 438–444.

18. Foote, RL, et al. Glomus jugulare tumor: tumor control and complications after stereotactic radiosurgery. *Head Neck,* 2002. 24(4): p. 332–338; discussion 338–339.

19. Urgosik, D, et al. Treatment of essential trigeminal neuralgia with gamma knife surgery. *J Neurosurg,* 2005. 102 Suppl: p. 29–33.

20. Kondziolka, D, et al. Stereotactic radiosurgery for trigeminal neuralgia: a multi-institutional study using the gamma unit. *J Neurosurg,* 1996. 84(6): p. 940–945.

21. Young, RF, et al. Gamma knife thalamotomy for treatment of tremor: long-term results. *J Neurosurg,* 2000. 93 Suppl 3: p. 128–135.

22. Spencer, SS. Long-term outcome after epilepsy surgery. *Epilepsia,* 1996. 37(9): p. 807–813.

23. McGarry, RC, et al. Stereotactic body radiation therapy of early-stage non-small cell lung carcinoma: phase I study. *Int J Radiat Oncol Biol Phys,* 2005. 63(4): p. 1010–1015.

24. Timmerman, R, et al. Extracranial stereotactic radioablation: results of a phase I study in medically inoperable stage I non-small cell lung cancer. *Chest,* 2003. 124(5): p. 1946–1955.

25. Schefter, TE, et al. A phase I trial of stereotactic body radiation therapy (SBRT) for liver metastases. *Int J Radiat Oncol Biol Phys,* 2005. 62(5): p. 1371–1378.

26. Herfarth, KK, et al. Stereotactic single-dose radiation therapy of liver tumors: results of a phase I/II trial. *J Clin Oncol,* 2001. 19(1): p. 164–170.

27. Chang, EL, et al. Phase I clinical evaluation of near-simultaneous computed tomographic image-guided stereotactic body radiotherapy for spinal metastases. *Int J Radiat Oncol Biol Phys,* 2004. 59(5): p. 1288–1294.

28. Ryu, S, et al. Patterns of failure after single-dose radiosurgery for spinal metastasis. *J Neurosurg,* 2004. 101 Suppl 3: p. 402–405.

29. Yamada, Y, et al. Multifractionated image-guided and stereotactic intensity-modulated radiotherapy of paraspinal tumors: a preliminary report. *Int J Radiat Oncol Biol Phys,* 2005. 62(1): p. 53–61.

30. Beitler, JJ, et al. Definitive, high-dose-per-fraction, conformal, stereotactic external radiation for renal cell carcinoma. *Am J Clin Oncol,* 2004. 27(6): p. 646–648.

31. Qian, G, Lowry J Silverman P, Grosman I Makara D, Lederman G. Stereotactic extra-cranial Radiosurgery for renal cell carcinoma. *International Journal of Radiation Oncology, Biology, and Physics,* 2003. 57(2): p. S283.

32. Koong, AC, et al. Phase I study of stereotactic radiosurgery in patients with locally advanced pancreatic cancer. *Int J Radiat Oncol Biol Phys,* 2004. 58(4): p. 1017–1021.

33. Koong, AC, et al. Phase II study to assess the efficacy of conventionally fractionated radiotherapy followed by a stereotactic radiosurgery boost in patients with locally advanced pancreatic cancer. *Int J Radiat Oncol Biol Phys,* 2005. 63(2): p. 320–323.

34. Hoyer, M, et al. Phase-II study on stereotactic radiotherapy of locally advanced pancreatic carcinoma. *Radiother Oncol,* 2005. 76(1): p. 48–53.

35. Madsen, BL, et al. Intrafractional stability of the prostate using a stereotactic radiotherapy technique. *Int J Radiat Oncol Biol Phys,* 2003. 57(5): p. 1285–1291.

# 7

# Palliation and Oncologic Emergencies

*Molly Gabel, MD*

## OVERVIEW

Although radiation is quite frequently used to palliate the disability and pain caused by advanced cancers, until recently the literature has reflected a paucity of data directing optimum care. This chapter separates emergent conditions from general palliation, but the overriding principle is the same: to offer rapid relief from symptoms while causing minimal toxicity. Two recent advances have resulted in significant improvement toward this goal: technologic advances within radiation oncology and emergence of palliative medicine as a science. These advances used together offer the clinician valuable data upon which to base treatment practices.

Technologic advances within the field include highly conformal delivery techniques designed to minimize normal tissue toxicity. Cranial and extracranial radiosurgery are being used with increasing frequency in the treatment of brain metastases, spinal metastases, and, most recently, liver metastases. Advances outside of our field, such as improved stenting techniques for relief of superior vena cava syndrome and dysphagia, allow clinicians to offer options that complement or replace radiation.

The field of palliative medicine has evolved greatly over the past decade. The American Board of Hospice and Palliative Medicine (ABHPM) defined palliative medicine as *"the medical discipline devoted to achieve the best possible quality of life of the patient and family throughout the course of a life-threatening illness through the relief of suffering and the control of symptoms."* Since 1996 the ABHPM has certified physicians, and it is anticipated that the first American Board of Medical Specialties (ABMS) exam in hospice and palliative medicine will be given in 2008. Training and credentialing requirements have promoted palliative medicine as a science and, as a result, current research efforts focus on detailed quality of life assessment in addition to the more standard outcomes of pain relief, local control, and survival.

This chapter will review the basis for standard palliative treatment options and describe promising new technologies and outcome measures that have led to current clinical trials.

# I. ONCOLOGIC EMERGENCIES

## Spinal Cord Compression

### Epidemiology

Malignancy-associated spinal cord compression is seen in approximately 5%–10% of all cancer patients. The vast majority are metastatic lesions from prostate, lung, and breast primaries, followed less frequently by other malignancies and primary spinal cord tumors.[1]

### Presenting Symptoms

Symptoms appear in characteristic frequency and order. Back pain is seen in almost all patients and, if undiagnosed, may progress to radicular pain, weakness, sensory deficits, loss of bladder and/or bowel control, and then paralysis. Assessment of the neurologic status of the cancer patient presenting with back pain is essential, with particular attention to the sensory examination because that will help identify the level of the lesion.

### Diagnosis

MRI has replaced myelography as the gold standard for diagnosis, primarily because it is non-invasive. Alternatively, CT myelogram may be used.

### Treatment Overview

Optimal management requires multidisciplinary input from neurosurgeon, medical, and radiation oncologist.

#### Steroids

Prompt initiation of steroids is essential. Standard clinical practice is to administer dexamethasone 10mg IV bolus followed by 16 mg per day in divided doses based on one small randomized study,[2] although strong data are lacking.[3]

#### Assessment for local treatment

- **Surgery:** Although older data did not show any advantage to combining a posterior surgical approach with radiation, recent data indicates that, in select patients, anterior decompressive laminectomy significantly improves the ambulation rate.[4,5] Surgery is indicated in patients presenting with:
  a. a single destructive lesion,
  b. life expectancy > 3 months,
  c. good performance status,
  d. limited or no visceral metastases.

Of course, surgery is also indicated to obtain tissue diagnosis for patients presenting with cord compression without a previous cancer diagnosis.

---

**BOX 7-1**

Prospective trial randomizing between surgery followed by radiation (n = 50) vs. radiation alone (n = 51). This study was stopped early because at a median follow-up of 3 months, surgery significantly improved ambulation rates (84% vs. 57%) and length of neurologic improvement (122 days vs. 13 days).

Patchell, R. et al. Direct decompressive surgical resection in the treatment of spinal cord compression caused by metastatic cancer: a randomized trial. Lancet (366): 643–48 2005.

*Radiation Therapy*

Radiation is indicated for most patients, whether used alone or to improve local control after surgery.

*Radiation Technique*   Treatment fields for the treatment of high grade or complete cord compression historically include the spinal lesion(s) plus two vertebral bodies above and below the lesion(s). Consideration may be given to decreasing this margin when radiologic studies clearly demarcate the extent of metastatic lesion(s) and when larger fields would result in significant toxicity.

Fraction size for standard therapy depends on field size, anatomic location and patient prognosis and comorbidities. Fractionation varies worldwide from delivering a single fraction of 800 cGy to 4000 cGy delivered in 20 fractions.[6,7] The most common fractionation schedules used in the United States are 3,000 cGy delivered in ten fractions or 3,500–3,750 cGy delivered in 14 to 15 fractions. Further discussion of fractionation is included in the Bone Metastases section.

For patients presenting with mild to moderate cord compression, extracranial radiosurgery has been shown to have promising results for both pain relief and improved neurologic status.[8,9]

*Outcome and Prognosis*

Significant reduction of back pain after radiation occurs in 80%–90% of patients. The return of neurologic function depends on pretreatment function, duration of motor deficits, and tumor cell type. In general, full neurologic function is obtained for >90% of patients who are ambulatory at the time of spinal cord compression presentation and treatment. In contrast, only 28% of patients presenting with paresis, and 21% of patients with paraplegia regain ambulatory capacity after treatment.[10]

## Superior Vena Cava Syndrome

### Epidemiology

In up to 70%–90% of cases, SVC syndrome is caused by malignancy. The most frequently seen histologies are small and non-small cell carcinomas of the lung, and lymphomas (particularly primary mediastinal large B-cell lymphoma with sclerosis, diffuse large cell and lymphoblastic lymphomas). It is estimated that 20% of patients with small cell carcinoma of the lung will develop SVC syndrome.[11,12]

SVC syndrome is said to be an emergency due to the risk of airway obstruction and/or cerebral edema. However, lack of data showing any correlation between duration of symptoms and treatment outcome has led many authors to conclude that although rapid palliation is warranted, timing of treatment has less importance than originally believed.[11,12]

### Presenting Symptoms

Dyspnea is the most common symptom, and some patients report a sensation of facial fullness and swelling which is exacerbated by bending down. Additional pathognomonic findings include distention of the jugular veins, presence of collateral circulation on the anterior chest wall, and facial edema.

### Diagnosis

Although CXR will reveal a lung or mediastinal mass in the majority of cases, CT scan of the chest is preferred because it can accurately localize the extent and level of the obstruction. MRI may also be used for patients unable to tolerate IV contrast.

### Treatment Overview

1. It is critical to make a histologic diagnosis to direct appropriate treatment.
2. Although many physicians prescribe steroids at the time of diagnosis (presumably due to the response rate seen in some tumor types), data are lacking to support the use of steroids.[11,12]

3. If a patient presents with thrombosis, consideration should be given to anticoagulation.
4. Intraluminal stenting can provide the quickest palliation (<48 hours) and does not inter-fere with systemic or radiation therapy delivered later.[11-13]
5. Chemosensitive tumors (lymphomas, germ cell, and small cell tumors) respond well to sys-temic therapy, and radiation is added to decrease local recurrence (lymphoma) and/or increase survival (small cell lung).[13]
6. Initially, radiation may be given (for non-chemosensitive tumors) alone or in combination with chemotherapy.

### Radiation Technique

Fractionation is dependent upon the rapidity and severity of symptom onset, as well as on field size. For patients presenting with acute symptom onset, initial fractions of 250–400 cGy × 3 fol-lowed by fraction size reduction yields excellent results, with palliation observed after only two to four fractions. Total dose should depend on the histology. Doses equivalent to 3,500–4,500 cGy delivered at standard fractionation should be used for lymphomas, while lung cancers require dose equivalents of 6,000 cGy or more.[14,15]

### Outcome/Prognosis

For chemo and radiosensitive tumors, local response rates range from 75%–90%, and radiation response does not appear to be related to fractionation. For non-small cell carcinomas, the range of local response with radiation ranges from 50%–90%, and does depend on both fraction size and total dose.[11,12] Overall survival after treatment is dependent upon the type and extent of disease.

## II. PALLIATION

### Overview

A significant proportion of patients receive radiation with palliative intent. Every effort should be made to offer rapid palliation with minimal toxicity and to consider the complexities inherent in evaluation of quality of life outcomes.[16-19]

### Brain Metastases

#### Epidemiology

Brain metastases are the most common type of intracranial tumor, occurring in up to 30% of all cancer patients. Frequent primary cancers metastasizing to the brain include lung, breast, colon, renal cell, and melanoma. Even with treatment, brain metastases cause significant morbidity and account for approximately one third of all cancer deaths.

#### Presenting Symptoms

Symptoms are related to cerebral edema and the location of the lesion, and include headache, decreased mentation, focal neurologic deficits, and new-onset seizures.

#### Diagnosis

Although CT scan may identify large lesions, MRI provides greater sensitivity in identifying sub-centimeter lesions. As discussed later in this section, treatment and prognosis are strongly corre-lated to the number of cerebral metastases; therefore, MRI is essential in the workup of patients presenting with limited metastatic disease.

## Treatment Overview

The goal of treatment is to provide symptomatic relief and local tumor control. The optimal therapy depends on the location, size and number of lesions, the extracranial tumor control, the patient's neurologic and general medical conditions, and the natural history of the primary tumor site.

### Pharmacologic

Steroids are indicated to reduce edema. In patients presenting with significant headache, nausea/vomiting, or severe neurologic impairment, doses similar to those used for treatment of spinal cord compression are advised. For patients with more stable conditions, consideration may be given to dose reduction or initiation of steroids only upon neurologic worsening. Anticonvulsants are indicated for patients presenting with seizures. For those patients presenting with brain metastases without seizure activity, the risk of future seizures is approximately 30%, but the toxicity and relative inefficacy of anticonvulsants in preventing seizures render their use unnecessary.

### Surgical

Craniotomy is of greatest value for patients requiring histologic diagnosis, immediate relief of symptoms, or for select patients for whom surgery confers a local control advantage (see below). Surgery is most often used when there is a single intracranial metastasis and controlled extracranial disease.

### Radiation

Radiation is the cornerstone of palliative treatment for brain metastases. Multiple studies have shown benefit whether used alone or in combination with surgery.

*Patients presenting with multiple brain metastases*    Whole brain radiotherapy is the standard treatment. Although fractionation has been the focus of several RTOG studies (doses ranging from 2000 cGy in five fractions to 4,000 cGy in 20 fractions), there appears to be no difference in symptomatic response rates or survival between regimens. The two most commonly prescribed schedules used in the United States are 3,000 cGy delivered in 10 fractions, or 3,750 cGy delivered in 15 fractions. Selection of fraction size depends mostly on patient comorbidity and prognosis.[20] To date, dose escalation, accelerated fractionation, and the use of radiosensitizers have not been shown to improve on the results of standard treatment.

Whole brain radiation is associated with both acute and chronic toxicities. Temporary effects include mild fatigue, hair loss, headache, and nausea/vomiting. The most critical chronic toxicity is radiation-associated dementia, best studied in lung cancer patients. Although early studies showed concerning rates of dementia one year after radiation, the dementia was found to be associated with high radiation fraction size ($>3$Gy per fraction).[21] Later studies introduced the concept of multifactorial causation for the dementia (comorbidities, paraneoplastic syndromes, and chemotherapy), and found no objective evidence of decline in mental status after radiotherapy.[22]

*Patients presenting with one to three brain metastases*    Over the past decade, this clinical presentation has been the focus of multiple clinical trials. There are five treatment options:

1. Whole brain radiotherapy: As described in the previous section.
2. Surgery followed by whole brain radiation: Several retrospective and randomized studies have shown that surgery added to whole brain radiotherapy confers both survival and local control advantage in select patients presenting with a single brain metastasis.[23,24]
3. Surgery without whole brain radiotherapy: Whole brain radiotherapy following surgery is standard of care, based largely on data from retrospective trials. Only one randomized trial has been performed comparing surgery alone to surgery followed by whole brain radiation.

Although there was no improvement in survival, patients in the radiotherapy arm experienced a decrease in local recurrence.[25] Surgery without whole brain radiotherapy is advised only for patients at particular risk for radiation-induced dementia, or for patients with histologies deemed radioresistant.

4. Whole brain radiation plus stereotactic boost: Two randomized trials compared whole brain radiotherapy versus whole brain radiotherapy followed by stereotactic boost. Kondziolka et al conducted a trial which stopped accrual early due to greater than expected results. Patients in the radiosurgical boost arm experienced both reduction in local failure (100% vs. 8%) and improved survival (7.5 months vs. 11.5 months).[26] This trial, however, included only 27 patients. A similar RTOG study randomized 333 patients. The group receiving the boost experienced a greater rate of stability or improvement in performance status at 6 months (27% vs. 43%) and a slight survival advantage (median survival 4.9 vs. 6.5 months).[27]

---

**BOX 7-2**

333 patients were randomized to whole brain radiation (3750 cGy delivered in 15 fractions) vs. whole brain radiation plus stereotactic boost (15–24Gy single fraction). The group receiving the boost experienced a greater rate of stability or improvement in performance status at 6 months (27% vs. 43%) and a slight survival advantage (median survival 4.9 vs. 6.5 months). The subgroup meeting criteria for RPA Class I had a median survival of 11.5 months.

Andrews, D. et al. Whole brain radiotherapy with or without stereotactic boost for patients with one to three brain metastases: phase III results of the RTOG 9508 randomized trial. *Lancet* 363(9422): 1665–72, 2004.

---

5) Radiosurgery without whole brain radiation: Several retrospective studies have shown no difference in survival, but a local control advantage to adding whole brain radiation to stereotactic radiosurgery (SRS). A QOL analysis showed decreased memory loss, depression and fatigue in patients receiving radiosurgery alone,[28] but the authors admit their results need validation. Sneed et al reported a retrospective comparison of outcomes in 569 patients treated at 10 institutions either with whole brain radiation plus SRS or with SRS alone. They found no survival difference, but patients in the SRS alone group required salvager treatment more often (37% vs. 7%).[29]

*Prognosis*

The 1 year survival is 15%, with median survivals ranging from 3 to 16 months and neurologic improvement in 50%–90% depending on treatment and patient factors. Using methodology that creates a regression tree according to prognostic significance, an analysis of results from RTOG trials has identified three classes of patients with median survivals of 7 (patients presenting with KPS >70, age <65 and controlled extracranial disease), 4, and 2 months (KPS <70) respectively.[30]

## Current Clinical Trials

- **Study Group:  EORTC**
    - Eligibility: One to three brain metastases
    - Trial Design: Phase III Randomized:
        **SRS/surgery alone vs. SRS/surgery + WBRT**
- **Study Group: RTOG 0320**
    - Eligibility: One to three Brain metastases secondary to non-small cell lung cancer
    - Trial Design: Phase III Randomized:
        **WBRT + SRS alone vs. WBRT + SRS + temozolomide vs. WBRT + SRS + erlotinib**

- **Study Group: ECOG**
  - Eligibility: Brain metastases secondary to non-small cell lung cancer
  - Trial Design:
    **Phase II WBRT + temozolomide**

## Patients Presenting with Leptomeningeal Metastases, Cranial Nerve Palsies, or Leukocytosis Associated with Acute Leukemia

For those patients presenting with carcinomatous metastases, intrathecal chemotherapy is the standard treatment. Radiation is used only to treat bulky areas of disease obstructing CSF outflow or causing focal neurologic symptoms.[31]

In patients presenting with cranial nerve palsies associated with lymphoma or leukemia, cranial radiation has an overall response rate of 95% with median time to response of 12 days. Although delayed radiation did not affect the response rate, earlier treatment (within 3 days) resulted in more rapid symptom resolution.[32]

Hyperleukocytosis (WBC >100,000) occurring in patients with acute leukemia is often associated with central nervous system and/or pulmonary infiltrate. Although randomized data are lacking, case reports and retrospective series have shown benefit in adding cranial and/or pulmonary irradiation in addition to antimetabolites.[33-35] Although it is imperative to start radiation as soon as possible in order to prevent cranial hemorrhage, care should be taken to limit cerebral edema with steroids, particularly in patients presenting with papilledema. Reported doses range from 1.5 Gy in one fraction to 15 Gy in 10 fractions and, from the limited literature, it appears that doses between 3 and 6 Gy in one to three fractions result in excellent outcomes.

## Bone Metastases

### Presenting Symptoms

The most common symptom is pain, occurring in 70% of patients with bony metastases. Although the majority of patients report pain levels of 7 to 9, almost one quarter report their pain as intolerable. Less than half of patients presenting for palliative radiation report measurable pain relief with prescribed analgesics.[36]

### Diagnosis

Bone scan is the most widely utilized method for detection of skeletal metastases, as it offers excellent sensitivity and evaluation of the entire skeleton. CT scan and MRI may be performed to help demarcate destructive lesions, but their expense prohibits routine use. Consideration of bone biopsy should be given when tissue diagnosis is needed.

### Treatment Overview

Bone metastases may be treated with systemic chemotherapy, radionuclides, or local field radiation. Bisphosphonates have been shown to significantly decrease the risk of pathologic fracture, the need for palliative radiation, and incidence of hypercalcemia, while offering a favorable toxicity profile.[37] The primary advantage of radioisotopes is their ability to treat multiple sites of metastatic disease, and the primary toxicity seen is pancytopenia, with counts reaching approximately 50% of pretreatment levels.[25] External beam radiation only causes significant pancytopenia when fields are large, and is therefore recommended for localized bony disease.

*Radiation Technique*

Radiation is delivered to bony lesions with margin given for daily motion and set-up variation. Care should be given to use techniques that shield oropharynx and bowel, thereby minimizing treatment-related morbidity.

As with all palliative radiation courses, the optimum fractionation depends on field size and anatomic location. In the United States, the most commonly prescribed fractionation schedules are 3,000 cGy delivered in 10 fractions or daily fractions of 250 cGy delivered in 14 or 15 fractions.

Several randomized studies[38-41] have compared palliation of bone metastases with a single 800 cGy fraction to the standard 3,000 cGy delivered in 10 fractions. These studies have shown similar pain control but higher retreatment rates (18% vs. 9%) in the single fraction arm. Similar results were obtained in a Dutch trial comparing 800 cGy ×1 with 400 cGy ×6.[42]

---

**BOX 7-3**

This was a prospective randomized trial of single 800 cGy fraction (n = 455) vs. fractionated (3,000 cGy in 10 fractions, n = 443). Although late toxicity (4% vs. 4%), complete pain relief (15% vs. 18%), and partial pain relief (50% vs. 48%) were not significantly different, the fractionated group demonstrated greater acute toxicity (10% vs. 17%) and decreased need for later retreatment (18% vs. 9%).

Hartsell WF et al. Randomized trial of short- vs. long-course radiotherapy for palliation of painful bone metastases. *Journal of the National Cancer Institute* 97(11): 798–804, 2005.

---

Retreatment of bony metastases has been reported, with pain relief in >80% and overall local control rates as high as 95%.[43-45]

### Prognosis/Outcome

Both radiopharmaceuticals and external beam radiation yield response rates of 75%, with 25% of patients obtaining a complete resolution of pain and 50% obtaining partial relief.[39] Maximal pain relief occurs most typically 4 to 12 weeks after completion of radiotherapy, indicating that re-ossification plays a role in pain reduction.

### Current Clinical Trials:

- **Study Group: CALGB**
  - Eligibility: Patients receiving androgen deprivation for bone metastases secondary to prostate cancer
  - Trial Design: Phase III Randomized:
    **Zoledronate vs. placebo**
- **Study Group: Canadian NCI and RTOG 0433**
  - Eligibility: Painful bone metastases s/p previous radiation
  - Trial Design: Phase III Randomized:
    **Single fraction vs. fractionated re-irradiation**

## Liver Metastases

### Epidemiology

Liver metastases are most commonly associated with colorectal cancer primary. Twenty percent of patients have liver metastases at the time of diagnosis, and 50%–60% of recurrences involve the liver.

*Diagnosis*

CT scan can detect lesions >1cm, and MRI may help to differentiate metastatic disease from cysts or hemangiomas. If nonsurgical treatment is planned, PET scan is a valuable tool used to assess treatment response.

*Treatment Options*

1. Surgical resection is potentially curative for select patients, resulting in survival rates as high as 40%.[46] Selection criteria include <4 lesions and size/anatomic location amenable to surgery with minimal resection of surrounding normal tissue. Unfortunately, due to poor baseline hepatic function, size, number, or location of the tumors, only 25% of patients are surgical candidates at the time of presentation.[47]
2. Chemotherapy is most commonly used when there is uncontrolled disease outside the liver or when liver lesions are numerous. Techniques include systemic and/or regional administration, or chemoembolization.
3. Radiofrequency ablation, whether done at the time of surgical resection or percutaneously, has reported ablation rates of 90% and 5-year survival of 26%.[48,49]
4. Radiation: There has been a recent resurgence of interest in using radiation to palliate liver lesions. Precise localization minimizes the amount of normal liver treated, and early studies show response rates of greater than 80% and survival rates comparable to surgery.

   It is widely accepted that the whole liver can tolerate only 30 Gy, and doses required to eradicate sizable liver lesions is 70–80 Gy at standard fractionation.

   a. **3D conformal technique:** Several small series have shown that doses >70 Gy to liver lesions can be achieved with 10% risk of radiation-induced liver toxicity.[50] Multivariate analysis of 203 patients undergoing conformal radiation to liver lesions showed that the mean liver dose > 31Gy, hepatobiliary rather than metastatic tumor and male gender predisposed patients to higher risk of radiation-induced liver damage.[51]
   b. **Extracranial stereotactic radiosurgery:** Optimal candidates for extracranial stereotactic radiosurgery have five or less lesions, all measuring <6 cm. Although this technique is limited by lesion location within the liver (and resultant movement upon inspiration), several Phase I/II trials have demonstrated excellent efficacy with favorable toxicity profiles using either single fraction or fractionated radiosurgery[52,53] (see Box 7-4). These data, combined with software to account for respiration, have encouraged investigators to study this technique on a larger scale. As information such as optimal dose and careful monitoring of liver function and toxicity are needed, readers are encouraged to offer SRS for liver lesions only as part of a clinical trial.
   c. **Other techniques:** Investigators in Europe have explored intraoperative placement of interstitial catheters and the role of sphere delivery. Most commonly sphere delivery entails delivery of Yttrium-90 (or other comparable radioisotope) through the hepatic artery.

**BOX 7-4**

Dose limiting toxicity was defined in this study as Grade 3 or 4 small bowel or liver toxicity. Eligibility criteria for study enrollment included lesion size < 6 cm and adequate pretreatment liver function. Dose escalation began with 12Gy × 3 fractions, and continued to 20Gy × 3 fractions. No patient experienced dose-limiting toxicity.

Sheffer et al. A clinical phase I dose escalation trial to determine maximum tolerable dose of stereotactic body radiation therapy (SBRT) for liver metastases.

### Outcome/Prognosis

Surgical resection, radiofrequency ablation, and radiation can each achieve an 80% or greater local control rate and prolongation of median survival in treated patients.[54,55] Surgery and radiation confer greater survival benefit, possibly due to selection bias.

### Current Clinical Trials:

- **Study Group: RTOG 0438**
  - Eligibility: Liver metastases <5 lesions, none >6 cm
  - Trial Design
    **Phase I highly conformal SRT**

## Splenic Radiation

Palliative splenic radiation therapy is used to relieve symptoms of pain and distention caused by splenomegaly associated with CML, AML, CLL, idiopathic myelofibrosis, polycythemia vera, and ITP. Treatment is usually administered in two to three fractions per week. Pretreatment assessment of blood counts is necessary to allow dose escalation. The most common fractionation scheme is 50 cGy per fraction, escalated to 100 cGy per fraction to a total dose of 350 to 600 cGy.[52] About one third of patients experience significant cytopenia (Hgb <7, WBC <1,000 and platelets <20,000) and treatment-related mortality is similar to that seen with splenectomy.[56] Care should be taken to monitor the dose to the ipsilateral kidney, especially when considering retreatment.

## Gynecologic Cancers

Patients presenting with bleeding gynecologic tumors may be treated with either high dose rate brachytherapy (should geometry prove favorable) or limited central external beam radiation. Careful consideration should be given to fractionation, for patients with no evidence of metastatic disease are at risk for late bowel and bladder toxicities with aggressive initial fraction sizes. For patients presenting with locoregional disease, consideration should be given to delivering three initial fractions of 3 Gy each to the central tumor, and continue treatment with whole pelvic radiation at standard fractionation.

## Ocular Tumors

Metastatic disease is the most common ocular malignancy, and response rates to external beam radiation depend on dose and primary site of disease. The most common fractionation schedule is 25 to 30 Gy delivered in 10 fractions. Dose and fractionation should be driven by the type of metastatic lesion. Response rates range from 60% (breast cancer primary) to 100% (lymphomas).

## Palliation of Recurrent Disease

Retreatment may offer short-term palliation but carries with it the risk of late toxicities. Patients suffering from uncontrolled systemic disease with localized symptomatology may benefit most because retreatment may reduce discomfort greatly during their last weeks of life.

### Respiratory Distress

Patients previously treated with external beam radiation and presenting with symptomatic endobronchial disease can be offered HDR intraluminal radiation with expected palliation of respiratory symptoms in 80%–90% of patients. Standard fractionation schemes include 7 Gy × 3, 10 Gy × 2 or one fraction of 20 Gy, prescribed to a depth of 1 cm from the catheter. Laser resection of intraluminal tumor should be considered if technical difficulty in placing the catheter or excessive edema is expected.[19]

## *Dysphagia*

A number of treatment options exist for patients presenting with symptomatic esophageal lesions. Placement of esophageal stents, limited field external beam radiation, or HDR radiation all are effective means of palliating pain and dysphagia. The most common fractionation schedule used after previous treatment is 6–8 Gy delivered in three fractions, although lower fraction size should be considered if patients have received prior radiation to the area. Toxicity from HDR treatment can be as high as 30%, occurring within 6 months of retreatment, with stricture and fistula most commonly seen. A patient presenting with painful dysphagia should be offered multidisciplinary evaluation to determine the optimal mode of palliation.

## *Locally Advanced Rectal Disease*

Either limited field external beam radiation or endorectal high dose rate radiation may be offered to relieve pain and obstruction form large rectal tumors. Palliation is achieved in 70% of patients, and when the two modalities are combined, the response rate may be higher. Typical fractionation for external beam treatment is six fractions of 5 Gy each, delivered twice per week. HDR fractionation is similar to that previously described for relief of dysphagia.

## ADDITIONAL SUGGESTED READING

### Spinal Cord Compression

1. Abraham J. Assessment and treatment of patients with malignant spinal cord compression. *Journal of Support Oncology* 2:377–401, 2004.
2. Vecht C et al. Initial bolus of conventional vs. high-dose dexamethasone in metastatic spinal cord compression. *Neurology* 39:1255, 1989.
3. Loblaw, D. Emergency treatment of malignant extradural spinal cord compression: An evidence-based guideline. *Journal of Clinical Oncology* 16:1613–24, 1998.
4. Van den Bent, M. Surgical resection improves outcome in metastatic epidural spinal cord compression. *Lancet* Aug 20–26 366(9484):609–610, 2005.
5. Patchell R et al. Direct decompressive surgical resection in the treatment of spinal cord compression caused by metastatic cancer: a randomized trial. Lancet (366):643–48 2005.
6. Janjan N. Radiotherapeutic management of spinal metastases. *Journal Pain Symptom Management,* Jan; 11(1); 47–56, 1996.
7. Rades D et al. Evaluation of five radiation schedules and prognostic factors for metastatic spinal cord compression. *Journal of Clinical Oncology* 23:3366–75, 2005.
8. Rock J et al. The evolving role of stereotactic radiosurgery and stereotactic radiation therapy for patients with spine tumors. *Journal of Neuro-Oncology* 69(1–3):319–34, 2004.
9. Ryu S et al. Image-guided and intensity-modulated radiosurgery for patients with spinal metastasis. *Cancer* 97(8):2013–8, 2003.
10. Helweg-Larsen S. Clinical outcome in metastatic spinal cord compression. A prospective study of 153 patients. *Acta Neurologica Scandinavica* 94(4):269–75, 1996 Oct.

### SVC Syndrome

11. Wilson LD, Detterbeck FC, Yahalom J. Clinical Practice. Superior vena cava syndrome with malignant causes. *N Engl J Med* 356:1862–1869, 2007.
12. Rowell NP et al. Steroids, radiotherapy, chemotherapy and stents for superior vena caval obstruction in carcinoma of the bronchus: a systematic review. *Clinical Oncology* 14:338–51, 2002.

13. Nicholson AA. et al. Treatment of malignant superior vena cava obstruction: metal stents or radiation therapy. *Journal of Vascular & Interventional Radiology* 8(5):781–8, 1997.
14. Chan RH et al. Superior vena cava obstruction in small-cell lung cancer. International *Journal of Radiation Oncology, Biology, Physics* 38(3):513–20, 1997.
15. Armstrong, BA et al. Role of irradiation in the management of superior vena cava syndrome. International *Journal of Radiation Oncology, Biology, Physics* 13(4):531–9, 1987.

## General Palliative Care

16. Chow E et al. Accuracy of survival prediction by palliative radiation oncologists. International Journal of Radiation *Oncology, Biology, Physics* 61(3):870–873, 2005.
17. Anderson P and Coia L. Fractionation and outcomes with palliative radiotherapy. *Seminars in Radiation Oncology* 10(3):191–9, 2000.
18. Barton M et al. Palliative radiotherapy of bone metastases: an evaluation of outcome measures. *Journal of Evaluation in Clinical Practice* 7(1):47–64, 2001.
19. Konski A, Feigenberg S and Chow E. Palliative Radiation Therapy. *Seminars in Oncology* 32(2):156–164, 2005.

## Brain Metastases

20. Coia LR. The role of radiation therapy in the treatment of brain metastases. International *Journal of Radiation Oncology, Biology, Physics* 23(1):229–38, 1992.
21. DeAngelis LM, Posner JB. Radiation-induced dementia in patients cured of brain metastases. *Neurology* 39:789–796, 1989.
22. Van Oosterhout AG, Boon PJ, Houx PJ et al. Follow-up of cognitive functioning in patients with small cell lung cancer. *International Journal of Radiation Oncology, Biology, Physics* 31:911–914, 1995.
23. Patchell RA et al. A randomized trial of surgery in the treatment of single metastases to the brain. *New England Journal of Medicine* 322(8):494–500, 1990 Feb 22.
24. Mintz AH et al. A randomized trial to assess the efficacy of surgery in addition to radiotherapy in patients with a single cerebral metastasis. *Cancer* 78(7):1470–6, 1996 Oct 1.
25. Patchell R et al. Postoperative radiotherapy in the treatment of single brain metastasis to the brain. *Journal of the American Medical Association* 280:1485, 1998.
26. Kondziolka D et al. Stereotactic radiosurgery plus whole brain radiotherapy versus radiotherapy alone for patients with multiple brain metastases. International Journal of *Radiation Oncology, Biology, Physics* 45(2):427–34, 1999 Sep 1.
27. Andrews DW et al. Whole brain radiation therapy with or without stereotactic radiosurgery boost for patients with one to three brain metastases: phase III results of the RTOG 9508 randomized trial. *Lancet* 363(9,422):1665–1672, 2004 May 22.
28. Kondziolka D et al. Radiosurgery with or without whole-brain radiotherapy for brain metastases: the patients' perspective regarding complications. *American Journal of Clinical Oncology* 28:173–179, 2005.
29. Sneed P et al. A multi-institutional review of radiosurgery alone vs. radiosurgery with whole brain radiotherapy as the initial management of brain metastases. *International Journal of Radiation Oncology, Biology, Physics* 53:519–526, 2002.
30. Gaspar L et al. Recursive partitioning analysis (RPA) of prognostic factors in three Radiation Therapy Oncology Group (TROG) brain metastases trials. *International Journal of Radiation Oncology, Biology, Physics* 37(4):745–751.
31. Kim L. Glantz MJ. Neoplastic meningitis. *Current Treatment Options in Oncology* 2(6):517–27, 2001 Dec.

32. Gray J, and Wallner K. Reversal of cranial nerve dysfunction with radiation therapy on adults with lymphoma and leukemia. *International Journal of Radiation Oncology, Biology, Physics* (19):439–444, 1990.
33. Dutcher J, Schiffer C and Wiernik P. Hyperleukocytosis in adult acute nonlymphocytic leukemia: impact on remission rate and duration, and survival. *Journal of Clinical Oncology* 5(9):1364–1372, 1987 Sep.
34. von Eyben F, Siddiqui M and Spanos G. High voltage irradiation and hydroxyurea for pulmonary leukostasis in acute myelogenous leukemia. *Acta Haematologica* 77(3):180–182, 1987.
35. Flasshove M et al. Pulmonary and cerebral irradiation for hyperleukocytosis in acute myelomonocytic leukemia. *Leukemia* 8(10):1792, 1994.

## Bone Metastases

36. Janjan NA et al. Presenting symptoms in patients referred to a multidisciplinary clinic for bone metastases. *Journal of Pain & Symptom Management* 16(3):171–178, 1998.
37. Krempien R. et al. Bisphosphonates and bone metastases: current status and future directions. *Expert Review of Anticancer Therapy* 5(2):295–305, 2005 Apr.
38. Silberstein, E. Teletherapy and radiopharmaceutical therapy of painful bone metastases. *Seminars in Nuclear Medicine* 35(2):152–158, 2005.
39. Janjan, N. Radiation for bone metastases. *Cancer Suppl* 80(8); 1628–1645, 1997.
40. Hartsell WF et al. Randomized trial of short- versus long-course radiotherapy for palliation of painful bone metastases. *Journal of the National Cancer Institute* 97(11):798–804, 2005.
41. Anonymous. 8 Gy single fraction radiotherapy for the treatment of metastatic skeletal pain: randomized comparison with a multi-fraction schedule over 12 months of patient follow-up. Bone Pain Trial Working Party. *Radiotherapy & Oncology* 52(2):111–121, 1999 Aug.
42. Steenland E et al. The effect of a single fraction compared to multiple fractions on painful bone metastases: a global analysis of the Dutch bone metastasis study. *Radiotherapy & Oncology* 52(2):101–109, 1999 Aug.
43. Mithal NP et al. Retreatment with radiotherapy for painful bone metastases. International *Journal of Radiation Oncology, Biology, Physics* 29(5):1011–1014, 1994.
44. Milker-Zabel S et al. Clinical results of retreatment of vertebral bone metastases by stereotactic conformal radiotherapy and intensity-modulated radiotherapy. *International Journal of Radiation Oncology, Biology, Physics* 55(1):162–167, 2003.
45. Ryu S et al. 'Full dose' re-irradiation of human cervical spinal cord. *American Journal of Clinical Oncology* 23(1):29–31, 2000.

## Liver Metastases

46. Liu LX, Zhang WH and Jiang HC. Current treatment for liver metastases from colorectal cancer. *World Journal of Gastroenterology* 9(2):193–200, 2003.
47. Fiorentini G et al. Global approach to hepatic metastases from colorectal cancer: indication an outcome of intra-arterial chemotherapy and other hepatic-directed treatments. *Medical Oncology* 17(3):163–173, 2000.
48. Chen MH et al. Treatment efficacy of radiofrequency ablation of 228 patients with malignant tumor and the relevant complications. *World Journal of Gastro-enterology* 11(40): 6395–6401, 2005.
49. Gillams AR and Lee WR. Radiofrequency ablation of colorectal liver metastases. *Abdominal Imaging* 30(4):419–426, 2005.
50. Greco C et al. Radiotherapy of liver malignancies from whole liver irradiation to stereotactic hypofractionated radiotherapy. *Tumori* 90(1):73–79, 2004.

51. Dawson L and Lawrence T. The role of radiotherapy in the treatment of liver metastases. *Cancer Journal* 10(2):139–144, 2004.

52. Schefter T et al. A phase I trial of stereotactic body radiation therapy (SBRT) for liver metastases. International *Journal of Radiation Oncology, Biology and Physics* 62(5): 1371–1378, 2005.

53. Herfarth K et al. Stereotactic single dose radiation therapy of liver tumors: results of a phase I/II trial. *Journal of Clinical Oncology* 19(1):164–170, 2001.

54. Stubbs R, Cannan R and Mitchell A. Selective internal radiation therapy with 90-yttrium microspheres for extensive colorectal liver metastases. *Journal of Gastrointestinal Surgery* 5(3):294–302, 2001.

55. Lim L et al. A prospective evaluation of treatment with selective internal radiation therapy (SIR-spheres) in patients with unresectable liver metastases from colorectal cancer previously treated with 5-FU based chemotherapy. *BMC Cancer,* 5:132, 2005.

## Splenic Radiation

56. McFarland, J. Palliative irradiation of the spleen. *American Journal of Clinical Oncology* 26(2):178–2003, 2003.

# 8

# Useful Tools for Radiation Oncology

*Anwar Khan, MD*
*Benjamin D. Smith, MD*

## OVERVIEW

For patients undergoing radiation therapy there are some general tools, that can aid the clinician in managing the patient?s overall care during their treatment course. These tools include an understanding of general principles, and details regarding performance status, toxicities, pain management, nutritional issues, and common approaches to management of treatment related toxicities and supportive care. In this chapter, we attempt to cover common overall management issues which can be used as a guide to caring for patients throughout their course of radiation.

## PERFORMANCE STATUS

Performance status refers to a patient's functional status. The two most commonly used performance status scales were developed by Karnofsky (KPS) and ECOG (Eastern Cooperative Oncology Group) (Tables 8-1 and 8-2). Numerous studies have demonstrated an association between impaired performance status and an increased risk of death. For example, KPS < 50 typically predicts a survival of less than 8 weeks for patients with metastatic cancer.

## RADIATION SIDE EFFECTS: ASSESSMENT AND MANAGEMENT

### Tolerance Doses and Toxicity

Table 8-3 presents commonly accepted tolerance doses for fractionated, external beam radiation therapy.[1] TD (toxic dose) 5/5 refers to the dose that results in a 5% risk of an adverse outcome at 5 years. TD 50/5 refers to the dose that results in a 50% risk of an adverse outcome at 5 years. The tolerance doses are presented as a function of the volume of organ irradiated, either 1/3, 2/3, or 3/3 (or a specific field size for skin and spinal cord).

The National Cancer Institute's Common Terminology Criteria for Adverse Events v3.0 are presented in Table 8-4 in an abbreviated form. This schema can be used to describe and report both acute and late toxicity attributed to radiation.

### Skin

Skin reactions are commonly encountered during radiotherapy (for grading of skin and other reactions, see Table 8-4). To help prevent and/or minimize skin reactions, patients should be advised

## TABLE 8-1 Karnofsky Performance Status

100. Normal, no complaints; no evidence of disease.
 90. Able to carry on normal activity; minor signs or symptoms of disease.
 80. Normal activity with effort; some signs or symptoms of disease.
 70. Cares for self; unable to carry on normal activity or to do active work.
 60. Requires occasional assistance, but is able to care for most of his personal needs.
 50. Requires considerable assistance and frequent medical care.
 40. Disabled; requires special care and assistance.
 30. Severely disabled; hospital admission is indicated although death not imminent.
 20. Very sick; hospital admission necessary; active supportive treatment necessary.
 10. Moribund; fatal processes progressing rapidly.
  0. Dead.

Schag CC, Heinrich RL, Ganz PA: Karnofsky performance status revisited: reliability, validity, and guidelines. *J Clin Oncol* 2:187–193, 1984.

## TABLE 8-2 ECOG Performance Status

0. Fully active, able to carry on all predisease performance without restriction.
1. Restricted in physically strenuous activity but ambulatory and able to carry out work of a light or sedentary nature, such as light house work, office work.
2. Ambulatory and capable of all selfcare but unable to carry out any work activities. Up and about more than 50% of waking hours.
3. Capable of only limited selfcare, confined to bed or chair more than 50% of waking hours.
4. Completely disabled. Cannot carry on any selfcare. Totally confined to bed or chair.
5. Dead.

Oken MM, Creech RH, Tormey DC, et al: Toxicity and response criteria of the eastern cooperative oncology group. *Am J Clin Oncol* 5:649–655, 1982.

to: (1) Gently wash their skin with lukewarm water and mild soap, such as Dove®, (2) Apply a non-scented, lanolin-free hydrophilic cream to irradiated skin two to three times daily, (3) Continue personal hygiene practices, such as the application of deodorant.

Management of acute skin reactions should be graded according to their severity. Pruritus associated with Grade 1 and 2 skin reactions may respond to topical corticosteroids, such as triamcinolone ointment 0.1% applied twice daily. Creams such as Biafene® or Trolamine should not be applied directly to areas of moist desquamation. Although there is limited evidence to define an optimal treatment strategy for moist desquamation, general principles of wound care such as promoting moisture and minimizing bacterial colonization apply. The following may be helpful:

1. Open Wet Dressings. A single layer of gauze moistened with saline is applied to the affected area and allowed to air dry for at least 10 minutes. This helps to remove serous exudates and relieve patient symptoms.
2. Hydrocolloid dressings. These dressings help to provide moisture, absorb exudate, prevent bacterial infection, and relieve patient symptoms. They adhere to the wound surface and should be changed every 1 to 4 days depending on the degree of exudate. Examples of hydrocolloid products include Vigilon,® Granuflex,® Comfeel,® and Tegasorb.® In our experience, Vigilon® provides the best symptomatic response.

**TABLE 8-3  Tolerance Doses[1]**

| Organ | TD 5/5 (cGy) Volume | | | TD 50/5 (cGy) Volume | | | Clinical Endpoint |
|---|---|---|---|---|---|---|---|
| | 1/3 | 2/3 | 3/3 | 1/3 | 2/3 | 3/3 | |
| **Gastrointestinal** | | | | | | | |
| Colon | 5500 | — | 4500 | 6500 | — | 5500 | Obstruction, perforation, ulceration, fistula |
| Liver | 5000 | 3500 | 3000 | 5500 | 4500 | 4000 | Liver failure |
| Rectum | — | — | 6000 | — | — | 8000 | Severe proctitis, necrosis, fistula, stenosis |
| Small intestine | 5000 | — | 4000 | 6000 | — | 5500 | Obstruction, perforation, fistula |
| Stomach | 6000 | 5500 | 5000 | 7000 | 6700 | 6500 | Ulceration, perforation |
| **Genitourinary** | | | | | | | |
| Bladder | — | 8000 | 6500 | — | 8500 | 8000 | Symptomatic bladder contracture and volume loss |
| Kidney | 5000 | 3000 | 2300 | — | 4000 | 2800 | Clinical nephritis |
| **Head and Neck** | | | | | | | |
| Ear mid/external | 3000 | 3000 | 3000 | 4000 | 4000 | 4000 | Acute serous otitis |
| Ear mid/external | 5500 | 5500 | 5500 | 6500 | 6500 | 6500 | Chronic serous otitis |
| Larynx | 7900 | 7000 | 7000 | 9000 | 8000 | 8000 | Cartilage necrosis |
| Larynx | — | 4500 | 4500 | — | — | 8000 | Laryngeal edema |
| Lens of eye | — | — | 1000 | — | — | 1800 | Cataract requiring intervention |
| Parotid | — | 3200 | 3200 | — | 4600 | 4600 | Xerostomia |
| Retina | — | — | 4500 | — | — | 6500 | Blindness |
| **Integumentary** | | | | | | | |
| Femoral head | — | — | 5200 | — | — | 6500 | Necrosis |
| | 10 cm² | 30 cm² | 100 cm² | 10 cm² | 30 cm² | 100 cm² | |
| Skin | 7000 | 6000 | 5500 | — | — | 7000 | Necrosis, ulceration |

(continues)

**TABLE 8-3** (continued)

| Organ | TD 5/5 (cGy) Volume | | | TD 50/5 (cGy) Volume | | | Clinical Endpoint |
|---|---|---|---|---|---|---|---|
| | 1/3 | 2/3 | 3/3 | 1/3 | 2/3 | 3/3 | |
| **Nervous System** | | | | | | | |
| Brachial plexus | 6200 | 6100 | 6000 | 7700 | 7600 | 7500 | Clinically apparent nerve damage |
| Brain | 6000 | 5000 | 4500 | 7500 | 6500 | 6000 | Necrosis, infarction |
| Brainstem | 6000 | 5300 | 5000 | 7500 | 6500 | 6000 | Necrosis, infarction |
| Cauda Equina | — | — | 6000 | — | — | 7500 | Clinically apparent nerve damage |
| Optic nerve and chiasm | — | — | 5000 | — | — | 6500 | Blindness |
| Spinal cord | 5 cm | 10 cm | 20 cm | 5 cm | 10 cm | 20 cm | Myelitis, necrosis |
| | 5000 | 5000 | 4700 | 7000 | 7000 | — | |
| **Thorax** | | | | | | | |
| Lung | 4500 | 3000 | 1750 | 6500 | 4000 | 2450 | Pneumonitis |
| Heart | 6000 | 4500 | 4000 | 7000 | 5500 | 5000 | Pericarditis |

Reprinted with permission Elsevier, Inc.

**TABLE 8-4  Common Terminology Criteria for Adverse Events v3.0**

| Toxicity | Grade 1 | Grade 2 | Grade 3 | Grade 4 | Grade 5 |
|---|---|---|---|---|---|
| **CARDIO-PULMONARY** | | | | | |
| Atelectasis | Asymptomatic | Symptomatic (dyspnea, cough), medical intervention indicated (bronchoscopic suctioning, chest physiotherapy, suctioning) | Operative (stent, laser) intervention indicated | Life-threatening respiratory compromise | Death |
| Dyspnea | Dyspnea on exertion, but can walk 1 flight of stairs without stopping | Dyspnea on exertion and unable to walk 1 flight of stairs or 1 city block (0.1km) without stopping | Dyspnea with ADL | Dyspnea at rest; intubation/ventilator indicated | Death |
| FEV-1 | 90–75% of predicted value | <75–50% of predicted value | <50–25% of predicted value | <25% of predicted | Death |
| Hypotension | No intervention | <24 hrs therapy (fluids, etc); no physiologic consequences | >24 hrs therapy (fluids, etc); no *persistent* physiologic consequences | Shock | Death |
| Left ventricular systolic dysfunction | Asymptomatic; resting EF <60–50% | Asymptomatic; resting EF <50–40% | Symptomatic CHF responsive to therapy; EF <40–20% | Symptomatic CHF poorly responsive to therapy; EF <20% | Death |
| Pericarditis | Asymptomatic, ECG or physical exam (rub) changes consistent with pericarditis | Symptomatic pericarditis (chest pain) | Pericarditis with physiologic consequences (pericardial constriction) | Life-threatening consequences; emergency intervention indicated | Death |
| Pulmonary fibrosis | Minimal radiographic findings (or patchy or bibasilar changes) with estimated radiographic proportion of total lung volume that is fibrotic of <25% | Patchy or bibasilar changes with estimated radiographic proportion of total lung volume that is fibrotic of 25–<50% | Dense or widespread infiltrates/consolidation with estimated radiographic proportion of total lung volume that is fibrotic of 50–<75% | Estimated radiographic proportion of total lung volume that is fibrotic is ≥75%; honeycombing | Death |
| **CONSTITUTIONAL** | | | | | |
| Hot flashes | Mild | Moderate | Severe | — | — |
| Fatigue | Mild | Moderate | Interfering with ADL | Disabling | — |

*(continues)*

**TABLE 8-4 (continued)**

| Toxicity | Grade 1 | Grade 2 | Grade 3 | Grade 4 | Grade 5 |
|---|---|---|---|---|---|
| Insomnia | Occasional and not affecting function or ADL | Affecting function but not ADL | Frequent, affecting ADL | Disabling | — |
| Obesity | — | BMI 25–29.9 | BMI 30–39.9 | BMI >40 | — |
| Weight loss | 5–10%; intervention not indicated | 10–20%; nutritional support indicated | >20%; TPN or TF needed | — | — |
| **GASTROINTESTINAL** | | | | | |
| Colitis | Asymptomatic, pathologic or radiographic findings only | Abdominal pain; mucus or blood in stool | Abdominal pain, fever, change in bowel habits with ileus; peritoneal signs | Life-threatening consequences (perforation, bleeding, ischemia, necrosis, toxic megacolon) | Death |
| Constipation | Occasional or intermittent symptoms; occasional use of stool softeners, laxatives, dietary modification, or enema | Persistent symptoms with regular use of laxatives or enemas indicated | Symptoms interfering with ADL; obstipation with manual evacuation indicated | Life-threatening consequences (obstruction, toxic megacolon) | Death |
| Diarrhea | Increase of <4 stools per day over baseline; mild increase in ostomy output compared to baseline | Increase of 4–6 stools per day over baseline; IV fluids indicated <24 hrs; moderate increase in ostomy output compared to baseline; not interfering with ADL | Increase of ≥7 stools per day over baseline; incontinence; IV fluids ≥24 hrs; hospitalization; severe increase in ostomy output compared to baseline; interfering with ADL | Life-threatening consequences (hemodynamic collapse) | Death |
| Esophagitis | Asymptomatic pathologic, radiographic, or endoscopic findings only | Symptomatic; altered eating/swallowing (altered dietary habits, oral supplements); IV fluids indicated <24 hrs | Symptomatic and severely altered eating/swallowing (inadequate oral caloric or fluid intake); IV fluids, tube feedings, or TPN indicated ≥24 hrs | Life-threatening | Death |
| Dysphagia | Symptomatic, able to eat regular diet | Symptomatic and altered eating/swallowing (altered dietary habits, oral supplements); IV fluids indicated <24 hrs | Symptomatic and severely altered eating/swallowing (inadequate oral caloric or fluid intake); | Life-threatening consequences (obstruction, perforation) | Death |

| | Grade 1 | Grade 2 | Grade 3 | Grade 4 | Grade 5 |
|---|---|---|---|---|---|
| **Gastritis** | Asymptomatic, radiographic or endoscopic findings only | Symptomatic; altered gastric function (inadequate oral caloric or fluid intake); IV fluids indicated <24 hrs | Symptomatic and severely altered gastric function (inadequate oral caloric or fluid intake); IV fluids, tube feedings, or TPN indicated ≥24 hrs | Life-threatening consequences; operative intervention requiring complete organ resection (gastrectomy) | Death |
| **Incontinence, anal** | Occasional use of pads required | Daily use of pads required | Interfering with ADL; operative intervention indicated | Permanent bowel diversion indicated | Death |
| **Obstruction, GI** | Asymptomatic radiographic findings only | Symptomatic; altered GI function (altered dietary habits, vomiting, diarrhea, or GI fluid loss); IV fluids indicated <24 hrs | Symptomatic and severely altered GI function (altered dietary habits, vomiting, diarrhea, or GI fluid loss); IV fluids, tube feedings, or TPN indicated ≥24 hrs; operative intervention indicated | Life-threatening consequences; operative intervention requiring complete organ resection (total colectomy) | Death |
| **Proctitis** | Rectal discomfort, intervention not indicated | Symptoms not interfering with ADL; medical intervention indicated | Stool incontinence or other symptoms interfering with ADL; operative intervention indicated | Life-threatening consequences | Death |
| **Vomiting** | 1 episode in 24 hrs | 2–5 episodes in 24 hrs; IVF for <24 hrs | >5 episodes in 24 hrs; IVF, or TPN for >24 hrs | Life-threatening consequences | Death |
| **GENITOURINARY/GYNECOLOGICAL** | | | | | |
| **Bladder spasms** | Symptomatic, intervention not indicated | Symptomatic, antispasmodics indicated | Narcotics indicated | Major surgical intervention indicated (cystectomy) | Death |
| **Cystitis** | Asymptomatic | Frequency with dysuria; macroscopic hematuria | Transfusion; IV pain medications; bladder irrigation indicated | Catastrophic bleeding; major non-elective intervention indicated | — |

(continues)

## TABLE 8-4 (continued)

| Toxicity | Grade 1 | Grade 2 | Grade 3 | Grade 4 | Grade 5 |
|---|---|---|---|---|---|
| **Erectile dysfunction** | Decrease in erectile function (frequency/rigidity of erections) but erectile aids not indicated | Decrease in erectile function (frequency/rigidity of erections), erectile aids indicated | Decrease in erectile function (frequency/rigidity of erections) but erectile aids not helpful | — | — |
| **Gynecomastia** | — | Asymptomatic breast enlargement | Symptomatic breast enlargement; intervention indicated | — | — |
| **Incontinence, urinary** | Occasional (with coughing, sneezing, etc.), pads not indicated | Spontaneous, pads indicated | Interfering with ADL; intervention indicated (clamp, collagen injections) | Operative intervention indicated (cystectomy or permanent urinary diversion) | — |
| **Obstruction, GU** | Symptomatic, radiographic or endoscopic findings only | Symptomatic but no hydronephrosis, sepsis or renal dysfunction; dilation or endoscopic repair or stent placement indicated | Symptomatic and altered organ function (sepsis or hydronephrosis, or renal dysfunction); operative intervention indicated | Life-threatening consequences; organ failure or operative intervention requiring complete organ resection indicated | Death |
| **Urinary frequency** | Increase in frequency or nocturia up to 2 × normal; enuresis | Increase >2 × normal but <hourly | ≥1 ×/hr; urgency; catheter indicated | — | — |
| **Vaginal mucositis** | Erythema; min symptoms | Patchy ulcerations; mod symptoms ordyspareunia | Confluent ulcerations; bleeding with minor trauma | Tissue necrosis; significant spontaneous bleeding; life-threatening consequences | — |
| **Vaginal stenosis** | Vaginal narrowing and/or shortening not affecting function | Vaginal narrowing and/or shortening affecting function | Complete obliteration; not surgically correctable | — | — |
| **HEAD & NECK** | | | | | |
| **Hearing loss** | — | Not affecting ADL or requiring hearing aid | Affecting ADL or requiring hearing aid | Profound bilateral loss >90 db | — |
| **Hypothyroidism** | Asymptomatic, intervention not indicated | Symptomatic, not interfering with ADL; thyroid replacement indicated | Symptoms interfering with ADL; hospitalization indicated | Life-threatening myxedema coma | Death |

| | Grade 1 | Grade 2 | Grade 3 | Grade 4 | Grade 5 |
|---|---|---|---|---|---|
| **Larynx edema** | Asymptomatic edema by exam only | Symptomatic edema, no respiratory distress | Stridor; respiratory distress; interfering with ADL | Life-threatening airway compromise; tracheotomy, intubation, or laryngectomy indicated | Death |
| **Otitis externa (non-infectious)** | Erythema or dry desquamation | Moist desquamation; tm perforation | Mastoiditis, stenosis or osteomyelitis | Tissue necrosis | |
| **Otitis media (non-infectious)** | Serous | Needs med intervention | Discharge and mastoiditis | Tissue necrosis | Death |
| **Mucositis/stomatitis** | Erythema of the mucosa | Patchy ulcerations or pseudomembranes | Confluent ulcerations or pseudomembranes; bleeding with minor trauma | Tissue necrosis; significant spontaneous bleeding; life-threatening consequences | Death |
| **Salivary gland changes** | Slightly thickened saliva; slightly altered taste (metallic) | Thick, ropy, sticky saliva; markedly altered taste; alteration in diet indicated; secretion-induced symptoms not interfering with ADL | Acute salivary gland necrosis; severe secretion-induced symptoms interfering with ADL | Disabling | — |
| **Tinnitus** | — | Not interfering with ADL | Interfering with ADL | Disabling | — |
| **Trismus** | Decreased range of motion without impaired eating | Decreased range of motion requiring small bites, soft foods or purees | Decreased range of motion with inability to adequately aliment or hydrate orally | — | — |
| **Xerostomia** | Symptomatic (dry or thick saliva) without significant dietary alteration; unstimulated saliva flow >0.2 ml/min | Symptomatic and significant oral intake alteration (copious water, other lubricants, diet limited to purees and/or soft, moist foods); unstimulated saliva 0.1 to 0.2 ml/min | Symptoms leading to inability to adequately aliment orally; IV fluids, tube feedings, or TPN indicated; unstimulated saliva <0.1 ml/min | — | — |
| | | >30% inter-limb discrepancy | | | |

**TABLE 8-4 (continued)**

| Toxicity | Grade 1 | Grade 2 | Grade 3 | Grade 4 | Grade 5 |
|---|---|---|---|---|---|
| **MUSCULOSKELETAL** | | | | | |
| Limb edema | 5–10% inter-limb discrepancy in volume or circumference at point of greatest visible difference; swelling or obscuration of anatomic architecture on close inspection; pitting edema | >10–30% inter-limb discrepancy in volume or circumference at point of greatest visible difference; readily apparent obscuration of anatomic architecture; obliteration of skin folds; readily apparent deviation from normal anatomic contour | >30% inter-limb discrepancy in volume; lymphorrhea; gross deviation from normal anatomic contour; interfering with ADL | Progression to malignancy (lymphangiosarcoma); amputation indicated; disabling | Death |
| Lymphedema-related fibrosis | Minimal to moderate redundant soft tissue, unresponsive to elevation or compression, with moderately firm texture or spongy feel | Marked increase in density and firmness, with or without tethering | Very marked density and firmness with tethering affecting ≥40% of the edematous area | — | — |
| Osteoporosis | Radiographic evidence of osteoporosis or Bone Mineral Density (BMD) t-score—to −2.5 (osteopenia) and no loss of height or therapy indicated | BMD t-score <−2.5; loss of height <2 cm; antiosteoporotic therapy indicated | Fractures; loss of height ≥2 cm | Disabling | — |
| **SKIN** | | | | | |
| Radiation dermatitis | Faint erythema or dry-desquamation | Moderate to brisk erythema; patchy moist desquamation, mostly confined to skin folds and creases; moderate edema | Moist desquamation other than skin folds and creases; bleeding induced by minor trauma or abrasion | Skin necrosis or ulceration of full thickness dermis; spontaneous bleeding | Death |
| Ulceration | — | Superficial ulceration <2 cm size; local wound care; medical intervention indicated | Ulceration ≥2 cm size; operative debridement, primary closure or other invasive intervention indicated (hyperbaric oxygen) | Life-threatening consequences; major invasive intervention indicated (complete resection, tissue reconstruction, flap, or grafting) | Death |

Adapted from the Cancer Therapy Evaluation Program, Common Technology Criteria for Adverse Events v3.0, DCTD, NCI, NIH, DHHS, December 12, 2003. NIH Publication #03-5410. http://ctep.cancer.gov/forms/CTCAEv3.pdf.

---

**BOX 8-1**

Trolamine, also known as Biafine®, is an oil-in-water emulsion with non-steroidal anti-inflammatory properties and is commonly used to prevent and treat radiation dermatitis. Calendula oil is made from a plant in the marigold family and has been used in the past to treat burn injuries. This phase III trial randomized 254 patients undergoing breast radiation to Biafine or Calendula oil applied twice daily during radiotherapy. Patients were evaluated by their radiation oncologist, who was blinded to the treatment received. Grade 2 or greater dermatitis was significantly lower in the Calendula oil arm (41% for Calendula oil versus 63% for Biafine, P <0.001). Skin pain and radiation treatment breaks were also reduced in the Calendula arm. However, patients did find Calendula more difficult to apply than Trolamine.

Pommier et al. Phase III randomized trial of Calendula Officinalis compared with trolamine for the prevention of acute dermatitis during irradiation for breast cancer. *J Clin Oncol* 22:1447–1453, 2004.

---

3. Hydrofera blue. This is a polyvinyl alcohol sponge complexed with two bacteriostatic pigments, gentian violet and methylene blue. Hydrofera blue should be moistened with sterile saline or water, applied to the wound, and held in place with a secondary dressing. It should be changed every 1–3 days. In our experience, this product provides substantial symptomatic relief and accelerates wound healing.

## Head and Neck

Treatment of H&N malignancies can be challenging for patients, particularly due to the common, significant acute and long-term side effects that impact their private and public lifestyles due to alteration of anatomy, speech, and swallowing function. However, it is worth emphasizing that some of the widely endorsed management strategies may not only help reduce the intensity of these adverse effects but also improve the treatment outcome for the patients. Table 8-4 lists CTC toxicity scale.

### H&N Adverse Effects and Management:

1. Mucositis—Inflammation of the mucous membranes is usually noticeable within 2–3 weeks of radiation therapy. It is adversely affected by use of induction or concurrent chemotherapy, poor nutritional status, and ongoing tobacco use. Ironically, pain from mucositis interferes with proper nutritional intake which in turn can slow the mucosal recovery.

    Management of pain is essential and must be frequently reassessed during therapy. In addition, oral discomfort can be reduced by swishing and swallowing/spitting 5–10cc of **Duke's Solution** (60cc of 2% viscous lidocaine, 120cc of Maalox, 120cc benadryl) every 3–4 hours as needed. Patients find it helpful to use this mixture about 15–20 minutes before a meal. They must not eat or drink immediately afterwards. **Miracle Mouthwash** (tetracycline, mycostatin, hydrocortisone, benadryl) is an alternative mixture that contains antibacterial plus antifungal agents and can be used similarly.

    Oral hygiene can be maintained by use of a homemade mouth wash consisting of 1 tsp baking soda and ½ tsp salt in a quart of water. About 10cc of this solution should be used to rinse the mouth and gargle several times daily. This mixture soothes the mucosa and normalizes the pH.

    Although not yet available in the United States, benzydamine is a topical NSAID (nonsteroidal anti-inflammatory drug) with analgesic, anti-inflammatory, anesthethic, and antimicrobial properties that is beneficial in patients receiving moderate dose radiation (about 50 Gy) and is recommended by the clinical practice guideline panel for prevention of mucositis.[2,3] The same panel advised against the use of chlorhexidine (Peridex) as a preventative agent.[3]

Smoking cessation is critical since continued use of tobacco worsens mucositis and lowers treatment outcomes. During concurrent chemoradiation, opportunistic infections including candida are common and must be recognized and treated, especially since concurrent radiation mucositis may make them less easily recognizable. As mentioned above, Miracle Mouthwash can also be used prophylactically.

2. Xerostomia—Major salivary glands are quite sensitive to radiation damage in a dose dependent fashion. The parotid glands provide the majority of saliva during mastication and mostly secrete *serous* content while the submandibular and sublingual glands provide the majority of resting saliva and mostly secrete *mucinous* content. Changes in the quantity and quality of saliva can be seen within a few weeks of radiation therapy. Compromise of normal salivary function not only interferes with swallowing but also increases risk for dental caries.

The best preventative strategy consists of excluding the parotid glands from the radiation port when feasible. Given the parallel architecture of the gland, sparing even parts of the glands is helpful. If IMRT is being used, the general criteria is to keep the median dose to at least one parotid gland below 26 Gy. This strategy has been clinically beneficial in several studies.

Amifostine (Ethyol) is a cytoprotector pro-drug that has been shown in some studies to be beneficial in sparing salivary function without protecting the tumor. However, this drug requires daily IV or SC administration about 30 minutes before radiation treatment. Side effects include significant emesis and hypotension and therefore patients must be aggressively premedicated with antiemetics and well hydrated.

Pilocarpine (Salagen) is a cholingeric agonist that can be used both during and after radiation to increase saliva production. It is typically administered at 5–10mg tid. Patients may not notice any immediate results. Side effects include possible excessive sweating, bronchospasm, bradycardia, and hypotension.

Artificial saliva (Salivert, Xerolube, Numoisyn) can be used to lubricate the oral cavity on an as-needed basis. There are no serious side effects.

Papain (papaya extract) and guaifenesin (such as Mucinex, an expectorant) are agents that can help reduce the viscosity of thick saliva and may assist in expectorating tenacious mucous.

In one study, acupuncture was shown to help with permanent xerostomia in patients not benefiting from pilocarpine.[4]

3. Hypothyroidism—The incidence of hypothyroidism in H&N cancer patients treated with radiation is high (about 50%) and increases with the dose. Interestingly, the risk is thought to be increased by neck surgery but not by use of chemotherapy. If mild, the condition may be asymptomatic. Patients with pre-existing borderline insufficiency might be more prone to develop overt hypothyroidism after radiation. In one study, the median time before this condition developed was between 1.4 and 1.8 years (range 0.3–7.2 years).[5]

Thyroid function should be checked routinely in all patients receiving H&N radiation if the low neck is treated. Unless prompted earlier by clinical symptoms, screening every 6 months is reasonable. Patients already taking a thyroid supplement might need titration of their dose and should also be checked.

The starting dose of levothyroxine (Synthroid) is usually 50 micrograms daily. Dose adjustments are usually made in increments of 25 micrograms every few weeks until adequate normalization of TSH is achieved.

4. Trismus—Patients receiving H&N radiation are at risk for developing limitation of jaw opening, particularly if the temporomandibular joints and the masticatory muscles receive a significant dose. Trismus is clinically assessed by measuring the vertical distance between the jaws anteriorly as the patient fully opens the mouth. Regular jaw exercises during and after radiation therapy can reduce the incidence and severity of trismus. Patients should receive appropriate physical therapy for both prevention and treatment of trismus.

5. Smoking—Most H&N cancers are related to tobacco use. Data suggests increase in risk of new primaries and higher treatment failures/recurrence rates in patients who continue to smoke.[6] Ongoing use of tobacco during radiation also increases the severity and duration of mucositis.[7]

Patients must be counseled about the risks of continued smoking and strongly urged to quit. The most commonly used interventions include use of alternate sources of nicotine (patch, gum, lozenge, nasal spray, inhaler) that are generally weaned gradually to facilitate easier physiological adjustment as well as non-nicotinic medications. The nicotine patches, gum, and lozenge are available over-the-counter. The daily Nicoderm CQ patches come in different strengths (21 mg/day, 14 mg/day, 7 mg/day) and are typically lowered sequentially every few weeks as tolerated. In contrast, Nicotrol patches do not require any tapering and should be worn for 16 hours daily over several weeks. As for the gums/lozenges, if a patient has been smoking more than 25 cigarettes daily, 1–2 gums/lozenges of 2mg each are typically needed every hour initially for several weeks followed by tapering as tolerated.

Bupropion (Zyban) is a prescription antidepressant that is an alternative to nicotine products. It works by modifying the serotonin receptors. It is prescribed as 150mg bid and should be started about 2 weeks before planned date of quitting. Although this medication is generally prescribed for 2–3 months, the optimum length of therapy is not well known. Bupropion may be used together with the nicotine patches for enhanced efficacy. Relative contraindications include history of seizures, anorexia, or heavy alcohol abuse.

Varenicline (Chantix) is another prescription drug that was approved by the FDA in 2006 for smoking cessation. Early data suggested superior outcome when compared to both bupropion and placebo. It acts as a partial agonist at the nicotinic acetylcholine receptors in the brain. The starting dose is 0.5mg daily for 3 days, followed by 0.5mg bid for 4 days, then 1mg bid for the rest of the therapy. It is prescribed about 1 week before planned date of quitting and is continued for about 12 weeks. A repeat course may be considered for an additional 12 weeks. Gastrointestinal side effects are common, particularly nausea which may be experienced by up to one third of the patients (Table 8-5).

## TABLE 8-5  Smoking Cessation Strategies—Brief Summary

|  | Dosage | Remark |
|---|---|---|
| **Nicotine Based** | | |
| Nicotine inhaler | 10 mg cartridge used over 20 minutes (typically 5–15 cartridges daily) | |
| Nicotine nasal spray | 1–2 sprays every hour (typically 10–40 sprays daily) | Throat/nasal irritation |
| Nicotine patch—OTC* | Nicodern CQ in different strengths; Nicotrol in single strength | Skin irritation |
| Nicotine gum—OTC* | 2, 4 mg tabs; tapered over 6 weeks | |
| **Non-Nicotone Based** | | |
| Bupropion (Zyban)* | 150mg bid | Possible anti-depressant benefit |
| Varenicline (Chantix)* | 1 mg bid maintenance after initial lower dose for 7 days | FDA approved in 2006 |

*Please see text for additional details.

6. Nutrition—Patients with advanced malignancies have several cancer-related mechanisms for weight loss, even in the presence of fair caloric intake. Metabolic derangements have been identified as the main basis of cancer cachexia. Certain cytokines including TNF-alpha, IL-1 beta, IL-6 are postulated to elevate the so-called Resting Energy Expenditure (REE) in cancer patients. In addition, the utilization of fats vs proteins is altered in a way that favors the preferential metabolism of proteins with resultant, disproportionately larger loss of lean body mass; this particular change in metabolism is the hallmark of cancer cachexia and distinguishes it from starvation.

In patients with H&N cancers, treatment-related side effects including mucositis, xerostomia, and trismus can further worsen their nutritional status by decreasing the caloric intake. It must be appreciated that recovery from acute radiation damage is linked to good nutrition. In patients being treated with large fields, concurrent chemotherapy, or who are otherwise in poor health, prophylactic advance placement of a percutaneous endoscopic gastrostomy (PEG) tube should be considered. An evaluation for removal of the PEG several weeks after completion of radiation therapy must take into account the patient's ability to consume total nutrition by mouth as well as any ongoing need for analgesics for odynophagia; this evaluation should incorporate a swallowing study to access recovery of function vis-à-vis risk of aspiration.

Generally, patients need 25–30 cal/kg for merely maintaining weight. This translates into approximately 2,000 calories per day for an average 70 kg adult. The suggested estimates of daily calories must include dietary protein at about 1.0–1.2 g protein/kg body weight. (Net protein synthesis or breakdown can be determined by calculating the so-called nitrogen balance, which compares protein intake versus urinary nitrogen excretion, and can roughly estimate protein need). These requirements are higher in patients with significant weight loss. Daily fluid requirements are typically 30–35 ml/kg body weight and must be adjusted for conditions with increased fluid loses.

If a PEG is being utilized, it can generally be used 1 day after placement. The choice of appropriate nutritional supplements must take into account the patient's individual needs, mode of administration, and underlying comorbid conditions. For instance, specialized preparations are available for patients with diabetes (Glucerna), renal insufficiency (Amin Aid), hepatic dysfunction (Hepatic Aid), pulmonary dysfunction (Pulmocare), and gastrointenstinal disorders (Citrotein). Guidance from a dietician can be extremely helpful in making these decisions and is strongly encouraged. Although bolus feeding is often less cumbersome, gravity drip may be appropriate for patients with small stomach volume or gastroparesis. Use of metoclopramide (Reglan) 10mg three times daily can help improve gastric motility. A few commonly used preparations are listed in Table 8-6.

7. Dental—After radiation therapy, there is a high risk for developing dental caries in the absence of normal salivary function. Dental work in these patients carries a high risk of infections and poor healing, which in turn increases the risk of osteonecrosis. Hence, pretreatment dental evaluation and extraction of decaying teeth must be performed before radiation. Fluoride prophylaxis for the remaining teeth is recommended for the patient's lifetime for which the dentist generally makes a custom tray to be used with fluoride gel for a few minutes daily. A period of 14–21 days must be allowed for tooth sockets to heal before radiation is started.

## Thorax

Radiation oncologists providing radiation therapy for thoracic malignancies must carefully consider the tolerance doses of different structures, particularly the heart, lung, and esophagus. Both acute and late adverse effects can occur (Table 8-4).

TABLE 8-6 **Common Tube Feedings**

| Formula | Nutrition | Remarks |
|---|---|---|
| Advera | 303 cal/8 oz, 14.2 g protein | Peptides for easier absorption |
| Boost | 240 cal/8 oz, 10 g protein | Hyperosmolar, no dietary fiber |
| Boost Plus | 360 cal/8 oz, 14 g protein | Hyperosmolar, no dietary fiber |
| Ensure | 253 cal/8 oz, 11 g protein | Hyperosmolar, no dietary fiber |
| Ensure Plus | 355 cal/8 oz, 13 g protein | Hyperosmolar, no dietary fiber |
| Jevity | 250 cal/8 oz, 10.5 g protein | Isomolar, 3.4 g dietary fiber |
| Osmolite | 250 cal/8 oz, 8.8 g protein | Isomolar, no dietary fiber |
| Osmolite HN | 355 cal/8 oz, 10.5 g protein | Isomolar, no dietary fiber |
| Sustacal | 240 cal/8 oz, 14.4 g protein | Hyperosmolar, no dietary fiber |
| Sustacal HN | 360 cal/8 oz, 14.4 g protein | Hyperosmolar, no dietary fiber |
| Ultracal | 250 cal/8 oz, 10.5 g protein | Isomolar, 3.4 g dietary fiber |

*Thoracic Adverse Effects and Management:*

1. Lung—The lung parenchyma is highly sensitive to radiation damage, as reflected by its relatively low TD 5/5 of about 17–18 Gy. Several distinct, sequential phases have been identified in the process of lung damage from radiation: most notably, the acute inflammatory phase occurring 1–3 months after radiation, followed by a phase of late fibrosis that can stabilize in 1–2 years and is permanent with no recovery thereafter. During the acute phase, patients may complain of a dry, hacking cough with dyspnea, pleuritic chest pain, and may in fact have low grade fever and even hemoptysis. Radiographically, the changes appear as patchy, alveolar, infiltrates which geometrically match the radiation ports (straight line effect), although negative scans are possible in early subacute phase. In contrast, the classic appearance of late lung injury consists of lung retraction and elevation of hemidiaphragm.

   A great deal of research has focused on identifying and validating reliable dosimetric parameters that may predict the likelihood of clinically symptomatic lung injury in patients undergoing lung radiation. In this regard, various quantities have been studied including V20 (percentage of lung receiving at least 20 Gy), MLD (mean lung dose to total lung), NTCP (normal tissue complication probability), etc., all of which estimate the risk of complications based on dose to the normal lung tissue. During the treatment planning phase, one should try to keep these quantities as low as possible. However, reported studies do not necessarily recommend consistently similar thresholds for these parameters in order to minimize the risk of pulmonary toxicity.[8] Arguably, *keeping V20 ≤ 30%, MLD < 20 Gy, and NTCP < 10% is a reasonable general strategy*, as seen in the University of Michigan data for dose escalation—although more conservative thresholds may be preferred if achievable.[9] In a recent study, V10 and V13 (percentage of lung receiving at least 10 Gy and 13 Gy respectively) were found to be more predictive of lung injury and the authors suggested using these parameters, especially in cases with IMRT where large volumes of lung receive low doses of radiation.[10] In terms of V20, in a series of patients treated with definitive three-dimensional conformal radiation for non-small cell lung cancer, the complication rate was 0% if the V20 was less than 20%. The complication rate was 16% if the V20 was between 20% and 31%. Several fatal complications were noted in patients whose V20 exceeded 35%.[11]

   Several other factors that increase the risk of radiation pneumonitis have been identified. These include smoking history, poor baseline lung function, COPD, steroid withdrawal during radiation therapy, lung collapse, younger age, female sex, and prior radiation therapy. The physician must assess these risks and discuss the implications with the patient, including the possible need for supplemental oxygen after treatment. Certain chemotherapeutic agents, such as bleomycin, taxanes, and adriamycin, also increase this risk. Concurrent chemotherapy is more toxic than sequential chemotherapy.

As discussed, the best preventative measure necessitates keeping dose to normal lung at a minimum, as measured by any of the stated dosimetric parameters. Interestingly, one randomized trial of 40 patients showed benefit with prophylactic use of pentoxyfylline 400mg tid during radiation resulting in 20% vs 50% incidence of grade 2–3 pneumonitis.[12]

Amifostine has also been studied for prevention of pneumonitis and esophagitis with some studies showing a benefit.

Once the diagnosis of pneumonitis is confirmed radiographically in symptomatic patients, treatment consists mainly of steroids that are slowly tapered over a period of several weeks. NSAIDs can be used for mild cases, but systemic steroids are generally used for symptomatic cases. A commonly used regimen consists of 60mg prednisone (about 1mg/kg) daily for 2–4 weeks followed by a slow taper over weeks as clinically guided. *It is worth noting that at the time of radiographic diagnosis, an infectious process must be ruled out before steroids are started, particularly if the findings are equivocal.* During the use of steroids, patients with diabetes might notice an increase in their blood sugar levels and some patients taking NSAIDs might develop dyspepsia. Diuretics and supplemental oxygen may also be used as clinically indicated.

In regards to late fibrosis—which is the ultimate, irreversible event—oxygen and brochodilators are the mainstay of therapy. In terms of the pulmonary function tests (PFT), diffusion capacity (DLCO) of the lung is the quantity that is most affected by late radiation damage although other quantities, including lung volumes and lung compliance, also change in a manner seen with typical fibrotic diseases consistent with restrictive pathology. The alveolar-arterial oxygen gradient (A-a gradient) might often be increased due to impaired diffusion of oxygen across the alveolus and the arterial blood.

2. Esophagus—Clinical symptoms of esophagitis are typically seen by the third week of radiation therapy. Patients complain of *non-exertional* chest pain, often worse with swallowing. It may be quite severe and even interfere with sleep. In patients with pre-existing mucosal irritation from conditions such as reflux disease, symptoms may be more intense and present earlier. Similarly, patients taking steroids, aspirin, or NSAIDs may be more prone to these symptoms. Use of *prophylactic* anti-secretory therapy with H2-blockers or proton pump inhibitors (Table 8-7) is appropriate in these patients and may delay the symptoms.

Once symptoms of acute esophagitis develop, the primary therapy consists of antisecretory agents, analgesics, and local anesthetics (Duke's Solution—see H&N section). Consider discontinuing NSAIDs, if possible, in patients taking them for conditions that can be treated alternatively.

Long term complications of radiation include risk for late esophageal strictures. One study showed this risk to be 2% with 50 Gy vs 15% with 60 Gy.[13] The same study showed an increased risk with use of doxorubicin chemotherapy. Treatment of symptomatic strictures may require endoscopic dilatation.

3. Heart—Radiation damage can injure different structures of the heart through the process of fibrosis, which is dose as well as volume dependent and is worsened by some chemotherapeutic agents. (For instance, the concurrent use of anthracycline-based chemotherapy is expressly avoided in breast cancer patients to minimize the known risk of cardiomyopathy.) The spectrum of possible disorders is vast and includes pericarditis, pancarditis, ventricular dysfunction, cardiomyopathy, conduction abnormalities, coronary artery disease, valvular dysfunction, etc.

## TABLE 8-7 Common Gastrointestinal Medications

### Acidity (anti-secretory agents)

| | |
|---|---|
| Cimetidine (Tagamet)—H2 blocker | 800–1200 mg daily in divided doses |
| | (100, 200, 300, 400, 800mg tabs; 300mg/5ml liq; 300mg/2ml inj) |
| Famotidine (Pepcid)—H2 blocker | 20 mg bid |
| | (40mg tabs; 40mg/5cc susp; 10, 20mg tabs OTC; 10mg/ml inj) |
| Lansoprazole (Prevacid)— Proton pump inhibitor | 15–30mg qd |
| | (15, 30 mg caps/tabs; 15, 30mg/packet powder; 30mg/vial inj) |
| Omeprazole (Prilosec)—Proton pump inhibitor | 20–40 mg qd |
| | (10, 20, 40mg caps; 20mg tabs OTC; 20mg/packet powder) |
| Pantoprazole (Protonix)—Proton pump inhibitor | 40 mg qd |
| | (20, 40 mg tabs, 40mg/vial inj) |
| Rabeprazole (Aciphex)—Proton pump inhibitor | 20 mg qd |
| | (20 mg tabs) |
| Ranitidine (Zantac)—H2 blocker | 150 mg bid |
| | (300mg tabs; 75, 150mg tabs OTC; 15mg/cc syrup; 25 mg/cc inj) |

### Constipation

| | |
|---|---|
| Biscodyl (Dulcolax)—OTC | 10–15 mg PO qd-tid; 10 mg PR qd |
| | (5 mg tab; 5, 10 mg supp) |
| Docusate (Colace)—OTC | 50–250 mg PO qd-bid |
| | (50, 100 mg tabs; 10, 50 mg/ml liq; 20, 50, 60 mg/5ml syrup) |
| Lactulose | 10–30 g daily |
| | (10, 20 g packets; 10g/15ml syrup) |
| Magnesium Citrate—OTC | $1/2$–1 bottle PO prn |
| | (10 oz bottle) |
| Polyethylene glycol (Miralax, GlycoLax) | 17 g in 8 oz water qd-bid |
| | (255, 527g bottles) |
| Sennakot | 1–3 tabs qd-tid |
| | Senekot-S has stool softener; SenekotXTRA is double strength |

### Diarrhea

| | |
|---|---|
| Diphenoxylate/atropine (Lomotil) | 2 tablets or 10 cc qam, then 1 tablet or 5 cc after each loose stool. Max 8 tabs or 40 cc daily |
| | (2.5 mg diphenoxylate/0.025mg atropine per tablet or per 5 cc ) |
| Loperamide (Imodium)—OTC | 2–4 mg initially then 2 mg after each loose stool Max 16 mg daily |
| | (2 mg caplets or 1 mg/5 cc) |

### Nausea/Vomiting

| | |
|---|---|
| Dolasetron (Anzemet) | 50–100 mg PO 1 hour before RT |
| | (50,100 mg tabs; 20mg/ml inj) |

(continues)

TABLE 8-7 (continued)

**Nausea/Vomiting** *(continued)*

| | |
|---|---|
| Granisetron (Kytril) | 1 mg PO bid |
| | (1 mg tab) |
| Metoclopramide (Reglan) | 10 mg tid |
| | (5, 10 mg tabs; 5mg/5cc syrup) |
| Ondansetron (Zofran) | 8 mg PO q8h |
| | (4, 8 mg tabs) |
| Prochlorperazine (Compazine) | 5–10 mg PO q6-8hrs; 5–10 mg IV (slowly, max 40 mg/day); 25 mg PR bid |
| | (5, 10, 25 mg tabs; 5mg/5ml syrup; 10mg/2ml injection; 2.5,5,25 mg suppository) |
| Promethazine (Phenergan) | 12.5–25mg PO/IM/PR q4-8hrs |
| | (12.5, 25, 50 mg tabs; 6.25mg/5cc, 25mg/5cc syrup; 12.5, 25, 50mg supp; 25mg/cc, 50mg/cc amp) |

However, in the present era marked by careful dose assessment and conformal planning, radiation is more commonly likely to produce the acute/subacute condition of pericarditis and the late condition of coronary artery disease through accelerated atherosclerosis. Therefore, these two conditions are further discussed here.

Patients may present with symptoms of pericarditis weeks to months after chest radiation. The risk is related to the volume of the heart treated and the dose delivered; a dose of <40 Gy is recommended to minimize this risk. Common symptoms include pleuritic chest pain and dyspnea. The pain might be alleviated by leaning forward, in contrast to pain of esophagitis. In severe cases, pericardial effusion can form and even cause hemodynamic compromise. On physical examination, a pericardial friction rub is pathognomonic but may not always be present. Diagnosis is facilitated by typical EKG changes if present: early stage changes consist of diffuse, concave upwards, ST segment elevations without reciprocal ST depression in opposite leads and absence of Q waves. During intermediate phase, ST segments return to baseline and T wave inversion develops in the same leads. Late phase involves resolution of the T wave changes.

Treatment of acute pericarditis includes mainly NSAIDs such as indomethacin 25–50mg bid-tid or naproxen 250–500mg bid-tid. Steroids may also be added as 30–60mg prednisone daily in severe cases. In severe cases complicated by symptomatic pericardial effusion, the risk of impending cardiac tamponade with resultant hemodynamic collapse may require a therapeutic pericardiocentesis and must be treated as an emergency. The classic findings of tamponade include Beck's triad: hypotension, distant heart sounds, distended neck veins. An ultrasound can accurately evaluate for pericardial effusion.

Constrictive pericarditis is a late complication that can develop months to years after radiation and may not be preceded by a recognizable episode of acute pericarditis. The normal pericardium is 1–2 mm; a thickness of 4 mm on a CT or MRI scan is diagnostic for this condition.[14] Due to characteristic compromise of the right side of the heart causing poor diastolic filling, treatment in the form of surgical pericardiectomy might be necessary.

As for the late risk of coronary disease, it is prudent to minimize dose to the heart, particularly the left ventricle *as well as* the aortic root (where the coronary arteries emerge). Use of smaller fraction sizes is also preferred because data has shown a higher risk for coronary disease with larger radiation fractions.[15] These preventative strategies are of particular relevance in patients with Hodgkins disease and breast cancer where high cure rates are possible, giving rise to long-term survivors. The vascular changes continue over a period of years and may not present clinically for a long time. The generally recognized risk factors for coronary disease, such as high cholesterol, smoking, poorly controlled hypertension or diabetes, etc., remain applicable and elevate the risk further. Therefore, these patients should be urged to observe general guidelines for lowering risk of cardiovascular disease by modifying their lifestyles. For accelerated coronary artery disease particularly involving the left descending artery, one study suggested that a dose of >24 Gy might be necessary.[16]

## Abdomen and Pelvis

Radiation therapy for many GI, GU, and GYN malignancies shares similar side effects (Table 8-4) and management strategies.

### Abdominal/Pelvic Adverse Effects and Management:

1. Stomach—Presenting symptoms and their management are similar for acute gastritis and esophagitis (previously discussed) and consists mainly of antisecretory therapy with H2 blockers or proton pump inhibitors. In addition, antiemetics may be used if nausea/vomiting is present. Use of prokinetic agents such as metoclopramide 10mg tid is beneficial if gastroparesis is suspected.

2. Small/large bowel—Abdominopelvic radiation often produces diarrhea, which is intensi-fied by concurrent chemotherapy. The risk for dehydration can be significant, particularly in the elderly.

   We routinely encourage meeting with a dietician at the start of radiation to discuss vari-ous dietary modifications such as restriction of high fiber food, fresh produce, deep fried meals, and various dairy products. If possible, during the treatment planning and simula-tion, the use of prone position with a belly board ought to be considered to minimize small bowel irradiation. Use of IMRT can also help minimize dose to the small bowel. *If a patient develops diarrhea during therapy and there is suspicion of a possible bowel infection, this latter condition must be investigated and treated before any antidiarrheals are prescribed!* Some commonly used gastrointestinal medications are listed in Table 8-7.

   The panel for clinical practice guidelines to prevent gastrointestinal mucositis recom-mended use of 500mg oral sulfasalazine bid for patients receiving pelvic radiation to decrease the risk of enteropathy, since this regimen was shown in one study to reduce the incidence of diarrhea in patients receiving pelvic radiation (55% vs 86%).[17,18] The same panel advised against the *prophylactic* use of oral sucralfate, mesalazine, and olsalazine in these patients.[18] Several randomized trials have failed to show preventative benefit from oral sucralfate or sucralfate enema (although data supports use of sucralfate enemas for *treatment* of established proctitis!).

   Some other preventative agents that have been evaluated as mucosal protectants include amifostine, misoprostol, and glutamine supplement.

3. Rectum/anus—Inflammation of the rectum and anus is common during radiation. The first step of any treatment must confirm that poorly-controlled diarrhea or constipation is not acutely exacerbating the condition. Presence of hemorrhoidal irritation should also be eval-uated. Maintaining soft, semi-formed stools appears to be least traumatic for patients under these circumstances.

   Most previously discussed preventative strategies to minimize bowel toxicity also apply here. The most common symptoms of proctitis include tenesmus or rectal urgency and bleeding. The acute symptoms may develop within a few weeks of radiation or shortly there-after and are mostly transient. Treatment of acute proctitis and perianal reaction during radiation therapy includes use of Sitz baths, steroid enemas, and creams. A few commonly used steroid-containing preparations include Analpram HC (cream/lotion), Anusol HC (cream/suppository), Cortifoam (foam), Cortenema (retension enema), Preparation H (cream/suppository), Proctofoam HC (foam).

Generally months to years elapse before chronic proctitis presents itself. Injury to mucosal surface with associated fibrosis generally leads to pain, urgency, bleeding, diarrhea, and less commonly incontinence or even obstruction due to stricture formation. The risk for chronic proctitis is related to the radiation dose and volume of rectum irradiated, as described extensively in the literature. In prostate cancer patients where total target dose is usually 75–80 Gy, it is critical to carefully evaluate dosimetry. The diagnosis of this complication requires an endoscopic evaluation to rule out other causes. Subsequent treatment options are based on severity of the symptoms. For instance, no specific therapy may be necessary in patients with only occasional, light rectal spotting as many of them may improve spontaneously.[19] For treatment of patients with more substantial bleeding, sucralfate enemas have been shown to be effective (though not useful for prevention).[20] In this setting, the use of sucralfate enemas was also recommended by the panel on clinical guidelines.[18] One study showed this therapy to be more effective than oral sulfasalazine even when combined with steroid enemas.[21] For refractory bleeding, other interventions include laser coagulation and electrocautery. Topical application of formaldehyde has been shown to be effective but carries a significant risk for subsequent serious complications, including strictures, fistula formation, and incontinence. Surgical intervention is typically reserved as the last resort.

In patients with chronic proctitis causing prominent symptoms of rectal discomfort and urgency only, use of sucralfate or corticosteroid enemas is appropriate. One study failed to show benefit of 5-aminosalicylic acid enemas in this setting.[21] Stool softeners should be considered when indicated.

4. Bladder—Acute, non-infectious cystitis/urethritis during radiation therapy is common and typically presents with dysuria, frequency, and urgency. This condition can also increase the risk for urinary tract infections, which must be evaluated and treated with appropriate antibiotics. Similarly, both indwelling and intermittent catherization of the bladder also increase this risk of infection. Once the possibility of an infection has been addressed, symptomatic relief from mucosal irritation can be achieved with frequently used analgesic and antispasmodic medications as listed in Table 8-8.

5. Prostate—Patients with urinary obstructive symptoms often experience worsening of their condition during radiation therapy. Various alpha adrenergic blockers are useful in improving urinary obstructive symptoms and represent the most frequently used pharmacological intervention (Table 8-8). The American Urologic Association (AUA) questionnaire for BPH symptoms is a reliable marker for assessing patient baseline and subsequent clinical response. A high AUA baseline score before commencement of radiation therapy should alert the physician for possible use of prophylactic pharmacological intervention, possibly in the form of hormonal therapy and/or alpha blockers. In patients with low blood pressure or those taking antihypertensive therapy, risk of orthostasis must be kept in mind, particularly at the time of initiation of medicine or whenever an upward dose titration is contemplated.

In patients with large prostate glands or baseline benign prostatic hypertrophy (BPH) symptoms, the incidence of acute urinary obstruction during radiation is also lowered by use of hormones that serve to achieve cytoreduction. However, flare-up of BPH symptoms can be observed if a GnRH *agonist* (Lupron) is started without a concomitant anti-androgen (Casodex) especially in patients with significant baseline obstructive symptoms. The underlying mechanism is thought to be stimulation of the pituitary gland, which increases the pro-

---

**TABLE 8-8 Common Genitourinary Medications**

**Irritative Symptoms**

| | |
|---|---|
| Phenazopyridine (Pyridium)* | 100–200 mg po tid |
| | (100, 200 mg tabs) |
| | *Note:* Azo-Standard is OTC equivalent; use 1–2 tabs tid; each tab is 95mg phenazopyridine |
| Prosed DS** | 1 tab po tid |
| | *Note:* contains analgesic, antiseptic, and atropine |
| Pyridium Plus* | 1 tab po tid |
| | *Note:* contains phenazopyridine, hyoscamine, and butabarbital |
| Urised** | 2 tabs po tid |
| | *Note:* contains analgesic, antiseptic, and atropine |

**Overactivity Symptoms**

| | |
|---|---|
| Flavoxate (Urispas) | 100–200 mg po tid |
| | (100 mg tabs) |
| Oxybutynin (Ditropan) | 5 mg po bid-tid; 36 mg patch twice per week |
| | (5 mg tab; 5mg/5ml syrup; 36 mg patch) |
| Tolterodine (Detrol) | 1–2 mg po bid |
| | (1, 2 mg tabs) |

**Obstructive Symptoms**

| | |
|---|---|
| Doxazosin (Cardura) | Start 1mg po qhs; Max up to 8mg qd if tolerated |
| | (1, 2, 4, 8 mg tabs) |
| Finasteride (Proscar) | 5 mg po qd |
| | (5 mg tab) |
| | *Note:* Prostate Specific Antigen levels may show a decrease |
| Terazosin (Hytrin) | Start 1mg po qhs; Max up to 10 mg qd if tolerated |
| | (1, 2, 5, 10 mg caps) |
| Tamsulosin (Flomax) | 0.4–0.8 mg po qd |
| | (0.4, 0.8 mg caps) |
| Alfuzosin (Uroxatral) | 10 mg po qd |
| | (10 mg caps) |

*Orange coloration of urine is expected.
**Various contraindications including glaucoma, bladder neck obstruction, sulfa drugs, etc.

---

duction of follicle-stimulating hormone (FSH) and leutinizing hormone (LH), resulting in a transient elevation in circulating testosterone level followed by a decline. (Similarly, in patients with symptomatic spinal metastasis from prostate cancer, exacerbation of symptoms can occur during this flare-up.) Ideally, a 2-week overlap of the two medications is recommended. Alternatively, monotherapy with a GnRH *antagonist* such as abarelix (Plenaxis) has been shown to be equally effective clinically without the associated risk for flare-up and is FDA approved for management of metastatic prostate cancer. However, allergic reactions causing hypotension can occur with this medication and reportedly increase with duration of use.

In patients with significant refractory obstructive symptoms despite optimal pharmacological intervention, an indwelling or intermittent catherization scheme might be necessary during the course of radiation. However, increased risk for a urinary tract infection must be kept in mind and consideration can be given to prophylactic antibiotics in select cases.

6. Penis—The risk of impotence is high in patients with prostate cancer who undergo radiation therapy. Presence of baseline erectile dysfunction, diabetes, advanced age, preceding prostatectomy, as well as use of hormonal therapy may further increase that risk. The complete workup and treatment of impotence often requires the involvement of a urologist. Available treatment options include pharmacological and mechanical interventions such as oral phosphodiesterase inhibitors (discussed in upcoming paragraphs), self-injection of vasodilators into penile tissue, vacuum devices, and implantable prostheses.

Phosphodiesterase-5 inhibitors (PDEi) constitute a class of drugs that are effective in combating impotence by enhancing penile vasodilatation via blocking the catabolism of cyclic GMP. These drugs are often prescribed as the first-line therapy due to ease of use and effectiveness. There are three available drugs from this class and they differ slightly in their characteristics (Table 8-9). Sildenafil and vardenafil are effective for up to 4 hours, while tadafil may be effective for up to 36 hours. Tadafil may also be taken with food while the other two require an empty stomach. The onset of action is also more rapid for Tadafil, although as a general guideline patients are often instructed to take a PDEi about 1 hour before anticipated sexual activity. The starting dose is usually the midpoint of the permitted dose range, with subsequent titrations to optimize benefit and minimize adverse effects.

Of the three discussed PDEi, sildenafil is the oldest and has the most data available. It was shown to be effective in about 50% of prostate cancer patients who received radiation.[22] In post-prostatectomy patients, it was found to be more effective in patients who had nerve-sparing surgery.[23]

All PDEi are contraindicated in patients taking nitrates because this combination can cause severe hypotension. Caution must be exercised in prescribing PDEi to patients with cardiovascular conditions including coronary ischemia, even if they are not taking nitrates. Similarly, concurrent use of alpha adrenergic antagonists is also generally avoided, although low doses of tamsulosin (Flomax) may be acceptable with tadafil. Some of the common side effects of PDEi include flushing, headache, dyspepsia, and visual disturbance.

7. Vulva/vagina—Concurrent infection with candida is common during chemoradiation therapy but may not be readily recognizable in context with radiation-related mucositis/dermatitis. Oral therapy with flucanazole (Diflucan) is a good choice, often with better patient compliance, especially if significant radiation-related mucositis/dermatitis is present. In terms of late effects, stenosis and dryness of vaginal mucosa can lead to dyspareunia and should be addressed. Use of artifical lubricants and graduated vaginal dilators is most helpful. The Cochrane review of pertinent literature supported use of dilators and intercourse as effective interventions but suggested a need for additional data to evaluate usefulness of topical estrogens and benzydamine douches.[24] Even in patients who are sexually inactive, stenosis of the vagina is undesirable because it limits thorough physical examinations for future surveillance.

## TABLE 8-9 Medications for Erectile Dysfunction

| Drug | Dose | With Food* | Interaction** | Duration |
|------|------|-----------|---------------|----------|
| Sildenafil (Viagra) | 25–100mg | Empty stomach | No alpha blocker | About 4 hours |
| Vardenafil (Levitra) | 2.5–20mg | Empty stomach | No alpha blocker | About 4 hours |
| Tadalafil (Cialis) | 2.5–20mg | OK | Tamsulosin may be OK | Up to 36 hours (half life 18 hrs) |

*Fat content of food affects drug absorption and delays time to peak plasma levels.
**Nitrates are contraindicated with all phosphodiesterase-5 inhibitors.

## Central Nervous System

### *Tumor-Related Edema and Use of Steroids*

Radiation therapy for primary or metastatic cancer involving the CNS often requires use of steroids for prevention and treatment of edema. Glucocorticoids are very effective in reducing tumor-induced edema within hours of administration. The degree of tumor edema and severity of clinical symptoms is used to guide the dose and duration of steroids. Although data from randomized trials showed benefit from high dose steroids in patients with cord compression, this was accompanied by significant side effects.[25,26] As a result, the most commonly used steroid regimen uses significantly lower doses of steroids for mildly symptomatic patients while the higher doses of steroids may be appropriate for patients with severe symptoms such as paraplegia. The steroid doses are tapered as clinically allowed with a close evaluation of the change in patients' symptoms once the radiotherapy course has commenced. In patients with other comorbidities that are exacerbated with steroids, there is an even more pressing need to initiate the steroid taper in a timely fashion without undue delay. At the same time, this tapering must not be rushed but be judiciously guided by the individual patient's progress. For instance, premature tapering of steroids in a patient with brain metastases and edema may exacerbate symptoms of headache, ataxia, paraparesis, diplopia, nausea, and vomiting.

Dexamethasone is the most commonly used glucocorticoid steroid, mainly due to its high potency and relatively little concomitant mineralocorticoid activity (Table 8-10). In symptomatic cases, a patient with brain or spinal cord metastasis is typically preferred to have been on steroids for 24–48 hours prior to initiating radiation therapy. If a very high dose of steroids is clinically indicated, one could use historic data to start with up to 96mg of dexamethasone bolus followed by 24mg q6 hours for 2–3 days, with eventual taper over an additional 8–10 days as guided by clinical response. In contrast, *the more commonly used regimen for mild neurologic symptoms consists of 10mg dexamethasone bolus (which may even be omitted) followed by 4mg q6 hours for a few days, with a complete taper over 10–14 days as clinically indicated.*

It is important to recognize that these are general guidelines only and progress of an individual patient truly determines the ideal rate of tapering. During steroid use, beware of elevated blood sugar level in patients with diabetes, dyspepsia in patients with reflux disease or taking NSAIDs, complaints of insomnia or mood lability, etc. Concerns about adrenal suppression are applicable in patients who require long steroid therapy over several weeks at substantial doses. These patients may need stress-dose steroids if they show signs of hemodynamic collapse under conditions of acute physiologic stress such as sepsis.

**TABLE 8-10  Comparison of Common Glucocorticoids**

| Glucocorticoid | Relative Potency | Equivalent Dose (mg) |
| --- | --- | --- |
| Cortisol | 1 | 20 |
| Prednisone | 4 | 5 |
| Dexamethasone | 30–150 | 0.75 |

## MEDICAL ISSUES AND SUPPORTIVE CARE

## Antibiotics for Common Infections

Table 8-11 presents management strategies for common infectious issues that may arise during or after a course of radiotherapy.

## TABLE 8-11 Common Infections and their Treatment

| Infection | Symptoms and Diagnosis | Treatment |
|---|---|---|
| **GENITOURINARY** | | |
| **Epididymitis** | Scrotal pain, point tenderness in the epididymis, with or without irritative voiding symtpoms and fever. Urine culture may identify causative organism. | Ciprofloxacin extended release 500 mg 1×/d for 10–14 days. |
| **Prostatitis** | Fever, dysuria, pelvic pain, cloudy urine, and physical exam revealing tender/edematous prostate. Urinalysis and culture should be obtained to confirm diagnosis and guide therapy. | Ciprofloxacin extended release 500 mg 1×/d or trimethoprim/sulfamethoxazole DS 2×/d for 4–6 weeks. |
| **Urinary tract infection** | Dysuria, frequency, urgency, suprapubic tenderness, and/or hematuria. Urinalysis and culture should be obtained to confirm diagnosis and guide therapy. Presence of fever and/or flank pain should raise clinical suspicion for pyelonephritis. | First-line: trimethoprim/sulfamethoxazole (TMP/SMX) DS 2×/d. If allergic to TMP/SMX, then ciprofloxacin extended release 500 mg 1×/d.<br>Treat for 7 days if any of the following: receiving or recently completed pelvic radiation, pelvic malignancy, male sex, or indwelling foley. Otherwise, treat for 3 days. |
| **Vaginal candidiasis** | Thick, white, cottage cheese-like discharge. Culture should be obtained to confirm diagnosis and guide anti-fungal therapy. | For patients receiving radiation therapy, fluconazole 150 mg days 1 and 4. |
| **HEAD/NECK** | | |
| **Oropharyngeal candidiasis** | White plaques with or without erythema on mucous membranes. | Clotrimazole 10 mg oral troches 5×/d, nystatin oral solution 100,000 U/ml 1 teaspoon swish and swallow 4×/d, or fluconazole (200 mg day 1 followed by 100 mg daily) × 7–14d. |
| **Sinusitis** | Nasal congestion, purulent nasal discharge, post-nasal drip, facial pain/headache, and fever. Although sinus CT and sinus aspiration are the gold standard for diagnosis, they are not recommended for uncomplicated community acquired sinusitis. | Viral infection accounts for approximately 98% of all cases of rhinosinusitis and typically improves within 7–10 days of diagnosis. Bacterial sinusitis should be suspected if (1) symptoms progress after 5–7 days or do not improve after 10 days, or (2) severe symptoms including fever, facial pain, or facial swelling regardless of duration. If bacterial sinusitis is suspected, then treat for 7–10 days with one of the following: Amoxicillin/Clavulanate 875/125 2×/d, Levofloxacin 500 mg 1×/d, Moxifloxacin 400 mg 1×/d. |
| **RESPIRATORY/THORACIC** | | |
| **Bronchitis** | Productive cough, no fever, normal chest radiograph | Supportive care. If cough persists greater than 14 days and pertussis is suspected, then azithromycin 500 mg day 1, 250 mg days 2–5. For bronchitis in setting of severe COPD exacerbation, consider azithromycin, cefuroxime 500 mg 2×/d, gatifloxacin 400 mg 1×/d, levofloxacin 500 mg 1×/d, or moxifloxacin 400 mg 1×/d × 5–10d. |

## TABLE 8-11 (continued)

| Infection | Symptoms and Diagnosis | Treatment |
|---|---|---|
| **Esophageal candidiasis** | May occur with or without concomitant oropharyngeal candidiasis. Hallmark is odynophagia yet diagnosis can only be confirmed with endoscopy and biopsy. Empiric treatment should be strongly considerd in patients who develop severe esophagitis early in the course of thoracic radiation. | Fluconazole (200 mg day 1 followed by 100 mg daily) × 14–21d. Topical agents should not be used. |
| **Influenza** | Abrupt onset of fever, myalgias, headache, malaise, and respiratory tract symptoms. Diagnose with rapid immunofluorescence assay performed on swab from nasopharynx. May confirm with viral culture. | Oseltamivir 75 mg bid × 5d, Zanamivir 2 inhalations bid × 5d. Must begin treatment within 36 hours of symptom onset. |
| **Pneumonia** | Fever, cough, and infiltrate on chest radiograph. For outpatients, sputum culture is rarely necessary. | For patients without significant comorbidity: azithromycin 500 mg day 1 followed by 250 mg daily.<br>For patients with significant comorbidity or post-obstructive pneumonia: gatifloxacin 400 mg 1×/d, levofloxacin 500 mg 1×/d, or moxifloxacin 400 mg 1×/d.<br>If aspiration pneumonia a strong concern (patients unable to protect airway and/or poor dentition), then clindamycin 450 mg 4×/d.<br>Treat until patient afebrile for at least 3 days. |
| **SKIN/SOFT TISSUE** | | |
| **Cellulitis** | Warm, tender, painful skin erythema. Consider blood cultures if febrile. | Cephalexin 500 mg 4×/d × 10–14d or Dicloxacillin 500 gm 4×/d × 10–14d. |
| **Cutaneous candidiasis** | Foul smelling, erythematous plaque in skin fold, such as inframammary or inguinal folds. Diagnosis may be confirmed by culture of skin scrapings. | Topical nystatin, clotrimazole, or amphotericin B cream applied 3–4×/d × 7–14d. |
| **Herpes simplex** | Prodrome of local pain and/or dysesthesias followed by vesicle formation. Classic sites include orolabial and genital. Diagnosis may be confirmed by viral culture of vesicular fluid and/or immunofluorescence staining of cells scraped from base of lesion. The sensitivity of these tests is low; a negative test does not rule out herpes simplex. | For oral:<br>Topical options include: Penciclovir 1% q2h × 4d, Docosanol 10% 5×/d until healed, Acyclovir 5% cream 6x/d × 7d.<br>Systemic options include Valacyclovir 2 gm 2×/d x 1d, Famciclovir 500 mg 2×/d x 7d, Acyclovir 400 mg 5×/d × 5d. Famciclovir may be most effective but is also most expensive.<br>For genital:<br>If an episodic recurrence: Acyclovir 400 mg 3x/d x× 5d, Famciclovir 125 mg 2×/d x 5d, Valacyclovir 500 mg 2×/d × 3d. If a primary episode then extend treatment duration to 7–10d. |

*(continues)*

TABLE 8-11 (continued)

| Infection | Symptoms and Diagnosis | Treatment |
|---|---|---|
| Herpes zoster | Prodrome of fever, headache, malaise, and dermatomal dysesthesias followed by eruption of dermatomal vesicular rash. Diagnosis may be made clinically. If doubt exists, pursue viral culture of vesicular fluid and/or immunofluorescence staining of cells scraped from base of lesion. | Valacyclovir 1000 mg 3×/d × 7d, Famciclovir 750 mg 1×/d × 7d, Acyclovir 800 mg 5×/d × 7–10d. For older patients with large number of lesions, prednisone may confer a symptomatic benefit (30 mg 2×/d days 1–7, 15 mg 2×/d days 8–14, and 7.5 mg 2×/d days 15–21). Involvement of the eye should prompt emergent opthalmology evaluation. Patients with disseminated zoster require hospitalization, IV medication, and airborne precautions. |
| Postoperative mastitis | Erythema, edema, and pain +/− fever. Any discharge should be sent for culture to guide antibiotic therapy. Patients should be carefully assessed for a fluctuant mass that would require drainage. | Initial therapy: Cephalexin 500 mg 4×/d OR Dicloxacillin 500 gm 4×/d × 10–14d. If no clinical response within 3 days, consider ultrasound to rule out abscess and switch to Levofloxacin 500 mg 1×/d PLUS Clindamycin 450 mg 3×/d. |
| Superinfected radiation dermatitis | Diagnosis is supported by moist desquamation with purulent exudate and erythema extending outside radiation field. Culture should be obtained to guide antibiotic therapy. | Head/neck or breast: Cephalexin 500 mg 4×/d ×10–14d OR Dicloxacillin 500 gm 4×/d until moist desquamation begins to heal. Groin/perineum: Amoxicillin/Clavulanate 875/125 2×/d OR the combination of Levofloxacin 500 mg 1×/d PLUS Clindamycin 450 mg 3×/d. Again, treat until moist desquamation begins to heal. |

## Pain Management

More than 80% of cancer patients will develop pain prior to death. With appropriate utilization of pharmacologic and non-pharmacologic interventions, cancer pain can be successfully managed for the majority of patients. Pharmacologic interventions are selected based on the severity and duration of pain. For patients with mild, intermittent pain, NSAIDs and/or acetaminophen may be adequate. For patients with moderate pain of variable duration, mild opioid analgesics such as codeine, hydrocodone, or tramadol are recommended (Table 8-12). Patients with severe, constant pain require potent opioid analgesics such as oxycodone, morphine, fetanyl, hydromorphone, or methadone. These patients typically require both fast-acting (rescue, Table 8-12) and long-acting (maintenance, Table 8-13) opioids. Guidelines for conversion of different opioid regimens are presented in Table 8-14. Adjuvant medications tailored to the patient's specific pain syndrome may provide an additional benefit when combined with opioid analgesics. Examples of adjuvant medications include NSAIDs or bisphosphonates for bony pain and tricyclic antidepressants or anticonvulsants for neuropathic pain. Corticosteroids may also provide substantial pain relief and, additionally, increase energy level and appetite.

Side effects of opiod analgesics are common. Constipation is the most common adverse effect and is not strongly dependant on dose. All patients receiving opioid analgesia should, therefore, initiate a bowel regimen (Table 8-15). Nausea and vomiting may occur shortly after initiation of opioids, although typically these symptoms improve with time. For patients with severe nausea, prochlorperazine or metoclopramide are usually effective. Other side effects of opioids may include sedation, mental status changes, respiratory depression, myoclonus, and urinary retention. Patients who develop mental status changes should be thoroughly evaluated for other potential

## TABLE 8-12 Short-Acting Opiates

| Medication | Dose* | Duration | Tablet Size and Elixir Concentrations |
|---|---|---|---|
| *For moderate pain* | | | |
| Codeine | 15–60 mg | 4–6h | 15, 30, 60 |
| Acetaminophen/Codeine | 1–2 tabs | 4–6h | 300/15, 300/30, 300/60, 120/12 per 5 mL |
| Ibuprofen/Hydrocodone | 1 tab | 4–6h | 200/7.5 |
| Acetaminophen/Hydrocodone | 1–2 tabs | 4–6h | 500/2.5; 325,500/5; 325,500,650,750/7.5; 325,500,650,660/10; 500/7.5 per 15 mL |
| Tramadol | 50–100 mg | 4–6h | 50 |
| Acetaminophen/Tramadol | 2 tabs | 4–6h | 325/37.5 |
| *For severe pain* | | | |
| Oxycodone | 5–10 mg | 4h | 5, 15, 30, 5 per 5 mL, 20 per mL |
| Acetaminophen/Oxycodone | 1–2 tabs | 4–6h | 325/2.5; 325,500/5; 325,500/7.5; 325, 650/10; 325/5 per 5 mL |
| Morphine Sulfate | 15–30 mg | 4–6h | 15, 30, 2 per mL, 4 per mL, 20 per mL |
| Hydromorphone | 2–4 mg | 4–5h | 2, 4, 8, 1 per mL |

*Doses are reported for opiate-naïve patients. For opiate-tolerant patients, the short-acting opiate dose should be approximately 10%–20% of the total daily opiate dose and should be administered every 2 hours as needed. For all patients, the 24-hour dose of acetaminophen should not exceed 4 gm. Morphine is cleared by the kidney and should not be used for patients with renal insufficiency.

## TABLE 8-13 Long-Acting Opiates

| Medication | Duration | Tablet Size |
|---|---|---|
| Oxycontin (long-acting oxycodone tablets) | 8–12h | 10, 20, 40, 80, 160 mg |
| Morphine Sulfate Sustained Release | 8–12h | 15, 30, 60, 100, 200 mg |
| Duragesic (fentanyl transdermal) | 48–72h | 12, 25, 50, 75, 100 mcg/hr |
| Methadone | 8h | 5, 10 mg |

Appropriate dosing for long-acting opiates depends on the patient's tolerance and prior exposure to short-acting opioids. Table 8-14 presents guidelines for converting the short-acting dose of one opioid to the long-acting dose of another.

## TABLE 8-14 Equianalgesic Table

| Drug | Oral Dose |
|---|---|
| Codeine | 200 mg |
| Oxycodone | 20 mg |
| Morphine Sulfate | 30 mg |
| Hydromorphone | 7.5 mg |

The above dosages are all equivalent to 10 mg of IM morphine sulfate. When converting from one opioid to another, the starting dose of the new opioid should be reduced by approximately 25% to account for incomplete cross-tolerance. Duragesic (fentanyl transdermal) 25 mcg/hr is equivalent to 1 mg/hr of IV morphine sulfate and 72 mg of oxycodone per day.

## TABLE 8-15 Recommended Bowel Regimen

1. Docusate (Colace) 100 mg 3×/d + senna (Senakot) 2 tablets 2×/d.
2. If ineffective, increase senna to 2 tablets 3×/d.
3. If still ineffective, assess for obstruction or impaction. If no evidence for obstruction or impaction, then consider polyethylene glycol (Miralax or GoLytely) or magnesium citrate.

causes such as metabolic derangements (hypercalcemia, hyponatremia, or uremia), metastatic disease to the brain, and drug-drug interactions.

## Hot Flashes

Hot flashes represent vasomotor instability that is possibly mediated at the hypothalamic level, although the clear mechanism is not well understood. Alteration in the balance of circulating hormones, as seen during menopause in women and androgen blockade in men, triggers hot flashes.

Estrogen replacement can be a very effective treatment for hot flashes in women, although there is concern that estrogen replacement may increase the risk of recurrence in patients with breast or endometrial cancer. Progestin (megesterol acetate, or Megace 20–80 mg/day) is also shown to be highly effective with about an 85% response rate. After initial response, dose can be lowered for maintenance. However, weight gain is a considerable side effect of progestins. Also, there is a theoretical risk of adrenal gland suppression upon discontinuation due to its similarity to glucocorticoids.

Both men and women can benefit from use of low dose selective serotonin reuptake inhibitors (SSRI) that may also give the added benefit of serving as anti-depressants. *This class of drugs is generally considered the first line therapy.* For example, Venlaxafine (Effexor), a selective serotonin and norepinephrine reuptake inhibitor, at 37.5–75mg daily is highly effective and, in fact, may be superior to some other SSRIs, including fluoxetine (Prozac). Side effects were seen more frequently at higher doses, including mouth dryness, anorexia, nausea, and constipation.[27]

Clonidine (Catapres), a centrally acting antihypertensive agent, can be given in 0.1–0.4 mg/day doses via oral pill or transdermal patch (patch is applied q7 days). Studies have shown varying response rates. This may be appropriate for patients with hypertension, but blood pressure should be closely monitored at least initially. Other, less commonly used options include vitamin E, soy products, and acupuncture.

## Appetite Stimulants

The cancer-related cachexia/anorexia syndrome is commonly encountered in patients with advanced malignancies. Not only do these patients have an elevated metabolic rate, but their poor appetites worsen the condition by lowering their nutritional intake. Available pharmacological interventions include appetite stimulants, anticatabolic agents, and anabolic agents. Although these agents can produce increased appetite and weight gain, they do *not* prolong survival.

Based on multiple studies, progestational agents (megesterol acetate) are considered the best choice overall. Although a dose-response was observed for daily doses of 160–800mg megesterol acetate (Megace), *the optimal dose recommendation is 480–800 mg daily.*[28] This medication is available in both tablet and liquid forms; the latter may be more convenient and should be considered. Possible side effects include risk for venous thrombosis and adrenal suppression.

Although corticosteroids (dexamethasone 2–4 mg/qd) have been shown to improve appetite and weight gain, the effectiveness of this therapy is felt to be rather short-lived. In addition, significant side effects of steroids are known, including myopathy, osteoporosis, gastritis, mood lability, insomnia, etc. For these reasons, steroids are felt to be a suitable intervention only for patients with very short life expectancy.

Several other less well-studied agents include oxandrolone 20 mg/qd (anabolic steroid), cyproheptadine 8mg tid (histamine and serotonin antagonist), dronabinol (active ingredient in marijuana), that have some supporting data and may be considered.

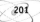

## Psychiatric Issues

Depression, anxiety, and insomnia are commonly encountered in cancer patients. Agents commonly used to treat these conditions are summarized in Table 8-16.

## Bone Health

Growing evidence suggests that men treated with gonadotropin-releasing hormone (GnRH) agonists experience an increased risk of osteoporosis and fracture. Patients who will receive a GnRH agonist should, therefore, be evaluated for osteoporosis risk factors, receive calcium plus vitamin D supplementation, and receive bisphosphonate therapy as indicated (Table 8-17).

## IV Contrast: Pertinent Medical Issues

Intravenous contrast is frequently used for both treatment planning and diagnostic CT scans. The following steps are necessary to safely administer intravenous contrast:

1. Identify patients at high risk for a contrast reaction and document baseline renal function for those at risk (Table 8-18).

---

**TABLE 8-16 Common Psychiatric Medications**

**Anti-depressants**

| | |
|---|---|
| Amitriptyline (Elavil)—TCA | 50–150mg qd (tabs 10, 25, 50,75, 100, 150mg); start low |
| Fluoxetine (Prozac)—SSRI | 20–80 mg qd (pulvules 10, 20mg; liquid 20mg/5cc) |
| Paroxetine (Paxil)—SSRI | 20–40 mg qd (tabs 10, 20, 30 40mg) |
| Sertraline (Zoloft)—SSRI | 50–200 mg qd (tabs 25, 50, 100mg) |
| Venlafaxine (Effexor)—SNRI | 37.5–100mg qd (tabs 25,37.5, 50, 75, 100mg) |

**Anxiolytics**

| | |
|---|---|
| Alprazolam (Xanax) | 0.25–1mg bid-tid (tabs 0.25, 0.5, 1, 2mg) |
| Diazepam (Valium) | 2–10mg bid-tid (tabs 2,5,10mg; liquid 5mg/5cc) |
| Lorazepam (Ativan) | 0.5–1mg bid-tid (tabs 0.5, 1, 2mg) |

**Sleep Aids**

| | |
|---|---|
| Diphenhydramine (Benadryl)—OTC | 25–50mg qhs (tabs 25mg) |
| Flurazepam (Dalmane) | 15–30mg qhs (caps 15, 30mg) |
| Temazepam (Restoril) | 7.5–30mg qhs (caps 7.5, 15, 30mg) |
| Zolpidem (Ambien) | 5–10mg qhs (tabs 5,10mg) |

Abbreviations: OTC (over-the-counter), SNRI (serotonin-norepinephrine reuptake inhibitor), SSRI (selective serotonin reuptake inhibitor), TCA (tricyclic antidepressant).

---

**BOX 8-2**

This retrospective observational cohort study examined the association between receipt of a GnRH agonist and risk of fracture among 50,613 men with prostate cancer identified in the SEER-Medicare cohort. The 5-year risk of fracture was 19.4% for men who received a GnRH agonist and 12.6% for men who did not. A dose response relationship was also noted, with a higher total number of GnRH agonist injections correlated with a higher risk of fracture.

Shahinian et al. Risk of Fracture after Androgen Deprivation for Prostate Cancer. *N Engl J Med* 352:154–164, 2005.

**TABLE 8-17 Management of Bone Health for Patients Receiving a GnRH Agonist**

### Recommendations for all patients receiving GnRH agonist therapy:
- Smoking and alcohol cessation.
- Moderate exercise regimen.
- Supplementation with one tablet twice daily calcium citrate/vitamin D (630 mg/400 IU). Note that a history of nephrolithiasis or renal insufficiency is a relative contraindication to calcium supplementation.

### If anticipated duration of GnRH agonist is greater than 6 months:
- Baseline bone density study
- If osteoporosis is present, then
    - Consider endocrinology referral.
    - Lab workup: Calcium, TSH, 25-hydroxyvitamin D, alkaline phosphatase, PTH.
    - Begin Alendronate 70 mg tablets one week.
        - Alendronate should not be given to patients with active upper gastrointestinal disease or severe renal impairment (CrCl < 35).
        - Alendronate should be discontinued in patients who develop any symptoms of esophagitis.
        - Alendronate should be taken on an empty stomach with at least 240 mL (8 oz) of water while sitting or standing to minimize the risk of the tablet getting stuck in the esophagus. Do not take alendronate at the same time calcium is taken, as this may decrease absorption.
        - Patients should remain upright for at least 30 minutes before eating, both to minimize the risk of reflux and improve absorption of the drug.
        - Contraindications: Severe renal failure with creatinine clearance less than 30 ml/min.
        - Cost is $70 per month.
- Follow bone density scan on a yearly basis. If patient subsequently develops osteoporosis, or if there is evidence of significant bone loss over time that does not yet meet criteria for osteoporosis, then alendronate should be initiated.

---

**TABLE 8-18 Risk Factors for an Adverse Event Following IV Contrast Administration**

1. Previous reaction to contrast
2. Renal insufficiency with a baseline creatinine > 1.5 mg/dL
3. Serious allergies and/or asthma
4. Significant cardiovascular disease
5. Hyperuricemia
6. Multiple myeloma
7. Hypertension
8. Age > 70 years
9. Diabetes mellitus
10. Currently taking metformin (Glucophage or Glucovance)

---

2. For patients with renal impairment:
   - Intravenous fluids 100 ml/hr for 4 hours before scan and 24 hours after scan.
   - N-acetylcysteine 600 mg po bid the day prior to the scan and the day of the scan.
3. Hold metformin, given the risk of lactic acidosis (Table 8-19).
4. Administer appropriate premedications for patients with a history of contrast reactions (Table 8-20).

**TABLE 8-19  Management of Metformin for Patients Receiving IV Contrast**

1. Stop metformin prior to IV contrast injection
2. Hold metformin for 48 hours after contrast administration
3. Confirm normal renal function prior to resuming metformin

**TABLE 8-20  Premedication for Patients with a History of IV Contrast Reactions**

1. Steroid Regimen
   a. Methylprednisolone 32 mg taken 12 and 2 hours prior to study.
      OR
   b. Prednisone 50 mg taken 12, 6, and 1 hour prior to study.
2. May add antihistamine: Diphenhydramine 50 mg taken 1 hour prior to study.

# References

1. Emami B, Lyman J, Brown A, et al. Tolerance of normal tissue to therapeutic irradiation. *Int J Radiat Oncol Biol Phys* 21:109–122, 1991.
2. Epstein JB, Silverman S, Jr., Paggiarino DA, et al. Benzydamine HCl for prophylaxis of radiation-induced oral mucositis: results from a multicenter, randomized, double-blind, placebo-controlled clinical trial. *Cancer* 92:875–885, 2001.
3. Rubenstein EB, Peterson DE, Schubert M, et al. Clinical practice guidelines for the prevention and treatment of cancer therapy-induced oral and gastrointestinal mucositis. *Cancer* 100:2026–2046, 2004.
4. Johnstone PA, Niemtzow RC, Riffenburgh RH. Acupuncture for xerostomia: clinical update. *Cancer* 94:1151–1156, 2002.
5. Garcia-Serra A, Amdur RJ, Morris CG, et al. Thyroid function should be monitored following radiotherapy to the low neck. *Am J Clin Oncol* 28:255–258, 2005.
6. Browman GP, Wong G, Hodson I, et al. Influence of cigarette smoking on the efficacy of radiation therapy in head and neck cancer. *N Engl J Med* 328:159–163, 1993.
7. Rugg T, Saunders MI, Dische S. Smoking and mucosal reactions to radiotherapy. Br J Radiol 63:554–556, 1990.
8. Rodrigues G, Lock M, et al. Prediction of radiation pneumonitis by dose-volume histogram parameters in lung cancer: a systematic review. *Radiother Oncol* 71:127–138, 2004.
9. Kong FM, Hayman JA, et al. Final toxicity results of a radiation-dose escalation study in patients with non-small cell lung cancer (NSCLC): Predictors for radiation pneumonitis and fibrosis. *Int J Radiat Oncol Biol Phys* 65:1075–1086, 2006.
10. Schallenkamp JM, Miller RC, et al. Incidence of radiation pneumonitis after thoracic irradiation: Dose-volume correlates. *Int J Radiat Oncol Biol Phys* 67:410–416, 2007.
11. Graham MV, Purdy JA, Emami B, et al. Clinical dose-volume histogram analysis for pneumonitis after 3D treatment for non-small cell lung cancer (NSCLC). *Int J Radiat Oncol Biol Phys* 45:323–329, 1999.
12. Ozturk B, Egehan I, Atavci S, et al. Pentoxifylline in prevention of radiation-induced lung toxicity in patients with breast and lung cancer: a double-blind randomized trial. *Int J Radiat Oncol Biol Phys* 58:213–219, 2004.
13. Coia LR, Myerson RJ, Tepper JE. Late effects of radiation therapy on the gastrointestinal tract. *Int J Radiat Oncol Biol Phys* 31:1213–1236, 1995.

14. Bull RK, Edwards PD, Dixon AK. CT dimensions of the normal pericardium. *Br J Radiol* 71:923–925, 1998.

15. Stewart JR, Fajardo LF, Gillette SM, et al. Radiation injury to the heart. *Int J Radiat Oncol Biol Phys* 31:1205–1211, 1995.

16. Carr ZA, Land CE, Kleinerman RA, et al. Coronary heart disease after radiotherapy for peptic ulcer disease. *Int J Radiat Oncol Biol Phys* 61:842–850, 2005.

17. Kilic D, Egehan I, Ozenirler S, et al. Double-blinded, randomized, placebo-controlled study to evaluate the effectiveness of sulphasalazine in preventing acute gastrointestinal complications due to radiotherapy. *Radiother Oncol* 57:125–129, 2000.

18. Rubenstein EB, Peterson DE, et al. Clinical practice guidelines for the prevention and treatment of cancer therapy-induced oral and gastrointestinal mucositis. *Cancer* 100 (9 Suppl): 2026–2046, 2004.

19. Gilinsky NH, Burns DG, Barbezat GO, et al. The natural history of radiation-induced proctosigmoiditis: an analysis of 88 patients. *Q J Med* 52:40–53, 1983.

20. Kochhar R, Sriram PV, Sharma SC, et al. Natural history of late radiation proctosigmoiditis treated with topical sucralfate suspension. *Dig Dis Sci* 44:973–978, 1999.

21. Kochhar R, Patel F, Dhar A, et al. Radiation-induced proctosigmoiditis. Prospective, randomized, double-blind controlled trial of oral sulfasalazine plus rectal steroids versus rectal sucralfate. *Dig Dis Sci* 36:103–107, 1991.

22. Schover, LR, Fouladi, RT, et al. The use of treatments for erectile dysfunction among survivors of prostate carcinoma. *Cancer* 95:2397–2407, 2002.

23. Zippe, CD, Kedia, AW, et al. Treatment of erectile dysfunction after radical protatectomy with sildenafil citrate (Viagra). *Urology* 52:963–966, 1998.

24. Denton AS, Maher EJ. Interventions for the physical aspects of sexual dysfunction in women following pelvic radiotherapy. The Cochrane Database of Systematic Reviews 2003, Issue 1. Art. No.: CD003750.

25. Sorensen PS, Helweg-Larsen S, et al. Effect of high-dose dexamethasone in carcinomatous metastatic spinal cord compression treated with radiotherapy: a randomised trial. *Eur J Cancer* 30A:22–27, 1994.

26. Heimdal K, Hirschberg H, et al. High incidence of serious side effects of high-dose dexamethasone treatment in patients with epidural spinal cord compression. *J Neurooncol* 12:141–144, 1992.

27. Loprinzi CL, Kugler JW, Sloan JA, et al. Venlafaxine in management of hot flashes in survivors of breast cancer: a randomised controlled trial. *Lancet* 356:2059–2063, 2000.

28. Loprinzi CL, Michalak JC, Schaid DJ, et al. Phase III evaluation of four doses of megestrol acetate as therapy for patients with cancer anorexia and/or cachexia. *J Clin Oncol* 11:762–767, 1993.

# 9

# Radioimmunotherapy and the Use of Unsealed Sources in Radiation Oncology

*Vipul V. Thakkar, MD*
*Roger M. Macklis, MD*

## Overview

Unsealed radioactive sources have been used in the treatment of disease for many decades. However, the recent development of advanced immunobiologic techniques has ushered in a new era of targeted therapies. This chapter focuses on the use of "naked" radioisotopes as well as radioimmunoconjugates in treatment of malignant disease.

## Introduction

The term radiopharmaceutical or "unsealed source" refers to delivery of a radioactive compound, either alone or in conjugated form, for treatment of medical conditions. The very first radiopharmaceuticals were merely soluble forms of radioactive isotopes that had an innate physiologic bias to accumulate in an organ or site of interest. Although effective, these agents had limited targeting ability and significant hematopoietic toxicity which precluded generalized use, thus limiting their role in oncology. The recent development of molecular targeted drug therapy has led to new classes of agents that combine the targeting specificity of the immune system with the cytotoxic effects of radiation therapy.[1] In addition to newer biologically targeted agents, the classic disease-avid radiopharmaceuticals are still indicated in selected patients. A list of the most commonly used agents for unsealed source therapy is presented in Table 9-1. The common link between these isotopes is a decay scheme that includes a high energy, short range beta emission. In some cases a gamma emission suitable for imaging is also present.

## Radioimmunotherapy in Non-Hodgkin's Lymphoma

In the United States alone, approximately 58,000 people were diagnosed with non-Hodgkin's lymphoma (NHL) in 2007 with a significant proportion of these patients falling into the low-grade or follicular, CD20+ B-cell subgroup of NHL.[3] Indolent NHL typically responds to initial therapy, but a pattern of multiple relapses at progressively shorter intervals occurs and eventually causes a slow, inexorable clinical decline leading to death at a median of 8–10 years after diagnosis.[4]

TABLE 9-1  Physical Properties of Commonly Used Isotopes in Unsealed Source Therapy[2]

| Radionuclide | Physical Half Life | Maximum Particle Energy (MeV) | Gamma Energy (MeV) | Maximum Range in Tissue (mm) |
|---|---|---|---|---|
| 32P | 14.3 days | 1.7 | None | 8.2 |
| 131I | 8.0 days | 0.6 | 0.36 | 2.3 |
| 90Y | 64.1 hours | 2.3 | None | 11.3 |
| 89Sr | 50.5 days | 1.5 | None | 7.0 |
| 153Sm | 1.9 days | 0.8 | 0.10 | 3.1 |

New approaches that specifically target cancer cells using antibody therapies, such as the chimeric anti-CD20 antibody rituximab, have proven to be highly effective and well tolerated.[5] Nevertheless, rituximab does not appear curative. Efforts to enhance the killing effect and thereby improve the clinical outcomes of antibody therapy have resulted in FDA approval for two compounds that link a radioactive isotope to murine monoclonal anti-CD20 antibodies. Addition of a radioisotope allows delivery of not only targeted, cell-specific immunotherapy, but also targeted molecular radiotherapy.

## The Target[6]

As a marker found on mature B lymphocytes and expressed by >90% of B-cell lymphomas, CD20 is considered an ideal molecule for targeted therapy. It is not present on plasma cells or stem cells, allowing immunoglobulin levels and precursor cells to remain unaffected after treatment with anti-CD20 therapy. Furthermore, the molecule is securely anchored in the plasma membrane and is not susceptible to detachment or internalization. Although its exact function is not known, CD20 is thought to play a role in cell cycle regulation, control of apoptosis, and calcium regulation.

## Pharmacology, Mechanism of Action, and Dosimetry

While rituxan is a chimeric antibody composed of both human and murine components, a pure murine monoclonal antibody appears better suited for RIT due to a shorter clearance time. This reduces the risk of overdose and subsequent marrow suppression when the antibody has an associated radionuclide. In fact, the anti-CD20 antibody ibritumomab is the murine monoclonal antibody genetically modified to produce the chimeric rituximab. Tositumomab has an alternate binding location on the CD20 molecule and its binding characteristics are somewhat different than rituximab/ibritumomab. Mechanistically, the binding of the antibody alone to the CD20 molecule on the outer surface of the B-lymphocyte may result in the death of the target cell through several distinct mechanisms including apoptosis, antibody-dependent cellular cytotoxicity, and complement-dependent cytotoxicity. Addition of a radionuclide allows targeting of cells that are in close proximity but not directly bound to the therapeutic compound. This is termed the "cross-fire" effect and is a major mechanism of action in RIT.[6] Although it was initially thought that general principles of radiation biology and dosimetry would apply to RIT, it became evident that this was not entirely true. The dose rate delivered by RIT is very low (~1–10 cGy/hour), and the cumulative absorbed doses from RIT often do not correlate well with clinical response. Thus, although the radiation dose absorbed by the target may be rather low, a greater than expected response is typically seen.[7]

## Indications for RIT in NHL

Relapsed or refractory low-grade, follicular, or transformed B-cell, CD-20 positive non-Hodgkin's lymphoma, including rituximab refractory follicular non-Hodgkin's lymphoma.

Work-up before administration of radioimmunotherapy includes:

- History and physical examination
- Bone marrow biopsy within 60 days of treatment
- Complete blood count (CBC) with differential white blood cell count

## Contraindications to RIT in NHL

Some protocol based exceptions are under study.

- Marrow involvement by lymphoma >25%
- Impaired bone marrow reserve (previous stem cell transplant or external beam radiation therapy to >25% of marrow)
- Platelet count <100,000 per μL
- Absolute neutrophil count <1500 per μL
- Altered biodistribution on pretreatment imaging
- Known hypersensitivity reaction to rituximab or murine proteins

## Agents

Food and Drug Administration (FDA) approval for the radioimmunotherapy compound yttrium-90 ibritumomab tiuxetan (Zevalin®) came in February of 2002, and similar clearance was provided in June of 2003 for iodine-131 tositumomab (Bexxar®). A comparison of the two agents is presented in Table 9-2.

### *Administration of Zevalin®[9-11]*

Radioimmunotherapy with either radiopharmaceutical is a multi-step process and occurs over 1–2 weeks. For Zevalin,® the patient first receives the unlabeled chimeric antibody rituximab at a dose of 250 mg/m$^2$. This "cold" antibody, delivered at a lower dose than when rituximab is given alone, improves the biodistribution of the radiolabeled antibody by clearing CD20 expressing B cells from the circulation and binding B lymphocytes in the spleen. Since $^{90}$Y is a pure beta emitter and cannot be used for imaging, the gamma emission of indium-111 is required for dosimetric analysis using a gamma camera single photon emission computed tomography (SPECT) scan. For this scan, 5 mCi of $^{111}$In ibritumomab tiuxetan is given intravenously after the cold antibody infusion. Currently, the FDA requires only a single scan, 48–72 hours after $^{111}$In administration, to confirm appropriate biodistribution. Additional SPECT images, typically at 0–24 hours and 96–120 hours, may be performed at the physician's discretion. Evaluation of the images to detect abnormal biodistribution is an essential safety step prior to therapy.

The activity of $^{90}$Y ibritumomab tiuxetan is then calculated using the patient's weight and baseline platelet count. For a platelet count equal to or greater than 150,000 per μL, a dose of 0.4 mCi/kg is recommended and 0.3 mCi/kg is given to patients with platelet counts between 100,000 and 149,000 per μL. Notably, for Zevalin® therapy the therapeutic dose is based solely on the patient's weight and pretreatment platelet count and the initial antibody scan is not a determi-nant in dose calculation. Approximately 1 week after the imaging dose, another dose of cold antibody is given, and within 4 hours the patient receives the therapeutic intravenous injection of Zevalin® over 10 minutes. Figure 9-2 graphically shows the dosing schedule for administration of Zevalin.®

### *Administration of Bexxar®[8,11]*

There are distinct differences in the administration of $^{131}$I-Bexxar® when compared to $^{90}$Y-Zevalin.® First, since iodinated compounds undergo some level of physiologic dehalogenation and are naturally taken up in the thyroid, a protective agent is required to minimize the risk of iatrogenic

**TABLE 9-2 Comparison of the Two Approved Radioimmunotherapy Compounds[8-10]**

| | 90Y Ibritumomab Tiuxetan (Zevalin®) | 131I Tositumomab (Bexxar®) |
|---|---|---|
| Antibody used for RIT | ibritumomab—murine IgG1-κ | tositumomab—murine IgG2a-λ |
| Specificity | CD20 | CD20 |
| Linker molecule | Tiuxetan | None (directly halogenated) |
| "Cold" antibody | Chimeric rituximab 250 mg/m² | Murine tositumomab 450 mg |
| Pretreatment imaging agent and dose | 111In ibritumomab tiuxetan – 5 mCi | 131I tositumomab – 5 mCi |
| Primary intent of imaging dose | Biodistribution safety assessment | Calculation of dose based on individual clearance patterns |
| Number of pretreatment scans | One* | Three |
| Therapeutic isotope | Yttrium-90 | Iodine-131 |
| Major emission spectra | 2.3 MeV β | 0.6 MeV β and 0.36 MeV γ |
| Dosing parameters | | |
| Platelets ≥ 150,000/μL | 0.4 mCi/kg | 75 cGy whole body dose |
| Platelets 100,000–149,000/μL | 0.3 mCi/kg | 65 cGy whole body dose |
| | Maximum 32 mCi | |
| Typical overall response rate (ORR) | 60–80% | 60–80% |
| Typical complete response rate (CR) | 20–40% | 20–40% |

* Additional scans are optional.

FIGURE 9-1 Pretreatmemt scan 24 hours after administration of $^{111}$In ibritumomab tiuxetan in a 59-year-old female with indolent NHL and minimal prior therapy.

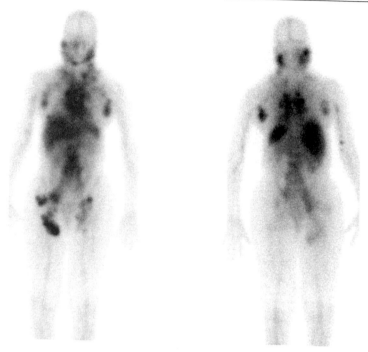

hypothyroidism. Either supersaturated potassium iodide (four drops daily), Lugol's solution (20 drops three times daily), or potassium iodide tablets (130 mg daily) are given, beginning at least 24 hours prior to the first dosimetric scan and continued for 2 weeks after the therapeutic injection. For the reasons previously discussed, an unlabeled 450 mg dose of tositumomab is initially administered, followed by the imaging dose of 5 mCi $^{131}$I tositumomab. The gamma emission of iodine-131 allows pretreatment imaging to be obtained without the use of a surrogate isotope as is necessary for Zevalin®. Three serial quantitative SPECT images with whole body radioactivity counts are then obtained.

The radioisotope clearance patterns are used to calculate the isotope residence time, which is then used to determine the total millicurie dose of $^{131}$I required to deliver the desired total body equivalent dose (TBED). Unlike $^{90}$Y ibritumomab tiuxetan, the wide variability in the clearance of $^{131}$I tositumomab requires these steps to be performed to ensure proper dosing. Thus, a higher absolute millicurie activity is required to deliver the equivalent TBED for "rapid clearance patients" compared to patients with slower clearance of the radiolabeled antibody. The ultimate goal is to achieve an equal area under the concentration times time curve.

The desired TBED is determined by evaluating the pretreatment platelet count of the patient. For a baseline platelet count of greater than 150,000 per μL, a whole body dose of 75 cGy is

TABLE 9-3 Examples of Altered Biodistribution in Radioimmunotherapy Treatment[8,10,11]

| Agent | Example of Altered Biodistribution |
|---|---|
| 90Y ibritumomab tiuxetan (scan performed using 111In as surrogate) | Inadequate visualization of the blood pool or intense uptake in the liver or spleen on image 1 (taken at 0–24 hours). |
| | Diffuse, intense uptake in the lung greater than the cardiac blood pool on image 1 or more intense than liver on image 2 (taken at 48–72 hours) or 3 (taken at 96–120 hours). |
| | Uptake suggestive of urinary obstruction, diffuse lung uptake greater than blood pool, or greater uptake by normal bowel than liver on images 2 or 3. |
| 131I tositumomab | Criteria similar to those listed above for 90Y ibritumomab tiuxetan. |
| | Total body residence times of <50 hours or >150 hours. |

FIGURE 9-2 Administration of yttrium-90 ibritumomab tiuxetan (Zevalin®).

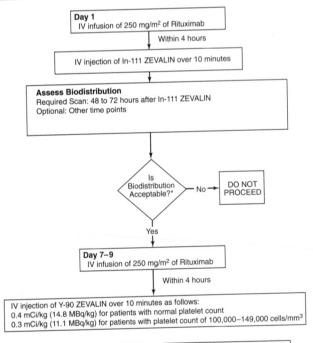

Used with permission, Zevalin Prescribing Information Packet, *Overview of Dosing Schedule*, p. 24, September 2005, Biogen Idec.

FIGURE 9-3  Pretreatment imaging with $^{131}$I labeled tositumomab for Bexxar® therapy.

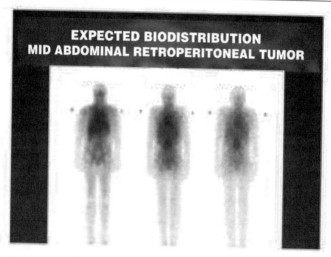

EXPECTED BIODISTRIBUTION
MID ABDOMINAL RETROPERITONEAL TUMOR

Used with permission of the GlaxoSmithKline Group of Companies.

recommended and 65 cGy is prescribed for patients with platelet counts between 100,000 and 150,000 per μL. As with Zevalin®, patients receive unlabeled tositumomab (450 mg) prior to the therapeutic injection of $^{131}$I tositumomab. The treatment schema for Bexxar® is given in Figure 9-5.

### Radiation Safety[8–13]

Nuclear Regulatory Commission (NRC) guidelines require inpatient stays for patients from whom radiation exposure to others is likely to exceed 5 mSv (500 mrem), but both radiolabeled compounds can typically be administered on an outpatient basis. Because $^{90}$Y is a pure beta emitter, its

FIGURE 9-4  Graph demonstrating the modification of treatment dose in patients with rapid and slow clearance, respectively, to obtain an equal area under the curve for Bexxar administration.

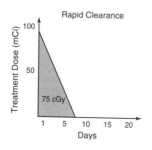
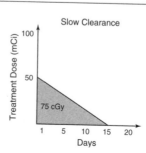

Used with permission of the GlaxoSmithKline Group of Companies.

**FIGURE 9-5** Administration of iodine-131 tositumomab (Bexxar®).

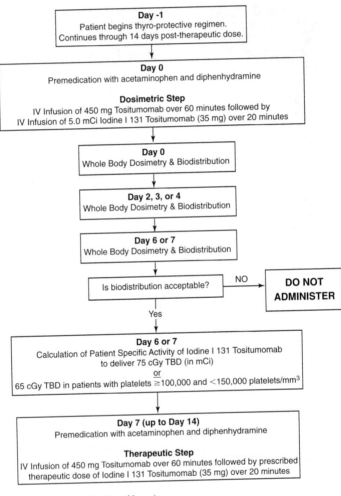

**Day -1**
Patient begins thyro-protective regimen.
Continues through 14 days post-therapeutic dose.

**Day 0**
Premedication with acetaminophen and diphenhydramine

**Dosimetric Step**
IV Infusion of 450 mg Tositumomab over 60 minutes followed by
IV Infusion of 5.0 mCi Iodine I 131 Tositumomab (35 mg) over 20 minutes

**Day 0**
Whole Body Dosimetry & Biodistribution

**Day 2, 3, or 4**
Whole Body Dosimetry & Biodistribution

**Day 6 or 7**
Whole Body Dosimetry & Biodistribution

Is biodistribution acceptable? — NO → **DO NOT ADMINISTER**

Yes

**Day 6 or 7**
Calculation of Patient Specific Activity of Iodine I 131 Tositumomab
to deliver 75 cGy TBD (in mCi)
or
65 cGy TBD in patients with platelets ≥100,000 and <150,000 platelets/mm³

**Day 7 (up to Day 14)**
Premedication with acetaminophen and diphenhydramine

**Therapeutic Step**
IV Infusion of 450 mg Tositumomab over 60 minutes followed by prescribed
therapeutic dose of Iodine I 131 Tositumomab (35 mg) over 20 minutes

Used with permission of the GlaxoSmithKline Group of Companies.

use requires fairly minimal post treatment radiation safety precautions other than standard "universal precautions." Only minimal risk of exposure to healthcare workers and patients' families occurs, and there is no need to determine dose rate limits prior to release of the patient. For $^{131}$I compounds, the more penetrating gamma emissions mandate full involvement of the radiation safety team. Although most patients can also be discharged after Bexxar® therapy, dose rate calculations must be performed and additional instructions given to the patient regarding radiation safety precautions.

TABLE 9-4 **Differences Between Y-90 Zevalin® and I-131 Bexxar® Post Treatment Radiation Safety Related Patient Instructions. The Recommendations for Bexxar® are to be Observed for a Period of 2 Weeks or Less Based on Post-Treatment Dosimetry**

| Agent | Radiation Safety Precautions |
|---|---|
| Zevalin® | • Radiation exposure to healthcare workers, family, and others is similar to background levels<br>• Patients can be released immediately<br>• Avoid contact with or exchange of body fluids for 3–7 days<br>• Wash hands thoroughly after urination<br>• Utilize condoms for 7 days after treatment and effective contraception for 12 months after treatment |
| Bexxar® | • Administer thyroid-blocking agent prior to treatment and continue for at least two weeks after treatment<br>• Most patients can be released on the same day as infusion<br>• Sleep in a separate bed (at least 6 feet from others)<br>• Avoid taking long trips while seated next to others in the first few days<br>• Airport radiation detectors may be activated after treatment<br>• Stay at least 6 feet from children and pregnant women<br>• Use separate bathroom, if possible<br>• Urinate while seated, flush three times with the lid closed<br>• Avoid sexual contact for 1–2 weeks and discontinue breast feeding before treatment<br>• Wash hands often and shower daily<br>• Drink plenty of liquids<br>• Use separate towels, washcloths, and toothbrush from others<br>• Avoid using disposable items that cannot be flushed down the toilet<br>• Use separate eating utensils and dishes<br>• Hold clothing and linen before laundering and wash these items separately |

## Morbidity[14–16]

Acute toxicity for both radiolabeled anti-CD20 radiopharmaceuticals is usually limited to an infusion reaction caused by a hypersensitivity to the murine components of the antibody. Premedication with acetaminophen and diphenhydramine is recommended to combat this and other common side effects in the immediate post-infusion setting such as asthenia, nausea, and chills. The dose-limiting, sub-acute toxicity from radioimmunotherapy is a reversible hematopoietic suppression, with cytopenias developing by week 4–6, reaching nadir values at weeks 7–9, and recovering within 1–4 weeks of nadir. The duration of hematologic toxicity is often longer in patients with thrombocytopenia (<150,000 platelets per μL) prior to treatment, and the severity of hematopoietic suppression increases with increasing marrow involvement by lymphoma. Weekly complete blood counts with differential are obtained to follow the nadir and subsequent recovery of the marrow. Supportive measures, particularly platelet transfusions, are occasionally required, but neutropenic fever occurs infrequently. For patients receiving Bexxar®, biochemical hypothyroidism is seen in 10%–20% of patients, despite pretreatment with a thyroid blocking agent. For this reason, an annual thyroid stimulating hormone (TSH) level is recommended at the time of follow-up. The murine antibodies used in RIT can themselves be immunogenic, and formation of human antimouse antibodies (HAMA) occurs in 1%–2% of patients treated with Zevalin® and approximately 10% of patients treated with Bexxar®. Circulating HAMAs can increase the risk of serious hypersensitivity and alter clearance of the antibody upon subsequent administration. The theoretical increased risk of second malignancy, including myelodysplastic syndrome, is not clearly established and is most certainly augmented by previous cytotoxic therapies.

## Outcomes

Although there are some differences between the two commercially approved agents, there are currently no direct data showing superiority of either compound. Given the heavily pretreated nature of these patients, some of whom have had four or more chemotherapy regimens, the overall and complete response rates after RIT are remarkable. The pivotal comparative studies for both agents in NHL are listed below.

---

**BOX 9-1**

Initial phase I/II study of yttrium-90 ibritumomab tiuxetan in 51 patients. Results established the maximum tolerated dose of 0.4 mCi/kg in patients with a platelet count $\geq$ 150,000. Overall response rate was 67% and 26% of patients achieved a complete response. Response was higher in low grade lymphoma compared to intermediate grade disease (82% vs. 43%). Adverse events were primarily hematologic and correlated with marrow involvement by NHL and baseline platelet count.

*Kaminski M et al. Pivotal study of Iodine 131 tositumomab for chemotherapy-refractory low-grade or transformed low-grade B-cell lymphomas. J Clin Oncol 19: 3918–3928, 2001.*

60 patients previously treated with at least two chemotherapy regimens with no response or progression were treated with a single course of iodine-131 tositumomab. Overall response rate was significantly improved with RIT compared to response after the last course of chemotherapy (65% vs. 28%). The median duration of response was also significantly increased, from 3.4 months after the last course of chemotherapy to 6.5 months after RIT.

Witzig TE et al. Phase I/II trial of IDEC-Y2B8 radioimmunotherapy for treatment of relapsed or refractory CD20(1) B-cell non-Hodgkin's lymphoma. *J Clin Oncol* 17: 3793–3803, 1999.

---

In addition, phase III data comparing the radioimmunotherapy compound to unlabeled antibody show an enhanced effect with the addition of a radionuclide to the anti-CD20 construct.

---

**BOX 9-2**

143 patients were randomized to a single treatment of Zevalin® versus rituximab weekly for four cycles. Overall response rate was significantly improved in the RIT arm (80% vs. 56%) as was the rate of complete response (30% vs. 16%). Duration of response and time to progression were not improved with RIT and the major toxicity was reversible myelosuppression.

Witzig T et al. Randomized controlled trial of yttrium-90-labeled ibritumomab tiuxetan radioimmunotherapy versus rituximab immunotherapy for patients with relapsed or refractory low-grade, follicular or transformed B-cell non-Hodgkin's lymphoma. *J Clin Oncol.* 20: 2453–2463, 2002.

*(continues)*

**BOX 9-2** (CONTINUED)

Multi-center, randomized study of 78 patients with refractory/relapsed non-Hodgkin's lymphoma randomized to tositumomab alone or I-131 tositumomab. Overall response rates were improved with RIT compared to immunotherapy alone (55% vs. 19%). Complete responses (33% vs. 8%) were also significantly increased with RIT. Median duration of response had not been reached in the RIT arm compared to 28 months in the tositumomab alone arm. Hematologic toxicity was more severe and non-hematologic events were more common in the RIT arm.

Davis T et al. The radioisotope contributes significantly to the activity of radioimmunotherapy. *Clin Cancer Res* 10: 7792–7798, 2004.

### Insights and Future Directions

Historically, radioimmunotherapy has been relegated to a late, often preterminal phase, usually after other agents have lost efficacy and the bone marrow is severely depleted. However, there is now increasing evidence that earlier treatment may be more effective.[17] This is highlighted by recently published work of Kaminski and others.

**BOX 9-3**

76 patients received a single course of tositumomab and I-131 tositumomab to a total body dose of 75 cGy as initial treatment for stage III/IV follicular lymphoma. With a median follow-up of 5.1 years, a response was seen in 95% of patients with 75% having a clinical complete response to Bexxar.® A molecular response was seen in 80% of patients with a clinical CR. Five year progression free survival (PFS) was 59% and median PFS was 6.1 years. No patients required transfusions or growth factors and no cases of myelodysplastic syndrome were noted.

Kaminski MS, et al. 131I-Tositumomab as initial therapy for follicular lymphoma. *New England Journal of Medicine* 352:441–449, 2005.

Along these lines, a current SWOG protocol is evaluating six cycles of CHOP chemotherapy followed by RIT versus six cycles of CHOP followed by rituximab as first line therapy for advanced low-grade follicular lymphomas. A large, multicenter study from Europe randomized patients after chemotherapy to consolidation with a single dose of Zevalin® versus no further treatment. Initial results reported in 2007 show a 2-year prolongation of progression-free survival. This improvement was statistically significant (p<0.01).[18]

The influence of a multitude of other factors on the effect of RIT is currently being elucidated. For example, data from our institution show that progression after RIT most often occurs in bulky sites (maximal diameter ≥ 5 cm).[19] Also, given the natural history of indolent lymphoma, RIT does not usually appear to "burn bridges" with regard to marrow reserve if additional systemic therapies are needed.[20] Retreatment with a second course of RIT (perhaps dose reduced) has also been shown to be feasible and effective as evidenced in a study of 32 patients retreated with 131-I tositumomab. An overall response rate of 56% and median duration of response of 15.2 months was reported by Kaminski and colleagues.[21] Additional studies are evaluating the therapeutic role of RIT in patients with relapsed aggressive NHL who are not suitable candidates for stem cell transplantation and as "liquid TBI" in preparation for transplant.

### The RIT Team[22]

The process of radioimmunotherapy delivery requires coordination across several departments: Hematology/Medical Oncology, Radiation Oncology, and Nuclear Medicine. A harmonious collaboration will result in optimal delivery and follow-up for the patient. The medical oncologist often has the longest relationship with the patient and plays an important role in identifying appropriate candidates for treatment. The medical oncologist also aids with administration of "cold" antibody, monitoring hematopoietic toxicity, and follow-up. Pretreatment image acquisition and interpretation is often best performed by the nuclear medicine physician who, in some institutions, may also administer the therapeutic dose. The typical primary roles of the radiation oncologist, which may overlap with those of both nuclear medicine and medical oncology, are in the initial triage and work-up of patients, the final therapeutic infusion, and follow up. In addition, considering the current multidisciplinary nature of residency training in radiation oncology, the radiation oncologist may be ideally positioned to discuss the relevant data, advantages, toxicities, and alternatives with the patient and other members of the RIT team.

## RADIOPHARMACEUTICAL THERAPY FOR BONE METASTASES[13,23–25]

The skeleton represents the third most common site of metastatic disease in cancer patients and an important cause of morbidity in the form of pain, pathologic fracture, hypercalcemia, and spinal cord compression. Effective palliation of bony metastases is a timely issue with increasing survival of patients with breast and prostate cancer. Treatment options range from medical therapy with analgesics, opioids, hormonal therapy, and bisphosphonates to a surgical approach for stabilization. In addition, both local and wide-field radiation therapy have well established roles in patient management. Often, a combination of treatments is required because a single modality is rarely successful at long-term palliation. Radiopharmaceuticals also have a role in the treatment of bone metastases, and samarium-153-EDTMP (Quadramet) and strontium-89 (Metastron) represent the two most commonly prescribed radionuclides.

### Advantages and Indications

Administration of radionuclides for bone pain has several advantages compared to other treatments. First, administration guidelines are straightforward and do not require expensive equipment. Further, radioisotopes treat multiple sites of blastic bone disease simultaneously with an acceptable toxicity profile.

The optimal patient for radiopharmaceutical therapy has:

- A life expectancy of >6 weeks.
- Multiple painful blastic metastases which show uptake on a recent bone scan.
- Adequate bone marrow reserve (leukocyte count >3,000 per μL and platelet count >60,000 per μL).

Additional workup should ensure sufficient renal and hepatic function and the absence of hypercalcemia.

Factors that generally preclude radionuclide therapy include:

- Impending pathologic fracture
- Spinal cord or nerve root compression
- Index lesions with poor uptake on bone scan
- A large extra-osseous component of disease
- Extensive areas of bone destruction

- Recent myelosuppressive chemotherapy
- Disseminated intravascular coagulation (DIC)

### Strontium-89

Elemental strontium is located just below calcium on the Periodic Table and is distributed by the body to sites of new bone formation. Studies with $^{89}$Sr chloride (Metastron®) have generally focused on men with metastatic prostate cancer and results show significant improvement in pain relief and quality of life while decreasing analgesic consumption. A trial in Canada studied the combination of local field radiation and strontium therapy in a prospective, randomized fashion. Results showed a reduction in analgesic use at 3 months as well as fewer new active sites of pain, but no difference in survival or pain reduction at the index site was noted. Additional randomized data has been conflicting. The typical prescribed dose for $^{89}$Sr is 40–60 μCi/kg with a maximum dose of 4.0 mCi and the drug is administered by intravenous infusion over 1–2 minutes.

### Samarium-153-EDTMP

Quadramet® is a complex of radioactive $^{153}$Sm attached to lexidronam, a tetra phosphonate chelate also known as ethylene diamine tetramethylene phosphonate (EDTMP). While its exact mechanism of action is not known, lexidronam allows selective accumulation in bone with specific targeting of osteoblastic lesions and low concentrations in normal bone. Compared to strontium-89, samarium-153 has a shorter half-life, lower energy beta particle, and is suitable for imaging due to its gamma emission (Table 9-1). Three randomized, phase III studies with nearly 400 patients have been performed using samarium-153 for bone metastases and show a significant improvement in pain compared to placebo as well as an optimal dosing schedule of 1.0 mCi/kg given intravenously over 1–2 minutes.

## Results

Overall, both agents used in the radioisotope therapy of bone metastases significantly improve pain control without improving survival. These agents show an overall response rate ranging from 40%–90% with a complete response rate of approximately 30%. Pain relief typically occurs in days to weeks and may last for several months. An initial intensification of pain occurs in about 15% of patients, lasts several days, and is commonly treated with analgesic medications.

## Toxicity and Safety

Radiopharmaceutical treatment of bone metastases is well tolerated, and the dose limiting toxicity for both radioisotopes is marrow suppression, often manifested as thrombocytopenia. While neutropenia is infrequently seen with these agents, additional systemic therapies should be

**TABLE 9-5  Comparison of Samarium-153 and Strontium-89 for Treatment of Bone Metastases**

|  | Strontium-89 | Samarium-153 |
|---|---|---|
| Brand name | Metastron® | Quadramet® |
| Agent | Strontium-89 chloride | Samarium-153 lexidronam |
| Dosing | 4.0 mCi or 40–60 μCi/kg, maximum 4.0 mCi | 1.0 mCi/kg |
| Typical response time | 14–28 days | 2–7 days |
| Typical response duration | 12–26 weeks | 8 weeks |
| Typical time to marrow nadir | 4 weeks | 2–4 weeks |
| Typical time to marrow recovery | 12 weeks | 8–12 weeks |

delayed until full recovery of marrow and blood counts should be monitored regularly until recovery. Patients treated with [89]Sr can be discharged immediately. For [153]Sm lexidronam, the previously discussed NRC regulations apply due to low energy gamma emission. After injection, universal precautions should be observed with all body fluids, particularly urine and feces, and incontinent patients should be temporarily catheterized to minimize the risk of contamination.

## Future Directions

Currently, radiopharmaceutical therapy for bony metastases is used most often in patients who have failed local therapy. However, there is increasing interest in their use as an adjunct to local-field radiation as well as in conjunction with systemic therapies.

## RADIONUCLIDE THERAPY FOR BENIGN AND MALIGNANT THYROID DISEASE[13,23,26]

The thyroid gland's exceptional ability to sequester iodine opens avenues in radioisotope administration for both imaging and therapeutic purposes. Accordingly,[131] I is indicated in the treatment of benign conditions such as hyperthyroidism, toxic nodular goiter, and solitary toxic nodule, as well as for differentiated thyroid carcinoma. For benign indications, pretreatment evaluation should include a radioiodine uptake test and an estimate of gland size. Importantly, at the time of scanning and treatment, the patient should be devoid of iodine-containing medications, contrast agents, exogenous thyroid hormone, and anti-thyroid medications. The dosing of iodine-131 for hyperthyroidism is 50–200 $\mu$Ci per gram of thyroid or a standard dose of 6.4 or 9.5 mCi. Often I-131 therapy for toxic nodular goiter and solitary toxic nodule requires a higher activity (up to 30+ mCi) due to the relative resistance of these conditions to radioiodine therapy.

## Malignant Indications

Radioiodine therapy is a mainstay in the treatment of differentiated thyroid carcinoma. For [131]I avid tumors, treatment is indicated in the postoperative setting as well as for recurrent and metastatic disease. In the adjuvant setting, [131]I is used to ablate residual thyroid tissue. Ablation is typically indicated for high risk histologic features such as tumor size (>1.0 –1.5 cm), invasion of the thyroid capsule, vascular invasion, multifocal disease, or soft tissue invasion. An assessment of residual [131]I avid thyroid tissue is performed at 2–6 months post thyroidectomy. Uptake in the thyroid bed, neck, or distant sites on this initial whole body scan is an indication for therapeutic [131]I administration. Dosing of [131]I in this setting varies based on the sites of disease and pathologic risk factors. Typically, an activity of 30–100 mCi is delivered in the postoperative, ablative setting. In addition to the clinical benefits of ablating residual thyroid tissue adjuvantly, treatment with [131]I removes additional sources of thyroglobulin (Tg), which enhances the ability to use the Tg level as a tumor marker in the future. Subsequent elevation of thyroid stimulating hormone (TSH) after postoperative ablation will also expose the presence of micro-metastatic foci on subsequent imaging since uptake of [131]I by malignant cells is augmented by maximal TSH stimulation. In addition to the ablative setting, [131]I is often used for treatment of recurrent or metastatic disease based on an abnormal diagnostic scan, rising thyroglobulin level, or both. Treatment for recurrent or metastatic disease requires an activity of 150–250 mCi and administration guidelines are similar to those for postoperative treatment. The calculated absorbed doses for this level of radiopharmaceutical may exceed 100 Gy.

## Radiation Safety and Toxicity

Patients must be given explicit instructions regarding radiation safety precautions and some occasionally require admission to the hospital in accordance with NRC guidelines. From a toxicity standpoint, radioiodine therapy is generally well tolerated. Acute side effects of treatment may include: transient thyroid storm, neck pain and swelling, fatigue, odynophagia, sialodenitis, and bone marrow suppression. Long term complications include hypothyroidism and a theoretical risk of second malignancy. Pulmonary fibrosis and pneumonitis have also been reported in patients with lung metastases from [131]I avid thyroid carcinoma.

## Therapeutic Indications for Phosporus-32[13,26]

Two distinct forms of the radioisotope [32]P have therapeutic indications. The sodium phosphate form, which accumulates in bone marrow, spleen, and liver, is used for treatment of myeloprolifer-ative disorders such as polycythemia vera and thrombocytosis. For these patients, pretreatment evaluation should ensure that patients have a platelet count $>100,000$ per $\mu L$ and leukocyte count $> 3,000$ per $\mu L$, and dosing is either standardized at 5 mCi or adapted to body surface area at 2.3 $mCi/m^2$ (maximum dose 5 mCi). The colloidal form of [32]P accumulates in intracavitary surfaces and is sometimes used for treatment of malignant ascites, pleural effusion, and intracavitary therapy of ovarian and endometrial carcinoma. This form of [32]P should not be administered intravenously. Typical activity for intra pleural therapy is 6–12 mCi, while 10–20 mCi is used for intraperitoneal disease. For intracavitary administration, the patient must be "rotated" to ensure distribution of the agent and a scan with [99]mTc should be performed to demonstrate adequate dispersal of the agent prior to treatment. Toxicity from the use of [32]P may include nausea, vomiting, diarrhea, abdominal pain, and bowel obstruction, and an augmentation of side effects has been noted with simultaneous external beam radiation to the pelvis.

## CONCLUSION

Use of unsealed source radiopharmaceutical therapy for the treatment of cancer is currently expe-riencing a revitalization through the approval of biologically targeted constructs such as the radioimmunoconjugates Zevalin® and Bexxar® for treatment of patients with non-Hodgkin's lym-phoma. Treatment with RIT is effective and well tolerated and further studies are expected to clar-ify and expand the role of these agents. The search for similar agents in the fight against breast, colon, and prostate cancer is ongoing. In addition to the newly developed radioimmunoconju-gates, traditional radiopharmaceuticals such as strontium-89, samarium-153, phosphorus-32, and iodine-131 continue to play an important role in the management of patients with malignancy.

## REFERENCES

1. Pohlman B, Sweetenham J, Macklis RM. Review of clinical radioimmunotherapy. Expert Rev Anticancer Ther 6: 445–462, 2006.
2. Kassis AI, Adelstein SJ. Radiobiologic principles in radionuclide therapy. J Nucl Med 46:S4–S12, 2005.
3. American Cancer Society: Cancer Facts and Figures 2006. http://www.cancer.org/docroot/STT/stt_0.asp.
4. Horning, SJ. Natural history of and therapy for the indolent non-Hodgkin's lymphomas. Semin Oncol 20(Suppl 5):75–8, 1993.
5. McLaughlin P, Grillo-Lopez AJ, Link BK, et al. Rituximab chimeric anti-CD20 monoclonal antibody therapy for relapsed indolent lymphoma: Half of patients respond to a four-dose treatment program. J Clin Oncol 16: 2825–2833, 1998.
6. Hernandez MC, Knox SJ. The radiobiology of radioimmunotherapy: Targeting CD20 B-cell anti-gen in non-Hodgkin's lymphoma. Int J Radiat Oncol Biol Phys 59: 1274–1287, 2004.
7. Macklis R. How and why does radioimmunotherapy work? Int J Radiat Oncol Biol Phys 59: 1269–1271, 2004.
8. Bexxar prescribing information 2005. Research Triangle Park, NC: GlaxoSmithKline.

9. Wagner H, Wiseman GA, Marcus CS, et al. Administration guidelines for radioimmunotherapy of non-Hodgkin's lymphoma with [90]Y-labeled anti-CD20 monoclonal antibody. J Nucl Med 43:267–272, 2002.

10. Zevalin prescribing information 2005. San Diego, CA: IDEC Pharmaceuticals Corporation.

11. Dillehay GL, Ellerbroek NA, Balon H, et al. Practice guideline for the performance of therapy with unsealed radiopharmaceutical sources. Int J Radiat Oncol Biol Phys 64:1299–1307, 2006.

12. Siegel JA, Kroll S, Regan D, et al. A practical methodology for patient release after tositumomab and (131)I-tositumomab therapy. J Nucl Med 43:354–63, 2002.

13. U.S. Nuclear Regulatory Commission: Part 35—Medical use of byproduct material. http://www.nrc.gov/reading-rm/doc-collections/cfr/part035/.

14. Witzig TE, White CA, Gordon LI, et al. Safety of yttrium-90 ibritumomab tiuxetan radioimmunotherapy for relapsed low-grade, follicular, or transformed non-Hodgkin's lymphoma. J Clin Oncol 21:1263–70, 2003.

15. Bennett JM, Kaminski MS, Leonard JP, et al. Assessment of treatment-related myelodysplastic syndromes and acute myeloid leukemia in patients with non-Hodgkin lymphoma treated with tositumomab and iodine I131 tositumomab. Blood 105: 4576–4582, 2005.

16. Gregory SA, Leonard JP, Knox SJ, et al. The iodine I-131 tositumomab therapeutic regimen: Summary of safety in 995 patients with relapsed/refractory low-grade (LG) and transformed LG non-Hodgkin's lymphoma (NHL). ASCO Annual Meeting 2004.

17. Gregory SA, Leonard JP, Vose JM, et al. Superior outcomes associated with earlier use: experience with tositumomab and iodine-131 tositumomab in 1,777 patients with low-grade, follicular, and transformed non-Hodgkin's lymphoma. ASCO Annual Meeting 2005.

18. Hagenbeek A, Bischof-Delaloye A, Radford JA, et al. Y90-ibritumomab tiuxetan consolidation of first remission in advanced stage follicular non-Hodgkin's lymphoma: First results of the international randomized phase 3 first-line indolent trial (FIT) in 414 patients. Abstract retrieved on January 17, 2008 from http://abstracts.hematologylibrary.org/cgi/content/abstract/110/11/643.

19. Gokhale AS, Mayadev J, Pohlman B, et al. Gamma camera scans and pretreatment tumor volumes as predictors of response and progression after Y-90 anti-CD20 radioimmunotherapy. Int J Radiat Oncol Biol Phys 63:194–201, 2005.

20. Ansell SM, Ristow KM, Habermann TM, et al. Subsequent chemotherapy regimens are well tolerated after radioimmunotherapy with yttrium-90 ibritumomab tiuxetan for non-Hodgkin's lymphoma. J Clin Oncol 20:3885–3890, 2002.

21. Kaminski MS, Radford JA, Gregory SA, et al. Re-treatment with I-131 tositumomab in patients with non-Hodgkin's lymphoma who had previously responded to I-131 tositumomab. J Clin Oncol 23: 7985–7993, 2005.

22. Macklis R. Radio-immunotherapy in a radiation oncology environment: Building a multi-specialty team. Int J Radiat Oncol Biol Phys, in press, 2006.

23. Perez C, Brady L, Halperin E, et al (eds). Principles and Practice of Radiation Oncology. Philadelphia, Lippincott, Williams, and Wilkins; Philadelphia, Pennsylvania, 2004.

24. Serafini AN. Therapy of metastatic bone pain. J Nucl Med 42: 895–906, 2001.

25. Bauman G, Charette M, Reid R, et al. Radiopharmaceuticals for the palliation of painful bone metastases—a systematic review. Radiother Oncol 75: 258–270, 2005.

26. Leibel SA, Phillips TL (eds). Textbook of Radiation Oncology. Saunders, Philadelphia, Pennsylvania, 2004.

# 10

# Central Nervous System

Jonathan P.S. Knisely, MD, FRCPC
John H. Suh, MD
Christina Tsien, MD

Tumors affecting the central nervous system (CNS) may be benign or malignant. If malignant, they may develop within the CNS or metastasize to the central nervous system. The behavior of various tumors differs; the clinical management, which frequently includes radiation therapy (RT), should be directed from knowledge of the likely patterns of spread and how various therapies may be used to benefit the afflicted individual.

## Brain Metastases

### Incidence

Although the exact incidence of brain metastases is unknown, hematogenous metastases from extracranial primary malignancies are the most commonly encountered intracranial tumors and are felt to occur in over 170,000 patients in the United States annually. Since brain metastases are a major cause of morbidity and mortality, they are among the most feared complications of systemic cancer. It is believed that their incidence has been on the rise due to better imaging techniques with MRI and CT, greater awareness among physicians, and greater patient survival from their primary cancers due to advances in cancer treatment.

### Pathology

The most common primary tumors responsible for brain metastases include lung cancers, breast cancers, melanomas, renal cell carcinomas, and unknown primaries. These tumors typically arise from hematogenous spread to the white matter of the watershed area of the brain at the junction of the gray and white matter. Brain metastasis distribution is based on the weight and blood supply of areas in the brain with 85% occurring in the cerebral hemisphere, 10%–15% in the cerebellum, and 1%–3% in the brain stem. They typically grow as spherical, well demarcated, solid masses that displace adjacent tissue with associated edema depending on size. Melanoma, renal cell, choriocarcinoma, and testicular cancers may be hemorrhagic. Lung and melanoma have greater tendency for multiple lesions.

### Presentation

Patients may present with generalized symptoms from increased intracranial pressure (headaches, nausea, vomiting, confusion) and may have focal symptoms from localized deposits that may affect specific functions of the brain. The discovery of asymptomatic lesions as part of restaging or staging is becoming more common.

## Management

Most patients with brain metastases die of metastatic cancer. Controlling brain metastases so as to reverse and prevent neurologic deterioration from uncontrolled growth is a primary goal. Class II evidence supports the standard management for more than a half-century for patients known to harbor brain metastases—whole brain radiation therapy (WBRT).[1] WBRT is known to improve neurologic dysfunction caused by macroscopic disease and can also prevent the development of subclinical metastatic foci into macroscopic and symptomatic disease. WBRT, as compared to supportive care alone, has not been studied in randomized clinical trials. Supportive care alone, without offering WBRT, may be appropriate for some patients, particularly those with advanced disease and/or a poor performance status.[2]

The most commonly used predictive instrument for patients with brain metastases is based on the Radiation Therapy Oncology Group (RTOG) recursive partitioning analysis (RPA) which analyzed 1,200 patients from three consecutive RTOG phase III trials performed from 1979 to 1993.[3] Factors that were most significant for survival were age, control of primary tumor, Karnofsky performance scale (KPS), and presence of extracranial metastatic disease. Based on this analysis, patients were categorized into three prognostic classes (Table 10-1).

In the past, treatment options for patients with brain metastases were limited to corticosteroids, RT, and surgery. However, recent technological and medical advances have expanded treatment options available to patients and physicians. The armamentarium now includes brachytherapy, stereotactic radiosurgery, chemotherapy, and radiation sensitizers. Given the increased number of treatment options, management of brain metastases has become more complicated and is an area of active research. Brachytherapy is not commonly used because of the requirement for an invasive surgical procedure, and radiation sensitizers have been evaluated in phase III clinical studies and have not demonstrated survival benefit to date. Chemotherapy is not felt to be of major benefit in most solid tumors metastatic to the brain; the blood-brain barrier presents problems in getting adequate drug delivery into this protected site.

### Whole Brain Radiation Therapy (WBRT)

This approach represents the primary treatment for the majority of patients with brain metastases, is available in all radiation oncology departments, and provides improvement of neurologic symptoms for most patients. Unfortunately local control is low, resulting in neurologic death in 25%–54% of patients.[3]

For simulation, patients are in the supine, neutral head position. Opposed lateral fields with collimation or divergent blocking are used to include coverage of the cribriform plate, middle cranial fossa, and foramen magnum. In simulating customized WBRT portals, using a posterior gantry tilt of 3–5 degrees will prevent divergence of the treatment beams through the contralateral lenses. When patients have leptomeningeal disease, the field may be modified to include coverage

TABLE 10-1  **RTOG RPA Classification for Brain Metastases[4]**

| RPA Class | Characteristics | Median Survival (mo) |
|---|---|---|
| I | KPS $\geq$ 70, age < 65, primary controlled, no extracranial metastases | 7.1 |
| II | All others | 4.2 |
| III | KPS < 70 | 2.3 |

of the posterior orbits. WBRT portals are commonly extended inferiorly to the junction of vertebral bodies C2 and C3. This facilitates the junctioning of these "helmet" portals with any palliative spinal radiation portals that may be required in the future.

No randomized controlled trial has shown any benefit in terms of overall survival, neurologic function, or symptom control for any abbreviated or more protracted fractionated scheme than 30.0 Gy in 10 fractions.[2] It may be reasonable to use a more protracted fractionation scheme (between 37.5 Gy in 15 fractions and 45.0 Gy in 25 fractions) for a patient who is expected to have a long-term survival (because of concerns about the potential for late, radiation-induced neurocognitive deficits), and an abbreviated fractionation scheme (20.0 Gy in 5 fractions) for patients who require palliative WBRT but have a short anticipated survival.

## Surgery

Given the low local control rates associated with WBRT alone, microsurgical resection of CNS metastases—particularly for single or symptomatic lesions—was explored in hopes of improving survival, quality of life, and local control. Surgery can also establish or confirm the diagnosis, especially for patients without primary tumor confirmation. In addition, surgery can provide immediate and effective palliation of symptomatic mass effect.

Two of three randomized studies provide class I data that demonstrate the benefit of surgery and WBRT vs. biopsy and WBRT.[5,6] The trial that failed to show a benefit of surgery was not well balanced for known prognostic factors such as extracranial disease activity, histology, and permitted the enrollment of patients with lower performance status.[7] These trial results are listed in Table 10-2.

## Stereotactic Radiosurgery (SRS)

Brain metastases have characteristics that make them ideal targets for SRS. Most are pseudospherical, noninfiltrative tumors located at the gray-white junction, and are diagnosed while still ≤4 cm in diameter. These features permit accurate target delineation and the planning and delivery of a high dose single fraction radiation treatment with various radiosurgery devices. In addition, a single large fraction of radiation appears to have an equal effect in all tumor types, even among the "radioresistant" tumors, such as renal cell carcinoma and melanoma.[8–10]

Because of the improved local control and survival benefit demonstrated with surgical resection of single metastasis, the use of SRS as an alternative focal strategy for brain metastases became appealing. This interest was based on the potential advantages of SRS, which include outpatient delivery, elimination of general anesthesia, minimal risk for bleeding or infection, lower costs, short convalescence time, and lower risk for complications. In addition, SRS is generally not limited by location, number of lesions, or medical comorbidities. For these various reasons, SRS has

**TABLE 10-2  Phase III Surgical Trials of WBRT Versus Surgery + WBRT**

| Trial | Treatment | # of Patients | Functional Independence* | Median Survival (wks) | P-value |
|---|---|---|---|---|---|
| Patchell[5] | S + WBRT | 25 | 38 | 40 | <0.01 |
| | WBRT | 23 | 8 | 15 | |
| Noordijk[6] | S + WBRT | 32 | 34 | 43 | 0.04 |
| | WBRT | 31 | 21 | 26 | |
| Mintz[7] | S + WBRT | 41 | — | 24 | ns |
| | WBRT | 43 | — | 27 | |

* Functional Independence: Patients had a KPS ≥70 for the indicated number of weeks.

become a viable alternative to surgery given the potential cost savings and quality-of-life benefits.[11-13] There have been no randomized controlled trials comparing microsurgical resection to radiosurgery in the management of brain metastases.

The potential benefit of SRS and WBRT compared to WBRT alone was assessed in a large phase III trial (RTOG 9508) that randomized 333 patients with one to three brain metastases newly diagnosed on MRI, each ≤4 cm in diameter, to WBRT (37.5 Gy in 15 fractions) and SRS vs. WBRT alone.[14] The SRS marginal dose was determined from a prior RTOG dose-escalation trial of SRS salvage treatment of primary and metastatic brain tumors recurrent after initial radiation management. Patients had a KPS ≥70 and were excluded if any metastasis was located in the brain stem or within 1 cm of the optic apparatus. Table 10-3 lists the results including some post-hoc analyses. Although the addition of SRS did not improve the overall survival for patients with two or three metastases, KPS at 6 months had stabilized or improved with the addition of SRS plus WBRT vs. WBRT alone (43% vs. 27%, respectively; P=0.03). Steroid use was also lower in the SRS and WBRT arm. Local control was improved at 1 year (82% vs. 71%; P=0.01). A similar, smaller single institution phase III trial also observed a statistically significant improvement in control of brain metastases in patients who received SRS in addition to WBRT.[15] Survival in both of these trials appeared to be predominantly controlled by extracranial metastatic disease activity.

---

**BOX 10-1**

The Sperduto Index was generated through a retrospective analysis of 1,960 patients with brain metastases enrolled on RTOG trials and was performed to identify subsets with varying prognoses.[16] Statistically different survival probabilities were identified for groups of patients based upon age, Karnofsky performance status (KPS), number of central nervous system (CNS) metastases, and the presence or absence of extracranial metastatic disease. Summing individual scores for each category provided a prognostic score between 0 and 4.0. The lowest level of statistical significance between Sperduto Index groups was p < 0.0001.[16]

|  | Score | | |
|---|---|---|---|
|  | 0 | 0.5 | 1 |
| Age | >60 | 50–59 | <50 |
| KPS | <70 | 70–80 | 90–100 |
| Number of CNS Metastases | >3 | 2 | 1 |
| Extracranial Metastases | Present | | None |

| Sperduto Index Score | Median Survival |
|---|---|
| 0–1.0 | 2.6 months |
| 1.5–2.5 | 3.8 months |
| 3.0 | 6.9 months |
| 3.5–4.0 | 11.0 months |

---

### Surgery or SRS Alone

Elimination of WBRT for patients with brain metastases who are treated with focal therapies such as SRS or microsurgical resection is controversial. Phase III studies document that the omission of WBRT in such cases results in higher intracranial relapse rates.[17,18] The addition of radiotherapy to a focal therapy does not appear to affect survival although the published phase III trials were not powered to determine this. One phase III study observed improvement in survival for patients with single brain metastasis who were treated with postresection WBRT.[19] Some physicians believe that routine use of WBRT in patients with oligometastatic brain metastases is unwarranted because WBRT may

**TABLE 10-3  Results from the Phase III RTOG 9508 for Patients with 1–3 Brain Metastases[14]**

| Survival Analyses | WBRT + RS (Months) | WBRT (Months) | P-value |
|---|---|---|---|
| Overall | 6.5 | 5.7 | 0.13 |
| 1 brain metastasis | 6.5 | 4.9 | 0.04 |
| **Post-hoc subsets** | | | |
| 1–3 mets & age <50 | 9.9 | 8.3 | 0.04 |
| 1–3 mets & NSCLC | 5.0 | 3.9 | 0.05 |
| 1–3 mets & RPA Class 1 | 11.6 | 9.6 | 0.05 |

cause side effects that reduce a patient's quality of life, but because the impact on neurologic function is a delicate balance between the potential for toxicities of WBRT and the negative consequences of tumor relapse, much controversy still exists regarding use of WBRT.[20] Table 10-4 lists local and regional control rates seen in two phase III studies of a focal therapy with or without WBRT.

---

**BOX 10-2**

Aoyama et al[18] reported on a randomized Japanese Radiation Oncology Study Group trial carried out over 4 years at 11 institutions in which 132 patients with 1–4 brain metastases ≤3 cm in diameter were all treated with radiosurgery, with the SRS doses determined by the diameter of the metastasis and whether or not the patient had been randomized to the arm that would receive WBRT to 30 Gray in 10 fractions prior to SRS (30% dose reduction if WBRT preceded SRS). The baseline characteristics of the enrolled patients were well balanced, but an inadequate number were enrolled to detect any survival difference. Neurologic functioning in each cohort was similar before and after treatment. Small numbers of patients in each arm had nonobligatory neurocognitive testing done with the mini-mental status examination (MMSE) and no differences were seen between the two arms with this instrument. An increased intracranial failure rate was seen in the cohort treated with SRS alone, but this did not apparently affect survival, MMSE testing, or neurocognitive functioning. This is the first phase III trial to be published on the results of deferring WBRT in patients with limited numbers of brain metastases; additional research needs to be done to better determine the risks and benefits of this approach.

---

**TABLE 10-4a  Result of Phase III Trial of Surgery Versus Surgery + WBRT[17]**

| Recurrence | Surgery Alone (46 Patients) | Surgery + WBRT (49 Patients) | Relative Risk | P-value |
|---|---|---|---|---|
| Any brain | 70% | 18% | 2.9 | <.001 |
| Surgical bed | 46% | 10% | 3.6 | <.001 |
| Distant brain | 37% | 14% | 1.6 | <.001 |

**TABLE 10-4b  Result of Phase III Trial of Radiosurgery vs. Radiosurgery + WBRT[18]**

| Recurrence | SRS Alone (67 Patients) | SRS + WBRT (65 Patients) | Hazard Ratio | P-value |
|---|---|---|---|---|
| Any brain | 76% | 47% | | <.001 |
| SRS site | 28% | 11% | 4.83 | .002 |
| Distant brain | 64% | 42% | .32 | .003 |

An NCI-funded phase III clinical trial (NCCTG 0574) that is open to accrual through the National Cancer Institute's Cancer Trials Support Unit (CTSU) and compares SRS to SRS followed by WBRT for patients with 1–3 brain metastases includes detailed neurocognitive testing of study participants and should help determine the nature of the risks to neurocognitive function of deferring or including WBRT in patients with 1–3 brain metastases treated with SRS.

## GLIOMAS

### LOW-GRADE GLIOMA

#### Incidence

The incidence of LGG is low; about 1/100,000 adults are diagnosed annually in North America with LGG.[21] An increased incidence of LGG is seen in association with neurofibromatosis type I and tuberous sclerosis.

#### Pathology

Low-grade gliomas (LGG) may be partitioned into those that are noninfiltrative and those that are diffusely infiltrative. The archetypal example of the former is pilocytic astrocytoma, and management of this type of grade I glioma is covered in the pediatric section. Those diffusely infiltrative primary brain tumors that are histopathologically determined to be Grade II tumors by the WHO grading system may be oligodendrogliomas, astrocytomas, mixed oligoastrocytomas, or rarer tumor types.[22]

LGG in adults tend to occur in the cerebral hemispheres, although they can occur in the midbrain, brainstem, or spinal cord. The cells of origin are specialized support cells in the CNS: astrocytes, oligodendrocytes, or rarely other cells that may have features of these or other histological lineages. The environmental and genetic factors that are associated with the development of an LGG are unclear.

#### Presentation

Patients with LGG may present in any of a number of ways, though seizures and gradually developing headache and focal neurologic deficits are perhaps most common. On CT, imaging will usually show an area of hypodensity. On MRI, there will be hypodensity relative to normal brain on T1 weighted pulse sequences and a bright area on T2 or FLAIR pulse sequences. Post-contrast tumor enhancement is not common in infiltrating low-grade gliomas, and has been described as being associated with a more aggressive clinical picture.[23]

#### Management

The increasingly routine use of MRI has led to early detection of LGGs in minimally symptomatic or asymptomatic patients with normal neurologic function. The appropriateness of aggressive surgical management and radiation treatment has been questioned. Additionally, although chemotherapy has not been felt to be effective for LGGs, for some LGGs, a response to chemotherapy may be seen, further complicating the clinical management picture.

LGGs have traditionally been felt to be slow growing and nonaggressive, leading some to advocate early treatment in the expectation that early treatment with surgery and radiation may be able to eradicate tumor clonogens capable of progression and causing death. Others have argued for a nonaggressive management approach, because of the morbidity that can be associated with surgery and radiation, and the uncertainty about the true benefit associated with early treatment. Conventional management includes surgery, RT, and, for some patients, chemotherapy.

#### Surgery

No class I data shows improved survival associated with a maximal safe resection of LGG. Class II data is provided by two studies. One reported improved survival associated with intraoperative MR-guided complete resection.[24] A complete resection could be achieved in only about one third of patients. The second study reported that image analysis of the degree of resection of LGG showed that more nearly complete resections were associated with lower recurrence rates.[25] From these data, it appears that as complete a resection as is feasible with acceptable neurosurgical morbidity should be performed, and consideration should be given to making a referral to a specialist neuro-oncological surgeon to achieve this goal.

### Radiotherapy

Phase III trials that provide class I data have been conducted to guide radiotherapeutic management of patients with LGG, but the data generated have been interpreted as supporting widely divergent management practices. Questions posed in these studies relate to the timing of RT and to the dose of radiation to use.

---

**BOX 10-3**

The European Organization for the Research and Treatment of Cancer (EORTC) trial 22845 evaluated the timing of RT in relation to the initial diagnosis of a grade II glioma in adults.[26] This randomized trial of 314 patients either used 54 Gray in 1.8 Gray fractions delivered to partial brain portals either at the time of diagnosis or at the time of progression. Only 65% of the patients randomized to delayed RT got radiotherapy at the time of progression. Despite no difference in survival between the two arms (7.4 vs. 7.2 years in the control arm), the improved seizure control rate at 1 year's time after radiotherapy and a better median progression-free survival rate (5.3 vs. 3.4 years) in the patients treated with early radiotherapy led those who reported the study to advocate for early irradiation as a matter of policy for patients with LGG. The lack of a survival benefit and the fact that over one third of the patients in the deferred treatment arm never got RT brings this conclusion into doubt.[27]

---

Class II evidence, possibly supporting a deferral of RT delivery in some patients, also comes from RTOG trial 98-02 for grade II gliomas. This study included an observation-only arm for patients under the age of 40 with completely resected grade II gliomas, in which the OS and PFS at 3 years was 97% and 73%, respectively.[28]

Therefore, it does not appear that there is a compelling reason to offer early RT to many patients diagnosed with LGG. Retrospective analyses in patients with LGG have been conducted by many researchers to try to identify risk factors for progression. A useful scoring system for predicting survival has been derived from EORTC trial data.[29] This study identified factors predictive of recurrence including age $\geq$40, astrocytoma histology, maximal tumor dimension $\geq$6 cm, tumor crossing midline, and the presence of a neurologic deficit prior to surgery. Risk factors and survival predictions based upon data from the EORTC low-grade glioma trials are listed in Table 10-5 and are the basis for the phase II RTOG 0424 trial. Patients with 0–2 of these factors are deemed to be low risk, and those with >2 factors are in the high-risk group. This report did not identify the degree of resection as a significant prognostic variable and did not collect data upon tumor enhancement, which other investigators have found to be an adverse prognostic feature in low-grade gliomas.[23,30] Few would argue with offering radiation treatment to patients who are neurologically compromised by their tumors or who have hard-to-control tumor-related epilepsy. Responses in these patients may provide a significant benefit in quality of life that far outweighs any possible adverse side effects from RT.

Because RT's adverse effects on the CNS are related to dose, volume, treatment duration, and fraction size, a smaller and more conformal treatment volume should decrease normal tissue irradiation and decrease morbidity if all other factors are kept constant. There are no class I data to guide radiotherapy treatment portal design. Careful use of ionizing radiation will minimize tumor-related or iatrogenic sequelae and will result in the best possible outcomes for patients.

---

**BOX 10-4**

Another series of phase III trials have been conducted to try to determine if there may be a dose-response relationship for LGG treated with external beam irradiation. EORTC study 22844 randomly assigned patients to receive partial brain RT to 45 Gray in 5 weeks or 59.4 Gray in 6.6 weeks time.[31] The 5-year progression-free survival rate was not significantly different between the two groups at 47% and 50%, respectively, and there was no difference in the survival rate. A North American Intergroup investigation randomized patients with LGG to partial brain RT to a dose of 50.4 Gray in 5.6 weeks time or 64.8 Gray in 7.2 weeks time. Similar to the European experience, the 5-year progression-free survival was not significantly different between the low and high dose arms (55% and 52%), with survival rates at 2 and 5 years for the low dose arm at 94% and 72% vs. 85% and 64% for the high dose arm. More grade 3 and 4 toxicities were seen in the high dose arm (10% vs. 2% at 5 years).[32] This class I data does not support prescribing a dose higher than 45–50.4 Gray in 1.8 Gray fractions for LGG using conventionally planned and delivered partial brain RT.

---

Guidelines for radiotherapy portal design on RTOG 9802 included the T2 signal abnormality from a postoperative MRI scan with a 2 cm margin to the block edge. Two-dimensional treatment planning was acceptable, and it is entirely likely that the technical limitations of radiotherapy treatment planning capabilities at the time the study was conducted led to the treatment planning recommendations in this study. It is likely that smaller volumes than these can be used without compromising local control. Analyses of the failure pattern for patients with low-grade gliomas treated with RT have shown that failures beyond the target volume are very rare unless the radiotherapy treatment portals are inadequate.[33–35] Treatment volumes for low-grade gliomas should respect barriers to anatomic spread such as dural surfaces or bone. Hemispheric gliomas are extremely unlikely to ever spread to the cerebellum or even to the contralateral hemisphere unless the corpus callosum is involved.[36]

---

TABLE 10-5a **EORTC LGG Risk Factors for Survival.**[29]

**Prognostic Factor (favorable vs. unfavorable)**
*(One Point is Scored for Each Adverse Prognostic Factor Present)*

Age (<40 vs. ≥40 years old)
Tumor largest diameter (<6 cm vs. ≥6 cm)
Tumor crossing midline (yes vs. no)
Histopathological tumor type (oligodendroglioma or mixed vs. astrocytoma)
Neurologic deficit present preoperatively (absent vs. present)

---

TABLE 10-5b **EORTC LGG Survival Prediction Based on LGG Risk Factor Score**

| Score | Predicted Survival in Years (95% CI) |
|---|---|
| 0 | 9.1 (9.1–NA) |
| 1 | 8.6 (7.4–NA) |
| 2 | 6.3 (5.3–7.8) |
| 3 | 4.4 (3.0–6.4) |
| 4 | 3.0 (1.9–NA) |
| 5 | 2.4 (0.7–NA) |
| Low risk (0–2) | 7.8 (6.8–8.9) |
| High risk (3–5) | 3.7 (2.9–4.7) |

To be able to design these smaller volumes for treatment, a volumetric CT scan of the head and neck in an immobilization device for treatment planning purposes is appropriate. A T2 weighted or FLAIR MR imaging study can be coregistered to this scan, reformatted, and redisplayed with the CT scan's geometric parameters.[37] With these steps, the MRI abnormality is defined as the GTV, a margin around this volume is designated to generate a CTV, and the PTV can be determined based upon the anticipated setup variation with the immobilization techniques being used. In dosimetric planning, beams may be chosen to develop a treatment plan that emphasizes conformity to the target volume, dose homogeneity within the target volume and minimal high dose delivery outside the target volume. This can be done with 3D conformal radiotherapy treatment (3DCRT) planning using several noncoplanar beams and selecting couch, gantry, and collimator rotations, beam energies, wedges, and weights to achieve this goal, or it can be done with intensity modulated radiation therapy (IMRT).

No clinical studies have compared IMRT and 3DCRT for LGG. IMRT's attractiveness includes simplifying the planning process to obtain a highly homogeneous dose distribution as well as sufficient sparing of critical normal structures that cannot be easily avoided. Appropriate development of planning constraints will permit a very homogeneous and conformal dose distribution to be generated, and many treatment planning systems will allow further adjustment of plans to optimize homogeneity or coverage. Noncoplanar plans can achieve better dose distributions in the CNS than coplanar plans.[38]

### Chemotherapy

Chemotherapy's role has been less important than that of surgery and RT in low-grade gliomas. One phase III trial conducted in the 1980s randomized patients with incompletely resected low-grade gliomas to radiotherapy $+/-$ CCNU. No statistical survival advantage was detected with use of chemotherapy, despite a difference in median survivals of 4.5 vs. 7.4 years.[39] The trial was likely to have been severely compromised by a lack of central pathology review and stratification by commonly recognized risk factors for progression in patients with LGG.

The identification of loss of heterozygosity (LOH) of chromosomes 1p and 19q in chemoresponsive anaplastic oligodendrogliomas[40] led to the evaluation of LOH and chemotherapy in LGG. LOH of chromosomes 1p and 19q is common and predicts for a longer survival.[41,42] Likelihood of a response to chemotherapy is higher in patients with oligodendroglioma than in astrocytoma, and those patients with a chromosomal loss of heterozygosity (LOH) for 1p and 19q have a higher likelihood of response to chemotherapy than those without this marker.[43]

For patients with LGG, administering chemotherapy before RT should be regarded as investigational. There is insufficient data to support concomitant use of chemotherapy and RT for LGG. In patients who are symptomatic from LGG who need therapy to prevent tumor progression-related neurologic complications, deferring chemotherapy until after RT is more appropriate because of an expected lower response rate to chemotherapy than RT. Clinical trials evaluating early use of chemotherapy in poor risk LGG have been mounted by both the RTOG and the EORTC. RTOG 0424 is a phase II study of RT (54Gy) with temozolomide both during and following RT, and EORTC 22033 is a phase III trial for high-risk supratentorial LGG that randomizes patients to RT (50.4 Gy) or temozolomide (no RT), after stratification by chromosome 1p deletion status (present vs. absent).

## HIGH-GRADE GLIOMA

Unlike the situation for patients with newly diagnosed LGG, where there is less consensus among specialists about best management practices, reasonable accord exists among specialists about the appropriate management of newly diagnosed malignant, or high-grade gliomas (HGG). This accord arises from the relatively larger number of patients diagnosed with anaplastic gliomas and glioblastoma multiforme and from the large number of clinical trials that have been conducted over past decades with patients having malignant gliomas.

## Incidence

Incidence of HGG in adults in North America is about 5/100,000/year. All HGG are infiltrative, and may be of oligodendroglial, astrocytic, or mixed histopathological character.[22] HGG may develop from previously diagnosed LGG or develop *de novo*.

## Pathology

Most gliomas are classified as astrocytomas or oligodendrogliomas or as mixed gliomas with varying proportions of these two different cell lineages. High grade gliomas may have cellular and nuclear atypia, increased cellular density, and vascular proliferation; necrosis may be seen with adjacent pseudopalisading of glioma cells. Current glioma classification schemes are based upon the histopathological appearance. Given the subjectivity in classifying these tumors, differences in opinion among neuropathologists are frequent. Because different molecular signatures are associated with different precursor pathways, molecular markers are already providing better diagnostic and prognostic information and may allow tailoring of therapies.[44]

## Presentation

Clinical manifestations of HGG are dependent upon the location and size of the lesion. Symptoms may arise from increased intracranial pressure or from local invasion or compression. Headache, nausea, and vomiting are common, as are subtle neurocognitive changes. Imaging will usually show an area of hypodensity on CT; mixed hyper- and hypodensities may be seen after iodinated contrast administration. On MRI, there will be a hypodensity relative to normal brain on T1 weighted pulse sequences that enhances in a heterogeneous pattern after gadolinium administration. Peritumoral edema may be seen on T2 or FLAIR pulse sequences. It is common to start steroids and anticonvulsants as a reflex when patients are diagnosed with an HGG. The benefit of anticonvulsants is questionable in the absence of a clear seizure history, and these should be discontinued if possible. Steroids should also be tapered to the lowest dose (or off) if there are no neurologic symptoms exacerbated by the steroid taper.

### Surgery

Many patients are unresectable at diagnosis, and for such cases, a simple debulking or diagnostic biopsy may be entirely appropriate surgical management to confirm diagnosis and permit appropriate nonsurgical therapy to start. However, several phase III trials provide class I evidence of the benefit of complete resection in patients with HGG.[45,46] If, through the integration of high tech-

---

**BOX 10-5**

322 patients with potentially resectable suspected malignant gliomas were randomized to receive a prodrug, 5-Aminolevulinic acid, that accumulates as fluorescent porphyrins in malignant gliomas.[46] A microsurgical resection was performed under either normal operative lighting or under conditions in which the fluorescence could be visualized. Immediate postoperative MR imaging showed that a gross total resection of all contrast-enhancing tumor was achieved in 65% of the patients who had fluorescence-guided resections, and 36% of those resected under standard operating room conditions. Postoperative neurological complications were similar in both arms. Progression-free survival at 6 months (41% vs. 21%) was significantly improved in the group having fluorescence-guided resections; the trial was not powered adequately to detect differences in survival between the two cohorts.

nology such as fMRI, intraoperative monitoring of eloquent cortex, image guided resection, etc., it is possible to achieve a gross total resection of tumor, this should be done, because it will likely result in a better outcome for patients with HGG.

### Radiation Therapy

Because of the grim prognosis for patients with HGG, despite the use of aggressive RT, several phase III trials were mounted in the 1970s to evaluate the use of radiotherapy and chemotherapy in patients with newly diagnosed HGG.[47,48] These trials showed a >2-fold survival advantage for patients receiving RT, and it has since been the predominant postsurgical adjuvant treatment.

Initial trials of RT for gliomas were conducted when imaging could not adequately address questions about the extent of disease, and patients were treated with WBRT to doses of 45–60 Gray. A subsequent trial has confirmed that there is no need to deliver RT to anything other than localized fields.[49]

Treatment volumes for HGG are generally much more conformal than they have been in the past. This has been facilitated by use of volumetric imaging studies that are coregistered to plan treatment.[37] An initial treatment volume is commonly designed much the same as would be done for an LGG, using the coregistered FLAIR or T2 weighted MRI to help define the initial GTV. A three-dimensional expansion of the GTV (conventionally using a margin of 2 cm, [based only on class III evidence]) generates a CTV that may then be adjusted to reflect anatomical barriers to tumor spread, such as the tentorium cerebelli or the cranial vault. Appropriate margins can then be added for daily setup variation to describe a PTV. This volume is treated to a dose of approximately 46 Gray, and a conedown volume that was generated from the coregistered gadolinium-enhanced T1 weighed imaging study and a similar volumetric expansion process is used to deliver the final 7–10 radiation treatments. As for LGG, dose homogeneity and conformality of the high-dose volumes may be emphasized because the predominant pattern of failure remains overwhelmingly dominated by local progression, despite increasingly tight conformal radiation volumes. Use of wedges, gantry, and collimator rotations together with the selection of beam energies and weighting can achieve this goal with 3DCRT. The use of IMRT may simplify the planning process, and for HGG, IMRT may also be able to direct higher doses of radiation to biologically more aggressive subvolumes of tumor identified with specialized imaging techniques. It has yet to be shown that such a strategy will result in better outcomes.

Clinical databases have been evaluated using a recursive partitioning analysis methodology to determine prognostic factors for patients with malignant gliomas.[50–52] The presently used RTOG RPA stratification variables and predicted survivals for patients with glioblastoma multiforme are listed in Table 10-6.

Local control of HGG is hard to achieve despite aggressive surgery and RT. It appeared from early trial data that RT doses of approximately 60 Gray were required for the best control.[53] This was confirmed in a phase III British trial.[54] Formal dose escalation trials of up to 82 Gray appeared to provide a survival advantage to conventionally delivered treatment escalation beyond approximately 60 Gray in 6 weeks' time.[55] However, a phase III trial conducted by the RTOG and the Eastern Cooperative Oncology Group (ECOG) did not confirm this finding.[56] Class I data exists supporting a hypofractionated regimen delivering 3 Gray fractions to a dose of 36–45 Gray in patients who have a poor prognosis, and it is also reasonable to withhold RT from those whose KPS (and anticipated survival) is extremely poor, just as it would be for any patient whose prognosis is profoundly grim.[57,58]

Modern technology has permitted a readdressing of the question of whether or not dose escalation for HGG confers any benefit. In a phase III trial mounted by the RTOG in glioblastoma, addition of stereotactic radiosurgery to radiotherapy and BCNU provided no survival advantage.[59,60] Similarly, two randomized trials of brachytherapy have shown no survival advantage in patients

TABLE 10-6  **RTOG RPA Classification for Glioblastoma**[52]

| RPA Class | Definition | Median Survival Time | 1-Year Survival Rate | 3-Year Survival Rate | 5-Year Survival Rate |
|---|---|---|---|---|---|
| III | Age < 50, KPS ≥ 90 | 17.1 mos | 70% | 20% | 14% |
| IV | Age < 50, KPS > 90 | 11.2 mos | 46% | 7% | 4% |
|  | Age ≥ 50, KPS ≥ 70, G/STR, W+ |  |  |  |  |
| V + VI | Age ≥ 50, KPS ≥ 70, G/STR, W− | 7.5 mos | 28% | 1% | 0% |
|  | Age ≥ 50, KPS ≥ 70, Biopsy |  |  |  |  |
|  | Age ≥ 50, KPS ≥ 70 |  |  |  |  |

KPS = Karnofsky Performance Status. G/STR = Gross/Subtotal Resection, W = Working

with HGG.[61,62] A phase II trial of accelerated RT incorporating a weekly stereotactic boost treatment also has shown no survival advantage compared to conventional treatment.[63] These data indicate that dose escalation for HGG should not be offered to patients outside a structured clinical trial.

All published phase III trials that attempted to increase the therapeutic ratio for RT for malignant gliomas by using accelerated fractionation have been negative.[64] A number of complementary modalities, including radiation sensitizers to improve the therapeutic ratio, have also shown little benefit. As new compounds are developed, they undoubtedly will also be tested to see if they add benefit to conventional management.

## Chemotherapy

Earlier phase III trials demonstrated an improvement in long-term survival, though no difference in median survival was noted for patients with HGG treated with concomitant RT and nitrosourea chemotherapy as compared to RT or chemotherapy alone.

### BOX 10-6

In a landmark randomized trial, Stupp et al reported on 573 patients with glioblastoma were randomly assigned to receive radiotherapy alone to a dose of 60 Gray in 30 fractions with or without continuous daily temozolomide (75 mg/m$^2$ of body-surface area per day, 7 days per week from the first to the last day of radiotherapy), followed by six cycles of adjuvant temozolomide (150 to 200 mg per square meter for 5 days during each 28-day cycle).[65] The unadjusted hazard ratio for death in the radiotherapy-plus-temozolomide group was 0.63 (95 percent confidence interval, 0.52 to 0.75; P<0.001 by the log-rank test) at a median follow-up of 28 months. Median survivals were 14.6 vs. 12.1 months, and the 2-year survival rate was 26.5% with radiotherapy plus temozolomide and 10.4% with radiotherapy alone. Temozolomide added to radiotherapy for newly diagnosed glioblastoma resulted in a clinically meaningful and statistically significant survival benefit with minimal additional toxicity.

A companion study to Stupp et al. showed that inactivation of a gene responsible for repair of alkylating damage done by temozolomide (MGMT) was responsible for the majority of the benefit from this drug's use in these patients.[66] Based on the results of these studies, the RTOG and EORTC have started a phase III trial (RTOG 0525), which randomizes patients after radiation therapy and temozolomide to standard versus dose dense adjuvant temozolomide. The methylation status of the MGMT promoter for all patients will be evaluated. Additional studies of the molecular mechanisms of resistance to conventional therapies and of the underlying genetic and biochemical alterations associated with HGG will undoubtedly clarify which patients are more appropriately managed with certain therapeutic strategies.

For patients with anaplastic oligodendrogliomas and anaplastic oligoastrocytomas, class I data show that use of chemotherapy as part of the initial management does not prolong survival, though it is associated with a progression-free survival benefit.[67,68] Compared to radiation alone, chemotherapy with procarbazine, CCNU, and vincristine as the initial therapy (as was used in these two studies) appears to increase toxicity. There is no similar phase III data evaluating the use of temozolomide in this setting, but it appears to have largely replaced other glioma chemotherapy regimens because of its tolerability and demonstrated activity.

## EPENDYMOMA

### Incidence

Ependymomas are rare glial tumors that account for 1%–3% of adult CNS tumors. Intra-medullary ependymomas are the most common spinal cord tumor in adults and account for 60% of cases. In contrast to pediatric patients, supratentorial sites occur more frequently in adults and can arise in the brain parenchyma from ependymal rests, lateral ventricle, and less commonly third ventricle. Infratentorial sites arise from the floor or roof of the fourth ventricle or cerebello-pontine angle (CPA) in the posterior fossa.[22]

### Pathology

Ependymomas arise from ependymal cells lining the CNS, including the cerebral ventricles, the central canal of the spinal cord, and the filium terminale, as well as cortical rests.[22] Histopathologically, ependymomas are characterized by perivascular pseudorosettes that surround a central vascular space.[69] The World Health Organization (WHO) grading scheme for ependymomas is based on histologic appearance. Grade I tumors are either subependymomas or myxopapillary ependymomas. The former are small and often incidentally discovered lesions more commonly found in adults, most commonly involving the lateral or fourth ventricles. Myxopapillary ependymomas are well circumscribed extramedullary tumors that arise strictly from the spinal cord's conus medullaris or filum terminale and have an excellent prognosis. WHO Grade II tumors are ordinary ependymomas and may be cellular, papillary, and clear cell variants. WHO Grade III tumors are anaplastic, characterized by the presence of increased cellularity, nuclear atypia, mitoses and micro-vascular proliferation.[22]

### Presentation

The most common symptoms from intracranial tumors are related to increased intracranial pressure from either mass effect or obstructive hydrocephalus. Spinal tumors are generally associated with an insidiously worsening neurologic deficit affecting the lower extremities and sphincter function. There may be back pain from dural irritation. Workup includes MRI of the complete spinal axis to rule out CSF dissemination, as well as a lumbar puncture for CSF cytology. Sub-arachnoid seeding with drop metastases is seen in approximately 5% of cases.[70]

### Surgery

Class II data suggests that the extent of tumor resection is the most consistent factor associated with local control as well as overall survival. Second-look surgery and re-operation is recommended in those patients with residual disease if associated with acceptable morbidity.[69] The impact of histologic grade on outcome in ependymomas remains controversial, but several large series have confirmed this finding.[71–73]

### Radiotherapy

Observation may be recommended in a select group of patients with gross total resection and negative wide margins. Rogers et al reported on a retrospective series that suggested improved local control with the addition of adjuvant radiotherapy even in patients with gross total resection.[73] Ten-year local control (LC) rate without RT was 50% compared to 100% in those with postoperative RT. Long-term follow-up is required in these patients because late recurrences can occur up to 12 years following surgery.[73] Postoperative radiotherapy should be given for anaplastic ependymomas, even in cases with gross total resection.[70]

Neuraxis dissemination predominantly occurs following local recurrence and rarely as an isolated event.[69,71–74] Class II and III data suggest a dose response for ependymoma.[70,71] Class II data show no benefit from hyperfractionated radiotherapy in pediatric ependymomas.[75] Class III data support completing radiotherapy promptly once commenced; a duration of treatment <50 days was associated with improved 5-year overall survival (86% vs. 46%) and local control (71% vs. 46%).[72]

Based upon these studies, the current recommendation for adult intracranial ependymomas is to deliver involved field radiation using image-based treatment planning to a dose of 59.4 Gy. Clinical target volume (CTV) is typically the postoperative tumor bed including residual disease (post-gadolinium MR T1 enhancing lesion) with a 1.0–1.5 cm margin. A further setup margin of 0.5 cm to the CTV defines the PTV. Target volumes should respect anatomic barriers to tumor spread.[70] Craniospinal irradiation (CSI) is indicated in patients with a positive CSF cytology or gross spinal metastases on MRI. The dose is typically 36–39.6 Gy followed by a boost to the primary (59.4 Gy) and metastatic sites (≥50.4Gy). Myxopapillary and spinal ependymomas are typically treated to an initial larger field to cover the tumor bed to 45 Gy followed by a boost to residual disease to 50.4–59.4 Gy depending on location of the disease.

### Chemotherapy

Response rates to single-agent chemotherapy are approximately 10%–15%. Cisplatin/carboplatin and etoposide appear to be the most active agents. There is no proven role for adjuvant or concomitant chemotherapy in the treatment of ependymoma.[70]

## PITUITARY ADENOMAS

### Incidence

These benign tumors represent about 10% of all intracranial tumors and may be broadly classified into macroadenomas (>1 cm diameter) and microadenomas (<1cm). Many never become clinically symptomatic.

### Pathology

Pituitary adenomas can be subdivided into secretory (~2/3 of cases) and nonsecretory tumors (~1/3). Hormone overproduction (and underproduction—from mass effect on normal pituicytes) can lead to a number of presentations, which are listed in Table 10-7.

### Presentation

Detection of hormone abnormalities controlled by the pituitary gland may lead to clinical diagnosis. The pituitary gland sits in the sella turcica and is in close proximity to a number of critical

TABLE 10-7  **Hormone-Secreting Pituitary Adenoma: Clinical Presentation and Medical Management**

| Hormone Secreted | Signs and Symptoms | Medical Therapy |
|---|---|---|
| Prolactin | Amenorrhea, galactorrhea, decreased libido, impotence | Cabergoline, bromocriptine (dopaminergic drugs) |
| Growth hormone (GH) | Gigantism, acromegaly (enlargement of hands and feet, coarse facial features, weight gain, arthritis, organomegaly, glucose intolerance, oily skin, skin tags, and colon polyps) | Octreotide, lanreotide (somatostatin analogues) |
| ACTH | Cushing's disease (truncal obesity, hypertension, skin striae, diabetes, hirsutism), Nelson's syndrome | Ketoconazole, metyrapone, mitotane (interference in steroid biosynthesis) |
| TSH | Hyperthyroidism | Octreotide, lanreotide (somatostatin analogues) |

structures including the hypothalamus, cavernous sinuses, internal carotids, and multiple cranial nerves (II–VI). Growth of an adenoma to a degree that adjacent structures are invaded or compressed leads to a number of possible clinical presentations including visual deficits, diplopia, ptosis, and headaches.

## Management

The goal of treatment is to remove or destroy the tumor, control hypersecretion, restore lost pituitary function, and minimize damage to surrounding normal brain. Treatment options include surgery, medical therapy, RT, and stereotactic radiosurgery. Depending on the type, size, symptoms, and patient age, any of these options are possibly beneficial, and multidisciplinary management is generally accepted as the standard of care.

### Surgery

In general, surgery is the treatment of choice, usually through a transsphenoidal approach. It is the best option to reduce mass effect and hypersecretion. In some cases, surgery is followed by adjuvant radiation and/or medical therapy.

### Drug Therapy

Medical therapy is generally not curative, and is conventionally used only for secretory tumors. It has traditionally been used only after a surgical intervention, but better therapeutic drugs have increased the potential for effective medical management of pituitary adenomas. Table 10-7 lists some medical options for secretory tumors.

### Radiation Therapy

Radiation options can be broadly classified into fractionated RT and SRS. Radiation can be used after incomplete resection, persistent hypersecretion after surgery or medical therapy, recurrent disease, and inoperable cases. For fractionated cases, doses of 45 to 54 Gy are delivered using 1.8 Gy/fraction. Introduction of fractionated radiosurgery, IMRT and image guided radiation therapy (IGRT) may minimize acute and long-term side effects.[76,77] For small discrete tumors 3–5 mm away from the optic chiasm and nerves, SRS, using a dose of 15–25 Gy delivered to the edge of the tumor, offers an attractive option because it is an outpatient procedure and normalizes excessive hormone production faster than fractionated therapy. There are no class I data comparing SRS and fractionated RT for pituitary adenomas. Class III evidence suggests that medical therapy for prolactinomas and growth hormone secreting adenomas should be limited when using radiation.[78,79] Although it appears that acute and long-term side effects such as hypopituitarism and secondary tumors appear to perhaps be lower with SRS than conventionally fractionated RT (Class II evidence), it is still too early to assess some of the late complications associated with SRS for pituitary adenomas. In the past, brachytherapy was used for patients with Cushing's disease, but unacceptably high complication rates were experienced, which limited enthusiasm for subsequent brachytherapy trials.

## MENINGIOMAS

### Incidence

Intracranial meningiomas account for 15%–30% of adult CNS tumors, with an overall incidence of ~6/100,000 that increases with age; women are more frequently affected than men (RR 2:1).[80] Leading sites include the cerebral convexities (20%–35%), parasagittal locations (20%), sphenoid ridge (20%), posterior fossa (10%), and parasellar regions (10%).[81]

### Pathology

Meningiomas are vascular, nonglial tumors that arise from the arachnoidal cells of the leptomeninges.[22] In 2000, the WHO classification for meningiomas was revised to include features of grade, histological subtype, proliferation index, and brain invasion. WHO Grade I tumors have a low proliferative index and limited invasiveness and account for the majority of meningiomas.[22] In comparison, WHO Grade II (atypical, chordoid, and clear cell histologies) and WHO Grade III (anaplastic, papillary, and rhabdoid histologies) meningiomas account for 15%–20% and 1%–3% of cases, respectively, and are associated with a higher risk of recurrence and worse prognosis.[82] Other prognostic factors associated with higher recurrence risks include prior resection, tumor size, and high mitotic index.[81,83] Mutations in the NF2 gene with loss of chromosome 22q are the most frequently noted genetic alteration.[84] Established risk factors include previous exposure to ionizing radiation and neurofibromatosis Type 2 (NF-2).[85]

### Presentation

Symptoms at presentation arise from mass effect or seizures, although an increasing number of patients have incidentally detected lesions.

### Management

Tumor location is a key factor in determining treatment. Other factors include tumor size, neurologic symptoms, and medical condition of the patient. Options include observation, resection, fractionated RT, and SRS, and these may be combined for some patients.

#### Surgery

Surgical resection is the primary treatment for the majority of meningiomas, allowing for acute relief of mass effect and signs or symptoms attributed to the lesion and providing a definitive diagnosis and grade. However, not all meningiomas can be resected without significant morbidity. A five-tier surgical grading system that related the extent of resection and the risk of clinical recurrence was described by Simpson et al. in a landmark paper in 1957.[86] This retrospective analysis provides class III evidence that has been used to advocate for postoperative RT in certain situations. Complete tumor excision including dural involvement was associated with the lowest rate of recurrence (9%), and higher recurrence rates (up to 44% or more) were observed in less complete resections.[86] The Simpson grading system is presented in Table 10-8.

Given control rates of 80%–95% in patients following total resection without radiation, adjuvant RT is generally considered only if there is residual or recurrent tumor, or if the histology is atypical or anaplastic (WHO II–III).[87,88] Benign asymptomatic meningiomas in suitable intracranial locations may simply be followed with periodic imaging evaluation in selected patients given the indolent natural history of many meningiomas.[81]

## Radiation

Incomplete resection may be appropriate if debulking is expected to relieve tumor-related symptoms. An exception is when a meningioma involves the optic nerve sheath, the cavernous sinus, or a major venous sinus. These tumors have excellent outcomes even without resorting to surgical intervention.[89,90] Improvements in vision for patients with optic nerve sheath meningiomas may occur even during RT.[91] In the majority of cases, adjuvant radiotherapy will not lead to significant additional changes in tumor volume. In less than 15% of cases, measurable decreases in visible tumor may occur, but often after several years.[88] Goldsmith et al reported on a retrospective series of 140 patients with subtotal resection and postoperative radiation. This management strategy achieved a 10-year progression-free survival of approximately 80%. Progression-free survival was improved to 90% with increased radiation doses above 53 Gy and use of CT/MRI in treatment planning to avoid geographic misses. This class III evidence supports offering postoperative RT following a subtotal resection to halt further tumor growth and provide a progression-free survival similar to patients who had a gross total resection.[87,88]

Current radiotherapy options in patients who require treatment include fractionated 3DCRT/IMRT external beam radiotherapy, stereotactic fractionated radiotherapy using a relocatable frame or image guidance, and single fraction stereotactic radiosurgery. There is no class I evidence to indicate one method of delivering radiotherapy is superior to another, but for these benign tumors, highly conformal treatment that avoids incidental irradiation of normal tissues is recommended. Even with contrast-enhanced MR imaging, it can be difficult to differentiate residual

TABLE 10-8  **Simpson's Classification of the Extent of Resection of Intracranial Meningiomas and Risk of Recurrence**[86]

| Simpson Grade | Extent of Surgery | Risk of Recurrence |
|---|---|---|
| I | Gross total resection of tumor, dural attachments, and abnormal bone | 9% |
| II | Gross total resection of tumor, coagulation of dural attachments | 19% |
| III | Gross total resection of tumor, without resection or coagulation of dural attachments, or alternatively of its extradural extensions (invaded sinus or hyperostotic bone) | 29% |
| IV | Partial resection of tumor | 44% |
| V | Simple decompression (biopsy) | |

meningioma from dural enhancement that occurs after a subtotal resection. This may be an issue if extremely conformal treatment such as SRS is being considered. Therapeutic decisions are based on patient and physician preference, tumor size, tumor location and extent, distance from the optic nerve/chiasm, and by equipment availability.

Single fraction stereotactic radiosurgery has been increasingly used but is typically limited to well circumscribed lesions <3 cm in diameter with sufficient distance from the optic nerve/chiasm or brainstem so as to spare these critical structures from treatment-related injury.[92] However, careful follow-up and further patient accrual is required to evaluate the long-term efficacy of stereotactic radiosurgery in comparison to surgical resection and fractionated radiotherapy. Several reports suggest excellent local control rates of more than 90% using SRS with limited complications.[92–94]

Reasonable treatment recommendations for patients treated with conventionally fractionated EBRT include careful targeting using MR and CT imaging to define the GTV (residual tumor volume) with a 1.0 cm margin to account for the CTV (clinical target volume). A further 0.3–0.5 cm margin is then added to account for setup uncertainty and to define PTV. This volume should be treated to a dose of 54 Gy in benign meningiomas and a dose of 59.4–63 Gy in those with atypical or anaplastic meningiomas. Dose homogeneity within the PTV may be critical in avoiding treatment-related complications.[95]

### Chemotherapy

Chemotherapy is not a generally accepted management strategy for meningiomas. Responses to hormonal manipulation and to hydroxyurea therapy have been reported, but the likelihood of benefit is small for most patients.

## VESTIBULAR SCHWANNOMA

### Incidence

Incidence of the benign, Schwann cell-derived tumors known as vestibular schwannoma (also called acoustic neuroma or acoustic neurinoma) is about 1/100,000/year in adults, with a median age at diagnosis in the sixth decade.

### Pathology

These usually indolent tumors represent 80%–90% of cerebellopontine angle tumors, and nearly all are unilateral and spontaneous; 5% are bilateral and associated with NF-2 (chromosome 22). Over 90% have extracanalicular extension into the cerebellopontine angle at the time of diagnosis.

### Presentation

The most common presenting symptoms are otologic (hearing loss, tinnitus, and gait unsteadiness or dizziness). As tumors enlarge, trigeminal or facial nerve symptoms arise, and brain stem symptoms occur for patients with the largest tumors. Hearing and facial nerve function can be graded with the Gardner-Robertson and House-Brackmann scales, respectively.[96,97] These grading scales are presented in Tables 10-9 and 10-10. Audiometry should be obtained in all patients with cerebellopontine angle tumors to establish a baseline for future comparisons no matter whether observation or active treatment may be contemplated.

### Management

Treatment options include observation, microsurgical resection, SRS, and FSRT. Class II and III evidence exists to support these therapeutic options. Observation is an appropriate option for some

TABLE 10-9 Gardner-Robertson Classification Scale of CN VIII Function[96]

| Class | Description | Pure-tone Audiogram (dB) | Speech Discrimination Score |
|---|---|---|---|
| I | Good | 0–30 dB | 70%–100% |
| II | Serviceable (can use telephone) | 31–50 dB | 50%–69% |
| III | Nonserviceable | 51–90 dB | 5%–49% |
| IV | Poor | 91–max | 1%–4% |
| V | None | Not testable | 0 |

TABLE 10-10 House-Brackmann Classification Scale of CN VII Function[97]

| Grade | Description |
|---|---|
| 1 | Normal facial muscle function. |
| 2 | Mild dysfunction. Complete eye closure. Facial symmetry at rest. |
| 3 | Moderate dysfunction. Complete eye closure. Facial asymmetry at rest. |
| 4 | Moderate to severe dysfunction. Incomplete eye closure, obvious facial asymmetry. |
| 5 | Severe dysfunction. Incomplete eye closure, barely perceptible facial movement. |
| 6 | Total facial paralysis. |

patients, such as advanced age, evidence of slow growth on serial MRI. Tumor growth rates vary, but generally average 1–2 mm per year.[98] Microsurgical resection via translabyrinthine, or middle cranial fossa approaches with the goal of complete tumor resection while preserving the facial nerve has been the gold standard of management until recently, when radiation approaches, including SRS delivering 12–13 Gray and fractionated stereotactic radiotherapy (FSR) using conventional fractionation to doses of approximately 50–60 Gray, have shown excellent tumor control rates and lower complication rates.[99–104] Anticipated iatrogenic injury for all therapeutic interventions relates to CN VIII injury (almost universal even with the most skilled microsurgical teams) and CN VII and V injury, which appear to be related to microsurgical skill and to the dose-volume relationship for patients treated with SRS.[105] There may be a less clear dose-volume relationship for conventionally fractionated FRS. It is unlikely a phase III trial will ever be conducted to compare FRS and SRS; no randomized trials have compared the results of surgery versus SRS or fractionated irradiation. Two separate prospective series evaluating the functional outcome of SRS versus surgery demonstrated better functional outcomes for the SRS patients.[105,106]

Class II evidence of comparability of hypofractionated FRS and SRS is provided by a prospective nonrandomized trial of SRS (10.0 and 12.5 Gy) and FRS (20.0 Gy/5 fractions and 25.0 Gy/5 fractions) that revealed comparable tumor control, hearing preservation, V and VII nerve preservation. In this single institution series, edentulous patients were treated with SRS and those with teeth had dental molds made that were used for guiding FRS.[107]

# CRANIOPHARYNGIOMA

## Incidence

Craniopharyngiomas comprise 1%–4% of adult brain tumors and 5%–10% of pediatric brain tumors. Their incidence is bimodal, with one peak occurring in childhood and another after the age of 50.

## Pathology

Craniopharyngiomas are benign neuroepithelial tumors that arise from the hypophyseal duct or Rathke's pouch and are frequently partly solid and partly cystic.[21]

## Presentation

These tumors often cause diabetes insipidus, pituitary and hypothalamic dysfunction, and visual symptoms.

## Management

Microsurgery, intracavitary irradiation, RT, and SRS all have appropriate roles and should be used adjunctively and interactively to provide the best patient outcomes.

### Surgery

Surgical resection can be curative, but these tumors are difficult to resect *in toto* because of frequent involvement of the pituitary stalk, the hypothalamus, adjacent blood vessels, and the optic apparatus. Attempts at radical resection are frequently followed by unacceptable neurologic, ophthalmological, and endocrine morbidity. Ten-year progression-free survival rates range from 30%–40% with surgery alone, and from 55%–90% with surgery and RT.

### Radiation Therapy

Radiation has been used for a number of decades with good results; the preponderance of data for the use of radiation in these benign tumors is class II and class III data obtained from single-institution series and retrospective reviews. There are no phase III studies comparing surgery to radiation, and no phase III studies comparing one or another method of delivering RT. External beam treatment can be delivered to localized portals, using conventional fractionation to deliver a dose above 54 Gray, if possible. The proximity of the optic apparatus is frequently the dose-limiting structure in treating these tumors. There is no conclusive data that one or another treatment technique (IMRT vs. 3DCRT vs. SRS) provides better outcomes, although there are encouraging early results (100% local control at 5 and 10 years) for SRS.[108] There are no published series on the results of IMRT for craniopharyngioma. An initial cohort of patients treated with proton beam therapy in Boston had 5- and 10-year local control rates of 93% and 85%.[109] SRS has been used for craniopharyngiomas adequately separated from the optic chiasm with control rates of approximately 85%–90%, when modern imaging and high speed computing are integrated into the treatment planning process.[110] Many radiosurgery series lack long-term follow-up, but one should expect good control rates if adequate coverage and dose delivery are achieved.

An alternate management strategy has been used for cystic craniopharyngiomas, in which a radiocolloid β-emitter ($^{90}$Y or $^{32}$P) is injected into the cyst to deliver a dose of 200–250 Gray to the cyst wall. Promising results with this strategy have been reported on by several groups, with best results for this technique seen with monocystic tumors without a significant solid component.[111,112]

## PARAGANGLIOMA

### Incidence

Paragangliomas, also known as glomus tumors or chemodectomas, are unusual tumors sometimes seen at skull base locations. They are not commonly seen, even in large tertiary care centers.

### Pathology

Paragangliomas are uncommon benign, though locally aggressive, vascular tumors that develop from neural crest origins. They are most commonly seen in the jugular bulb (glomus jugulare), the middle ear (glomus tympanicum), and along the carotid artery (carotid body tumor). Histopathologically, clumps of round and polygonal cells are seen in a vascular stroma, and staining for chromogranin and synaptophysin can help make the diagnosis.[22]

## Presentation

Some paragangliomas are metabolically active and can secrete vasoactive substances; most lack this capacity. Hypertension in a patient with a paraganglioma may be related to catecholamine secretion, and can be worked up with plasma and urinary studies for metanephrines. Other patients seek medical attention because of their awareness of pulsatile blood flow through the tumor. Specialized nuclear medicine imaging with metaiodobenzylguanidine (MIBG) may be useful in identifying whether or not a suspected paraganglioma may be one of multiple tumors. There are kindreds with familial paragangliomas, and in such kindreds, these tumors are inherited in an autosomal dominant fashion and can be multiple.[113]

## Management

Paragangliomas can be technically difficult to resect in certain locations with acceptable morbidity; RT has been used for unresectable and residual tumors with control of growth in approximately 90% of patients, even with unsophisticated treatment techniques.[114] There have been no phase III studies comparing surgery with RT or one form of delivering RT to another.

Embolization is frequently used to treat a paraganglioma prior to a planned resection. There is no evidence that it benefits a patient to be treated with SRS or RT. Embolization has been proposed as a palliative treatment for patients unable to undergo surgical resection. There have been no phase III trials comparing outcomes for such patients treated with embolization or RT.

Class III data appears to show improved control rates for combined modality therapy to surgery alone.[115] This should not be viewed as justification for planned subtotal resection of a paraganglioma to be followed by RT which would subject the patient to risks of both procedures when RT alone would suffice.

It is occasionally difficult to discern the exact location of residual skullbase paraganglioma after a microsurgical procedure. Differentiation of residual contrast-enhancing tumor from surgical effect may confound targeting for a focal procedure such as SRS. Fractionated RT does not require such accurate target delineation, and may therefore be able to better cover the surgical bed and any residual paraganglioma. IMRT can be used to conformally avoid structures adjacent to a skull base paraganglioma, such as the ipsilateral parotid, carotid artery, and the brainstem while still covering the volume at risk. One experienced center has reported worse outcomes with SRS than with fractionated RT for paragangliomas.[116] The follow-up for SRS for these benign tumors is still inadequate to assess the long-term control.

## PINEAL REGION TUMORS

### Incidence

Pineal tumors account for fewer than 1% of CNS tumors in adults.[22]

### Pathology

Germinomas are the most common pineal region tumors. Nongerminomatous germ cell tumors such as teratoma, endodermal sinus tumors, mixed germ cell, and less commonly, choriocarcinoma and embryonal carcinoma, account for the remaining 1/3 of CNS germ cell tumors.[22] Germinomas contain admixed syncytiotrophoblastic giant cells that stain positively for β-HCG. Endodermal sinus tumors stain positively for alpha-fetoprotein (AFP). Choriocarcinomas stain strongly positive for β-HCG.

Pineal parenchymal tumors account for less than 15% of pineal region tumors and include pineoblastoma and pineocytoma. Pineocytomas are slow-growing tumors and rarely disseminate in the CSF, but can behave more aggressively if less-differentiated. Pineoblastoma is an aggressive subtype of primitive neuro-ectodermal tumors (PNET) and is generally managed like other PNETs such as medulloblastoma. Tumors of other cell origin include astrocytoma, glioma, meningioma, and metastases; vascular malformations and pineal cysts are also included in the differential diagnosis.

## Presentation

Neurologic symptoms result from obstruction of the cerebral aqueduct with progressive hydrocephalus. Compression of the tectum leads to Parinaud's syndrome (supranuclear impairment of upward gaze, loss of convergence, and slow pupillary response to light).

## Management

Standard workup should start with a preoperative craniospinal MRI, measurement of serum and CSF alpha-fetoprotein, total β-HCG, and CSF cytology. Although adequate tissue sampling is an issue for stereotactic biopsy, if a tissue diagnosis of a germinoma can be obtained, no further surgical therapy is required. Open microsurgical resection may be helpful (and potentially curative) for many other tumors arising in this location. SRS may allow definitive treatment to be delivered to discrete and well demarcated tumors while avoiding the risks of a craniotomy, but determining the histopathology is critical for appropriate management, because treatments will differ, sometimes considerably, depending on underlying pathology, thus making a definitive diagnosis (without unacceptable operative morbidity) quite important in overall management. The following discussion focuses only on management of germ cell tumors.

### GERMINOMAS

Optimal treatment for localized germinoma continues to evolve. A common pattern of failure is via subependymal spread along the third and fourth ventricles with intraventricular relapses prior to further spinal dissemination. CSI has been a standard of care for decades, but the current standard is to use localized radiotherapy and limit the use of CSI to those with a disseminated disease. A Class II recommendation regarding radiation treatment volume and dose for localized germinoma receiving radiation also is to deliver whole ventricular field RT of 24–30 Gy followed by IF RT to a total dose of 45 Gy is based upon retrospective and prospective studies carried out at major institutions.[117,118]

Initial clinical studies with chemotherapy alone show a substantially increased risk of mortality as well as an inferior long-term disease-free survival rate compared to those achieved using RT.[119] Therefore, chemotherapy alone remains an experimental treatment option.

Although the outcome with radiation alone is excellent, current prospective studies assess the potential benefit of a combined modality approach to safely limit the radiation treatment volume and dose and therefore late treatment-related CNS toxicities.

In a prospective phase II study, 56 of 67 patients (85%), achieved a complete remission to induction carboplatin/etoposide followed by involved field RT to 24 Gy. There was a 12% relapse rate with the majority of relapses outside the RT field but within a whole ventricular RT field.[119] A randomized phase III COG trial comparing radiation alone to induction carboplatin and etoposide chemotherapy followed by radiotherapy is currently ongoing. Patients are stratified by disease extent at diagnosis and the response to initial therapy will determine the radiation dose and treatment volume. Localized germinoma patients treated with radiation alone will receive whole ventricular radiation irradiation to 24 Gy plus a boost to the primary tumor to a total dose of 45 Gy. Patients randomized to the combined modality arm will receive two cycles of carboplatin and etoposide followed by involved field radiation to a total dose of 30 Gy if a complete response is achieved.

## NONGERMINOMATOUS GERM CELL TUMORS

Combination chemotherapy with carboplatin, etoposide, and ifosfamide followed by CSI of 30.6–36 Gy with a boost to 50.4 Gy may be used in patients with an intermediate prognosis. Combination chemotherapy needs to be delivered before CSI to allow adequate dose intensity and hematologic recovery. The optimal drug schedules and regimens are unknown. Those with poor-prognosis tumors receive more aggressive chemotherapy.[118,121] CSI cannot be omitted for patients with nongerminomatous germ cell tumors. There still appears to be a predominance of local failures as a component of first failures with current management practices, suggesting a higher dose of RT to the primary site may be needed to achieve adequate local control for nongerminomatous germ cell tumors.

## PRIMARY CNS LYMPHOMAS

### Incidence

Primary CNS lymphoma (PCNSL) is an uncommon form of extranodal NHL confined to the brain, leptomeninges, spinal cord, or eyes, and accounts for <2% of all NHL. It is more common in patients with immune deficiencies. Since this is an uncommon tumor the data regarding treatment are small.

### Pathology

On pathology, the vast majority are diffuse large B-cell (90%), with T-cell or low-grade histology rarely seen.[22] Since the CNS and eyes lack native lymphocytes, lymphatics, or lymph nodes, evidence suggests malignant cells arise peripherally, are sequestered, and thrive in the immune-privileged CNS, while systemic cells are eliminated by the intact immune system.

### Presentation

Patients may present with focal neurologic symptoms, symptoms from increased intracranial pressure, confusion, or with a seizure.[122] PCNSL tumors are typically supratentorial (frontal most common) and periventricular in location and can traverse the corpus callosum and ependyma to involve the ventricular surface. Tumors tend to be diffuse; 30% are multifocal and 25%–40% have frank meningeal involvement. On brain MRI with contrast, the tumor is isodense on T1, enhancing after gadolinium administration, and slightly bright on T2. Some lesions will exhibit a "cotton-wool" appearance.

### Management

Other workup should include HIV serology, serum LDH, a dilated eye exam w/slit lamp, KPS or ECOG assessment, and MMSE testing. The International PCNSL Collaborative Group (IPCG) recently published guidelines suggesting immunophenotyping, CT w/contrast of chest, abdomen, and pelvis, bone marrow biopsy, and testicular U/S in older males.[123] These studies may reveal occult, systemic NHL in up to 8% of patients. One should attempt assessment of CSF cytology via a lumbar puncture although the yield is only 15%. Since these tumors are very sensitive to steroids, one should, if possible, avoid steroids prior to staging procedures.

The Ann Arbor staging system has no value for PCNSL patients. Memorial Sloan-Kettering Cancer Center performed a recursive partitioning analysis on their patients with non-HIV-associated PCNSL that identified three distinct prognostic classes. This model was validated on patients enrolled on RTOG clinical trials.[124] Three distinct prognostic classes were identified. The first included all patients under age 50, the second included patients ≥50 with a KPS >70, and the third was all patients ≥50 with a KPS < 70. Median survivals were 8.5, 3.2, and 1.1 years, respectively.[124]

Class II data supports a number of treatment options for patients with PCNSL, including systemic chemotherapy alone or with blood-brain barrier disruption. RT may be used alone, or after chemotherapy, but RT alone has yielded poor outcomes.[122,125] The most important advance has been the recognition of the contribution of high-dose methotrexate therapy.[126] Combined modality therapy has yielded better results than WBRT alone.[127] No consensus exists regarding optimal treatment, although methotrexate-based systemic therapy is increasingly regarded as important. Most current clinical research activity in PCNSL is focused on phase I and II studies of the addition of agents such as temozolomide or rituximab to existing chemotherapy regimens with or without irradiation. No phase III trials evaluating the role of radiation therapy in addition to systemic chemotherapy in the management of PCNSL have been conducted.

## REFERENCES

1. Chao JH, Phillips R, Nickson JJ. Roentgen-ray therapy of cerebral metastases. *Cancer* 7:682–689, 1954.
2. Tsao MN, Lloyd N, Wong R, et al. Whole brain radiotherapy for the treatment of multiple brain metastases. *Cochrane Database Syst Rev* 2006 Jul 19;3:CD003869.
3. Borgelt B, Gelber R, Kramer S, et al. The palliation of brain metastasis: final results of the first two studies by the Radiation Therapy Oncology Group. *Int J Radiat Oncol Biol Phys* 6:1–9, 1980.
4. Gaspar L, Scott C, Rotman M, et al. Recursive partitioning analysis (RPA) of prognostic factors in three Radiation Therapy Oncology Group (RTOG) brain metastases trials. *Int J Radiat Oncol Biol Phys* 37:745–751, 1997.
5. Patchell RA, Tibbs PA, Walsh JW, et al. A randomized trial of surgery in the treatment of single metastases to the brain. *N Engl J Med* 322:494–500, 1990.
6. Noordijk EM, Vecht CJ, Haaxma-Reiche H, et al. The choice of treatment of single brain metastasis should be based on extracranial tumor activity and age. *Int J Radiat Oncol Biol Phys* 29:711–717, 1994.
7. Mintz AH, Kestle J, Rathbone MP, et al. A randomized trial to assess the efficacy of surgery in addition to radiotherapy in patients with a single cerebral metastasis. *Cancer* 78:1470–1476, 1996.
8. Flickinger JC, Kondziolka D, Lunsford LD, et al. A multi-institutional experience with stereotactic radiosurgery for solitary brain metastasis. *Int J Radiat Oncol Biol Phys* 28:797–802, 1994.
9. Yu C, Chen JCT, Apuzzo MLJ, et al. Metastatic melanoma to the brain: prognostic factors after gamma knife radiosurgery. *Int J Radiat Oncol Biol Phys* 52:1277–1287, 2002.
10. Goyal LK, Suh JH, Reddy CA, et al. The role of whole brain radiotherapy and stereotactic radiosurgery on brain metastasis from renal cell carcinoma. *Int J Radiat Oncol Biol Phys* 47:1007–1012, 2000.
11. Rutigliano MJ, Lunsford LD, Kondziolka D, et al. The cost-effectiveness of stereotactic radiosurgery vs. surgical resection in the treatment of solitary metastatic brain tumors. *Neurosurgery* 37:445–453, 1995.
12. Sperduto PW, Hall WA. Radiosurgery, cost-effectiveness, gold standards, the scientific method, cavalier cowboys, and the cost of hope. *Int J Radiat Oncol Biol Phys* 36:511–513, 1996.
13. Mehta M, Noyes W, Craig B, et al. A cost-effectiveness and cost-utility analysis of radiosurgery vs. resection for single brain metastases. *Int J Radiat Oncol Biol Phys* 39:445–454, 1997.
14. Andrews DW, Scott CB, Sperduto PW, et al. Whole brain radiation therapy with or without stereotactic radiosurgery boost for patients with one to three brain metastases: phase III results of the RTOG 9508 randomised trial. *Lancet* 363:1622–1672, 2004.
15. Kondziolka D, Patel A, Lunsford LD, et al. Stereotactic radiosurgery plus whole brain radiotherapy versus radiotherapy alone for patients with multiple brain metastases. *Int J Radiat Oncol Biol Phys* 45:427–434, 1999.

16. Sperduto PW, Berkey B, Gaspar LE, et al. A new prognostic index and comparison to three other indices for patients with brain metastases: an analysis of 1960 patients in the RTOG database. *Int J Radiat Oncol Biol Phys.* 70:510–514, 2008.
17. Patchell RA, Tibbs PA, Regine WF, et al. Postoperative radiotherapy in the treatment of single metastases to the brain: a randomized trial. *JAMA* 280:1485–1489, 1998.
18. Aoyama H, Shirato H, Tago M, et al. Stereotactic radiosurgery plus whole brain radiation therapy vs. stereotactic radiosurgery alone for treatment of brain metastases. *JAMA* 296:2483–2491, 2006.
19. Vecht CJ, Haaxma-Reiche H, Noordijk EM, et al. Treatment of single brain metastasis: radiotherapy alone or combined with neurosurgery? *Ann Neurol* 33:583–590, 1993.
20. Regine WF, Huhn JL, Patchell RA, et al. Risk of symptomatic brain tumor recurrence and neurologic deficit after radiosurgery alone in patients with newly diagnosed brain metastases: results and implications. *Int J Radiat Oncol Biol Phys* 52:333–338, 2002.
21. Claus EB, Black PM. Survival rates and patterns of care for patients diagnosed with supratentorial low-grade gliomas: data from the SEER program, 1973–2001. *Cancer* 106:1358–1363, 2006.
22. Kleihues P, Cavenee WK, eds. World Health Organization classification of tumours: pathology and genetics of tumours of the nervous system. Lyon: IARC Press, 2000.
23. Piepmeier JM. Observations on the current treatment of low-grade astrocytic tumors of the cerebral hemispheres. *J Neurosurg* 67:177–181, 1987.
24. Claus EB, Horlacher A, Hsu L, et al. Survival rates in patients with low-grade glioma after intraoperative magnetic resonance image guidance. *Cancer* 103:1227–1233, 2005.
25. Berger MS, Deliganis AV, Dobbins J, Keles GE. The effect of extent of resection on recurrence in patients with low-grade cerebral hemisphere gliomas. *Cancer* 74:1784–1791, 1994.
26. van den Bent MJ, Afra D, de Witte O, et al. Long-term efficacy of early vs. delayed radiotherapy for low-grade astrocytoma and oligodendroglioma in adults: the EORTC 22845 randomised trial. *Lancet* 366:985–90, 2005. Erratum in: *Lancet* 367:1818, 2006.
27. Knisely J. Early or delayed radiotherapy for low-grade glioma? *Lancet Oncol* 6:921, 2005.
28. Shaw EG, Won M, Brachman DG et al. Preliminary results of RTOG protocol 9802: a phase II study of observation in completely resected adult low-grade glioma. World Federation of Neuro-Oncology Second Quadrennial Meeting Abstract 7. *Neurooncology* 2005 7(3): 284.
29. Pignatti F, van den Bent M, Curran D, et al. Prognostic factors for survival in adult patients with cerebral low-grade glioma. *J Clin Oncol* 20:2076–2084, 2002.
30. Lote K, Egeland T, Hager B, et al. Survival, prognostic factors, and therapeutic efficacy in low-grade glioma: a retrospective study in 379 patients. *J Clin Oncol* 15:3129–3140, 1997.
31. Karim AB, Maat B, Hatlevoll R, et al. A randomized trial on dose-response in radiation therapy of low-grade cerebral glioma: European Organization for Research and Treatment of Cancer (EORTC) Study 22844. *Int J Radiat Oncol Biol Phys* 36:549–556, 1996.
32. Shaw E, Arusell R, Scheithauer B, et al. Prospective randomized trial of low- vs. high-dose radiation therapy in adults with supratentorial low-grade glioma: initial report of a North Central Cancer Treatment Group/Radiation Therapy Oncology Group/Eastern Cooperative Oncology Group study. *J Clin Oncol* 20:2267–2276, 2002.
33. Knisely JP, Haffty BG, Christopher SR. Early vs. delayed radiotherapy in a small cohort of patients with supratentorial low-grade glioma. *J Neurooncol* 34:23–9, 1997.
34. Pu AT, Sandler HM, Radany EH, et al. Low-grade gliomas: preliminary analysis of failure patterns among patients treated using 3D conformal external beam irradiation. *Int J Radiat Oncol Biol Phys* 31:461–466, 1995.

35. Rudoler S, Corn BW, Werner-Wasik M, et al. Patterns of tumor progression after radiotherapy for low-grade gliomas: analysis from the computed tomography/magnetic resonance imaging era. *Am J Clin Oncol* 21:23–27, 1998.

36. Morris DE, Bourland JD, Rosenman JG, Shaw EG. Three-dimensional conformal radiation treatment planning and delivery for low- and intermediate-grade gliomas. *Semin Radiat Oncol* 11:124–137, 2001.

37. Knisely JPS, Yue N, Chen Z, et al. Automatic three-dimensional co-registration of diagnostic MRI and treatment planning CT for brain tumor radiotherapy treatment planning. *Int J Radiat Oncol Biol Phys* 45:3 (Suppl. 1):190, 1999.

38. Besa de Carcer P, Venencia D. Intensity modulated radiation therapy (IMRT) with noncoplanar beams for brain tumor treatment, clinical experience. *Radiotherapy & Oncology.* 73S1 pS331 abstract 768, 2004.

39. Eyre HJ, Crowley JJ, Townsend JJ, et al. A randomized trial of radiotherapy vs. radiotherapy plus CCNU for incompletely resected low-grade gliomas: a Southwest Oncology Group study. *J Neurosurg* 78:909–914, 1993.

40. Cairncross G, Macdonald D, Ludwin S, et al. Chemotherapy for anaplastic oligodendroglioma. National Cancer Institute of Canada Clinical Trials Group. *J Clin Oncol* 12:2013–2021, 1994.

41. Okamoto Y, Di Patre PL, Burkhard C, et al. Population-based study on incidence, survival rates, and genetic alterations of low-grade diffuse astrocytomas and oligodendrogliomas. *Acta Neuropathol* (Berl) 108:49–56, 2004.

42. J. C. Buckner, K. V. Ballman, B. W. Scheithauer, et al. NCCTG 94–72-53: Diagnostic and prognostic significance of 1p and 19q deletions in patients (pts) with low-grade oligodendroglioma and astrocytoma. *J Clin Oncol,* 2005 ASCO Annual Meeting Proceedings. Vol 23, No 16S (June 1 Supplement) 1502, 2005.

43. Hoang-Xuan K, Capelle L, Kujas M, et al. Temozolomide as initial treatment for adults with low-grade oligodendrogliomas or oligoastrocytomas and correlation with chromosome 1p deletions. *J Clin Oncol* 22:3133–3138, 2004.

44. Fuller CE, Perry A. Molecular diagnostics in central nervous system tumors. *Adv Anat Pathol* 12:180–194, 2005.

45. Vuorinen V, Hinkka S, Farkkila M, Jaaskelainen J. Debulking or biopsy of malignant glioma in elderly people—a randomized study. *Acta Neurochir* (Wien) 145:5–10, 2003.

46. Stummer W, Pichlmeier U, Meinel T, et al. Fluorescence-guided surgery with 5-aminolevulinic acid for resection of malignant glioma: a randomized controlled multicentre phase III trial. *Lancet Oncol* 7:392–401, 2006.

47. Walker MD, Green SB, Byar DP, et al. Randomized comparisons of radiotherapy and nitrosoureas for the treatment of malignant glioma after surgery. *N Engl J Med* 303:1323–1329, 1980.

48. Kristiansen K, Hagen S, Kollevold T, et al. Combined modality therapy of operated astrocytomas grade III and IV. Confirmation of the value of postoperative irradiation and lack of potentiation of bleomycin on survival time: a prospective multicenter trial of the Scandinavian Glioblastoma Study Group. *Cancer* 47:649–652, 1981.

49. Kita M, Okawa T, Tanaka M, Ikeda M. Radiotherapy of malignant glioma–prospective randomized clinical study of whole brain vs. local irradiation. *Gan No Rinsho* 35:1289–1294, 1989.

50. Curran WJ Jr, Scott CB, Horton J, et al. Recursive partitioning analysis of prognostic factors in three Radiation Therapy Oncology Group malignant glioma trials. *J Natl Cancer Inst* 85:704–710, 1993.

51. Lamborn KR, Chang SM, Prados MD. Prognostic factors for survival of patients with glioblastoma: recursive partitioning analysis. *Neuro-oncol* 6:227–235, 2004.

52. Shaw EG, Seiferheld W, Scott C, et al. Reexamining the Radiation Therapy Oncology Group recursive partitioning analysis for glioblastoma multiforme patients. *Int J Radiat Oncol Biol Phys* 57:S135–S136, Abstract 20, 2003.

53. Walker MD, Strike TA, Sheline GE. An analysis of dose-effect relationship in the radiotherapy of malignant gliomas. *Int J Radiat Oncol Biol Phys* 5:1725–1731, 1979.

54. Bleehen NM, Stenning SP. A Medical Research Council trial of two radiotherapy doses in the treatment of grades 3 and 4 astrocytoma. The Medical Research Council Brain Tumour Working Party. *Br J Cancer* 64:769–774, 1991.

55. Salazar OM, Rubin P, Feldstein ML, Pizzutiello R. High dose radiation therapy in the treatment of malignant gliomas: final report. *Int J Radiat Oncol Biol Phys* 5:1733–1740, 1979.

56. Chang CH, Horton J, Schoenfeld D, et al. Comparison of postoperative radiotherapy and combined postoperative radiotherapy and chemotherapy in the multidisciplinary management of malignant gliomas. A joint Radiation Therapy Oncology Group and Eastern Cooperative Oncology Group study. *Cancer* 52:997–1007, 1993.

57. Phillips C, Guiney M, Smith J, et al. A randomized trial comparing 35Gy in ten fractions with 60Gy in 30 fractions of cerebral irradiation for glioblastoma multiforme and older patients with anaplastic astrocytoma. *Radiother Oncol* 68:23–26, 2003.

58. Roa W, Brasher PM, Bauman G, et al. Abbreviated course of radiation therapy in older patients with glioblastoma multiforme: a prospective randomized clinical trial. *J Clin Oncol* 22:1583–1588, 2004.

59. Souhami L, Seiferheld W, Brachman D, et al. Randomized comparison of stereotactic radiosurgery followed by conventional radiotherapy with carmustine to conventional radiotherapy with carmustine for patients with glioblastoma multiforme: report of Radiation Therapy Oncology Group 93-05 protocol. *Int J Radiat Oncol Biol Phys* 60:853–860, 2004.

60. Tsao MN, Mehta MP, Whelan TJ, et al. The American Society for Therapeutic Radiology and Oncology (ASTRO) evidence-based review of the role of radiosurgery for malignant glioma. *Int J Radiat Oncol Biol Phys* 63:47–55, 2005.

61. Laperriere NJ, Leung PM, McKenzie S, et al. Randomized study of brachytherapy in the initial management of patients with malignant astrocytoma. *Int J Radiat Oncol Biol Phys* 41:1005–1011, 1998.

62. Selker RG, Shapiro WR, Burger P, et al. The Brain Tumor Cooperative Group NIH Trial 87-01: a randomized comparison of surgery, external radiotherapy, and carmustine vs. surgery, interstitial radiotherapy boost, external radiation therapy, and carmustine. *Neurosurgery* 51:343–355, 2002.

63. Cardinale R, Won M, Choucair A, et al. A phase II trial of accelerated radiotherapy using weekly stereotactic conformal boost for supratentorial glioblastoma multiforme: RTOG 0023. *Int J Radiat Oncol Biol Phys* 65:1422–1428, 2006.

64. Nieder C, Andratschke N, Wiedenmann N, et al. Radiotherapy for high-grade gliomas. Does altered fractionation improve the outcome? *Strahlenther Onkol* 180:401–407, 2004.

65. Stupp R, Mason WP, van den Bent MJ, et al. Radiotherapy plus concomitant and adjuvant temozolomide for glioblastoma. *N Engl J Med* 352:987–996, 2005.

66. Hegi ME, Diserens AC, Gorlia T, et al. MGMT gene silencing and benefit from temozolomide in glioblastoma. *N Engl J Med* 352:997–1003, 2005.

67. Cairncross G, Berkey B, Shaw E, et al. Phase III trial of chemotherapy plus radiotherapy compared with radiotherapy alone for pure and mixed anaplastic oligodendroglioma: Intergroup Radiation Therapy Oncology Group Trial 9402. *J Clin Oncol* 24:2707–2714, 2006.

68. van den Bent MJ, Carpentier AF, Brandes AA, et al. Adjuvant procarbazine, lomustine, and vincristine improves progression-free survival but not overall survival in newly diagnosed

anaplastic oligodendrogliomas and oligoastrocytomas: a randomized European Organisation for Research and Treatment of Cancer phase III trial. *J Clin Oncol* 24:2715–2722, 2006.

69. Merchant TE, Jenkins JJ, Burger PC, et al. Influence of tumor grade on time to progression after irradiation for localized ependymoma in children. *Int J Radiat Oncol Biol Phys* 53:52–57, 2005.

70. Merchant TE, Fouladi M: Ependymoma: new therapeutic approaches including radiation and chemotherapy. *J Neurooncol* 75:287–299, 2005.

71. Shaw EG, Evans RG, Scheithauer BW, et al. Postoperative radiotherapy of intracranial ependymoma in pediatric and adult patients. *Int J Radiat Oncol Biol Phys* 13:1457–1462, 1987.

72. Paulino AC, Wen BC, Buatti JM, et al. Intracranial ependymomas: an analysis of prognostic factors and patterns of failure. *Am J Clin Oncol* 25:117–122, 2002.

73. Rogers L, Pueschel J, Spetzler R, et al. Is gross-total resection sufficient treatment for posterior fossa ependymomas? *J Neurosurg* 102:629–636, 2005.

74. Mansur DB, Perry A, Rajaram V, et al. Postoperative radiation therapy for grade II and III intracranial ependymoma. *Int J Radiat Oncol Biol Phys* 61:387–391, 2005.

75. Massimino M, Gandola L, Giangaspero F, et al. Hyperfractionated radiotherapy and chemotherapy for childhood ependymoma: final results of the first prospective AIEOP (Associazione Italiana di Ematologia-Oncologia Pediatrica) study. *Int J Radiat Oncol Biol Phys* 58:1336–1345, 2004.

76. Colin P, Jovenin N, Delemer B, et al. Treatment of pituitary adenomas by fractionated stereotactic radiotherapy: a prospective study of 110 patients. *Int J Radiat Oncol Biol Phys* 62:333–341, 2005.

77. Mackley HB, Reddy CA, Lee SY, et al. Intensity-modulated radiotherapy for pituitary adenomas: The preliminary report of the Cleveland Clinic experience. *Int J Radiat Oncol Biol Phys* 67:232–239, 2007.

78. Landolt AM, Haller D, Lomax N, Scheib S, Schubiger O, Siegfried J, Wellis G. Octreotide may act as a radioprotective agent in acromegaly. *J Clin Endocrinol Metab* 85:1287–1289, 2000.

79. Landolt AM, Lomax N. Gamma knife radiosurgery for prolactinomas. J Neurosurg. 93 Suppl 3:14–18, 2000.

80. Longstreth WT, Dennis LK, McGuire VM, et al. Epidemiology of intracranial meningioma. *Cancer* 72:639–648, 1993.

81. Stafford SL, Perry A, Suman VJ, et al. Primarily resected meningiomas: outcome and prognostic factors in 581 Mayo Clinic patients, 1978 through 1988. *Mayo Clin Proc* 73:936–942, 1998.

82. Riemenschneider MJ, Perry A, Reifenberger G. Histological classification and molecular genetics of meningiomas. *Lancet Neurol* 5(12):1045–1054, 2006.

83. Perry A, Stafford SL, Scheithauer BW, et al. The prognostic significance of MIB-1, and DNA flow cytometry in completely resected primary meningiomas. *Cancer* 82:2262–2269, 1998.

84. Perry A, Stafford SL, Scheithauer BW, et al. Meningioma grading: an analysis of histologic parameters. *Am J Surg Path* 21:1455–1465, 1997.

85. Harrison MJ, Wolfe DE, Lau TS, et al. Radiation-induced meningiomas: experience at the Mount Sinai Hospital and review of the literature. *J Neurosurg* 75:564–574, 1991.

86. Simpson D. The recurrence of intracranial meningomas after surgical treatment. J *Neurol Neurosurg Psychiatry* 20:22–39, 1957.

87. Goldsmith BJ, Wara WM, Wilson CB, et al. Postoperative irradiation for sub-totally resected meningiomas: a retrospective analysis of 140 patients treated from 1967 to 1990. *J Neurosurg* 80:195–201, 1994.

88. Wilson CB. Meningiomas: genetics, malignancy, and the role of radiation in induction and treatment. The Richard C. Schneider Lecture. *J Neurosurg* 81:666–675, 1994.

89. Narayan S, Cornblath WT, Sandler HM, et al. Preliminary visual outcomes after three-dimensional conformal radiation therapy for optic nerve sheath meningioma. *Int J Radiat Oncol Biol Phys* 56:537–543, 2003.

90. Dufour H, Muracciole X, Metellus P, et al. Long-term tumor control and functional outcome in patients with cavernous sinus meningiomas treated by radiotherapy with or without previous surgery: is there an alternative to aggressive tumor removal? *Neurosurgery* 48:285–294; discussion 294–296, 2001.

91. Vagefi MR, Larson DA, Horton JC. Optic nerve sheath meningioma: visual improvement during radiation treatment. *Am J Ophthalmol* 142(2):343–344, 2006.

92. Stafford SL, Pollock BE, Foote RL, et al. Meningioma radiosurgery: tumor control, outcomes, and complications among 190 consecutive patients. *Neurosurgery* 49:1029–1037; discussion 1037–1038, 2001.

93. Kondziolka D, Levy EI, Niranjan A, et al. Long-term outcomes after meningioma radiosurgery: physician and patient perspectives. *J Neurosurg* 91:44–50, 1999.

94. DiBiase SJ, Kwok Y, Yovino S, et al. Factors predicting local tumor control after gamma knife stereotactic radiosurgery for benign intracranial meningiomas. *Int J Radiat Oncol Biol Phys* 60:1515–1519, 2004.

95. Uy NW, Woo SY, Teh BS, et al. Intensity-modulated radiation therapy (IMRT) for meningioma. *Int J Radiat Oncol Biol Phys* 53:1265–1270, 2002.

96. Gardner G, Robertson JH. Hearing preservation in unilateral acoustic neuroma surgery. *Ann Otol Rhinol Laryngol* 97:55–66, 1998.

97. House WF, Brackmann DE. Facial nerve grading system. *Otolaryngol Head Neck Surg* 93:184–193,1985.

98. Rosenberg SI. Natural history of acoustic neuromas. *Laryngoscope* 110:497–508, 2000.

99. Chan AW, Black P, Ojemann RG, et al. Stereotactic radiotherapy for vestibular schwannomas: favorable outcome with minimal toxicity. *Neurosurgery* 57(1):60–70, (2005).

100. Combs SE, Volk S, Schulz-Ertner D, et al. Management of acoustic neuromas with fractionated stereotactic radiotherapy (FSRT): long-term results in 106 patients treated in a single institution. *Int J Radiat Oncol Biol Phys* 63:75–81, 2005.

101. Maire JP, Huchet A, Milbeo Y, et al. Twenty years experience in the treatment of acoustic neuromas with fractionated radiotherapy: a review of 45 cases. *Int J Radiat Oncol Biol Phys* 66:170–178, 2006.

102. Friedman WA, Bradshaw P, Myers A, Bova FJ. Linear accelerator radiosurgery for vestibular schwannomas. *J Neurosurg* 105:657–661, 2006.

103. Lunsford LD, Niranjan A, Flickinger JC, Maitz A, Kondziolka D. Radiosurgery of vestibular schwannomas: summary of experience in 829 cases. *J Neurosurg* 102 Suppl:195–199, 2005.

104. Flickinger JC, Barker FG 2nd. Clinical results: Radiosurgery and radiotherapy of cranial nerve schwannomas. *Neurosurg Clin N Am* 17:121–128, 2006.

105. Regis J, Pellet W, Delsanti C, et al. Functional outcome after gamma knife surgery or microsurgery for vestibular schwannomas. *J Neurosurg* 97:1091–1100, 2002.

106. Pollock BE, Driscoll CL, Foote RL, et al. Patient outcomes after vestibular schwannoma management: a prospective comparison of microsurgical resection and stereotactic radiosurgery. *Neurosurgery* 59:77–85, 2006.

107. Meijer OW, Vandertop WP, Baayen JC, et al. Single-fraction vs. fractionated linac-based stereotactic radiosurgery for vestibular schwannoma: a single-institution study. *Int J Radiat Oncol Biol Phys* 56:1390–1396, 2003.

108. Schulz-Ertner D, Frank C, Herfarth KK, et al. Fractionated stereotactic radiotherapy for craniopharyngiomas. *Int J Radiat Oncol Biol Phys* 54:1114–1120, 2002.

109. Fitzek MM, Linggood RM, Adams J, Munzenrider JE. Combined proton and photon irradiation for craniopharyngioma: long-term results of the early cohort of patients treated at Harvard Cyclotron Laboratory and Massachusetts General Hospital. *Int J Radiat Oncol Biol Phys* 64:1348–1354, 2006.

110. Suh JH, Gupta N. Role of radiation therapy and radiosurgery in the management of craniopharyngiomas. *Neurosurg Clin N Am* 17:143–148, 2006.

111. Voges J, Sturm V, Lehrke R, et al. Cystic craniopharyngioma: long-term results after intracavitary irradiation with stereotactically applied colloidal beta-emitting radioactive sources *Neurosurgery* 40:263–269, (1997).

112. Hasegawa T, Kondziolka D, Hadjipanayis CG, Lunsford LD. Management of cystic craniopharyngiomas with phosphorus-32 intracavitary irradiation. *Neurosurgery* 54:813–820, 2004.

113. Plouin PF, Gimenez-Roqueplo AP. Initial workup and long-term follow-up in patients with phaeochromocytomas and paragangliomas. *Best Pract Res Clin Endocrinol Metab* 20:421–434, 2006.

114. Zabel A, Milker-Zabel S, Huber P, et al. Fractionated stereotactic conformal radiotherapy in the management of large chemodectomas of the skull base. *Int J Radiat Oncol Biol Phys* 58:1445–1450, 2004.

115. Powell S, Peters N, Harmer C. Chemodectoma of the head and neck: results of treatment in 84 patients. *Int J Radiat Oncol Biol Phys* 22:919–924, 1992.

116. Feigenberg SJ, Mendenhall WM, Hinerman RW, et al. Radiosurgery for paraganglioma of the temporal bone. *Head Neck* 24:384–389, 2002.

117. Rogers SJ, Mosleh-Shirazi MA, Saran FH. Radiotherapy of localised intracranial germinoma: time to sever historical ties? *Lancet Oncol* 6:509–519, 2005.

118. Haas-Kogan DA, Missett BT, Wara WM, et al. Radiation therapy for intracranial germ cell tumors. Int J Radiat Oncol Biol Phys 56:511–518, 2003. Erratum in: *Int J Radiat Oncol Biol Phys* 57:306, 2003.

119. Balmaceda C, Heller G, Rosenblum M, et al. Chemotherapy without irradiation—a novel approach for newly diagnosed CNS germ cell tumors: results of an international cooperative trial. The First International Central Nervous System Germ Cell Tumor Study. *J Clin Oncol* 14:2908–2915, 1996.

120. Aoyama H, Shirato H, Ikeda J, et al. Induction chemotherapy followed by low-dose involved-field radiotherapy for intracranial germ cell tumors. *J Clin Oncol* 20:857–865, 2002.

121. Matsutani M. Japanese Pediatric Brain Tumor Study G: Combined chemotherapy and radiation therapy for CNS germ cell tumors—the Japanese experience. *J Neuro-Oncol* 54:311–316, 2001.

122. Laperriere NJ, Cerezo L, Milosevic MF, et al. Primary lymphoma of brain: results of management of a modern cohort with radiation therapy. *Radiother Oncol* 43:247–252, 1997.

123. Abrey LE, Batchelor TT, Ferreri AJ, et al. Report of an international workshop to standardize baseline evaluation and response criteria for primary CNS lymphoma. *J Clin Oncol* 23:5034–5043, 2005.

124. Abrey LE, Ben-Porat L, Panageas KS, et al. Primary central nervous system lymphoma: the Memorial Sloan-Kettering Cancer Center prognostic model. *J Clin Oncol* 24:5711–5715, 2006.

125. Nelson DF, Martz KL, Bonner H, et al. Non-Hodgkin's lymphoma of the brain: can high dose, large volume radiation therapy improve survival? Report on a prospective trial by RTOG 8315. *Int J Radiat Oncol Biol Phys* 23:9–17, 1992.

126. Batchelor T, Carson K, O'Neill A, et al. Treatment of primary CNS lymphoma with methotrexate and deferred radiotherapy: a report of NABTT 96–07. *J Clin Oncol* 21:1044–1049, 2003.

127. Deangelis LM, Iwamoto FM. An update on therapy of primary central nervous system lymphoma. *Hematology Am Soc Hematol Educ Program*. 311–316, 2006.

# 11

# Current Management of Oral Cavity/Oropharynx/Hypopharynx Cancer

*Kenneth Hu, MD*
*Peter Han, MD*
*Louis B. Harrison, MD*

## OVERVIEW

Cancers of the oropharynx, hypopharynx, and oral cavity are located in central locations which can severely impact speech, mastication, taste, swallowing, and cosmesis. Eradicating disease and preserving organ function represent important goals of treatment. For early stage disease, single modality therapy is preferred, whereas complex multidisciplinary evaluation is needed for locoregionally advanced disease. Important advances have been made with altered fractionation and incorporation of chemotherapy to improve disease control. More recent advances involve better targeting of tumor either through better imaging, radiation delivery, or biologic therapies. Oropharyngeal cancers are more amenable to nonsurgical organ preservation therapy than hypopharynx and oral cavity lesions, but further improvements in treatment of all three are necessary to improve cure rates. Preservation of quality-of-life and organ function are crucial endpoints which tailor selection of the optimal treatment for the individual patient.

## ANATOMY

The oral cavity is comprised of the lips, hard palate, oral tongue (anterior two thirds of the tongue), alveolar ridge, retromolar tigone, floor of mouth, and the buccal mucosa. The primary lymphatic drainage of the oral cavity is to levels I, II, and III.

The oropharynx is comprised of four different sites: soft palate, tonsillar region (fossa and pillars), base of tongue, and posterior and lateral pharyngeal wall between the nasopharynx and the pharyngoepiglottic fold.[1]

The hypopharynx is comprised of the piriform sinuses, post-cricoid area, and posterior pharyngeal wall from the level of the hyoid to the cricopharyngeus.

The primary lymphatic drainage of the oropharynx and hypopharynx is to jugulodigastric node(s) located in the upper deep jugular chain and often drain directly to retropharyngeal and parapharyngeal nodes.[2]

**FIGURE 11-1** Anatomy of oral cavity and pharynx.

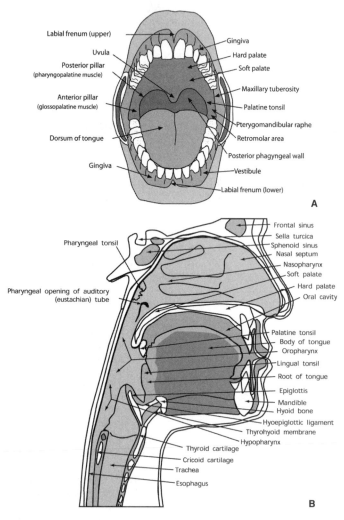

Yarbro, et al. *Cancer Nursing,: Principles and Practice,* 6e, copyright 2005. Jones and Bartlett Publishers, Sudbury, MA.

Skip nodal drainage to the lower level III and IV nodal stations is uncommon but lesions of the hypopharynx and posterior pillar lesions may drain directly to the level V nodal basin.[3]

Regional lymph nodes have been divided into levels I–V as follows:

Level I: submental and submandibular nodes

Level II: upper jugular nodes above the hyoid bone to skull base

Level III: mid-jugular nodes between the hyoid and cricoid cartilages under the sternocleoido-mastoid muscle

Level IV: lower jugular nodes

Level V: posterior triangle nodes outlined by the trapezius muscle and posterior border of the sternocleidomastoid muscle

## Pathology

Greater than 90% of all oral cavity, oropharyngeal, and hypopharyngeal cancers are squamous cell carcinomas (SCC).[4] The remainder includes minor salivary gland carcinomas, lymphoma, sarcoma, and melanoma.

## Presentation/Workup

Cancer of the oral cavity can present as a nonhealing ulcer, pain, bleeding, or ill-fitting dentures. These lesions can also be preceded and/or associated with leukoplakia and erythroplakia which represent premalignant epithelial changes. More advanced lesions may present with trismus, dysphagia, otalgia, hypersalivation, speech difficulties, and neck masses.

Oropharyngeal carcinomas present differently depending on their site of origin. Soft palate tumors often present in early stages due to their easy visualization. Cancers of the base of tongue often remain occult due their remote location and because the tongue base is devoid of pain fibers. They commonly present with an asymptomatic neck node. However, symptoms may include foreign body sensation in the throat, otalgia due to referred pain from cranial nerve involvement, dysphagia, and changes in voice/articulation due to tongue fixation. Tonsillar lesions may present with pain, dysphagia, trismus, and ipsilateral neck mass. Hypopharynx lesions usually present with sore throat, hoarseness, otalgia, and foreign body sensation. Progressive dysphagia, initially for solid foods and later for liquids, is a hallmark symptom for tumors of the lower hypopharynx and cervical esophagus.

## Staging

The clinical anatomic staging of oral cavity/oropharyngeal/hypopharyngeal cancers depend on both physical examination and imaging. The AJCC sixth edition staging for the oropharynx groups tumors by size and resectability as well as by nodal involvement. Large tumors are further characterized by their extent of invasion into adjacent critical boundaries involving bone, cartilage, or vessels.

### Stage Grouping

Stage 0 TisN0M0

Stage I T1N0M0

## TABLE 11-1 Oral Cavity, Primary Tumor (T) Staging

| | |
|---|---|
| Tis | Carcinoma in situ |
| T1 | Tumor 2 cm or less in greatest dimension |
| T2 | Tumor >2cm but ≤4cm |
| T3 | Tumor >4 cm |
| T4 (Lip) | Tumor invades through cortical bone, inferior alveolar nerve, floor of mouth, or skin of face, (chin or nose) |
| T4a (Oral Cavity) | Tumor invades through cortical bone, into deep [extrinsic] muscle of tongue, maxillary sinus or skin of face |
| T4b | Tumor involves masticator space, pterygoid plates, or skull base and/or encases internal carotid artery |

### TABLE 11-2 Oropharynx T-Staging

| | |
|---|---|
| T1 | Tumor 2 cm or less in greatest dimension |
| T2 | Tumor >2 cm but ≤4 cm |
| T3 | Tumor >4 cm |
| T4a | Tumor invades the larynx, deep, extrinsic muscle of tongue/medial pterygoid/ hard palate or mandible |
| T4b | Tumor invades lateral pterygoid muscle, pterygoid plates, lateral nasopharynx, skull base or encases carotid artery |
| Nx | Regional nodes cannot be assessed |
| N1 | Metastasis in a single ipsilateral node 3 cm or less in greatest dimension |
| N2a | Single ipsilateral node >3 cm and ≤6 cm |
| N2b | Multiple ipsilateral nodes, all ≤6 cm |
| N2c | Multiple bilateral or contralateral neck nodes, all ≤6 cm |
| N3 | Nodes >6 cm |
| M1 | Distant metastasis |

Stage II T2N0M0
Stage III T1-3N1, T3N0
Stage IVa (resectable) T4aN0-1M0 or T1-T4aN2M0
Stage IVb (unresectable) T4bM0
Stage IVc M1

## INTRODUCTION

Each year, approximately 31,000 cases of pharynx and oral cavity tumors are newly diagnosed in the United States with 7,430 leading to deaths.[5] Oropharynx cancer, hypopharynx, and oral cavity comprise the majority of such patients and commonly present with locoregionally advanced disease. For pharyngeal cancers, radical resection followed by postoperative radiation was once the accepted standard treatment. However, with high rates of locoregional control and function preservation, radiation therapy is now most often considered first line treatment. Patients with oral cavity and bulky hypopharynx tumors are better controlled with a primary surgical approach. Improvements in radiation therapy delivery techniques and fractionation schedules, the incorporation of concomitant chemotherapy, as well as the use of targeted biologic agents allow the majority of patients to achieve excellent locoregional control, function preservation, and maintenance of quality-of-life outcomes.

### TABLE 11-3 The Clinical Staging of Hypopharynx Cancer is Likewise an Estimation of Tumor Volume

| | |
|---|---|
| T1 | Tumor limited to one subsite and 2 cm or less in greatest dimension |
| T2 | Tumor invades more than one subsite without vocal cord fixation and >2 cm but ≤4 cm |
| T3 | Tumor >4 cm or with vocal cord fixation |
| T4a | Tumor invades thyroid/cricoid cartilage/hyoid bone, thyroid gland, esophagus, or central compartment |
| T4b | Tumor invades prevertebral fascia, encases carotid artery, or involves mediastinal structures |
| N/M staging | Same as for oral cavity and oropharynx |

## Risk Factors and Prognostic Markers

Tobacco or alcohol use is the major risk factor for these tumors with tobacco use having the greatest impact. Men typically make up about two thirds of patients and have worse prognosis than women and average age is greater than 50 years.[5] Human papillomavirus (HPV) is implicated in the transformation of tonsil cancer with the subtype HPV-16 most associated with malignancy.[6] HPV-positive oropharyngeal cancers may have an improved prognosis either related to the biology of these tumors or may be related to the lack of significant smoking history in many of these patients.[7] In addition, chewing areca or betel nuts, paan, and tobacco are risk factors for oral cancer, contributing to the high incidence found in Southern Asian countries.[8,9]

Biologic markers demonstrated to have prognostic value include p53 and epidermal growth factor receptor (EGFR). Koch has shown that locoregional recurrence is higher in head and neck cancer patients with p53 mutations after definitive or postoperative radiation.[10] EGFR overexpression has been associated with poorer locoregional control in patients treated with definitive radiation therapy.[11]

## MANAGEMENT OF ORAL CAVITY CANCER

The overall approach will depend upon the extent of disease, tumor characteristics, maximizing functional outcome, minimizing treatment morbidities, patient preferences/factors, and obviously cure of the disease. A multidisciplinary approach is crucial to obtain optimal oncological outcomes. In general, early stage oral cavity cancer can be treated by either radiation therapy or surgery alone. Typically, for T1-2 lesions, surgery is generally preferred with or without reconstruction. However, if the expected functional sequelae are significant, radiation therapy can be employed, usually incorporating brachytherapy with or without external beam radiation therapy. In one large series, Lefebvre et al reported 579 patients with early oral cavity cancers including 429 treated with brachytherapy alone with a local control rate of 82%.[12]

---

**FIGURE 11-2** Flow diagram workup with suspicious oral cavity lesion.

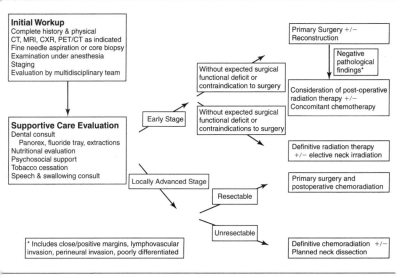

Single modality approach is usually preferred to minimize treatment morbidities. Patients with locally advanced disease usually need combined modalities incorporating surgery and radiation therapy.

## ORAL TONGUE

One of the largest series with definitive radiation treatment, comprised of more than 600 patients, is from the Curie Institute in Paris.[13] Most of the T1 and T2 lesions were treated with brachytherapy alone (6,000–7,000 cGy over 6–9 days). Larger T2 and T3 tumors were treated with a combination of EBRT (5,000–5,500 cGy) and LDR interstitial brachytherapy (2,000–3,000 cGy). The local control for T1, T2, and T3 lesions were 86%, 80%, and 68%, respectively. Mazeron et al reported on 166 patients with early staged T1-2 lesions with interstitial brachytherapy.[14] One hundred and fifty-five node negative patients had a 5-year local control rate of 87%. This compares favorably to a surgical series from Memorial Sloan-Kettering Cancer Center in New York, with local control rates of 85%, 77% and 50% for T1, T2, and T3 lesions, respectively.[15] Patients who have undergone primary surgery may need postoperative therapy due to close/positive margins, lymphovascular invasion, perineural invasion. In select cases, there are reports with using brachytherapy alone with excellent local control.[16,17,18]

## FLOOR OF MOUTH

Similarly, early stage tumors can be treated with either surgery or radiation therapy, typically with utilization of brachytherapy. However, these lesions are principally managed with primary surgery especially if the lesion is in close proximity to the mandible, which can result in high incidence of osteoradionecrosis with interstitial brachytherapy. When definitive radiation therapy is employed, many reports support the use of brachytherapy alone or with EBRT. Chu and Fletcher reported the outcomes of patients with floor of mouth cancer who were treated with definitive radiation therapy using EBRT alone, brachytherapy alone, or a combination of EBRT and brachytherapy for the treatment of oral tongue and floor of mouth.[19] Significant improvement was seen with the use of brachytherapy either with EBRT or alone, resulting in local controls of 98%, 93%, and 86% for T1, T2, and T3 lesions, respectively. Pernot et al reported the outcomes of 207 patients with FOM cancers treated with definitive EBRT and brachytherapy or brachytherapy alone. The 5-year local control was 97%, 72%, and 51% for T1, T2, and T3, respectively.[20] Wang et al also reported excellent results with the use of an intra-oral cone electron boost without brachytherapy.[21] In addition, patients who have undergone primary surgery may need postoperative therapy due to close/positive margins, lymphovascular invasion, perineural invasion. In select cases, patients may undergo brachytherapy alone with close/positive margins.[18]

## BUCCAL MUCOSA

Small lesions can be equally managed with surgery or radiation therapy. If the lesion is accessible intra-orally without significant functional sequelae, surgery is generally preferred. Select lesions can be treated with radiation therapy, which may include interstitial brachytherapy, intra-oral cone, ipsilateral electrons, or conformal EBRT with photons. Lapeyre et al compared two techniques in T1-3 patients with a median dose of 6,550 cGy.[22] The authors reported improved local control with a loop technique with only 1 out of 22 patients with local recurrence with a 5-year actuarial local control of 91%. One of the largest series on buccal mucosa cancers is by the European Group of Curietherapy.[23] Seven hundred and forty-eight patients were treated by either brachytherapy alone, brachytherapy with EBRT, or EBRT alone. Local control rates were 81% for brachytherapy alone, 65% for combined treatment, and 66% for external radiation alone. Results from surgical series varies with incidence of locoregional failure. Diaz et al reported on 119 patients of all stages with 71% of patients treated with surgery alone.[24] There was 45% incidence of locoregional recurrence with 32% of failures including the primary location. Dixit et al compared outcomes of 176 patients treated with either surgery alone or with postoperative radiation therapy with the latter improving locoregional control in patients with close surgical margins, tumor thicker than 10 mm, high-grade tumors, positive node, and bone invasion.[25] The actuarial 3-year locoregional control for stage III/IV was 11% and 48% in favor of postoperative radiation therapy.

## LIP

Most lesions can be treated with either surgery or radiation alone. Surgery is preferred for small lesions without significant functional deficits. Lesions involving the commissure should be irradiated. Jorgensen et al reported a large radiation treatment series of 869 patients with lip cancer with 766 patients treated with LDR interstitial brachytherapy alone (2,500–5,600 cGy).[26] The local control rate was 93%, 87%, and 75% for T1, T2, and T3 lesions, respectively. The European Group of Brachytherapy reported their results of over 1,800 cases of lip cancer, which were treated with a radioactive implant.[27] The local control was 98.4%, 96.6%, and 89.9% for T1, T2, and T3 lesions, respectively. Electron and orthovoltage beams have been reported with local control from 94%–100% for T1-2 lesions.[28,29]

## POSTOPERATIVE RADIATION THERAPY FOR EARLY STAGE ORAL CAVITY CANCER

Early stage lesions, after undergoing primary surgery, may have pathologic factors associated with high risk of recurrence, including positive close margins. Such patients may be considered for concomitant chemotherapy. Select oral tongue and floor of mouth cancers can be treated with brachytherapy alone for positive margins with excellent local control.[16,17,18]

---

**FIGURE 11-3** Clinical example of oral tongue cancer treated with external beam radiation therapy and brachytherapy.

---

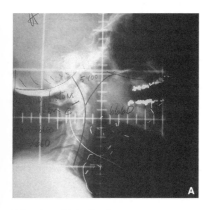 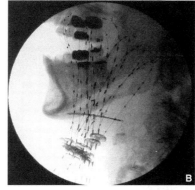

**(A)** Patient with locally advanced oral tongue cancer with positive margins. A total dose of 6,660 cGy was given with 180 cGy per fraction to the primary site and involved neck nodes. A tongue depressor was used to allow sparing of the hard palate. A low anterior neck was matched for a total dose of 5,000 cGy with a laryngeal block.
**(B)** Patient with persistent positive margins after partial glossectomy and neck dissection for early stage oral tongue cancer. A plastic loop technique was used for postoperative interstitial brachytherapy with LDR Ir-192. A total dose of 5,000 cGy was delivered at 1,000 cGy per day. A custom designed lead-lined mandibular shield was used during the irradiation.

## ADVANCED DISEASE IN ORAL CAVITY CANCER

Patients will need to undergo a combined modality approach, typically incorporating primary surgery and postoperative therapy. Two major landmark trials demonstrated a benefit with the use of post-operative concomitant chemotherapy with external beam radiation therapy for high-risk head and neck squamous cell carcinomas including oral cavity cancers. Additionally, patients may undergo definitive chemoradiation therapy, especially patients with unresectable disease with a planned neck dissection.

---

### BOX 11-1

(RTOG 95-01/Intergroup Trial) 459 patients with squamous cell carcinoma of the head and neck arising in the oral cavity, oropharynx, larynx, or hypopharynx who underwent complete macroscopic resection with high-risk features were randomized to postoperative external beam radiation therapy (60–66 Gy) with or without concurrent chemotherapy using cisplatin 100 mg/m$^2$ given every 3 weeks.

High-risk factors included:
1. two or more regional metastatic lymph nodes
2. extracapsular nodal disease
3. or microscopic involved mucosal margins of resection.

After a median follow-up of 45.9 months, the 2-year locoregional control rates were 82% in the chemoradiation arm and 72% in the radiation alone arm. The hazard ratio of 0.78 for disease-free survival (DFS) favored the combined arm. There was no statistical difference in overall survival or incidence of distant metastasis. There was also a statistically significant increase in incidence of acute grade 3 or higher adverse effects (77% vs 34%, respectively). There was a 2% incidence of treatment related deaths in the combined arm and none in the radiation therapy alone arm.

Cooper JS et al. Postoperative concurrent radiotherapy and chemotherapy for high-risk squamous cell carcinoma of the head and neck. *N Engl J Med.* 2004 May 6;350(19):1937–44.

(EORTC 22931) 334 patients with squamous cell carcinoma of the head and neck arising in the oral cavity, oropharynx, larynx, or hypopharynx who underwent primary surgical resection with high-risk factors were randomized to postoperative external beam radiation therapy (66 Gy) with or without concurrent chemotherapy using cisplatin 100 mg/m$^2$ given every 3 weeks.

Eligible patients included:
1. pathological tumor stage, pT3-4 and any nodal stage (except pT3N0 larynx with negative margins),
2. tumor stage 1–2 with nodal stage 2–3
3. T1-2 and N0-1 with extranodal spread, positive surgical margins, perineural or lymphvascular invasion. In addition, oral cavity or oropharyngeal tumors with involved lymph nodes at level IV or V.

After a median follow-up of 60 months, there was significantly statistically improvement in overall survival, progression-free survival, local/regional control rates, with concomitant chemoradiation therapy in comparison to radiation therapy alone. The 5-year Kaplan-Meier overall survival was 53% and 40%, respectively. The 5-year Kaplan-Meier progression-free survival was 47% and 36%, respectively. The 5-year estimated local or regional relapses was 18% and 31%, respectively. There was also a statistically significant increase in incidence of acute grade 3 or higher adverse effects (41% vs 21%, respectively). One patient in each group died from treatment related adverse effects.

Bernier J et al. Postoperative irradiation with or without concomitant chemotherapy for locally advanced head and neck cancer. N Engl J Med. 2004 May 6;350(19):1945–52.

## MANAGEMENT OF OROPHARYNGEAL/HYPOPHARYNGEAL CANCER

Due to the central location of the oropharynx/hypopharynx and their integral role in swallowing, speech and phonation, management of oropharynx/hypopharynx cancers require complex, multidisciplinary evaluation. Treatment decisions depend upon both the ability of a particular modality to control disease at the primary tumor and neck and associated morbidity. In general, early-stage disease is treated by a single modality, either radiation therapy (RT) or surgery, to avoid the morbidity of both, whereas more advanced lesions often are treated with combined modality therapy. RT is chosen more often than surgery for most early lesions because the control rates are high and the functional outcome is better. Chemotherapy generally is combined with radiation for patients with advanced disease. Special methods of delivering radiation, such as brachytherapy or intensity modulated radiation, further improve upon treatment outcomes.

### EARLY STAGE

#### Oropharynx

##### Surgery for Early Stage

Selected patients with small oropharyngeal lesions and a clinically negative neck can be managed with primary resection and elective neck dissection. Surgical results for early base of tongue tumors reflect relatively high local control rates from 75%–85%.[30,31] A significant percentage will be found to harbor positive microscopic nodes, often necessitating postoperative RT. Given the significant likelihood of

---

**FIGURE 11-4** Treatment algorithm for oro- and hypopharynx cancer.

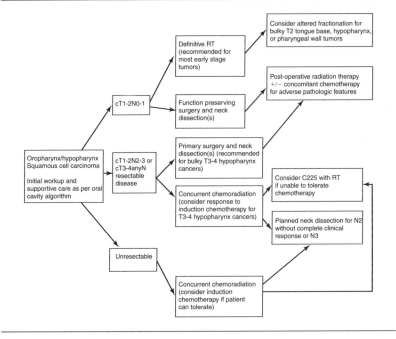

**TABLE 11-4 Tonsillar Carcinoma: Local Control and Survival with External Beam Radiation Therapy**

| Study and Institution | No. of Patients | Median Follow-Up (Mos) | % T3–4 | Percentage Local Control | | | | Percentage Local Control | | | | 5-Year Survival (%) | |
|---|---|---|---|---|---|---|---|---|---|---|---|---|---|
| | | | | T1 | T2 | T3 | T4 | N0 | N1 | N2 | N3 | DFS | Overall |
| **MDAC | 112 | 50 | 63 | 100 | 89 | 68 | 24 | 95 | 95 | 95 | 95 | 48 | 85 |
| ***UFla503 | 24 (minimum) | | 94 | 79 | 59 | 50 | NS | NS | NS | NS | NS | — | — |
| †Institut Curie | 698 | 60 | 72 | 89 | 84 | 63 | 43 | NS | NS | NS | NS | NS | NS |
| ‡Centre Alexis | 277 | 36 | 36 | 89 | 86 | 69 | — | NS | NS | NS | NS | 62 | NS |
| §Henri Mondor | 165 | 60 | 0 | 100 | 94 | — | — | NS | NS | NS | NS | 71 | 53 |

DFS, disease-free survival; NS, not significant.

*With implant.

**Remmler D, Medina JE, Byers RM, et al: Treatment of choice for squamous carcinoma of the tonsillar fossa. *Head Neck Surg* 1985; 7:206.

***Mendenhall WM, Morris CB, Amdur RJ, et al. Definitive radiotherapy for tonsillar squamous cell carcinoma. *Am J Clin Oncol* 2006; 29 (3):290–297.

†Bataini JP, Asselain B, Jaulery C, et al: A multivariate primary tumour control analysis in 465 patients treated by radical radiotherapy for cancer of the tonsillar region: clinical and treatment parameters as prognostic factors. *Radiother Oncol* 1989; 14:265.

‡Pernot M, Malissard L, Taghian A, et al. Velotonsillar squamous cell carcinoma: 277 cases treated by combined external irradiation and brachytherapy—results according to extension, localization, and dose rate. *Int J. Radiat Oncol Biol Phys* 1992; 23: 715–723.

§Mazeron JJ, Crook J, Martin M, et al: Iridium 192 implantantion of squamous cell carcinomas of the oropharynx. *Am J. Otolaryngol* 1989; 10:317.

nodal disease and spread into nodal basins that are difficult to address surgically, primary RT is often the preferred strategy. Laccouyre recently reported a large experience using a mandibultomy-sparing transoral approach for early stage tonsillar lesions with excellent local control rates but with a large percentage treated with induction chemotherapy and postoperative radiation.[31]

### External Beam Radiation Therapy for Early Stage

Conventionally fractionated radiation therapy (CF) alone controls the majority of early stage oropharyngeal lesions but may be suboptimal for T2 base of tongue and posterior pharyngeal wall cancers.

For tonsil cancers, several large single institutional series show excellent local control after conventional fractionated radiation alone (1.8–2.0Gy/dose over 6.5–7 weeks to doses of 65–70Gy), approximating 80%–90% for T1–T2 lesions and 63%–74% for T3.

For early-stage soft palate and pharyngeal wall cancers, many lesions are near midline leaving bilateral neck and retropharyngeal nodes at risk. Therefore, external beam radiation (EBRT) is often preferable because of comprehensive nodal coverage with high rates of control for T1-T2 lesions similar to that of tonsil cancers. Also, functional deficits after surgery, such as uvulo-palatal insufficiency requiring prosthetic obturators to prevent reflux into the nasopharynx/nasal cavity, can be avoided. Large single institution series show similar high rates of local control after EBRT alone.[32,33,34]

### Brachytherapy for Oropharynx Cancer

Brachytherapy has been a mainstay treatment for oropharyngeal cancers for decades and excellent results have been reported. Brachytherapy (BT) implantation of radioactive seeds directly into the target volume offers dose escalation to tumor and sparing of surrounding normal tissue by inverse square attenuation, producing excellent dose conformality. Normal tissue toxicity is further lessened because the dose of external beam radiation is reduced which is advantageous, especially in those receiving concurrent chemotherapy.

Near identical results using this approach for base of tongue have been reported by Puthawala et al and Goffinet et al.[35,36] Equally excellent local control for early-stage tonsil and soft palate cancers treated with combined EBRT and BT boost.[37,38,39]

### Ipsilateral EBRT for Early-Stage Tonsil Cancer

In general, most lateralized T1 to T2 lesions in patients with an N0 or N1 neck can be treated with ipsilateral radiation fields (Figure 11-5). Lesions that cross the midline, extensively involve the tongue base or soft palate, or associated with N2 or more advanced neck disease, should receive comprehensive bilateral neck therapy. Such an approach minimizes irradiation to the contralateral salivary glands and reduces the incidence of xerostomia. Eisbruch has demonstrated that patients treated unilaterally experience less xerostomia and better quality-of-life compared to those treated with intensity modulated radiotherapy delivery of bilateral radiation with contralateral parotid sparing.[40]

## Early-Stage Hypopharynx

Early-stage patients constitute about 25% of all those who present with hypopharynx cancers.[41] Important goals in patients with T1 and T2 resectable disease are to obtain local control while optimizing swallowing and voice preservation, which can be accomplished with either conservation surgery or radiation therapy. Only patients with early tumors of the pharyngeal walls or piriform sinus may be considered for laryngeal conservation surgical procedures. Tumors involving the piriform apex, anterior wall ("anterior angle"), or postcricoid area, causing any impairment in vocal cord mobility or a favorable tumor in a patient with poor lung function often will require total laryngectomy.[42] Neck management is indicated for N0 patients who will have a 30%–40% risk of occult neck metastases.[43]

**TABLE 11-5 Base-of-Tongue Carcinoma: Local Control and Survival with External-Beam Radiation Therapy Alone**

| Institution | No. of Patients | Median F/U (Yrs) | % T3/T4 | Percentage Local Control | | | | Percentage Local Control | | | | 5-Year Overall Survival (%) | | | |
|---|---|---|---|---|---|---|---|---|---|---|---|---|---|---|---|
| | | | | T1 | T2 | T3 | T4 | N0 | N1 | N2 | N3 | T1 | T2 | T3 | T4 |
| *Institut Curie | 166 | 5 | 58 | 96 | 57 | 45 | 23 | 86 | 79 | 58 | 61 | 49 | 29 | 23 | 16 |
| **MDAC | 174 | 10[a] | 54 | 91 | 71 | 78 | 52 | NS | NS | NS | NS | 100 | 58 | 38 | 20 |
| †U of Fla | 84 | 8 | 54 | 89 | 88 | 77 | 36[b] | NS | NS | NS | NS | 100 | 86 | 56 | 36[b] |
| ‡Hospital Necker | 54 | 8 | 0 | 78 | 47 | — | — | 4 | 9 | — | 40 | 17 | 17 | — | — |

NS, not significant.

[a]Extrapolated.

[b]Average of stages IVa and IVb.

*Spanos WJ Jr, Shukovsky LJ, Fletcher GH: Time, dose and tumour volume roleationships in irradiation of squamous cell carcinomas of the base of the tongue. Cancer 1976; 37:2591.

**Jaulerry c, Rodgriguez J, Brunin F, et al: Results of radiation therapy in carcinoma of the base of the tongue. The Curie Institute experience with about 166 cases. Cancer 1991; 67:1532.

†Foote RL, Parsons JT, Mendenhall WM, et al: Is interstitial implantation essential for successful radiotherapeutic treatment of base of tongue carcinoma. Int J. Radiat Oncol Biol Phys 1990; 18: 1293.

‡Housset M, Baillet F, Dessard-Diana b, et al: A retrospective study of three treatment techniques for T1-T2 base of tongue lesions: surgery plus postoperative radiation, external radiation plus interstitial implantation and external radiation alone. Int J. Radiat Oncol Biol Phys 1987; 15: 511.

## BOX 11-2

Base of tongue lesions are particularly ideal candidates for brachytherapy (BT) because local control is suboptimal after CF for even early-stage lesions.

BT is typically used as a boost (20–30 Gy) after a reduced dose of conventional fractionated EBRT that treats the bilateral necks and primary site (50–54 Gy to the primary site , 54–60 Gy to regional neck nodes). Harrison et al have reported long-term results of 68 patients treated in this manner combined with planned neck dissection for patients presenting with involved nodes. At 5-year actuarial estimate, local control is as follows: T1 (n = 17) 87%, T2 (n = 32) 93%, T3 (n = 17) 82%, regional control is 96% and overall survival is 86%.

Harrison LB, Zelefsky MJ, Sessions RB, et al. Base-of-tongue cancer treated with external beam irradiation plus brachytherapy: oncologic and functional outcome. *Radiology* 1992; 184: 267–270.

Harrison, LB, Lee H, Kraus DH, et al. Long-term results of primary radiation therapy for squamous cancer of the base of tongue. *Radiother Oncol.* 1996; 39:S6.

**FIGURE 11-5** Tonsil cancer: unilateral neck treatment.

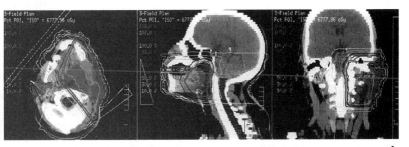

A

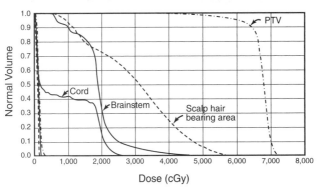

B

**(See Color Plate 1). (A)** Tonsil cancer. Unilateral neck treatment technique. The patient is a 50-year-old female who had a T2N0 left tonsil cancer and was treated unilaterally. She was treated with a three-field plan to minimize dose to the contralateral parotid.
**(B)** Dose-volume histogram of this plan showing good coverage of the target volume and adequate protection of the surrounding normal structures.

## External Beam Radiotherapy

Early-stage patients including T1 or low-bulk T2 hypopharyngeal squamous cell carcinomas may be effectively treated with EBRT, especially when the tumors are exophytic and don't involve the apex. Radiation has the advantage of sterilizing occult and early cervical metastases, obviating the need for extensive nodal dissections and their associated morbidity. The local control rates for T1-2 lesions treated with radiation therapy alone vary widely depending on the series, radiation technique/dose, patient selection factors, and neck staging.[44,45,46,47] Taken together, local control varies between 47%–90% and 5-year survival varies from 11%–52%. In general the best results have been obtained with conventional fractionation to doses >65Gy for T1 lesions and hyperfractionated radiation for T2 lesions in large single institution series.

---

### BOX 11-3

Two hundred twenty-eight patients with tonsillar carcinomas were treated with ipsilateral radiotherapy at Princess Margaret Hospital. Eligible patients typically had T1 or T2 tumors (191 T1-2, 30 T3, 7 T4) with N0 (133 N0, 35 N1, 27 N2-3) disease. Radiation was typically delivered with wedged pair cobalt beams and ipsilateral low anterior neck field delivering 50Gy in 4 weeks to the primary volume. At a median follow-up of 5.7 years, the 3-year local control rate was 77%, regional control 80%, and cause-specific survival 76%. Contralateral neck failure occurred in 3% (8/228). All patients with T1 lesions or N0 neck status had 100% contralateral neck control. Patients with a 10% or greater risk of contralateral neck failure included those with T3 lesions, lesions involving the medial 1/3 of the of the soft hemi palate, tumors invading the middle third of the ipsilateral base of tongue, and patients with N1 disease.

O'Sullivan B, Warde P, Grice B, et al. The benefits and pitfalls of ipsilateral radiotherapy in carcinoma of the tonsillar region. *Int J Radiat Oncol Biol Phys* 2001 Oct 1;51(2):332–43.

---

### BOX 11-4

Amdur updated the UF experience with 101 T1 or T2 lesions involving the pyriform sinus. T1 hypopharynx lesions are well controlled with CF while T2 lesions require altered fractionation based on two single institutional experiences at the University of Florida and MD Andersen Cancer Center. Conventional fractionation to a mean dose of 67 Gy was given in 54 patients while the rest received 1.2Gy bid to a mean dose of 75 Gy. With a minimum follow-up of 5-years in 87% of patients, the 5-year actuarial local control for T1 and T2 were 90% and 80%, respectively. Univariate analysis showed apical involvement by tumor resulted in lower control for T1 lesions [33% (1/3) vs. 100% (14/14), p = .02] while there was an apparent improvement in local control for T2 lesions with hyperfractionation [89% (33/37) vs. 73% (22/30), p = .09)] compared to CF.

Garden also reported that T2 hypopharynx lesions treated with hyperfractionation (n = 40) had improved local control compared to conventional fractionation (n = 23) (86% vs. 60%, p = .004).

Amdur RJ, Mendenhall WM, Stringer SP, et al. Organ preservation with radiotherapy for T1-T2 carcinoma of the piriform sinus. *Head Neck* 2001; 23:353.

Garden AS, Morrison WH, Ang KK, et al. Hyperfractionated radiation in the treatment of squamous cell carcinomas of the head and neck. *Int J. Radiaiat Oncol Biol Phys* 1995; 31:493.

---

## ADVANCED STAGE OROPHARYNX/HYPOPHARYNX

For most patients with advanced oropharynx and selected hypopharynx tumors, combined modality therapy with primary chemoradiation is recommended to maximize organ and function preservation. Radiation alone provides less optimal rates of local control in T3-4 lesions or patients with advanced N2/3 neck disease due to high rates of persistent disease after treatment compared to combined treatment but may be considered in patients with intermediate stage cancers T1-2N1 or T2N0. Advanced, bulky hypopharyngeal cancers are more often considered for upfront primary resection because tumor control/organ preservation is suboptimal after nonsurgical therapy and patients often have morbidity such as chronic aspiration due to destruction of normal tissues by the tumor or treatment. In such setting, total laryngectomy with partial or total pharyngectomy must be considered mandatory followed by adjuvant radiation with or without chemotherapy. Locoregional failure is the primary pattern of failure after any treatment approach for advanced oropharynx/hypopharynx patients. In an effort to improve locoregional control, major strides have been achieved with the incorporation of altered fractionated radiation, chemotherapy, and biologic therapy.

## ALTERED FRACTIONATED RADIATION

Altered fractionated radiation therapy attempts to improve tumor control either by accelerating radiation treatment to overcome tumor repopulation or by dose escalation with hyperfractionation to utilize the radiation repair advantage of normal tissues over tumor. Analyzing 676 tonsil cancers treated with widely different dose-fractionation radiation regimens, Withers demonstrated that an apparent delayed accelerated tumor repopulation appeared to occur 30 days after the beginning of radiation and could be overcome by increasing total dose or shortening treatment duration.[48] Radiation therapy can be successfully accelerated by delayed concomitant boost or a Danish regimen of six conventional treatments per week while dose escalation is best accomplished by hyperfractionation.[49,50,51] Metanalysis indicate a survival advantage of hyperfractionation (HF) with dose escalation compared to conventional fractionation (CF), but no advantage is noted for accelerated radiation compared to CF.[52]

Altered fractionated radiation represents a reasonable treatment option for T2N1 hypopharynx/base of tongue cancers or patients with T3 tonsil lesions who cannot tolerate chemotherapy.

## CONCURRENT RADIATION AND CHEMOTHERAPY

Numerous overviews demonstrate the advantage of adding chemotherapy to radiation.[54,55,56] A metanalysis by Monnerat concludes that concurrent chemotherapy offers an 8% survival benefit, induction chemotherapy 2%, and adjuvant therapy a 1% benefit.[55]

## COMBINING CHEMOTHERAPY WITH ALTERED FRACTIONATED RADIATION

Efforts to further improve locoregional control and survival have explored combining concurrent chemotherapy with altered fractionated radiation as both approaches independently improve outcome for head and neck cancer patients. The present challenge is to find the optimal chemoradiation regimen(s), which offer high rates of locoregional control and organ function preservation with acceptable morbidity and the possibility of integration with new biologic agents or additional chemotherapy.

### Phase III Studies

The majority of phase III trials show a benefit of the addition of concurrent chemotherapy to altered fractionated radiation either with HF or DCB compared to the same radiation regimen alone. Budach estimates a 12% 2-year survival benefit from the addition of chemotherapy to either hyperfractionation or accelerated radiation.[52]

## ROLE OF INDUCTION CHEMOTHERAPY

Induction chemotherapy has been utilized to reduce tumor burden and predict successful treatment of tumors to organ preservation therapy.[57] This is particularly evident for patients with hypopharynx cancers and may be the best way to select appropriate patients for nonsurgical therapy. With regard

## BOX 11-5

A landmark trial conducted by Radiation Therapy Oncology Group (RTOG-90-03) compared the leading U.S. altered fractionated regimens[50,52,53] (mendenhall, gwodz, wang) for cancers primarily stage III/IV head and neck cancers or stage II hypopharynx or base of tongue cancers. A total of 1,073 patients were randomized to a) conventional fractionation (CF) 70Gy/7weeks b) split course accelerated fractionation (S-AF) with 1.6 Gy bid to 67.2 Gy over 6 weeks with an intentional 2-week break after 38.4 Gy c) accelerated radiation by delayed concomitant boost (DCB) 72 Gy/6 weeks with bid last 12 days of treatment and d) pure hyperfractionation (HF) with 1.2 Gy twice daily 81.6 Gy/7 weeks. At 8 years median follow-up, the DCB and HF arms had significantly better 8-year locoregional control compared to CF (48% vs. 49% vs. 41%, respectively) and improved disease-free survival (30% vs. 31% vs. 21%, respectively) without significant difference in distant metastases (27% vs. 29% vs. 29%, respectively). Overall survival was 34% vs. 37% vs. 30%, respectively.

Fu KK, et al. A radiation therapy oncology group (RTOG) phase III randomized study to compare hyperfractionation and two variants of accelerated fractionation to standard fractionation radiotherapy for head and neck squamous cell carcinomas. First report of RTOG 9003. *Int J Radiat Oncol Biol Phys* 2000 Aug 1;48(1):7–16.

Trotti A, Fu K, Pajak T, et al. Long-term outcomes of RTOG 90-03: a comparison of hyperfractionation and two variants of accelerated fractionation to standard fractionation radiotherapy for head and neck squamous cell carcinoma. *Int J. Radiat Oncol Biol Phys* 2005; 63:S70.

## BOX 11-6

Horiot reported results of the EORTC 22791 randomized trial comparing a hyperfractionation regimen of 1.15 cGy bid (4–6 hour between fractions) to 80.5 Gy over 7 weeks versus conventional fractionation of 1.8–2.0 Gy to 70 Gy over 7–8 weeks in the treatment of 356 pts with T2-3N0-1 oropharyngeal cancers excluding the base of tongue with a mean follow-up of about 4 years, hyperfractionation improved 5-year actuarial locoregional control compared to conventional fractionation (59% vs. 40%, respectively p = 0.02) with a trend toward improved survival (38% vs. 29%, respectively, p = 0.08). T3 tumors benefited from hyperfractionation but not T2 lesions.

Horiot JC, et al. Hyperfractionation versus conventional fractionation in oropharyngeal carcinoma: final analysis of a randomized trial of the EORTC cooperative group of radiotherapy. *Radiother Oncol* 1992; 25: 231–241.

## BOX 11-7

The French intergroup (GORTEC 94-01) phase III randomized trial established concurrent chemoradiation as the standard treatment for locoregionally advanced oropharynx cancer over conventional radiation alone. Two hundred twenty-six patients with stage III (32%) and IV (68%) were randomized to 70 Gy/7 weeks or 70 Gy with three cycles of concurrent carboplatin(70mg/m2/dx4)/5-fluorouracil (600mg/m2/dx4) (week 1, 4, and 7). The initial report with a median follow-up of 35 months showed that patients in the combined modality arm had an about a 20% improvement in 3-year locoregional control (66% vs. 42%, p = .03), disease-free survival (42% vs. 20%, p = .04), and overall survival (51% vs. 31%, p = .02) but no difference in rate of distant metastases (11% vs. 11%, respectively). Long-term follow-up with a median follow-up of 5.5 years, confirms a 5-year overall survival (22.4% vs. 15.8%), disease-free survival (26.6% vs. 14.6%), and locoregional control (47.6% vs. 24.7%,) advantage with combined therapy. Still, despite such intensive therapy, over 50% of patients failed locoregionally.

Calais G, Alfonsi M, Bardet E, et al. Randomized trial of radiation therapy versus concomitant chemotherapy and radiation therapy for advanced-stage oropharynx carcinoma. *J Natl Cancer Inst* 1999; 91:2081–2016.

Denis F, Garaud P, Bardet E, et al. Final results of the 94-01 French Head and Neck Oncology and Radiotherapy Group randomized trial comparing radiotherapy alone with concomitant radiochemotherapy in advanced-stage oropharynx carcinoma. *J Clin Oncol* 2004 Jan 1;22(1):69–76.

to survival benefit, multiple metanalysis show only a minor benefit of induction chemotherapy.[53,54,54] However, recent data show that the addition of taxotere to induction cisplatin/5FU followed by radiation or concurrent chemoradiation improves survival and locoregional control.

Most recently, the addition of taxotere to cisplatin/5 fluorouracil (TPF) has been shown to improve survival and organ preservation in patients treated with subsequent radiation or concurrent chemoradiation.

The addition of taxotere to induction PF also increases larynx preservation. GORTEC Trial 2000-01 randomized 220 patients with hypopharynx or larynx cancer for whom total laryngectomy would be required to either TPF or PF followed by conventionally fractionated radiation to 70 Gy. The complete response rate was higher in patients with TPF 60.6% vs. 46.7% as was the overall response rate, 82.8% vs. 57.6%, respectively. At a median follow-up of 35 months, 3-year larynx preservation was 73% vs. 63%.

**TABLE 11-6  Randomized Trials of Chemotherapy and Altered Fractionated Radiation**

| Study | # Pts | 2Yr OS Diff | 2Yr LRC Diff |
|---|---|---|---|
| [*]Brizel<br>HF vs HF+CDDP/5FU | 116 | 18% | 26% |
| [**]Wendt<br>SC-AF vs SC-AF+CDDP/5FU | 270 | 25% | 19% |
| [***]Jeremic<br>HF vs HF+daily CDDP or CBCDA | 130 | 22% | 15% |
| [†]Starr<br>DCB vs DCB+CBCDA/5FU | 270 | 8% | 6% |
| [††]Dobrowsky<br>CHART vs CHART+MMC | 161 | 18% | 16% |
| [§]Budach<br>HART vs HART+MMC/5FU | 384 | 7% | 15% |
| [§§]Bensadoun<br>HF vs HF+5FU/CDDP | 163 | 18% | 31% |

OS diff: Overall survival difference, LRC diff: Locoregional control difference; HF: Hyperfractionation; SC-AF: Split course accelerated fractionation; DCB: Accelerated radiation by delayed concomitant boost; CHART: Continuous hyperfractionated accelerated radiation therapy; HART: Hyperfractionated accelerated radiation therapy; CDDP: Cisplatin, 5FU: 5-fluorouracil; CBCDA: Carboplatin, MMC: Mitomycin-C

[*] Brizel DM, Albers ME, Fisher SR, Scher RL, Richtsmeier WJ, Hars V, et al. Hyperfractionated irradiation with or without concurrent chemotherapy for locally advanced head and neck cancer. N Engl J Med. 1998 Jun 18;338(25):1798–804.
[**] Wendt TG, Grabenbauer GG, Rodel CM, et al. Simultaneous radiochemotherapy versus radiotherapy alone in advanced head and neck cancer: a randomized multicenter study. J Clin Oncol. 1998 Apr;16(4):1318–24.
[***] Jeremic B, Shibamoto Y, Milicic B, et al. Hyperfractionated radiation therapy with or without concurrent low-dose daily cisplatin in locally advanced squamous cell carcinoma of the head and neck: a prospective randomized trial. J Clin Oncol. 2000 Apr;18(7):1458–64.
[†] Starr S, Rudat V, Stuetzer H, et al. Intensified hyperfractionated accelerated radiotherapy limits the additional benefit of simultaneous chemotherapy—results of a multicentric randomized German trial in advanced head and neck cancer. Int J Radiat Oncol Biol Phys. 2001 Aug 1;50(5):1161–71.
[††] Dobrowsky W, Naude J. Continuous hyperfractionated accelerated radiotherapy with/without mitomycin C in head and neck cancers. Radiother Oncol. 2000 Nov;57(2):119–24.
[§] Budach V, Stuschke M, Budach W, et al. Hyperfractionated accelerated chemoradiation with concurrent fluorouracil-mitomycin is more effective than dose-escalated hyperfractionated accelerated radiation therapy alone in locally advanced head and neck cancer: final results of the radiotherapy cooperative clinical trials group of the German Cancer Society 95-06 Prospective Randomized Trial. J Clin Oncol. 2005 Feb 20;23(6):1125–35.
[§§] Bensadoun RJ, Benezery K, Dassonville O, et al. French multicenter phase III randomized study testing concurrent twice-a-day radiotherapy and cisplatin/5-fluorouracil chemotherapy (BiRCF) in unresectable pharyngeal carcinoma: results at 2 years (FNCLCC-GORTEC). Int J Radiat Oncol Biol Phys. 2006 Mar 15;64(4):983–94.

---

**BOX 11-8**

Two randomized trials included only patients with oropharynx or hypopharynx carcinoma in comparing the benefit of combining chemotherapy with altered fractionation versus the same altered fractionation alone.[4,7]

Bensadoun investigated the benefit of chemotherapy with hyperfractionated radiation (HF) for 163 unresectable oropharynx (n = 123) or hypopharynx carcinoma (n = 40) randomized to receive HF (1.2 bid to 80.4 Gy) with or without cisplatin (100mg/m2 day 1, 22,43)/5FU (750mg/m2/5days on day 1, 430mg/m2/5days day 22,43).[4] Actuarial 2-year locoregional control, disease-free, and overall survival were better in the patients receiving concurrent chemoradiation: 59% vs. 27.5% (p = 0.0003), 48.2% vs. 25.2% (p = 0.002) and 37.8% vs. 20.1% (p = 0.038), respectively.

Starr reported a benefit of the addition of chemotherapy to DCB in a German randomized trial of 246 stage III/IV oropharyngeal (n = 178) and hypopharynx (n = 62).[7] In a 2 × 2 study, all patients were treated with delayed concomitant boost (69.6 Gy/5 1/2 weeks) randomized to receive carboplatin (70mg/m2) /5FU (600mg/m2/d × 5d) on weeks 1 and 5 of RT and then randomized again to receive G-CSF or not. At a median follow-up of 22 months, the 1- and 2-year rates of locoregional control were 69% and 51% after CT/RT compared to 58% and 45% after RT (p = 0.14). Patients receiving G-CSF had reduced locoregional control (55% vs. 38%, p = .0072) and decreased mucositis (p = .06), raising the issue of possible tumor radioprotection with G-CSF.

For both trials, the addition of chemotherapy sharply increased acute mucositis, hematologic toxicity, and feeding tube dependence.

---

**BOX 11-9**

This landmark trial randomized 202 patients with selected locally advanced hypopharyngeal cancer (T2 to T4 tumors limited to the piriform sinus or hypopharyngeal aspect of the aryepiglottic fold excluding T2 exophytic lesions) to radical resection and postoperative irradiation (5,000 to 7,000 cGy; 200-cGy fractions) versus induction chemotherapy with two to three cycles of cisplatin/5-fluorouracil (100mg/m2 and 1000mg/m2 over 5 days), followed by conventional fractionated radiation (70Gy/7 weeks) if patients had a clinical complete response after induction chemotherapy. Complete response was defined as total resolution of all macroscopic disease and complete return of laryngeal mobility. At a median follow-up of 51 months, there was no statistical difference between the arms in either of the rates of local and regional failures. The 3-year survival rates (43% vs. 57%) favored the larynx preservation arm; however, at 5 years there was no significant survival difference (34% vs. 29%). For all patients entered in the organ-preservation arm, the 3-year organ preservation rate was 42%. Among complete responders, the larynx preservation rate increased to 64%.

Lefebvre JL, Chevalier D, Luboinski B, et al. Larynx preservation in pyriform sinus cancer: preliminary results of a European Organizaion of Reseach and Treatment of Cancer phase III trial. *J Natl Cancer Inst* 1996; 88:890.

## BIOLOGIC THERAPY

### C225

Epidermal growth factor receptor (EGFR) is commonly expressed on head and neck cancer cell lines. Ang reported in a study of a cohort of RTOG 90-03 patients that a greater than median level of EGFR expression correlated with a greater risk for 2-year locoregional relapse (74% vs. 45%, respectively, p = 0.0031), lower 2-year disease-free survival (18% vs. 29%, p = 0.0016) and lower 2-year overall survival

**BOX 11-10**

EORTC #24971 randomized 358 locally advanced head and neck cancer patients to receive TPF (75mg/m2d1, 750mg/m2 CI d1-5, respectively) or PF (100mg/m2 day 1, 1000mg/m2 CI d1-5), respectively followed by conventional or altered fractionated radiation. Patients in the TPF arm demonstrated superior response rate (68% vs. 54%, p = 0.007). and increased 3-year overall survival (36.5% vs. 23.9% ) at 51 month median follow-up. Patients who received TPF had less grade 3–4 toxicity and fewer toxic deaths (3.7% vs. 7.8%) compared to those receiving PF due to the reduced doses of platinum and 5FU in the TPF regimen.

Posner reports a benefit of adding taxotere to PF followed by concurrent chemoradiation. Four hundred ninety-four were randomized to three cycles of induction TPF (75/mg/m2, 100mg/m2, 1000mg/m2) or three cycles of PF (100mg/m2, 1000mg/m2) followed by concurrent chemoradiation (70Gy/7 weeks and weekly carboplatin AUC 1.5). At a median follow-up of 42 months, 3 years OS (62% vs 48%, p = 0.0058), and PFS were increased (49% vs. 37%, p = 0.004) after TPF compared to PF.

Vermorken J, Remenar E, van Herpen C, et al. Standard cisplatin/infusional 5-fluorouracial (PF) vs. docetaxel (T) plus PF (TPF) as neoadjuvant chemotherapy for nonresectable locally advanced squamous cell carcinoma of the head and neck (LA-SCCHN): a phase III trial of the EORTC head and neck cancer group (EORTC #24971). *J. Clin Oncol* 2004; 22:490S.

Remenar E, Van Herpen C, Germa Lluch J, et al. A randomized phase III multicenter trial of neoadjuvant docetaxel plus cisplatin and 5-fluorouracial (TPF) versus neoadjuvant PF in patients with locally advanced unresectable squamous cell carcinoma of the head and neck (SCCHN). Final analysis of EORTC 24971. *J Clin Oncol* 2006; 24:18S. Posner, ASCO 2006.

**BOX 11-11**

A pivotal phase III trial reported by Bonner demonstrated the benefit of adding cetuximab (C225), the monoclonal antibody targeting EGFR, to radiation. Four hundred twenty-four patients with stage III/IV head and neck cancer (oropharynx/hypopharynx cancer comprised 85% of patients enrolled) were randomized to 7 weeks of C225 plus radiation (CF or altered fractionation) or radiation alone. At a median follow-up of 38 months, the C225/RT arm was superior to RT alone with respect to 2 year locoregional control (56% vs. 48%), 2-year overall survival (62% vs. 55%) and median overall survival (54 month vs. 28 months, p = 0.02). With regard to toxicity, C225, unlike the addition of concurrent chemotherapy or the acceleration of radiation, did not significantly increase grade 3/4 mucositis (55% vs. 52%, respectively) but was associated with increased dermatitis (34% vs. 18%, p = 0.0003) and infusion reaction (3%).

Bonner J, Harari P, Giralt J, et al. Radiotherapy plus cetuximab for squamous cell carcinoma of the head and neck. *N Engl J Med* 2006 Feb 9;354(6):567–78.

(30% vs. 59%, p = 0.0006) compared to those patients with tumors expressing less or equal to the median EGFR expression.[11] No difference in distant metastases were noted between the two groups.

## ADVANCED STAGE SURGERY AND POSTOPERATIVE RADIATION

For patients with advanced lesions where primary resection offers the best chance for locoregional control, adjuvant radiation is usually required. With regard to hypopharynx cancer, multiple single institution studies show an improvement of approximately 28%–43% in locoregional control when radiation therapy is added to surgery.[58,59] For high-risk patients, trials conducted by the RTOG and EORTC show a significant benefit for the addition of concurrent chemotherapy to conventional fractionated postoperative radiation. (See oral cavity sec-tion). For high-risk cases in which patients are unable to tolerate chemotherapy, post-operated accelerated radiation by delayed concomitant boost or conventional fractionated radiation starting within 4 weeks after surgery improves locoregional control and should be considered.[60]

## IMRT

Recent efforts to improve radiation dose conformality and reduce toxicity have been made with 3D and intensity modulated radiation therapy (IMRT) techniques to treat complex, irregularly shaped head and neck tumors. IMRT has generated tremendous enthusiasm because it allows exquisite dose conformality with sparing of adjacent organs. Each radiation field is divided into a number of beamlets with the aid of an intensity modulator and inverse treatment planning. The different beamlets are added to form a cumulative dose distribution tailored to the shape of the tumor and respecting designated normal tissue tolerance constraints. IMRT also offers the possibility of differential dosing to the elective nodal basin, high-risk nodal areas, and primary tumor sites with resultant modest accelerated radiation.

Cancers of the oropharynx are ideal sites for IMRT since the tumors often present in close proximity to sensitive normal tissues such as the parotid glands or involve the pharyngeal wall/retropharyngeal nodes close to the spinal cord. Locoregional control of 87%–89% appears similar and possibly better than conventional technique based on initial single institution series.[61,62,63,64] IMRT regimens of 70 Gy in 33 fractions or 37 fractions are well tolerated, even with concurrent chemotherapy. A multi-institutional RTOG 0022 protocol has completed and the results are pending.

To date, the greatest benefit of IMRT in reducing toxicity has been the reduction of severe xerostomia compared to standard techniques. Eisbruch et al showed that stimulated salivary flow can be preserved if the mean dose to one parotid is ≤26 Gy using IMRT with full recovery occurring up to 2 years after treatment.[65]

Chao et al showed that if the parotid glands received a mean dose of 32 Gy, approximately 25% of the stimulated salivary flow at 6 months could be preserved and at 16 Gy, approximately 50% or more of the baseline salivary flow could be retained.[66] This is clearly an important advance because xerostomia represents the primary quality-of-life complaint among long-term head and neck cancer survivors treated with radiation.

### TECHNIQUE

### Conventional Technique

Pre-irradiation dental evaluation includes panorex, dental extractions if indicated, and fluoride tray. Patients should be immobilized in an aquaplast mold with neck extension and shoulder board to separate the oropharynx site from the larynx or hyopharynx cancers from the shoulders. For tongue cancers, a bite block may be used to depress the tongue downward and away from the palate, allowing easier blocking of the palate. Palpable neck disease should be outlined with wire. The target volume of the parallel opposed fields should include the primary with margin, plus draining lymph nodes of the upper neck with a high match above the arytenoids for oropharynx lesions, and a low match below the cricoid cartilage for hypopharyngeal lesions. Owing to the high probability of lymph node metastasis, these portals also will include the retropharyngeal lymph node groups up to the skull base. Fields are matched to a low anterior neck using a split isocenter technique with a spinal cord/vocal cord block in the LAN for oropharynx cancer or a lateral field cord block in patients with hypopharynx cancer.

Initial lateral fields are treated to 40–45 Gy followed by an off cord cone down to the primary and upper neck to a dose of 50–54 Gy and a final cone down to gross disease to a dose of 66–70 Gy for T3 and 70–80 Gy for a T4 lesion. Posterior necks are treated with electron strips using 6 to 9MeV electrons to appropriate doses of 50–70 Gy. For lesions involving the posterior pharyngeal wall or retropharygeal nodes, careful attention should be paid regarding the posterior border of the off cord block. Fein has shown that moving the posterior border from the middle to the posterior edge of the vertebral body improves local control.[33]

## Brachytherapy

The dose with LDR Ir-192 interstitial brachytherapy ranges from 2,000–3,000 cGy at 40–60 cGy/hour which is done approximately 3 weeks after the completion of EBRT. Mandibular lead-lined shields can be used to decrease the incidence of osteoradionecrosis. Ideally, interstitial brachytherapy should not be performed with lesions abutting/tethering mandible due to risk of osteoradionecrosis. Morrish et al reported that doses of greater than 7,500 cGy resulted in 50% or higher rates of osteoradionecrosis.[67] HDR has also been used, including treatments without EBRT.[68,69] See Figure 11-3A for clinical example of postoperative brachytherapy for oral tongue cancer.

## Postoperative Radiation

When postoperative radiation is administered, patients should be set up similarly as described previously. The match line should be above the arytenoids for oropharynx cancer and above the stoma for hypopharynx cancers. A typical dose and fractionation schedule would be 6,300–6,600 cGy to high-risk areas, 5,760–5,940 cGy to intermediate regions of the neck (in 180-cGy fractions), and 5,000–5,400 cGy to low-risk areas. The low anterior neck is treated to a dose of 5,000 cGy; the stoma (when present) often is boosted with electrons to 6,000 cGy. See Figure 11-3A for clinical example of postoperative EBRT for oral tongue cancer.

## IMRT Technique

IMRT should be considered particularly for oropharyngeal/hypopharyngeal tumors near the spinal cord such as those involving the posterior pharyngeal wall or nasopharynx as well as for those where significant parotid sparing can be attained, such as those patients with negative contralateral neck nodes.

The patient should be immobilized with neck extended as described earlier. An isocenter should be selected to treat the primary and upper neck nodes for oropharyngeal cancers with a lower border matched to a low anterior neck field to treat the lower cervical and supraclavicular node. An extended field treating the primary and all regional nodes should be considered for hypopharyngeal tumors. Treatment planning CT using 3mm slice thickness should be performed over the primary and regional nodes. IV contrast is recommended. Fusion with PET and MRI should be considered. CTV encompassing gross tumor volume, microscopic disease, and potential for tumor spread should be outlined and stratified according to burden of disease—high risk: gross disease; intermediate risk: areas with high likelihood of nodal disease or tumor spread and low risk: elective nodal treatment. Care must be taken not to underdose regional nodes near the parotid, as well as to evaluate dose at the match line. If a patient has a clinically negative neck, the superior border of regional node delineation can end at the bottom of the C1 transverse process, sparing significant parotid tissue.

### IMRT

70 Gy to high-risk CTV; 5,940 cGy to intermediate risk and 5,000–5,400 cGy to elective risk.

### Normal dose constraint guidelines

Parotid glands: V50 26 Gy; Brainstem: <54 Gy V1<60 Gy; Spinal cord 45 Gy V1<50 Gy; Mandible: <70 Gy and V1<75 Gy; Temporal lobes: <60 Gy; Optic nerves and chiasm: <50 Gy V1<54 Gy.

**FIGURE 11-6** Clinical example of base of tongue cancer treated with radiation therapy.

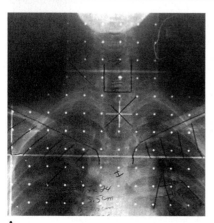
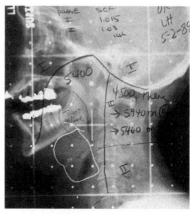

A

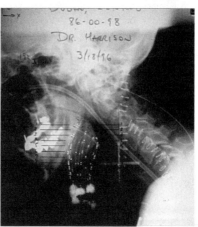

B

**(A)** Base of tongue cancer. Technique using external beam plus brachytherapy. The patient had a T2N2aM0 squamous cell cancer of the tongue base. The patient was simulated and treated with external beam radiation first using opposed laterals and low anterior neck. The patient received 5,400 cGy to the primary site, 5,940 cGy for ipsilateral nodes, and 5,400 cGy to contralateral neck.
**(B)** Approximately 3 weeks after external beam radiation is completed, the patient is brought to the operating room for planned dissection and a brachytherapy implant. She received a 2,200 cGy brachytherapy Ir-192 implant.

## Toxicity

### Acute

Mucositis, pain, phlegm production, xerostomia, dysphagia, dysgeusia, dermatitis, weight loss, laryngeal edema, lhermitte's.

**FIGURE 11-7** Intensity modulated radiation therapy for oropharynx cancer.

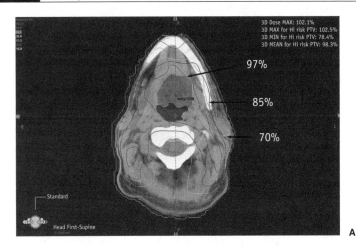

3D Dose MAX: 102.1%
3D MAX for Hi risk PTV: 102.5%
3D MIN for Hi risk PTV: 78.4%
3D MEAN for Hi risk PTV: 98.3%

97%

85%

70%

Standard

Head First-Supine

A

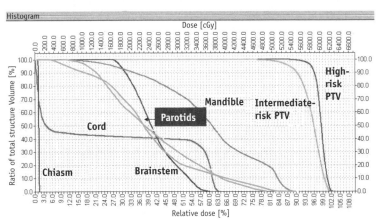

B

(See Color Plate 2). (A) Intensity modulated radiation therapy for oropharynx cancer. The patient is a 62-year-old male with a T2N2bM0 squamous cell carcinoma of the left base of tongue who received chemoradiation with IMRT to a dose of 60 Gy to the primary and involved nodes and 54 Gy elective treatment to the contralateral neck and three cycles of concurrent cisplatin. Subsequently, he underwent planned neck dissection and brachytherapy implant boost to 20 Gy.
(B) Dose volume histogram shows that 95% of the PTV's received the intended dose, respecting the dose tolerance of the parotids and normal critical structures.

## Chronic

Xerostomia, hypothyroidism, cervical fibrosis, dental decay, osteoradionecrosis, chondronecrosis, dysphagia/PEG dependence, cricopharyngeal stricture, fistula, epilation.

## Radiation Therapy

The major sequelae of RT can be divided into acute and chronic side effects. These depend on total dose, fraction size, fractionation, prior or concomitant therapy (surgery or chemotherapy), and target volume. Mucositis is the major dose-limiting toxicity of radiation. Severe mucositis can result in treatment breaks, which can compromise locoregional control and cause infection in patients compromised by chemotherapy. Based on RTOG 90-03, altered fractionation increases acute grade 3–4 toxicity by 20%, primarily mucositis.[70] Addition of chemotherapy steeply increases mucositis, feeding tube dependence, dermatitis, hematologic suppression, and infection. Addition of C225 increases infusion reaction and dermatitis.[71]

With regard to chronic toxicity, the major issues after definitive radiation therapy are xerostomia which represents the main quality-of-life complaint, as well as feeding tube dependence. The incidence of feeding tube dependence appears to be increased with concurrent chemoradiation, particularly after addition of cisplatin chemotherapy to DCB. In the Starr trial, patients in the CT/RT had had more swallowing problems and continuous need for feeding tube (51% vs. 25%, p = .02). Other important side effects to consider include soft tissue and bone ulceration and necrosis, neck fibrosis, trismus, dental caries, epilation, and hypothyroidism.

### Brachytherapy

Complications after the implant and EBRT include soft tissue ulcer, osteoradionecrosis, infection, and bleeding.

### FOLLOW-UP

Close follow-up of the patient is required, especially during the first 2 years of treatment because locoregional failure is most likely to occur during this period. The risk of developing a secondary malignancy in the aerodigestive tract is 6%–8%/year and may be decreased by half if patients cease smoking or consuming alcohol.[41] Even, if controlled at 2 years after treatment, patients with hypopharynx cancers are at high risk for the development of not only secondary primary tumors, but also of delayed locoregional recurrence and distant metastases.[41]

Follow-up every 1–2 months first year, every 2–3 months second year, every 3–6 months years 3–5, then annually. TSH q 6 months first 2 years, then yearly afterward. Baseline cross-sectional imaging post-treatment. Yearly CXR and additional studies as indicated. Dental prophylaxis and speech/swallowing evaluation as needed.

### RESEARCH

A number of ongoing studies should identify the optimal chemoradiation regimen and whether induction chemotherapy and biologic therapy can and should be integrated.

### RTOG H-0129

The Radiation Therapy Oncology Group (RTOG) H-0129 trial investigates whether accelerated radiation by delayed concomitant boost 72 Gy in 6 weeks with two cycles of high-dose cisplatin (100mg/m$^2$ weeks 1 and 4 of radiation) is superior to the control arm of concurrent chemoradiation with conventional fractionation (70 Gy/7 weeks) with three cycles of high dose CDDP (weeks 1, 4, and 7 of radiation).

### RTOG H-5022

The follow-up trial will test, in a randomized fashion, whether the addition of C225 to the accelerated radiation by delayed concomitant boost with two cycles of CDDP improves outcome versus the same regimen without the biologic therapy.

# Paradigm Trial

A randomized study will compare the AFX-Cb and two cycles of CDDP versus induction TPF (three cycles), followed by concurrent chemoradiation if there is at least a partial tumor response. Patients with a partial response will proceed to AFX-CB plus taxotere, while patients undergoing a complete response at the primary site will receive conventionally fractionated radiation with weekly carboplatin.

Given the extensive concomitant morbidities resulting from intensification of treatment, future studies will also be needed to identify radioprotectants and improve treatment techniques which will maintain organ function preservation and allow patients to complete treatment and maintain quality-of-life. For example, IMRT is being studied to reduce the risk of long-term tube feeding dependence after chemoradiation by decreasing dose to structures important in swallowing.[72]

## REFERENCES

1. Rouviere H. Anatomy of the human lymphatic system. Ann Arbor, *MI Edward Brothers,* 1938.
2. Candela FC, Kothari K, Shah JP. Patterns of cervical node metastases from squamous carcinoma of the oropharynx and hypopharynx. *Head Neck* 12:197–203, 1990.
3. Lindberg R. Distribution of cervical lymph node metastases from squamous cell carcinoma of the upper respiratory and digestive tracts. *Cancer* 29:1446–1449, 1972.
4. Crawford BE, Callihan MD, Corio RL, et al. Oral pathology. *Otolaryngol Clin North Am* 12:29–43; 1979.
5. American Cancer Society: Facts & Figures 2006. Atlanta, ACS; 2006.
6. Dahlstrand HM and Dalinis T. Presence and influence of human papillomaviruses (HPV) in tonsillar cancers. *Adv Cancer Res* 93:59–89, 2005.
7. Weinberger P, Yu Z, Haffty B, et al. Molecular classification identifies a subset of human papillomavirus—associated oropharyngeal cancers with favorable prognosis. *J Clin Oncol* 24(5) 736–747, 2006.
8. Balaram P, Sridhar H, Rajkumar T, et al. Oral cancer in southern India: the influence of smoking, drinking, paan-chewing and oral hygiene. *Int J Cancer* 98(3):440–445, 2002.
9. Merchant A, Husain SS, Hosain M, et al. Paan without tobacco: an independent risk factor for oral cancer. *Int J Cancer* 86(1):128–131, 2000.
10. Koch wM, Breenan JA, Zhurak M, et al. p53 mutation and locoregional treatment failure in head and neck squamous cell carcinoma. *J Natl Cancer Inst* 88:1580–1586, 1996.
11. Ang KK, Andratschke NH and Milas L. Impact of epidermal growth factor receptor expression on survival and pattern of relapse in patients with advanced head and neck carcinoma. *Cancer Res* 62 (24):7350–7356, 2002.
12. Lefebvre JL, Coche-Dequeant B, Buisset E, et al. Management of early oral cavity cancer. experience of centre oscar lambret. *Eur J Cancer B Oral Oncol* 30B(3):216–220, 1994.
13. Decroix Y, Ghossein NA. Experience of the Curie Institute in treatment of cancer of the mobile tongue: I. Treatment policies and result. *Cancer* 47(3):496–502, 1981.
14. Mazeron JJ, Crook JM, Benck V, et al. Iridium 192 implantation of T1 and T2 carcinomas of the mobile tongue. *Int J Radiat Oncol Biol Phys* 19:1369–1376, 1990 .
15. Spiro RH, Strong EW. Epidermoid carcinoma of the mobile tongue. treatment by partial glossectomy alone. *Am J Surg* 122:707–710, 1971.
16. Hu KS, Sachdeva G, Harrison LB. Adjuvant interstitial Iridium 192 brachytherapy for resected T1 and T2 cancers of the oral cavity with close or positive margins. Presented at 6th international head and neck conference, Washington, D.C. Aug 2004.

17. Ange DW, Lindberg RD, Guillamondegui OM. Management of squamous cell carcinoma of the oral tongue and floor of mouth after excisional biopsy. *Radiology* 116(1):143–146, 1975.

18. Lapeyre M, Hoffstetter S, Peiffert D, et al. Postoperative brachytherapy alone for T1-2 N0 squamous cell carcinomas of the oral tongue and floor of mouth with close or positive margins. *Int J Radiat Oncol Biol Phys* 48(1):37–42, 2000.

19. Chu A, Fletcher GH. Incidences and causes of failure to control by irradiation the primary lesion in squamous cell carcinomas of the anterior two thirds of the tongue and floor of mouth. *Am J Roentgenol* 117:502–508, 1973.

20. Pernot M, Hoffstetter S, Peiffert D, et al. Epidermoid carcinomas of the floor of mouth treated by exclusive irradiation: statistical study of a series of 207 cases. *Radiother Oncol* 35(3):177–185, 1995.

21. Wang CC, Doppke KP, Biggs PJ. Intra-oral cone radiation therapy for selected carcinomas of the oral cavity. *Int J Radiat Oncol Biol Phys* 9(8):1185–1189, 1983.

22. Lapeyre M, Peiffert D, Malissard L, et al. An original technique of brachytherapy in the treatment of epidermoid carcinomas of the buccal mucosa. *Int J Radiat Oncol Biol Phys* 33(2): 447–454, 1995.

23. Gerbaulet A, Pernot A. Cancer of the buccal mucosa. Proceedings of the 20th annual meeting of the European Curietherapy Group. *J Eur Radiother* 6: 1–4, 1985.

24. Diaz EM Jr, Holsinger FC, Zuniga ER, et al. Squamous cell carcinoma of the buccal mucosa: one institution's experience with 119 previously untreated patients. *Head Neck* 25(4):267–273, 2003.

25. Dixit S, Vyas RK, Toparani RB, et al. Surgery versus surgery and postoperative radiotherapy in squamous cell carcinoma of the buccal mucosa: a comparative study. *Ann Surg Oncol* 5(6): 502–510, 1998.

26. Jorgensen K, Elbronad O, Anderson AP. Carcinoma of the lip. A series of 869 cases. *Acta Radiol Ther Phys Biol* 12:177–190, 1973.

27. Mazeron JJ, Richaud P. Lip cancer. Report of the 18th annual meeting of the European Curietherapy Group. *J Eur Radiother* 5: 50–56, 1984.

28. Petrovich Z, Parker RG, Luxton G, et al. Carcinoma of the lip and selected sites of head and neck skin. A clinical study of 896 patients. *Radiother Oncol* 8(1):11–17, 1987.

29. Sykes AJ, Allan E, Irwin C. Squamous cell carcinoma of the lip: the role of electron treatment. *Clin Oncol* (R Coll Radiol) 8(6):384–386, 1996.

30. Weber RS, Gidley P, Morrison WH, et al. Treatment selection for carcinoma of the base of the tongue. *Am J Surg* 160:415–419, 1990.

31. Laccourreye O, Hans S, Menard M, et al. Transoral lateral oropharyngectomy for squamous cell carcinoma of the tonsillar region: II. An analysis of the incidence, related variables and consequences of local recurrence. *Arch Otolaryngol Head Neck Surg* 131(7):592–599, 2005.

32. Fein DA, Mendenhall WM, Parsons JT, et al. Pharyngeal wall carcinoma treated with radiotherapy: impact of treatment technique and fractionation. *Int J Radiat Oncol Biol Phys* 26; 751, 1993.

33. Amdur RJ, Mendenhall WM, Parsons JT, et al. Carcinoma of the soft palate treated with irradiation: analysis of results and complications. *Radiother Oncol* 9:185, 1987.

34. Weber RS, Peters LJ, Wolf P, et al. Squamous cell carcinoma of the soft palate, uvula and anterior faucial pillar. *Otolaryngol Head Neck Surg* 99:16, 1988.

35. Goffinet DR, Fee WE Jr., Wells J, et al. 192Ir pharyngoepiglottic fold interstitial implants. The key to successful treatment of base of tongue carcinoma by radiation therapy. *Cancer* 55: 941–948, 1985.

36. Puthawala AA, Syed AM, Eads DL, et al. Limited external beam and interstitial 192 iridium irradiation in the treatment of carcinoma of the base of the tongue: a ten-year experience. *Int J Radiat Oncol Biol Phys* 14:839–848, 1988.

37. Pernot M, Hoffstetter S, Peiffer D, et al. Role of interstitial brachytherapy in oral and oropharyngeal carcinoma: reflection of a series of 1344 patients treated at the time of initial presentation. *Otolaryngol Head Neck Surg* 115:519, 1996.

38. Mazeron JJ, Belkacemi Y, Simor JM, et al. Place of iridium 192 implantantion in definitive irradiation of faucial arch squamous cell carcinomas. *Int J Radiat Oncol Biol Phys* 1993; 27: 251–257.

39. Esche BA, Haie CM, Gerbaulet AP, et al. Interstitial and external radiotherapy in carcinoma of the soft palate and uvula. *Int J Radiat Oncol Biol Phys* 15: 619–662, 1988.

40. Eisbruch, et al. Xerostomia and its predictors following parotid-sparing irradiation of head and neck cancer. *Int J Radiat Oncol Biol Phys* 50:332–343, 2001.

41. Spector JG, Sessions DG, Haugher BH, et al. Delayed regional metastases, distant metastases and second primary malignancies in squamous cell carcinomas of the larynx and hypopharynx. *Laryngoscope* 111:1079, 2001.

42. Laccourreye O, Merite-Drancy A, Brasnu D, et al. Supracricoid hemilaryngopharyngectomy in selected pyriform sinus carcinoma staged as T2. *Laryngoscope* 103:1373, 1993.

43. Ogura JH, Biller HF, Weete R. Elective neck dissection for pharyngeal and laryngeal cancers: an evaluation. *Ann Oral Rhinol Laryngol* 8:646, 1971.

44. Bataini P, Brugere J, Bernier J, et al. Results of radical radiotherapeutic treatment of carcinoma of the pyriform sinus: experience of the Insitut Curie. *Int J Radiat Oncol Biol Phys* 8; 1277, 1982.

45. Amdur RJ, Mendenhall WM, Stringer SP, et al. Organ preservation with radiotherapy for T1-T2 carcinoma of the piriform sinus. *Head Neck* 23:353, 2001.

46. Garden AS, Morrison WH, Ang KK, et al. Hyperfractionated radiation in the treatment of squamous cell carcinomas of the head and neck. *Int J Radiat Oncol Biol Phys* 31:493, 1995.

47. Johansen LV, Grau C, Overgaard J. Hypopharyngeal squamous cell carcinoma—treatment results in 138 consecutively admitted patients. *Acta Oncol* 39–529, 2000.

48. Withers HR, et al. Local control of carcinoma of the tonsil by radiation therapy: an analysis of patterns of fractionation in nine institutions. *Int J Radiat Oncol Biol Phys* 33:549–562, 1995.

49. Gwozdz JT, et al. Concomitant boost radiotherapy for squamous carcinoma of the tonsillar fossa. *Int J Radiat Oncol Biol Phys* 39:127–135, 1997.

50. Overgaard J, Hansen HS, Specht L, et al. Five compared with six fractions per week of conventional radiotherapy of squamous cell carcinoma of head and neck: DAHANCA 6 and 7 randomized controlled trial. *Lancet* 362(9388):933–940, 2003.

51. Million RR, Parsons JT, Cassisi NJ. Twice-a-day irradiation technique for squamous cell carcinomas of the head and neck. *Cancer* 55(suppl)2096–2099, 1985.

52. Budach W, Hehr T, Bucah V, et al. A metanalysis of hyperfractionated and accelerated radiotherapy and combined chemotherapy and radiotherapy regimens in unresected locally advanced squamous cell carcinoma of the head and neck, *BMC Cancer* 6:28, 2006.

53. Wang, CC. Local control of oropharyngeal carcinoma after two accelerated hyperfractionation radiation therapy schemes. *Int J Radiat Oncol Biol Phys* 14;1143–1146, 1988.

54. Pignon JP, et al. Chemotherapy added to locoregional treatment for head and neck squamous cell carcinomas: three metanalyses of updated individual data. MACH-NC Collaborative Group. Metanalysis of chemotherapy on head and neck cancer. *Lancet* 355:949–955, 2000.

55. El-Sayed S, Nelson N. Adjuvant and adjunctive chemotherapy in the management of squamous cell carcinoma of the head and neck region. A metanalysis of prospective and randomized trials. *J Clin Oncol* 14:838–847, 1996.

56. Monnerat C, Faivre S, Temam S, et al. End points for new agents in induction chemotherapy for locally advanced head and neck cancers. *Ann Oncol* 13(7):995–1006, 2002.

57. Urba, S, Wolf, G Eisbruch, et al. Single cycle induction chemotherapy selects patients with advanced laryngeal cancer for combined chemoradiation: a new treatment paradigm. *J Clin Oncol.* 1;24(4):593–598, 2006.

58. Frank JL, Garb JL, Kay S, et al. Postoperative radiotherapy improves survival in squamous cell carcinoma of the hypopharynx. *Am J Surg* 168:476, 1994.

59. Slotman BJ, Kralendonk JH, Snow GB, et al. Surgery and postoperative radiotherapy and radiotherapy alone in T3-T4 cancers of the pyriform sinus. Treatment results and patterns of failure. *Acta Oncol* 33:55, 1994.

60. Ang, KK, et al. Randomized trial addressing risk features and time factors of surgery plus radiotherapy in advanced head and neck cancer. *Int J Radiat Oncol Biol Phys* 51:571–578, 2001.

61. Chao KS, Ozyigit G, Blanco AI, et al. Intensity-modulated radiation therapy in the treatment of oropharyngeal cancer: impact of tumor volume. *Int J Radiat Oncol Biol Phys* 59:43–50, 2004.

62. Eisbruch A, Marsh L, Dawson LA, et al. Recurrences near the base of skull following IMRT of head and neck cancer: implications for target delineation in the high neck and for parotid gland sparing. *Int J Radiat Oncol Biol Phys* 59:28–42, 2004.

63. de Arruda FF, Puri DR, Zhung J, et al. Intensity-modulated radiation therapy for the treatment of oropharyngeal carcinoma: the Memorial Sloan-Kettering Cancer Center experience. *Int J Radiat Oncol Biol Phys* 64(2):363–373, 2006.

64. Huang K, Lee N, Xia P, et al. Intensity-modulated radiotherapy in the treatment of oropharyngeal carcinoma: a single institutional experience. *Int J Radiat Oncol Biol Phys* 57 S2:2303, 2003.

65. Eisbruch A, Kim HM, Terrell JE. Xerostomia and its predictors following parotid-sparing irradiation of head and neck cancer. *Int J Radiat Oncol Biol Phys* 50(3):695–704, 2001.

66. Chao KS, Deasy JO, Markman J, et al. A prospective study of salivary function sparing in patients with head and neck cancers receiving intensity-modulated or three-dimensional radiation therapy: initial results. *Int J Radiat Oncol Biol Phys* 49:907–916, 2001.

67. Morrish RB Jr, Chan E, Silverman S Jr, et al. Osteonecrosis in patients irradiated for head and neck carcinoma. *Cancer* 47(8):1980–1983, 1981.

68. Inoue T, Inoue T, Teshima T, et al. Phase III trial of high- and low-dose rate interstitial radiotherapy for early oral tongue cancer. *Int J Radiat Oncol Biol Phys* 36(5):1201–1204, 1996.

69. Yamazaki H, Inoue T, Yoshida K, et al. Brachytherapy for early oral tongue cancer: low-dose rate to high-dose rate. *J Radiat Res* (Tokyo) 44(1):37–40, 2003.

70. Fu KK, et al. A radiation therapy oncology group (RTOG) phase III randomized study to compare hyperfractionation and two variants of accelerated fractionation to standard fractionation radiotherapy for head and neck squamous cell carcinomas. First report of RTOG 9003. *Int J Radiat Oncol Biol Phys.* 48(1):7–16, 2000.

71. Bonner J, Harari P, Giralt J, et al. Radiotherapy plus cetuximab for squamous cell carcinoma of the head and neck. *N Engl J Med* 354(6):567–578, 2006.

72. Eisbruch, Schwartz M, Rasch C, et al. Dysphagia and aspiration after chemoradiotherapy for head and neck cancer: which anatomic structures are affected and can they be spared by IMRT? *Int J Radiat Oncol Biol Phys* 60(5):1425–1439, 2004.

# 12

# Laryngeal Cancer

*Ömür Karakoyun Çelik, MD*
*Paul M. Busse, MD, PhD*

## OVERVIEW

When diagnosed in its early stage, glottic cancer is a curable disease with single modality therapy of either surgery or radiation. Advanced stages require more aggressive treatment and a multidisciplinary approach for organ preservation.

## INTRODUCTION

Of all the anatomic regions within the upper aerodigestive tract, the larynx is the most common site for the development of squamous cell carcinoma. In the United States, the incidence of laryngeal carcinoma is approximately 10,000 new cases per year with 4,000 deaths. The 5-year survival for all stages is 65%, making the laryngeal cancer one of the more curable cancers of the upper aerodigestive tract. Disease is 4.5-fold more common in men. In women, supraglottic cancers are more common than glottic cancers. The incidence increases with age, with a peak in the sixth and seventh decades.[1] The primary risk factors and presenting symptoms are listed in Tables 12-1 and 12-2.

## ANATOMY

The larynx is divided into three distinct sites, each with a staging system:

- Supraglottis (SGL)
- Glottis
- Subglottis

The supraglottic larynx consists of the epiglottis, aryepiglottic fold, arytenoid, false vocal cord, and ventricle. The inferior border of the SGL is the lateral wall of the ventricle. Anterior to the SGL is the pre-epiglottic space (a potential pattern of spread), which is defined by the thyrohyoid membrane, the hyoid bone, and the vallecula. The glottic larynx represents a relatively small anatomic volume that is restricted to the true vocal cords and the anterior and posterior commissures. The subglottic larynx has no subsites and begins 5 mm below the true vocal cords and extends inferiorly to the bottom of the cricoid cartilage.

TABLE 12-1  Risk Factors

Risk Factors
- Tobacco use
- Gastro esophageal reflux disease (GERD)
- Alcohol use
- Nutritional deficiencies
- Exposure to wood dust, nitrogen mustard, asbestos, and ionizing radiation
- Human papilloma virus (HPV)

TABLE 12-2  Presenting Symptoms

Symptoms depend mainly on the size and location of the tumor.
- Hoarseness or other change in voice quality
- Pain
- Sore throat
- Earache (referred otalgia)
- Neck node metastases
- Airway obstruction/stridor

**FIGURE 12-1** Larynx.

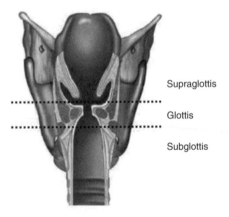

Supraglottis

Glottis

Subglottis

## PATHOLOGY

More than 95% of all primary laryngeal cancers are squamous cell carcinomas or variants thereof, with the remainder being sarcomas, adenocarcinomas, neuroendocrine tumors, and other types. The management of nonsquamous cell types should reflect current therapeutic principles that are based on histology rather than the anatomic site of origin. Some examples of this would be combined modality therapy for neuroendocrine tumors and lymphoma and surgical resection with adjuvant radiation therapy for soft tissue sarcomas.[2]

## EVALUATION

It is important to perform a proper physical examination and the first step is to position the patient such that the oropharynx and larynx can be completely visualized. This can be achieved either indirectly through the use of an examination mirror or directly with a fiberoptic endoscope. Once the larynx is visualized, all of the mucosal surfaces should be examined, including the pyriform sinuses. Phonation of the vowel "e" brings the vocal cords to apposition in the midline. Note should be made if the vocal cords are altered in their mobility or fixed. The cornerstone of staging for any head and neck cancer is a thorough examination. This includes a careful and systematic visual inspection and palpation of the oral cavity and oropharynx as well as indirect or fiberoptic examination of the nasopharynx, larynx, and hypopharynx. Attention is paid to the presence of premalignant lesions, mobility of the tongue and vocal cords, and contour of the mucosal surfaces. When examining the primary lesion, the specific location and extent of disease are noted. In addition, the tumor's gross appearance (exophytic, ulcerative, infiltrative, etc.) is described and the depth of invasion is estimated. It is useful for treatment planning as well as for follow-up to document the tumor location on anatomic diagrams. It is generally recognized that most squamous cell carcinomas of the head and neck are associated with a long history of tobacco and alcohol use and that whatever carcinogen initiated the known carcinoma also exposed the remainder of the upper aerodigestive tract. The incidence of synchronous carcinomas has been reported to be as high as 5% and, because of this, patients are evaluated under anesthesia by direct laryngoscopy, bronchoscopy, and esophagoscopy. These studies are referred to as triple endoscopy. While the yield may be low for some tumors, such as those arising in the anterior oral cavity, the consequences of missing a synchronous second tumor are significant and it is a rare exception that these studies should be deferred. Every patient should receive a chest X-ray or CT as part of their initial evaluation. Pretreatment referral to a dentist for a complete evaluation, prophylactic therapy, and long-term follow-up is recommended. Dental extractions, when indicated, should precede the start of radiation therapy.

## IMAGING

An accurate assessment of the amount and location of disease is essential in order to correctly stage and make the right therapeutic decision. The larynx is difficult to evaluate by clinical examination alone and the inaccuracy (understaging) can be as high as 40%–50%. A complete evaluation should include either CT or MRI. Each has relative strengths and weaknesses as an imaging modality. There is little controversy with regards to the ability of CT or MRI to image the paraglottic and pre-epiglottic spaces and to determine the extent of soft tissue spread outside the larynx. There is debate as to which modality to use to accurately predict invasion of the laryngeal cartilages. A very systematic study of this problem was conducted by Zbaren.[3] In this study, 40 consecutive patients underwent clinical and endoscopic staging then both CT and MRI evaluation. These patients then underwent a planned laryngectomy that involved a very detailed pathologic evaluation of the resected larynx. It was found that the clinical staging accurately revealed the full extent of disease only 45% of the time. MRI was more sensitive than CT in detecting cartilage invasion, however, it tended to overestimate the frequency of invasion. CT was more specific than MRI but underestimated the frequency of invasion. The best preclinical assessment was obtained from both studies, however the combined staging accuracy does not significantly exceed that of clinical evaluation and CT alone.

Radiographic assessment of lymphatics appears to be equivalent with either modality. Lymph nodes that show rim enhancement and central necrosis are considered to be abnormal regardless of size, as are lymph nodes that exhibit extranodal extension and obliteration of facial planes between the lymph node and an adjacent structure. Small volume lymphatic disease is detected by size criteria, >1.5 cm for the jugulodigastric region and >1 cm elsewhere, a criteria that can be determined either by CT or MRI.[4] As a rule, whichever modality best suits the assessment of the primary is used to also assess the neck. The role of positron emission tomography (PET) scanning in the evaluation of laryngeal cancer is an area of evolving interest and could aid in more precise target definition. PET may also be a useful tool for the detection of early recurrent or persistent diseases after radiotherapy or chemo-radiotherapy.[5,6]

## STAGING

The following (Tables 12-5 to 12-7) are the AJCC criteria for primary tumor and lymphatic staging.[7] Physical examination, as well as information from radiographic studies, is used in determining stage.

One of the deficiencies of the AJCC staging system for laryngeal carcinoma is its reliance on tumor location and local spread rather than size in the determination of T-stage. While this is important in determining the best surgical approach for early stage tumors, it is less important for therapeutic decisions regarding radiation. The probability of disease control following radiation depends more on the number of clonogenic tumor cells than on the location within the larynx. This is best reflected in tumor size. Data from the University of Florida support this contention[8,9] and suggest that larger tumors may benefit from more aggressive therapy even if they have a less advanced T-stage (Table 12-8).

---

TABLE 12-3 **T-Stage, Supraglottic Larynx**

T-Stage, Supraglottic Larynx
TX:  Minimum requirements to assess the primary tumor cannot be met
T0:  No evidence of primary tumor
Tis: Carcinoma *in situ*
T1:  Tumor limited to one subsite of supraglottis with normal vocal cord mobility
T2:  Tumor invades more than one subsite of supraglottis or glottis, normal cord mobility
T3:  Tumor limited to larynx with either vocal cord fixation, involvement of the postcricoid area,
       medial wall of the pyriform sinus, preepiglottic space, or minor thyroid cartilage invasion
T4a: Tumor completely invades the thyroid cartilage and/or extends to other tissues beyond larynx
T4b: Tumor invades prevertebral space, encases carotid artery, or invades the mediastinum

---

TABLE 12-4 **T-Stage, Glottic Larynx**

T-Stage, Glottic Larynx
TX:  Minimum requirements to assess the primary tumor cannot be met
T0:  No evidence of primary tumor
Tis: Carcinoma *in situ*
T1:  Tumor limited to vocal cords with normal mobility
       T1a: Tumor limited to one vocal cord
       T1b: Tumor involves both vocal cords
T2:  Tumor extends to supraglottis and/or subglottis and/or with impaired cord mobility
T3:  Tumor limited to larynx with vocal cord fixation, invasion of the paraglottic space, or minor
       thyroid cartilage invasion
T4a: Tumor completely invades the thyroid cartilage and/or extends to other tissues beyond larynx
T4b: Tumor invades prevertebral space, encases carotid artery, or invades the mediastinum

---

TABLE 12-5 **T-Stage Subglottic Larynx**

T-Stage, Subglottic Larynx
TX:  Minimum requirements to assess the primary tumor cannot be met
T0:  No evidence of primary tumor
Tis: Carcinoma *in situ*
T1:  Tumor limited to the subglottis
T2:  Tumor extends to vocal cords with normal or impaired cord mobility
T3:  Tumor limited to larynx with vocal cord fixation
T4a: Tumor invades cricoid or thyroid cartilage and/or extends to other issues beyond the larynx
T4b: Tumor invades prevertebral space, encases carotid artery, or invades the mediastinum

## NATURAL COURSE OF DISEASE

### Local Spread

#### Supraglottic Larynx

Squamous cell cancers that arise in the supraglottic larynx tend to spread superficially and involve other sites within the supraglottic larynx. Sometimes the site of origin is difficult to ascertain because an exophytic mass may involve more than one supraglottic subsite. Fortunately, for exophytic tumors it is easy to appreciate the extent of disease and to follow the clinical progress during a course of

**TABLE 12-6  N and M-Stages for Head and Neck Cancer**

Lymphatics and Metastatic disease

NX:  Minimum requirements to assess the regional nodes cannot be met

N0:  No clinically positive node

N1:  Single ipsilateral node, 3 cm or less

N2:

   N2a: Single ipsilateral node, >3 cm ≤ 6 cm

   N2b: Multiple ipsilateral nodes, none more than 6 cm

   N2c: Bilateral or contralateral nodes, none more than 6 cm

N3:  Any lymph node >6 cm

MX:  Presence of distant metastasis cannot be assessed

M0:  No distant metastasis

M1:  Distant metastasis

therapy. A second pattern of spread, much more insidious, is invasion of the soft tissue deep to the mucosa and extension superiorly and inferiorly within the paraglottic space. This can manifest itself as seemingly innocent appearing mucosa but with an irregular contour of the laryngeal lumen. Paraglottic space involvement can be best appreciated with reconstructed coronal views from CT or MRI. Anterior extension through the laryngeal surface of the epiglottis will lead to invasion of the pre-piglottic space. More extensive involvement can give rise to destruction of the thyroid cartilage, fixation of the vocal cords, or invasion into the hypopharynx.

### Glottic Larynx

By definition, T1 tumors of the true vocal cord remain localized to that structure, although the entire length of the vocal cord may be involved, including the anterior commissure. This is a troublesome area because it is difficult to examine by indirect methods and is a location where a minimal amount of anterior invasion could lead to involvement of the thyroid cartilage. T2-4 glottic tumors behave like their counterparts that arise in the supraglottic or subglottic larynx. The pattern of spread and proclivity for lymphatic involvement is dependent upon the location and extent of disease for tumors that arise in those sites.

### Subglottic Larynx

This site comprises a relatively small proportion of laryngeal tumors, less than 1%. When encountered, it is most likely an inferior extension of disease from the glottic larynx. This anatomic site cannot be

**TABLE 12-7  Stage Grouping**

| Stage | T | N | M |
|---|---|---|---|
| 0 | T in situ | N0 | M0 |
| I | T1 | N0 | M0 |
| II | T2 | N0 | M0 |
| III | T3 | N0 | M0 |
| | T1 | N1 | M0 |
| | T2 | N1 | M0 |
| | T3 | N1 | M0 |
| IVa | T4 | N0 | M0 |
| | T4 | N1 | M0 |
| | Any T | N2 | M0 |
| IVb | Any T | N3 | M0 |
| IVc | Any T | Any N | M1 |

**TABLE 12-8  Relationship between Tumor Volume and Local Control**

| T-Stage/Site | Amount of Disease | Local Control |
|---|---|---|
| T1a Larynx | <5 mm | 12/12 (100%) |
| T1a Larynx | 5–15 mm | 73/78 (94%) |
| T1a Larynx | >15 mm | 45/50 (90%) |
| T1-4 Supraglottis | <6 cm² | 15/18 (83%) |
| T1-4 Supraglottis | >6 cm² | 6/13 (46%) |

adequately examined by indirect or fiberoptic laryngoscopy and an EUA is necessary to complete the physical examination. Because it is a clinically silent area and difficult to visualize, subglottic primaries can be advanced by the time they are detected and may extend into the cricoid cartilage, trachea, and soft tissue of the neck.[10,11]

## Regional Spread

Except for T1 and perhaps some very early T2 tumors of the glottic larynx, regional disease must be taken into account. The larynx has an extensive lymphatic drainage pattern and because of its midline nature, consideration must be given to the possibility of bilateral regional involvement. The most common lymphatic levels involved in laryngeal cancer are Level II, III, and Level IV. Levels I and V are rarely involved unless disease is present in Levels II or III. The risk of lymphatic disease increases with stage and, probably more importantly, with the size of the primary lesion. Less well differentiated tumors carry a higher likelihood of lymphatic spread. Data regarding the incidence of regional spread are derived from a number of sources. The percentage of patients who present with clinically positive nodes, the incidence of positive lymph nodes from elective neck dissection specimens, and the frequency of nodal relapse after treatment of the primary and observation of clinically negative necks. Some of the most detailed information on regional disease comes from a long clinical experience at the M.D. Anderson Hospital.[12] Table 12-9 shows the percentage of patients who presented with clinically positive lymph nodes as a function of primary site and institutional (MDAH) T-stage.

Additional information on the incidence of occult disease in a clinically negative neck is displayed Table 12-10.[13]

The overall incidence of occult lymph node metastases in all stages of supraglottic laryngeal carcinoma is approximately 27%. Some of the lower incidences in T3-4 primaries may be due to the increased likelihood of these tumors initially presenting with palpable disease. As disease becomes more advanced in the neck, the risk of involvement of other lymphatic groups, both ipsilateral and bilateral, increases. This risk of occult nodal disease dictates the scope of the comprehensive radiation fields used for the treatment of laryngeal cancer, which can extend from Level II through Level IV. Involvement of mediastinal lymph nodes is rare, even for subglottic carcinoma and when present is considered as distant metastases.

**TABLE 12-9 Incidence of Clinical Adenopathy**

| Primary Site | T-Stage | Nodal Disease (%) |
|---|---|---|
| Supraglottic larynx | T1 | 39 |
| | T2 | 42 |
| | T3 | 64 |
| | T4 | 59 |
| Hypopharynx | T1 | 63 |
| | T2 | 70 |
| | T3 | 79 |
| | T4 | 74 |

**TABLE 12-10 Incidence of Occult Adenopathy**

| Primary Site | T-Stage | Nodal Disease (%) |
|---|---|---|
| Supraglottic larynx | T1-2 | 31 |
| | T3-4 | 25 |
| Glottic larynx | T1-2 | 21 |
| | T3-4 | 14 |
| Pyriform sinus | T1-2 | 67 |
| | T3-4 | 55 |
| Pharyngeal wall | T1-2 | 20 |
| | T3-4 | 63 |

## Distant Spread

The most common site for distant metastases is the lung and, given the risk of lung as a second primary, tissue confirmation should be obtained. Factors associated with an increased risk of distant spread are a supraglottic primary, bulky adenopathy, and extracapsular extension.

# Management

Surgery and radiotherapy are the two major modalities for the local treatment of laryngeal cancer. Treatment options depend upon the stage and the location of the tumor within the larynx as well as other factors such as the likelihood of regional spread, comorbidities, and chances for functional organ preservation. In general, every effort is made to preserve function while not sacrificing chances for survival. Bilateral lymphatic treatment is part of every treatment plan except for T1 tumors of the glottic larynx. Bulky T4B disease is rarely controlled with radiation alone or combined modality therapy, and such advanced disease is best treated with surgery followed by postoperative radiation or chemoradiation.[14,15]

## Carcinoma in situ

In order to define the *in situ* lesion completely, the entire lesion and whole basement membrane is subjected to surgical stripping. In some cases, this can be therapeutic but falls short of a true cancer operation. Additional measures are required in order to assure the disease is completely eradicated. Further stripping or ablative procedures such as endoscopic laser resection can lead to long-term changes in voice quality and for that reason we recommend early radical radiation therapy rather than repeat microlaryngoscopies. The technique and the dose are basically similar to those for T1 glottic cancer and carry the same high local control rates, in excess of 90%.[16-19]

## T1 N0 Glottis

Perhaps one of the most straightforward treatment techniques in radiation oncology is for early-stage carcinoma of the true vocal cord. The volume of disease is small, the incidence of regional spread remote, and the anatomy is very reproducible; yet, patients still fail because of a marginal miss or an underdose of either total dose, dose per fraction, or both. Because this disease is potentially curable and the consequence for treatment failure so significant (laryngectomy), it is worth reviewing treatment technique. As with all head and neck patients, the simulation is in the supine position with a facemask to facilitate reproducibility and minimize inadvertent motion. A reproducible landmark for the larynx is the anterior thyroid cartilage which, when viewed on a lateral radiograph, gives the appearance of a figure of eight. This is seen particularly well in older patients where the cartilage is partially calcified. A 5 × 5 or 6 × 6 cm field is used to encompass the true vocal cords, lower half of the supraglottic larynx, and subglottic larynx. This corresponds to the thyroid and cricoid cartilages. The central axis of the simulated field should pass directly through the figure of eight. This assures the vocal cords will be in the center of the field. Anteriorly, the field edge extends beyond the skin margin. Posteriorly, the field edge is at or slightly behind the anterior border of the vertebral body. This is particularly important for tumors that may involve the entire length of the vocal cord. If the treatment field is offset such that the vocal cords are close to either field edge, the buildup region could lead to an underdose (a marginal miss).

A contour or set of CT images is taken through the central axis and an individual treatment plan is generated. Unless the patient has an unusually thick anterior neck, wedges are used as tissue compensators. The posterior vocal cord receives 100% of the prescribed dose and the anterior vocal cords as well as anterior commissure typically receive between 105%–107%. Head and neck cancer at the MGH is treated on 6 MV linear accelerators. Concern was raised that an underdose of anterior structures could occur from this energy due to insufficient tissue for dose buildup,[20] although the magnitude of this effect may be less than anticipated.[21] While the potential for an anterior underdose may be true for some patients treated with parallel-opposed open lateral fields, when appropriate treatment planning measures are taken with individual contours and tissue compensation, 6 MV photons can be used to treat laryngeal carcinoma as effectively as can $^{60}$Co or 4 MV photons. The issue of field size is occasionally raised. Since the volume of disease is small and very well defined, even a

**FIGURE 12-2** T1 Laryngeal treatment field.

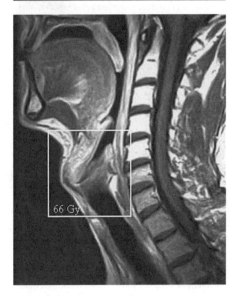

66 Gy

$5 \times 5$ cm field is more than sufficient.[22] Theoretically, swallowing during therapy could move the vocal cords and result in a reduced dose; however, this has been studied as well and the total dose would be decreased by only 0.5%, an insignificant change.[23] Two factors that do appear to have a great deal of importance with respect to the likelihood of achieving local control are the dose per fraction and the overall total dose.[24] It is generally accepted that the minimum daily dose is 2 Gy and the total dose is 66 Gy with no treatment breaks. Consideration could also be given to daily doses of 2.25 Gy to a total of 61–65 Gy.[25] Fractionation schedules of 1.8 Gy should be avoided even when a patient is experiencing a moderate amount of acute reaction because of the lower rate of disease control.

### T1-2 N0 SGL, T2N0 Glottic Larynx

Once tumor has spread beyond the glottic larynx, it behaves in a similar fashion to the area it has just invaded, particularly with respect to the probability and location of lymphatic involvement. Thus, T2 carcinoma of the glottis is treated similarly to T1 and T2 tumors that originated in the SGL. In this setting, the entire supraglottic larynx and pre-epiglottic space are treated along with the first echelon regional lymphatics, which are the jugulodigastric and jugular (Levels II and III) lymph nodes. Essentially, the entire larynx is encompassed within lateral fields that extend from above the angle of the jaw to the base of the neck. It is not necessary to treat with a low-neck field. In order to cover the jugular lymphatics (which lie along the jugular vein and course below the sternocleidomastoid muscle) the spinal cord is almost always within the original field. A field reduction is made or cord block is placed at 44–45 Gy. At approximately 54–56 Gy, the field size is reduced to include just the primary site and treated to the final dose of 66–74 Gy, depending upon the fractionation schedule. The decision to use an alternative fractionation schedule, in this case BID, for T2 disease and greater is derived from the diminished ability of once-daily radiation to control more advanced disease[26] and the improvement in disease control seen with accelerated fractionation schedules.[27]

### T3 Larynx

Historically, once-daily radiation of T3 (fixed vocal cord) carcinoma of the larynx was associated with a primary control rate of 30%–40%[28] with surgical salvage bringing the final control rate to only 60%. For this reason, the standard of care for fixed vocal cord lesions was total laryngectomy followed by postoperative radiation to the laryngeal bed and bilateral lymphatics. The cure rate was overshadowed by the life-changing morbidity of a total laryngectomy and the larynx became the site for clinical trials using accelerated fractionation and combined modality therapy in order to increase the rate of organ preservation while not sacrificing overall survival. The success of these approaches has altered the management of this disease, reducing the role of surgery for primary management. Two single institution clinical experiences paved the way for a more widespread use of accelerated fractionation as a means to increased laryngeal preservation, the MGH[26,29] and the University of Florida.[30] From the latter institution comes a notable study regarding the role of BID radiation in the management of patients with T3 carcinoma of the glottic larynx.[30] Three important issues that frequently arise when deliberating as to whether a patient is best served by surgery and post-operative radiation or radiation as a single modality were addressed in this paper. The first is the level of primary site control achieved with BID radiation alone which, in this series, is 71%. Second, at 81%, the overall local control is the same whether patients were treated with primary radiation therapy and surgical salvage or underwent a total laryngectomy followed by postoperative radiation. Third, the presence of fixed vocal cords after radiation therapy does not necessarily indicate a radiation

**FIGURE 12-3** T1-2 Supraglottic larynx, T2 glottic larynx treatment fields.

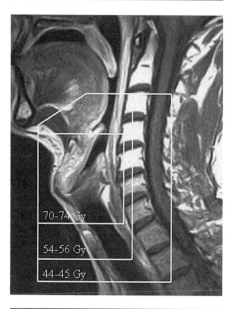

70-74 Gy

54-56 Gy

44-45 Gy

failure, as 61% of patients with persistent fixed vocal cords 1 month after radiation therapy remained free of disease. It is important to note that the single institution experiences, while offering improved laryngeal preservation rates over historical controls, had not been formally compared until RTOG 90–03.[27] This trial compared three alternative fractionation schedules against 70 Gy in 35 daily fractions. Both an accelerated fractionation schedule with 1.2 Gy BID throughout and a concomitant boost schedule were superior to the other two arms and now represent the standard of care for radiation alone for disease other than T1.

## Combined Modality Therapy for Larynx Preservation

As previously noted, advanced stage laryngeal cancer has traditionally been treated with total laryngectomy and postoperative radiotherapy. However, recent studies have demonstrated that combined modality therapy is as effective as surgery (total laryngectomy) with respect to overall survival.[31-34] Combined modality therapy can consist of many forms: induction or neo-adjuvant therapy, concurrent chemo-radiation, and adjuvant chemotherapy. Each has its specific rationale and chemotherapeutic regimen. In general, cis-platinum is the centerpiece of the regimen although interest in the use of taxanes is growing. Two prospective randomized trials have changed the management of advanced laryngeal cancer: the VA Larynx trial[32] and RTOG 91–11.[31] The VA larynx trial demonstrated that induction chemotherapy followed by definitive radiotherapy yields a 64% larynx preservation rate at 2 years in patients with advanced stage laryngeal cancers. What makes this trial notable is the proof that patients who elect to undergo a form of therapy that offers the prospect of laryngeal preservation do not compromise their chances for survival. The 2-year survival rate was 68% in both groups, induction chemotherapy followed by radiation or surgery followed by postoperative radiotherapy. Another randomized trial was conducted by the EORTC with hypopharyngeal tumors treated in the same fashion, either induction chemotherapy followed by 70 Gy or standard surgery followed by postoperative radiation.[33] The results were quite similar to the VA larynx trial in that patients who received induction therapy achieved a comparable level of laryngeal preservation and comparable survival in both treatment arms. An argument is frequently raised that these trials do not prove the merit of induction therapy because radiation alone might have fared as well, although that is unlikely given the historical ability of conventionally fractionated radiation to control T3 laryngeal carcinoma. Both trials demonstrate lower rates of organ preservation in more advanced tumors.

---

**BOX 12-1**

First major randomized trial designed to ask the question as to whether laryngeal preservation following induction chemotherapy and radiotherapy afforded the same survival likelihood as total laryngectomy and postoperative radiation therapy. The actuarial survival rates were the same in both arms, 68% at 3 years with a 64% rate of laryngeal preservation. These conclusions were confirmed by an identical study on hypopharyngeal cancer conducted by the EORTC.[33]

Department of Veterans Affairs Laryngeal Cancer Study Group. Induction chemotherapy plus radiation compared with surgery plus radiation in patients with advanced laryngeal *Cancer. N Engl J Med* 1991 324:1685–1690.

---

RTOG 91-11 investigated the role of chemotherapy in the treatment of laryngeal cancer with the goal of organ preservation.[31] Patients with stage III and IV SCC of the larynx were randomly assigned to one of the three treatments: induction cis-platinum plus fluorouracil followed by radiotherapy, radiotherapy concurrent with cis-platinum, or conventionally fractioned radiotherapy alone. Nonresponders after two cycles of chemotherapy underwent salvage total laryngectomy and postoperative radiotherapy. The rationale for the use of concurrent chemo-radiation was based on the radiosensitizing effects of cis-platinum and the success of this regimen in nasopharynx.[35] The rate of laryngeal preservation at a median follow-up of 3.8 years was significantly higher in the concurrent chemo-radiotherapy group (84%). Induction chemotherapy followed by radiotherapy was not significantly better than radiotherapy alone. Overall survival was 75% at 2 years with no significant difference among the treatment arms.

---

**BOX 12-2**

A prospectively randomized Intergroup study (RTOG 91-11) designed to compare induction chemotherapy followed by radiation therapy vs. concurrent chemo-radiotherapy vs. radiation alone in stage III and IV supraglottic and glottic carcinoma. Laryngeal preservation rates were 88% for the concurrent chemo-radiation arm, 75% for the induction chemotherapy-radiation arm, and 70% for the radiation only arm. The improvement for concurrent combined modality was significant. Locoregional control was also statistically improved in the concurrent arm, 78% vs. 61% induction arm vs. 56% radiation arm. Toxicity was acceptable in all arms. This study built upon the VA larynx trial in demonstrating the feasibility of laryngeal preservation in advanced disease and that concurrent chemo-radiation was superior to sequential.

Forastiere AA, Goepfert H, Mao M, et al. Concurrent chemotherapy and radiotherapy for organ preservation in advanced laryngeal cancer. *N. Engl J Med* 2003 349:2091–2098.

Examination of the acute and chronic toxicities as well as quality-of-life experienced by patients in the three treatment arms revealed that induction chemotherapy followed by radiotherapy was as toxic as concurrent therapy. Chemotherapy-related toxic effects were seen during the induction phase although the rate of acute toxic effects such as neutropenia, severe nausea and vomiting, as well as mucosal and skin reactions, were seen more in the concurrent arm. Late toxic effects were similar in all three arms.

## Technical Aspects of Radiation for T3 Larynx

Because of the relatively high incidence of lymphatic spread, the larynx and entire neck are treated comprehensively. Irrespective of the method of treatment, IMRT or a conventional 3-field arrangement, the GTV and CTVs are the same, specifically, the entire larynx and levels II through IV and V bilaterally. N2 or N3 disease may warrant additional superior extension of the CTV into the junctional area at the level of C1 and jugular foramen. With conventional fields, the upper neck and larynx are encompassed by opposed lateral fields that cover Levels II, III, and V. Level IV is treated with single anterior (supraclavicular) field and the junction is as low into the neck as possible. Even with nondivergent fields, it is prudent to include either an anterior or lateral junction block over the spinal cord in order to minimize the risk of divergent or overlapping radiation that could exceed spinal cord tolerance. Whether the treatment is daily with chemotherapy or hyperfractionation alone, fields are basically the same, comprehensive coverage to a dose of 44–45 Gy after which a cord block is placed at 44–45 Gy. Level V radiation can continue with electrons and at approximately 54–56 Gy, the field size is reduced to include just the larynx and any lymphatic GTV. The final dose is 70–72 Gy when given in daily fraction sizes of 2 Gy or 74–76 Gy when delivered in 1.2 Gy fractions BID.

### Subglottic Larynx

Unlike other laryngeal sites, the lymphatic drainage of the subglottic larynx does not include the jugulodigastric (Level II) lymph nodes unless there is advanced disease or nodal disease in Level III. The treatment fields should include the larynx, upper trachea, and lower lymphatics from the inferior jugular nodes through the superior mediastinum. The same fractionation schedule is used as for T3 larynx. In order to have a continuous laryngeal dose at the junction of the lateral fields and the anterior supraclavicular field junctional cord, blocks are placed on the inferior lateral fields from the beginning. CT-guided, 3-D planing is useful to design treatment fields that will treat the inferiorly-based laryngeal GTV.

### Postoperative Radiation

In the setting of advanced disease, typically a T4 primary, surgery is frequently the first line of therapy. Because of the extensive local disease and the high risk of failure either in the laryngeal bed or regional lymphatics, most of these cases also receive postoperative radiation, which may or may not include concurrent chemotherapy, depending upon the assessment of risk.[14,15] The CTV and conventional radiation fields are very similar to that demonstrated in Figure 12-4 with the notable exception of the inferior extent of the lateral fields. This field edge is placed above the tracheostomy stoma and the stoma itself is included in the low anterior neck field. Bolus material is also placed over the tracheostomy site in order to assure that full dose is delivered to this site. Fraction sizes vary from 1-8–2.0 Gy and the total dose to the CTV is 60 Gy, with appropriate attention paid to spinal cord tolerance. Depending upon risk, the laryngeal bed may receive 66 Gy.

### Management of Nodal Disease

For laryngeal carcinoma, the preferable treatment for subclinical disease is radiation alone because surgery would require a bilateral neck dissection. Except for T1 tumors of the glottic

**FIGURE 12-4** T3-T4a larynx treatment fields.

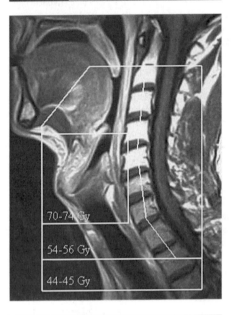

70-74 Gy

54-56 Gy

44-45 Gy

larynx, almost all patients with laryngeal carcinoma have a sufficient risk of harboring occult regional disease that some form of neck irradiation is warranted. The extent of this coverage has already been demonstrated. A comprehensive dose to clinically occult nodal CTVs can range from 44 to 60 Gy, depending upon proximity to the larynx and likelihood of harboring disease. For a clinically occult neck, doses are typically 44–45 Gy to the posterior neck and supraclavicular fossae and 50–60 Gy for more proximal lymphatics in the jugulodigastric region and mid-jugular chain (Levels II and III). Both sides of the neck are treated. Radiation can be used as a single modality for N1 disease and low-volume N2 disease. With aggressive combined modality regimens and CT-based treatment planning, patients who have gross nodal disease treated to doses of 70–72 Gy can realize a complete clinical and radiographic response obviating the need for radical surgery. Whether PET imaging plays a role in determining which patients need surgery after radiation is still an open question. A more conservative approach for nodal disease greater than 3 cm is for neck dissection in conjunction with 50–60 Gy. It is not necessary for the patient to receive surgery first, particularly if the primary site is being managed by radiation.

## Quality-of-Life Outcomes

It is becoming increasingly important to include quality-of-life (QOL) assessments in treatment protocols. Organ preservation with severe dysfunction or chronic pain is not an acceptable therapeutic outcome and can lead to a lower QOL than an upfront laryngectomy. For early stage laryngeal cancer, conservative surgical procedures and radiotherapy each provide good quality-of-life outcomes and functional results. In general, patients who maintained their larynx have a higher QOL compared with patients who undergo a laryngectomy. In a study that investigated speech and voice quality in the management of early laryngeal carcinoma, it was found that speech and voice were significantly better in patients treated by irradiation than in those treated by conservative surgical methods.[36]

Interest has also been directed to the QOL of patients with advanced laryngeal cancer who underwent particular organ preservation protocols. Terrel et al reported the long-term QOL results of VA larynx trial.[37] Patients who had successful organ preservation had significantly better QOL scores, better emotional well-being, and a lower incidence of depression. Results of other QOL studies generally demonstrate that patients who have undergone laryngectomy are more depressed and socially isolated than patients who were treated by organ preservation protocols.[38,39]

TABLE 12-11 Treatment Guidelines

| Disease Site | Stage | Chemotherapy | Treatment to Lymph Nodes | Faction-ation | Dose/ Fraction (Gy) | Total Dose (Gy) |
|---|---|---|---|---|---|---|
| SGL | T1 | No | Yes (limited) | Daily | 2.0 | 66–68 |
| | T2 | No | Yes (limited) | BID* | 1.2 | 72–74 |
| | T3 | Yes | Yes (full) | Daily | 2.0 | 70–72 |
| (Resection) | T4 | Yes | Yes (full) | Daily | 2.0 | 60–66 |
| Glottic Lx | T1 | No | No | Daily | 2.0 | 66 |
| | T2 | No | Yes (limited) | BID* | 1.2 | 72–74 |
| | T3 | Yes | Yes (full) | Daily | 2.0 | 70–72 |
| (Resection) | T4 | Yes | Yes (full) | Daily | 2.0 | 60–66 |
| Subglottic Lx | T1 | No | Yes (limited) | Daily | 2.0 | 64–66 |
| | T2 | No | Yes (limited) | BID* | 1.2 | 72–74 |
| | T3 | Yes | Yes (full) | Daily | 2.0 | 70–72 |
| (Resection) | T4 | Yes | Yes (full) | Daily | 2.0 | 60–66 |
| Hypopharynx | T1 | No | Yes (full) | BID* | 1.2 | 72 |
| | T2 | Yes | Yes (full) | Daily | 2.0 | 70–72 |
| | T3 | Yes | Yes (full) | Daily | 2.0 | 70–72 |
| | T4 | Yes | Yes (full) | Daily | 2.0 | 70–72 |

*BID fractionation has a 6-hour intertreatment interval.

## Treatment Guidelines

Table 12-11 shows the treatment guidelines currently in practice at the MGH for primary carcinoma of the larynx and hypopharynx. Stage I and II is generally treated with radiation alone and Stage III and IV with concurrent chemo/radiation. The regimen is once-daily radiation and weekly carboplatinum (1.5 AUC) and paclitaxel (45 mg/m2). These guidelines are subject to modification based on a patient's performance status, presence of comorbid disease, willingness to comply with the proposed treatment schedule, etc. With proper nursing, nutritional support, and encouragement, most patients are able to complete therapy without treatment breaks. When BID radiation is utilized the fractions are given at least 6 hours apart.

## REFERENCES

1. Jemal, A., et al. Cancer statistics, 2006. *CA Cancer J Clin,* 2006. 56(2): 106–130.
2. Hamlyn, P.J., C.J. O'Brien, and H.J. Shaw. Uncommon malignant tumors of the larynx: A 35 year review. *Journal of Laryngology and Otology,* 1986. 100: 1163–1168.
3. Zbaren, P., M. Becker, and H. Lang. Pretherapeutic staging of laryngeal carcinoma. *Cancer,* 1995. 77: p. 1263–1273.
4. Som, P.M. and R.T. Bergeron, eds. Head and Neck Imaging, second ed. 1991, Mosby Year Book: St. Louis, MO.
5. Lowe, V.J., et al. Primary and recurrent early stage laryngeal cancer: preliminary results of 2-[Fluorine 18]fluoro-2-deoxy-D-glucose PET imaging. *Radiology,* 1999. 212(3): 799–802.
6. Gordin, A., et al. Fluorodeoxyglucose-positron emission tomography/computed tomography imaging in patients with carcinoma of the larynx: diagnostic accuracy and impact on clinical management. *Laryngoscope,* 2006. 116(2): 273–278.

7. Greene, F.L., et al., eds. American Joint Committee on Cancer Manual for Staging of Cancer. Sixth ed. 2002, Springer: Cambridge, MA.

8. Freeman, D.E., et al. Irradiation alone for supraglottic larynx carcinoma: can CT findings predict treatment results? *International Journal of Radiation Oncology Biology Physics,* 1990. 1 485–490.

9. Mendenhall, W.M., et al. T1-T2 vocal cord carcinoma: a basis for comparing the results of radi therapy and surgery. *Head and Neck Surgery,* 1988. 10: 373–377.

10. Shaha, A.R. and J.P. Shah. Carcinoma of the subglottic larynx. *American Journal of Surger* 1982(144): 456–458.

11. Warde, P., et al. Carcinoma of the subglottis. *Archives of Otolaryngology Head and Ne Surgery,* 1987. 113: 1228–1229.

12. Lindberg, R.D. Distribution of cervical lymph node metastases from squamous cell carcinor of the upper respiratory and digestive tracts. *Cancer,* 1972. 29: 1446–1449.

13. Byers, R.M., P.F. Wolf, and A.J. Ballantyne. Rationale for elective modified neck dissectio *Head and Neck Surgery,* 1988. 10: 160–167.

14. Bernier, J., et al. Postoperative Irradiation with or without concomitant chemotherapy f locally advanced head and neck Cancer. *N Engl J Med,* 2004. 350(19): 1945–1952.

15. Cooper, J.S., et al. Postoperative concurrent radiotherapy and chemotherapy for high-ri squamous cell carcinoma of the head and neck. *N Engl J Med,* 2004. 350(19): 1937–1944.

16. Elman, A.J., et al. In situ carcinoma of the vocal cords. *Cancer,* 1979. 43: 2422–2428.

17. Le, Q.-T., et al. Treatment results of carcinoma in situ of the glottis: an analysis of 82 case *Arch Otolaryngol Head Neck Surg,* 2000. 126(11): 1305–1312.

18. MacLeod, P.M. and F. Daniel. The role of radiotherapy in in situ carcinoma of the larynx. *Inte national Journal of Radiation Oncology Biology Physics,* 1990. 18: 113–117.

19. Smitt, M.C. and D.R. Goffinet. Radiotherapy for carcinoma in situ of the glottic larynx. *Inte national Journal of Radiation Oncology Biology Physics,* 1994. 28: 251–255.

20. Million, R.R. The larynx... so to speak: everything I wanted to know about layngeal cance learned in the last 32 years. *International Journal of Radiation Oncology Biology Physi* 1992. 23: 691–704.

21. Sombeck, M.O., et al. Radiotherapy for early vocal cord cancer: a dosimetric analysis of 60 versus 6 MV photons. *Head and Neck,* 1996. 18: 167–173.

22. Teshima, T., M. Chatani, and T. Inoue. Radiation therapy for early glottic cancer (T1N0M0): prospective randomized study concerning radiation field. *International Journal of Radiatio Oncology Biology Physics,* 1990. 18: 119–123.

23. Hamlet, S., G. Ezzell, and A. Aref. Larynx motion associated with swallowing during radiatio therapy. *International Journal of Radiation Oncology Biology Physics,* 1993. 28: 467–470.

24. Schwaibold, F., et al. The effect of fraction size on control of early glottic cancer. *Internation Journal of Radiation Oncology Biology Physics,* 1988. 14: 451–454.

25. Mendenhall, W.M., et al. T1-T2 squamous cell carcinoma of the glottic larynx treated with ra ation therapy: relationship of dose-fractionation factors to local control and complicatior *International Journal of Radiation Oncology Biology Physics,* 1988. 15: 1267–1273.

26. Wang, C.C. Radiation Therapy for Head and Neck Neoplasms. 1997, New York: Wiley-Liss.

27. Fu, K.K., et al. A radiation therapy oncology group (RTOG) phase III randomized study to co pare hyperfractionation and two variants of accelerated fractionation to standard fractior tion radiotherapy for head and neck squamous cell carcinomas: first report of RTOG 90C *International Journal of Radiation Oncology Biology Physics,* 2000. 48(1): 7–16.

28. Wang, C.C. Factors influencing the success of radiation therapy for T2 and T3 glottic carcin mas. *American Journal of Clinical Oncology,* 1986. 9: 517–520.

29. Wang, C.C., et al. Local control of T3 carcinomas after accelerated fractionation: a look at the gap. *International Journal of Radiation Oncology Biology Physics,* 1996. 35(3): 439–441.

30. Mendenhall, W.M., et al. Stage T3 squamous cell carcinoma of the glottic larynx: a comparison of laryngectomy and irradiation. *International Journal of Radiation Oncology Biology Physics,* 1992. 23: 725–732.

31. Forastiere, A.A., et al. Concurrent chemotherapy and radiotherapy for organ preservation in advanced laryngeal cancer. *N Engl J Med,* 2003. 349(22): 2091–2098.

32. Group., D.o.V.A.L.C.S. Induction chemotherapy plus radiation compared with surgery plus radiation in patients with advanced laryngeal cancer. *New England Journal of Medicine,* 1991. 324: 1685–1690.

33. Lefebvre, J.L., et al. Larynx preservation in pyriform sinus cancer: preliminary results of a european organization for research and treatment of cancer phase III trial. *Journal of the National Cancer Institute,* 1996. 38: 890–898.

34. Weber, R.S., et al. Outcome of salvage total laryngectomy following organ preservation therapy: the radiation therapy oncology group trial 91-11. *Arch Otolaryngol Head Neck Surg,* 2003. 129(1): 44–49.

35. Al-Sarraf, M., et al. Chemo-radiotherapy versus radiotherapy in patients with advanced nasopharyngeal cancer: phase III randomized Intergroup study 0099. *J Clin Oncol,* 1998. 16(4): 1310–1317.

36. Jones, A.S., et al. The treatment of early laryngeal cancers (T1-T2 N0): surgery or irradiation? *Head and Neck,* 2004. 26: 127–135.

37. Terrell, J.E., et al. Long-term quality-of-Life after treatment of laryngeal Cancer. *Arch Otolaryngol Head Neck Surg,* 1998. 124(9): 964–971.

38. Hanna, E., et al. Quality-of-Life for patients following total laryngectomy vs. chemoradiation for laryngeal preservation. *Arch Otolaryngol Head Neck Surg,* 2004. 130(7): 875–879.

39. Lee-Preston, V., et al. Optimizing the assessment of quality-of-life after laryngeal cancer treatment. *J Laryngol Otol,* 2004. 118(6): 432–438.

# 13

# Nasopharynx and Sinuses

*William P. O'Meara, MD*
*Nancy Lee, MD*

## NASOPHARYNX

### Overview

Cancer of the nasopharynx is a distinct entity from other head and neck cancers of the aerodigestive tract. Given its relationship to the base of skull and difficulty of complete surgical resection in this region, radiation therapy has historically played a central role in the definitive management of nasopharyngeal cancer. Early-stage node negative disease can be managed with RT alone. Cisplatin-based concurrent chemo-radiotherapy followed by adjuvant chemotherapy is the standard of care for locally advanced disease. Neck dissection is reserved for persistent or recurrent neck node metastasis. IMRT has replaced conventional RT as the treatment technique of choice. A multidisciplinary effort is underway to explore more effective systemic therapy to improve rates of distant metastasis.

### Anatomy

The nasopharynx is an open cuboidal chamber below the base of skull and behind the nasal cavity. The upper boundary is the base of skull. The lower boundary is the superior surface of the soft palate. The posterior boundary is the posterior pharyngeal wall anterior to C1 and C2. The anterior boundary is the posterior choana of the nasal cavity. The lateral boundary is the eustachian tube orifice, torus tubarius, and fossa of Rosenmuller.

### Pathology

Carcinomas of the nasopharynx are classified into three histological types by the WHO:

- WHO type 1—Squamous cell carcinoma (keratinizing SCC)
- WHO type 2a—Differentiated non-keratinizing carcinoma
- WHO type 2b—Undifferentiated carcinoma

WHO type 1 occurs most often in U.S.-born whites, while WHO type 2b is most common in Asians. WHO type 2b was previously classified as type 3. Lymphoepithelioma is a subset of WHO type 2b and is distinguished by numerous lymphocytes among the tumor cells.

## Epidemiology and Risk Factors

Nasopharynx cancer is uncommon in the United States but prevalent in Southeast Asia, among Inuits of Alaska, and in North Africa. Pertinent epidemiological facts about nasopharyngeal cancer include the following:

- Average Age    ~45–55 years but can be seen in teenagers
- Male:Female    2–3:1
- Race           Higher incidence in Southeast Asian, Inuits of Alaska, and North African

Risk factors appear to be multifactorial and include the following:

- Genetic predisposition
- Viral: Epstein-Barr Virus
- Environmental: smoking
- Diet: salt-cured fish

## Presentation/Workup

A neck mass is the most frequent presenting sign and symptom in nasopharynx cancer. However, it is not uncommon for U.S.-born whites to present with unilateral ear problems. Common signs and symptoms at presentation include the following:

- Neck mass
- Refractory serous otitis media
- Epistaxis
- Unilateral hearing impairment
- Nasal obstruction
- Referred ear pain
- Cranial neuropathy (cranial nerves V and VI are the most commonly involved)

The most common site of the primary mass is within the fossa of Rosenmuller. The incidence of lymphadenopathy is 80%–90% at presentation, and bilateral neck disease occurs 50% of the time. Retropharyngeal nodes are the most common site of nodal involvement and level II nodes are the second most common. The following pretreatment diagnostic evaluations are recommended:

- Complete history and physical examination including a fiberoptic endoscopic examination and detailed cranial nerve examination
- MRI (preferred unless medically contraindicated) and/or CT scan with bone windows of the nasopharynx and neck. Imaging should include the base of skull, nasal cavity, paranasal sinuses, and the neck down to the clavicles.
- PET scan
- CBC, liver function tests, EBV titers
- Pretreatment dental evaluation and initiation of dental prophylaxis

Data are emerging to support the utility of PET scan,[1,2] however, from the practical standpoint, PET scan has already replaced CXR, CT scan of chest, MRI scan of liver, and bone scan in the initial metastatic workup.

## Staging

Staging is specific to nasopharyngeal cancer and different from other head and neck sites.

## TABLE 13-1  2002 AJCC TNM Staging System for the Nasopharynx

**Primary Tumor (T)**

| | |
|---|---|
| T1 | Tumor confined to the nasopharynx |
| T2 | Tumor extends to soft tissues |
| T2a | Tumor extends to the oropharynx and/or nasal cavity without parapharyngeal extension |
| T2b | Any tumor with parapharyngeal extension |
| T3 | Tumor invades bony structures and/or paranasal sinuses |
| T4 | Tumor with intracranial extension and/or involvement of cranial nerves, infratemporal fossa, hypopharynx, orbit, or masticator space |

**Regional Lymph Nodes (N)**

| | |
|---|---|
| N0 | No regional lymph node metastasis |
| N1 | Unilateral metastasis in lymph node(s), 6 cm or less in greatest dimension, above the supraclavicular fossa |
| N2 | Bilateral metastasis in lymph node(s), 6 cm or less in greatest dimension, above the supraclavicular fossa |
| N3 | Metastasis in a lymph node(s) more than 6 cm and/or to supraclavicular fossa |
| N3a | More than 6 cm in dimension |
| N3b | Extension to the supraclavicular fossa |

**Distant Metastasis (M)**

| | |
|---|---|
| M0 | No distant metastasis |
| M1 | Distant metastasis |

Used with the permission of the American Joint Committee on Cancer (AJCC), Chicago, Illinois. The original source for this information is the *AJCC Cancer Staging Manual, Sixth Edition* (2002) published by Springer-Verlag New York, www.springer-ny.com.

## Management

Because of the difficulty in obtaining adequate surgical margins, radiotherapy is the primary treatment modality in both early and advanced stage disease. Concurrent chemotherapy is added for advanced disease as established by Intergroup 0099.[3,4]

In response to the Intergroup 0099 trial, five Asian institutions initiated similar phase III studies to evaluate the role of concurrent chemoradiation in nasopharyngeal carcinoma in their populations, and they have all confirmed the benefit of the addition of chemotherapy in locally advanced disease.[5-10] In addition, a number of meta-analyses have been performed which all

### BOX 13-1

Intergroup 0099 is the landmark trial for nasopharynx cancer that demonstrated improved progression-free and overall survival with the addition of chemotherapy to conventional radiation therapy in the treatment of locally advanced nasopharyngeal cancer. Patients were randomized to RT alone vs. chemo-radiotherapy. Radiotherapy was identical in both arms and consisted of 70 Gy delivered via standard opposed laterals using daily fractions of 1.8 to 2 Gy. The investigational arm also received chemotherapy with cisplatin 100 mg/m$^2$ on days 1, 22, and 43 during radiotherapy. Following concurrent treatment, adjuvant chemotherapy with cisplatin 80 mg/m$^2$ on day 1 and fluorouracil 1,000 mg/m$^2$/d on days 1 to 4 was administered every 4 weeks for three courses.

Al-Sarraf et al. Chemoradiotherapy versus radiotherapy in patients with advanced nasopharyngeal cancer: phase II randomized Intergroup study 0099. *J Clin Oncol.* 1998 Apr 1; 16(4):1310–1317.

TABLE 13-2 **Results of Concurrent Chemoradiation Arms in Randomized Trials of Nasopharyngeal Cancer**

| Study | Time Point (years) | Treatment Arm | Regional Control | Progression-Free Survival | Metastasis-Free Rate | Overall Survival |
|---|---|---|---|---|---|---|
| Al-Sarraf et al (United States)[3,4] | 5 | ChemoRT | | 58%* | | 67%* |
| | | RT | | 29%* | | 37%* |
| Chan et al (Hong Kong)[5,6] | 5 | ChemoRT | | 60% | | 70%* |
| | | RT | | 52% | | 59%* |
| Lin et al (Taiwan)[9] | 5 | ChemoRT | | 72%* | 79% | 72%* |
| | | RT | | 53%* | 70% | 54%* |
| Kwong et al (Hong Kong)[7] | 3 | ChemoRT | 80% | 69% | 85%* | 87%† |
| | | RT | 72% | 58% | 71%* | 77%† |
| Wee et al (Singapore)[10] | 3 | ChemoRT | | 72%* | 87%* | 80%* |
| | | RT | | 53%* | 70%* | 65%* |
| Lee et al (Hong Kong)[8] | 3 | ChemoRT | 92%* | 72%* | 76% | 78% |
| | | RT | 82%* | 62%* | 73% | 78% |

Abbreviations: NPC = nasopharyngeal cancer. ChemoRT = chemo-radiation. RT = radiotherapy.
*Statistically significant difference.
†ChemoRT arm had trend towards survival benefit with p = 0.06.
Used with permission from Lippincott Williams & Wilkins. This table is a modification of one originally published in *Curr Opin Oncol.* 2005 May;17(3):227.

similarly demonstrate an absolute survival benefit of approximately 5% with the addition of concurrent chemotherapy to definitive RT.[11,12]

Tumor control in nasopharynx cancer has been highly correlated with higher doses of radiation delivered to the tumor. However, because of the anatomic location of the nasopharynx in proximity to many critical normal structures, one of the challenges of designing radiation fields using conventional techniques is delivery of an adequate dose to disease without causing potentially serious complications. As a result of the desire for dose escalation to tumor but increased sparing of normal

---

**BOX 13-2**

These recent metanalyses explored the role of adjuvant chemotherapy to radiotherapy and reached similar conclusions. This addition of chemotherapy led to an absolute survival benefit of 4%–6% at 5 years. The benefit was greatest when chemotherapy was administered concurrently with RT.

Baujat et al. Chemotherapy in locally advanced nasopharyngeal carcinoma: an individual patient data metanalysis of eight randomized trials and 1,753 patients. *Int J Radiat Oncol Biol Phys* 2006 Jan 1; 64(1): 47–56.

Langendijk et al. The additional value of chemotherapy to radiotherapy in locally advanced nasopharyngeal carcinoma: a metanalysis of the published literature. *J Clin Oncol* 2004 Nov 15; 22(22): 4,604–4,612.

TABLE 13-3  **Management Flow Chart by TNM Staging**

| T1-T2a, N0, M0 | → | ≥70 Gy to nasopharynx<br>50–60 Gy to bilateral neck<br>No chemotherapy |
|---|---|---|
| T1, N1-3 | → | ≥70 Gy to primary and gross nodal disease |
| T2b-T4, any N | | 50–60 Gy to bilateral neck<br>Concurrent cisplatin (100 mg/m$^2$) on days 1, 22, and 43, followed by adjuvant cisplatin (80 mg/m$^2$) on day 1 + 5-FU (1,000 mg/m$^2$) on days 1 through 4 every 4 weeks × 3 cycles |
| M1 | → | Combination chemotherapy<br>Consider RT to the primary and neck if a complete response to chemotherapy is obtained |

structures, nasopharynx cancer was one of the first sites where IMRT was applied. Although there has not been a randomized study demonstrating the superiority of IMRT over conventional radiotherapy, IMRT has still emerged as the standard of care based on single-institution reports of excellent control rates and reduced toxicities.[13–16] UCSF has utilized IMRT in treating nasopharynx cancers for over a decade and has published the largest clinical series to date. With IMRT, excellent local and regional control was achieved with 4-year actuarial rates of 97% and 98%, respectively. However, distant metastases remained high with a distant metastasis-free rate of only 66% at 4 years.

## Radiation Therapy

Radiation therapy treatment design will be described as performed in RTOG 0225, a study on IMRT in nasopharyngeal cancer. The immobilization device should include neck and shoulder immobilization; a head mask alone is not sufficient. CT scan thickness should be 3 mm or smaller through the region that contains the primary target volumes. MRI scans assist in definition of target volumes.

The GTV is defined as all known gross disease. Two different CTVs are defined: CTV70 for the gross tumor volume and CTV59.4 for the high risk regions. The margin between GTV and CTV should

---

**BOX 13-3**

These single-institution studies are the earliest published experiences on utilizing IMRT in the treatment of nasopharyngeal cancer and provide data to support IMRT as the standard of care. These studies demonstrated excellent target coverage while sparing the parotids and minimizing the rates of xerostomia. Excellent rates of local and regional control were obtained in each study with the use of IMRT, but patients still failed distally at rates similar to that seen in the combined modality randomized trials where conventional radiotherapy was used.

Kam et al. Treatment of nasopharyngeal carcinoma with intensity-modulated radiotherapy: the Hong Kong experience. *Int J Radiat Oncol Biol Phys.* 2004 Dec 1;60(5):1,440–1,450.

Kwong et al. Intensity-modulated radiotherapy for early-stage nasopharyngeal carcinoma: a prospective study on disease control and preservation of salivary function. *Cancer.* 2004 Nov 1; 101(7):1,584–1,593.

Lee et al. Intensity-modulated radiotherapy in the treatment of nasopharyngeal carcinoma: an update of the UCSF experience. *Int J Radiat Oncol Biol Phys.* 2002 Jun 1;53(1):12–22.

Wolden et al. Intensity-modulated radiation therapy (IMRT) for nasopharynx cancer: update of the Memorial Sloan-Kettering experience. *Int J Radiat Oncol Biol Phys.* 2006 Jan 1;64(1):57–62.

**TABLE 13-4 Results from Series Treating Nasopharyngeal Carcinoma with IMRT ± Chemotherapy**

| Study | N | Characteristics | Median Follow-Up (months) | Time Point (years) | Local Control | Regional Control | Distant Metastasis-Free Rate | Overall Survival |
|---|---|---|---|---|---|---|---|---|
| Lee et al (United States) | 87 | All stages | 31 | 4 | 97% | 98% | 66% | 73% |
| Kwong et al (Hong Kong) | 33 | T1N0-1 | 24 | 3 | 100% | 92% | 100% | 100% |
| Kam et al (Hong Kong) | 64 | All stages | 29 | 3 | 92% | 98% | 79% | 90% |
| Wolden et al (United States) | 74 | All stages | 35 | 3 | 91% | 93% | 78% | 83% |

Abbreviations: NPC=nasopharyngeal cancer, IMRT = intensity-modulated radiation therapy.
Used with permission from Lippincott Williams & Wilkins. This table is a modification of one originally published in *Curr Opin Oncol.* 2005 May;17(3):228.

have a minimum of 5 mm except in cases where GTV is adjacent to brainstem where the CTV margin can be as small as 1 mm. CTV59.4 includes the entire nasopharynx, retropharyngeal lymph nodal regions, clivus, base of skull, pterygoid fossae, parapharyngeal space, inferior sphenoid sinus, and posterior third of the nasal cavity and maxillary sinuses. Regarding lymph nodes, CTV59.4 includes levels IB through V bilaterally and the retropharyngeal nodes bilaterally. However, level I lymph nodes can be spared when patients present with node negative disease. In general, CTVs are expanded by 5 mm to create PTVs. The low neck or supraclavicular field may be treated with a conventional AP field that is beam split to the IMRT fields.

A dose painting technique is utilized in treatment planning and delivery. Gross disease (PTV70) receives 70 Gy in 33 fractions at 2.12 Gy per fraction. High-risk regions (PTV59.4) receive 59.4 Gy in 33 fractions at 1.8 Gy per fraction. If using a conventional AP field, the low neck receives 50.4 Gy in 28 fractions at 1.8 Gy per fraction. Treatment is delivered once daily, five fractions per week over 6.5 weeks. Breaks should be minimized.

## Follow-Up

Follow-up is similar to other head and neck sites. The patient should have a physical examination every 3 months during the first year, every 4 months during the second, every 6 months during years 3–5, and every year thereafter. Post-RT imaging may include both anatomical (MRI or CT) and functional (PET) imaging. The first anatomical scan may be obtained 3 months after completing RT, and, in order to avoid false positives secondary to treatment-induced inflammation, the first follow-up PET scan should be obtained no earlier than 4 months after completing RT.[17] Physical examination should include a fiberoptic endoscopic examination at every visit. Thyroid function should be evaluated every 6–12 months. Follow-up visits should have a shorter interval if the patient requires active management of treatment sequelae.

## Future Directions

RTOG 0225 is a phase II study of IMRT ± chemotherapy for stage I-IVB nasopharyngeal cancer where the primary purpose is to test the feasibility and transportability of delivering IMRT in a multi-institutional setting. This study closed to accrual in 2005 and results are anticipated to be released in the near future when there is meaningful follow-up for all patients. Since most nasopharyngeal cancer patients fail distantly, one rationale for the use of IMRT is to reduce RT-related toxicities and thus allow for increased systemic treatments. The follow-up to RTOG 0225 is currently in development and will be exploring this concept with the addition of a novel systemic therapy regimen.

## NASAL CAVITY AND PARANASAL SINUSES

### Overview

The sinonasal tract includes the nasal cavity and paranasal sinuses which include the ethmoid, frontal, maxillary and sphenoid sinuses. Sinonasal cancers are uncommon and represent a heterogenous group of head and neck malignancies. Patients usually present with locally advanced disease. The most common anatomical site is the maxillary sinus, and the most common histology is squamous cell carcinoma. Resection followed by RT is the standard of care. Unresectable patients should get chemoradiotherapy. Prophylactic lymph node irradiation to the node negative neck is controversial but should be considered for T3–4 patients, particularly with squamous cell carcinoma histology. IMRT minimizes serious toxicity while maintaining tumor dose.

### Pathology

The most common histology is squamous cell carcinoma which is found in up to 80% of cases. Other histologies include minor salivary gland histologies (adenocarcinoma, adenoid cystic carcinoma), neuroendocrine histologies (esthesioneuroblastoma, sinonasal undifferentiated carcinoma),

**FIGURE 13-1**

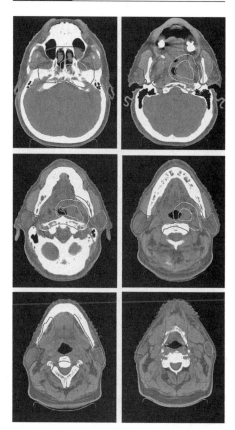

**(See Color Plate 3).** Target delineation for a T2bN0M0 nasopharyngeal carcinoma receiving definitive IMRT.

From Bortfeld T, Schmidt-Ulrich, De Neve W, Wazer D: Image-Guided IMRT. Springer Berlin Heidelberg 2006: 324.

melanoma, sarcoma, and lymphoma. Although nonsquamous cell carcinoma histologies are rare, approximately 20% of all head and neck adenoid cystic carcinomas arise in the sinonasal region.

### Epidemiology and Risk Factors

Current epidemiological data regarding sinonasal cancers are limited. The male:female ratio is about 2:1, and these tumors tend to occur between the sixth to eighth decade of life. Esthesioneuroblastoma, however, occurs over a wider age range with a bimodal distribution with peaks around 20-years-old and 60-years-old.[18]

Risk factors are poorly understood but appear to be associated with exposure to a variety of dusts and chemicals. Known environmental risk factors include nickel exposure for squamous cell carcinoma of the maxillary sinus and wood dust exposure for adenocarcinoma of the nasal cavity and ethmoid sinus. Although study results are conflicting, smoking has been implicated as a risk factor.

## Presentation

Cancer of the nasal cavity and paranasal sinuses is usually diagnosed in advanced stage due to the fact that early symptoms are vague and mimic sinusitis symptoms. Patient presentation depends on site of disease. About 60%–70% of sinonasal cancers occur in the maxillary sinus, 20%–30% in the nasal cavity, 10%–15% in the ethmoid sinuses and <5% in the frontal and sphenoid sinuses.[19] Maxillary sinus tumors grow with little or no symptoms and present in advanced stage when there is involvement of adjacent structures, causing oral symptoms such as pain in the maxillary teeth and cheek paresthesias. Advanced ethmoid sinus tumors tend to cause orbital symptoms such as proptosis, eye pain, and visual disturbance from involvement of cranial nerves III, IV, and VI. Primary nasal cavity tumors and paranasal sinus tumors that extend into the nasal cavity present with sinus congestion, unilateral nasal obstruction, rhinorrhea, and epistaxis. Sphenoidal sinus tumors tend to cause cranial neuropathy from involvement of cranial nerves V and VI. Frontal sinus tumors tend to cause frontal headaches.

## Workup

Although usually locally advanced at diagnosis, nodal and distant metastases are uncommon in sinonasal cancers. The following pretreatment diagnostic evaluations are recommended:

- Complete history and physical examination, including a fiberoptic endoscopic examination and detailed cranial nerve examination
- MRI scan with/without gadolinium and/or CT scan with contrast and bone windows of sinuses
- CXR
- Pretreatment dental evaluation and initiation of dental prophylaxis

CT and MRI scans are complementary in sinonasal cancers. CT scan defines early bone erosion of the thin bony structures of the nasal cavity, paranasal sinus and orbit more clearly than MRI scan; however, MRI scan is better at base of skull involvement. MRI scan better delineates soft tissue and can differentiate among opacification of the sinuses due to fluid, inflammation, or tumor. MRI scan is also useful in defining intracranial, intraorbital, and perineural involvement.

## Staging

There are two subsites for the T-stage in the AJCC TNM staging system for cancers of the nasal cavity and paranasal sinuses. The maxillary sinus falls under one T-stage system, and the nasal cavity and ethmoid sinus fall under another. There is no T-stage for frontal or sphenoid sinus tumors. N- and M-staging is the same for all sites. Ohngren's line is a theoretical line of demarcation between the medial canthus of the eye and the angle of the mandible that separates the maxillary sinus into an anteroinferior zone (infrasturcture-better prognosis) and a superoposterior zone (suprastructure).

## Prognosis

Locoregional control and incidence of distant metastasis are dependent on both T-stage and tumor histology. Regional lymph node involvement and distant metastasis are uncommon, even in advanced cases. About 10% of patients with cancer of the nasal cavity or paranasal sinus present with cervical lymph node metastasis and another 10% develop regional nodal metastasis in follow-up. The incidence of cervical lymph node metastasis is higher in esthesioneuroblastoma and sinonasal undifferentiated carcinoma (SNUC) at up to 20%–30%. Perineural spread is a concern with all histologies but occurs most commonly with adenoid cystic carcinomas.

---

**TABLE 13-5 2002 AJCC TNM Staging System for the Nasal Cavity and Paranasal Sinuses**

**Primary Tumor (T)**

*Maxillary Sinus*

T1   Tumor limited to the maxillary sinus mucosa with no erosion or destruction of bone

T2   Tumor causing bone erosion or destruction, except extension to the posterior wall of maxillary sinus and pterygoid plates

T3   Tumor invades any of the following: bone of the posterior wall of maxillary sinus, subcutaneous tissues, floor or medial wall of orbit, pterygoid fossa, ethmoid sinuses

T4a  Tumor invades anterior orbital contents, skin of cheek, pterygoid plates, infratemporal fossa, cribriform plate, sphenoid or frontal sinuses

T4b  Tumor invades any of the following: orbital apex, dura, brain, middle cranial fossa, cranial nerves other than maxillary division of trigeminal nerve V2, nasopharynx, or clivus

*Nasal Cavity and Ethmoid Sinus*

T1   Tumor restricted to one subsite, with or without bony invasion

T2   Tumor invading two subsites in a single region or extending to involve an adjacent region within the nasoethmoidal complex, with or without bony invasion

T3   Tumor extends to invade the medial wall or floor of the orbit, maxillary sinus, palate, or cribriform plate

T4a  Tumor invades any of the following: anterior orbital contents, skin of nose or cheek, minimal extension to anterior cranial fossa, pterygoid plates, sphenoid or frontal sinuses

T4b  Tumor invades any of the following: orbital apex, dura, brain, middle cranial fossa, cranial nerves other than maxillary division of trigeminal nerve V2, nasopharynx, or clivus

**Regional Lymph Nodes (N)**

N0   No regional lymph node metastasis

N1   Metastasis in a single ipsilateral lymph node(s), 3 cm or less in greatest dimension

N2a  Metastasis in a single ipsilateral lymph node(s), more than 3 cm but not more than 6 cm in greatest dimension

N2b  Metastasis in multiple ipsilateral lymph nodes, none more than 6 cm in greatest dimension

N2c  Metastasis in bilateral or contralateral lymph nodes, none more than 6 cm in greatest dimension

N3   Metastasis in a lymph node, more than 6 cm in greatest dimension

**Distant Metastasis (M)**

M0   No distant metastasis

M1   Distant metastasis

---

## Management

Due to a lack of randomized trials, the optimal management of sinonasal cancers is not known. Traditionally, surgery has been the primary treatment modality, and advances in resection and reconstructive techniques have resulted in functional and cosmetic improvements. Post-operative adjuvant radiotherapy is used in advanced stage and for close or positive margins. When patients are medically unfit for surgery or have unresectable disease, radiotherapy $\pm$ concurrent chemotherapy is utilized. Contraindications to surgery include involvement of nasopharynx, base of skull, sphenoidal sinus, brain, and optic chiasm. Outcomes with T4 tumors are poorer, but there are few specific

TABLE 13-6 Expected Outcomes in Contemporary Sinonasal Series

| Author | Institution | N | 5-yr Local Control | 5-yr Survival |
|---|---|---|---|---|
| Blanco et al[20] | Washington U. | 106 | 58% | 27% |
| Katz et al[21] | Florida | 78 | 60% | 56% |
| Porceddu et al[22] | MacCallum | 60 | 49% | 40% |
| Myers et al[23] | UT Southwestern | 141 | 49% | 52% |
| Le et al[24] | Stanford/UCSF | 97 | 43% | 34% |
| Dulguerov et al[25] | UCLA/Geneva | 220 | 57% | 63% |
| Hoppe et al[26] | MSKCC | 85 | 62% | 67% |

data on tumors with unresectable (T4b) disease. Such tumors are typically being treated with concur rent chemoradiotherapy, where efficacy has been demonstrated in general head and neck cancers.

## Radiation Delivery

The complexity of the sinonasal tract and its close proximity to critical normal structures such a the optic nerves, optic chiasm, brain, brainstem, and salivary glands make tumors well suited fc IMRT. Consequently, IMRT should be utilized to minimize dose to normal tissue. In preparation fc accurate target delineation, the operative node must be scrutinized and a discussion with th operating surgeon should take place to identify any areas at high risk for local recurrence. In th definitive setting or in a post-operative case with gross residual disease, obtaining an MRI scan i addition to a CT scan will greatly aid in target delineation of the GTV. In the post-operative settin with no gross residual disease, the CTV should encompass the entire post-operative bed. I perineural invasion is present on pre-operative workup or on pathology, the CTV must include th affected nerve up to the base of skull. Standard dosing is 60 Gy in two Gy fractions to the pos operative bed and 66 Gy in 2 Gy fractions to gross disease.

Based on the low prevalence of neck involvement and theoretical lack of lymphatic drainage standard practice is not to electively treat the node negative neck. In a series from UCSF an Stanford, Le et al reported a 5-year risk of nodal relapse of 12%, and all recurrence occurred in T3– tumors of squamous cell carcinoma histology.[24] However, Paulino et al observed a much higher rat of neck failure at 29% in a smaller series.[27] At the very least, one should consider lymph node irra diation in cases of locally advanced disease and squamous cell carcinoma histology. Porceddu et a found that most patients with a neck relapse also fail locally or distantly.[22] Therefore, there ma not be a survival benefit to elective nodal irradiation.

## Follow-Up

Follow-up is similar to other head and neck sites. The patient should have a physical examinatio every 3 months during the first year, every 4 months during the second, every 6 months durin years 3–5, and every year thereafter. Routine post-treatment imaging should be obtained n sooner than 3 months after all treatment has been completed. Physical examination should includ a fiberoptic endoscopic examination. Follow-up visits should have a shorter interval if the patier requires active management of treatment sequelae. Unfortunately, treatment options for sinonas. tumors that recur are limited.

## Future Directions

Resection of tumors involving the nasal cavity and paranasal sinuses frequently involves orbit exenteration. Radiotherapy with concurrent chemotherapy is being explored as definitive trea ment in place of surgery for the sake of eye preservation. Recently, the North American Skull Base Society opened a clinical trial on management of advanced paranasal sinus cancers utilizing preoperative chemoradiation followed by surgery.

## RARE SINONASAL TUMORS

### Esthesioneuroblastoma

Esthesioneuroblastoma, also known as olfactory neuroblastoma, is a rare malignancy of neuroendocrine histology with its own staging system and management approach.[18] Esthesioneuroblastoma tends to arise from the upper nasal cavity. Staging is much simpler than the AJCC staging system and defined according to the Kadish staging system:

- A: Tumor confined to the nasal cavity
- B: Tumor extending to the paranasal sinus
- C: Direct extension beyond the paranasal sinus, including the cribriform plate, base of skull, orbit, or intracranial cavity

Two separate management approaches have emerged, one surgery-based and the other nonsurgical. The standard surgical management is as follows:

- Stage A: Surgery alone
- Stage B: Surgery + post-operative RT
- Stage C: Surgery + post-operative RT ± chemotherapy

The nonsurgical approach treats stage A with RT alone and stages B-C with concurrent chemoradiotherapy; surgery may be utilized for salvage. In a retrospective series from Florida, there was a 44% rate of nodal failure in patients who did not receive elective neck irradiation.[28] Therefore, elective RT to the neck should be highly considered.

### Sinonasal Undifferentiated Carcinoma (SNUC)

Sinonasal undifferentiated carcinoma is a rare, aggressive malignancy which is also thought to be a neuroendocrine carcinoma and which also has its own management approach.[29] These tumors are most commonly found in the nasal cavity, and the rates of local, regional, and distant failure are relatively high compared to other sinonasal malignancies. Patients are staged according to the AJCC staging system. Surgery alone is considered for T1N0M0 disease. However, post-operative chemoradiotherapy is utilized for all other stages of nonmetastatic disease. Definitive chemo-radiotherapy is utilized in unresectable or medically inoperable situations. Unlike other sinonasal malignancies, the clinically node negative neck should always be irradiated due to the high risk of regional metastases.

## REFERENCES

1. Chang JT, Chan SC, Yen TC, et al. Nasopharyngeal carcinoma staging by (18)F-fluorodeoxyglucose positron emission tomography. *Int J Radiat Oncol Biol Phys* 2005;62(2):501–507.
2. Liu FY, Chang JT, Wang HM, et al. [18F]fluorodeoxyglucose positron emission tomography is more sensitive than skeletal scintigraphy for detecting bone metastasis in endemic nasopharyngeal carcinoma at initial staging. *J Clin Oncol* 2006;24(4):599–604.
3. Al-Sarraf M, LeBlanc M, Giri PG, et al. Superiority of five-year survival with chemo-radiotherapy (ct-rt) vs. radiotherapy in patients with locally advanced nasopharyngeal cancer (NPC). Intergroup (0099) (SWOG 8892, RTOG 8817, ECOG 2388) Phase III Study: Final Report [abstract]. *Proc ASCO* 2001;20:226a. Abstract 905.

4. Al-Sarraf M, LeBlanc M, Giri PG, et al. Chemo-radiotherapy versus radiotherapy in patient with advanced nasopharyngeal cancer: phase III randomized Intergroup study 0099. *J Cli Oncol* 1998;16(4):1310–1317.

5. Chan AT, Leung SF, Ngan RK, et al. Overall survival after concurrent cisplatin-radiotherap compared with radiotherapy alone in locoregionally advanced nasopharyngeal carcinoma *J Natl Cancer Inst* 2005;97(7):536–539.

6. Chan AT, Teo PM, Ngan RK, et al. Concurrent chemotherapy-radiotherapy compared with radic therapy alone in locoregionally advanced nasopharyngeal carcinoma: progression-free sun vival analysis of a phase III randomized trial. *J Clin Oncol* 2002;20(8):2038–2044.

7. Kwong DL, Sham JS, Au GK, et al. Concurrent and adjuvant chemotherapy for nasopharyngea carcinoma: a factorial study. *J Clin Oncol* 2004;22(13):2643–2653.

8. Lee AW, Lau WH, Tung SY, et al. Preliminary results of a randomized study on therapeutic gai by concurrent chemotherapy for regionally-advanced nasopharyngeal carcinoma: NPC-990( Trial by the Hong Kong Nasopharyngeal Cancer Study Group. *J Clin Oncol* 2005;23(28 6966–6975.

9. Lin JC, Jan JS, Hsu CY, Liang WM, Jiang RS, Wang WY. Phase III study of concurrent chemc radiotherapy versus radiotherapy alone for advanced nasopharyngeal carcinoma: positiv effect on overall and progression-free survival. *J Clin Oncol* 2003;21(4):631–637.

10. Wee J, Tan EH, Tai BC, et al. Randomized trial of radiotherapy versus concurrent chemc radiotherapy followed by adjuvant chemotherapy in patients with American Joint Committe on Cancer/International Union against cancer stage III and IV nasopharyngeal cancer of th endemic variety. *J Clin Oncol* 2005;23(27):6730–6738.

11. Baujat B, Audry H, Bourhis J, et al. Chemo-therapy in locally advanced nasopharyngeal carc noma: an individual patient data metanalysis of eight randomized trials and 1753 patients. *Ir J Radiat Oncol Biol Phys* 2006;64(1):47–56.

12. Langendijk JA, Leemans CR, Buter J, Berkhof J, Slotman BJ. The additional value of chemc therapy to radiotherapy in locally advanced nasopharyngeal carcinoma: a meta-analysis of th published literature. *J Clin Oncol* 2004;22(22):4604–4612.

13. Kam MK, Teo PM, Chau RM, et al. Treatment of nasopharyngeal carcinoma with intensity modulated radiotherapy: the Hong Kong experience. *Int J Radiat Oncol Biol Phys* 2004;60(5 1440–1450.

14. Kwong DL, Pow EH, Sham JS, et al. Intensity-modulated radiotherapy for early-stage nasopha ryngeal carcinoma: a prospective study on disease control and preservation of salivary fun( tion. *Cancer* 2004;101(7):1584–1593.

15. Lee N, Xia P, Quivey JM, et al. Intensity-modulated radiotherapy in the treatment of nasopha ryngeal carcinoma: an update of the UCSF experience. *Int J Radiat Oncol Biol Phys* 200. 53(1):12–22.

16. Wolden SL, Chen WC, Pfister DG, Kraus DH, Berry SL, Zelefsky MJ. Intensity-modulated radi tion therapy (IMRT) for nasopharynx cancer: update of the Memorial Sloan-Kettering exper ence. *Int J Radiat Oncol Biol Phys* 2006;64(1):57–62.

17. Fischbein NJ, OS AA, Caputo GR, et al. Clinical utility of positron emission tomography wit 18F-fluorodeoxyglucose in detecting residual/recurrent squamous cell carcinoma of the hea and neck. *AJNR Am J Neuroradiol* 1998;19(7):1189–1196.

18. Klepin HD, McMullen KP, Lesser GJ. Esthesioneuroblastoma. *Curr Treat Options Oncol* 200 6(6):509–518.

19. Maghami E, Kraus DH. Cancer of the nasal cavity and paranasal sinuses. *Expert Rev Anticanc( Ther* 2004;4(3):411–424.

20. Blanco AI, Chao KS, Ozyigit G, et al. Carcinoma of paranasal sinuses: long-term outcomes with radiotherapy. *Int J Radiat Oncol Biol Phys* 2004;59(1):51–58.
21. Katz TS, Mendenhall WM, Morris CG, Amdur RJ, Hinerman RW, Villaret DB. Malignant tumors of the nasal cavity and paranasal sinuses. *Head Neck* 2002;24(9):821–829.
22. Porceddu S, Martin J, Shanker G, et al. Paranasal sinus tumors: Peter MacCallum Cancer Institute experience. *Head Neck* 2004;26(4):322–330.
23. Myers LL, Nussenbaum B, Bradford CR, Teknos TN, Esclamado RM, Wolf GT. Paranasal sinus malignancies: an 18-year single institution experience. *Laryngoscope* 2002;112(11):1964–1969.
24. Le QT, Fu KK, Kaplan MJ, Terris DJ, Fee WE, Goffinet DR. Lymph node metastasis in maxillary sinus carcinoma. *Int J Radiat Oncol Biol Phys* 2000;46(3):541–549.
25. Dulguerov P, Jacobsen MS, Allal AS, Lehmann W, Calcaterra T. Nasal and paranasal sinus carcinoma: are we making progress? A series of 220 patients and a systematic review. *Cancer* 2001; s92(12):3012–3029.
26. Hoppe BS, Lee N, Rosenzweig K, et al. Post-operative radiotherapy in the treatment of paranasal sinus and nasal cavity and cancer. *Int J Radiat Oncol Biol Phys* 2005;63(Supplement 1): S377–S378.
27. Paulino AC, Fisher SG, Marks JE. Is prophylactic neck irradiation indicated in patients with squamous cell carcinoma of the maxillary sinus? *Int J Radiat Oncol Biol Phys* 1997;39(2): 283–289.
28. Monroe AT, Hinerman RW, Amdur RJ, Morris CG, Mendenhall WM. Radiation therapy for esthesioneuroblastoma: rationale for elective neck irradiation. *Head Neck* 2003;25(7):529–534.
29. Mendenhall WM, Mendenhall CM, Riggs CE, Jr., Villaret DB, Mendenhall NP. Sinonasal undifferentiated carcinoma. *Am J Clin Oncol* 2006;29(1):27–31.

# 14

# Management of the Neck

*Daniel T. Chang, MD*
*Russell W. Hinerman, MD*
*William M. Mendenhall, MD*

## ANATOMY

The cervical lymph nodes are divided into different levels based on surgical anatomy (Figure 14-1).[1]

They include the following: level I, submental (IA) and submandibular (IB) nodes; level II, upper internal jugular nodes, from the skull base to the level of the hyoid bone; level III, middle internal jugular nodes, from the level of the hyoid bone to the omohyoid muscle; level IV, inferior internal jugular nodes, from the level of the omohyoid muscle to the clavicle; level V, spinal accessory lymph nodes; and level VI, anterior neck nodes, bounded by the hyoid bone, the sternum, and the common carotid arteries. Included in level VI are the paratracheal, pretracheal, precricoid (Delphian), and tracheoesophageal groove nodes. Level II can also be further divided into IIA and IIB by the spinal accessory nerve. Because many of the landmarks used to define these nodal levels are not easily visualized on radiographic imaging, Computed Tomography (CT)-based nodal classifications have been proposed.[2] The current consensus guidelines for lymph node level classification in the node negative neck is shown in Table 14-1.[3]

According to these guidelines, level II extends up to the transverse process of C1. In the node positive neck, the space superior to the transverse process of C1 and inferior to the base of skull is defined as the retrostyloid space.[4] These guidelines have important implications in defining the clinical target volume (CTV) for intensity-modulated radiotherapy (IMRT).

## NATURAL HISTORY

The risk of lymph node metastases is influenced by the location of the primary tumor, the degree of histologic differentiation, the size of the primary tumor, and the surrounding capillary lymphatic network.[5] The N-stage distribution according to T-stage and primary site are shown in Table 14-2.

Recurrent lesions have a higher risk of lymphatic involvement than untreated lesions. The most commonly involved lymph nodes in the head and neck are the subdigastric lymph nodes, followed by the midjugular lymph nodes. Lesions that are well lateralized almost always spread first to the ipsilateral neck nodes. Lesions on or near the midline, as well as lateralized base of tongue and nasopharyngeal lesions, may spread bilaterally.

**FIGURE 14-1 Lymph node levels.**[13]

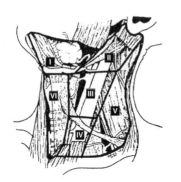

Ipsilateral lymph node metastases may theoretically increase the risk for contralateral lymph node spread if the metastatic disease produces significant obstruction of the lymphatic trunks. Furthermore, previous surgery on one side of the neck may cause shunting of lymph flow across the submental region to the contralateral neck. When contralateral lymph node metastases occur, level II is the region most frequently involved, followed by level III. The risk of clinically and pathologically involved nodal levels varies by primary site and is shown in Tables 14-3 and 14-4.

Tumor spread along the lymphatics of the neck usually follows an orderly and predictable pattern, first appearing in the upper neck and then in the lower neck and supraclavicular fossa. Distant metastases without lower neck level involvement or advanced neck disease is unusual.[6] However, because of normal lymphatic channel shunting, drainage may bypass certain neck levels altogether, which may lead to the development of discontiguous or skip metastases. Byers and coworkers showed that 15.8% of patients with oral tongue primaries had either level III or IV as the sole site of neck disease in the absence of level I or II involvement.[7]

As a tumor enlarges in the lymph nodes, it may eventually penetrate through the capsule and invade surrounding structures. The risk of capsular penetration increases with increasing lymph node size (Table 14-5).[8]

The risk of retropharyngeal lymph node involvement is related to primary site and neck involvement (Table 14-6).[9]

## DIAGNOSTIC WORKUP

### Physical Examination

Patients should be examined in the sitting position with the examiner behind them. The examiner should have one hand on the occiput to flex the patient's head forward and the other hand on the side of the neck to be examined. To examine the internal jugular lymph nodes, which lie deep to the sternocleidomastoid muscle along the internal jugular vein, the examiner's thumb and index finger are placed around the sternocleidomastoid muscle in the form of a C and then gently proceed from the sternal notch to the angle of the mandible. Both sides of the neck should not be examined simultaneously. The submandibular and submental nodes may be evaluated by direct palpation of these areas as well as by a bimanual examination with the index finger placed in the floor of the mouth.[10] The examiner should record the anatomic location, size, consistency, tenderness, mobility, and clinical impression of the node to determine whether it is involved.

### Radiographic Evaluation

CT, Magnetic Resonance Imaging (MRI), and ultrasound may all be used to evaluate cervical metastatic disease.[11] CT and MRI are comparable in terms of sensitivity and predictive value.[12] At the University of Florida, CT remains the primary method of examining most carcinomas arising in

TABLE 14-1 Consensus Guidelines for the Radiological Boundaries of the Neck Node Levels[3]

| Level | Cranial | Caudal | Anterior | Posterior | Lateral | Medial |
|---|---|---|---|---|---|---|
| | | | Anatomical Boundaries | | | |
| Ia | Geniohyoid m., plane tangent to basilar edge of mandible | Plane tangent to body of hyoid bone | Symphysis menti, platysma m. | Body of hyoid bone | Medial edge of anterior belly of digastric m. | n.a.[a] |
| Ib | Mylohyoid m., cranial edge of submandibular gland | Plane through central part of hyoid bone | Symphysis menti, platysma m. | Posterior edge of submandibular gland | Basilar edge/innerside of mandible, platysma m., skin | Lateral edge of anterior belly of digastric m. |
| IIa | Caudal edge of lateral process C1 | Caudal edge of the body of hyoid bone | Posterior edge of submandibular gland; anterior edge of internal carotid artery; posterior. edge of posterior belly of digastric m. | Posterior border of internal jugular vein | Medial edge of sternocleidomastoid | Medial edge of internal carotid artery, paraspinal (levator scapulae) m. |
| IIb | Caudal edge of lateral process C1 | Caudal edge of the body of hyoid bone | Posterior border of internal jugular vein | Posterior border of the sternocleidomastoid m. | Medial edge of sternocleidomastoid | Medial edge of internal carotid artery, paraspinal (levator scapulae) m. |
| III | Caudal edge of the body of hyoid bone | Caudal edge of cricoid cartilage | Postero-lateral edge of the sternohyoid m.; anterior edge of sternocleidomastoid m. | Posterior edge of the sternocleidomastoid m. | Medial edge of sternocleidomastoid | Interior edge of carotid artery, paraspinal (scalenius) m. |
| IV | Caudal edge of cricoid cartilage | 2 cm cranial to sternoclavicular joint | Anteromedial edge of sternocleidomastoid m. | Posterior edge of the sternocleidomastoid m. | Medial edge of sternocleidomastoid | Medial edge of internal carotid artery, paraspinal (scalenius) m. |

(continues)

**TABLE 14-1 (continued)**

| Level | Cranial | Caudal | Anterior | Anatomical Boundaries Posterior | Lateral | Medial |
|-------|---------|--------|----------|---------------------------------|---------|--------|
| V | Cranial edge of body of hyoid bone | CT slice encompassing the transverse cervical vessels[b] | Posterior edge of the sternocleidomastoid m. | Anterior-lateral border of the trapezius m. | Platysma m., skin | Paraspinal (levator scapulae, splenius capitis) m. |
| VI | Caudal edge of body of thyroid cartilage[c] | Sternal manubrium | Skin; platysma m. | Separation between trachea and esophagus[d] | Medial edges of thyroid gland, skin, and anterior-medial edge of sternocleidomastoid m. | n.a. |
| Retro-pharyngeal | Base of skull | Cranial edge of body of hyoid bone | Fascia under the pharyngeal mucosa | Prevertebral m. (longus colli, longus capitis) | Medial edge of the internal carotid artery | Midline |

[a] Midline structure lying between the medial borders of the anterior bellies of the digastric muscles.

[b] For NPC, the reader is referred to the original description of the UICC/AJCC 1997 edition of the Ho's triangle. In essence, the fatty planes below and around the clavicle down to the trapezius muscle.

[c] For paratracheal and recurrent nodes, the cranial border is the caudal edge of the cricoid cartilage.

[d] For pretracheal nodes, trachea and anterior edge of cricoid cartilage.

Modified from Gregoire V, Levendag P, Ang KK, Bernier J, Braaksma M, Budach V, Chao C, Coche E, Cooper JS, Cosnard G, Eisbruch A, El Sayed S, Emami B, Grau C, Hamoir M, Lee N, Maingon P, Muller K, Reychler H. CT-based delineation of lymph node levels and related CTVs in the node negative neck: DAHANCA, EORTC, GORTEC, NCIC, RTOG consensus guidelines. *Radiother Oncol* 2003;69:227–36.

**TABLE 14-2 Clinically Detected Nodal Metastases on Admission Correlated with T Stage[36]**

| Primary Site | T stage | N0 (%) | N1 (%) | N2–3 (%) |
|---|---|---|---|---|
| Oral tongue | T1 | 86 | 10 | 4 |
| | T2 | 70 | 19 | 11 |
| | T3 | 53 | 17 | 31 |
| | T4 | 24 | 10 | 67 |
| Floor of mouth* | T1 | 89 | 9 | 2 |
| | T2 | 71 | 19 | 10 |
| | T3 | 57 | 20 | 24 |
| | T4 | 47 | 11 | 43 |
| Retromolar trigone/ | T1 | 88 | 3 | 9 |
| anterior tonsillar pillar[†] | T2 | 63 | 18 | 20 |
| | T3 | 46 | 21 | 33 |
| | T4 | 33 | 18 | 50 |
| Soft palate[†] | T1 | 92 | 0 | 8 |
| | T2 | 64 | 12 | 25 |
| | T3 | 35 | 26 | 39 |
| | T4 | 33 | 11 | 56 |
| Tonsillar fossa[†] | T1 | 30 | 41 | 30 |
| | T2 | 33 | 14 | 54 |
| | T3 | 30 | 18 | 52 |
| | T4 | 11 | 13 | 77 |
| Base of tongue[†] | T1 | 30 | 15 | 55 |
| | T2 | 29 | 15 | 57 |
| | T3 | 26 | 23 | 52 |
| | T4 | 16 | 9 | 76 |
| Oropharyngeal walls[†] | T1 | 75 | 0 | 25 |
| | T2 | 70 | 10 | 20 |
| | T3 | 33 | 23 | 45 |
| | T4 | 24 | 24 | 52 |
| Supraglottic larynx[‡] | T1 | 61 | 10 | 29 |
| | T2 | 59 | 16 | 26 |
| | T3 | 36 | 25 | 40 |
| | T4 | 41 | 18 | 41 |
| Hypopharynx[§] | T1 | 37 | 21 | 42 |
| | T2 | 31 | 21 | 49 |
| | T3 | 21 | 26 | 54 |
| | T4 | 27 | 15 | 59 |
| Nasopharynx[‖] | T1 | 8 | 11 | 82 |
| | T2 | 16 | 13 | 72 |
| | T3 | 12 | 9 | 80 |
| | T4 | 17 | 6 | 78 |

Data are those of 2,044 patients, M.D. Anderson Hospital, Houston, TX, 1948–1965.

*T stage defined by Lindberg.[36]
[†]T stage defined by Fletcher et al.[37]
[†]T stage defined by Fletcher et al.[38]
[§]T stage defined by McComb et al.[39]
[‖]T stage defined by Chen and Fletcher.[40]

Modified from Lindberg R. Distribution of cervical lymph node metastases from squamous cell carcinoma of the upper respiratory and digestive tracts *Cancer* 29:1446–1449, 1972.

**TABLE 14-3 Distribution of Clinical Metastatic Neck Nodes from Head and Neck Squamous Cell Carcinomas[41-44]**

| Tumor Site | Patients with N+ | Distribution of Metastatic Lymph Nodes Per Level (percentage of the node positive patients) | | | | | |
|---|---|---|---|---|---|---|---|
| | | I | II | III | IV | V | Other[a] |
| Oral cavity (n = 787) | 36% | 42 (3.5%[b]) | 79 (8%) | 18 (3%) | 5 (1%) | 1 (0%) | 1.4 (0.3%) |
| Oropharynx (n = 1479) | 64% | 13 (2%) | 81 (24%) | 23 (5%) | 9 (2.5%) | 13 (3%) | 2 (1%) |
| Hypopharynx (n = 847) | 70% | 2 (0%) | 80 (13%) | 51 (4%) | 20 (3%) | 24 (2%) | 3 (1%) |
| Supraglottic larynx (n = 428) | 55% | 2 (0%) | 71 (21%) | 48 (10%) | 18 (7%) | 15 (4%) | 2 (0%) |
| Nasopharynx (n = 440) | 80% | 9 (5%) | 71 (56%) | 36 (32%) | 22 (15%) | 32 (36%) | 15 (10%) |

[a]Parotid, buccal nodes.
[b]Ipsilateral/contralateral nodes.

Modified from Gregoire V, Coche E, Cosnard G, Hamoir M, Reychler H. Selection and delineation of lymph node target volumes in head and neck conformal radiotherapy. Proposal for standardizing terminology and procedure based on the surgical experience. *Radiother Oncol* 2000;56:135–50; JP, Bernier J, Brugere J, Jaulerry C, Picco C, Brunin F. Natural history of neck disease in patients with squamous cell carcinoma of oropharynx and pharyngolarynx. *Radiother Oncol* 1985;3:245-55; Lindberg R. Distribution of cervical lymph node metastases from squamous cell carcinoma of the upper respiratory and digestive tracts. *Cancer* 1972;29:1446-9; Shah JP. Cervical lymph node metastases—diagnostic, therapeutic, and prognostic implications. *Oncology* (Williston Park) 1990;4:61-9.

the upper aerodigestive tract and regional lymphatics. On the other hand, MRI is the primary method used for nasopharyngeal malignancies. MRI may also be used if the patient has an allergy to intravenous contrast medium.

Ultrasound and MRI may be useful in evaluating tumor extension to the carotid if suggested on CT, however, MRI tends to be better at excluding extension to the neurovascular bundle when it is suspected on CT, whereas ultrasound can help show invasion of the vessel wall—thus confirming focal extension to the artery.

Positron emission tomography (PET) is rarely used in the initial staging of patients with head and neck cancer at our institution. It may be useful in the occasional patient with a synchronous peripheral pulmonary nodule to determine whether it is malignant.

## Staging

The staging system is similar for all head and neck sites except for nasopharyngeal carcinoma (Table 14-7).

## TREATMENT

### Surgery

Radical neck dissection involves removal of the superficial and deep cervical fascia with its lymph nodes from levels I–V, the sternocleidomastoid muscle, the omohyoid muscle, the internal and external jugular veins, the spinal accessory nerve, and the submandibular gland. Very few patients currently undergo this procedure at our institution.

Modified radical neck dissection removes the superficial and deep cervical fascia with its enclosed lymph nodes and leaves the sternocleidomastoid/digastric muscles, internal jugular vein, and/or spinal accessory nerve.

**TABLE 14-4 Incidence (%) of Pathologic Lymph Node Metastasis in Squamous Cell Carcinomas of the Oral Cavity, Oropharynx, Hypopharynx, and Larynx[41; 45–47]**

Distribution of Metastatic Lymph Nodes per Level (percentage of the neck dissection procedures)

| | Prophylactic RND[a] | | | | | | Therapeutic (immediate or subsequent) RND | | | | | |
|---|---|---|---|---|---|---|---|---|---|---|---|---|
| Tumor Site | No. of RNDs | I[b] | II | III | IV | V | No. of RNDs | I | II | III | IV | V |
| **Oral Cavity** | | | | | | | | | | | | |
| Tongue | 58 | 14 | 19 | 16 | 3 | 0 | 129 | 32 | 50 | 40 | 20 | 0 |
| Floor of mouth | 57 | 16 | 12 | 7 | 2 | 0 | 115 | 53 | 34 | 32 | 12 | 7 |
| Gum | 52 | 27 | 21 | 6 | 4 | 2 | 52 | 54 | 46 | 19 | 17 | 4 |
| Retromolar trigone | 16 | 19 | 12 | 6 | 6 | 0 | 10 | 50 | 60 | 40 | 20 | 0 |
| Cheek | 9 | 44 | 11 | 0 | 0 | 0 | 17 | 82 | 41 | 65 | 65 | 0 |
| Total | 192 | 20 | 17 | 9 | 3 | 1 | 323 | 46 | 44 | 32 | 16 | 3 |
| **Oropharynx** | | | | | | | | | | | | |
| Base of tongue + vallecula | 21 | 0 | 19 | 14 | 9 | 5 | 58 | 10 | 72 | 41 | 21 | 9 |
| Tonsillar fossa | 27 | 4 | 30 | 22 | 7 | 0 | 107 | 17 | 70 | 42 | 31 | 9 |
| Total | 48 | 2 | 25 | 19 | 8 | 2 | 165 | 15 | 71 | 42 | 27 | 9 |
| **Hypopharynx** | | | | | | | | | | | | |
| Pyriform sinus | 13 | 0 | 15 | 8 | 0 | 0 | 79 | 6 | 72 | 72 | 47 | 8 |
| Pharyngeal wall | 11 | 0 | 9 | 18 | 0 | 0 | 25 | 20 | 84 | 72 | 40 | 20 |
| Total | 24 | 0 | 12 | 12 | 0 | 0 | 104 | 10 | 75 | 72 | 45 | 11 |
| **Larynx** | | | | | | | | | | | | |
| Supraglottic larynx | 65 | 6 | 18 | 18 | 9 | 2 | 138 | 6 | 62 | 55 | 32 | 5 |
| Glottic larynx | 14 | 0 | 21 | 29 | 7 | 7 | 45 | 9 | 42 | 71 | 24 | 2 |
| Total | 79 | 5 | 19 | 20 | 9 | 3 | 183 | 7 | 57 | 59 | 30 | 4 |

[a]Radial neck dissection.
[b]I–V are in percentages.

Modified from Gregoire V, Coche E, Cosnard G, Hamoir M, Reychler H. Selection and delineation of lymph node target volumes in head and neck conformal radiotherapy. Proposal for standardizing terminology and procedure based on the surgical experience. *Radiother Oncol* 2000;56:135–50; Shah JP, Candela FC, Poddar AK. The patterns of cervical lymph node metastases from squamous carcinoma of the oral cavity. *Cancer* 1990;66:109–13; Candela FC, Kothari K, Shah JP. Patterns of cervical node metastases from squamous carcinoma of the oropharynx and hypopharynx. *Head Neck* 1990;12:197–203; Candela FC, Shah J, Jaques DP, Shah JP. Patterns of cervical node metastases from squamous carcinoma of the larynx. *Arch Otolaryngol Head Neck Surg* 1990;116:432–5.

TABLE 14-5 **Relationship Between Node Size, the Presence of Tumor in the Node, and Capsular Penetration in 519 Nodes*[8]**

|  | Size of Node (cm) | | | | |
|---|---|---|---|---|---|
| Size of node (cm) | 1 | 2 | 3 | 4 | $\geq$ 5 |
| Percent positive | 33 | 62 | 81 | 88 | 100 |
| Percent positive with capsular penetration | 14 | 26 | 49 | 71 | 76 |

*Institut Gustave-Roussy, Villejuif, France.
Modified from Richard JM, Sancho-Garnier H, Micheau C. Prognostic factors in cervical lymph node metastasis in upper respiratory and digestive tract carcinoma. Study of 1,713 cases during a 15-year period. *Laryngoscope* 97:97–101, 1987.

TABLE 14-6 **Incidence of Positive Retropharyngeal Nodes for Various Primary Sites and Clinical Neck Stages (794 Tumors)[9]**

|  | Clinical Neck Stage | | |
|---|---|---|---|
| **Primary Site** | **N0 Neck** | **N+ neck** | **Overall** |
| Nasopharynx | 2/5 (40%) | 12/14 (86%) | 74% |
| Pharyngeal wall | 6/37 (16%) | 12/56 (21%) | 19% |
| Soft palate | 1/21 (5%) | 6/32 (19%) | 13% |
| Tonsillar region | 2/56 (4%) | 14/120 (12% | 9% |
| Pyriform sinus or postcricoid area | 0/55 (0%) | 7/81 (9%} | 5% |
| Base of tongue | 0/31 (0%) | 5/90 (6%) | 4% |
| Supraglottic larynx | 0/87 (0%) | 4/109 (4%) | 2% |

N+ = neck nodes clinically involved (stages N1–3B).

TABLE 14-7 **2002 American Joint Committee on Cancer Staging for Neck Lymph Nodes**

| Stage | Definition |
|---|---|

NX   Regional lymph nodes cannot be assessed
N0   No regional lymph node metastasis
N1   Metastasis in a single ipsilateral lymph node, 3 cm or less in greatest dimension
N2   Metastasis in a single ipsilateral lymph node, more than 3 cm but not more than 6 cm in greatest dimension; or in multiple ipsilateral lymph nodes, none more than 6 cm in greatest dimensions; or in bilateral or contralateral lymph nodes, none more than 6 cm in greatest dimension
N2a  Metastasis in single ipsilateral lymph node more than 3 cm but not more than 6 cm in greatest dimension
N2b  Metastasis in multiple ipsilateral lymph nodes, none more than 6 cm in greatest dimension
N2c  Metastasis in bilateral or contralateral lymph nodes, none more than 6 cm in greatest dimension
N3   Metastasis in a lymph node more than 6 cm in greatest dimension

Nasopharynx
NX   Regional lymph nodes cannot be assessed
N0   No regional lymph node metastasis
N1   Unilateral metastases $\leq$ 6 cm in greatest dimension, without involvement of the supraclavicular fossa
N2   Bilateral metastases $\leq$ 6 cm in greatest dimension, without involvement of the supraclavicular fossa
N3a  Metastasis in a lymph node more than 6 cm in greatest dimension
N3b  Extension to the supraclavicular fossa

For a selective neck dissection, one or more of lymph node groups I–V are spared. See Figure 14-2A-E for the different types of neck dissection.[13]

Supraomohyoid neck dissection removes levels I–III and is most commonly used for patients with small oral cavity cancers and a clinically negative neck. A lateral neck dissection removes level II–IV nodes and is most often used in the treatment of laryngeal, oropharyngeal, and hypopharyngeal cancers. If significant metastatic adenopathy is encountered during a selective neck dissection, the procedure should be converted to a radical or modified radical dissection. A posterolateral neck dissection removes levels II–V and is used for skin cancers involving the posterior scalp or upper neck.

An extended radical neck dissection implies removal of additional lymph node groups or nonlymphatic structures in addition to the structures removed in a radical neck dissection. Bilateral neck dissections may be performed simultaneously or separately (staged) in patients with bilateral neck disease, but one internal jugular vein must be preserved.

Complications of neck dissection include hematoma, seroma, lymphedema, wound infection, wound dehiscence, chyle fistula, carotid exposure, carotid rupture, and damage to cranial nerves VII, X, XI, and XII. There are even more complications when neck dissection is combined with resection of the primary lesion or when it follows a course of radiation therapy.

## Elective Treatment of the Neck

The decision to irradiate the neck electively is based on several criteria: site and size of the primary lesion, histologic grade, difficulty in neck examination, relative morbidity for adding lymph node coverage, likelihood of the patient returning for follow-up examinations, and suitability of the patient for a radical neck dissection if disease should arise in the neck at a later date. A patient with a primary lesion to be treated by radiation therapy and a clinically negative neck that has a 20% or greater risk of subclinical disease should receive elective neck irradiation to a minimum dose equivalent to 45–50 Gy over 4.5–5 weeks. Lesions arising in the lip, nasal vestibule, nasal cavity, or paranasal sinuses have a low risk of neck involvement, and the neck is not treated electively unless the lesion is recurrent, advanced, or poorly differentiated. The risk of occult neck disease is essentially zero for T1 and 1.7% for T2 glottic carcinomas, and elective neck radiation therapy is not indicated.[14]

The lateral radiation portals for treating tumors of the oropharynx, supraglottic larynx, and hypopharynx include the upper jugular and often the midjugular chain lymph nodes. For primary lesions of the oral cavity, nasopharynx, glottis, nasal cavity, and paranasal sinuses, the portals must be enlarged to include the lymph nodes. The treatment portals for irradiation of the neck must be designed to minimize additional mucosal irradiation. A common error in irradiating oropharyngeal and nasopharyngeal cancers is to enlarge the lateral portals inferiorly to unnecessarily include the entire larynx in the lateral portals (Figures 14-3A–D).[15]

Treatment portals used at the University of Florida are shown in Figures 14-4 A–B.

Because the mid-neck is smaller in circumference than the upper neck, the total dose and dose per fraction are higher in the larynx than along the central axis of the beam. Although a field junction through a positive node may be avoided with IMRT, the larynx still receives a substantially higher dose compared with a separate anterior low neck portal with a midline laryngeal block junctioned at the thyroid notch.

Treating an unnecessarily large field increases the acute effects of radiation therapy, which increases the risk of an unplanned split, thereby reducing the probability of disease control.[15,16]

Knowledge of the spread pattern from various head and neck sites is essential in determining which nodal levels need to be included with the target volumes. As the use of IMRT becomes more commonplace, understanding of the anatomic boundaries of each level is required. The recommended nodal levels to be included electively for each primary site are shown in Table 14-8A.

**FIGURE 14-2** Lymph node levels.[13]

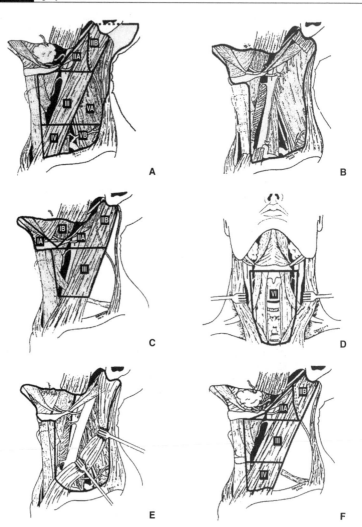

(A) Radical neck dissection. (B) Modified radical neck dissection with preservation of the sternocleido mastoid muscle, spinal accessory nerve, and/or internal jugular vein. (C) Selective neck dissectio (SND) for oral cavity cancer: SND (I-III) or supraomohyoid neck dissection. (D) SND for oropharyngeal hypopharyngeal, and laryngeal cancer: SND (II-IV) or lateral neck dissection. (E) SND for thyroid can cer: SND (VI) or anterior neck dissection. (F) SND for posterior scalp and upper posteriolateral nec cutaneous malignancies: SND (II-V), postauricular, suboccipital, or posterolateral neck dissection.[13]

*Arch Otolaryngol,* 2002, 128: 751-58. Copyright c. 2002. American Medical Association. All rights reserved.

**FIGURE 14-3** Carcinoma of the base of the tongue: large radiation portals.

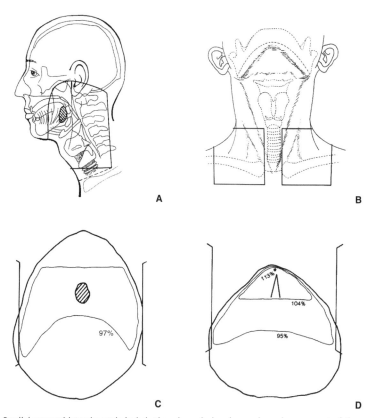

A

B

C

D

(A) Parallel-opposed lateral portals include the primary lesion, larynx, hypopharynx, most of the cervical spinal cord, and the upper portion of the trachea and cervical esophagus. Treatment through this portal tangentially irradiates the skin of the anterior neck unnecessarily. If an anterior field is not used to irradiate the low neck, the inferior border of the lateral field may be placed near the clavicle (dashed line). **(B)** Anterior low-neck portal. The wide midline tracheal block partially shields the low internal jugular lymph nodes, which are located adjacent to the trachea. The supraclavicular lymph nodes, which are less likely to be involved with tumor than the low jugular nodes, are adequately covered. **(C)** Central axis dosimetry at the level of the base of tongue primary lesion. The contours were obtained from a RANDO phantom using parallel 60Co fields weighted equally. The base of tongue tumor is outlined, and the tumor dose is specified at 97% of maximum dose. **(D)** Off-axis contour through larynx. The minimum dose to the entire larynx is 104% of the maximum dose specified at the central axis, and the maximum dose on this off-axis contour is 113%. If the base of tongue tumor dose is specified as 50 Gy at 2 Gy per fraction, the minimum larynx dose is 53.61 Gy at 2.14 Gy per fraction, and the maximum larynx dose is 58.25 Gy at 2.33 Gy per fraction. If the tumor dose is specified as 60 Gy at 2 Gy per fraction, the minimum larynx dose is 64.33 Gy at 2.14 Gy per fraction, and the maximum larynx dose is 69.9 Gy at 2.33 Gy per fraction.[15]

---

**FIGURE 14-4** Carcinoma of the base of the tongue.

---

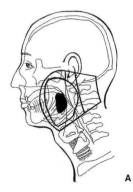
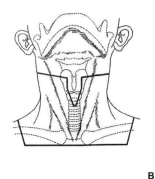

**A**                    **B**

**(A)** Lateral treatment portals for oropharynx primary tumors as used at the University of Florida. **(B)** Low anterior neck field for oropharynx primary tumors as used at the University of Florida.

---

## Treatment of the Clinically Positive Neck

Historically, neck dissection following radiotherapy has been employed for advanced nodal disease to increase regional control over either modality alone.[17,18] The dose required to control a clinically positive lymph node depends on the size of the node,[19,20] and is not reduced when early complete

---

**TABLE 14-8A  University of Florida IMRT Guidelines for Coverage of Nodal Levels According to Primary Site for an N-0 Neck**

| | N-0 bilaterally | | | | | | | | | | | | |
|---|---|---|---|---|---|---|---|---|---|---|---|---|---|
| | IA | IB | | II | | III | | IV | | V | | VI | RP | |
| | — | Ip | C | Ip | C | Ip | C | Ip | C | Ip | C | — | Ip | C |
| Nasopharynx | | | | X | X | X | X | X | X | X | X | | X | X |
| Palate | | | | X | X¹ | X | X | X | X | | | | X | X |
| Tonsil† | | | | X | X¹ | X | X | X | X | | | | X | |
| Base of tongue | | | | X | X¹ | X | X | X | X | | | | X | |
| Posterior pharynx wall | | | | X | X | X | X | X | X | | | ** | X | X |
| Pyriform sinus | | | | X | X | X | X | X | * | | | ** | X | * |
| Postcricoid space | | | | X | X | X | X | X | X | | | ** | X | X |
| Supraglottic larynx | | | | X | X | X | X | X | X | | | ** | | |
| Glottic larynx‡ | | X¹ | X¹ | X | X | X | X | | | | ** | | |

Ip-Ipsilateral; C-Contralateral

¹To transverse process of C1 to cover jugulo-digastric node.
*Cover only if tumor extends to or past midline.
**Cover only if esophagus or apex of pyriform sinus involved, but attempt to spare larynx.
†Lateralized T₁–T₂ tonsillar cancers received treatment to the ipsilateral neck and primary site.
‡The neck is not irradiated for T₁–T₂ glottic carcinomas.

regression occurs during treatment. The control rates after radiotherapy with 1.8 Gy per fraction are not as good as those obtained with 2 Gy per fraction.[21] Preoperative doses of 50 Gy are sufficient for mobile lymph nodes 3–4 cm in size, but 60 Gy or more is recommended for 5- to 6-cm nodes and/or fixed nodes. Lymph nodes measuring 7–8 cm are almost always fixed to adjacent structures and often require doses of 70–75 Gy for the surgeon to achieve a complete resection. If the lymph node lies behind the plane of the spinal cord, electrons may be used to boost the dose after the primary fields have been reduced off the spinal cord.[22]

After spinal cord tolerance has been reached and the treatment to the primary lesion is completed, another technique commonly used for boosting the dose to the neck mass is opposed anterior and posterior fields with wedges. The final dose to the neck node (not to the entire neck) may be 70–80 Gy without exceeding the spinal cord tolerance (Figure 14-5).

The anterior and posterior wedge-pair technique is preferable to an appositional electron boost field because high-energy electron beams increase the skin and mucosal dose. Depending on the situation, IMRT may also be used. Table 14-8B-C shows the nodal levels to be covered in the target volume for patients with clinically positive nodes according to primary site.

Patients with bilateral neck disease require joint planning by the radiation oncologist and surgeon. If disease is minimal on one side, radiation therapy alone may be used to control the disease on that side of the neck, and a neck dissection may be needed only on the side with more advanced disease. If major bilateral disease is present, bilateral neck dissections should be performed.

In select cases, the neck may be observed following complete clinical and radiologic regression of nodal disease to spare the morbidity of neck dissection. Some studies have shown that these patients have a low risk of neck recurrence,[23–25] while others suggest a benefit to adding a neck dissection.[26,27] Predicting the risk of residual nodal disease using physical exams such as CT, MRI, and PET has been an area of extensive investigation. PET offers unique advantages over conventional radiologic studies, but the time interval needed before it can provide accurate results may not coincide with the time window in which the morbidity of a neck dissection is minimal (which lies between 1–8 weeks following radiotherapy, when acute inflammation has resolved but late fibrosis has not developed). Data suggest that PET may not be able to provide a reliable predictive value until 4 months post-radiotherapy.[28] Waiting this long before surgery may add morbidity as well as compromise outcome if the residual tumor is allowed to repopulate, since neck recurrences are rarely salvaged.[29]

Previous data have examined the use of CT to evaluate the need for neck dissection. A recent study by Liauw et al suggests that simple radiographic features can reliably predict residual nodal disease and the probability of neck control.[30] As a result, the policy at the University of Florida is to observe all patients who have a complete response by physical exam and CT 4–6 weeks following completion of radiotherapy (those thought to have

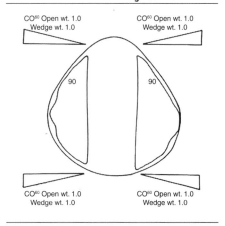

**FIGURE 14-5** Dose distribution for anterior and posterior wedge $^{60}$Co portals, both fields weighted 1.0.

CO$^{60}$ Open wt. 1.0
Wedge wt. 1.0

CO$^{60}$ Open wt. 1.0
Wedge wt. 1.0

90

90

CO$^{60}$ Open wt. 1.0
Wedge wt. 1.0

CO$^{60}$ Open wt. 1.0
Wedge wt. 1.0

---

**BOX 14-1**

211 patients treated with primary RT at the University of Florida for head and neck cancer had post-RT CT scans reviewed for neck nodal response and correlated with pathologic findings. The findings of any lymph node >1.5 cm in size and presence of focal abnormality predicted best for residual disease on neck dissection. In the absence of both of these findings on CT, the negative predictive value (NPV) was 94% for residual disease. The neck control rate for these patients who do not undergo neck dissection was 97%.

Liauw, SL et al. Post-radiotherapy neck dissection for lymph node positive head and neck cancer: the use of computed tomography to manage the neck. *J Clin Oncol.* 2006 Mar 20;24(9):1421–7.

---

≤5% risk of residual disease). Because the likelihood of successful salvage of a neck recurrence in an initially positive neck is low, a neck dissection is still recommended in borderline cases.

## CERVICAL LYMPH NODE METASTASIS FROM AN UNKNOWN PRIMARY TUMOR

Approximately 3% of patients present with enlarged cervical lymph nodes and the primary lesion cannot be found after full diagnostic workup. Patients with enlarged lymph nodes in the upper neck have a better prognosis when treated aggressively compared to those with involved nodes in the low internal jugular chain or supraclavicular fossa, which more likely arise from a primary tumor below the clavicles. The majority of patients have either squamous cell or poorly differentiated carcinoma. Those with adenocarcinoma almost always have a primary lesion below the clavicles, but if the nodes are located in the upper neck the salivary gland, thyroid, or parathyroid primary tumor must be excluded. Squamous cell carcinoma found in the parotid gland is almost

---

**TABLE 14-8B** University of Florida IMRT Guidelines for Coverage of Nodal Levels According to Primary Site for Unilateral Neck Disease

| | N1, N-2a-b, or Ipsilateral N3 | | | | | | | | | | | | |
|---|---|---|---|---|---|---|---|---|---|---|---|---|---|
| | IA | IB | | II | | III | | IV | | V | | VI | RP | |
| | — | Ip | C | Ip | C | Ip | C | Ip | C | Ip | C | — | Ip | C |
| Nasopharynx | | *** | | X | X | X | X | X | X | X | X | | X | X |
| Palate | | *** | | X | X[1] | X | X | X | X | X | | | X | X |
| Tonsil[†] | | *** | | X | X[1] | X | X | X | X | X | | | X | |
| Base of tongue | | *** | | X | X[1] | X | X | X | X | X | | | X | |
| Posterior pharynx wall | | *** | | X | X | X | X | X | X | X | | ** | X | X |
| Pyriform sinus | | *** | | X | X | X | X | X | X | X | | ** | X | * |
| Postcricoid space | | *** | | X | X | X | X | X | X | X | | X | X | X |
| Larynx | | *** | | X | X[1] | X | X | X | X | X | | X | X | * |
| Ip-Ipsilateral; C-Contralateral | | | | | | | | | | | | | | |

[1]To transverse process of C1 to cover jugulo-digastric node.

[2] Cover up to base of skull/jugular foramen if positive nodes in level II, V, or RP.

* Cover only if tumor extends to or past midline.

** Cover only if esophagus or apex of pyriform sinus involved, but attempt to spare larynx.

*** In the absence of high volume level II disease, cover only the posterior level IB, 1 cm anterior to the submandibular gland.

[†]Lateralized $T_1$-$T_2$ tonsillar cancers receive radiotherapy to the primary site and ipsilateral neck.

TABLE 14-8C  **University of Florida IMRT Guidelines for Coverage of Nodal Levels According to Primary Site for Bilateral Neck Disease**

| | N-2c (bilateral neck nodes) | | | | | | | | | | | | |
|---|---|---|---|---|---|---|---|---|---|---|---|---|---|
| | IA | IB | | II[1] | | III | | IV | | V | | VI | RP | |
| | — | Ip | C | Ip | C | Ip | C | Ip | C | Ip | C | — | Ip | C |
| Nasopharynx | | *** | | X | X | X | X | X | X | X | X | | X | X |
| Palate | | *** | | X | X | X | X | X | X | X | X | | X | X |
| Tonsil | | *** | | X | X | X | X | X | X | X | X | | X | X |
| Base of tongue | | *** | | X | X | X | X | X | X | X | X | | X | X |
| Posterior pharynx wall | | *** | | X | X | X | X | X | X | X | X | **** | X | X |
| Pyriform sinus | | *** | | X | X | X | X | X | X | X | X | **** | X | X |
| Postcricoid space | | *** | | X | X | X | X | X | X | X | X | X | X | X |
| Larynx | | *** | | X | X | X | X | X | X | X | X | X | X | X |

IP-Ipsilateral; C-Contralateral

Note: IMRT is rarely used with bilateral adenopathy. The situation where we have used IMRT with N2c disease is a nasopharynx primary and low volume adenophathy confined to level II-III and the RP nodes.
[1]Cover up to base of skull/jugular foramen if positive nodes in level II, V, or RP.
*** In the absence of high volume level II disease, cover only the posterior level IB, 1 cm anterior to the submandibular gland.
**** Cover but attempt to spare larynx.

exclusively from a primary skin lesion. This section deals with patients presenting with squamous cell or poorly differentiated carcinoma in the upper or middle neck.

Patients should undergo careful examination of the head and neck. A fine-needle aspiration biopsy of the lymph node should be performed. After chest roentgenography, a CT or MRI of the head and neck is obtained to detect an unknown primary lesion arising from the mucosa of the head and neck. The utility of fluorodeoxyglucose (FDG) single-photon emission computed tomography (SPECT) or PET scans in identifying primary lesions that would not otherwise be identifiable is unclear.[31] The available data suggest that few patients will benefit from these studies. In a series from the University of Florida, only 1/24 patients (4%) had FDG-SPECT as the sole test that correctly identified the primary site. Therefore, SPECT or PET is not routinely incorporated into the workup of these patients at our institution. If PET is used, it should be done prior to panendoscopy so that suspicious sites can be biopsied without post-biopsy inflammation obscuring the results of the scan. For patients with bulky nodal disease or multiple nodes involving the lower neck, a chest CT should be done to evaluate for the presence of lung metastases. Direct laryngoscopy and examination under anesthesia are performed with directed biopsies of the nasopharynx, tonsils, base of the tongue, and pyriform sinuses as well as any abnormalities noted on CT or MRI or suspicious mucosal lesions noted on laryngoscopy. Patients with adequate lymphoid tissue in their tonsillar fossae should undergo an ipsilateral tonsillectomy. The diagnostic evaluation for the patient with cervical metastasis from an unknown head and neck primary lesion is summarized in Table 14-9.

The results of a diagnostic evaluation for an unknown primary site in 130 patients at the University of Florida are depicted in Table 14-10.

In the University of Florida series, the primary site was discovered in over 40% of patients and was most often located in the tonsillar fossa or base of tongue (Table 14-11).

Treatment directed only to the involved area of the neck may be sufficient for cure,[32] although we usually irradiate the nasopharynx and oropharynx as well as both sides of the neck. The hypopharynx and larynx were irradiated until 1997, at which time these sites were eliminated

---

TABLE 14-9 **Diagnostic Workup for Cervical Lymph Node Metastases: Unknown Primary Tumor**

---

**General**
  History
  Physical examination
  Careful examination of the neck and supraclavicular regions
  Examination of oral cavity, pharynx, and larynx (indirect laryngectomy)
**Radiographic Studies**
  Chest roentgenogram
  Computed tomography or magnetic resonance imaging scans of head and neck (special attention to nasopharynx, pharynx, and larynx)
**Laboratory Studies**
  Complete blood cell count
  Blood chemistry profile
**Direct Laryngoscopy and Directed Biopsies**
  Nasopharynx, both tonsils, base of tongue, both pyriform sinuses, and any suspicious or abnormal mucosal areas
  Fine-needle aspirate or core needle biopsy of the cervical node
  Tonsillectomy

---

because they are rarely the site of the primary cancer and because the morbidity of treatment increases when they are included. Early data with this approach at our institution suggest decreased toxicity with favorable disease control.[33] Irradiating these sites should be considered if isolated level III or IV nodal involvement is present. Alternatively, a neck dissection alone and close observation may be considered. The nasopharynx could likely be excluded from treatment,

---

TABLE 14-10 **Biopsy-Proven Primary Site Versus Physical and Radiographic Findings and Number of Panendoscopies[22]**

---

| | No. of Patients with Biopsy-Proven Primary Site/No. Patients Evaluated* | | | |
| | Number of Panendoscopies | | | |
| Patient group | 1 | 2 | 3 | Total Patients |
|---|---|---|---|---|
| PE∅/RAD∅ | 6/34 (18%) | 0/7 | 1/1 | 7/42 (17%) |
| PE∅/RAD⊕ | 19/34 (56%) | 9/21 (43%) | 1/1 | 29[†]/56 (52%) |
| PE⊕/RAD∅ | 4/6 | 1/3 | No data | 5/9 (56%) |
| PE⊕/RAD⊕ | 11/16 (69%) | 4/7 | No data | 15[‡]/23 (65%) |
| Total | 40/90 (44%) | 14/38 (37%) | 2/2 | 56/130 (43%) |

Significance levels: 7/42 vs. 34/65, $p = .00023$; 7/42 vs. 15/23, $p = .00012$; 34/65 vs. 15/23, $p = .20413$.
[†]One of 29 patients had a positive FDG-SPECT scan and a negative CT of the head and neck; the remaining 28 patients had a positive CT and/or MR scan.
[‡]Two of the 15 patients had a positive FDG-SPECT scan and a negative CT of the head and remaining 13 patients had a positive CT scan and/or MR scan.
Key: PE∅ = no suggestive findings on physical examination; PE⊕ = suggestive of a primary site, but not definitely positive; RADΔ = no suggestive findings on radiographic findings; RAD∅ = radiographic studies suggestive of primary site.

Modified from Mendenhall WM, Mancuso AA, Parsons JT, Stringer SP, Cassisi NJ. Diagnostic evaluation of squamous cell carcinoma metastatic to cervical lymph nodes from an unknown head and neck primary site. *Head Neck* 1998;20:739-44.

**TABLE 14-11  Results of Diagnostic Evaluation of 130 Patients with Squamous Cell Carcinoma for an Unknown Head and Neck Primary Site—Location of the Primary Lesion (58 Lesions in 56 Patients)[22]**

| Primary Site | Number of Patients (%) |
| --- | --- |
| Tonsillar fossa | 25 (43) |
| Base of tongue | 23 (39) |
| Pyriform sinus | 5 (9) |
| Posterior pharyngeal wall | 2 (3) |
| Lateral pharyngeal wall | 1 (2) |
| Vallecula | 1 (2) |
| Suprahyoid epiglottis | 1 (2) |

Modified from Mendenhall WM, Mancuso AA, Parsons JT, Stringer SP, Cassisi NJ. Diagnostic evaluation of squamous cell carcinoma metastatic to cervical lymph nodes from an unknown head and neck primary site. *Head Neck* 1998;20:739–44.

but because the retropharyngeal nodes are at risk, radiation portals need to extend to the base of the skull, which includes most of the nasopharynx by default. Therefore, little morbidity is added by slightly enlarging the field to include the entire nasopharynx. It is not necessary to irradiate the oral cavity, unless the patient has submandibular adenopathy, in which case we either do a neck dissection and observe the patient or irradiate the oral cavity and oropharynx and not the nasopharynx. It must be remembered that the base of tongue is a midline structure with a propensity to spread to both sides of the neck, and it harbors the undetected primary site as often as does the tonsillar fossa. Therefore, it is the policy at the University of Florida to treat both sides of the neck. Patients are treated with parallel-opposed fields at 1.8 Gy per fraction to a midline dose of 64.8 Gy with reduction of the spinal cord at 45 Gy tumor dose (Figure 14-6).

The lower neck is treated through a separate anterior field. IMRT has recently been employed as a means to treat the bilateral neck to reduce morbidity from permanent xerostomia. The results of treatment in various series can be seen in Table 14-12.

The incidence of metachronous mucosal primary lesions was compared by Erkal and coworkers[34] between 1,112 patients with a known primary site (oropharynx, hypopharynx, and supraglottis) and 126 patients treated for an unknown primary site at the University of Florida. The incidence of a subsequent mucosal head and neck cancer was similar (9% vs. 13%, respectively, p = 0.81), suggesting either that mucosal irradiation significantly reduced the risk of primary site failure or that patients with unknown primary sites have a much lower risk of developing a second primary head and neck cancer.[34]

Open biopsy of a clinically positive neck node before definitive treatment potentially spills tumor cells along tissue planes that may not be removed with a radical neck dissection. McGuirt and McCabe reported that incisional or excisional biopsy of positive neck nodes before definitive surgery increased the risk of neck failure and worsened the prognosis for patients with squamous cell carcinoma of the head and neck.[35] The University of Florida experience showed that after excisional biopsy of a single lymph node, radiation therapy alone to the primary lesion and to the neck resulted in a 95% rate of neck control.[29] If residual disease remained in the neck after biopsy, radiation therapy followed by neck dissection was more successful than radiation therapy alone for controlling neck disease.

If there is no palpable disease remaining in the neck after excisional biopsy of a positive node, the neck may be treated with radiation therapy alone. If an incisional biopsy of the node has been performed (leaving gross disease) or if other positive nodes remain after an excisional neck node

**FIGURE 14-6** Radiation therapy portals used since 1997 to treat head and neck mucosal sites and upper cervical lymph nodes.

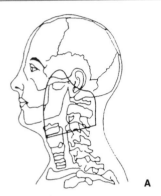 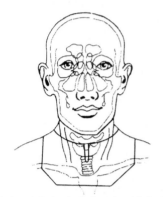

**(A)** and lower cervical and supraclavicular lymph nodes **(B)** The inferior border for lateral portals is placed at the superior anterior border of the thyroid cartilage, shielding the hypopharynx and larynx.[34]

A. *International Journal of Radiation Oncology Biology Physics*, V18:1531-1533, Mendenhall WM et al. Unnecessary irradiation of . . . c. 1990, with permission of Elsevier.
B. *International Journal of Radiation Oncology Biology Physics*, V50: 55-63, Erkal HS et al. Squamous cell carcinoma . . . c.2001, with permission of Elsevier.

biopsy, radiation therapy may be followed by a neck dissection. The dose of radiation preceding a neck dissection depends on the amount of gross disease in the neck and the degree of fixation.[22]

The main complication of radiation therapy for patients treated for an unknown head and neck primary tumor is xerostomia, which can be ameliorated, in part, by using IMRT. The complications

**TABLE 14-12 Results of Treatment for Unknown Primary of the Head and Neck**

|  | N | Treatment | Neck Control | Mucosal Control | FFDM | 5-yr CSS | 5-yr OS |
|---|---|---|---|---|---|---|---|
| Erkal et al[34] | 126 | RT—bilateral neck and mucosa | 78% | 87% | 86% | 67% | 47% |
| Colletier et al[48] | 136 | RT—bilateral neck and mucosa | 91% | 90% | 85% | 74% | 60% |
| Reddy and Marks[49] | 36 | RT—bilateral neck and mucosa | 69% | 92% |  |  | 53% |
|  | 16 | RT—ipsilateral neck | 81% | 56% |  |  | 47% |
| Grau et al[50] | 224 | RT—bilateral neck and mucosa | 52% | 87% |  | 47% | 34% |
|  | 26 | RT—ipsilateral neck | 43% | 77% |  | 32% | 22% |
|  | 23 | Surgery alone | 58% | 45% |  |  |  |

RT = radiotherapy
OS = overall survival
CSS = cause-specific survival
FFDM = freedom from distant metastases

of treatment of the neck, which have been discussed previously, depend on whether a neck dissection is added.

# REFERENCES

1. Robbins KT, Medina JE, Wolfe GT, Levine PA, Sessions RB, Pruet CW. Standardizing neck dissection terminology. Official report of the Academy's Committee for Head and Neck Surgery and Oncology. *Arch Otolaryngol Head Neck Surg* 1991;117:601–605.
2. Som PM, Curtin HD, Mancuso AA. An imaging-based classification for the cervical nodes designed as an adjunct to recent clinically based nodal classifications. *Arch Otolaryngol Head Neck Surg* 1999;125:388–396.
3. Gregoire V, Levendag P, Ang KK, Bernier J, Braaksma M, Budach V, Chao C, Coche E, Cooper JS, Cosnard G, Eisbruch A, El Sayed S, Emami B, Grau C, Hamoir M, Lee N, Maingon P, Muller K, Reychler H. CT-based delineation of lymph node levels and related CTVs in the node-negative neck: DAHANCA, EORTC, GORTEC, NCIC, RTOG consensus guidelines. *Radiother Oncol* 2003; 69:227–236.
4. Gregoire V, Hamoir M, Levendag P, Eisbruch A. CT-based delineation of lymph node levels and related CTVS in the node-positive and the postoperative neck. *Int J Radiat Oncol Biol Phys* 2004; 60:S497–S498 (Abstract)
5. Mendenhall WM, Million RR. Elective neck irradiation for squamous cell carcinoma of the head and neck: analysis of time-dose factors and causes of failure. *Int J Radiat Oncol Biol Phys* 1986;12:741–746.
6. Al-Othman MOF, Morris CG, Hinerman RW, Amdur RJ, Mendenhall WM. Distant metastases after definitive radiotherapy for squamous cell carcinoma of the head and neck. *Head Neck* 2003;25:629–633.
7. Byers RM, Weber RS, Andrews T, McGill D, Kare R, Wolf P. Frequency and therapeutic implications of skip metastases in the neck from squamous carcinoma of the oral tongue. *Head Neck* 1997;19:14–19.
8. Richard JM, Sancho-Garnier H, Micheau C, Saravane D, Cachin Y. Prognostic factors in cervical lymph node metastasis in upper respiratory and digestive tract carcinomas: study of 1,713 cases during a 15-year period. *Laryngoscope* 1987;97:97–101.
9. McLaughlin MP, Mendenhall WM, Mancuso AA, Parsons JT, McCarty PJ, Cassisi NJ, Stringer SP, Tart RP, Mukherji SK, Million RR. Retropharyngeal adenopathy as a predictor of outcome in squamous cell carcinoma of the head and neck. *Head Neck* 1995;17:190–198.
10. Million RR, Cassisi NJ, Mancuso AA, Stringer SP, Mendenhall WM, Parsons JT. Management of the neck for squamous cell carcinoma. In: Million RR, Cassisi NJ. *Management of Head and Neck Cancer: A Multidisciplinary Approach*. Philadelphia: J.B. Lippincott Company, 1994:75–142.
11. Mancuso AA, Hanafee WN. *Computed Tomography and Magnetic Resonance Imaging of the Head and Neck*. Baltimore, MD: Williams & Wilkins, 1985.
12. Curtin HD, Ishwaran H, Mancuso AA, Dalley RW, Caudry DJ, McNeil BJ. Comparison of CT and MR imaging in staging of neck metastases. *Radiology* 1998;207:123–130.
13. Robbins KT, Clayman G, Levine PA, Medina J, Sessions R, Shaha A, Som P, Wolf GT. Neck dissection classification update: revisions proposed by the American Head and Neck Society and the American Academy of Otolaryngology-Head and Neck Surgery. *Arch Otolaryngol Head Neck Surg* 2002;128:751–758.
14. Mendenhall WM, Parsons JT, Stringer SP, Cassisi NJ, Million RR. T1-T2 vocal cord carcinoma: a basis for comparing the results of radiotherapy and surgery. *Head Neck Surg* 1988;10:373–377.
15. Mendenhall WM, Parsons JT, Million RR. Unnecessary irradiation of the normal larynx [Editorial]. *Int J Radiat Oncol Biol Phys* 1990;18:1531–1533.

16. Amdur RJ, Li JG, Liu C, Hinerman RW, Mendenhall WM. Unnecessary laryngeal irradiation in the IMRT era. *Head Neck* 2004;26:257–264.

17. Mendenhall WM, Parsons JT, Stringer SP, Cassisi NJ, Million RR. Squamous cell carcinoma of the head and neck treated with irradiation: Management of the neck. *Semin Radiat Oncol* 1992;2:163–170.

18. Barkley HT, Jr., Fletcher GH, Jesse RH, Lindberg RD. Management of cervical lymph node metastases in squamous cell carcinoma of the tonsillar fossa, base of tongue, supraglottic larynx, and hypopharynx. *Am J Surg* 1972;124:462–467.

19. Dubray BM, Bataini JP, Bernier J, Thames HD, Lave C, Asselain B, Jaulerry C, Brunin F, Pontvert D. Is reseeding from the primary a plausible cause of node failure? *Int J Radiat Oncol Biol Phys* 1993;25:9–15.

20. Taylor JMG, Mendenhall WM, Lavey RS. Time-dose factors in positive neck nodes treated with irradiation only. *Radiother Oncol* 1991;22:167–173.

21. Mendenhall WM, Million RR, Bova FJ. Analysis of time-dose factors in clinically positive neck nodes treated with irradiation alone in squamous cell carcinoma of the head and neck. *Int J Radiat Oncol Biol Phys* 1984;10:639–643.

22. Mendenhall WM, Mancuso AA, Parsons JT, Stringer SP, Cassisi NJ. Diagnostic evaluation of squamous cell carcinoma metastatic to cervical lymph nodes from an unknown head and neck primary site. *Head Neck* 1998;20:739–744.

23. Peters LJ, Weber RS, Morrison WH, Byers RM, Garden AS, Goepfert H. Neck surgery in patients with primary oropharyngeal cancer treated by radiotherapy. *Head Neck* 1996;18:552–559.

24. Johnson CR, Silverman LN, Clay LB, Schmidt-Ullrich R. Radiotherapeutic management of bulky cervical lymphadenopathy in squamous cell carcinoma of the head and neck: is post-radiotherapy neck dissection necessary? *Radiat Oncol Investig* 1998;6:52–57.

25. Chan AW, Ancukiewicz M, Carballo N, Montgomery W, Wang CC. The role of post-radiotherapy neck dissection in supraglottic carcinoma. *Int J Radiat Oncol Biol Phys* 2001;50:367–375.

26. Brizel DM, Prosnitz RG, Hunter S, Fisher SR, Clough RL, Downey MA, Scher RL. Necessity for adjuvant neck dissection is setting of concurrent chemoradiation for advanced head and neck cancer. *Int J Radiat Oncol Biol Phys* 2004;58:1418–1423.

27. Lavertu P, Adelstein DJ, Saxton JP, Secic M, Wanamaker JR, Eliachar I, Wood BG, Strome M. Management of the neck in a randomized trial comparing concurrent chemotherapy and radiotherapy with radiotherapy alone in resectable stage III and IV squamous cell head and neck cancer. *Head Neck* 1997;19:559–566.

28. Greven KM, Williams DW, III, McGuirt WF, Sr., Harkness BA, D'Agostino RB, Jr., Keyes JW, Jr., Watson NE, Jr. Serial positron emission tomography scans following radiation therapy of patients with head and neck cancer. *Head Neck* 2001;23:942–946.

29. Mabanta SR, Mendenhall WM, Stringer SP, Cassisi NJ. Salvage treatment for neck recurrence after irradiation alone for head and neck squamous cell carcinoma with clinically positive neck nodes. *Head Neck* 1999;21:591–594.

30. Liauw SL, Mancuso AA, Amdur RJ. Post-radiotherapy neck dissection for lymph node positive head and neck cancer: the use of computed tomography to manage the neck. *J Clin Oncol* 2006;24:1421–1427.

31. Mukherji SK, Drane WE, Mancuso AA, Parsons JT, Mendenhall WM, Stringer SP. Occult primary tumors of the head and neck: detection with 2-[F-18] fluoro-2-deoxy-D-glucose SPECT. *Radiology* 1996;199:761–766.

32. Coster JR, Foote RL, Olsen KD, Jack SM, Schaid DJ, DeSanto LW. Cervical nodal metastasis of squamous cell carcinoma of unknown origin: indications for withholding radiation therapy. *Int J Radiat Oncol Biol Phys* 1992;23:743–749.

33. Barker CA, Morris CG, Mendenhall WM. Larynx-sparing radiotherapy for squamous cell carcinoma from an unknown head and neck primary site. *Am J Clin Oncol* 2005;28:445–448.
34. Erkal HS, Mendenhall WM, Amdur RJ, Villaret DB, Stringer SP. Squamous cell carcinomas metastatic to cervical lymph nodes from an unknown head and neck mucosal site treated with radiation therapy alone or in combination with neck dissection. *Int J Radiat Oncol Biol Phys* 2001;50:55–63.
35. McGuirt WF, McCabe BF. Significance of node biopsy before definitive treatment of cervical metastatic carcinoma. *Laryngoscope* 1978;88:594–597.
36. Lindberg RD. Distribution of cervical lymph node metastases from squamous cell carcinoma of the upper respiratory and digestive tracts. *Cancer* 1972;29:1446–1449.
37. Fletcher GH, Jesse RH, Healey JE, Jr., Thoma GW, Jr. Oropharynx. In: MacComb WS, Fletcher GH. *Cancer of the Head and Neck*. Baltimore: Williams & Wilkins, 1967:179–212.
38. Fletcher GH, Jesse RH, Lindberg RD, Koons CR. The place of radiotherapy in the management of the squamous cell carcinoma of the supraglottic larynx. *Am J Roentgenol Radium Ther Nucl Med* 1970;108:19–26.
39. MacComb WS, Healey JE, Jr., McGraw JP, Fletcher GH, Gallager HS, Paulus DD. Hypopharynx and cervical esophagus. In: MacComb WS, Fletcher GH. *Cancer of the Head and Neck*. Baltimore: Williams & Wilkins Company, 1967:213–240.
40. Chen KY, Fletcher GH. Malignant tumors of the nasopharynx. *Radiology* 1971;99:165–171.
41. Gregoire V, Coche E, Cosnard G, Hamoir M, Reychler H. Selection and delineation of lymph node target volumes in head and neck conformal radiotherapy. Proposal for standardizing terminology and procedure based on the surgical experience. *Radiother Oncol* 2000;56:135–150.
42. Bataini JP, Bernier J, Brugere J, Jaulerry C, Picco C, Brunin F. Natural history of neck disease in patients with squamous cell carcinoma of oropharynx and pharyngolarynx. *Radiother Oncol* 1985;3:245–255.
43. Lindberg R. Distribution of cervical lymph node metastases from squamous cell carcinoma of the upper respiratory and digestive tracts. *Cancer* 1972;29:1446–1449.
44. Shah JP. Cervical lymph node metastases—diagnostic, therapeutic, and prognostic implications. *Oncology (Williston Park)* 1990;4:61–69.
45. Shah JP, Candela FC, Poddar AK. The patterns of cervical lymph node metastases from squamous carcinoma of the oral cavity. *Cancer* 1990;66:109–113.
46. Candela FC, Kothari K, Shah JP. Patterns of cervical node metastases from squamous carcinoma of the oropharynx and hypopharynx. *Head Neck* 1990;12:197–203.
47. Candela FC, Shah J, Jaques DP, Shah JP. Patterns of cervical node metastases from squamous carcinoma of the larynx. *Arch Otolaryngol Head Neck Surg* 1990;116:432–435.
48. Colletier PJ, Garden AS, Morrison WH, Goepfert H, Geara F, Ang KK. Postoperative radiation for squamous cell carcinoma metastatic to cervical lymph nodes from an unknown primary site: Outcomes and patterns of failure. *Head Neck* 1998;20:674–681.
49. Reddy SP, Marks JE. Metastatic carcinoma in the cervical lymph nodes from an unknown primary site: results of bilateral neck plus mucosal irradiation vs. ipsilateral neck irradiation. *Int J Radiat Oncol Biol Phys* 1997;37:797–802.
50. Grau C, Johansen LV, Jakobsen J, Geertsen P, Andersen E, Jensen BB. Cervical lymph node metastases from unknown primary tumours: results from a national survey by the Danish Society for Head and Neck Oncology. *Radiother Oncol* 2000;55:121–129.

# 15

# Salivary Gland Tumors

*Daniel T. Chang, MD,*
*Russell W. Hinerman, MD,*
*William M. Mendenhall, MD*

## ANATOMY

### Major Salivary Glands

The three major salivary glands are the parotid, submandibular, and sublingual glands.

### *Parotid*

The parotid gland lies superficial to the ramus of the mandible overlying the masseter muscle, partially extending posteriorly to the anterior border of the sternocleidomastoid (SCM). Superiorly, it abuts the zygomatic arch and lies adjacent to the anterior and inferior portions of the external auditory canal and then extends to the tip of the mastoid. The inferior border approaches the upper border of the posterior belly of the digastric muscle. Deep to the anterior portion of the parotid gland are the masseter muscle and the horizontal ramus of the mandible. The retromandibular portion of the gland extends between the horizontal ramus of the mandible and the mastoid tip. The deep portion is in relationship to the styloid process with its three attached muscles (the stylohyoid, styloglossus, and stylopharyngeus), the lateral process of C1, the internal pterygoid muscle, and the contents of the parapharyngeal space.

The superficial and deep lobes are separated by the facial nerve, which enters as a single trunk and divides into its five main branches within the gland. The nerves are tightly interwoven within the tissue, requiring meticulous care when dissecting during parotid surgery. The auriculotemporal nerve, a branch of the trigeminal nerve, extends from the upper masticator space into the deep and superficial lobe of the gland with branches that contain parasympathetic fibers. This nerve provides one route of perineural spread to the base of the skull and cavernous sinus. Severing these branches may contribute to the development of Frey's syndrome (gustatory sweating).

The superficial preauricular nodes, usually one or two in number, lie outside the fascia of the parotid gland, immediately in front of the tragus in the subcutaneous fat and in close relationship to the superficial temporal vessels. These lymph nodes drain the skin of the ear, temple, and upper face, including the eye and the nose. They are most frequently involved by metastatic skin cancer (carcinoma and melanoma) and lymphoma, but not usually by parotid neoplasms. Secondary invasion of the gland and facial nerve may occur. The preauricular lymph nodes drain either to the superficial lymph nodes (inferior parotid lymph nodes) along the external jugular vein as it crosses the sternocleidomastoid muscle, or directly to the internal jugular nodes.

The true parotid lymph nodes are composed of two groups within the fascia of the parotid gland. One group, lying within the substance of the parotid gland, contains 4–10 small lymph nodes scattered along the retromandibular, posterior facial, and jugular veins. Thus, some of them lie deep to the facial nerve and may not be removed by a superficial parotidectomy. A second group lies between the gland and the superficial fascia. One or two nodes lie in front of the ear, and one or two between the tail of the parotid and the anterior border of the SCM, in association with the external jugular vein. These latter lymph nodes are referred to as the subparotid or tail-of-parotid lymph nodes. An enlarged subparotid node is difficult to distinguish from a mass originating in the tail of the parotid gland.

### Submandibular

The normal submandibular gland is about the size of a walnut. Most of the gland rests on the external surface of the mylohyoid muscle in the niche between the mandible and the insertion of the mylohyoid, between the anterior and posterior bellies of the digastric muscle. The submandibular duct (Wharton's duct) is about 5 cm long. It courses between the sublingual gland and the genioglossus muscle and exits in the anterior floor of the mouth near the midline.

## EPIDEMIOLOGY

Salivary gland malignancies are uncommon and comprise less than 3% of newly diagnosed head and neck cancers in North America annually.[1] The incidence varies from 1.5–4.0 per 100,000 persons per year.[1] Men and women are affected equally.[1,2] Approximately one fourth of parotid tumors and one half of submandibular tumors are malignant. The majority of salivary gland cancers (~80%) occur in the parotid.[1,2] Parotid tumors are more likely to be benign, compared with those arising in other sites where the probability of malignancy is 50% or higher.[1] The average age of patients with malignant neoplasms is 55 years, and for benign tumors it is about 40 years.

## PATHOLOGY

A large variety of benign and malignant neoplasms occur in the major salivary glands. Table 15-1 depicts the relative frequency of parotid neoplasms.

The initial diagnosis for parotid masses is most often made by a frozen section at the time of exploration. It may be difficult to distinguish between benign and malignant neoplasms on frozen section, and the patient must be advised of this difficulty.[3]

## PATTERNS OF SPREAD

### Benign Mixed Tumors

Benign mixed tumors infiltrate locally, but due to their slow rate of growth, rarely cause facial nerve palsy. Large masses may, however, cause severe stretching of the nerve. When incompletely excised, multiple tumor nodules may develop within the surgical bed. The skin may become involved in recurrent lesions. Bone invasion rarely occurs. A sudden increase in the growth rate may indicate a malignant change, although a few benign mixed tumors may intermittently grow rapidly. Facial nerve palsy is an almost certain sign of malignant change.

### Malignant Tumors

Malignant neoplasms infiltrate the parotid gland, invade the facial nerve or the auriculotemporal nerve, and spread along nerve sheaths. Tumor may invade the adjacent skin, muscles, and bone.

Adenoid cystic carcinoma, for example, widely infiltrates adjacent tissues without respect for anatomical planes. The external jugular vein may become thrombosed, and the external carotid artery may be compressed. Obstruction of the parotid duct is rarely seen. Deep lobe tumors invade the parapharyngeal space and base of the skull and compromise cranial nerves. The rate of lymph node metastases varies with the grade, the size, the T stage, and the salivary gland involved. There is little difference in the rate of lymph node metastases among the various high-grade histologies; the risk increases with recurrent disease.

TABLE 15-1  **Relative Frequency of Parotid Neoplasms**

| Histology | Incidence (%) |
|---|---|
| Benign mixed tumors (pleomorphic adenoma) | 65 |
| Miscellaneous benign tumors | 15 |
| Malignant mixed tumors | 4 |
| Mucoepidermoid carcinoma | 6 |
| Adenoid cystic carcinoma | 3 |
| Acinic cell carcinoma | 3 |
| Adenocarcinoma | 3 |
| Miscellaneous malignant tumors | 1 |

From Million RR, Cassisi NJ, Manucso AA. Major Salivary Gland Tumors. In: *Management of Head and Neck Cancer: A Multidisciplinary Approach,* 2nd Ed. Philadelphia: JB Lippincott, 1994: 711–735.

## DIFFERENTIAL DIAGNOSIS

### Parotid

- Primary parotid neoplasm
- Metastatic cancer, lymphoma, or leukemia involving parotid area lymph nodes
- Reactive lymphadenopathy
  - Fatty replacement, tail of parotid
- Chronic parotitis
- Sarcoidosis
- HIV infection
- Stone in duct
- Cysts (branchial cleft, dermoid)
- Hypertrophy associated with diabetes
  - Hypertrophy of masseter muscle, unilateral or bilateral
- Neoplasms of the mandible
- Prominent transverse process of C1 (atlas)
- Penetrating foreign bodies
- Hemangioma/lymphangioma
- Lipoma

### Submandibular

- Primary submandibular neoplasm
- Inflammatory disease
- Sialolithiasis
- Metastatic lymph node

## DIAGNOSTIC IMAGING

Magnetic resonance imaging (MR) and computed tomography (CT) are the radiographic studies used to evaluate parotid region masses. Ultrasound may be used for the evaluation of parotid inflammatory disease or masses. Imaging for a parotid mass is used to determine if the mass is intrinsic or extrinsic to the parotid gland, to determine its relationship to the facial nerve if intrinsic, and assess whether morphology is suggestive of invasive disease. If the mass is intrinsic, confined to the superficial lobe, and nonaggressive appearing, then superficial parotidectomy is indicated for initial diagnosis and management.

Although the parotid is encapsulated, there are several natural routes of spread that can be visualized on CT and MR studies, including:

1. the external carotid artery branches, especially the internal maxillary artery;
2. the junction of the pterygoid venous plexus and deep veins with the retromandibular vein;
3. the course of the auriculotemporal nerve in the masticator space of the parotid gland;
4. the facial nerve;
5. the interface of the gland with the cartilages of the external ear.

The facial nerve is the one most frequently in question and is usually best evaluated with gadolinium-enhanced MR in multiple planes. The surgical landmarks for identifying and dissecting the facial nerve are all visible on imaging studies. The descending facial canal, the stylomastoid foramen, the fat pad below the stylomastoid foramen, the tragal pointer, the digastric groove and posterior belly of the digastric muscle, and the external carotid artery and retromandibular vein are all used to track the course of the facial nerve.

## BIOPSY TECHNIQUE

### Parotid Gland

Excisional and incisional biopsies are not recommended because they increase the risk of recurrence and facial nerve damage and also increase the surgical morbidity by necessitating a wide removal of the biopsy site. Use of fine-needle aspiration is recommended but requires a pathologist skilled in its interpretation.

### Submandibular Gland

Needle biopsy may be indicated and useful if a malignant tumor is diagnosed. But, if negative, is often misleading and may delay diagnosis. If a careful search of the head and neck area fails to reveal a primary mucosal lesion, the submandibular triangle may be dissected as the biopsy procedure. Incisional or excisional biopsy increases the risk of tumor recurrence, even when followed by appropriate treatment, and increases surgical morbidity by requiring wide excision of the biopsy site.

## MANAGEMENT

Surgical resection is the mainstay of treatment for major salivary gland tumors.

### Surgery

#### Parotid Gland

*Benign mixed tumors*

Surgical removal with a rim of normal tissue, which can be accomplished by a superficial lobectomy in most cases, is the treatment of choice. Postoperative radiation therapy (RT) is considered when there is a positive margin and/or multifocal recurrent tumors. We no longer use tumor "spill" as an indication for adding RT. The few recurrences after operation alone are usually successfully managed by further resection, but the risk of facial nerve damage is increased. Routine use of postoperative RT is not advised, especially in younger patients, because of the risk of an RT-induced malignancy and other late complications. However, these factors must be balanced against the substantial risk of facial nerve loss that is associated with operating for recurrent disease.

## Low- to intermediate-grade malignancies

Most low- to intermediate-grade malignancies can be treated adequately by a superficial lobectomy, but total parotidectomy may be required in some cases. Postoperative RT is usually not needed but may be indicated if there is a positive or close margin, rupture of the capsule, surgical dissection close to the facial nerve, or recurrent tumor.

## Adenoid cystic carcinoma

Microscopically, adenoid cystic carcinoma may appear to be a low-grade malignancy but its growth may be variable. Therefore, it is best approached as a high-grade malignancy. Metastases to regional lymph nodes and distant sites do occur. Perineural involvement is a characteristic finding, and facial nerve palsy may be present at the time of diagnosis.

Management of this malignancy can be one of the most frustrating experiences in oncologic practice because the tumor frequently demonstrates an unpredictable behavior with late recurrences and distant metastases. Therefore, a treatment strategy that provides maximum local-regional control and survival rates with acceptable morbidity is needed. The usual approach is wide surgical resection followed by RT to a generous volume including the perineural pathways. Wide surgical excision may be difficult to perform, and positive margins are frequent. Borderline resectable lesions should be considered for preoperative RT or even RT alone. Patients presenting with asymptomatic slowly evolving lung metastases may live several years. The local-regional management in these patients may not differ markedly from that used in patients without distant metastasis at presentation.

## High-grade carcinomas

Because of their aggressive nature, high-grade neoplasms are usually managed by parotidectomy and postoperative RT. The risk for local recurrence is 35%–55% after surgery alone, and the addition of postoperative RT can reduce the risk to about 10%–15%. If the tumor grossly invades the facial nerve, one or more branches must be sacrificed. Otherwise, the nerve may usually be spared. The surgeon should not attempt to save a functioning facial nerve that is invaded by the tumor in the hope that postoperative RT will adequately treat residual disease, as this situation is unfavorable for cure even with very high doses of radiation.

The lymph nodes adjacent to the parotid gland are removed in continuity with the specimen. A neck dissection is added only if the neck lymph nodes are clinically positive. Postoperative RT is added in nearly all cases, regardless of the margins, and includes the entire ipsilateral neck.

Preoperative RT should be considered for patients with unresectable disease. Unresectable tumors are treated by RT alone, sometimes with a combination of external beam and interstitial implant brachytherapy; a modest proportion of these patients are cured.

## Submandibular Gland

Dissection of the submandibular triangle is used to make the diagnosis. If a frozen-section diagnosis shows a malignant lesion and there is no involvement of nerves, the mandible, or soft tissues, the surgeon need not proceed further, and postoperative RT is then delivered to the surgical bed and ipsilateral neck for high-grade malignancies.

If there has been simple excision of the malignant mass and the margins are negative, RT is recommended without further surgery. If, however, positive margins, perineural invasion, bone invasion, clinical involvement of a cervical lymph node(s), or extension to contiguous soft tissues are present, then the resection is enlarged to encompass the involved areas. This resection may include the removal of the mylohyoid muscle, digastric muscle, adjacent floor of the mouth or tongue, involved nerves, part of the mandible, and also a neck dissection. If the lesion is fixed to the mandible but not frankly invading bone, the inferior border of the mandible may be resected, and postoperative RT added. Unresectable lesions are treated with preoperative RT or RT alone.

## Irradiation Technique

### Parotid Gland

Postoperative RT is indicated for most high-grade lesions, close or positive margins, lesions involving the deep lobe, recurrent disease, or involvement of multiple regional lymph nodes.

The minimum treatment volume includes the parotid bed and upper cervical lymph nodes. If perineural invasion is present, the treatment portals are enlarged to encompass the nerve pathways. RT of the entire ipsilateral neck is indicated for high-grade lesions with a clinically negative neck and for clinically positive nodes after a neck dissection specimen. The dose to the primary site is 6,000 cGy over 6 weeks if no gross residual is present. Higher doses are used for gross disease or positive margins; altered fractionation should be considered in these situations. No conclusive data are available to show a difference in dose required for the various histologies, although the treatment failure rate for malignant mixed tumors may be greater.[4,5]

Two basic techniques are used for parotid radiation. One is an anterior-posterior photon beam "wedge pair," with the portals angled sufficiently to direct the beam path away from the orbits and oral cavity. The disadvantage of this technique is the inability to avoid irradiation of a portion of the posterior fossa contents.

A second technique employs a mixed beam of high-energy photons and high-energy electrons shaped to fit the anatomy, which produces a homogeneous dose distribution and delivers 3,000 cGy or less to the opposite salivary glands (Figure 15-1).[6] The disadvantage of this technique is that the dose falls off rapidly at a 4–4.5 cm depth and tumors involving the skull base at the stylomastoid foramen may be underdosed.

For perineural spread, the intraosseous pathway of the facial nerve and the auriculotemporal nerve must be included. The tumor may spread antegrade as well as retrograde along the facial nerve, making adequate coverage along the peripheral distribution necessary. When the tumor involves the deep lobe or otherwise extends near the midline, a wedge pair is necessary to provide adequate target coverage. The physician must be cognizant of the dose to the brainstem and spinal cord.

**FIGURE 15-1**

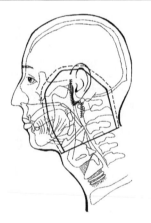

The anterior border is usually at the anterior border of the masseter muscle; the inferior border is at the top of the thyroid cartilage. Superiorly and posteriorly, the entire parotid and surgical bed are included. Electron portal (dashed lines) is 1 cm larger than photon portals because of the constriction of electron isodose lines at depth. An intra-oral stent made of lead or Lipowitz's metal will further reduce contralateral RT. About 2–3 cm of the distal facial canal is included in this example. The doses to the temporal lobe and posterior fossa must be calculated.

*Submandibular Gland*

Ipsilateral external beam portals are tailored to the extent of disease found in the surgical dissection. Possible sites of local recurrence include the submandibular triangle, adjacent oral cavity, pterygomaxillary fossa, base of the skull, and neck. When major nerve trunks are involved, the nerves are included beyond the margin of dissection to the skull base, even if the final nerve margin is clear. Skip lesions along nerves are common. The entire ipsilateral neck is typically included, but the contralateral neck is not usually at risk. The beam energy depends on the depth of the target volume. An electron beam, photon beam, or a combination may be used, depending on the situation. Intensity-modulated radiotherapy (IMRT) may be employed in situations where there is gross perineural invasion and it is necessary to create an irregular dose distribution to include the submandibular triangle and the nerve pathways to the skull base. The postoperative dose is 6,000 cGy–6,500 cGy over 6–6.5 weeks if there is no gross residual disease and margins are negative. Higher doses are used if there is microscopic or gross residual disease. An interstitial implant may be added to the tumor bed if residual disease is suspected.

## MANAGEMENT OF RECURRENCE

### Benign Mixed Tumors

Recurrent benign tumors can be reresected, but the risk of permanent damage to the facial nerve is higher because of scar tissue from previous procedures. RT is added on an individualized basis, especially when recurrence is multinodular or margins are positive. In patients with incompletely resectable benign mixed tumors, salvage may be achieved by RT alone, but the likelihood of cure is reduced if gross disease is present. Dose-fractionation schedules similar to those employed for carcinomas are used. Observation is appropriate in certain cases.

### Malignant Tumors

Malignant tumors that recur after an operation are managed by another operation and postoperative RT or, if unresectable, by RT alone.

## RESULTS OF TREATMENT

Table 15-2 shows the 5-year survival rates for various histologies of salivary gland malignancies. Table 15-3 shows the results of standard treatment for major salivary gland cancers.

**TABLE 15-2** **Parotid Carcinoma: Absolute 5-Year Survival Rates (120 Patients)**

| Histology | No. of Patients | 5-Year Survival (%) |
|---|---|---|
| Acinic cell | 12 | 92 |
| Mucoepidermoid (low grade) | 28 | 76 |
| Adenocarcinoma | 12 | 66 |
| Malignant mixed | 27 | 50 |
| Adenoid cystic | 10 | 50 |
| Squamous cell | 6 | 50 |
| Mucoepidermoid (high grade) | 13 | 46 |
| Undifferentiated | 12 | 33 |

Note: M.D. Anderson Hospital data; patients treated 1944–1965.
From Guillamondegui OM, Byers RM, Luna MA, Chiminazzo H Jr, Jesse RH, Fletcher GH. Aggressive surgery in treatment for parotid cancer: the role of adjunctive postoperative radiotherapy. *Am J Roentgenol Radium Ther Nucl Med* 123:49–54, 1975. Copyright © 1975, American Roentgen Ray Society. Table I, p. 50.

TABLE 15-3  Results of Standard Therapy for Cancer of the Parotid

| Investigator | No. of Patients | Treatment | 5-Year Survival Rate | 10-Year Survival Rate | Local Control Rate |
|---|---|---|---|---|---|
| King and Fletcher[a;5] | 93 | R, S + R | 34% (NED) | 62% | 75% |
| Spiro et al[33] | 288 | S | 62% | 54% | 73% |
| Guillamondegui et al[34] | 120 | S (n=104), S + R (n=10), R (n = 6) | 33%–92% (depends on histology) | | 74% |
| Guillamondegui et al[34] | 29 | S + R | | | 80% |
| Kagan et al[b;35] | 130 | S | | | 49% |
| Rafla[b,36] | 62 | S ± R | 21% (NED) | | 34% |
| Fu et al[37] | 63 | S, S ± R, R | 68% | 54% | 73% |
| Beahrs et al[38] | 162 | S | 38%–85% | | 28%–50% |
| McNaney et al[39] | 77 | S + R | | | 87% |
| Matsuba et al[40] | 21 | S | 52% | | 33% |
| | 26 | S + R | 65% | | 73% |
| Spiro[26] | 623 | S | 55% | 47% | |
| Spiro et al[41] | 62 | S + R | 77% (NED) | 65% (NED) | 95% 5-y actuarial; 84% 10-y actuarial |

S, surgery; R, irradiation; NED, no evidence of disease.
[a]Parotid, 88%; submandibular, 12%.
[b]Malignant.

## SPECIFIC HISTOLOGIES

### Pleomorphic Adenomas

Pleomorphic adenomas are the most common benign tumors and account for 80% of parotid neoplasms. They first appear in patients in their early 20s, with a mean age at presentation of 40 years. Benign mixed tumors may grow to enormous size, but they are usually 2 cm–7 cm in diameter. Consistency of the mass varies with the relative amount of connective tissue, cartilage, vascular stoma, and cystic degeneration. They are discrete, slow-growing neoplasms surrounded by an imperfect pseudocapsule that is traversed by the fingers of the tumor. Enucleation or removal with a narrow cuff of normal tissue results in recurrence in at least 20% of patients.

The histologic distinction between benign and malignant mixed (carcinoma ex-pleomorphic adenoma) tumors is only occasionally difficult. Lesions considered benign for many years may unexpectedly become clearly malignant and develop metastases. Some benign mixed tumors recur innumerable times and display a locally aggressive behavior in spite of a benign histologic appearance.

The goal of treatment is local tumor control with minimal morbidity; facial nerve preservation is key for patients with parotid tumors. Surgery is the treatment of choice.[7-11] Although an excision with wide margins is the goal, depending on the location of the tumor, this may not be possible. Because pleomorphic adenomas usually occur in the parotid, issues relating to surgery pertain mostly to the extent of parotidectomy and facial nerve preservation. Harney et al and Witt have observed that the mean thickness of the thinnest part of the capsule in superficial lobe tumors is about 0.035 mm and that focal capsular exposure occurs in virtually all parotid operations for pleomorphic adenoma.[12,13] In addition, dissecting a pleomorphic adenoma from the facial nerve leads to positive margins in approximately 25% of cases.[12,13] Obtaining wide circumferential margins with facial nerve preservation is not possible in most cases because there is no parotid tissue between the tumor–nerve interface. Despite these limitations, the likelihood of local recurrence after parotidectomy alone is very low. Therefore, RT is used only in situations where the probability of recurrence is thought to be high,[14–19] or when salvage surgery for local recurrence would be associated with an increased risk of facial nerve injury.[14,20,21]

Indications for postoperative RT include microscopically positive margins and recurrent multifocal tumors. Although gross residual disease may sometimes be controlled long term with RT alone, the probability of local control is improved if gross total resection precedes RT.[22,23] Therefore, gross tumor should be resected prior to RT, if feasible. Although intra-operative spill was once used as a sole indication for postoperative RT, this is no longer the case.[17] Similarly, close margins are no longer an indication for postoperative RT. Dose fractionation schedules are similar to those used for carcinomas. Because of the risk of RT complications, particularly in young patients, RT should be used only when complete resection with acceptable morbidity is not possible. Pleomorphic adenomas may rarely progress to a carcinoma in the absence of previous RT. Olsen and Lewis[24] reported on 73 patients treated at the Mayo Clinic (Rochester, MN) for carcinoma ex-pleomorphic adenoma; 70 of these patients (96%) had no history of prior radiotherapy to the site of the tumor. Although the risk of a malignant transformation is probably increased minimally by the use of RT, it would be nearly impossible to definitively address this issue because of the paucity of data.

The limited data pertaining to the efficacy of treatment indicates that the local control rates are >90%.[16,18] Local control and survival are worse if gross residual disease is present. Researchers at the University of Washington reported that 15-year local control rates were as follows: gross tumor, 76%; subclinical disease, 100%; and overall, 85%.[25] A series from Princess Margaret Hospital showed that 10-year relapse-free survival rates were 62% for those treated with RT for gross disease compared with 93% for those treated for subclinical disease ($p = 0.0005$).[14]

## Adenoid Cystic Carcinoma

Adenoid cystic carcinoma is a relatively uncommon malignancy that accounts for approximately 22% of all salivary gland cancers.[26] The peak incidence is in the sixth and seventh decades of life with a wide age range; there is a slight female preponderance.[27] Adenoid cystic carcinoma occurs most often in the minor salivary glands of the head and neck.[26,28,29] About two thirds occur in the minor salivary glands, while 19% occur in the parotid and 16% in the submandibular gland. The most common minor salivary gland site is the palate.[26]

Data comparing surgery alone with surgery and adjuvant RT are limited because adenoid cystic carcinomas are considered to be high-grade neoplasms and are often treated with combined modality therapy. It has been our policy to use adjuvant RT after surgery regardless of margin status in essentially all patients. The occasional patient with a grade 1 T1N0 lesion resected with widely negative margins may be observed.

The incidence of clinically positive neck nodes at diagnosis is relatively low; the risk of pathologically positive nodes was ~10% in a series from the MD Anderson Cancer Center.[29–32] Thirty-three patients with a clinically negative neck treated at the University of Florida received no elective neck treatment; the 5- and 10-year rates of neck control were 97% and 90%, respectively. However, it would seem to be prudent to electively treat the first echelon nodes for patients with primary tumors in sites that are rich in capillary lymphatics, such as the base of tongue and nasopharynx.

See Table 15-4 for results of treatment.

**TABLE 15-4 Results of Treatment for Adenoid Cystic Carcinoma**

|  | N | Treatment | 5-Yr Local Control | 10-Yr Local Control | Distant Metastases | 5-Yr DFS | 5-Yr OS |
|---|---|---|---|---|---|---|---|
| Matsuba et al[40] | 36 | Surgery/RT |  | 83% | 50%[a] |  |  |
|  | 24 | Surgery |  | 25% |  |  |  |
|  | 11 | RT |  | 41% |  |  |  |
| Miglianico et al[30] | 43 | Surgery/RT | 78% |  | 31%[a] | 54% | 72% |
|  | 38 | Surgery | 44% |  |  | 49% | 83% |
|  | 21 | RT | 66% |  |  | 47% | 79% |
| Garden et al[29] | 198 | Surgery/RT | 95% | 86% | 37%[a] | 52% | 65% |
| Cowie and Pointon[27] | 41 | Surgery/RT | 86% |  |  |  |  |
|  | 41 | RT | 37% |  |  |  |  |
| Mendenhall et al[42] | 59 | Surgery/RT | 94% | 91% | 39%[b] |  | 77% |
|  | 42 | RT | 56% | 42% |  |  | 57% |

[a]crude incidence
[b]5-yr actuarial rate
RT = radiotherapy
DFS = disease-free survival
OS = overall survival

In general, compared with single-modality therapy, combined-modality therapy appears to improve local control with no clear benefit in survival. These data, however, are subject to selection bias.

## FOLLOW-UP

Late recurrences develop in the benign mixed tumors, acinic cell carcinomas, and adenoid cystic carcinomas, requiring lifetime follow-up. Neurologic symptoms or signs in the absence of physical findings of recurrent disease are often the harbinger of perineural recurrence. MR is the preferred method of imaging as it can differentiate between postoperative changes, fibrosis, and recurrent disease. Recurrences near the base of skull can be imaged with MR and CT.

## COMPLICATIONS

Surgical complications include loss of sensation in the earlobe, gustatory sweating (Frey's syndrome) in 5%–25% of patients after parotidectomy, and temporary paresis of the facial nerve. The latter occurs in approximately 50% of uncomplicated lateral lobectomies because of intra-operative nerve manipulation, but usually resolves within 1–6 months.

RT complications mainly include xerostomia, which can usually be avoided by techniques that spare the contralateral salivary tissues. Other complications include trismus due to fibrosis of the masseter and pterygoid muscles, ankylosis of the temporomandibular joint, serous otitis media, dry ear canal, localized hair loss, and osteoradionecrosis.

## REFERENCES

1. Foote RL, Olsen KD, Bonner JA, Lewis JE. Salivary gland cancer. In: Gunderson LL, Tepper JE. *Clinical Radiation Oncology*. Philadelphia: Churchill Livingstone—A Harcourt Health Sciences Company, 2000:518–534.
2. Yu GY, Ma DQ. Carcinoma of the salivary gland: a clinicopathologic study of 405 cases. *Semin Surg Oncol* 1987;3:240–244.

3. Miller RH, Calcaterra TC, Paglia DE. Accuracy of frozen section diagnosis of parotid lesions. *Ann Otol Rhinol Laryngol* 1979;88:573–576.

4. Katz AD. Unusual lesions of the parotid gland. *J Surg Oncol* 1975;7:219–235.

5. King JJ, Fletcher GH. Malignant tumors of the major salivary glands. *Radiology* 1971; 100:381–384.

6. Parsons JT, Mendenhall WM, Bova FJ, Million RR. Head and neck cancer. In: Levitt SH, Khan FM, Potish RA. *Levitt and Tapley's Technological Basis of Radiation Therapy: Practical Clinical Applications*. Philadelphia: Lea & Febiger, 1992:203–231.

7. Laccourreye H, Laccourreye O, Cauchois R, Jouffre V, Menard M, Brasnu D. Total conservative parotidectomy for primary benign pleomorphic adenoma of the parotid gland: A 25-year experience with 229 patients. *Laryngoscope* 1994;104:1487–1494.

8. Renehan A, Gleave EN, Hancock BD, Smith P, McGurk M. Long-term follow-up of over 1000 patients with salivary gland tumours treated in a single centre. *Br J Surg* 1996;83: 1750–1754.

9. Stevens KL, Hobsley M. The treatment of pleomorphic adenomas by formal parotidectomy. *Br J Surg* 1982;69:1–3.

10. Niparko JK, Beauchamp ML, Krause CJ, Baker SR, Work WP. Surgical treatment of recurrent pleomorphic adenoma of the parotid gland. *Arch Otolaryngol Head Neck Surg* 1986;112: 1180–1184.

11. Woods JE, Weiland LH, Chong GC, Irons GB. Pathology and surgery of primary tumors of the parotid. *Surg Clin North Am* 1977;57:565–573.

12. Harney MS, Murphy C, Hone S, Toner M, Timon CV. A histological comparison of deep and superficial lobe pleomorphic adenomas of the parotid gland. *Head Neck* 2003;24:649–653.

13. Witt RL. The significance of the margin in parotid surgery for pleomorphic adenoma. *Laryngoscope* 2002;112:2141–2151.

14. Liu FF, Rotstein L, Davison AJ, Pintilie M, O'Sullivan B, Payne DG, Warde P, Cummings B. Benign parotid adenomas: a review of the Princess Margaret Hospital experience. *Head Neck* 1995;17: 177–183.

15. Ravasz LA, Terhaard CH, Hordijk GJ. Radiotherapy in epithelial tumors of the parotid gland: case presentation and literature review. *Int J Radiat Oncol Biol Phys* 1990;19:55–59.

16. Barton J, Slevin NJ, Gleave EN. Radiotherapy for pleomorphic adenoma of the parotid gland. *Int J Radiat Oncol Biol Phys* 1992;22:925–928.

17. Buchman C, Stringer SP, Mendenhall WM, Parsons JT, Jordan JR, Cassisi NJ. Pleomorphic adenoma: effect of tumor spill and inadequate resection on tumor recurrence. *Laryngoscope* 1994;104:1231–1234.

18. Dawson AK, Orr JA. Long-term results of local excision and radiotherapy in pleomorphic adenoma of the parotid. *Int J Radiat Oncol Biol Phys* 1985;11:451–455.

19. Spraggs PD, Rose DS, Grant HR, Gallimore AP. Post-irradiation carcinosarcoma of the parotid gland. *J Laryngol Otol* 1994;108:443–445.

20. Fee WE, Jr., Goffinet DR, Calcaterra TC. Mixed tumors of the parotid gland—results of surgical therapy. *Laryngoscope* 1978;88:265–273.

21. Maran AG, Mackenzie IJ, Stanley RE. Recurrent pleomorphic adenomas of the parotid gland. *Arch Otolaryngol* 1984;110:167–171.

22. Ghosh S, Panarese A, Bull PD, Lee JA. Marginally excised parotid pleomorphic salivary adenomas: risk factors for recurrence and management. A 12.5-year mean follow-up study of histologically marginal excisions. *Clin Otolaryngol* 2003;28:262–266.

23. Samson MJ, Metson R, Wang CC, Montgomery WW. Preservation of the facial nerve in the management of recurrent pleomorphic adenoma. *Laryngoscope* 1991;101:1060–1062.

24. Olsen KD, Lewis JE. Carcinoma ex-pleomorphic adenoma: a clinicopathologic review. *Head Neck* 2001;23:705–712.

25. Douglas JG, Einck J, Austin-Seymour M, Koh WJ, Laramore GE. Neutron radiotherapy for recurrent pleomorphic adenomas of major salivary glands. *Head Neck* 2001;23:1037–1042.

26. Spiro RH. Salivary neoplasms: overview of a 35-year experience with 2,807 patients. *Head Neck Surg* 1986;8:177–184.

27. Cowie VJ, Pointon RCS. Adenoid cystic carcinoma of the salivary glands. *Clin Radiol* 1984;35:331–333.

28. Douglas JG, Laramore GE, Austin-Seymour M, Koh W, Stelzer K, Griffin TW. Treatment of locally advanced adenoid cystic carcinoma of the head and neck with neutron radiotherapy. *Int J Radiat Oncol Biol Phys* 2000;46:551–557.

29. Garden AS, Weber RS, Morrison WH, Ang KK, Peters LJ. The influence of positive margins and nerve invasion in adenoid cystic carcinoma of the head and neck treated with surgery and radiation. *Int J Radiat Oncol Biol Phys* 1995;32:619–626.

30. Miglianico L, Eschwege F, Marandas P, Wibault P. Cervico-facial adenoid cystic carcinoma: study of 102 cases. Influence of radiation therapy. *Int J Radiat Oncol Biol Phys* 1987;13:673–678.

31. Frankenthaler RA, Byers RM, Luna MA, Callender DL, Wolf P, Goepfert H. Predicting occult lymph node metastasis in parotid cancer. *Arch Otolaryngol Head Neck Surg* 1993;119:517–520.

32. Armstrong JG, Harrison LB, Thaler HT, Friedlander-Klar H, Fass DE, Zelefsky MJ, Shah JP, Strong EW, Spiro RH. The indications for elective treatment of the neck in cancer of the major salivary glands. *Cancer* 1992;69:615–619.

33. Spiro RH, Koss LG, Hajdu SI, Strong EW. Tumors of minor salivary origin: a clinicopathologic study of 492 cases. *Cancer* 1973;31:117–129.

34. Guillamondegui OM, Byers RM, Luna MA, Chiminazzo HJr, Jesse RH, Fletcher GH. Aggressive surgery in treatment for parotid cancer: the role of adjunctive postoperative radiotherapy. *Am J Roentgenol Radium Ther Nucl Med* 1975;123:49–54.

35. Kagan AR, Nussbaum H, Handler S, Shapiro R, Gilbert HA, Jacobs M, Miles JW, Chan PY, Calcaterra T. Recurrences from malignant parotid salivary gland tumors. *Cancer* 1976;37:2600–2004.

36. Rafla S. Malignant parotid tumors: natural history and treatment. *Cancer* 1977;40:136–144.

37. Fu KK, Leibel SA, Levine ML, Friedlander LM, Boles R, Phillips TL. Carcinoma of the major and minor salivary glands: analysis of treatment results and sites and causes of failures. *Cancer* 1977;40:2882–2890.

38. Beahrs OH, Woolner LB, Carveth SW, Devine KD. Surgical management of parotid lesions: review of seven hundred sixty cases. *Arch Surg* 1960;80:890–904.

39. McNaney D, McNeese MD, Guillamondegui OM, Fletcher GH, Oswald MJ. Postoperative irradiation in malignant epithelial tumors of the parotid. *Int J Radiat Oncol Biol Phys* 1983;9:1289–1295.

40. Matsuba HM, Thawley SE, Devineni VR, Levine LA, Smith PG. High-grade malignancies of the parotid gland: effective use of planned combined surgery and irradiation. *Laryngoscope* 1985;95:1059–1063.

41. Spiro IJ, Wang CC, Montgomery WW. Carcinoma of the parotid gland: analysis of treatment results and patterns of failure after combined surgery and radiation therapy. *Cancer* 1993;71:2699–2705.

42. Mendenhall WM, Morris CG, Amdur RJ, Werning JW, Hinerman RW, Villaret DB. Radiotherapy alone or combined with surgery for adenoid cystic carcinoma of the head and neck. *Head Neck* 2004;26:154–162.

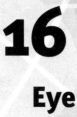

# 16

## Eye

*Sung Kim, MD*

## Overview

The eye and orbit are susceptible to a variety of both malignant and nonmalignant conditions. Radiation often plays a central role in curing or palliating these conditions while preserving useful vision. The use of radiation in this region must be tempered with knowledge of many sensitive normal structures, and the relative risks and benefits of radiation.

## Anatomy

The *eyeball* is comprised of three layers:

- Sclera: tough, fibrous outer layer, continuous with the cornea anteriorly
- Uvea: middle layer is vascular, contains melanocytes, and includes the choroid, ciliary body, and iris
- Retina: inner, delicate, light sensing layer

The optic nerve enters the retina at the optic disk. The optic disk contains only nerve fibers and no photoreceptor cells, so it is insensitive to light (a blind spot).[1] Lateral to the optic disk is a small, oval area called the macula, the central part of which (fovea) is the site of most acute vision. The functional part of the retina terminates anteriorly at the ora serrata, just posterior to the ciliary body. The central retinal artery (branch of the ophthalmic artery) and the central vein of the retina travel with the optic nerve.

The *bony orbit* is made up of seven bones and is shaped like a four-sided pyramid, its apex pointed posteriorly. It contains the globe, six extraocular muscles, supporting vasculature and nerves, and fat. Important nerves and vasculature enter the orbit as follows:

- Optic foramen —transmits CN II (optic nerve), ophthalmic artery, central vein of retina
- Superior orbital fissure —transmits CN III (oculomotor), CN IV (trochlear), CN VI (abducens), and CN V(1) (ophthalmic), superior and inferior ophthalmic veins
  —communicates between the orbit and middle cranial fossa (cavernous sinus)

- Inferior orbital fissure  –transmits CN V(2) (maxillary) and its zygomatic branches
  –communicates between the orbit and the pterygopalatine/ infratemporal fossae

## RESPONSE OF ORBITAL STRUCTURES TO RADIATION

A. The **lens** is the most radiosensitive organ in the body. Cataract development is a deterministic late effect, there is a minimum threshold below which they do not occur. The lens has decreased radiation tolerance with 1) single vs. multiple fractions and 2) shorter vs. longer time of delivery:

| fractionation and time of delivery | minimum dose to cause cataract |
|---|---|
| single fraction | 2 Gy |
| multiple fractions over 3 weeks–3 months | 4 Gy |
| multiple fractions over > 3 months | 5.5 Gy |

Clinically, there is a huge distinction between small, stationary cataracts that cause little visual impairment and progressive cataracts causing significant visual loss. The higher the dose, the more likely the cataract is to be progressive, and the shorter the latent period until it develops.[2]

| dose | latent period | probability cataract will be progressive |
|---|---|---|
| 2.5–6.5 Gy | 8 years | $1/3$ |
| 6.51–11.5 Gy | 4 years | $2/3$ |

B. **Eyelashes** help initiate a protective blink reflex, so their loss can result in irritation of the conjunctivae and cornea. There can be temporary loss of eyelashes with a dose around 10 Gy delivered over a few days. Hungerford reported loss of eyelashes at 20-30 Gy in 2-3 Gy fractions.[3] Any eyelashes that regrow may be shorter or lighter in color, and there is a risk of trichiasis (lashes grow toward the cornea and cause irritation).[2]

C. **Lacrimal gland.** Tear film is made up of three layers:

- Outer lipid layer from sebaceous glands reduces evaporation
- Middle aqueous layer from major and accessory lacrimal glands
- Inner mucinous layer from conjunctival goblet cells

The toxicity of radiation to the lacrimal gland is dry eye syndrome, which can result in visual loss secondary to corneal opacification, ulceration, and vascularization. The cornea is richly enervated, so pain from a dry eye can be considerable, resulting in sensitivity to light or wind.

Parsons used University of Florida data and a literature search to report the incidence of severe dry eye complications sufficient to cause visual loss:[4]

| dose | incidence severe dry eye |
|---|---|
| <30 Gy | 0% |
| 30–39 Gy | 5%–25% |
| 40–49 Gy | 23%–50% |
| >57 Gy | 100% |

D. **Corneal** complications are a result of 1) direct effect of radiation on the cornea and 2) indirect effect of radiation causing lacrimal gland dysfunction. Corneal injury occurs as a progression of insults, and antibiotics and steroids may be helpful in recovery:

- Punctate keratitis is development of tiny ulcers, apparent on fluorescein or Bengal rose staining. They usually occur after 30–50 Gy delivered over 4–5 weeks. It can occur during or months after treatment. In most cases, keratitis will subside over 4–6 weeks.
- Corneal edema occurs with 40–50 Gy. It can be a transient condition, but can also persist indefinitely, most frequently with doses >50 Gy, and usually around 70–80 Gy.
- Corneal ulceration is essentially coalescence of the tiny ulcers of punctate keratitis. It has been reported with doses as low as 20 Gy delivered in a single dose, but Merriam notes that most corneas will tolerate 40–50 Gy delivered over 4–5 weeks. Late toxicity appears with doses over 50 Gy.[2]

E. **Retinal** toxicity is caused by damage to retinal capillary endothelium. Findings on ophthalmic examination include retinal hemorrhages, microaneurysms, hard exudates, cotton wool spots, telangiectasias.

Parsons reported on 68 retinae in 64 patients treated with fractionated external beam radiation. When dose was <45 Gy, no one experienced decrease in vision to worse than 20/200. Above 45 Gy, toxicity rose sharply with dose.

| dose | vision decreased to 20/200 or worse |
|------|------|
| <45 Gy | 0% |
| 45–55 Gy | 50% |
| 55–65 Gy | 83% |
| >65 Gy | 100% |

There was a trend toward increased risk with fraction size >1.9 Gy, and they recommended fraction size not exceeding 1.8–1.9 Gy. The median time to onset of symptoms was 2.5 years.[5]

F. **Optic nerve and chiasm.** Parsons reported on 215 optic nerves in 131 patients receiving EBRT with daily or BID fractionation, and total doses ranging from <30 Gy to >75 Gy. No optic neuropathy developed in 106 optic nerves receiving less than 59 Gy. For those patients receiving ≥60 Gy, the risk of optic neuropathy depended more heavily on fraction size than total dose. Median time to development of symptoms was protracted, at over 2 years.[6]

| fraction size | vision decreased to 20/100 or worse |
|------|------|
| <1.9 Gy | 11% |
| ≥1.9 Gy | 47% |

Jiang similarly reported dramatically increased risk of optic nerve/chiasm injury above 60 Gy. Median fraction size for the optic nerve and chiasm were 2.2 Gy (1.1–2.5 Gy) and 2 Gy (0.43–2.6 Gy) respectively.[7]

| | no injury below | injury at 50–60 Gy | injury at >60 Gy |
|------|------|------|------|
| Optic nerve | 56 Gy | 3% | 34% |
| Optic chiasm | 50 Gy | 8% | 24% |

Considering that in these two studies, only one patient developed optic nerve or chiasm injury at doses <55 Gy, 54 Gy would seem a very reasonable limit for these structures in treatment planning. When dose must be escalated for tumor control, patients must be advised of the possibility of visual impairment.

G. The **Sclera** is extremely radio resistant, as evidenced by the large radiation doses it is subject to during radioactive plaque treatment for melanoma. Atrophy of the sclera involves areas of thinning that allow the uvea to be seen through them. They produce no symptoms, and doses of 200-300 Gy are most likely to cause this condition.[2]

## CHOROIDAL MELANOMA

Ocular melanoma constitutes about 5% of all melanomas.[8] They occur rarely in the conjunctivae or orbit, the vast majority originating in the uvea. The most common uveal site is the choroid, followed by ciliary body, and least commonly, the iris. It is a disease of an older population, with a peak incidence around age 70, and a slight male predominance. Among risk factors, race is the most important. Uveal melanoma is about 150 times more common in whites than blacks, and is also less common among Asians.[9] Though not as established as in cutaneous melanoma, there is accumulating evidence that sunlight exposure is a risk factor.[10] Blue or grey eye color is reported to be a risk factor for uveal melanoma, and also for subsequent development of metastases.[11,12] The diagnosis is made clinically via indirect ophthalmoscopy and ancillary studies like fluorescein angiography and ultrasound. The accuracy of clinical diagnosis among Collaborative Ocular Melanoma Study patients was reported as greater than 99%.[13]

The growth pattern of choroidal melanomas may be inward toward the vitreous, involving first Bruch's membrane (between the choroid and retina) and then the retina. They can also grow outward, into sclera and then orbital tissues. As there are no lymphatic channels within the eye metastasis occurs hematogenously. When lymph node metastases do occur, it is usually after extensive extraocular spread to the conjunctivae, adnexae, or orbital lymphatics.[14]

While roughly 50% of patients with posterior uveal melanoma will develop liver metastases within 15 years, metastases at initial presentation are rare, perhaps indicating subclinical metastases at the time of local treatment.[15] Per SEER data, the relative 5-year survival rate from 1973 to 1997 was 77%–84%, with no significant variation from year to year. Singh writes that the consistency of survival rates indicates that 1) recent treatment advances have not improved survival and 2) neither has the trend toward eye-sparing treatment compromised it.[9]

---

### BOX 16-1

T1  ≤10 mm greatest diameter and ≤2.5 mm thickness
   a. without extraocular extension
   b. with microscopic extraocular extension
   c. with macroscopic extraocular extension
T2  >10 mm but ≤16 mm in greatest diameter and between 2.5–10 mm thickness
   a. without extraocular extension
   b. with microscopic extraocular extension
   c. with macroscopic extraocular extension
T3  >16 mm in greatest diameter and/or >10 mm thickness, without extraocular extension
T4  >16 mm in greatest diameter and/or >10 mm thickness, with extraocular extension

Green FL, Page DL, Fleming ID et al, eds. *AJCC Cancer Staging Handbook From the AJCC Staging Manual Sixth Edition*. Springer-Verlag, 2002.

---

## TREATMENT

Historically, the treatment of choice was enucleation, but the trend is toward eye preserving therapies. Options include:

- observation (for small lesions that have a borderline classification between large benign nevus and early melanoma)

- radiation therapy (episcleral plaque brachytherapy or charged particle radiation with helium ions or protons)
- transpupillary thermotherapy and local resection are used less frequently
- enucleation is usually reserved for treatment failure, when vision is already lost, or when the lesion is large enough that the chance of retaining useful vision is minimal

Though eye-sparing treatments have decreased the morbidity of local treatment, perhaps the more important issue is of systemic metastases, and this has not been improved. To date, no specific local treatment has proven superior in terms of preventing metastases.[16]

## Observation for Small Melanomas

A central problem in treating small choroidal lesions is that clinical diagnosis is uncertain, compared to medium or large lesions where clinical diagnosis is extremely accurate. A clinician may have difficulty differentiating between a benign choroidal nevus vs. small choroidal melanoma. Growth of the lesion is a presumed indicator of malignant potential, though there are documented cases of stable melanomas and conversely, of growing nevi.[17]

Shields relates the important finding that in small pigmented choroidal lesions, growth is related to metastatic risk (not surprising considering that growth increases the odds of malignancy vs. nevus), and then outlines risk factors for growth.

---

### BOX 16-2

First paper was a retrospective review of 1,329 patients with small melanocytic choroidal lesions ≤3 mm thick. Tumor growth occurred in 18%, metastases in 3%, and were related in that growth conferred a 3 times risk of metastases vs. no growth. Risk factors for growth included:

- thickness >2 mm
- posterior tumor margin touching optic disc
- visual symptoms
- orange pigment
- subretinal fluid

Second paper details risk of growth, given the number of positive risk factors:

| # risk factors | 5-year risk of tumor growth |
| --- | --- |
| 0 | 4% |
| 1 | 36% |
| 2 | 45% |
| 3–5 | 50%–56% |

The authors conclude that observation is reasonable for patients with none, or even one risk factor, especially if the tumor is in a visually important location.

Shields CL, Shields JA, Kiratli H et al. Risk factors for growth and metastasis of small choroidal melanocytic lesions. *Ophthalmology* 102(9):1351–61, 1995.

Shields CL, Cater J, Shields JA et al. Combination of clinical factors predictive of growth of small choroidal melanocytic tumors. *Arch Ophthalmology* 118: 360–364, 2000.

---

Proponents of early treatment could argue that clearly, larger lesions are associated with more metastases and worse survival. Proponents of observation could rightly claim that there is no definitive proof that treating early lesions prior to growth improves survival, and that any treatment has associated toxicity (in practice, most small melanomas are observed for growth). Given the opposing viewpoints, and lack of randomized data, the decision to treat seems reasonably made on the basis of risk factors for growth.

## Plaque Brachytherapy for Medium Size Melanomas

Plaque brachytherapy (usually with [125]I) is a common treatment modality for medium size lesions (2.5–10 mm thickness and ≤16 mm diameter).[18] A COMS trial compared plaque brachytherapy vs. enucleation.

### BOX 16-3

1,317 patients with medium size choroidal melanomas (2.5–10 mm height and 16 mm diameter) were randomized to [125]I plaque brachytherapy vs. enucleation.

No difference in overall survival. In the brachytherapy arm, 5-year local failure was 10.3% and enucleation rate was 12.5%. The most common cause of enucleation over the Fist 3 yers was local recurrence and afterward was ocular pain. Risk factors for recurrence were:

• older age
• greater tumor thickness
• proximity of tumor to the foveal avascular zone

By 3 yers, 49% had lost six lines or more of visual acuity, most strongly associated with greater apical height and shorter distance to foveal avascular zone. Diabetes, tumor associated retinal detachment, tumors that were not dome shaped were also risk factors for loss of vision.

Jampol LM, Moy CS, Murray TG et al. The COMS randomized trial of Iodine 125 brachytherapy for choroidal melanoma IV. Local Treatment failure and enucleation in the first 5 years after brachytherapy. COMS Report No. 19. *Ophthalmology* 109(12): 2197–2206, 2002.

Collaborative Ocular Melanoma Study (COMS) randomized trial of I-125 brachytherapy for medium choroidal melanoma. I. Visual acuity after 3 years. COMS Report No. 16. *Ophthalmology* 108 (2): 348–366, 2001.

The American Brachytherapy Society notes that peripapillary (close to optic disc) lesions have worse local control and worse visual outcome. Patients with gross extrascleral invasion, ring melanoma, and involvement of more than half the ciliary body are not candidates for plaque brachytherapy. They recommend a minimum [125]I dose of 85 Gy delivered to the apex at a rate of 0.6–1.05 Gy/hr using AAPM TG-43 formalism in 3–7 consecutive days.[18]

## Charged Particle Radiation

Both protons and helium ions have been used successfully to treat uveal melanomas. Their associated Bragg peak allows for highly localized treatment, making them very good options to treat lesions near the optic disc or macula. There is randomized data favoring charged particle radiation over plaque brachytherapy.

In a randomized trial of proton doses, Gragoudas compared lower (50 Gy) vs. standard (70 Gy) doses in patients more likely to have functional disability related to treatment than to tumor (small to medium size tumors close to the optic disc or macula). At 5 years, there was no difference in local or systemic control, or visual acuity. They did report less visual field loss in the 50 Gy arm.[19]

## Enucleation

The trend is away from enucleation. The American Brachytherapy Society notes that enucleation is employed for those patients with blind, painful eyes, with tumor involving >40% of intraocular

---

**BOX 16-4**

184 patients with uveal melanomas <10 mm thick and <15 mm diameter were randomized to helium ion radiation vs $^{125}$I brachytherapy. All patients received 70 Gy equivalents (relative biologic effect for helium was 1.3 and for $^{125}$I was 1.0). At a median follow up of 55 months, the following was reported:

|  | tumor regrowth | enucleation | visual loss >4 lines | metastatic death |
|---|---|---|---|---|
| helium ion | 0% | 9.3% | 69% | 8% |
| brachytherapy | 13.3% | 17.3% | 69% | 8% |

Note that all the helium arm enucleations were due to complications, not local recurrence.

In general, anterior segment complications (neovascular glaucoma, dry eye, eyelash loss, epiphora) were more common in the helium arm. Vitreous hemorrhage and secondary strabismus were more common in the $^{125}$I arm. 7/13 local failures in the brachytherapy arm were relatively large, flat melanomas <1 mm from the optic nerve. The authors conclude that these tumors would have better local control with helium ions, though visual acuity would remain poor.

Char DH, Quivey JM, Castro JR et al. Helium ions versus iodine 125 brachytherapy in the management of uveal melanoma: a prospective, randomized, dynamically balanced trial. *Ophthalmology* 100(10): 1547–1554, 1993.

---

volume, eyes with neovascular glaucoma, or patients with medium/large lesions who do not want an organ sparing approach.[18]

Because of the high rate of eventual metastases (particularly to the liver), it has been hypothesized that manipulation of the globe during enucleation disseminates tumor cells, resulting in increased metastases. A COMS randomized trial asked whether preoperative radiation would decrease the rate of metastases.

---

**BOX 16-5**

1,003 patients with large choroidal melanomas >10 mm thickness or >16 mm diameter were randomized to enucleation ± pre-enucleation radiation to 20 Gy in 4 Gy fractions. There was no difference in 5-year overall survival: 62% for pre-enucleation RT arm vs 57% for enucleation alone. On MV analysis, only age and diameter correlated to survival.

The Collaborative Ocular Melanoma Study (COMS) randomized trial of pre-enucleation radiation of large choroidal melanoma II: initial mortality findings COMS report No. 10. *Am J Ophthalmol* 125(6):779–96, 1998.

---

## SUMMARY

- trend is for eye-sparing local therapy.
- though controversial, observation may be appropriate treatment for small, low-risk choroidal lesions.
- in medium size choroidal lesions, plaque brachytherapy vs enucleation does not compromise survival. Nearly 90% will retain their eye, but there is significant risk of visual acuity loss.
- charged particle radiation may offer better local control than plaque brachytherapy in medium size uveal lesions.
- enucleation is appropriate when vision is already lost, or when the tumor is large with little hope of retaining useful vision.

- eventual systemic metastasis is of great concern in this disease.
  - no local treatment has been demonstrated to be superior in this regard.
  - systemic adjuvant treatment has not been well evaluated.

## CHOROIDAL METASTASES

Metastases are the most common intraocular tumors. Autopsy studies of solid tumors of all types indicate a 4%–12% incidence of asymptomatic choroidal metastases.[20] The incidence of symptomatic lesions is much lower, estimated at about 2%. One might expect that as systemic therapy and survival for metastatic disease improve in the future, we may see even more uveal metastases.

As in uveal melanoma, diagnosis is typically a clinical one, and rarely is biopsy required. Overall survival is generally poor. In the Wiegel study which follows, median survival was about 7 months, while breast primaries did slightly better at 10 months. The Shields data presented in Box 16-6 are instructive regarding epidemiology.

---

### BOX 16-6

This was a report of 950 uveal metastases in 420 patients. Regarding location in the uvea:

- 88%  choroid
- 9%  iris
- 2%  ciliary body

Initially, 34% had no prior diagnosis of malignancy. Of those with known primaries, breast and lung were by far the most common, accounting for 47% and 21%, respectively. About 24% of patients had bilateral lesions. Symptoms were blurred vision (70%), flashes and floaters (12%), pain (7%), none (11%).

Shields CA, Shields JA, Gross NE et al. Survey of 520 eyes with uveal metastases. *Ophthalmol* 104: 1265–76, 1997.

---

Options for treatment include:

- systemic treatment, with local therapy held in reserve
- external beam radiation with photons or electrons
- less typically, charged particle radiation or plaque brachytherapy

**Systemic therapy** is a reasonable first line treatment. Letson reported on eight eyes (in six patients) with choroidal metastases from breast cancer treated with chemotherapy, without radiation. The chemotherapy regimens included cyclophosphamide and fluorouracil, along with other combinations of drugs. Tumor regressed in all eight eyes, with vision improving in five, and maintained in three eyes with good initial vision.[21]

**External beam radiation** can offer excellent palliation, with a high rate of visual stabilization. Typical doses are around 30–40 Gy in 2–3 Gy fractions.

The most common complication with external beam radiation is dry eye. Other complications such as development of cataracts or retinopathy are rare, likely due to poor survival time.[22]

**Charged particle radiation** is also a reasonable option. Tsina reported on 76 eyes treated with focal proton beam radiation with two fractions of 14 cobalt grey equivalents. Forty-seven percent of patients had stable or improved vision, 84% of tumors regressed completely, and 82% of retinal detachments resolved. Complications occurred in 56%, but no treated eyes required enucleation. They point out that requiring only two radiation treatments is very advantageous in this population with short survival.[23]

**Plaque brachytherapy** may be helpful in selected cases. Shields reported on 36 patients selected for having solitary metastases measuring 10 mm or less in thickness and 16 mm or less in diameter. They additionally had either failed other treatments (six had failed external beam radiation) or had no active systemic disease. Visual acuity improved in 19%, was stable in 39%, and decreased in 42%. Plaque brachytherapy was able to salvage 5/6 eyes failing external beam radiation.[22]

## SUMMARY

- uveal metastases are relatively common, and by far the most common primaries are breast and lung cancer.
- they can be treated with systemic therapy, if vision remains stable.
- external beam radiation with photons or electrons improves or stabilizes vision in the vast majority of cases. Typical dose is 30-40 Gy in 2-3 Gy fractions, and unilateral radiation may be helpful in prophylaxing the contralateral eye.
- charged particle radiation may be advantageous because of a short treatment time.
- plaque brachytherapy is a reasonable choice in solitary metastases that are not too large, and have failed other treatments.

## ORBITAL LYMPHOMA

One can roughly categorize ocular lymphoma as intraocular vs. orbital.

Lymphoid tumors are the most common *primary* orbital malignancies in adults. A large French series of orbital and intraocular lymphomas is instructive regarding histology and location:[24]

- 82% were low-grade NHL, the majority being MALT
- 18% were high-grade NHL, the majority being diffuse large B cell lymphoma
- Site of disease was intra-orbital 42%, conjunctival 35%, palpebral 9%, lacrimal 8%, intra-ocular 5%.

## Orbital Lymphomas

Primary orbital lymphomas can be subdivided into low-(MALT, follicular grade 1,2) vs. high-grade (DLBCL). Low-grade disease is very successfully treated with radiation alone. Zhou reported on 62 eyes in 56 patients with orbital lymphoma, predominantly MALT (48%) or follicular (30%) subtype. They were treated to a median dose of 30 Gy in 1.5–2.5 Gy, with 98% local control (100% for indolent lymphomas).[25] Primary high-grade orbital lymphomas are treated similarly to their

**FIGURE 16-1** Eye lymphoma flowchart.

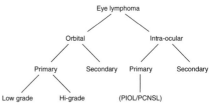

nodal counterparts, with systemic chemotherapy followed by radiation.[26] Bolek recommends a dos
tailored to chemotherapy response, 30 Gy for complete response and 40 Gy for partial response.[27]

In contrast to primary orbital lymphoma, most secondary orbital lymphomas are intermediat
to high grade. MDACC reported a series of 15 patients with secondary orbital NHL. Thirteen wer
treated with systemic therapy, plus or minus radiation and 11 achieved complete regression of th
orbital tumor, and another had partial regression. Five patients (33%) presented with optic nerv
compression and visual loss. Three were diagnosed early enough that chemotherapy was institute
and vision was saved; one had irreversible loss of vision; one died shortly thereafter.[28]

## Primary Intra-ocular Lymphoma

Primary CNS lymphoma (PCNSL) is typically a diffuse large B cell lymphoma. Primary intra-ocula
lymphoma (PIOL) is a subset of PCNSL where disease is detected in the eye but not in the rest of th
CNS. The majority of PIOL (about 2/3) will have undiagnosed CNS spread at the time of diagnosis
Conversely, 15%–25% of patients with PCNSL will have ocular involvement at the time of diagnosis
These diseases are relatively rare, with about 1,000 cases of PCNSL/year and 100 new cases/3 year
of PIOL in the United States. AIDS is a risk factor, and there is a slight male predominance. Media
age of diagnosis is the late 50s and 60s.

The most common sites of ocular involvement are the vitreous, retina, and subretinal pigmen
epithelium. Patients will often complain of floaters and mildly decreased vision. Distribution i
bilateral in at least 80% of cases. As PIOL often involves the CNS and very rarely metastasizes else
where, staging centers around neuroimaging and cytologic analysis of CSF. PIOL diagnosis is patho
logic, so if CSF cytology is negative, a vitreous biopsy is required.[29]

In the past, radiation to the posterior 2/3 of both globes has been a mainstay of treatment for PIOL
but prognosis was poor. Even when prophylactic brain radiation was added to globe radiation for PIOL
it often did not prevent CNS spread. Freeman reported two cases in which prophylactic whole brain R
(to 44.7 Gy in one pt) was offered in addition to globe radiation, and CNS spread occurred anyway
Recent treatment for PIOL has paralleled that for PCNSL, shifting away from primary radiation, an
more toward primary methotrexate-based chemotherapy, with or without local radiation therapy.[29-3]

## SUMMARY

- primary intraocular lymphoma is most commonly DLBCL; primary orbital lymphomas are
  usually low-grade NHL, though they can be high grade also.
- trend in PIOL or PCNSL with ocular involvement is away from radiation and towar
  methotrexate-based chemotherapy.
- primary low-grade orbital lymphomas are very successfully treated with radiation alone to
  about 30 Gy.
- primary high-grade orbital lymphomas are treated similarly to their nodal counterparts
  with sequential chemotherapy and radiation.
- in contrast to primary orbital lymphomas, most secondary orbital lymphomas are aggressive
  vigilance and early treatment (often chemotherapy) for optic nerve compression can preven
  permanent visual loss.

## GRAVES' OPHTHALMOPATHY

Graves' disease is an autoimmune condition associated with the clinical triad of hyperthyroidism
ophthalmopathy, pretibial dermopathy (rare). There is increasing evidence that the target of the
autoimmune response in the orbit is the TSH receptor.[32] The net result is deposition of gly
cosaminoglycans into the orbital fat and muscles, swelling of the orbital contents, and resultan
compressive symptoms. Most patients suffer only minor congestive signs such as chemosis, injec

ion, and lid edema that are self-limited to several months in duration. In some, the disease will progress to exophthalmos, extraocular muscle dysfunction, and periorbital edema. Rarely, optic neuropathy can cause visual deficits.[33] Classic imaging finding is enlargement of the belly of the extraocular muscles. Typical sparing of the tendinous attachment at the orbital apex can help differentiate from orbital pseudotumor.[34]

About 20%–25% of patients with Graves' hyperthyroidism will develop clinical Graves' ophthalmopathy. Interestingly, the timing of ophthalmopathy usually does not coincide with hyperthyroidism. Bartley reported a series in which the majority of ophthalmopathy occurred after, some prior, and only 20% concurrent with hyperthyroidism.[35] One must be careful not to confuse the proptosis and periorbital edema of Graves' ophthalmopathy with the lid lag and stare associated with excess thyroid hormone (due to contraction of the levator palpebrae muscle). Risk factors for developing Graves' ophthalmopathy include:

- smoking
- gender (more common in women, but may be more severe in men)
- genetics
- type of treatment (radioiodine, but not antithyroid medication or thyroidectomy, can hasten or exacerbate ophthalmopathy)

Possible treatment options for Graves' ophthalmopathy include corticosteroids, surgery, and radiation. Oral prednisone is typically first line treatment. Optimal dose is unclear, and Rx range is from 30–40 mg/day up to around 100 mg/day. Indications for surgery include:

- progressive disease despite corticosteroids or radiation
- vision-threatening changes to optic nerve, retina, cornea
- cosmetic correction of severe proptosis[36]

Goh reported on 57 decompressions for optic neuropathy, and 94% had improvement or stabilization of vision. Significantly, 30% had new or worse diplopia following decompression, probably due to asymmetric displacement of already hypertrophied extraocular muscles.[37]

Radiation is typically reserved for patients who are unresponsive to or intolerant of steroids. Though some authors offer ipsilateral radiation, paired laterals are typical, as this condition is often bilateral. A typical dose is 20 Gy in 2 Gy fractions. Peterson noted no advantage to 30 Gy compared to 20 Gy. He also reported that proptosis and eye muscle function responded less well to radiation than soft tissue signs, corneal involvement, and sight loss. Corrective surgery was still required in 29% after RT, usually for eye muscle dysfunction.[38]

A surprisingly large number of randomized trials have investigated the role of radiation in Graves' ophthalmopathy. EBRT was compared to sham radiation in mild Graves' ophthalmopathy, and was found to improve extraocular movement and diplopia, but not proptosis.[39] In a negative trial, Gorman treated one orbit with EBRT and the other with sham RT, then reversed therapies 6 months later.[40] EBRT has been found to be equally efficacious as prednisone, and the combination of the two is better than either modality alone.[41,42,43] When combining EBRT and steroids, IV methylprednisolone was more efficacious and better tolerated than oral prednisone.[44] Kahaly compared 20 Gy in 20 wks, 10 Gy in 2 weeks, 20 Gy in 2 weeks, and reported improved efficacy in the 20 week regimen.[45]

# SUMMARY

- First line treatment for Graves' ophthalmopathy is typically corticosteroids, with EBRT (typical dose 20 Gy in 2 Gy fractions) employed when the patient is unresponsive to or intolerant of steroids.
- corticosteroids and EBRT are similarly efficacious, and the combination of steroids (IV better than oral) and EBRT is better than either modality alone.

- EBRT may be more effective in alleviating soft tissue signs, corneal involvement and sight loss than proptosis or extraocular muscle motility.

## PTERYGIUM

Pterygium is a benign growth on the ocular surface, typically originating at the nasal conjunctivae and extending across to the cornea. It is so named (G. pteryos) for its typical wing shape. Reported risk factors include sun exposure, male gender, outdoor work, low education level, older age, black race.[46,47,48] The diagnosis is clinical and made by the classic appearance of a wedge-shaped lesion extending from the conjunctiva to the cornea. Pterygia can be differentiated from pinguecula by the latter's tendency to stay confined to the conjunctivae.

The natural history of pterygium varies tremendously from case to case. They can be active (red and thickened) and grow over months to years, or inactive (white and flat) and remain stable for decades. Pterygium can threaten vision by blocking the visual axis, or by inducing irregular astigmatism.

Recurrence following excision alone is frequent, reported between 35%–68%. There are multiple means to reduce the risk of recurrence including:

- conjunctival flap (sliding, rotational, free)
- mitomycin C (intra-operative or postoperative)
- B radiation ($^{90}$Sr)
- amniotic membrane transplantation

There are more than 30 reported series of postoperative $^{90}$Sr radiation, with widely varying doses from 10–70 Gy. They report 0%–20% recurrence rate, most commonly around 5%–8%.[50] A large series was reported by the North Florida Pterygium Study Group.

There is also a randomized controlled trial confirming the value of a single postoperative radiation dose vs. sham radiation. $^{90}$Sr was used to deliver 25 Gy to the scleral surface at 2–2.5 Gy/min. At 18 months, radiation reduced recurrence from 67% to 7%.[50]

---

### BOX 16-8

Eight hundred twenty-five pterygia in 690 patients were treated with surgery and $^{90}$SR. Dose was 60 Gy in 6 weekly fractions, starting within 24 hours of surgery. At a median of over 8 years there were only 1.7% recurrences (of the 14 recurrences, nine had undergone less than five treatments). They reported no major complications.

Paryani SB, Scott WP, Wells JW et al. Management of pterygium with surgery and radiation therapy. *Int J Radiat Oncol Biol Physics* 28:101–103, 1994.

---

Pajic reported on *primary* radiation for early pterygium. They treated 54 pterygia in 43 patients using $^{90}$Sr to 50 Gy in 4 weekly fractions. At a median of 96 months, they report no recurrences (defined as progressive growth), and no major complications. The local radiation did result in a thin grey avascular pannus.[49]

## SUMMARY

- rates of recurrence of pterygium following bare sclera surgery are unacceptably high, and adjunctive therapy is required.
- the reported radiation doses and schemes for postoperative B radiation vary greatly, but a reasonable schedule might be the one used by North Florida Pterygium Study Group (60 Gy in 6 weekly fractions). This has the advantage of being a large series, long follow-up, with excellent control.
- an emerging modality is primary B radiation, and further study is required.

## Orbital Pseudotumor

Orbital pseudotumor, otherwise known as idiopathic orbital inflammatory syndrome (IOIS), is a benign, inflammatory condition. As a diagnosis of exclusion, by definition it requires an involved workup. Orbital cellulitis and Graves' ophthalmopathy are the conditions most often confused with pseudotumor, but one must also exclude sarcoid, lymphoma, metastases, rheumatologic disease such as Wegener's granulomatosis.[51]

It can involve any orbital structure from the lacrimal gland to the cavernous sinus. Presenting symptoms are typically *acute* onset of pain, photophobia, proptosis, eyelid swelling, chemosis, conjunctival injection, diplopia, and sometimes, visual loss. It is usually unilateral but may be bilateral.

Diagnosis is typically a clinical one. Acute onset of pain, typically good response to corticosteroids, neuroimaging, ophthalmologic exam all contribute to the diagnosis. Biopsy is sometimes performed in case of a poor response to steroids. Typical findings include a mixed infiltrate with plasma cells, lymphocytes, macrophages, and polymorphonuclear cells. On imaging, orbital pseudo-tumor can involve any orbital structure, but the two most common appearances are solitary intraorbital mass and diffuse muscle thickening (including tendinous attachment at globe, unlike Graves' ophthalmopathy).[34]

Treatment options include corticosteroids, radiation therapy, and low-dose chemotherapy. Corticosteroids are first line treatment, and relief of pain and proptosis can occur as early as 1–2 days. Typical dose is 60–100 mg daily, followed by a slow taper. About 50% will have a durable response to steroids.[52]

Radiation therapy is indicated in patients who are unresponsive to or intolerant of steroids. Lanciano treated 26 orbits with 20 Gy in 10 fractions. They reported 66% durable local control and steroid independence.[53] Orcutt treated 24 orbits with 25 Gy in 12 fractions. They reported that 75% had a CR or PR, with no recurrences at average follow-up of 22 months.[54] Sergott reported on 21 orbits treated to 10–20 Gy over 10–15 days. Seventy-one percent had a favorable, durable response.

### Summary

- orbital pseudotumor is a diagnosis of exclusion, requiring extensive workup.
- first line treatment is corticosteroids, with EBRT reserved for patients unresponsive or intolerant to corticosteroids.
- EBRT has been given in varying doses ranging from 10 Gy to around 25 Gy. It appears to be very effective, with around 70% durable response.

## Eyelid

*Basal cell carcinoma* is the most common tumor of the eyelid, about 39 times more common than squamous cell carcinoma.[56] They occur most often on the lower eyelid. While it very rarely metastasizes, BCC can be locally destructive. The main risk factor is sun exposure, so BCC occur commonly in the head and neck regions. Most patients are in their 60s and 70s. Rarely, patients may carry a diagnosis of basal cell nevus syndrome, and radiation is contraindicated in these cases. Medial canthus lesions can be especially deceptive in their extent of involvement, so imaging with CT or MRI is warranted.

Mohs' surgery should be considered first line treatment for periocular BCC. Numerous authors report a 5-year cure rate of between 97% and 99% with Mohs' surgery.[57] Cryotherapy is an excellent option for small, localized lesions without involvement of underlying tissues. Recurrence rate is slightly higher than with Mohs' surgery, but still less than 10% for suitably selected patients.[58]

Radiation alone offers excellent local control (over 90%) in smaller BCCs (≤2 cm). As size increases, one must weigh the anticipated disfigurement of surgery vs. lower control rate of radiation when deciding on a treatment modality. Therefore, intermediate sized lesions (2–5 cm) may be treated with either Mohs' surgery or radiation. Larger lesions >5 cm treated with primary radiation will recur in over 40%, so most will benefit from excision followed by postoperative RT. If surgery will be disfiguring, it may be reasonable to attempt a trial of radiation, with surgery held in reserve for recurrence.[59]

When radiating upper eyelid BCC, there is some small risk of corneal ulceration/irritation. Anscher recommends that when a tumor is located in the middle two-thirds of the upper eyelid and easily resectable (superficial <5 mm), excision is preferable.[59]

Radiation doses and fractionation in BCC are widely varying. Char uses orthovoltage radiation to about 45 Gy in 3 Gy fractions. At our institution, we normally treat to about 60 Gy in 2 Gy fractions to optimize cosmesis. In patients who are debilitated or need to finish quickly, a scheme similar to Char's would be employed.

*Sebaceous carcinomas* are often referred to as Meibomian gland carcinomas, after the most common site of origin on the tarsal plate of the eyelids. However, they can originate from other sebaceous glands, such as those associated with eyelashes (glands of Zeis), caruncle, and eyebrows. They make up 1%–5.5% of eyelid malignancies.[60] They occur more often in women, the elderly, and in the Far East, and there is an association with prior radiation exposure. Unlike BCC, the upper eyelid is involved 2–3 times as often as the lower lid (likely due to predominance of Meibomian glands). About 32% will have nodal involvement, more often when the diagnosis is delayed (as it usually is). Metastases can occur to the parotid gland, cervical and preauricular LN, lungs and brain. They have a tendency toward multicentricity, which may contribute to recurrences. Mortality at 5 years is between 15%–30%.[58]

These tumors tend to be unimpressive at the external eyelid, while they involve deeper structures. It is no wonder that they often masquerade as benign conditions such as chalazion (inflammation of Meibomian gland resulting in chronic granuloma), conjunctivitis, blepharitis, keratoconjunctivitis. Therefore, persistent or unusual presentations of these benign conditions (especially chalazion) must be biopsied.

First line treatment is wide surgical excision, with exenteration reserved for orbital disease or diffuse intraepithelial neoplasia. In case of lymph node involvement, neck dissection, superficial parotidectomy, and postoperative radiation is recommended.[60]

Historically, these tumors have been thought to be radio resistant. Armed Forces Institute of Pathology reported a 4-year mortality of 78% for patients undergoing primary radiation vs. 33% for simple tumor excision and 7% for wide surgical excision. However, the authors concede a likely selection bias in this study. Yen et al reported on 20 cases of ocular sebaceous carcinomas treated with primary radiation in the English literature. Of the 13 cases before 1989, only five were cured, but since 1989, 7/7 have remained tumor free. They note that no recurrences occurred at doses >55 Gy.[62] While they similarly recommend surgical excision as first line therapy, they consider primary radiation a viable option for those who refuse or cannot tolerate surgery.

## SUMMARY

- first line therapy for BCC of the eyelid is Mohs' surgery, which offers excellent local control.
- radiation offers local control similar to Mohs' for small BCCs (≤2 cm), but in larger lesions, one must weigh the anticipated disfigurement of surgery vs. the lower control rate of radiation.
- sebaceous cell carcinomas are characterized by delayed diagnosis, multicentricity, and lymph node metastases.
- surgical resection is first line therapy for sebaceous carcinoma, with postoperative radiation indicated for residual disease or lymph node involvement.
- primary radiation is a reasonable option in sebaceous cell carcinoma when patient refuses or cannot tolerate surgery. A dose >55 Gy may be optimal.

# RADIATION TECHNIQUES

## Treating with Laterals

- when treating posterior structures as in Graves' ophthalmopathy or choroidal metastases, the anterior edge is often placed just posterior to lens.
- can spare C/L lens by half-beam blocking the anterior edge, or by rotating gantry posteriorly roughly 5 degrees.

## Eyes Open or Closed

- If treating with an anterior field, and superficial structures are to be spared, treat with eyes open to avoid the "bolus" effect of the eyelid on structures like the cornea and lacrimal glands.
- When superficial structures are to be treated, closing the eyelids can provide some bolus effect, which may or may not be adequate due to their thinness.

## Shielding Lens/Lacrimal Gland in an Anterior Field

- When location of the tumor allows, shielding of the cornea-lens, lacrimal gland, or both may minimize corneal injury. Jiang reported visual impairment due to corneal opacification, scarring, perforation, or neovascularization in 24/49 patients with no shielding, 2/8 with lacrimal shielding, 2/12 with cornea-lens shielding, and none with both cornea-lens and lacrimal shielding.[63]
- Shielding of lens can be accomplished via a metallic eye shield (placed directly on cornea) or a hanging block.

## Metallic Eye Shields

- Tungsten eye shields may be more appropriate than lead for shielding electrons.
  - Lead eye shields are designed for orthovoltage machines. To adequately shield 6 and 9 MeV electrons would require about 3 and 4.5 mm lead (plus 2–3 mm external coating). Most commercially available lead eye shields are around 1.5 mm in thickness, which is clearly inadequate. Shiu reported that transmission of 6 MeV electrons through a 1.7 mm lead shield at the cornea (surface) was 50% and at the lens (6 mm depth) was 27%. On the other hand, there was <5% transmission through a prototype 2.8 mm thick tungsten shield with both 6 and 9 MeV electrons.[64]
- Metallic eye shields must have adequate paraffin (or similarly low Z material) coating on the external surface to minimize back scatter from the shield to the eyelid. Backscatter is even more of a problem with tungsten than lead.

## Electrons vs Orthovoltage for Superficial Lesions

- Both have been used successfully for superficial lesions such as eyelid BCC.
- Advantages of orthovoltage
  - 100% surface dose, so does not require bolus like electrons
  - easier to shield normal structures from standpoint of less transmission through metallic eye shields and less "bowing out" compared to electrons
  - requires less margin than electrons, "less bowing out" (though surface collimation may widen isodose curves for electrons somewhat)[65]
- Advantages of electrons
  - has sharper dose fall-off, so will not penetrate as deeply into normal tissues as orthovoltage
  - will not preferentially deliver as much dose to cartilage and bone (hi Z) as orthovoltage

358 Eye

# REFERENCES

1. Moore KL, Dalley AF and Kelly PJ, eds. *Clinically Oriented Anatomy,* fourth edition Philadelphia, PA Lippincott, Williams & Williams, 1999.
2. Merriam G et al. The effects of ionizing radiation on the eye, in Vaeth JM, ed. *Radiation Effects and Tolerance, Normal Tissue.* Baltimore, Md, University Park Press, 1972.
3. Hungerford J. Current management of choroidal malignant melanoma. *Br J Hosp Med* 34 287–293, 1985.
4. Parsons J, Bova FJ, Fitzgerald CR et al. Severe dry-eye syndrome following external beam irradiation. *Int J Radiat Oncol Biol Phys* 30:775–780, 1994.
5. Parsons JT, Bova FJ, Fitzgerald CR et al. Radiation retinopathy after external beam irradiation analysis of time-dose factors. *Int J Radiat Oncol Biol Phys* 30:765–773, 1994.
6. Parsons JT, Bova FJ, Fitzgerald CR et al. Radiation optic neuropathy after megavoltage external-beam irradiation: analysis of time-dose factors. *Int J Radiat Oncol Biol Phys* 30 755–763, 1994.
7. Jiang GL, Tucker SL, Guttenberger R et al. Radiation-induced injury to the visual pathway. *Radiother Oncol* 30:17–25, 1994.
8. Chang AE, Karnell LH, Menck HR. The National cancer database report on cutaneous and noncutaneous melanoma: a summary of 84,836 cases from the past decade. The American College of surgeons commission on cancer and the American Cancer Society. *Cancer* 83(8): 1664–1678, 1998.
9. Singh AD, Bergman L, Seregard S et al. Uveal melanoma: epidemiologic aspects. *Ophthalmology Clinics of North America* 18:75–84, 2005.
10. Tucker MA, Shields JA, Hartge P et al. Sunlight exposure as risk factor for intraocular malignant melanoma. *NEJM* 313(13):789–792,1985.
11. Vajdic CM, Kricker A, Giblin M et al. Eye color and cutaneous nevi predict risk of ocular melanoma in Australia. *Int J Cancer* 92:906–912, 2001.
12. Regan S, Judge HE, Gragoudas ES et al. Iris color as a prognostic factor in ocular melanoma *Arch Ophthalmol* 117:811–814, 1999.
13. Anonymous. Accuracy of diagnosis of choroidal melanomas in the Collaborative Ocular Melanoma Study. COMS report no. 1. *Arch Opthalmol* 108(9):1268–1273, 1990.
14. Greene FL, Page DL, Fleming ID et al, eds: *AJCC Cancer Staging Handbook,* sixth edition. New York, NY, Springer, 2002.
15. Kujala E, Makitie T, Kivela T. Very long-term prognosis of patients with malignant uveal melanoma. *Invest Opthalmol Vis Sci* 44(11): 4651–4659, 2003.
16. Shields JA. Management of posterior uveal melanoma: past, present, future. *Retina* 22(2): 139–142, 2002.
17. The Collaborative Ocular Melanoma Study Group. Factors predictive of growth and treatment of small choroidal melanoma. COMS Report No. 5. *Arch Ophthalmol* 115: 1537–1544, 1997.
18. Nag S, Quivey JM, Earle JD et al. The American Brachytherapy Society recommendations for brachytherapy of uveal melanomas. *Int J Radiat Oncol Biol Phys* 56(2):544–555, 2003.
19. Gragoudas ES, Lane AM, Regan S et al. A randomized controlled trial of varying radiation doses in the treatment of choroidal melanoma. *Arch Ophthalmol* 118: 773–778, 2000.
20. Rudoler SB, Corn BW, Shields CL et al. External beam irradiation for choroid metastases: identification of factors predisposing to long-term sequelae. *Int J Radiat Oncol Biol Phys* 38(2): 251–256, 1997.
21. Letson AD, Davidorf FH, Bruce RA et al. Chemotherapy for treatment of choroidal metastases from breast cancer. *American Journal of Ophthalmology* 93:102–106, 1982.
22. Shields CL, Shields JA, De Potter P et al. Plaque radiotherapy for the management of uveal metastasis. *Archives of Opthalmol* 115(2): 203–209, 1997.

3. Tsina EK, Lane AM, Zacks DN et al. Treatment of metastatic tumors of the choroid with proton beam irradiation. *Opthalmol* 112(2): 337–343, 2005.

4. Meunier J, Rouic LL, Vincent-Salomon A et al. Ophthalmologic and intraocular Non-Hodgkin's lymphoma: a large single centre study of initial characteristics, natural history, and prognostic factors. *Hematological Oncology* 22:143–158, 2004.

5. Zhou P, Ng AK, Silver B et al. Radiation therapy for orbital lymphoma. *Int J Radiat Oncol Biol Physics* 63(3):866–871, 2005.

6. Briggs JH, Algan O, Miller TP et al. External beam radiation therapy in the treatment of patients with extranodal stage IA Non-Hodgkin's Lymphoma. *A J Clin Oncol* 25:34–37, 2002.

7. Bolek TW, Moyses HM, Marcus RB et al. Radiotherapy in the management of orbital lymphoma. *Int J Radiat Oncol Biol Physics* 44(1): 31–36, 1999.

8. Esmaeli B. Clinical presentation and treatment of secondary orbital lymphoma. *Ophthalmic Plastic and Reconstructive Surgery* 2002; 18(4): 247–253.

9. Levy-Clarke GA, Chan C, Nussenblatt RB et al. Diagnosis and management of primary intraocular lymphoma. *Hematology/Oncology Clinics N Am* 19: 739–749, 2005.

0. Freeman LN, Schachat, AP, Knox DL et al. Clinical features, laboratory investigations, and survival in ocular reticulum cell sarcoma. *Ophthalmology* 94:1631–1639, 1987.

1. Batara JF, Grossman SA. Primary central nervous system lymphomas. *Current Opinion in Neurology* 16:671–675, 2003.

2. Spitzweg C, Joba W, Hunt N et al. Analysis of human thyrotropin receptor gene expression and immunoreactivity in human orbital tissue. *Eur J Endocrinol* 136(6):599–607, 1997.

3. Bahn RS, Heufelder AE. Pathogenesis of Graves' Ophthalmopathy. *NEJM* 329: 1468–1475, 1993.

4. Haaga JR, Lanzieri CF, Gilkeson RC in Duerk JL, Sunshine JL, eds. *CT and MR Imaging of the Whole Body,* vol one-fourth edition. St Louis, MO, Mosby, 2003.

5. Bartley GB, Fatourechi V, Kadrmas EF et al. Chronology of Graves' ophthalmopathy in an incidence cohort. *Am J Ophthalmol* 121(4):426–434, 1996.

6. Lyons CJ, Rootman J. Orbital decompression for disfiguring exophthalmos in thyroid orbitopathy. *Ophthalmol* 101:223, 1994.

7. Goh MSY, McNab AA. Orbital decompression in Graves' orbitopathy: efficacy and safety. *Internal medicine journal* 35:586–591, 2005.

8. Peterson IA, Kriss JP, McDougall IR et al. Prognostic factors in the radiotherapy of Graves' ophthalmopathy. *Int J Radiat Oncology Biol Phys* 19:259–264, 1990.

9. Prummel MF, Terwee CB, Gerding MN et al. A randomized controlled trial of orbital radiotherapy versus sham irradiation in patients with mild Graves' ophthalmopathy. *J of Clinical Endocrinology & Metabolism* 89(1):15–20, 2004.

0. Gorman CA, Garrity JA, Fatourechi V et al. A prospective, randomized, double-blind, placebo-controlled study of orbital radiotherapy for Graves' ophthalmopathy. *Ophthalmol* 108(9): 1523–1534, 2001.

1. Prummel MF, Mourits M. Randomized double-blind trial of prednisone versus radiotherapy in Graves' ophthalmopathy. *Lancet* 342:949–954, 1993.

2. Marcocci C, Bartalena L, Bogazzi F et al. Orbital radiotherapy combined with high dose systemic glucocorticoids for Graves' Ophthalmology is more effective than radiotherapy alone: results of a prospective randomized study. *J Endocrinol Invest* 14(10):853–860, 1991.

3. Bartalena L, Marcocci C, Chiovato L et al. Orbital cobalt irradiation combined with systemic corticosteroids for Graves' ophthalmopathy: comparison with systemic corticosteroids alone. *J Clin Endocrinol Metab* 56(6):1139–1144, 1983.

4. Marcocci C, Bartalena L, Tanda ML et al. Comparison of the effectiveness and tolerability of intravenous or oral glucocorticoids associated with orbital radiotherapy in the management of

severe Graves' ophthalmopathy: results of a prospective, single-blind, randomized study. *J o, Clinical Endocrin & Metabolism* 86(8):3562–3567, 2001.

45. Kahaly GJ, Rosler HP, Pitz S et al. Low- versus high-dose radiotherapy for Graves' ophthalmopathy: a randomized, single blind trial. *J Clin Endocrinol Metab* 85:102–108, 2000.

46. Luthra R, Nemesure BB, Wu SY et al. Frequency and risk factors for pterygium in the Barbados eye study. *Arch Ophthalmol* 119:1827–1832, 2001.

47. Wong TY, Foster PJ, Johnson GJ et al. The prevalence and risk factors for pterygium in an adult Chinese population in Singapore: The Tanjong Pagar Surgey. *Am J of Ophthalmol* 131:176–183, 2001.

48. Threlfall TJ, English DR. Sun exposure and pterygium of the eye: a dose-response curve. *Am J of Ophthalmol* 128:280–287, 1999.

49. Pajic B, Greiner RH. Long term results of non-surgical, exclusive strontium-/yttrium-90 beta-irradiation of pterygia. *Radiotherapay & Oncology* 74:25–29, 2005.

50. Jurgenliemk-Schulz IM, Hartman LJ, Roesink JM et al. Prevention of pterygium recurrence by postoperative single-dose B-irradiation: a prospective randomized clinical double-blind trial. *Int J Radiat Oncol Biol Phys* 59(4):1138–1147, 2004.

51. Jacobs D, Galetta S. Diagnosis and management of orbital pseudotumor. *Current Opinion in Ophthalmology* 13:347–351, 2002.

52. Leone C, Lloyd W. Treatment protocol for orbital inflammatory disease. *Ophthalmology* 92: 1325–1331, 1985.

53. Lanciano R, Fowble B, Sergott RC. The results of radiotherapy for orbital pseudotumor. *Int J Radiat Oncol Biol Phys* 18:407–411, 1990.

54. Orcutt JC, Garner A, Henk JM et al. Treatment of idiopathic inflammatory orbital pseudo-tumours by radiotherapy. *British Journal of Ophthalmology* 67:570–574, 1983.

55. Sergott RC, Glaser JS, Charyulu K. Radiotherapy for idiopathic inflammatory orbital pseudotumor indications and results. *Arch Ophthalmol* 99:853–856, 1981.

56. Kwitko ML, Boniuk M, Zimmerman LE. Tumors of the eyelid with special reference to lesions often confused with squamous cell carcinoma. I. Incidence and errors in diagnosis. *Arch Ophthalmol* 63:693–697, 1963.

57. Leshin B, Yeatts P. Management of periocular basal cell carcinoma: Moh's micrographic surgery versus radiotherapy I. Mohs' micrographic surgery. *Survey of Opththalmology* 38:193–203, 1993.

58. Char DH. The management of lid and conjunctival malignancies. *Survey of Ophthalmology* 24(6):679–689, 1980.

59. Anscher M, Montano G. Management of periocular basal cell carcinoma: Mohs' micrographic surgery versus radiotherapy II. Radiotherapy. *Survey of Opththalmology* 38(2):203–210, 1993.

60. Kass LG, Hornblass A. Sebaceous carcinoma of the ocular adnexa. *Survey of Ophthalmology* 33(6):477–490, 1989.

61. Rao NA, McLean IW, Zimmerman LE. Sebaceous carcinoma of the eyelid and caruncle: correlation of clinicopathologic features with prognosis, in Jakobiec FA, ed. Ocular and Adnexal Tumors. Birmingham: *Aesculapius* 461–476, 1978.

62. Yen MT, Tse DT, Wu D et al. Radiation therapy for local control of eyelid sebaceous cell carcinoma Report of two cases and review of the literature. *Ophthalmic Plastic and Reconstructive Surgery* 16(3):211–215, 2000.

63. Jiang GL, Tucker SL, Guttenberger R. Radiation-induced injury to the visual pathway. *Radiotherapy and Oncology* 30:17–25, 1994.

64. Shiu AS, Tung SS, Gastorf RJ. Dosimetric evaluation of lead and tungsten eye shields in electron beam treatment. *Int J Radiat Oncol Biol Phys* 35:599–604, 1996.

65. Amdur RJ, Kalbaugh KJ, Ewald LM et al. Radiation therapy for skin cancer near the eye: kilovoltage X-rays versus electrons. *Int J Radiat Oncol Biol Phys* 23:769–779, 1992.

# 17

# Esophagus Cancer

*Jeffrey C. Haynes, MD*
*James M. Metz, MD*

## Overview

Esophageal cancer is an aggressive disease with one of the highest mortality rates of all reported cancers in the United States. The death rate approaches the yearly incidence rate. Multimodality management of this disease is increasing and is described in this chapter.

## Introduction

The American Cancer Society estimates that 15,560 Americans were diagnosed with esophageal cancer in 2007, of whom 13,940 died of their disease. Incidence varies dramatically worldwide with geography; rates are 10–100 times higher in India, Iran, southern Africa, and northern China than in the United States.[1]

## Anatomy

The esophagus can be described based on the anatomic region and distance from the incisors (Table 17-1). Understanding the location of the primary lesion is important for developing an appropriate treatment plan. Measurements are given based on distance from the incisors at endoscopy. The esophagus is approximately 26 cm in length and begins at the epiglottis and travels through the posterior mediastinum to insert in the stomach at the gastroesophageal junction. Along its course, it is in close proximity to a number of important structures in the mediastinum including the trachea, great vessels, and heart.

### Lymphatic Drainage

The esophagus has a rich lymphatic network, which makes lymphatic involvement common in this disease. Importantly, the ample lymphatics of the esophagus allow esophageal cancer cells to travel many centimeters before settling in a node; consequently, more distant nodes can be involved without the involvement of nearer nodes. Nevertheless, nodal involvement is most often in close proximity to the primary lesion, particularly with lower T stage. Lesions of all regions of the esophagus drain to mediastinal nodes. Cervical and upper thoracic lesions often drain to the cervical and supraclavicular lymph nodes. Distal thoracic lesions frequently drain to the celiac nodes.

TABLE 17-1 **Anatomical Divisions of the Esophagus**

| Section | Top | Bottom | From Incisors |
|---|---|---|---|
| Cervical | Cricoid cartilage | Thoracic inlet | 15–18cm |
| Upper thoracic | Thoracic inlet | Carina | 18–24cm |
| Mid thoracic | Carina | Inferior pulmonary veins | 24–32cm |
| Lower thoracic | Inferior pulmonary veins | GE junction | 32–40cm |

## PATHOLOGY

Sixty percent of esophageal cancers in the United States are adenocarcinoma; 40% are squamous cell carcinoma.[2] Worldwide, squamous cell carcinoma is much more common than adenocarcinoma. Squamous cell carcinoma tends to be more proximal, adenocarcinoma more distal. Interestingly, in the past several years there has been a significant shift in the histology in the United States. Previously squamous cell carcinomas were the most common histology, but their incidence has been decreasing with decreased tobacco use. At the same time, the incidence of adenocarcinoma has been increasing. This increase is only partly explained by increasing obesity and gastroesophageal reflux disease.

Survival is similar for the two histologies.[3] Many studies lump the two histologies together, though it is not clear that the optimal treatment approach is the same for each. Small-cell carcinomas, leiomyosarcoma, lymphoma, and Kaposi's sarcoma can, rarely, originate in the esophagus, but their management is beyond the scope of this chapter.

## RISK FACTORS:[4]

### Adenocarcinoma

- Barrett's esophagus
- GERD
- Obesity
- Diet low in fruits and vegetables

### Squamous Cell Carcinoma

- Alcohol consumption
- Tobacco use
- Diet low in fruits and vegetables
- Tylosis
- Caustic injury
- Achalasia
- Prior aerodigestive tract malignancy

## SCREENING

There is no serum marker for either type of esophageal cancer. Even among patients with Barrett's esophagus, no survival benefit has been demonstrated for regular screening endoscopy, likely due to the low incidence of adenocarcinoma even among such patients.[5-7] Given the small but real risk of perforation, aspiration, or cardiopulmonary events, routine endoscopic screening cannot be recommended for widespread use. Unfortunately, medical therapy using proton pump inhibitors has not been shown to be beneficial either.

## PRESENTATION

- Dysphagia, first to solids then to liquids
- Odynophagia

- Retrosternal pain, if invasion of mediastinal structures
- Cough or hoarseness, if recurrent laryngeal nerve involved

## WORKUP

### In All Patients

- Upper endoscopy with biopsy
- CT scan of chest, abdomen, and pelvis[8]
  - Accurate for lung, liver, and peritoneal metastases as well as aortic and tracheobronchial involvement
  - Insensitive for lymph node involvement
- PET[8]
  - 80%–90% accurate for distant metastasis
  - Changes management in 20% of cases
- Endoscopic Ultrasound (EUS)[9]
  - T staging 85% accurate
  - N staging 75% accurate

### Special Cases

- Barium swallow: if endoscope can't pass, to define distal extent of lesion
- Bronchoscopy: if suspicious disease above carina, to rule out tracheoesophageal fistula
- Bone scan: if bone pain

## STAGING

### TABLE 17-2  AJCC 2002 TNM Classification[10]

| Primary Tumor | TX | Cannot be assessed |
|---|---|---|
| | T0 | No evidence of primary tumor |
| | Tis | Carcinoma *in situ* |
| | T1 | Invades lamina propria or submucosa |
| | T2 | Invades muscularis propria |
| | T3 | Invades adventitia |
| | T4 | Invades adjacent structures |
| Regional Lymph Nodes | NX | Cannot be assessed |
| | N0 | No nodal metastases |
| | N1 | Nodal metastases |
| Distant Metastases | MX | Cannot be assessed |
| | M0 | No distant metastases |
| | M1a | Cervical node metastases from upper thoracic lesions |
| | | Celiac node metastases from lower thoracic lesions |
| | M1b | Other distant metastases |

Adapted from Greene FL, et al. *AJCC Cancer Staging Handbook*. 6th ed., 2002.

## BIOLOGY

Adenocarcinoma of the esophagus arises from mucosa that has become progressively more dysplastic as the cells acquired additional oncogenic mutations. Adenocarcinoma of the esophagus occurs more frequently in patients with Barrett's esophagus, in which columnar-lined epithelium replaces the

**TABLE 17-3  AJCC 2002 TNM Classification[10]**

| Stage | T | N | M |
|---|---|---|---|
| Stage 0 | Tis | N0 | M0 |
| Stage I | T1 | N0 | M0 |
| Stage IIA | T2 | N0 | M0 |
|  | T3 |  |  |
| Stage IIB | T1 | N1 | M0 |
|  | T2 |  |  |
| Stage III | T3 | N1 | M0 |
|  | T4 |  |  |
| Stage IV | Any T | Any N | M1 |
| Stage IVA | Any T | Any N | M1a |
| Stage IVB | Any T | Any N | M1b |

Adapted from Greene FL, et al. *AJCC Cancer Staging Handbook*. 6th ed., 2002.

normal stratified squamous mucosa. However, it is not clear that Barrett's esophagus represents the first step in the transformation to adenocarcinoma. Barrett's esophagus and adenocarcinoma may be coincident processes created independently by reflux.

Squamous cell carcinoma of the esophagus is associated with other squamous cell carcinomas of the aerodigestive tract. Exposure to carcinogens such as tobacco smoke and alcohol gives rise to successive mutations that result in dysplasia, which can progress to invasive cancer. The common etiology of squamous cell carcinomas of the esophagus and those of the head and neck accounts for the high rate of second cancers among these patients. The incidence of synchronous aerodigestive primary tumor in these patients is 7%.[11]

## MANAGEMENT

### Surgery

Although surgery alone has never been compared against chemoradiation alone in a randomized trial, nearly all patients with resectable disease will undergo esophagectomy. The mid and distal esophagus is removed entirely and gut continuity is re-established with either a gastric pull-up or colon interposition. In either case, if postoperative radiation is required, the entire surgical bed must be irradiated because tumor cells may have contaminated the surgical bed during the creation of the neoesophagus.

The most common surgical approaches are the Ivor-Lewis approach and the transhiatal approach. The Ivor-Lewis entails a right thoracotomy and an upper abdominal incision. The anastomosis is made in the upper to mid thoracic cavity. In the transhiatal approach, a cervical incision replaces the thoracotomy. Consequently, the anastomosis is made in the low neck. The Ivor-Lewis allows a more thorough dissection at the expense of more frequent postoperative complications; the largest randomized trial showed a trend toward improved survival with the Ivor-Lewis approach.[12] Because the transhiatal esophagectomy has fewer complications, most surgeons have gravitated toward this procedure for the majority of esophagectomies today. It must be remembered that the transhiatal approach requires a longer postoperative radiation field if the anastamosis is to be covered.

### Adjuvant Chemoradiation

Single-modality adjuvant therapy has not demonstrated clear benefit. Nevertheless, the high rate of local and distant recurrence following surgery alone has driven the pursuit of effective adjuvant therapy. Many esophageal patients are treated with concurrent chemoradiation. Four trials have randomized esophageal cancer patients to preoperative concurrent chemoradiation versus surgery alone.

While none of the randomized trials of neoadjuvant chemoradiation provide the highest level of evidence for the addition of chemoradiation, collectively they lend strong support to the practice.

### Definitive Chemoradiation

For patients who cannot undergo surgery, definitive chemoradiation is the optimal treatment approach. RTOG 85-01 demonstrated the superiority of chemoradiation over radiation alone.

## BOX 17-1

This study randomized 282 patients with stage I or II squamous cell cancer of the esophagus to a split course of 18.5 Gy in five daily 3.7 Gy fractions twice, with cisplatin (80mg/m2) 0–2 days before each week of radiation followed by en-bloc esophagectomy or surgery alone. At a median follow-up of 55 months, chemoradiation improved disease-free survival (RR = 0.6, P = 0.003) and freedom from local recurrence (RR = 0.6, P = 0.01) but not overall survival. Postoperative mortality was worse following chemoradiation (12% vs. 4%, P = 0.01) due to respiratory insufficiency and infection.

Bossett JF, Gignoux M, Triboulet JP, et al. Chemoradiotherapy followed by surgery compared with surgery alone in squamous cell cancer of the esophagus. *N Engl J Med.* 1997 Jul 17; 337(3): 161–167.

## BOX 17-2

This study randomized 100 patients with esophageal carcinoma to neoadjuvant cisplatin (20mg/m2/d d1-5 & 17-20), 5-fluorouracil (300mg/m$^2$/d d1-21), and vinblastine (1mg/m$^2$/d d1-4 & d 17-20) with radiation 45 Gy in twice daily 1.5 Gy fractions followed by esophagectomy or surgery alone. With median follow-up of 8.2 years, chemoradiation gave a trend towards improved survival at 3 years (30% vs. 16%, P = 0.15); operative mortality was similar (2% vs. 4%).

Urba S, Orringer M, Turrisi A, et al. Randomized trial of preoperative chemoradiation versus surgery alone in patients with locoregional esophageal carcinoma. *J Clin Oncol.* 19(2): 305–313, 2001 Jan 15.

## BOX 17-3

This study randomized 113 patients to radiation (40 Gy in 15 daily fractions) with cisplatin (75mg/m$^2$) on days 7 and 37 as well as 5 days of 5-fluorouracil (15mg/kg/day) in weeks 1 and 6 followed by esophagectomy or surgery alone versus higher dose radiation alone (64 Gy). Chemoradiation improved median survival (16 vs. 11 months, P = 0.01), and 3-year survival (32% vs. 6%, P = 0.01). However, the unusually low survival rate in the surgical arm of this study precludes drawing firm conclusions.

Walsh T, Noonan N, Hollywood D, et al. A comparison of multimodal therapy and surgery for esophageal adenocarcinoma. *N Engl J Med.* 1996 Aug 15; 335(7): 462–467.

## BOX 17-4

This study was designed to randomize 500 patients but was closed early due to poor accrual. Prior to closure, this study randomized 56 patients to cisplatin (100mg/m$^2$) and 5-fluorouracil (1000mg/m$^2$/d × 4d) weeks 1 and 5 concurrent with radiation (50.4 Gy in 1.8 Gy daily fractions) followed by esophagectomy with lymph node dissection vs. surgery alone. At 6 years median follow-up, neoadjuvant chemoradiation significantly improved median survival (4.5 vs. 1.8 years, P = 0.02) with a trend towards improved 5-year overall survival (39% vs. 16%). The neoadjuvant chemoradiation arm trended towards more hematopoietic complications and dysphagia but fewer surgical complications and deaths.

Krasna M, Tepper JE, Niedzwiecki D, et al. Trimodality therapy is superior to surgery alone in esophageal cancer: Results of CALGB 9781. Abstract presented at 2006 Gastrointestinal Cancers Symposium of ASCO.

---

**BOX 17-5**

This study randomized 123 patients with mostly squamous cell esophageal cancer to two cycles of cisplatin (75mg/m$^2$ d1) and 5-fluorouracil (1000mg/m$^2$ d1-4) concurrent with radiation (50Gy) followed by two cycles of cisplatin and fluorouracil versus higher dose radiation (64Gy). Chemoradiation improved median survival (14 vs. 9 months) and 5-year survival (27% vs. 0%, P < 0.0001). Systemic side effects including nausea, vomiting, renal complications, and myelosuppression occurred more often with chemoradiation, but local side effects were the same.

al-Sarraf M, Martz K, Herskovic A, et al. Progress report of combined chemoradiotherapy versus radiotherapy alone in patients with esophageal cancer: an intergroup study. *J Clin Oncol.* 1997 Jan; 15(10): 277–284.

---

## Palliative Radiation

Radiation therapy is effective in palliating dysphagia in 70% of patients.[13–15] With concurrent chemotherapy, 88% of patients can be palliated.[16] Median time to relief is 4 weeks, and dysphagia returns in only one third of patients.[17] Unfortunately, doses of radiation similar to those used in definitive therapy are needed for effective palliation, which necessitates more than one month of treatment visits for the patient. Thus one should always consider stent placement, because in some patients this can relieve dysphagia immediately. Brachytherapy can offer similar rates of palliation in fewer visits, though high doses have been associated with ulcers and even fistulas.

Tracheoesophageal fistula is traditionally viewed as a contraindication to radiation therapy. However, modern data support the safety and efficacy of radiation in the palliation of tracheoesophageal fistulas.[18]

## Supportive Care

Many of these patients are nutritionally deficient at the time of presentation. Multimodality therapy is a difficult treatment course requiring aggressive supportive measures. All patients receiving neoadjuvant therapy or definitive chemoradiotherapy should be considered for enteral feeding support. For those receiving neoadjuvant chemotherapy and radiation therapy, a jejunal feeding tube (J-tube) is placed prior to initiating treatment. For those receiving definitive chemotherapy and radiation therapy, a gastric feeding tube (G-tube) is placed prior to initiating treatment. Nutritional counseling should begin prior to starting treatment. Patients' nutritional status should be followed regularly though body weight, albumin, and pre-albumin levels.

## Prognosis

Patients often ask about the likely outcome of their treatment. In addition, predicted survival shapes treatment decisions. For both of these reasons, approximate survival rates by stage are useful.

**TABLE 17-4 Survival by Stage[19]**

| Stage | 5-Year Survival |
|-------|-----------------|
| 0 | >90% |
| I | >70% |
| IIA | 15–30% |
| IIB | 10–30% |
| III | <10% |
| IV | Rare |

## TECHNIQUE/DOSE

### Simulation

It is preferable to simulate the patient in the prone position to allow the esophagus to fall slightly anterior which may minimize the dose to the spinal cord. This is most effective for mid thoracic lesions. However the benefit is small, so if a J-tube or infusaport will make prone treatment uncomfortable, it is reasonable to simulate the patient supine. The patient should be placed in some form of cast for immobilization with the arms above the head. Thick oral contrast improves visualization of the esophageal mass and strictures and thereby helps with GTV contouring. CT/PET fusion may improve the accuracy of GTV contouring. At one institution, the addition of PET altered the GTV by ≥25% in 6 out of 34 patients.[20]

## Field Borders and Dose

For patients who have not undergone esophagectomy, field borders on the GTV should include a 2 cm margin anteriorly, posteriorly, and laterally to account for setup error and to treat any disease penetrating beyond the muscular wall of the esophagus or involving the periesophageal lymph nodes. For the first 45 Gy of treatment, the fields should extend 5 cm superior and inferior to the lesion to account for the ease with which cancer can travel through the rich lymphatics of the esophagus. Regardless of whether radiation is preoperative or postoperative, the celiac nodes should be included for lesions below the carina, and the supraclavicular nodes should be included for lesions above the carina. Subsequently, a conedown to a 2 cm margin on the GTV and any grossly involved lymph nodes for an additional 5.4 Gy boost is performed. A total dose of 50.4 Gy to the GTV is delivered when the patient will be undergoing subsequent surgery. There remains some controversy regarding the total dose in patients who are receiving definitive chemoradiation therapy without surgical resection. At our institution, when chemoradiation is the sole treatment, we deliver a total of 59.4 Gy to the GTV to maximize local control. While the Intergroup 0123 trial did not demonstrate an improvement in survival with dose greater than 50.4 Gy, its data are difficult to interpret.

---

**BOX 17-6**

This study randomized 218 patients to four cycles of cisplatin ($75mg/m^2$ d1) and 5-fluorouracil ($1000mg/m^2$ d1-4) concurrent with either 50.4 Gy or 64.8 Gy. The higher dose of radiation produced no significant improvement in median survival (13 vs. 18 months), 2-year survival (31% vs. 40%), or locoregional recurrence/persistence (56% vs. 52%). There were more treatment-related deaths in the high dose arm, but 7 out of 11 of these deaths occurred at radiation doses of less than 50.4 Gy. Further bias against the high dose arm came from the larger number of toxicity-related treatment breaks and the lower dose of flourouracil delivered in the high dose arm.

Minsky BD, Pajak TF, Ginsberg RJ, et al. INT 0123 (Radiation Therapy Oncology Group 94-05) phase III trial of combined-modality therapy for esophageal cancer: high-dose versus standard-dose radiation therapy. *J Clin Oncol.* 2002 Mar; 20(5):1167–1174.

---

Post-esophagectomy patients require somewhat different fields. Many physicians lengthen their fields to cover the surgical bed and anastomosis. However, for patients with a low lesion and a high anastomosis, a shorter field is likely adequate. For GE junction tumors, the CALGB 80101 protocol requires that the medial left hemi-diaphragm and adjacent body of pancreas be included in the fields for tumors invading into or beyond the subserosa. If the volume of normal tissue irradiated is acceptable, inclusion of the remaining stomach is appropriate, particularly if the surgical margins are less than 5 cm. The celiac nodes may be excluded from the fields if the tumor was pathologically T2N0. Anterior, posterior, and lateral borders should include a 2 cm margin on the surgical bed. These fields are treated to 45 Gy without subsequent conedown.

## Sparing the Spinal Cord

Some radiation oncologists deliver 41.4 Gy using AP/PA fields and then spare the cord on subsequent fractions with opposed oblique fields. We reduce the lung dose by sparing the spinal cord with an anterior field and a pair of posterior oblique fields, as illustrated in Figures 17-1 through

**FIGURE 17-1** Initial field arrangement for preoperative or definitive radiation.

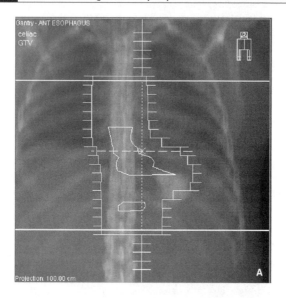

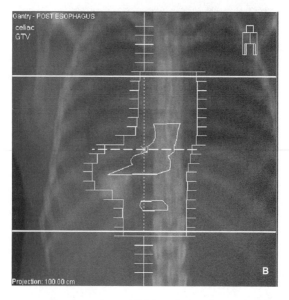

Initial field arrangement for preoperative or definitive radiation. GTV, spinal cord, and celiac nodes are outlined. Anterior **(A)** and posterior **(B)** fields.

**FIGURE 17-2** Off-cord three-field arrangement for preoperative or definitive radiation.

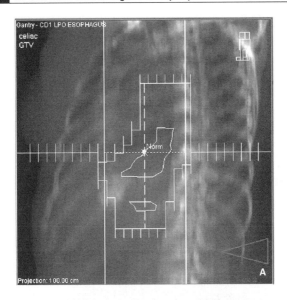

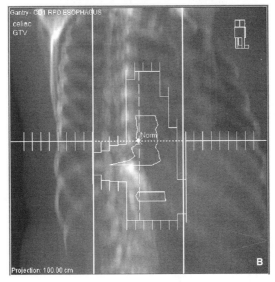

Off-cord three-field arrangement for preoperative or definitive radiation. GTV, spinal cord, and celiac nodes are oulined. Anterior field is as in Figure 17-1A; posterior field is replaced by left posterior oblique **(A)** and right posterior olique **(B)** fields.

**FIGURE 17-3** Conedown field arrangement for preoperative or definitive radiation.

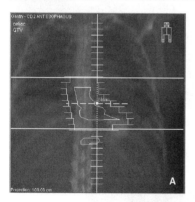
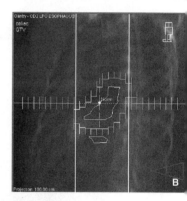
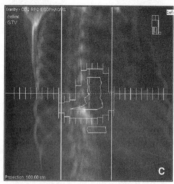

Conedown field arrangement for preoperative or definitive radiation. GTV, spinal cord, and celiac nodes are outlined. Anterior **(A)**, left posterior oblique **(B)**, and right posterior oblique **(C)** fields.

17-5. Because of the proximity of our oblique fields to the spinal cord, we switch from AP/PA to AP/LPO/RPO at 36 Gy.

## Sparing Vital Organs

On the basis of the experience at our institution, we use specific guidelines in judging whether a plan's toxicity will be acceptable.[21] We attempt to limit the median heart dose to 40 Gy, the median kidney dose to 18 Gy, and the median liver dose to 30 Gy. We try to limit the V20 of the lungs to 20%. We prefer to keep the maximum spinal cord dose below 45 Gy, though we sometimes accept doses as high as 50 Gy.

## FOLLOW-UP

Patients who have received radiation therapy for esophageal cancer should be seen by a member of the treatment team every 3 months for the first 2 years. We prefer to alternate amongst medical

FIGURE 17-4 **FIGURE 17-4** Dose volume histogram for the summation of the doses delivered by these fields in this case of neoadjuvant preoperative chemoradiation.

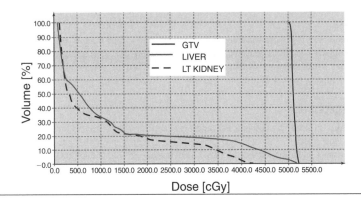

**FIGURE 17-5** Minimum, maximum, and average doses to target and organs at risk for the summation of the doses delivered by these fields in this case of neoadjuvant preoperative chemoradiation.

|  | Min [cGy] | Max [cGy] | Median [cGy] | Average [cGy] |
|---|---|---|---|---|
| GTV | 5038.087 | 5199.970 | 5100.411 | 5103.825 |
| celiac | 4508.741 | 4604.294 | 4561.837 | 4557.858 |
| Cord | 92.643 | 4485.137 | 394.375 | 1611.278 |
| External | 0.000 | 5225.177 | 162.497 | 739.832 |
| LT LUNG | 111.292 | 5097.327 | 301.211 | 782.942 |
| RT LUNG | 110.344 | 5194.827 | 458.974 | 836.229 |
| CARINA | 259.313 | 335.761 | 323.618 | 308.568 |
| HEART | 387.958 | 5209.435 | 3888.342 | 3190.556 |
| RT KIDNEY | 104.344 | 2112.312 | 211.620 | 489.179 |
| LT KIDNEY | 119.801 | 4373.181 | 300.096 | 985.219 |
| LIVER | 84.372 | 5225.177 | 544.929 | 1242.471 |

oncology, radiation oncology, and surgery in order to bring each specialty's expertise to the follow-up of the patient. Chest imaging should be obtained prior to each follow-up visit. Alternating between chest CT and chest X-ray every 3 months provides a balance between cost and benefit. An endoscopy 6 months after the completion of therapy verifies the absence of local recurrence. Subsequently, endoscopy is necessary only when symptoms indicate.

## MORBIDITY

### Acute Toxicity

Esophagitis is the most difficult symptom for patients undergoing treatment. Resultant dysphagia, odynophagia, and loss of appetite can lead to substantial weight loss during treatment. Topical anesthetics, narcotics, H2 blockers, and proton pump inhibitors can be helpful. The placement of a feeding tube prior to the start of radiation therapy improves the nutritional status and allows the patient to tolerate the treatment better. Some patients will experience skin reactions or, rarely, pneumonitis.

## Late Toxicity

Benign stricture occurs in approximately 15% of patients and can be treated with dilatation.[16] Decreased esophageal motility, delayed gastric emptying, and reflux can occur as well. Care must be taken at the time of radiation planning to reduce dose to the kidneys, liver, spinal cord, heart, and lungs to minimize the risk of resultant late toxicity to these organs.

## FUTURE DIRECTIONS

Much of the current research in esophageal cancer is evaluating the addition of targeted biologic therapies to the multimodality approach of radiation therapy, chemotherapy, and surgical resection. The most promising approaches target Epidermal Growth Factor Receptor (EGFR), which is overexpressed in 71% of squamous cell carcinomas of the esophagus.[22] As with any disease with such a poor predicted survival, much of the current research is in the phase I and phase II setting.

## REFERENCES

1. How Many People Get Cancer of the Esophagus? Vol 2006; 2005:1 http://www.cancer.org/docroot/CRI/content/CRI_2_2_1X_How_many_people_get_esophagus_cancer_12.asp?sitearea=.
2. Blot WJ. *Epidemiology and genesis of esophageal cancer in thoracic oncology*. Philadelphia: WB Saunders; 1995.
3. Altorki NK, Skinner DB. Occult cervical nodal metastasis in esophageal cancer: preliminary results of three-field lymphadenectomy. *Journal of Thoracic & Cardiovascular Surgery.* 1997; 113(3):540–544.
4. DeVita VTJ, Hellman S, Rosenberg SA. *Cancer: Principles & Practice of Oncology*. 17th ed. Philadelphia: Lippincott, Williams & Wilkins; 2004.
5. Volker F, Eckardt MD, Kanzler G, Bernhard G. Life expectancy and cancer risk in patients with Barrett's esophagus: a prospective controlled investigation. 2001;111:33–37.
6. Macdonald CE, Wicks AC, Playford RJ. Final results from 10 year cohort of patients undergoing surveillance for Barrett's oesophagus: observational study. 2000;321:1252–1255.
7. Gerson LB, Triadafilopoulos G. Screening for esophageal adenocarcinoma: an evidence-based approach. 2002;113(6):499–505.
8. Kole AC, Plukker JT, Nieweg OE, et al. Positron emission tomography for staging of oesophageal and gastroesophageal malignancy. 1998;78:521.
9. Rosch T. Endosonographic staging of esophageal cancer: a review of literature results. 1995;5:537.
10. Greene FL, Page DL, Fleming ID, et al. *AJCC Cancer Staging Handbook*. 6th ed. New York: Springer; 2002.
11. Poon RT, Law SY, Chu KM, Branicki FJ, Wong J. Multiple primary cancers in esophageal squamous cell carcinoma: incidence and implications. *Annals of Thoracic Surgery.* 1998;65(6):1529–1534.
12. Hulscher JB, van Sandick JW, de Boer AG, et al. Extended transthoracic resection compared with limited transhiatal resection for adenocarcinoma of the esophagus. *N Engl J Med.* Nov 21 2002;347(21):1662–1669.
13. Wara WM, Mauch PM, Thomas AN, Phillips TL. Palliation for carcinoma of the esophagus. *Radiology.* 1976;121(3 Pt. 1):717–720.

14. O'Rourke IC, McNeil RJ, Walker PJ, Bull CA. Objective evaluation of the quality of palliation in patients with oesophageal cancer comparing surgery, radiotherapy, and intubation. *Australian & New Zealand Journal of Surgery.* 1992;62(12):922–930.

15. Hayter CR, Huff-Winters C, Paszat L, Youssef YM, Shelley WE, Schulze K. A prospective trial of short-course radiotherapy plus chemotherapy for palliation of dysphagia from advanced esophageal cancer. *Radiotherapy & Oncology.* 2000;56(3):329–333.

16. Coia LR, Soffen EM, Schultheiss TE, Martin EE, Hanks GE. Swallowing function in patients with esophageal cancer treated with concurrent radiation and chemotherapy. *Cancer.* 1993;71(2):281–286.

17. Coia LR, Engstrom PF, Paul AR, Stafford PM, Hanks GE. Long-term results of infusional 5-FU, mitomycin-C, and radiation as primary management of esophageal carcinoma. *International Journal of Radiation Oncology, Biology, Physics.* 1991;20(1):29–36.

18. Gschossmann JM, Bonner JA, Foote RL, Shaw EG, Martenson JA, Jr., Su J. Malignant tracheo-esophageal fistula in patients with esophageal cancer. *Cancer.* 1993;72(5):1513–1521.

19. Paz BI, Hwang JJ, Iyer R, Coia L. Esophageal cancer. In: Pazdur R, Coia LR, Hoskins WJ, Wagman LD, eds. *Cancer Management: A Multidisciplinary Approach*. 9th ed. Lawrence, KS: CMP United Business Media; 2005:262.

20. Moureau-Zabotto L, Touboul E, Lerouge D, et al. Impact of CT and 18F-deoxyglucose positron emission tomography image fusion for conformal radiotherapy in esophageal carcinoma. *International Journal of Radiation Oncology, Biology, Physics.* 2005;63(2):340–345.

21. Emami B, Lyman J, Brown A, et al. Tolerance of normal tissue to therapeutic irradiation. *International Journal of Radiation Oncology, Biology, Physics.* 1991;21(1):109–122.

22. Itakura Y, Sasano H, Shiga C, et al. Epidermal growth factor receptor overexpression in esophageal carcinoma. An immunohistochemical study correlated with clinicopathologic findings and DNA amplification. *Cancer.* Aug 1 1994;74(3):795–804.

# 18

# Lung Cancer

*Ronald McGarry, MD, PhD*
*Andrew T. Turrisi, III, MD*

## GENERAL ASPECTS

### Epidemiology

In the United States, lung cancer represents 12% of all malignant tumors, but results in 29% of all cancer deaths each year. It is the leading cause of cancer deaths in both men and women, exceeding the four other leading causes of cancer deaths (colorectal/breast/prostate/pancreas) combined. In men, the incidence rate decreased from 102.1 per 100,000 in 1984 to 77.7 in 2001; however, in women it rose sharply from 6/per 100,000 in 1960 to 52.8/per 100,000 in 1998 to 49.1/per 100,000 in 2001.[1]

There will be an estimated 213,380 new cases with 160,390 deaths in 2008 with a high case fatality rate. The 5-year survival rate remains only 15% in the United States and 8% in Europe and developing nations. It is hoped that the success of smoking prevention efforts will result in reduction in lung cancer mortality in this century.[2]

### Risk Factors

Eighty-five percent to 95% of patients have a history of direct smoking of tobacco, but many cases may be multifactorial.[1]

#### Tobacco

- Smoking history is usually related in the average number of packs smoked per day times the number of years of consumption.
- Cigarette smoke has more than 40 carcinogenic agents. Two of the major carcinogens are N-nitrosamines and polycyclic aromatic hydrocarbons (benzopyrene and dimethylbenzanthracene).
- Smoking is most strongly associated with squamous cell and small-cell carcinoma.
- Predominant cell type in nonsmokers is adenocarcinoma.
- Smoking remains strongly associated with each of the four major types of lung cancer (squamous cell, adenocarcinoma, large cell, and small cell).
- 3,000 lung cancer deaths each year are attributed to secondhand smoke.[3]

### Occupational and Secondhand Exposure

Occupational exposure is related to asbestos and metals including arsenic, chromium, and cadmium. Radon gas decays to short-lived daughter particles (alpha emitters) which deposit in the lung tissues. Underground miners have a significant risk due to radon, but residential radon exposure adds a small increase in risk, similar to secondhand smoke with a relative risk of about 1.2.

### Genetic Factors

Family clusters of lung cancer have been documented with first relatives of lung cancer patients having 2- to 6-fold increases in their risk of developing lung cancers.

## HISTOLOGIC CLASSIFICATION[4,5]

### Squamous Cell Carcinoma

- Smoking a strong risk factor
- Mostly in proximal bronchi in origin
- Keratin pearl formation if well differentiated
- Variants include papillary, clear cell, basaloid

### Adenocarcinoma

- Mostly peripheral origin
- Most common cell type in nonsmokers
- Most common cell type in women
- Increasing incidence, 40% of all lung cancer
  - Possibly due to improving technology in pathology, identifying fewer undifferentiated large cell tumors
  - Pronounced increase in women

#### Variants

Acinar, papillary
- Bronchioloalveolar carcinoma (BAC)
  - Includes non-mucinous, mucinous, mixed, solid with mucinous formation
  - 3 major different presentations
    - solitary peripheral nodule
    - multifocal disease
    - progressive pneumonic form which spread from lobe to lobe by postulated airway spread, ultimately encompassing both lungs

### Adenocarcinoma with Mixed Subtypes

#### Variants

Well differentiated fetal adenocarcinoma, mucinous or colloid adenocarcinoma, mucinous cystadenocarcinoma, signet ring adenocarcinoma, clear cell adenocarcinoma

### Large Cell Carcinoma

- Least common of all NSCL due to better pathological techniques. The overall incidence is decreasing.

#### Variants

Large cell neuroendocrine carcinoma, combined large cell neuroendocrine carcinoma, basaloid carcinoma, lymphoepithelioma-like carcinoma, clear cell carcinoma, large cell carcinoma with rhabdoid phenotype

# LUNG CANCER STAGING[4]

## TABLE 18-1 TNM Staging of Lung Cancer

**TNM Definitions**

Primary Tumor (T)

| | |
|---|---|
| TX | Primary tumor cannot be assessed, or tumor proven by the presence of malignant cells in sputum or bronchial washings but not visualized by imaging or bronchoscopy |
| T0 | No evidence of primary tumor |
| Tis | Carcinoma *in situ* |
| T1 | Tumor 3 cm or less in greatest dimension, surrounded by lung or visceral pleura, without bronchoscopic evidence of invasion more proximal than the lobar bronchus,* (not in the main bronchus) |
|   T1a | $</= 2$ cm |
|   T1b | $>2$ cm to $</= 3$ cm |
| T2 | Tumor $>3$ cm but $</= 7$ cm or tumor with any of the following features (T2 tumors with these features are classified as T2a if $</=5$ cm) |

Involves main bronchus, 2 cm or more distal to the carina
Invades the visceral pleura
Associated with atelectasis or obstructive pneumonitis that extends to the hilar region but does not involve the entire lung

| | |
|---|---|
|   T2a | $>3$ cm to $</= 5$ cm |
|   T2b | $>5$ cm to $</= 7$ cm |
| T3 | Tumor $>7$ cm or one that directly invades any of the following: chest wall (including superior sulcus tumors), phrenic nerve, diaphragm, mediastinal pleura, parietal pericardium; or tumor in the main bronchus less than 2 cm distal to the carina*, but without involvement of the carina; or associated atelectasis or obstructive pneumonitis of the entire lung or separate nodules in the same lobe. |
| T4 | Tumor of any size that invades any of the following: mediastinum, heart, great vessels, trachea, recurrent laryngeal nerve, esophagus, vertebral body, carina; or separate tumor nodule(s) in a different ipsilateral lobe. |

*The uncommon superficial spreading tumor of any size with its invasive component limited to the bronchial wall, which may extend proximal to the main bronchus, is also classified T1.

**Regional Lymph Nodes (N)**

| | |
|---|---|
| NX | Regional lymph nodes cannot be assessed |
| N0 | No regional lymph node metastasis |
| N1 | Metastasis to ipsilateral peribronchial and/or ipsilateral hilar lymph nodes, and intrapulmonary nodes including involvement by direct extension of the primary tumor |
| N2 | Metastasis to ipsilateral mediastinal and/or subcarinal lymph nodes(s) |
| N3 | Metastasis to contralateral mediastinal, contralateral hilar, ipsilateral or contralateral scalene, or supraclavicular lymph nodes(s) |

**Distant Metastasis (M)**

| | |
|---|---|
| MX | Distant metastasis cannot be assessed |
| M0 | No distant metastasis |
| M1 | Distant metastasis present |
|   M1a | Separate tumor nodule(s) in a contralateral lobe, tumor with pleural nodules or malignant pleural effusion** |
|   M1b | Distant metastasis |

**Most pleural and pericardial effusions with lung cancer are due to tumor. If repeat cytologic exam shows fluid negative for tumor, nonbloody and an exudate, effusion may not be due to tumor. Based on these elements and clinical judgment, the effusion should be excluded from staging and the patient classified by the appropriate T stage.

**TABLE 18-2  Stage Grouping of Lung Cancer Based on the AJCC Staging System**

| T/M | N0 | N1 | N2 | N3 |
|-----|-----|------|------|------|
| T1a | IA | IIA | IIIA | IIIB |
| T1b | IA | IIA | IIIA | IIIB |
| T2a | IB | IIA | IIIA | IIIB |
| T2b | IIA | IIB | IIIA | IIIB |
| T3 | IIB | IIIA | IIIA | IIIB |
| T4 | IIIA | IIIA | IIIB | IIIB |
| M1a | IV | IV | IV | IV |
| M1b | IV | IV | IV | IV |

**TABLE 18-3  Regional Nodal Definitions and Station Number in Thoracic Anatomy**

| Location | Nodal Station Number |
|----------|----------------------|

**N1 Nodes**—All N1 nodes lie distal to the mediastinal pleural reflection and within the visceral pleura

| | |
|---|---|
| Hilum | 10 |
| Interlobar | 11 |
| Lobar nodes bronchi | 12 |
| Segmental | 13 |
| Subsegmental | 14 |

**N2 Nodes**—All N2 nodes lie within the mediastinal pleural envelope on the ipsilateral side

| | |
|---|---|
| Highest mediastinal | 1 |
| Upper para-tracheal | 2 |
| Pre-vascular and retro-tracheal | 3 |
| Lower para-tracheal | 4 |
| Sub-aortic (aorto-pulmonary window) | 5 |
| Para-aortic nodes (ascending aorta or phrenic) | 6 |
| Subcarinal | 7 |
| Para-esophageal (below carina) | 8 |
| Pulmonary ligament | 9 |

**N3 Nodes**

Contralateral mediastinal nodes, contralateral hilar, ipsilateral or contralateral scalene or supraclavicular lymph nodes constitute N3.

## IASLC LUNG CANCER STAGING PROJECT

Staging of non-small cell lung cancer has followed the 1997 revisions of the American Joint Committee on Cancer in the standard T (tumor), N (lymph node), M (metastatic deposit) format as presented in the 6th edition since 2002. More recently, evaluation of 100,869 patients treated for primary lung cancer between 1990 and 2002 were submitted to the Cancer Research and Biostatistics office in Seattle Washington for statistical analysis. Unlike previous staging systems, this database was international and may reflect outcomes more accurately than previous editions. This effort has culminated in the publication of revisions to the staging system for lung cancer to be published in the upcoming 7th edition of the *TNM Classification for Lung Cancer*. The new staging system will more accurately express the prognostic significance of both the T and N stage in lung cancer outcome.

T stage has been subdivided primarily based on size of the primary tumor. More advanced T stages will include additional nodules in the lung or pleural dissemination, both issues not well addressed in the previous staging system.

Staging of the lymph nodes will continue unchanged, although an effort to define nodal "zones" with respect to outcome is proceeding and may be incorporated into future editions.

### Pancoast Tumor

Pancoast tumor refers to a complex symptom caused by a tumor arising in the superior sulcus of the lung that involves the inferior branches of the brachial plexus (C8 and/or T1) and the sympathetic nerve trunks including the stellate ganglion. If the tumor invades a vertebral body or spinal canal, encases the subclavian vessels, or there is unequivocal involvement of the superior branches of the brachial plexus (C8 or above), then the tumor is classified as T4. If none of these criteria are met, then the tumor is staged T3.

Attribution to Pancoast from a report by Henry K. Pancoast in the 1930s in essence, said it was incurable. The first report was by Hare in the *London Medical Gazette* about 100 years earlier.

## Clinical Presentation

Most lung cancers present at advanced stages. Only approximately 25% present with stage I/II disease, 40% with stage III and 35% patients present with stage IV.[6]

### Locoregional Symptoms

- Local symptoms in the chest: cough/wheeze/stridor/dyspnea/hemoptysis
- Airway obstruction: atelectasis, pneumonia, and possible abscess
- Pain or pleural effusion suggests pleural or chest wall involvement
- Symptoms of Pancoast syndrome (see above) in the setting of an apical mass on radiograph, classical symptoms include lower brachial plexopathy, (T1, C8 root involvement), Horner's syndrome (ptosis, myosis and anhydrosis, sympathetic ganglion involvement), and shoulder pain
- SVC syndrome
  - Secondary to mediastinal lymphadenopathy compressing the SVC
  - Symptoms include periorbital edema, facial plethora (particularly when recumbent), dyspnea, superficial collateral vessels occasionally noted on chest
- Hoarseness: recurrent laryngeal nerve involvement
- Diaphragmatic paralysis: phrenic nerve involvement

### Nonmetastatic Features

Nonspecific systemic features include anorexia, cachexia, weakness, and fatigue. Unintended weight loss of more than 10% is a consistently negative prognostic factor.

Many paraneoplastic syndromes are associated with lung cancer and symptoms may disappear after effective definitive treatment of primary lesion. Hypercalcemia of malignancy is the most commonly seen paraneoplastic syndrome in non-small cell lung carcinoma, linked specifically to squamous cell carcinoma. Nonspecific gyneocomastia is most frequently associated with large cell lung carcinoma. Hypertrophic pulmonary osteoarthropathy refers to a spectrum of skeletal features and may include finger clubbing, periosteal bone formation, and symmetrical painful arthritis. Paraneoplastic syndromes are particularly common with small cell lung cancer due to its neuroendocrine nature. Most commonly seen symptoms include inappropriate ADH, Eaton-Lambert syndrome, and multiple subtypes of neurologic syndromes including subacute sensory neuropathy, subacute cerebellar degeneration, and others.

## DIAGNOSIS AND WORKUP

- Routine history and physical including smoking (# of packs/day × # of years = pack-years) and other risk factors
- Imaging: chest X-ray, computerized tomography of chest through liver and adrenals, Positron Emission Tomography (PET)
- Pulmonary function tests
  - Volumes (FEV1)
  - Diffusion of carbon monoxide from gas in lung to the blood [DLCO]—a measure of gas transmission, altered in "benign" interstitial and fibrotic conditions, worsened by radiotherapy, or combined modality. This measure is often corrected for relative hemoglobin content in the blood.

- Sputum cytology can diagnose 80% of central lesions and fewer than 20% for peripheral tumors.
  - Diagnosis increases from 60% after one sample to 90% after three samples.
  - Sensitivity of 70% for central disease and 45% for peripheral disease
- Bronchoscopy
  - Assesses the proximal tracheobronchial tree up to 2nd or 3rd subsegmental division.
  - At the time of bronchoscopy, cytologic (brushing, irrigation, and lavage cytology) or histologic specimens (biopsy forceps or transbronchial fine needle biopsy) should be obtained.
  - Sensitivity of 85% for central disease, 70% for larger peripheral disease, and only 33% for small ($</=2$ cm) peripheral lesions
- Mediastinoscopy
  - The procedure of choice to evaluate superior mediastinal nodes residing in the pretracheal space. The aortico-pulmonary window, a frequent location of nodes in the left-sided lesions, may require mediastinotomy rather than mediastinoscopy.
- Positron Emitted Tomography (PET): PET scanning has become an accepted staging tool to assess local extent of lung cancers and metastatic spread. Sensitivity has been reported to be between 85%–91% with specificity of 86%–90% compared to CT scanning alone with sensitivity of 61%–75% and specificity of 66%–79% for the primary tumor.[7,8] Detection of metastasis reportedly had a 95% sensitivity and 83% specificity for both mediastinal and distant metastatic disease.[8]
- Esophageal Endoscopic Ultrasound: Provides easy, less invasive access or confirmation of any node adjacent to, or where esophageal traction can assess mediastinal nodes. These are any nodes behind or under the airways (especially 7), but never anterior to the airway.

## Natural History and Screening for Non-Small Cell Lung Cancer

Little is known about the course of untreated lung cancer. In the early screening trials done at Memorial Sloan-Kettering, Johns Hopkins, and the Mayo Clinic, 10,000 high-risk patients were randomized to either chest radiography every 12 months vs. chest radiography and sputum cytology every 12 months with additional sputum cytology every 4 months. Within this study, there was a cohort of 45 patients diagnosed with stage I lung cancer who received no treatment. It was reported that most died of their lung cancers with only two patients surviving more than 5 years.[9] Similarly, McGarry et al[10] reviewed 49 patients who received no treatment for stage I lung cancer due to medical comorbidities and found that the median survival was 14.2 +/− 2.37 months with cause of death reported as lung cancer in 53% of patients. These results suggest that observation may be a poor choice if a treatment option is available for patients with early-stage lung cancer.

Screening remains controversial. The early multi-institutional study, the Mayo Lung Project, showed no survival advantage to screening with chest radiography or sputum cytology. Several earlier trials likewise showed no benefit to screening. Multiple explanations of causes of bias in these studies, including "length of time bias" have been postulated.[11]

The introduction of helical CT imaging held promise for the early diagnosis and enhanced curability of lung cancer. In 1993, the Early Lung Cancer Action Project (ELCAP) was initiated and experimentally screened a cohort of 1,000 high-risk persons. Recommendations for following detected nodules has resulted in 94% of biopsied nodules being positive for cancer and a preliminary report (abstract only) suggests an 8-year survival outcome of 95% when nodules were removed. Smaller cancers were detected on serial screening with the median diameter of the screen-diagnosed cases on repeat screening being 8 mm (vs. 15 mm at baseline screening). These results suggest that screening of high-risk individuals will prove cost-effective and potentially life-saving.[12]

| BOX 18-1 | HENSCHKE PAPER |
|---|---|

The object of this study was to determine the frequency and natural course of mediastinal masses in asymptomatic people at high risk for lung cancer who were undergoing computed tomographic (CT) screening in the ELCAP study. All documented mediastinal masses among the 9,263 baseline and 11,126 annual repeat screenings performed in the Early Lung Cancer Action Project (ELCAP) and its successor project, the New York ELCAP, were identified. Seventy-one patients had a mediastinal mass seen at baseline screening (prevalence of 0.77%). Of the 71 masses, 41 were thymic, 16 were thyroidal, two were esophageal cancers, six were tracheal-esophageal diverticula, and six were other masses. Among the 11,126 annual repeat screenings, only one new mediastinal mass was identified (incidence of 0.01%). This suggested a long average duration for mediastinal masses in asymptomatic people. Among the 41 thymic masses, five were larger than 3.0 cm in diameter, and all five were resected; of these five, one was a thymic carcinoma and four were noninvasive thymomas. Of the remaining 36 thymic masses, 25 were evaluated at follow-up CT 1 year later. Five had increased in diameter, two had decreased, and 18 remained unchanged. All 16 thyroid masses were due to goiter; none of these were changed at follow-up CT 1 year later. The authors concluded that, in the context of CT screening for lung cancer in asymptomatic people masses detected should be approached in a "conservative" manner; this includes thymic masses smaller than 3 cm in diameter, as most of these remained unchanged or even decreased in size.

Henschke, C.I., Lee, I., Wu, N., et al. For the ELCAP and NYELCAP Investigators 2006. CT Screening for Lung Cancer: Prevalence and Incidence of Mediastinal Masses. *Radiology.* 239: 586–590.

## TREATMENT OF NON-SMALL CELL LUNG CANCER BY STAGE

### Stage I/II (node negative)

Treatment options for early stage non-small cell lung carcinoma depend on patient factors such as pulmonary reserve to determine whether or not a patient is a surgical candidate. Typically, standard "cut-off" medical guidelines regarding surgical resection of NSCLC include the following: baseline FEV1 <40%, postoperative predicted FEV1 <30%, severely reduced diffusion capacity, baseline hypoxemia and/or hypercapnia, and exercise oxygen consumption <50% predicted. For surgical candidates, standard of care usually consists of radical surgery (lobectomy, pneumonectomy).

For patients who are considered high risk for surgery, treatment options include limited or sublobar resection, conventionally fractionated local radiation therapy, radiofrequency ablation or stereotactic body radiation therapy. We will review each option.

### Surgery

Details of surgical procedures will not be reviewed here. Commonly, the goal of surgical resection is to obtain a complete resection of the primary tumor. For those patients who are considered surgical candidates, surgery with either lobectomy or pneumonectomy leaving clear margins is considered the gold standard. Although mediastinal lymph node dissection at the time of surgery is mandatory, the degree of dissection is controversial. Lymph node dissection plays a role in staging of patients and an uncertain role therapeutically. At least one randomized trial comparing mediastinal lymphadenectomy versus mediastinoscopy plus intra-operative lymph node sampling revealed no significant difference in survival.[13] In most surgical series, pathological staging of clinically staged I patients results in upstaging of patients to higher stages in approximately 20%–30% of cases. Results of radical surgery for stage I lung cancer reveal 5-year survivals of

50%–80% depending on size of the mass. This is reflected in the 1997 AJCC staging system in which T-stage was subdivided based on size into stages Ia and Ib. In an analysis of 598 patients who received radical surgery with mediastinal lymph node dissection in the majority (560 patients), 5-year survival was 82% for pT1N0M0 patients and 68% for pT2N0M0 patients. The overall incidence of local or regional recurrence was low at 7% with systemic relapse much more common, occurring in up to 20% of patients.[14]

For those patients with marginal pulmonary reserve, limited resection (commonly known as a wedge or segmental resection) may be considered as a substitute for lobectomy, but local failure is higher. Few randomised studies have examined the role of limited surgery. The Lung Cancer Study Group[15] examined 276 patients with early-stage (T1N0M0) non-small cell lung carcinoma randomized into limited resection vs. lobectomy. They concluded that, compared with lobectomy, limited pulmonary resection does not confer improved perioperative morbidity, mortality, or late postoperative pulmonary function. Because of the higher death rate and locoregional recurrence rate associated with limited resection, lobectomy was still considered the surgical procedure of choice for patients with peripheral T1 N0 non-small cell lung cancer.

### Adjuvant Chemotherapy in Stage IB and Higher

As one might expect, the concern remains that both microscopic regional and distant metastasis occurs which may be missed by clinical staging. The report of The International Adjuvant Lung Cancer Trial (IALT) has suggested that chemotherapy may play a significant role in these patients.[16]

---

**BOX 18-2**

The IALT trial was designed to evaluate the effect of cisplatin-based adjuvant chemotherapy on survival after complete resection of non-small-cell lung cancer. Patients were randomly assigned either to three or four cycles of cisplatin-based chemotherapy or to observation. A total of 1,867 patients underwent randomization; 36.5% had pathological stage I disease, 24.2% stage II, and 39.3% stage III. Patients assigned to chemotherapy had a significantly higher survival rate than those assigned to observation (44.5% vs. 40.4% at 5 years [469 deaths vs. 504]; hazard ratio for death, 0.86; 95% confidence interval, 0.76 to 0.98; P <0.03). Patients assigned to chemotherapy also had a significantly higher disease-free survival rate than those assigned to observation (39.4% vs. 34.3% at 5 years [518 events vs. 577]; hazard ratio, 0.83; 95% confidence interval, 0.74 to 0.94; P <0.003).

The International Adjuvant Lung Cancer Trial Cooperative Group. 2004. Cisplatinum-Based Adjuvant Chemotherapy in Patients with Completely Resected Non-Small Cell Lung Cancer. *N.Eng. J. Med.* 350: 351–360.

---

In 2004, results from the NCI-Canada, reported that the use of adjuvant vinorelbine and cisplatin in patients with completely resected stage IB and II NSCLC, improved median (94 months vs. 73 months) and 5-year survival (69% vs. 54%) compared with observation.[17] In addition, the CALGB 9633 trial evaluating adjuvant chemotherapy with paclitaxel and carboplatin following resection of stage IB NSCLC demonstrated a significant improvement in the 4-year survival rate (71% vs. 59%) compared to an observation arm.[18] In these studies, patients received adjuvant platinum-based chemotherapy for four cycles. Collectively, these studies have established chemotherapy as having possible long-term benefits in patients with stage IB-IIIA NSCLC who have undergone a complete surgical resection, although the exact regimens, timing, and patient selection are still under active investigation. Internationally platinum based trials are embraced, particularly those employing vinorelbine, and the carboplatinum fancied in the United States is rarely used, especially with retraction of the survival data from Strauss and the CALGB.

## Conventionally Fractionated Radiation Therapy

While some may continue to embrace larger volume, elective nodal irradiation treatment (ENI), involved-field irradiation (IFI) is generally considered the treatment of choice for locally advanced NSCLC. The reports by Yuan et al examining ENI vs. IFI with concurrent radiotherapy certainly showed no defect in omitting clinically uninvolved nodes, and report a modest survival gain with slightly higher doses.[19a] Rosenzweig details a large Memorial Sloan Kettering series with a similar strategy of treating nodes only 1cm or larger.[19b] This is more pertinent for those patients with stage I lung cancer who cannot undergo surgery[19,20] but 5-year survival following radiotherapy alone is less than approximately half of that achieved by radical surgical resection. Typically, for those patients who are not surgical candidates, due to poor pulmonary reserve (FEV$_1$ <800cc) radiation fields usually encompass the mass with no real attempt at prophylactic nodal coverage. Doses traditionally have ranged between 60–70 Gy in fraction sizes of 180–200 cGy depending on volume of lung irradiated.

Consideration of the beam energy should be taken. As the photons traverse the low density lung, modeling shows a loss of electronic equilibrium on the periphery of high energy (18 Mv) beams which may result in underdosing of the tumor as electronic equilibrium is reestablished. While no randomized data have shown a negative outcome with high energy vs. lower energy beams, theoretically the lowest acceptable energy should be used.[22] General disagreement over

---

**FIGURE 18-1** "Postage stamp field."

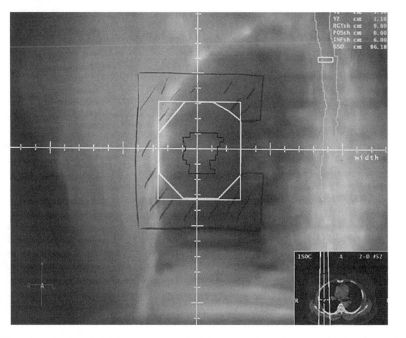

The patient was diagnosed with a 2 cm non-small cell lung cancer. The field was treated AP:PA to a total of 66 Gy.

the merits of algorithms used for correction of inhomogeneities in commercial planning systems remains and no single standard currently exists. The use of inhomogeneity correction, while now possible almost every place, remains left to the discretion of the treating physician because of confidence in the uniform density method, and uncertaintly about safety and applicability of corrected doses.

In multiple studies of outcome following definitive radiotherapy for medically inoperable NSCLC, survival was superior for patients with tumors under 3 cm. Sandler et al[23] reviewed 77 patients with stage I lung cancer treated with definitive radiation therapy to a median dose of 60 Gy. They reported a 22% actuarial disease free survival, but 3-year disease-free survival for patients with tumors less than 3 centimeters, 3–6 centimeters and >6 centimeters was 30%, 17% and 0%, respectively. Patients reviewed in this study were treated from 1970 through 1987 in an era spanning the development of CT and PET scanning, but the survival differences related to tumor size is striking.

In a review of the literature, Sibley[24] reviewed the results of 10 studies of the treatment of medically inoperable early stage NSCLC with radiotherapy. All patients received megavoltage radiotherapy to doses >55 Gy and a median dose of 66 Gy. Grade 3–5 complications occurred in <2% patients. Patients in these studies generally had a 15% median long-term survival (5 years), 25% dying of intercurrent disease, and 30% dying of metastatic disease. The 5-year cause-specific survival was 32%. On patterns of failure analysis, 42% were local-only and 38% were distant-only.

### Dose Escalation

As previously discussed, stage I lung cancer masses are commonly treated to doses of 66–70 Gy in the absence of chemotherapy with a significant risk of local recurrence. Most studies of dose escalation have included patients with higher stage disease. Due to the high risk of local recurrence, several studies have undertaken dose escalation using different strategies to maintain toxicity at acceptable levels. Most strategies try to equate dose/fractionation schemes by employing linear quadratic normalization (biological effective doses ([BED]). This is somewhat difficult because it does not take into account the lengths of treatment time in hypofractionated schemes. Applying the linear quadratic equation (BED=nd[1+d/a/b]) where n=the number of fractions, d=the dose/fraction and a/b ratio of 10 for acute reacting tissue and tumor cells), 70 Gy will have a BED of approximately 84 Gy. Using a mathematical model, Martel et al[25] predicted that for NSCLC patients, the dose to achieve significant probability of tumor control may be at least 84 Gy for longer (>30 months) local progression-free survival. RTOG 9311 was a multi-institutional trial in which a total of 179 patients were enrolled in a Phase I-II three-dimensional radiotherapy dose-escalation fashion.[26] Patients were stratified at escalating radiation dose levels depending on percentage of total lung volume that received >20 Gy with the treatment plan V(20). Patients with a V(20) <25% (Group 1) received 70.9 Gy in 33 fractions, 77.4 Gy in 36 fractions, 83.8 Gy in 39 fractions, and 90.3 Gy in 42 fractions, respectively. Patients with a V(20) of 25%–36% (Group 2) received doses of 70.9 Gy and 77.4 Gy, respectively. V(20) has been used as an indicator of risk for pneumonitis (see below). The radiation dose was safely escalated using three-dimensional conformal techniques to 83.8 Gy for patients with V(20) values of <25% (Group 1) and to 77.4 Gy for patients with V(20) values between 25% and 36% (Group 2), using fraction sizes of 2.15 Gy. The 90.3-Gy dose level was too toxic, resulting in dose-related deaths in two patients. Elective nodal failure occurred in <10% of patients. This study showed that, for patients receiving RT alone or radiation following induction chemotherapy, doses of 83.8 Gy using three-dimensional conformal RT techniques were tolerable, with excess mortality observed at 90.3 Gy. When concurrent chemotherapy and three-dimensional conformal RT are used, the maximum tolerated dose of radiation is reduced, and current indications suggest that the maximum tolerated dose in this setting is in the range of 70 to 74 Gy.[27] Nonetheless, it has not been prospectively demonstrated that dose escalation has produced superior outcomes and careful planning is needed to avoid toxicities. Willner et al[28] retrospectively examined the influence of total dose and tumor volumes on local control and survival in primary radiotherapy of non-small cell lung cancer. They concluded that there is a dose effect on local control and survival with doses of at least 70 Gy (standard fractionation) and that tumors with volumes >/= 100cc may require higher doses.

It thus stands to reason that improved local control may result from higher local radiation doses and studies are ongoing examining hypofractionated stereotactically delivered radiation therapy (see Box 18-4). In an analysis of various hypofractionated stereotactic-delivered radiation schemes, Wulf et al[29] reports that for an optimal control of a stage I lung cancer, a BED of >100 Gy is required. It is apparent that our current treatment regimens may be responsible for the high local recurrence rates, but when one considers the dose-limiting organs in the chest, dose escalation becomes difficult.

---

**BOX 18-4**

The authors present an example of the techniques and assumptions in determining the radiation doses which may theoretically be effective in cancer treatment. Tumor control probability (TCP) model calculations may be used in a relative manner to evaluate and optimize three-dimensional (3-D) treatment plans. Using a mathematical model which makes a number of simplistic assumptions, TCPs can be estimated from a 3-D dose distribution of the tumor given the dose required for a 50% probability of tumor control ($D_{50}$) and the normalized slope ($\gamma$) of the sigmoid-shaped dose–response curve at $D_{50}$. The purpose of this work was to derive $D_{50}$ and $\gamma$ from our clinical experience using 3-D treatment planning to treat non-small cell lung cancer (NSCLC) patients. The results suggest that for NSCLC patients, the dose to achieve significant probability of tumor control may be large (on the order of 84 Gy) for longer (>30 months) local progression-free survival.

Martel, M.K., Ten Haken, R.K., Hazuka, M.B., et al. 2003. Estimation of tumor control probability model parameters from 3-D dose distributions of non-small cell lung cancer patients. *Radiotherapy and Oncology*. 66:119–126.

---

## Stereotactic Body Radiation Therapy (SBRT)

SBRT is a newer technique for dose-escalating lung cancer in which the tumor target is carefully localized in three dimensions and treated with 3–5 large fractions of radiation therapy. In 2000, a phase I dose escalation trial was undertaken at Indiana University.[30] Patients with stage IA and IB (up to 7.0 cm) non-small cell lung cancer who were declared medically inoperable were treated. Preliminary results of this study have been published. Dose-limiting toxicity was not reached for stage IA cancers, but dose escalation was stopped with tumors at 2,000 cGy per fraction (6,000 cGy total dose, given in three fractions). For the stage IB cancers (3.0–7.0 cm), a separate dose escalation was continued to 2,400 cGy/fraction (7,200 cGy) at which dose was felt to be limiting based on the toxicity of pneumonitis appearing. A phase II trial of this treatment at Indiana University was completed with stage IA non-small cell lung cancers receiving 6,000 cGy and stage IB receiving 6,600 cGy delivered in three fractions.[31] With 2-year median follow-up, local control for all patients was >95% with median survival of 32 months for these fragile patients. A multi-institution phase II trial conducted by the RTOG (Radiation Therapy Oncology Group 0236) has been completed and results are pending. As a follow-up, RTOG has now opened a phase II trial to assess SBRT in healthy patients with stage I/II non-small cell lung cancer (RTOG 0618). In this trial, patients who are surgical candidates will be offered SBRT with surgery reserved for treatment failure.

While the stereotactic radiation was well tolerated, a minority of patients had what appears to be partial lung atelectasis downstream from the treated areas. Most of the atelectasis has been clinically insignificant; however, a decision was made in the development of the RTOG to designate a "safety zone" of 2 cm around the major airways which the primary tumor cannot encroach upon. In contrast, Hiraoka et al[32] recently reported on a feasibility study of hypofractionated stereotactic body radiation therapy in patients with solitary non-small cell lung cancers less than 4 cm. The eligibility criteria for primary lung cancer were: (1) solitary tumor less than 4 cm; (2) inoperable, or the patient refused operation; (3) histologically confirmed malignancy; (4) no necessity for oxygen support; (5) performance status equal to or less than 2; and (6) the tumor was not close to the spinal cord. A total dose of 48 Gy was delivered in four fractions in 2 weeks in most patients. Lung toxicity was minimal. No grade II toxicities for spinal cord, bronchus, pulmonary artery, or esophagus were observed. Overall survival for 29 patients with stage IA, and 14 patients with stage IB disease was 87% and 80%, respectively. No local recurrence was observed in a follow-up of 3–5 months. Regional lymph node recurrence developed in one patient, and distant metastases developed in four patients. A total dose of 48 Gy was delivered in four fractions in 2 weeks in most patients. Reported lung toxicity was minimal. No grade II or higher toxicities for spinal cord, bronchus, pulmonary artery, or esophagus were observed. Overall survival for 29 patients with stage IA, and 14 patients with stage IB disease was 87% and 80%, respectively. No local recurrence was observed in a follow-up of 3–5 months. Regional lymph node recurrence developed in one patient, and distant metastases developed in four patients. This fractionation regimen is now being used in a Japan-wide protocol to assess outcome in a multi-institutional trial.

### Toxicity of Radiation Therapy

As in any radiation therapy, one must define potential toxicities for organs at risk. Often these organs have a dose-volume relationship. Recently, analyses of organ function related to toxicity have become a useful means of predicting toxicity. Organs have been described as "serial functioning" or "parallel functioning," examples of which are spinal cord and lung respectively. As the model suggests, a break in a serial functioning organ results in malfunction of the entire organ (transverse myelitis in the spinal cord). In a parallel functioning organ, destruction or removal of one portion, within limits, does not prevent the organ from functioning. Thus in serial functioning organs point or small volumes of high doses can be critical and must be examined. One must also consider late effects and early effects separately.

As an outgrowth of the need to more uniformly define and describe toxicities, the National Cancer Institute produced the Common Terminology Criteria for Adverse Events (CTCAE) which can be accessed electronically at http://ctep.cancer.gov.

**FIGURE 18-2** Conceptual organ function.

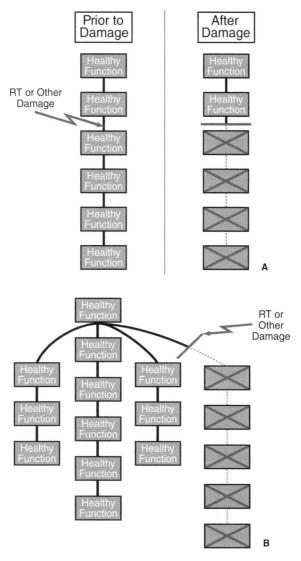

Organs can sometimes be thought of as "serial functioning" **(A)** or "parallel functioning" **(B)** As can be seen from the schematic, damage (by radiotherapy or other toxic insult) in the continuity of the serial functioning organ leaves it non-functional (spinal cord), whereas paraellel functioning organs have many non-interdependent subunits which can tolerate at least partial loss and still function on the organ level (lung).

## BOX 18-5

The authors (33) present the opinions and experience of the clinicians from four universities of normal tissue organs to irradiation. An NCI task force, chaired by the primary author, was formed and an extensive literature search was carried out to address this issue. This remains as a reference containing basic information on both whole and partial organ tolerances defining the TD 5/5 and 5/50 (5% or 50% organ complication at 5 years). It also emphasized the need to define an endpoint when trying to estimate toxicities.

Emami B. Lyman J. Brown A. Coia L. Goitein M. Munzenrider JE. Shank B. Solin LJ. Wesson M. 1991. Tolerance of normal tissue to therapeutic irradiation. Int. J. Rad. Oncol. Biol. Phy. 21(1):109–122.

TABLE 18-4  **Dose Limits to Organs in Stereotactic Body Radiation Therapy for Early-Stage Lung Cancer (RTOG 0236)**

| Organ | Volume | Dose (cGy) |
|---|---|---|
| Spinal Cord | Any point | 18 Gy (6 Gy per fraction) |
| Esophagus | Any point | 27 Gy (9 Gy per fraction) |
| Ipsilateral Brachial Plexus | Any point | 24 Gy (8 Gy per fraction) |
| Heart | Any point | 30 Gy (10 Gy per fraction) |
| Trachea and Ipsilateral Bronchus | Any point | 30 Gy (10 Gy per fraction) |

Within clinical trials there are often tables of dose limits defining the doses given to organs. For example, limits set within RTOG 0236 are shown in Table 18-3.

Pneumonitis is a challenging problem in the radiation therapy of early stage non-small cell lung carcinoma and it appears to represent a dose/volume relationship. Prediction of the risk of pneumonitis is an ongoing subject of research. Investigators often consider the "V(20)" and more recently, mean lung dose. Graham et al[34] reported the correlation between V(20) and the actuarial incidence of $>/=$ Grade 2 pneumonitis. The greater the volume of total lung (that is both lung volumes minus GTV) encompassed by the 20 Gy isodose line, the higher the risk of pneumonitis.

Typically, pneumonitis presents as a dry cough. Radiological examination will show an infiltrate within the radiation portal. Pneumonitis can be troublesome and is treated with tapering doses of prednisone. In severe cases, hospitalization will be necessary.

Esophageal toxicity, both acute (early) and late can be problematic in the therapy of lung cancer. Typically, with fractionated radiotherapy using 180–200 cGy fractions, patients begin to detect changes at 2,000 cGy with complaints of a "lump in my throat." From there, esophagitis can gradually worsen, although individual patient complaints are extremely variable. It is unclear how much concurrent chemotherapy adds to the severity of esophagitis. Emami et al[33] report a $TD_{5/5}$ for late effects defined as perforation/strictures between 5,500 and 6,000 cGy depending on volume radiated. Symptomatic strictures at doses commonly employed for non-small cell lung cancer are relatively rare. As dose escalation studies progress, this represents an important end organ toxicity to be considered. Strategies

TABLE 18-5  **Dose/Volume Considerations in the Risk of Developing Pneumonitis**

| V20 (%) | Grade 2 (%) | Grade 3 (%) |
|---|---|---|
| <22 | 0 | 0 |
| 22–31 | 7 | 0 |
| 32–40 | 13 | 5 (1 fatal) |
| >40 | 36 | 23 (3 fatal) |

for the management of esophagitis may include various local anesthetics ("Mary's Magic Mouthwash"), various opiate pain relievers and in extreme cases, implanted tube feeding devices.

## *Stage III*

The mountain staging system derives from the retrospective surgical experience of about 10,000 cases at MD Anderson. The International Association for the Study of Lung Cancer (www.IASLC.org) will elaborate a new staging system before this handbook is out of date.

Stage III is regarded mostly in surgical terms, but it is far from clear that surgery is the critical factor in either Stage IIIA or B.

In the early 1980s, the CALGB developed a project that employed chemotherapy first, which they called "proto-adjuvant." Brilliantly, and before their time, they based the treatment on two cycles of cis-platinum and four weekly doses of vinorelbine—no alkylating agents. The landmark, paradigm shifting trial widely known as the Dillman trial altered the course of non-surgical therapy by demonstrating that only brief courses of chemotherapy were significantly better than radiotherapy alone. The study was stopped early because of evidence that made continuing unreasonable. The median survival was nearly 14 months with the chemotherapy and only in the range of 9 months with radiotherapy alone to 60 Gy.[35] The study was replicated by an Intergroup effort that confirmed the fact that the same drugs as before were qualitatively, but not quantitatively, as good as CALGB announced.[36] The theory and apparent fact were that these tactics reduced distant metastasis, but did not alter local control.[37]

Contemporaneously, a Dutch trial randomized daily and weekly cisplatinum as a single agent comparing it to the common split course radiotherapy alone.[38] This trial supported a benefit of daily or weekly platinum as opposed to the 55 Gy split course radiotherapy delivered in somewhat larger doses per fraction.

These studies set the stage for the next 20 years of research, mostly distracted by a trainload of new drugs delivered in the early 1990s. Clearly, chemotherapy plus radiotherapy is better than radiotherapy alone. What chemotherapy and the fundamental issues of radiotherapy to what dose, over what time, and with what fractionation remain ill-defined. Furthermore, the timing issues, chemotherapy first, or chemotherapy after in a so-called sequential fashion, versus concurrent therapy are controversial issues. There have been too many phase II trials to list. The following facts are points to ponder:

1. Two drugs, platinum and another agent, work; three drugs are more toxic and no better.
2. The old combinations have been tested more thoroughly, platinum plus either vinblastine, vindesine, or VP-16 (etoposide)—the "V drugs." The addition of mitomycin, which has a low response rate in advanced disease, and causes pulmonary toxicity, may be associated with excess mortality, and quite clearly no longer has a place.
3. None of the new drugs in combination is superior, but they have been widely adopted, particularly carboplatinum-paclitaxel in the United States, gemcitabine and platinum in some European countries, and vinorelbine and platinum in other European countries and Canada. This is based on successful marketing, not scientific data.
4. Concurrent appears to be slightly better than sequential, but clearly is more toxic. The selection process for concurrent trials mandates a more fit patient.
5. The bloom is off the rose for "up-front" chemotherapy. LAMP, a Bristol-funded study, fails to show benefit with upfront strategies. Concurrent, followed by "adjuvant," also called "consolidation," currently is very popular based on very thin data.
6. We like to believe that a bigger dose of thoracic radiotherapy is better. We have anecdotes and demonstration projects, but no prospective data.

7. Elective nodal irradiation has never been subjected to trial about benefit or liability; it is controversial. Some do it because they were trained to and there is a frequency of failure. We did an early dose escalation trial and chose to omit the nodes. It does not compromise survival, and node-only failure is distinctly unusual.

The main controversy has been the value of "converting" a stage III patient into a patient relegated to no surgery to one that might benefit from surgery. Two trials fueled this concept: Rosell from Spain and Roth from MD Anderson. However, the pioneers of chemotherapy followed by surgery were the memorial team, which did not conduct randomized trials, but treated patients with mitomycin (M) vinblastine (V) and cisplatin (P).[39-42]

Two recent trials fail to convince doubters that surgery truly benefits IIIA as a category [43,44]; however, believers in surgery cling to the significant improvement in progression-free survival and post hoc subset "exploratory" analyses that point to liability for those requiring surgery and benefit to those resectable by lobectomy.[43]

### Postoperative Radiotherapy

Although there are legion retrospective studies before and after the PORT meta-analysis.[45,45a] There is no category A evidence to support the use of postoperative radiotherapy in any stage. The forest plots from this paper do not exclude the possibility of a small benefit to postoperative radiotherapy in N-2 patients or Stage III. Although this report generated a heated response, no prospective trials establishing radiotherapy have been done. The PORT seemed to cause late mortality, and this was attributed to dose and volume; however, safer doses and appropriate safer volumes are not described or established by trial. Experts do not agree on the appropriate use of postoperative radiotherapy.

The case of "accidental surgery" needs to be excluded. The majority of thoracic surgery is not done by board certified thoracic surgeons focusing on lung surgery. Inadequate preoperative staging and intra-operative nodal sampling and dissection can lead to a patient who has had an operation, a lobectomy, or a wedge resection without proper assessment of mediastinal nodes. If these prove to be positive by PET or endoscopic ultrasound, the inadequate accidental surgery should not prevent definitive chemoradiotherapy to full dose. Compounding the accident and leaving the patient without standard therapy is a mistake. On the other hand, finding a solitary node, immuno-histochemistry positive, after preoperative PET or mediastinoscopy may have a frequency of local failure, but the risk of systemic failure is larger. Some believe this justifies local therapy.

Until a prospective trial establishes safety and efficacy, the role of postoperative radiotherapy in lung cancer is speculative and not evidence-based.

## Small Cell Lung Cancer

Small cell lung cancer appears to be decreasing in clinical frequency (may be as low as 15% of lung cancer).[46] Classically one third had limited disease and two thirds extensive. Workup is similar to NSCLC, with the exception that brain evaluation is mandated in all cases, and PET scan is not paid for in initial evaluation.

Chemotherapy provides the cornerstone in management. Cisplatin etoposide [PE] remains the standard for the past 25 years, despite intensive interest and study of the "new" drugs from the early 1990s. The trial of Sundstrom put to rest with evidence the debate about the equivalency of alkylators/anthracycline regimens to this regimen. However, the meta-analyses still includes the older trials with this less effective chemotherapy at their foundation.[47-49] PE can be used concurrently in full dose without reduction in thoracic radiotherapy dose. As with NSCLC, the benefit may be small, and the toxicity also increases, but no other combination or addition of another drug has proven better.

Radiotherapy factors include total dose (and dose per fraction), target volume (what to include, as well as critical organ/structure dose), fractionation or delivery of dose per unit of time, and timing of radiotherapy with chemotherapy. These are nicely summarized and reviewed by Murray and Turrisi.[50]

Standard treatment is based on the randomized Intergroup study initiated in 1988, and published in 1999.[51] This trial compared two cooperative group pilots, and at the time of study conception, no one used doses of higher than 50 Gy. The trial was the first trial using upfront cisplatin etoposide and immediate concurrent therapy with 45 Gy, one group receiving daily therapy for 5 weeks, the other twice daily 1.5 Gy fractions for 3 weeks. The accelerated, twice-daily group produced significant survival benefit, with an absolute difference of 10% (26% vs. 16%) at 5 years, and a 60% relative improvement. The frequency of grade III esophagitis was doubled with accelerated concurrent therapy, 27% BID vs. 13% QD. Esophagitis always healed without stricture.

## Dose

Although doses have been escalated to 70 Gy, and 60 Gy is commonly used, these protract therapy, and overlap with multiple cycles of chemotherapy. No prospective trial establishes higher dose to be superior to 45 Gy BID in 3 weeks. A concept of concentration of the chemoradiotherapy package has been expressed by De Ruysscher and colleagues, and it suggests that protracting the start (S) to end (E) of radiotherapy (R) [SER] beyond 30 days results in worse outcome.[52]

The Intergroup study was conceived and carried out before the availability of three-dimensional or IMRT capabilities. The development of these has naturally led to explorations of higher doses. Doses have been probed at the same time new chemotherapeutics have been tested, so the two variables confound one another, and clear trials of one or the other have not been done. The cooperative group pilots have embarked on projects using doses between 60 and 63 Gy concurrently with PE, but using taxanes and topoisomerase drugs before or after. CALGB used a dose of 70 Gy after induction for two cycles with paclitaxel and topotecan.[53] It is unlikely that any of these will be tested because the 2- and 5-year assessments are not superior to the Intergroup result.

A hypothesis-oriented phase III study has been proposed in the United States (it has failed to inspire support by drug companies or the NCI's CTEP), and steps have been taken in Britain and the EU to look at a once daily dose in this range versus the 45 Gy in 3 weeks standard.

As dose and volume confound each other, so do dose and fractionation, or dose and timing. The Mayo Clinic initially, and then the North Central Cancer Treatment Group attempted to test the value of fractionation, and increased the comparative daily dose slightly.[54] However, the twice daily dose's liability of increased esophagitis caused them to install a planned treatment break midway through two courses, each of 24 Gy in 8 treatment days. So, the total twice daily treatment time took a minimum of 30 treatment days, and likely 40 elapsed days with the breaks and weekends included, nearly double the time of the 45 Gy twice daily treatment. Also, these studies included induction chemotherapy which further extends SER. Despite increasing the once daily dose to 54 Gy in 1.8 Gy fractions, the two treatments seem to produce equivalent survival, neither superior to the standard.

The Massachusetts General Hospital group has a series of patients, some of whom were assigned to high-dose daily therapy as high as 70 Gy and others to the accelerated short course of 45 Gy in 3 weeks. Their results have been summarized by Roof.[55] Retrospectively, these observations make the case for a prospective trial so that unanticipated variables could be checked by a process of randomization rather than assignment.

## Volume

This issue has two parts. Is there a standard volume regardless of response to chemotherapy, and is there evidence that bulk reduced by chemotherapy can be the sole target? There are few data to this point, and some expert opinion. The data are retrospective, again from Mayo.[56] These data largely address the second issue and find nothing lost by targeting just the volume found after chemotherapy reduces the target size. Older studies used a rather large traditional volume including supraclavicular nodes, both hilar areas, at least two vertebral bodies below the carina, and all of the nodes to the gastro-esophageal hiatus in lower lobe lesions. Such large volumes expose tremendous volumes of lung and esophagus and seem to add to toxicity. The Intergroup study forbade the treatment of supraclavicular nodes except when an ipsilateral one was clinically involved or treated in passing because the primary extended either from or to the area above the clavicle. Today, I urge inclusion only of nodes that measure ≥1 cm on a treatment planning CT scan. Others continue large volume, but there are no clear studies addressing the issue.

### Timing

Concurrent early therapy, preferably at cycle one, but commonly cycle two can be done safely to best outcome with cisplatin etoposide. This assertion gains support from the trans-Canada study[57] and the Intergroup Trial.[51] Against this proposition are the meta-analyses, which remember to include the older trials using alkylators and anthracyclines, which are ineffective or incompatible, respectively, with thoracic radiotherapy. Many continue to wish for benefit with upfront chemotherapy, a failed strategy in the PE era, but continued with fervent adherents. The difference is not overwhelming, but in the most fit patients of any age it seems the best chance for long-term survival. It is a mistake for unfit patients of any age. If chemotherapy is not offered or possible, treatment is palliative. Do not waste resources or their time, which is indeed limited. Long-term survival is anecdotal.

### Fractionation

Rather than debate the merits of once a day or twice a day in both sections, I will tackle the issue here. Frankly, speaking of it that simplistically is a fundamental error. It matters little if the delivery is once, twice, or three times each day, weekends included or weekends off, it is a biological issue of proliferating clonagens and short cell cycle times versus the kinetics and the ability of the tumor and irradiated normal tissues to repair damage. The short answer is that accelerated treatments have proven benefit in terms of survival in proof of principle studies. Hyperfractionation using 1.2 Gy per fraction has been done for too many years in RTOG pilots, and then added as a third "spoiler" arm, without ever demonstrating that using low dose per fraction delivered twice daily provides the intended protection to late effect tissues, and that the smaller fraction sizes actually are capable of killing cancer permanently (leading to adequate survival and local control). In prospective trials, 1.2 Gy to 69.6 Gy (why this anointed dose?) has never been isolated as a variable that makes the difference.

On the other hand, when an accelerated test is compared directly to a more protracted course, the accelerated course improves local control and survival at the price of increased acute responding tissue toxicity. Many argue that convenience (for the patients or for the equipment) or this toxicity (principally esophagitis, which while severe in about 25%–30% of cases, always reversible without long-term sequellae) are excuses to not use accelerated schemes which are too long, too unproven for too long, and more expensive.

## SPECIAL CASES

### Superior Vena Cava Syndrome

A common scenario most often resulting from locally advanced lung cancer in the chest is superior vena cava obstruction (SVCO) distal to the azygos vein leading to a symptomatic syndrome characterized by swelling of the head, face, and upper extremities. It is often exaggerated when the patient first arises from decumbency. In a review of 78 patients with SVCO syndrome, small cell and non-small cell lung cancer accounted for 17 (22%) and 19 (24%) cases, respectively, but a higher percentage of patients with small-cell lung cancer developed the syndrome (6% vs. 1%).[58] The most frequent signs and symptoms were face or neck swelling (82%), upper extremity swelling (68%), dyspnea (66%), cough (50%), and dilated chest vein collaterals (38%). Dyspnea at rest, cough, and chest pain were more frequent in the patients with malignancy. Besides lung cancer other malignancies which can be responsible for SVCO syndrome include lymphoma, thymic carcinomas, and germ cell tumors.

Treatment is aimed at rapid relief of symptoms. Mechanical stenting has been used in the setting of anticoagulation, steroids, and supplemental oxygen to provide rapid relief of symptoms in severe cases. Rowell and Gleeson[59] examined the effectiveness of several approaches to the management of SVCO syndrome in patients entered on several separate clinical trials of lung cancer. Superior vena cava obstruction was present at diagnosis in 10% of patients with small cell lung cancer (SCLC) and 1.7% of patients with non-small cell lung cancer (NSCLC). In SCLC, chemotherapy and/or radiotherapy relieved SVCO in 77%; 17% of those treated had a recurrence of SVCO. In NSCLC, 60% had relief of SVCO following chemotherapy and/or radiotherapy; 19% of those treated had a recurrence of SVCO. Insertion of an SVC stent relieved SVCO in 95%; 11% of those treated had further SVCO but recanalization was possible in the majority resulting in a long-term patency rate of 92%.

Radiotherapy treatment will vary depending on the goals and severity of presentation. It is always wise to delay treatment until pathology is obtained since it is rarely a life-threatening situation. Often it is considered a palliative condition and typical treatment will encompass the bulk of the mass to total doses of 30 Gy in 10 fractions of 3 Gy. Nonetheless, in the setting of potentially curative approaches to non-small cell lung cancer, more curative doses of radiotherapy could be considered. In small cell lung cancer, chemotherapy is often given up front and if the patient is considered limited stage, more conventional approaches can be undertaken.[60]

## Bronchial Invasion: Hemoptysis and Atelectasis

Central or hilar masses are very common and patients may present with symptoms secondary to local effects of tumor. Diagnostically, bronchoscopy become very important since biopsies may be obtained from tumor in the airway. If obstruction is present, the pulmonologist may be able to debulk tumor in an effort to begin palliation. Similarly, hemoptysis may be cauterized at the time of bronchoscopy. In palliative settings, endobronchial brachytherapy may be useful for palliation, but since prescription doses may only be 1–2 cm depth, long-term tumor control is not common, especially with masses of cancer >3 cm. We will not consider brachytherapy in detail here.

Patients who present with partial or complete atelectasis of the lung may benefit from PET scanning in an effort to distinguish tumor from collapsed lung. Depending on the bulk of disease or concomitant metastasis, radiotherapy may be short course/large fraction or more prolonged. Common palliative doses include 20 Gy in 400 cGy fractions or 30 Gy in 300 cGy fractions. For the patient with very limited life expectancy, Indiana University has used a multiple arc technique to give fractions of 1,000 cGy to limited fields with good success in opening airways (not published). In our experience, the success in re-inflating atelectatic lungs varies depending on the length of time they have been collapsed (>30 days is a negative factor), but is about 30% successful with radiation alone. Hemoptysis is treated similarly. It is often self-limiting as tumor erodes bronchial blood vessels; however, massive hemoptysis can occur resulting in death. Either by bronchoscopy or by CT, an effort should be made to localize the area where the blood is originating and targeted by the radiation oncologist. Depending on whether one is in a palliative or curative setting, the dose of radiation is chosen as previously described. For brisk bleeding, larger doses (small treatment volume), 400 cGy+ fractions are chosen. Often the bleeding decreases rapidly once radiotherapy is initiated.

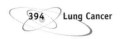 

## REFERENCES

1.  American Cancer Society. Cancer facts and figures. Atlanta; *2006*.
2.  Brown CC, and Kessler LG. Projections of lung cancer mortality in the United States 1985–2025. *JNCI.* 80:43–51.
3.  Centers for Disease Control and Prevention. *Annual smoking attributable mortality, years o potential life lost and economic costs—United States,* 1997–2001, MMWR Morb. *Mortal. Wkl Rep.* 54:625–628. 2005.
4.  American Joint Committee on Cancer. *AJCC Cancer Staging Manual,* 6th Edition. New York Springer-Verlag, 2002 Goldstraw P, Crowley J, Chansky MS, et al. The IASLC Lunc Cance Staging Project: proposals for the revision of the TNM stage groupings in the forthcomin (seventh) edition of the *TNM Classification of Malignant Tumours. J Thorac Oncol* 2007 2:706–714.
5.  Travis WD, Colby TV, Corrin B, et al. Histologic typing of lung and pleural tumors. In *Worl Health Organization Pathology Panel: World Health Organization Histological Classificatio of Tumors*, 3rd edition. Berlin: Springer-Verlag, 1999
6.  Bulzebruck H, Bopp R, Drings P, et al. 1992. New aspects in the staging of lung cancer Prospective validation of the international union against cancer TNM classification. *Cancer* 70:1102–1110.
7.  Pieterman RM, et al. Preoperative staging of NSCLC with PET. *N. Eng. J. Med.* 343:254–261. 2000
8.  Gould MK, Kuschner WG, Rydzak CE, et al. Test performance of *Ann Intern Med.* 139 879–892. 2003.
9.  Flehinger BJ, Kimmel M, et al. Screening for lung cancer. The Mayo Lung Project revisited *Cancer* 72:1573–80. 1993.
10. McGarry RC, Song G, DesRosiers P and Timmerman R. Observation-only management of earl stage, medically inoperable lung cancer: poor outcome. *Chest.* 121:1155–1158. 2002.
11. Fontana RS, Sanderson DR, Woolner LB, Taylor WF, Miller WE, Muhm JR, Bernatz PE. Payn WS. Pairolero PC. Bergstralh EJ. Screening for lung cancer. A critique of the Mayo Lun Project. *Cancer.* 67 (4. Suppl):1155–64. 1991.
12. Henschke CI, Lee I, Wu N, et al. For the ELCAP and NYELCAP investigators CT screening for lun cancer: prevalence and incidence of mediastinal masses. *Radiology.* 239:586–590. 2006.
13. Izbicki JR, Thetter O, Habekost M, et al. Radical systematic mediastinal lymphadenectomy in non-small cell lung cancer: a Randomised Controlled Trial. *Br. J. Surg.* 81:229. 1994.
14. Martini N, Bains MS, Burt ME, et al. Incidence of local recurrence and second primary tumor in resected stage I lung cancer. *J. Thor. Cardiov. Surg.*109:120–129. 1995.
15. Ginsberg RJ and Rubenstein LV for the Lung Cancer Study Group. Randomized trial of lobec tomy versus limited Resection for T1, N0 non-small cell lung cancer. *Ann. Thorac. Surg* 60:615–623. 1995.
16. The International Adjuvant Lung Cancer Trial Cooperative Group. Cisplatinum-based adjuvan chemotherapy in patients with completely resected non-small cell lung cancer. *N. Eng. J Med.* 350:351–360. 2004.
17. Winton T, Livingston D, Jonson J, et al. A prospective randomized trial of adjuvant vinorel bine (VIN) and cisplatin (CIS) in completely resected stage 1B and II non-small cell lung can cer (NSCLC) Intergroup JBR.10. *J. Clin. Oncol.* 22:7018. 2004.
18. Strauss G, Hernson J, Maddaus M, et al. Randomized clinical trial of adjuvant chemotherap with paclitaxel and carboplatin following resection in Stage IB non-small cell lung cance (NSCLC): Report of Cancer and Leukemia Group B (CALGB) Protocol 9633. *J. Clin. Oncol* 22:7019. 2004.

9.  Cheung PCF, MacKillop WJ, Dixon P, et al. Involved field radiotherapy alone for early stage non-small-cell lung cancer. *Int. J. Rad. Oncol. Biol. Phys.* 48:703–710. 2000.

9a. Yuan S, Sun X, Li M, et al. A randomized study of involved-field irradiation versus elective nodal irradiation in combination with concurrent chemotherapy for inoperable stage III non-small cell lung cancer. *Amer J Clin Oncol.* 30:239–244; 2007.

9b. Rosenzweig KE, Sura S, Jackson A, Yorke E. Involved-field radiation therapy for inoperable non-small cell lung cancer. *J Clin Oncol.* 25(35):5557–5561. 2007.

0.  Gail MH, Eagan RT, Feld R, et al. Prognostic factors in patients with resected stage I NSCLC: a report from the Lung Cancer Study Group. *Cancer* 54:1802–1813. 1984.

1.  Giraud P, Antoine M, Larrouy A, et al. Evaluation of microscopic formal radiotherapy planning. *Int. J. Rad. Oncol. Biol. Phys.* 48:1015–1024. 2000.

2.  Ekstrand KE and Barnes MS. Pitfalls in the use of high energy X-rays to treat tumors in the lung. *Int. J. Rad. Oncol. Biol. Tumor Extension in Non-Small Cell Lung Cancer for Three Dimensional ConPhys* 18:249–252. 1990.

3.  Sandler HM, Curran WJ and Turrisi AT. The influence of tumor size and pre-treatment staging on outcome following radiation therapy alone for stage I non-small cell lung cancer. *Int. J. Rad. Onc. Biol. Phys.* 19:9–13. 1990.

4.  Sibley GS, Jamieson TA, Marks,LB., et al. Radiotherapy alone for medically inoperable stage I non-small cell lung cancer: the Duke experience. *Int. J. Rad. Onc. Biol. Phys.* 40:49–154. 1998.

5.  Martel M, Ten Haken R, Hazuka M, et al. Estimation of tumor control probability from 3-D dose distributions of non-small cell lung cancer patients. *Lung Cancer.* 24:31–37. 1999.

6.  Bradley J, Graham MV, Winter K, Purdy JA, Komaki R, Roa WH, Ryu J K, Bosch W, Emami B. Toxicity and outcome results of RTOG 9311: a phase I-II dose-escalation study using three-dimensional conformal radiotherapy in patients with inoperable non-small cell lung carcinoma. *Int. J. Rad. Onc. Biol. Phys.* 61(2):318–328. 2005.

7.  Bradley J. A review of radiation dose escalation trials for non-small cell lung cancer within the Radiation Therapy Oncology Group. *Sem. Oncol.* 32 (2 suppl 3):S111–113. 2005.

8.  Willner J, Baier K, Caragiani E., et al. Dose, volume and tumor control reductions in primary radiotherapy of non-small cell lung cancer. *Int. J. Rad. Onc. Biol. Phys.* 52:382–389. 2002.

9.  Wulf J, Baier K, Mueller G, Flentje MP. Dose-response in the stereotactic irradiation of lung tumors. *Radiother. and Oncol.* 77:83–87. 2005.

0.  Timmerman R, Papiez, L, McGarry, R, Likes, L, DesRosiers, C, Bank, M, Frost, S, Randall, M, and Williams, M. Extracranial stereotactic radioablation: results of a phase I study in medically inoperable stage I non-small cell lung cancer patients. *Chest.* 124:1946–1955. 2003.

1.  McGarry, RC, Papiez L, Williams M, et al. Stereotactic body radiation therapy of early stage non-small cell lung carcinoma: phase I study. *Int. J. Rad. Onc. Biol. Phys.* 63:1010–1015. 2005.

2.  Hiraoka M, Nagata Y. Stereotactic body radiation therapy for early-stage non-small-cell lung cancer. *Int. J Clin. Oncol.* 9:352–355. 2004.

3.  Emami B, Lyman J, Brown A, Coia L, Goitein M, Munzenrider JE, Shank B, Solin LJ, Wesson M. Tolerance of normal tissue to therapeutic irradiation. *Int. J. Rad. Oncol. Biol. Phy.* 21(1):109–122. 1991.

4.  Graham MV, Purdy JA, Emami BE, et al. Clinical dose volume histogram analysis for pneumonitis after 3D treatment for non-small cell lung cancer (NSCLC). *Int J Rad. Oncol. Biol. Phys.* 45(2):323–329. 1999.

5.  Dillman RO, Herndon J, Seagren S, et al. Improved survival in stage III non-small cell lung cancer: seven-year follow-up of cancer and leukemia group B (CALGB) 8433 trial. *J Natl Cancer Inst* 88:1210–1215. 1996.

36. Sause W, Kolesar P, Taylor S, et al. Final results of a phase III trial in regionally advanced unresectable non-small cell lung cancer: Radiation therapy oncology group, eastern cooperative oncology group, and southwest oncology group. *Chest* 117:358–364. 2000.

37. Arriagada R, LeChevalier T, Quoix E, et al. ASTRO (American Society of Therapeutic Radiatio. Oncology) plenary: effect of chemotherapy on locally advanced non-small cell lung carcinoma: a randomized study of 353 patient. *Int J Radiat Oncol Biol Phys* 1183–1190. 1991.

38. Schaake Koning C, van den Bogaert W, Dalesio O, et al. Effects of concomitant cisplatin and radiotherapy on inoperable non-small cell lung cancer. *New Engl J Med* 326:524–530. 1992

39. Ng K, Kris K, Ginsberg RJ, et al. Induction chemotherapy employing dose intense cisplatin with mitomycin and vinblastine (MVP-400), followed by thoracic surgery or irradiation, for patients with stage III non-small cell lung cancer. *Cancer* 86:1189–1197. 1999.

40. Rosell R, Gomez-Codina J, Camps C, et al. Preresectional chemotherapy in stage IIIa non-small-cell lung cancer: a seven year assessment of a randomized controlled trial. *Lung Cancer* 26:7–14. 1999.

41. Roth J, Fossella F, Komaki R, et al. A randomized trial comparing perioperative chemotherapy and surgery with surgery alone in resectable IIIA non-small-cell lung cancer. *J Nat Cancer Inst* 86:673–680. 1994.

42. Albain K, Rusch V, Crowley J, et al. Concurrent cisplatin/etoposide plus chest radiotherapy followed by surgery for stages III A (N-2) and III B non-small cell lung cancer: mature results of Southwest Oncology Group phase II study 8805. *J Clin Oncol* 13:1880–1892, 1995.

43. Albain K, Swann S, Rusch V, et al. Phase III study of concurrent chemotherapy and radiotherapy (CT/RT) vs. CT/RT followed by surgical resection for stage III A (pN2) non-small cell lung cancer (NSCLC): outcomes update of North American Intergroup 0139 (RTOG 9309). *J Clin Oncol* 23(suppl 16s):624s (Abstr 7014). 2005.

44. Van Meerbeck J, Kramer G, Van Schil P, et al. A randomized trial of radical surgery versus thoracic radiotherapy after response to induction chemotherapy in patients with histo-/cytologically proven irresectable stage IIIA-N2 NSCLC (EORTC 08941). *J Clin Oncol* 23 (suppl 1. s):624s (Abstr 7015 LBA). 2005.

45. PORT Meta-analysis Trialist Group. Postoperative radiotherapy in non-small-cell lung cancer systematic review and meta-analysis from individual patient from nine randomized controlled studies. *Lancet* 352:257–274. 1998.

45a. Lally BE, Zelterman D, Colasanto, et al. Postoperative radiotherapy for stage II or III non-small-cell lung cancer using the surveillance, epidemiology, and end results database. *J Clin Oncol.* 24:2998–3006, 2006.

46. Page NC, Reed WL, Tierney RM, et al. The epidemiology of small cell lung carcinoma. *Proc Amer Soc Clin Oncol* 21:305a (abstract 1216). 2002.

47. Sundstrom S, Bremnes R, Kaasa S, et al. Cisplatin and etoposide regimen is superior to cyclophosphamide, epirubicin, and vincristine regimen in small cell lung cancer: results from randomized phase III trial with 5 years' follow-up. *J Clin Oncol* 20:4665–4672. 2002.

48. Pignon JP, Arriagada R, Ihde DC, et al. A meta-analysis of thoracic radiotherapy for small-cell lung cancer. *N Engl J Med* 327(23):1618–1624. 1992.

49. Warde P, and Payne D. Does thoracic irradiation improve survival and local control in limited stage small cell lung carcinoma of the lung? A metanalysis. *J Clin Oncol.* 1992.

50. Murray N and Turrisi AT. A review of first-line treatment of small-cell lung cancer. *J Thorac Oncol* 1:270–278. 2006.

51. Turrisi AT, 3rd, Kim K, Blum R, et al. Twice-daily compared with once-daily thoracic radiotherapy in limited small cell lung cancer treated concurrently with cisplatin and etoposide. *N Engl J Med* 340(4):265–271. 1999.

52. DeRuysscher D, Pijls-Johannesma M, Bentzen S, et al. Time between the first day of chemotherapy and the last day of chest radiation is the most important predictor of survival in limited-disease small cell lung cancer. *J Clin Oncol* 24:1057–1063. 2006.
53. Bogart JA, Herndon JE, Lyss AP, et al. 70 Gy thoracic radiotherapy is feasible concurrent with chemotherapy for limited-stage small cell lung cancer: analysis of cancer and leukemia group b study 39808 study. *Int J Radiat Oncol Biol Phys.* 59:460–468. 2004.
54. Schild S, Bonner JA, Shanahan TG, et al. Long-term results of a phase III trial comparing once-daily with twice-daily radiotherapy in limited-stage small cell lung cancer. *Int J Radiat Oncol Biol Phys* 59:943–951. 2004.
55. Roof K, Fidias P, Lynch T, et al. Radiation dose intensification in limited-stage small cell lung cancer. *Clin Lung Cancer* 4:339–346. 2003.
56. Liengswangswong V, Bonner JA, Shaw E, et al. Limited-stage small cell lung cancer: patterns of intrathoracic recurence and implications for thoracic radiotherapy. *J Clin Oncol* 12:496–502. 1994.
57. Murray N, Coy P, Pater JL, et al. Importance of timing for thoracic irradiation in the combined modality treatment of limited-stage small-cell lung cancer. The National Cancer Institute of Canada Clinical Trials Group. *J Clin Oncol* 11:336–344. 1993.
58. Rice TW, Rodriguez RM, Light RW. The Superior vena cava syndrome: clinical characteristics and evolving etiology. *Medicine.* 85: 37–42. 2006.
59. Rowell NP and Gleeson FV. Steroids, radiotherapy, chemotherapy, and stents for superior vena caval obstruction in carcinoma of the bronchus: a systematic review. *Clinical Oncology.* 14:338–351. 2002.
60. Wilson LD, Detterbeck FC, Yahalom J. Clinical practice. Superior vena cava syndrome with malignant causes. *N Engl J Med.* 356:1862–1869, 2007.

# 19

# Thyroid, Trachea, and Mediastinum

*Joseph Colasanto, MD*
*Richard Tsang, MD*
*James D. Brierley, MB*

## TUMORS OF THE THYROID

### Overview

Although thyroid cancer is uncommon, it is an important cancer because of its increasing incidence, unique clinical features, indolent natural history, molecular genetics, and the therapeutic effectiveness of radioactive iodine. The most common types of thyroid cancer, papillary and follicular types (differentiated thyroid carcinoma) have a high cure rate, unlike the highly aggressive anaplastic carcinoma, which remains a challenge to surgical and radiation oncologists. The management of thyroid cancer is primarily determined by the histology, age, and extent of disease as reflected by the stage. Because of the high survival rate in thyroid cancer (5-year relative survival rate of 97%),[1] an important goal of therapy for low-risk disease is to minimize the long-term toxicity of therapy. Surgery, with or without radioactive iodine remains the mainstay treatment for low-risk disease. The involvement of experienced thyroid surgeons is essential for best results. High-risk disease often requires a multi-disciplinary approach with participation of surgeons, endocrinologists, nuclear medicine physicians, and radiation oncologists to optimally control the disease. A limited role for medical oncology in the management of thyroid cancer remains.

### Epidemiology and Risk Factors

Thyroid cancers accounts for only 1% of all malignancies, and 0.2% of cancer deaths in the United States. Approximately 37,340 persons (28,410 females and 8,930 males) will be diagnosed with thyroid cancer in 2008, with approximately 1,590 deaths (females 910, males 680) in the same year.[1] A rising incidence has been reported in many countries, including the United States, although the cause of the increase is still debated. Increased use of accurate diagnostic tests, changes in pathologic criteria, and radiation exposure (therapeutic and non-therapeutic) probably all contribute to the increasing incidence trend. A female to male ratio of 3:1 is observed for differentiated thyroid cancer, and the incidence increases with age. Radiation exposure is the strongest risk factor for development of thyroid cancer, particularly with exposures occurring in childhood. The incidence of childhood thyroid cancer in Belarus increased 100-fold (0.3 to 30, per 100,000 from 1,981 to 1,985 to 1,991 to 1,994) due to the Chernobyl accident in April, 1986.[2] It is estimated that by the year 2065, the total number of excess thyroid cancers diagnosed in Europe due to that accident will reach 16,000 cases.[3] Radiation therapy to the neck, for Hodgkin's Lymphoma, is also a well-documented risk factor. Several rare genetic syndromes (Gardner syndrome, Cowden's disease, and adenomatous polyposis coli) are also associated with an increased risk of thyroid cancer. Medullary thyroid cancer occurring as part of multiple endocrine neoplasia type 2A or 2B, is almost always associated with germline mutations of the RET oncogene on chromosome 10.

## Anatomy and WorkUp

The thyroid gland is butterfly shaped (connected by the isthmus), located anterior to the second and third tracheal rings. Each lobe is about 3–4 cm in height, 2 cm wide, and 3–4 mm in thickness. Occasionally a pyramidal lobe is present and located just above the isthmus. A fibrous capsule covers the gland; therefore, tumor infiltrating through this capsule represents extrathyroidal extension of disease. This is distinct from the "capsule" sometimes described for tumor nodules within the thyroid gland, which is usually a "pseudocapsule" of compressed thyroid tissue. Anatomically relevant critical structures adjacent to the thyroid gland include the trachea, recurrent laryngeal nerves, carotid artery and jugular vein, esophagus, and the parathyroid glands. Identification and preservation of these structures are critical for successful surgery. Lymphatic drainage is in the following order: central compartment (level VI), other anterior deep cervical (level III, IV, and infrequently level II), posterior cervical (level V), superior mediastinum, and rarely level I.

## Thyroid Nodule—Investigations

In general thyroid nodules with size >1 cm should be evaluated. History should focus on neck symptoms (hoarseness of voice, dysphagia), possible family history, and prior radiation exposure. Physical examination focuses on the size and possible fixity of the nodule, cervical lymphadenopathy, and assessing for vocal cord palsy. Investigations flow chart is shown (Figure 19-1). If the TSH is low, a radionuclide scan should be done to assess for a hyperfunctioning ("hot") nodule, which occurs in ~5%. For other patients, ultrasound is most useful to document size, location, cystic component, and multifocality of lesions. The probability of a palpable thyroid nodule being malignant is about 10% to 15%, and the risk increases with size of the nodule. Fine needle aspirate (FNA) is the next step, either by palpation or ultrasound-guided. There are four possible outcomes of FNA results, with the following suggested management:

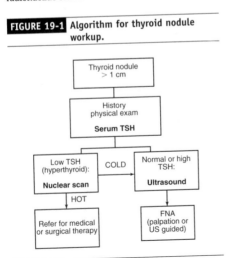

**FIGURE 19-1** Algorithm for thyroid nodule workup.

- Inadequate: attempt repeat FNA
- Benign: follow-up only (false negative rate <5%)
- Malignant: referral for surgery
- Indeterminate (includes follicular neoplasm/lesion, or "suspicious") action depends on clinical suspicion of malignancy

**BOX 19-1**

A comprehensive, up-to-date guideline document produced by the American Thyroid Association (ATA) Guidelines Task Force, and endorsed by the ATA. It deals with workup and management of thyroid nodules, and differentiated thyroid cancer, including surgery, RAI, and follow-up procedures. Recommendations are rated based on the evidence being good (A), fair (B) or from expert opinion (C). Excellent reference list.

Cooper, DS, et al. Management guidelines for patients with thyroid nodules and differentiated thyroid cancer. *Thyroid* 2006 (Feb); 16:109–142.

In general, thyroxine hormone is not recommended for suppression of a benign thyroid nodule.

## Staging

The UICC/AJCC staging classification for thyroid cancer[4] is unique in that it differs depending on patient age as well as histology (Tables 19-1 and 19-2). Those under the age of 45 are classified as stage I and if distant metastasis is present, stage II. Anaplastic carcinoma is stage IV regardless of local disease extent. For differentiated thyroid cancer, a number of alternative staging and prognostic indices exist, attempting to separate patients into low-risk and high-risk categories. The most common in North America is AGES (age, grade, extrathyroid extent, size), later evolving into MACIS, and also clinical class. MACIS is dependent on metastasis (M), age (A), completeness of excision (C), invasion beyond the thyroid (I), and size (S).

## Pathology and Clinical Behavior

The thyroid gland contains two main cell types: follicular cells and the calcitonin-secreting C Cells. Most cancers are of follicular origin (differentiated thyroid cancer), including papillary and follicular subtypes. The poorly differentiated types are of follicular origin and represent malignant transformation from differentiated thyroid cancer (also known as "de-differentiation").[5] In contrast, medullary thyroid cancer (MTC) originates from the C cells and is distinct from the other types.

### Papillary Carcinoma

- Most common type, includes mixed papillary-follicular, "follicular variant", or diffuse sclerosing subtypes
- Nuclear crowding, ground glass nuclei, psammoma bodies
- Frequently multifocal
- Tall cell variant is more aggressive
- Microscopic lymph node involvement frequent (50%–70%)
- Distant spread rare
- Excellent prognosis

### Follicular Carcinoma

- Invasion into surrounding normal thyroid tissue through the tumor

### TABLE 19-1  TNM Staging (UICC 6th Edition, 2002)

**Papillary, Follicular, and Medullary carcinomas**

| | |
|---|---|
| T1 | ≤ 2 cm, intrathyroidal |
| T2 | > 2 cm to 4 cm, intrathyroidal |
| T3 | > 4 cm or minimal extrathyroidal extension |
| T4a | Subcutaneous, larynx, trachea, esophagus, recurrent laryngeal nerve |
| T4b | Prevertebral fascia, mediastinal vessels, carotid artery |

**For Anaplastic/Undifferentiated Carcinoma**

| | |
|---|---|
| T4a | Tumor limited to thyroid |
| T4b | Tumor beyond thyroid capsule |

**All types**

| | |
|---|---|
| N1a | Level VI |
| N1b | Other regional |

TABLE 19-2 TNM Stage Grouping

**Papillary or Follicular, Age Under 45 Years**

| I  | Any T | Any N | M0 |
|----|-------|-------|----|
| II | Any T | Any N | M1 |

**Papillary or Follicular, Age 45 Years or Older, and Medullary**

| I   | T1      | N0     | M0 |
|-----|---------|--------|----|
| II  | T2      | N0     | M0 |
| III | T3      | N0     | M0 |
|     | T1,2,3  | N1a    | M0 |
| IVA | T1,2,3  | N1b    | M0 |
|     | T4a     | N0, N1 | M0 |
| IVB | T4b     | Any N  | M0 |
| IVC | Any T   | Any N  | M1 |

**Anaplastic/Undifferentiated (all are stage IV)**

| IVA | T4a   | Any N | M0 |
|-----|-------|-------|----|
| IVB | T4b   | Any N | M0 |
| IVC | Any T | Any N | M1 |

capsule, or into blood vessel distinguishes carcinoma from the benign follicular adenoma
- Lymph node involvement infrequent (10%–15%)
- Significant risk of distant spread
- Intermediate prognosis, especially for poorly differentiated tumors

### Hürthle Cell Carcinomas

- Synonymous with oncocytic carcinomas
- Abundant granular cells due to eosinophilic staining from mitochondria
- Can occur to variable extent in papillary carcinoma, or follicular carcinoma
- In its pure form considered a follicular carcinoma, typically not avid for iodine, hence may have worse prognosis[5]

### Insular Carcinomas

- Poorly differentiated carcinomas of follicular cell origin
- Represent part of a continuum from differentiated to anaplastic thyroid cancer
- Homogenous small cells, in sheets, may have areas of necrosis
- Stains positively for cytokeratin and thyroglobulin
- Clinically aggressive with tendency to locoregional invasion and distant spread
- Poor prognosis[5]

### Anaplastic Carcinoma

- Synonymous with undifferentiated carcinoma
- Spindle cell pattern, or giant cell, sarcomatoid morphology
- High mitotic rate, areas of necrosis

---

**BOX 19-2**

A cohort of 382 patients with differentiated thyroid cancer from Princess Margaret Hospital, Canada, was analyzed for clinical outcome by using 10 different classification systems (EORTC, AGES, TNM, AMES, MACIS, Clinical class, Ohio, MSK, Noguchi, and SAG). It was demonstrated that the AJCC/UICC TNM classification (4th edition) was as effective in predicting thyroid cancer-specific mortality as AGES and MACIS and better than the others. Since the TNM classification is universally available, and widely accepted for other disease sites, it should be used for all reports of treatment and outcome in thyroid cancer.

Brierley, J, et al. A comparison of different staging systems predictability of patient outcome. Thyroid carcinoma as an example. *Cancer* 1997; 79:2414–2423.

- Stains for cytokeratins (confirms not a lymphoma), but thyroglobulin staining is variable
- Highly fatal

## Medullary Thyroid Cancer

- Derived from C cells (parafollicular cells)
- Uniform nests of round and oval cells, separated by fibrovascular stroma
- Amyloid deposits found in the majority (Congo red stain)
- Stains for calcitonin, carcinoembryonic antigen (CEA), and neuroendocrine markers
- Lymph node metastasis frequent
- Hereditary cases
  - Have germline RET oncogene mutation
  - Have C cell hyperplasia in the same thyroid gland
  - May have familial MEN 2A syndrome (pheochormocytoma and hyperparathyroidism)
  - May have familial MEN 2B syndrome (pheochormocytoma, mucosal and/or gastrointestinal ganglioneuromas, marfanoid body habitus)

---

**BOX 19-3**

Clinical features are compared between the two subtypes of differentiated thyroid cancer in Hong Kong (N = 1057). Patients with papillary carcinoma when compared to patients with follicular carcinoma are younger, with higher female to male ratio, smaller sized primary tumors, higher tendency to multifocal disease (28% vs. 18%) and local extrathyroidal extension (39% vs. 14%), more frequent lymph node metastasis (33% vs. 12%), but less frequent distant metastasis (9% vs. 29%). Clinical outcomes are also better with papillary histology, with 10 year CSS of 92% (follicular: 81%), and freedom from distant metastasis of 91% (follicular 72%). Locoregional recurrence rates were similar. This study nicely illustrates the different biology of the two diseases.

Chow, SM, et al. Differentiated thyroid carcinoma: comparison between papillary and follicular carcinoma in a single institution. *Head Neck.* 2002 July; 24: 670–677.

---

## Treatment for Differentiated Thyroid Carcinoma

Differentiated thyroid cancer has a high cure rate. In one series of 1,353 patients, the cancer-specific survival rate is 94% at 20 years.[6] Age is the most important prognostic factor in determining survival[6,7] with older patients often presenting with other high-risk factors.[8] Other independent factors for cause-specific survival include tumor size, histologic grade, extrathyroidal extension of disease, postoperative presence of macroscopic residual disease, and presence of distant metastasis.[7,9] For locoregional recurrence, the most significant factor remains age, with additional factors being tumor size, multifocality within the thyroid gland, lymph node involvement, surgery less than a total thyroidectomy, and lack of use of radioactive iodine.[7] Younger patients (age <20) have high recurrence rates but survival remains excellent.[6]

## Surgery, Partial vs. Total, Nodal Disease Management

Many aspects of managing differentiated thyroid carcinoma are controversial because large phase II randomized trials have not been performed to guide therapy. The minimum surgical procedure is thyroid lobectomy and isthmusectomy, while some centers routinely perform total thyroidectomy. Sampling of level VI lymph nodes is recommended, although a modified neck dissection is not required unless lymph nodes are clinically enlarged. Young patients (age <45 years) with intrathyroidal tumor measuring <4 cm have excellent prognosis, with virtually 100% cause-specific survival at 10 years with limited surgery and no radioactive iodine.[7,10,11] However there is still a risk of locoregional recurrence, most frequently in cervical lymph nodes, in up to 10% of patients managed conservatively.[7,10,11] This risk can be reduced with an initial treatment plan of total thyroid ablation, with surgical total thyroidectomy, followed by routine postoperative remnant ablation with radioactive iodine.[6,12] These two approaches have not been compared in a randomized trial. The concern regarding total thyroidectomy for low-risk patients is the small but not negligible risk of recurrent laryngeal nerve paralysis (1%–4%, depending on surgical expertise), and a 5%–10% risk of permanent hypoparathyroidism requiring lifelong calcium therapy. In general, if surgical expertise is available and the philosophy of management is to minimize the long-term recurrence rate, total thyroid ablation is used.

## Radioactive Iodine (RAI)

There are no data to support the benefit of radioactive iodine (RAI) in very low-risk patients (those younger than 45, with unifocal papillary carcinoma <1.5 cm, completely resected without extrathyroidal extension or lymph node metastasis).[6,9] For tumors from 1.5 cm to 4 cm, the potential benefits of RAI remain controversial because the prognosis with surgery alone remains excellent. However, if total thyroid ablation is the goal, total thyroidectomy is followed by RAI to ablate any remnant tissue. For patients who have undergone lobectomy only, RAI is not optimal in achieving ablation of the remaining lobe[13] and it is preferable to perform a completion thyroidectomy, then followed by RAI. The activity of RAI ($^{131}$Iodine) when used routinely in this setting varies from 1,100 MBq (30 mCi) to 7,400 MBq (200 mCi), with the most common approach being an empiric activity of 3,700 MBq (100 mCi). Successful management requires appropriate preparation with thyroid hormone withdrawal to achieve a high TSH level, low iodine diet, and a gamma camera scan (either before or after therapy) to document the location of abnormal areas of uptake and screen for metastasis. The availability of recombinant TSH (rTSH) allows scanning and treatment without thyroid hormone withdrawal, and some studies have shown similarly high rates of ablation with rTSH stimulation compared with thyroid hormone withdrawal.[14] The advantages of rTSH are a better quality-of-life due to maintenance of the euthyroid state, and a lower blood dose.[14] However, there are still no long-term data ascertaining a low tumor recurrence rate with this approach. Until such data is available, it is still common practice for patients to undergo thyroid hormone withdrawal prior to receiving RAI, particularly for high-risk or metastatic disease.

The short-term toxicities of RAI include parotid swelling, altered taste and dryness of mouth, and, infrequently, nausea. Reversible bone marrow depression is maximal at 6 weeks, and chronic bone marrow depression is rare. Second malignancies, such as leukemia, have been associated with cumulative doses of greater than 29,400 MBq (800 mCi), and an increased risk of other solid cancers has been reported. Gonadal failure in men can occur after high cumulative doses (>200 mCi) and this may be irreversible. For women in a series of 2,113 pregnancies, there was no increased rate of adverse birth outcomes, compared to pregnancies after thyroid surgery without RAI.[15] Radiation pneumonitis or fibrosis is rare, but care should be exercised for patients with diffuse lung involvement.

---

**BOX 19-4**

This study evaluated the risk of second malignancies after a diagnosis of thyroid cancer in three European countries. Among 6,841 patients, 62% received RAI and 17% received RT. Comparison was made with the general population. In the whole cohort, an increased risk of second malignancy of 27% was

*(continues)*

seen, which included tumors from the GI tract, bone and soft tissues, skin melanoma, kidney, CNS, other non-thyroid endocrine glands, female breast, male genitalia, and leukemia. The risk of second malignancy in relation to RAI showed increased relative risk for the bone and soft tissue (RR = 4.0), female genital organs (RR = 2.2), CNS (RR = 2.2), and leukemia (RR = 2.5), with a dose-response relationship demonstrated. No significant association was found between RT and risk of second malignancy.

Robino, C, et al. Second primary malignancies in thyroid cancer patients. *Br J Cancer.* 2003, 89: 1638–1644.

Following RAI therapy, patients require lifelong thyroid replacement therapy to suppress TSH to prevent stimulation of tumor growth. Suppressed TSH was shown to associate with improved survival.[6] Overly aggressive TSH suppression should be avoided because it may lead to cardiac arrhythmias and osteopenia. For low-risk patients the aim is to suppress TSH to below normal range, and for high-risk patients an undetectable TSH level. TSH suppression may be relaxed after 10 years of disease-free survival. Patients are followed with regular physical examination, TSH, free T3, and thyroglobulin (TG), supplemented by ultrasound of the neck. Six to 12 months following a first RAI treatment, a repeat total body scan should be performed with tracer dose of $^{131}$Iodine, preferably under rTSH stimulation without stopping thyroxine. The TG level in the blood should be undetectable after complete thyroid ablation and, if raised, is a strong predictor for persistence or recurrence of disease.[16] Some TG assays are interfered by the presence of thyroid antibodies, and this can give rise to a false positive result. Some patients have undetectable TG levels despite active disease, due to de-differentiation into higher histologic grade.

**BOX 19-5**

This study evaluated the risk of thyroid cancer after a diagnosis of any invasive cancer and the risk of second cancers after a first diagnosis of thyroid cancer. A two-way, positive association was found between thyroid cancer and cancers of the breast, prostate, kidney, salivary glands, CNS, scrotum, and leukemia. RAI treatment for the thyroid cancer appears to result in a higher risk of subsequent stomach cancer, and non-CLL leukemia. It was concluded that enhanced medical surveillance likely plays a role, but the general increased risks for many types of invasive cancer → thyroid cancer, and thyroid cancer → other invasive cancer suggest etiologic similarities (still unidentified). Also possible are treatment effects with respect to RAI due to its preferential uptake in some organs such as the GI tract, salivary glands, urinary bladder, and bone marrow (for the combined group of cancers in these organs, the RR = 2, 95% CI, 1.29 − 2.76).

Ronckers, CM, et al. Thyroid cancer and multiple primary tumors in the SEER cancer registries. *Int J Cancer.* 2005, 117: 281–288.

**BOX 19-6**

A cohort of 729 patients with differentiated thyroid cancer at the Princess Margaret Hospital in Canada was analyzed for clinical outcome focusing on the effect of RAI and external beam RT on prognosis. It was demonstrated that the extent of surgery, RAI, and RT did not influence cause-specific survival, but RAI was associated with a lower risk of locoregional recurrence but not in the low-risk group (stage I, < age 45). In a high risk-group defined by age >60, and extrathyroidal extension of disease

*(continues)*

---

**BOX 19-6** (CONTINUED)

(n=70), the use of RT resulted in improved 10-year cause-specific survival (RT: 81.0%, no RT 64.6%, p = 0.04), and local relapse free rate (RT: 86.4%, no RT 65.7%, p = 0.01).

Brierley, J, et al. Prognostic factors and the effect of treatment with radioactive iodine and external beam radiation on patients with differentiated thyroid cancer seen at a single institution over 40 years. *Clin. Endocrinol.* (Oxf) 2005; 63:418–427.

---

**BOX 19-7**

Among 1,098 patients with differentiated thyroid cancer in Korea, 68 (6%) had tracheal invasion, treated surgically with thyroidectomy and "shave" excision. Twenty-five patients received RT, with 10-year local progression-free survival of 89%, compared with 38% (p <0.01) in the group who did not receive RT (n = 43). RT benefits patients with residual microscopic or gross disease following "shave" excision.

Keum, KC, et al. The role of postoperative external-beam radiotherapy in the management of patients with papillary thyroid cancer invading the trachea *Int. J. Radiat. Onocl. Biol. Phys.* 2006; 65(2):474–480.

---

## External Beam Radiotherapy (RT)

Locally invasive thyroid cancers usually do not concentrate RAI at the time of recurrence.[17] Adjuvant RT to optimally control the local disease should be considered for patients judged to have a high risk of local recurrence. Extensive extrathyroidal invasion (ETI), defined as disease infiltration into one or more of the critical structures of the neck such as carotid sheath, recurrent laryngeal nerve, larynx, trachea, and esophagus is a poor prognostic factor.[7,18,19] Mazzaferri and Jhiang[6] found that local tumor invasion was associated with an increase in 20-year recurrence rate (38% vs. 25%, p <0.001) and increased cancer mortality (20% vs. 5%, p =0.001). In a review of 262 patients with ETI, 53% had muscle invasion, 47% laryngeal nerve, 37% trachea, 21% esophagus, and 12% laryngeal involvement.[20] If possible, all gross disease should be removed surgically, and shave excision is preferred as the clinical outcome is comparable to radical excision, provided that residual gross disease is not present.[19,21] Adjuvant external beam RT has not been subjected to a randomized trial, but its benefit can be inferred from institutional series of patients with adverse risk, with a comparison of treated patients versus those that were not.[22,23]

Candidates for adjuvant external RT include the following: postoperative gross residual disease or an older patient ( >age 45 years) with an extensive ETI (T4) lesion after thyroidectomy with or without gross residual disease. Lymph node involvement by itself is not an indication to give external RT, as regional control is achieved with initial neck dissection, in combination with postoperative RAI. When RT is recommended, it should be given following RAI, to avoid the theoretical problem of "stunting." However, this "stunting" effect has not been adequately studied, and in fact recent in vitro data reported the opposite, with increased RAI uptake following exposure to radiation in cell culture.[24]

## Gross Residual Disease

RAI is unlikely to eradicate gross disease in the neck. These patients will benefit from planned combined therapy with RAI followed by external RT. In a series of 46 patients with postoperative gross disease, such an approach gave a 5-year CCS and local control rate of 65% and 62%, respectively.[7]

ther authors reported disease control rates of 30%–60%.[25,26] The RT volume should cover the gross disease generously to a dose of at least 60–70 Gy. After therapy, the time to response can be long, up to 8–12 months following RT.

## Local or Regional Recurrence of Thyroid Cancer

The most common location of recurrent disease is in the cervical lymph nodes (regional) rather than in the thyroid bed (local).[7,8] Lymph node recurrence is treated with a combination of neck dissection and additional RAI, resulting in a high probability of tumor control.[8] RAI alone without surgery may be adequate for small volume nodal disease (nodes <2 cm), provided that it is iodine-avid. External RT is recommended only if the nodal disease is persistent or recurrent, despite a modified neck dissection and RAI. In this situation, the RT volume covers bilateral cervical and superior mediastinal lymph nodes to a total dose of 50 Gy, with consideration of a boost to the main areas of involvement or extranodal extension of disease for a further 10–16 Gy.

Local recurrent disease in the thyroid bed is more ominous. The probability of the disease concentrating RAI is low.[17] This typically occurs in older patients with T4 lesions at initial diagnosis, not previously treated with RAI (or not iodine-avid) or RT. The treatment at the time of recurrence is a combination of surgical resection (if resectable), followed by RAI and RT. The volume and dose would be similar to the treatment of gross residual disease as previously described. Because survival may be prolonged even in the presence of metastatic disease,[8,27] surgical management to achieve local control may still be appropriate.

## RT Technique

The thyroid bed adopts a U-shaped volume, curving around the vertebral body and including the air column in the trachea. The challenge is to produce a technique that adequately treats this volume and yet spares the spinal cord. A variety of techniques have been described to overcome the difficulties,[28] with IMRT being the best in terms of adequate PTV coverage and minimizing dose to spinal cord.[29,30]

### Thyroid Bed Alone

- Superior limit: hyoid bone.
- Inferiorly just below the suprasternal notch (adjust superior and inferior limits depending on the operative and pathology findings).
- Planning computed tomography (CT) with neck extended and immobilization mask.
- CTV to cover thyroid bed, jugular and posterior cervical lymph nodes within the limits defined above, including level III, IV, VI, and partially level V nodal regions.
- Define spinal canal as dose avoidance structure with adequate margin (0.5 cm, depending on immobilization device), to generate a three-dimensional conformal plan or IMRT. Spinal cord dose typically <45 Gy.
- Dose prescription: 50 Gy in 1.8–2 Gy fractions, with boost 10–16 Gy for any gross residual disease or high risk area.

### Cervical and Superior Mediastinal Lymph Nodes and Thyroid Bed

- CTV to cover thyroid bed and lymph nodes, including levels II, III, IV, V, VI, and superior mediastinum
- For medullary thyroid cancer, and for differentiated thyroid cancer or anaplastic thyroid cancer where the lymph nodes are being treated, traditionally, the technique would consist of a minimum of two phases. The initial volume (phase I) includes the regional lymph nodes

**FIGURE 19-2** IMRT distribution on axial perspective and DVH.

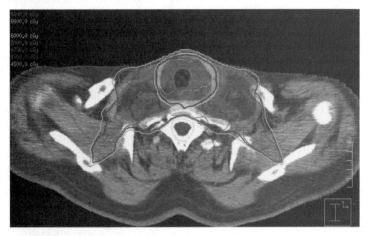

A

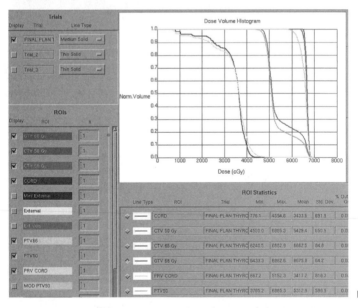

B

(See Color Plate 4). A 58-year-old man with 5 cm papillary thyroid carcinoma, invading into the trachea (pT4N1aM0), treated with total thyroidectomy, shave excision of disease from trachea, and RAI (150 mCi). External beam IMRT plan, for 50 Gy to thyroid bed and adjacent lymph nodes, with boost 16 Gy to area of tracheal invasion. Seven fields of 6 MV at the following gantry angles: 0, 40, 120, 160, 200, 240, and 320. **(A)** Axial Isodose Distribution. **(B)** Dose Volume Histograms for the Clinical Target Volumes, and Spinal Cord.

from the mastoid tip to the carina, including the thyroid bed. Parallel opposing AP/PA fields to 45–46 Gy, with phase II technique off the spinal cord for another 14 Gy (cumulative total dose of 60 Gy), while keeping the maximum spinal cord dose to 50 Gy.
- Best treated with IMRT with phase I dose 50 Gy for microscopic disease and a phase II reduced volume (shorter superior-inferior extent) for gross/high-risk disease to a further 10–16 Gy

## Metastatic Disease

Survival of patients with metastatic disease is dependent on age, histology, site of involvement, and the tumor burden. Patients under the age of 20 have a 100% survival at 10 years, but for those over the age of 40 years it falls to 20%. Survival is longer with diffuse lung metastasis concentrating RAI.[31,32] The mainstay of therapy is RAI, but this will be effective only if a total thyroidectomy has been performed. For diffuse lung metastasis, the complete response rate to RAI is 50% and the 10-year survival 60%, compared with bone metastasis where they are 10% and 20%, respectively.[32] Occasionally, surgical resection of a solitary bone lesion may be appropriate. Others will benefit from RT in addition to RAI, and in view of indolent disease in younger patients, a higher dose of RT is given to maximize the duration of local control (45–50 Gy in 1.8–2 Gy fractions). Patients who present with distant metastatic disease may have a prolonged survival. In one series of 111 such patients, the 10-year CSS was 31%.[27] Ideally treatment should be total thyroidectomy followed by RAI.

## Thyroglobulin-Positive, Scan-Negative Patients

If a high TG is detected but a [131]I scan is negative following an adequate RAI treatment, an FDG-PET scan can be helpful to distinguish local versus systemic location of disease,[33] hence guiding surgical therapy or consideration of RT, cervical lymph nodes, or a localized bone site. Stimulation with rTSH prior to FDG-PET scan increases sensitivity. There is little effective therapy for patients who have not responded to combination treatment with surgery, RAI, and external RT. Single agent doxorubicin with a response rate of 25%–40% is the most effective agent, and combination chemotherapy is generally not more effective.

## Medullary Thyroid Carcinoma (MTC)

Surgery is the main curative treatment modality. Since regional lymph node involvement is common (approximately 50%), meticulous neck and superior mediastinal dissections are often required. RAI has no role in the management of MTC. For those who have normal calcitonin and CEA levels following surgery, especially if obtained following pentagastrin and calcium stimulation, the prognosis is excellent.[34] However, a significant number of patients will have postoperative residual disease as evidenced by high serum calcitonin and CEA levels.[35] Other poor prognostic factors include extrathyroidal invasion, postoperative gross residual disease,[36] and clinical stage.[34,35] In these patients,

**TABLE 19-3  Medullary Thyroid Cancer: Results of Adjuvant RT in High-Risk Disease**

| First Author | No. Patients | 10-year Locoregional Recurrence Rate | |
|---|---|---|---|
| | | Surgery | Surgery + RT |
| Brierley | 73 | 86% | 52% |
| Fersht | 51 | 59% | 29% |
| Mak | 62 | 76% | 16% |
| Nguyen | 59 | — | 30% |

further investigation to locate regional and/or metastatic disease is required, with CT scans, somatostatin and bone scans, and/or FDG-PET.[33] Subclinical nodal disease in the neck and superior mediastinum is relatively common. In this situation, adjuvant external RT to the thyroid bed and regional nodal tissue may be considered if no systemic spread of disease has been identified. Without further treatment, approximately half of these high-risk patients will recur in the neck. Radiation doses of 40–50 Gy in 2 Gy fractions to lymph nodes in the neck and upper mediastinum followed by a boost to the thyroid bed to a total of 50 Gy resulted in a locoregional control rate of 86% at 10 years.[36] The treatment does not affect overall survival, but locoregional control is important because cervical relapse can have a deleterious impact on the patient's quality-of-life. Other investigators have confirmed similar results.[37–40] There is no established role for adjuvant chemotherapy.

Patients who test positive for a germline mutation in the RET oncogene should have genetic counseling, with screening of first-degree relatives (siblings, parents) and their children. The clinical probability of developing MTC in a RET mutation-positive person identified through screening is very high (>90% lifetime risk), and prophylactic thyroidectomy is recommended to prevent development of malignancy.[34]

The most frequent sites of metastatic disease are liver, lung, and bone. The treatment is palliative and chemotherapy is documented to have a response rate of 15%–30% including doxorubicin either as single agent or with cisplatin, 5-FU containing combinations. Hormonal therapy consists of somatostatin analogues (octreotide), with or without interferon alpha.[41] Local radiation is indicated for symptomatic osseous metastasis. Radioimmunotherapy approaches (anti-CEA, or [111]Indium-octreotide) are under active study.[42]

## Anaplastic Thyroid Carcinoma (ATC)

Patients with ATC typically present with a rapidly enlarging anterior neck mass, with symptoms of extrathyroidal invasion. Metastatic disease is frequently present at the time of diagnosis (30%–50%), typically in the lung. It is important to evaluate the integrity of the upper airway, and the need for tracheostomy. Chest radiographs or CT scan and a bone scan will help screen for metastatic disease. Complete surgical resection is rarely possible and those amenable to thyroidectomy usually have predominantly differentiated thyroid carcinoma and only a small focus of ATC.[43] Radical surgery is not warranted in patients with extensive ETI.[44] The treatment for ATC is unsatisfactory, as RAI has no role, and external beam RT, given with the aim of improving local control, often does not even achieve this goal. The expected 5-year survival is approximately 5% with any currently available treatments.[43,44] The suboptimal result with radiation alone has led to the

TABLE 19-4 **Anaplastic Thyroid Cancer: Local Control and Survival Following Fractionated RT and Concurrent Chemotherapy (series reporting >20 patients)[46–51]**

| First Author | No. Patients | Local Control | 2-year Survival | Fractionation | Concurrent Chemotherapy |
|---|---|---|---|---|---|
| Haigh | 33 | — | 20% | Not stated | Yes |
| Heron | 32 | — | 48%* | Daily | in 15 |
| Juror | 91 | 28% | 11%** | Daily | in 18 |
| McIver | 29 | — | 9%* | Daily | in 13 |
| Tennvall | 55 | 60% | 9% | Hyperfractionated | Yes |
| Wong | 32 | 22% | 18% | Accelerated/hyperfractionated | Yes |

* at 1 year
** at 3 years

development of novel fractionation schedules and concurrent chemotherapy, sometimes in combination with surgical resection. A study of hyperfractionated RT in 17 patients (60.8 Gy in 32 fractions, bid over 20 to 24 days) documented complete response in 3 patients (17.6%) and a partial response in 7 (41.2%).[45] Despite this, the majority of patients developed grade 3 or 4 toxicity, and in grade 5, death occurred before the toxicity resolved.

The most successful regimen in obtaining local control is that described by a Swedish group[46] using combined preoperative RT, chemotherapy, followed by surgical resection. Despite a local control rate of 60%, only 5 of 55 patients (9%) survived for 2 years or more,[46] leading one to question the value of such an aggressive approach. The problem has been the inevitable development of metastatic disease that responds poorly to chemotherapy. Innovative approaches are needed for this disease.

For patients with a good performance status and no metastasis, a reasonable approach is to use accelerated hyperfractionated RT without chemotherapy, 60 Gy in 40 fractions (1.5 Gy/fraction given bid) over 4 weeks, planned with IMRT. To avoid significant toxicity, regional lymph nodes may not be covered if uninvolved. For others, RT is given for local symptom relief (20 Gy in five fractions) with the option of a second course for responding patients 4 weeks later.

# THYMIC TUMOR

## Overview

The thymus is involved in the maturation of lymphocytes and releases T-lymphocytes in the circulation. Tumors of the thymus gland are known as thymomas. Thymomas are rare tumors of the mediastinum that progress locally but rarely metastasize outside of the thorax. There is a wide variety of histological appearance and clinical behavior. Surgery is the primary treatment option, while adjuvant chemotherapy or radiation therapy (discussed subsequently) also play a role in the management of this disease.

## Epidemiology and Risk Factors

Thymomas are associated with several comorbid conditions.[52] The most common condition is myasthenia gravis. Approximately 75% of patients with myasthenia gravis have a thymic abnormality, and 15% of this subgroup have thymomas.[53] Conversely, approximately 10%–64% of patients with thymomas have myasthenia gravis.[52,54,55] Other comorbid conditions include pure red cell aplasia (rare condition of profound anemia) (3%), adult-onset hypogammaglobulinemia (3%), and systemic lupus erythematosus (3%).[55,56,58] On the other hand, about 50% of patients with pure red cell aplasia have thymoma, while 10% of patients with hypogammaglobulinemia have thymoma.[55]

Gender is evenly distributed for thymoma.[56,57] The average age is approximately 50 years, with a wide range.[56,59] It is a rare tumor in children.

## Anatomy

Embryologically, the thymus is derived from the third pharyngeal pouch. The thymus reaches its maximum size at puberty and then will slowly atrophy. It is situated in the superior-anterior mediastinum and located anterior to the pericardium and the great vessels.

## Presentation/Workup

Thymic tumors are typically indolent and present with symptoms that are slowly progressive. Presenting symptoms are frequently related to the locoregional extension of the tumor and may cause chest pain, cough, dyspnea, dysphagia, odynophagia, or superior vena cava syndrome. However, 25%–63% of patients can be asymptomatic.[56,58,60,61]

Workup should include diagnostic imaging of the chest. Sensitivity of chest X-rays is variable, reported to range from 50% to 94%, while CT scan has a sensitivity of 97%.[62,63,64] Typically, thymic tumor is a well-defined round or oval mass. There is little support that seeding of a needle tract or incisional biopsy can occur; therefore, pathology should be obtained by fine needle aspirate or open surgical biopsy.

## Staging

There is no staging system designated by the American Joint Committee on Cancer. Bergh et al classified stage I as noninvasive thymomas, stage II as thymomas that invade the mediastinal fat, and stage III as thymomas that have metastasized or invade surrounding structures.[65] Masaoka et al developed a widely accepted staging system published in 1981 (Table 19-5).[66] More recent studies suggest dividing stage I into Stage IA and Stage IB subgroups based on surgery with stage IA showing no evidence of adherence to surrounding structures and stage IB with evidence of adherence to surrounding structures, but no invasion identified microscopically.[54,67]

## Pathology

Most thymomas are composed of cytologically bland thymic epithelial cells, although there is a wide spectrum of morphologic features. Histological classification systems vary and there is no system that is widely accepted or well correlated with outcome. Verley et al described four distinct histological variants of thymic carcinoma, including spindle or oval cell type, lymphocyte-rich, differentiated epithelial, and undifferentiated epithelial. Undifferentiated tumors are of poor prognosis.[54,67] Snover et al described five distinct histological variants, including mixed small cell undifferentiated squamous type, basaloid, mucoepidermoid, clear cell, and sarcomatoid carcinomas.[68] A more recent classification system published by the World Health Organization in 1999 includes six subtypes of thymic tumor.[69] Type A are epithelial cells that appear spindle-shaped or oval without atypia or lymphocytes. Type AB are epithelial cells that appear spindle-shaped or oval with neoplastic lymphocytes. Type B are epithelial cells that appear dendritic or plump. Type B is further subdivided into type B1, B2, and B3 based on increasing atypia in the neoplastic cells. Type C is considered thymic carcinoma and is histologically dissimilar to thymic tissue. Emerging data suggest that the WHO classification is an independent prognostic factor correlating with outcome.[70,71]

## Management

The primary modality of therapy is surgical resection with complete tumor removal because the tumor is localized in the majority. The type of surgery (complete resection, partial resection/debulking, or biopsy only) correlates with local control[72] and survival.[73] Maggi et al reported an 8-year overall survival of 82%, 72%, and 27% for complete resection, partial resection/debulking, and biopsy only, respectively.[73] Local recurrence following surgical resection is 4%–6%, 7%–36%, 16%–47% and 38%–80% for Masaoka stage I, II, III, and IV, respectively.[54,56,67] Adjuvant radiotherapy is controversial with no consensus from the literature. Some authors suggest

---

TABLE 19-5  **Masaoka Staging System**[105]

| | |
|---|---|
| Stage I | Macroscopically encapsulated with no microscopic capsular invasion |
| Stage II | Macroscopic invasion into surrounding fatty tissue or mediastinal pleura, or microscopic invasion into the capsule |
| Stage III | Macroscopic invasion into surrounding organs |
| Stage IVA | Pleural or pericardial metastases |
| Stage IVB | Lymphogenous or hematogenous metastasis |

adjuvant radiotherapy for all stages because a majority of recurrences are local. However, others suggest adjuvant radiotherapy for stages II/III and/or residual disease since the local recurrence rate is approximately 5% for completely resected Masaoka stage I disease. Chemotherapy is typically reserved for palliation. However, neoadjuvent chemotherapy may be considered to allow or improve resectability. Also, chemotherapy and radiotherapy should be considered for unresectable disease.[74]

## Technique/Dose

The classic adjuvant radiotherapy technique includes treatment to the tumor bed, entire mediastinum with or without the supraclavicular fossa. However, there are data indicating an increased risk of radiation pneumonitis and a lack of local control benefit with extended field radiotherapy for completely resected tumors.[72] Clinical target volume includes the tumor or surgical bed including any pathologically involved structures based on presurgical diagnostic imaging with 1–2 cm margin.

A wide variety of radiotherapy doses is reported in the literature. Adjuvant radiotherapy for completely resected tumors includes a total of 40 to 60 Gy given in 20–30 fractions 5 days per week. Currently, there is a paucity of data to support a dose-response relationship. However, Zhu et al reported a 5-year survival advantage on multivariate analysis for radiation doses of >50 Gy resulting in 82%, 5-year survival, versus 70% for total dose $\leq$50 Gy.[72] If there is residual disease following resection, or the patient is not a surgical candidate, then a higher total dose of 60–66 Gy is recommended.

## PRIMARY TUMOR OF THE TRACHEA

### Overview

Primary tumors of the trachea are rare. They are indolent tumors that are typically diagnosed following a long history of progressive symptoms. Surgery is the primary treatment modality while adjuvant chemotherapy or radiation therapy (discussed in following paragraphs) also plays a role in the management of this disease.

### Anatomy

The trachea is located in the mediastinum just anterior to the esophagus. The trachea extends from the level of the C6 vertebral body to the level of the T4/5 vertebral bodies. Superiorly, it is connected to the cricoid cartilage by the cricotracheal ligament. It bifurcates into the right and left mainstem bronchi at the carina. Minor salivary glands are abundant in the submucosa of the trachea. Primary tumors of the trachea occur most frequently in the distal third of the trachea.

### Pathology

The most common histological subtypes include squamous cell carcinoma (SCC) and adenoid cystic carcinoma (ACC). SCC is the most common histology and accounts for about half of all primary tracheal tumors.[75] SCC are more commonly found involving the distal trachea. ACC accounts for approximately 25% of all primary tracheal tumors and occurs more commonly in the upper third of the trachea. Other histological subtypes include adenocarcinoma, sarcoma, mucoepidermoid, or neuroendocrine tumors.

### Epidemiology and Risk Factors

Primary tumors of the trachea are most common in the sixth decade, although adenoid cystic carcinoma tends to occur more frequently at a slightly younger age. There is no gender predominance.

## Presentation/Workup

The trachea consists of sturdy tracheal rings with a relatively large diameter to allow for adequate ventilation. Therefore, primary tumors of the trachea are typically locally advanced for symptoms to occur. Patients may initially present with dyspnea, prolonged expiratory phase, cough and/or wheezing often mistaken initially as asthma. As the tumor progresses, the patient may develop stridor or hemoptysis. Bronchoscopy should be performed, but with caution to prevent airway obstruction. Rarely, the tumor is diagnosed with diagnostic imaging of an asymptomatic patient. Computed tomography scan or magnetic resonance imaging is helpful to determine the extent of the tumor and for surgical planning but can underestimate the longitudinal spread of disease. Endoscopy with biopsy and endotracheal ultrasound provide information regarding longitudinal tumor progression or extension through the trachea.

## Staging

There is no universal staging system.

## Management

Surgery is the primary treatment modality. Gaissert et al have reported a 5-year overall survival of 52% for resected ACC and 39% for resected SCC. For unresected disease, there was a 33% (ACC) and 7% (SCC) 5-year overall survival.[76] Endoscopic resections in select patients with a yttrium-argon-garnet (YAG) laser have been reported.[77] Adjuvant radiation therapy may also play a role in the management of this disease because tumor tends to spread submucosally, resulting in positive margins. Retrospective studies have reported improved survival with adjuvant radiotherapy for incomplete and completely resected tumors.[78] As an alternative to surgical resection, radiotherapy should be considered for unresectable disease or for those who refuse surgery. However, definitive radiotherapy alone has shown inferior survival in several retrospective reviews, although, patient selection and techniques may contribute to these results. The role of elective nodal irradiation is unclear. The tumor rarely spreads to locoregional lymph nodes. In fact, positive local-regional lymph nodes have not been clearly defined as a poor prognostic factor. Therefore, routine elective nodal irradiation is not advised. In addition, adjuvant chemotherapy has not been well studied.

## Technique/Dose

Target volume should include the trachea (preoperative or gross tumor volume with 1–2 cm margin), paratracheal region, and subcarinal region when appropriate. Routine elective nodal irradiation is not recommended; however, treatment of pathologically positive or enlarged local-regional lymph nodes should be considered. There is no consensus on total dose because there is a wide range reported in the literature. A total dose of >50 Gy in 2 Gy fractions for postoperative radiotherapy and at least 60 Gy in 2 Gy fractions for definitive radiotherapy should be considered. As an alternative, radiotherapy alone with endobronchial high dose rate radiotherapy boost may be considered. This has shown promising results that are comparable to surgery with adjuvant radiotherapy in some studies, although based on small retrospective reviews.

## REFERENCES

1. American Cancer Society. Cancer Facts and Figures. http://www.cancer.org/docroot/stt/stt_0.asp, 2008.
2. Stsjazhko VA, Tsyb AF, Tronko ND, et al. Childhood thyroid cancer since accident at Chernobyl. *Bmj* 310:801, 1995.
3. Cardis E, Krewski D, Boniol M, et al. Estimates of the cancer burden in Europe from radioactive fallout from the Chernobyl accident. *Int J Cancer*, 2006.

4. Sobin LH, Wittekind C. *UICC TNM Classification of Malignant Tumours,* 6th ed. New York, John Wiley & Sons, 2002.

5. Freschi G, Landi L, Castagnoli A, et al. Advanced thyroid carcinoma: An experience of 385 cases. *Eur J Surg Oncol,* 2006.

6. Mazzaferri EL, Jhiang SM. Long-term impact of initial surgical and medical therapy on papillary and follicular thyroid cancer. *Am. J. Med.* 97:418–428, 1994.

7. Tsang RW, Brierley JD, Simpson WJ, et al. The effects of surgery, radioiodine and external radiation therapy on the clinical outcome of patients with differentiated thyroid cancer. *Cancer* 82:375–388, 1998.

8. Coburn M, Teates D, Wanebo HJ. Recurrent thyroid cancer. Role of surgery versus radioactive iodine (I131). *Ann Surg* 219:587–593; discussion 593–595, 1994.

9. Hay ID, Thompson GB, Grant CS, et al. Papillary thyroid carcinoma managed at the Mayo Clinic during six decades (1940–1999): temporal trends in initial therapy and long-term outcome in 2,444 consecutively treated patients. *World Journal of Surgery.* 26:879–885, 2002.

10. Shaha AR, Shah JP, Loree TR. Low-risk differentiated thyroid cancer: the need for selective treatment. *Ann Surg Oncol* 4:328–333, 1997.

11. Sanders LE, Cady B. Differentiated thyroid cancer: reexamination of risk groups and outcome of treatment. *Arch Surg* 133:419–425, 1998.

12. Mazzaferri EL, Kloos RT. Clinical review 128: current approaches to primary therapy for papillary and follicular thyroid cancer. *J Clin Endocrinol Metab* 86:1447–1463, 2001.

13. Logue JP, Tsang RW, Brierley JD, et al. Radioiodine ablation of residual thyroid tissue in thyroid cancer: relationship between administered activity, neck uptake, and outcome. *British Journal of Radiology* 67:1127–1131, 1994.

14. Pacini F, Ladenson PW, Schlumberger M, et al. Radioiodine ablation of thyroid remnants after preparation with recombinant human thyrotropin in differentiated thyroid carcinoma: results of an international, randomized, controlled study. *J Clin Endocrinol Metab* 91:926–932, 2006.

15. Dottorini M, Lomuscio G, Mazzucchelli L, et al. Assessment of female fertility and carcinogenesis after iodine:131 therapy for differentiated thyroid cancer. 36:21–27, 1995.

16. Toubeau M, Touzery C, Arveux P, et al. Predictive value for disease progression of serum thyroglobulin levels measured in the postoperative period and after (131)I ablation therapy in patients with differentiated thyroid cancer. *J Nucl Med* 45:988–994, 2004.

17. Vassilopoulou-Sellin R, Schultz PN, Haynie TP. Clinical outcome of patients with papillary thyroid carcinoma who have recurrence after initial radioactive iodine therapy. *Cancer* 78: 493–501, 1996.

18. Brierley JD, Panzarella T, Tsang RW, et al. A comparison of different staging systems predictability of patient outcome. Thyroid carcinoma as an example. *Cancer* 79:2414–2423, 1997.

19. Segal K, Shpitzer T, Hazan A, et al. Invasive well-differentiated thyroid carcinoma: effect of treatment modalities on outcome. *Otolaryngol Head Neck Surg* 134:819–822, 2006.

20. McCaffrey TV, Bergstralh EJ, Hay ID. Locally invasive papillary thyroid carcinoma: 1940–1990. *Head Neck* 16:165–172, 1994.

21. McCaffrey JC: Aerodigestive tract invasion by well-differentiated thyroid carcinoma: diagnosis, management, prognosis, and biology. *Laryngoscope* 116:1–11, 2006.

22. Kim TH, Yang DS, Jung KY, et al. Value of external irradiation for locally advanced papillary thyroid cancer. *Int J Radiat Oncol Biol Phys* 55:1006–1012, 2003.

23. Meadows KM, Amdur RJ, Morris CG, et al. External beam radiotherapy for differentiated thyroid cancer. *Am J Otolaryngol* 27:24–28, 2006.

24. Meller B, Deisting W, Wenzel BE, et al. Increased radioiodine uptake of thyroid cell cultures after external irradiation. *Strahlenther Onkol* 182:30–36, 2006.

25. O'Connell M, Hern R, Harmer CL. Results of external beam radiotherapy in differentiated thyroid carcinoma: a retrospective study from the Royal Marsden Hospital. *Eur J Cancer* 30A:733–739, 1994.
26. Glanzmann C, Lutolf UM. Long-term follow-up of 92 patients with locally advanced follicular or papillary thyroid cancer after combined treatment. *Strahlenther Onkol* 168:260–269, 1992.
27. Haq M, Harmer C. Differentiated thyroid carcinoma with distant metastases at presentation: prognostic factors and outcome. *Clin Endocrinol (Oxf)* 63:87–93, 2005.
28. Harmer C, Bidmead M, Shepherd S, et al. Radiotherapy planning techniques for thyroid cancer. *Br J Radiol* 71:1069–1075, 1998.
29. Rosenbluth BD, Serrano V, Happersett L, et al. Intensity-modulated radiation therapy for the treatment of nonanaplastic thyroid cancer. *Int J Radiat Oncol Biol Phys* 63:1419–1426, 2005.
30. Nutting CM, Convery DJ, Cosgrove VP, et al. Improvements in target coverage and reduced spinal cord irradiation using intensity-modulated radiotherapy (IMRT) in patients with carcinoma of the thyroid gland. *Radiotherapy & Oncology.* 60:173–180, 2001.
31. Vassilopoulou-Sellin R, Goepfert H, Raney B, et al. Differentiated thyroid cancer in children and adolescents: clinical outcome and mortality after long-term follow-up. *Head Neck* 20:549–555, 1998.
32. Schlumberger M, Challeton C, De Vathaire F, et al. Radioactive iodine treatment and external radiotherapy for lung and bone metastases from thyroid carcinoma. *J Nucl Med* 37:598–605, 1996.
33. Crippa F, Alessi A, Gerali A, et al. FDG-PET in thyroid cancer. *Tumori* 89:540–543, 2003.
34. Modigliani E, Cohen R, Campos JM, et al: Prognostic factors for survival and for biochemical cure in medullary thyroid carcinoma: results in 899 patients. The GETC Study Group. Groupe d'etude des tumeurs a calcitonine. *Clin Endocrinol (Oxf)* 48:265–273, 1998.
35. Dottorini ME, Assi A, Sironi M, et al. Multivariate analysis of patients with medullary thyroid carcinoma: prognostic significance and impact on treatment of clinical and pathologic variables. *Cancer* 77:1556–1565, 1996.
36. Brierley JD, Tsang RW, Gospodarowicz MK, et al. Medullary thyroid cancer—analyses of survival and prognostic factors and the role of radiation therapy in local control. *Thyroid* 6:305–310, 1996.
37. Fife KM, Bower M, Harmer CL. Medullary thyroid cancer: the role of radiotherapy in local control. *Eur J Surg Oncol* 22:588–591, 1996.
38. Mak A, Morrison W, Garden A, et al. The value of postoperative radiotherapy for regional medullary carcinoma of the thyroid. *Int J Radiat Oncol Biol Phys* 30 (Suppl):234, 1994.
39. Nguyen TD, Chassard JL, Lagarde P, et al. Results of postoperative radiation therapy in medullary carcinoma of the thyroid: a retrospective study by the French Federation of Cancer Institutes—the Radiotherapy Cooperative Group. *Radiother Oncol* 23:1–5, 1992.
40. Fersht N, Vini L, A'Hern R, et al. The role of radiotherapy in the management of elevated calcitonin after surgery for medullary thyroid cancer. *Thyroid.* 11:1161–1168, 2001.
41. Vitale G, Tagliaferri P, Caraglia M, et al. Slow release lanreotide in combination with interferon-alpha2b in the treatment of symptomatic advanced medullary thyroid carcinoma. *J Clin Endocrinol Metab* 85:983–988, 2000.
42. Chatal JF, Campion L, Kraeber-Bodere F, et al. Survival improvement in patients with medullary thyroid carcinoma who undergo pretargeted anti-carcinoembryonic antigen radioimmunotherapy: a collaborative study with the French Endocrine Tumor Group. *J Clin Oncol* 24:1705–1711, 2006.
43. Voutilainen PE, Multanen M, Haapiainen RK, et al. Anaplastic thyroid carcinoma survival. *World J Surg* 23:975–978; discussion 978–979, 1999.

44. Passler C, Scheuba C, Prager G, et al. Anaplastic (undifferentiated) thyroid carcinoma (ATC): a retrospective analysis. *Langenbecks Arch Surg* 384:284–293, 1999.

45. Mitchell G, Huddart R, Harmer C. Phase II evaluation of high dose accelerated radiotherapy for anaplastic thyroid carcinoma. *Radiother Oncol* 50:33–38, 1999.

46. Tennvall J, Lundell G, Wahlberg P, et al. Anaplastic thyroid carcinoma: three protocols combining doxorubicin, hyperfractionated radiotherapy, and surgery. *British Journal of Cancer.* 86:1848–1853, 2002.

47. Haigh PI, Ituarte PH, Wu HS, et al. Completely resected anaplastic thyroid carcinoma combined with adjuvant chemotherapy and irradiation is associated with prolonged survival. *Cancer.* 91:2335–2342, 2001.

48. Heron DE, Karimpour S, Grigsby PW. Anaplastic thyroid carcinoma: comparison of conventional radiotherapy and hyperfractionation chemoradiotherapy in two groups. *Am J Clin Oncol* 25:442–446, 2002.

49. Junor E, Paul J, Reed N. Anaplastic thyroid carcinoma: 91 patients treated by surgery and radiotherapy. *European Journal of Surgery* 18:83–88, 1992.

50. McIver B, Hay ID, Giuffrida DF, et al. Anaplastic thyroid carcinoma: a 50-year experience at a single institution. *Surgery.* 130:1028–1034, 2001.

51. Wong CS, Van Dyk J, Simpson WJ. Myelopathy following hyperfractionated accelerated radiotherapy for anaplastic thyroid carcinoma. *Radiotherapy and Oncology* 20:3–9, 1991.

52. Drachman DB. Myasthenia gravis. *New England Journal of Medicine.* 330(25): 1797–1810, 1994.

53. Souadjian JV, Enriquez P, Silverstein MN, Pepin JM. The spectrum of diseases associated with thymoma: coincidence or syndrome? *Arch Intern Med.* 134(2):374–379, 1974.

54. Regnard JF, Magdeleinat P, Dromer C, Dulmet E, de Montpreville V, Levi JF, Levasseur P. Prognostic factors and long-term results after thymoma resection: a series of 307 patients. *J Thorac Cardiovasc Surg.* 112(2):376–384, 1996.

55. Rosenow EC 3rd, Hurley BT. Disorders of the thymus: a review. *Arch Intern Med.* 144(4): 763–770, 1984.

56. Blumberg D, Port JL, Weksler B, Delgado R, Rosai J, Bains MS, Ginsberg RJ, Martini N, McCormack PM, Rusch V, et al. Thymoma: a multivariate analysis of factors predicting survival. *Ann Thorac Surg.* 60(4):908–913; discussion 914, 1995.

57. Morgenthaler TI, Brown LE, Colby TV, Harper Jr CM and DT Coles. Thymoma. *Mayo Clin Proc.* 68:1110–1123, 1993.

58. Lewis JE, Wick MR, Scheithauer BW, Bernatz PE, Taylor WF. Thymoma: a clinicopathologic review. *Cancer.* 60(11):2727–2743, 1987.

59. Curran WJ Jr, Kornstein MJ, Brooks JJ. Turrisi AT 3rd: Invasive thymoma: the role of mediastinal irradiation following complete or incomplete surgical resection. *Clin Oncol.* 6(11):1722–1727, 1988.

60. Ogawa K, Uno T, Toita T, Onishi H, Yoshida H, Kakinohana Y, Adachi G, Itami J, Ito H, Murayama S. Postoperative radiotherapy for patients with completely resected thymoma: a multi-institutional, retrospective review of 103 patients. *Cancer.* 1;94(5):1405–1413, 2002.

61. Moore KH, McKenzie PR, Kennedy CW, McCaughan BC. Thymoma: trends over time. *Ann Thorac Surg.* 72(1):203–207, 2001.

62. Ellis K, Austin JH, Jaretzki A 3rd. Radiologic detection of thymoma in patients with myasthenia gravis. *AJR Am J Roentgenol.* 151(5):873–881, 1988.

63. Brown LR, Muhm JR, Gray JE. Radiographic detection of thymoma. *AJR Am J Roentgenol.* 134(6):1181–1188, 1980.

64. Chen JL, Weisbrod GL, Herman SJ. Computed tomography and pathologic correlations of thymic lesions. *J Thorac Imaging.* 3(1):61–65, 1988.

65. Bergh N, Gatzinsky P, Larsson S, Lundin P, Ridell B. Tumors of the thymus and thymic region: clinicopathological studies on thymomas. *Ann Thorac Surg.* 25(2):91–98, 1978.
66. Masaoka A, Monden Y, Nakahara K, Tanioka T. Follow-up study of thymomas with special reference to their clinical stages. *Cancer.* Dec 1;48(11):2485–2492, 1981.
67. Verley JM, Hollmann KH. Thymoma. A comparative study of clinical stages, histologic features, and survival in 200 cases. *Cancer.* 55(5):1074–1086, 1985.
68. Snover DC, Levine GD, Rosai J. Thymic carcinoma: five distinctive histological variants. *Am J Surg Pathol.* 6(5):451–470, 1982.
69. Rosai J, Sobin L. Histological typing of tumours of the thymus. *International Histological Classification of Tumours,* 2nd Ed. New York, Springer, 1999.
70. Detterbeck FC: Clinical value of the WHO classification system of thymoma. *Ann Thorac Surg.* 81(6):2328–3234, 2006.
71. Lucchi M, Basolo F, Ribechini A, Ambrogi MC, Bencivelli S, Fontanini G, Angeletti CA, Mussi A. Thymomas: clinical-pathological correlations. *J Cardiovasc Surg.* 47(1):89–93, 2006.
72. Zhu G, He S, Fu X, Jiang G, Liu T. Radiotherapy and prognostic factors for thymoma: a retrospective study of 175 patients. *Int J Radiat Oncol Biol Phys.* 60(4):1113–1119, 2004.
73. Maggi G, Casadio C, Cavallo A, Cianci R, Molinatti M, Ruffini E. Thymoma: results of 241 operated cases. *Ann Thorac Surg.* 51(1):152–156, 1991.
74. Loehrer PJ Sr, Chen M, Kim K, Aisner SC, Einhorn LH, Livingston R, Johnson D. Cisplatin, doxorubicin, and cyclophosphamide plus thoracic radiation therapy for limited-stage unresectable thymoma: an intergroup trial. *J Clin Oncol.* 15(9):3093–3099, 1997.
75. CM Gelder and MR Hetzel. Primary tracheal tumours: a national survey *Thorax.* 48: 688–692, 1993.
76. Gaissert HA, Grillo HC, Shadmehr MB, Wright CD, Gokhale M, Wain JC, Mathisen DJ: Long-term survival after resection of primary adenoid cystic and squamous cell carcinoma of the trachea and carina. *Ann Thorac Surg.* 78(6):1889–1896, 2004.
77. Okahara M, Segawa Y, Takigawa N, Maeda Y, Takata I, Kataoka M, Mandai K, Fujii M. Primary adenoid cystic carcinoma of the trachea effectively treated with the endoscopic Nd-YAG laser followed by radiation. *Intern Med.* 35(2):146–149, 1996.
78. Regnard JF, Fourquier P, Levasseur P. Results and prognostic factors in resections of primary tracheal tumors: a multicenter retrospective study. The French Society of Cardiovascular Surgery. *J Thorac Cardiovasc Surg.* 111(4):808–813, 1996.

# 20

# Early-Stage Breast Cancer

*Bruce G. Haffty, MD*

## OVERVIEW

Radiation therapy plays a critical role in the management of early-stage breast cancer. The role of radiation in the management of noninvasive and early-stage invasive cancer will be presented in this chapter. Post-mastectomy radiation and radiation for more advanced disease is discussed in the following chapter.

## EPIDEMIOLOGY AND RISK FACTORS

Breast cancer is a common malignancy, affecting more than 200,000 women annually in the United States.[1] From the radiation oncologist's perspective, breast cancer typically represents 10%–20% of the caseload in a general practice. Pertinent epidemiological facts about breast cancer include:

- Incidence:     >200,000 cases annually in the United States
- Deaths     >40,000 annually in the United States
- Female: Male     100:1
- Average Age     54 years
- Race     Lower incidence in African American, Hispanic, and Asian

Risk factors known to be associated with breast cancer are summarized in subsequent paragraphs. The history of the breast cancer patient should include a thorough assessment of all potential risk factors so that appropriate guidance and counseling can be provided. Although less than 5% of breast cancers are associated with the breast cancer susceptibility genes, (BRCA1 or BRCA2), women with strong family histories of early onset breast and/or ovarian cancer are more likely to be carriers of BRCA1 or BRCA2.[2] BRCA1/2 carriers may be appropriately treated with breast-conserving therapy and radiation and there is no evidence of radiotherapy resulting in more severe tissue reactions in carriers than non-carriers. However, the radiation oncologist needs to be aware of the risks of second malignancies and risk reduction strategies for BRCA carriers.

## Risk Factors for Breast Cancer

- Age     Incidence increases with age
- Race/Ethnicity     Higher in Caucasians, Ashkenazi Jewish,
     Lower in African American, Hispanic, Asian

- Family History      Relative risk with affected first degree—1.7
- Parity      Higher in nulliparous or late first pregnancy
       First pregnancy <30 protective
- Menstrual      Higher if menarche <age 12 yrs
- Prior breast disease      Increased with atypical ductal hyperplasia (ADH) (4–5 fold)
       Lobular carcinoma *in situ* (LCIS) (8–10 fold)
       Increased with personal history of breast cancer
- Radiation Exposure      Increased with chest radiotherapy (RT)(<20–25 yrs age)
       Increased in survivors of atomic bomb in Japan
- Hormonal Use      Increased with long-term replacement
- Diet      High fat diets associated with increased risk
- Obesity      Increased risk with postmenopausal obesity

## WORKUP

The history and physical examination and bilateral mammography remain the cornerstone of the workup for the breast cancer patient. Given the widespread utilization of screening mammography, an increasing number of women present with nonpalpable, mammographically detected cancers of the breast. Bilateral mammography is essential to rule out diffuse multicentric disease or a synchronous contralateral malignancy. The current classification scheme for mammographic findings (BI-RADS-Breast Imaging Reporting Data System) is summarized below. Mammography and physical examination are often complemented by ultrasound and MRI. However, these studies are generally considered complementary and their role in routine screening has not been established. Ongoing studies may further refine the roles of ultrasound and MRI in routine screening in subsets of women.

---

**BOX 20-1 MRI SCREENING IN HIGH RISK WOMEN**

This prospective study compared MRI with mammography in 1,909 high-risk women. The overall discriminating capacity of MRI was superior to that of mammography and clinical examination. The authors conclude that MRI is more sensitive than mammography in detecting tumors in women with an inherited susceptibility to breast cancer.

Kriege et al., Efficacy of MRI and mammography for breast-cancer screening in women with a familial or genetic predisposition. *N Engl J Med*. 2004 Jul 29;351(5):427–437.

---

### Bi-Rads Category and Recommendations

| BI-RAD | Description | Recommended Follow-up |
|---|---|---|
| 0 | Needs Additional Evaluation | Diagnostic mammogram, ultrasound |
| 1 | Normal Mammogram | Yearly screening |
| 2 | Benign Lesion | Yearly screening |
| 3 | Probably Benign Lesion | Short 3–6 month follow-up |
| 4 | Suspicious for Malignancy | Biopsy |
| 5 | Highly Suspicious | Biopsy |
| 6 | Known Malignancy | |

For patients with early stage breast cancer, sentinel lymph node mapping has gained widespread acceptance.[3] For patients with DCIS, sentinel node sampling is generally not indicated, though some would consider it for extensive DCIS, or if there is any question regarding a component of invasion (or if mastectomy is planned, in the event there is a component of invasive cancer

**TABLE 20-1 American Joint Committee on Cancer Staging of Breast Cancer**

## Primary Tumor (T)

Definitions for classifying the primary tumor (T) are the same for clinical and for pathologic classification. If the measurement is made by physical examination, the examiner will use the major headings (T1, T2, or T3). If other measurements, such as mammographic or pathologic measurements, are used, the subsets of T1 can be used. Tumors should be measured to the nearest 0.1-cm increment.

| | |
|---|---|
| TX | Primary tumor cannot be assessed |
| T0 | No evidence of primary tumor |
| Tis | Carcinoma *in situ* |
| Tis (DCIS) | Ductal carcinoma *in situ* |
| Tis (LCIS) | Lobular carcinoma *in situ* |
| Tis (Paget's) | Paget's disease of the nipple with no tumor |

*Note:* Paget's disease associated with a tumor is classified according to the size of the tumor.

| | |
|---|---|
| T1 | Tumor 2 cm or less in greatest dimension |
| T1mic | Microinvasion 0.1 cm or less in greatest dimension |
| T1a | Tumor more than 0.1 cm but not more than 0.5 cm in greatest dimension |
| T1b | Tumor more than 0.5 cm but not more than 1 cm in greatest dimension |
| T1c | More than 1 cm but not more than 2 cm in greatest dimension |
| T2 | Tumor more than 2 cm but not more than 5 cm in greatest dimension |
| T3 | Tumor more than 5 cm in greatest dimension |
| T4 | Tumor of any size with direct extension to chest wall or skin, only as described below |
| T4a | Extension to chest wall, not including pectoralis muscle |
| T4b | Edema (including *peau d'orange*) or ulceration of the skin of the breast or satellite skin nodules confined to the same breast |
| T4c | Both (T4a and T4b) |
| T4d | Inflammatory carcinoma |

## Regional Lymph Nodes (N)

| | |
|---|---|
| NX | Regional lymph nodes cannot be assessed (previously removed) |
| N0 | No regional lymph node metastasis |
| N1 | Metastasis to movable ipsilateral axillary lymph node(s) |
| N2 | Metastasis to ipsilateral axillary lymph node(s) fixed or matted or in clinically apparent ipsilateral internal mammary nodes in the absence of clinically evident axillary lymph node metastasis |
| N2a | Metastasis in ipsilateral axillary lymph nodes fixed to one another (matted) or to other structures |
| N2b | Metastasis only in clinically apparent ipsilateral internal mammary nodes and in the absence of clinically evident axillary lymph node metastasis |
| N3 | Metastasis to ipsilateral mammary lymph node(s) with or without axillary lymph node involvement, or in clinically apparent ipsilateral internal mammary lymph node(s) and in the presence of clinically evident axillary lymph node metastasis; or metastasis in ipsilateral supraclavicular lymph node(s) with or without axillary or internal mammary lymph node involvement |

*(continues)*

**TABLE 20-1 (continued)**

**Regional Lymph Nodes (N)(continued)**

| | |
|---|---|
| N3a | Metastasis in ipsilateral infraclavicular lymph node(s) |
| N3b | Metastasis in ipsilateral internal mammary lymph node(s) and axillary lymph node(s) |
| N3c | Metastasis in ipsilateral supraclavicular lymph node(s) |

**Pathologic Classification (pN)**

| | |
|---|---|
| pNX | Regional lymph nodes cannot be assessed (previously removed or not removed for pathologic study) |
| PN0 | No regional lymph node metastasis histologically, no additional examination for isolated tumor cells (ITC) |

*Note:* ITC are defined as single tumor cells or small cell clusters not greater than 0.2 mm, usually detected only by immunohistochemical (IHC) or molecular methods but which may be verified on hematoxylin-and-eosin stains. ITCs do not usually show evidence of malignant activity (proliferation or stromal reaction).

| | |
|---|---|
| pN0 (i−) | No regional lymph node metastasis histologically, negative IHC |
| pN0 (i+) | No regional lymph node metastasis histologically, positive IHC, no IHC cluster greater than 0.2 mm |
| pN0 (mol−) | No regional lymph node metastasis histologically, negative molecular findings (reverse transcriptase polymerase chain reaction [RT-PCR]) |
| pN0 (mol+) | No regional lymph node metastasis histologically, positive molecular findings (RT-PCR) |
| pN1 | Metastasis in one to three axillary lymph nodes, and/or in internal mammary nodes with microscopic disease detected by sentinel lymph node dissection but not clinically apparent |
| pN1mi | Micrometastasis (greater than 0.2 mm, none larger than 2 cm) |
| pN1a | Metastasis in one to three axillary lymph nodes |
| pN1b | Metastasis in internal mammary nodes with microscopic disease detected by sentinel node dissection but not clinically apparent |
| pN1c | Metastasis in one to three axillary lymph nodes and in internal mammary lymph nodes with microscopic disease detected by sentinel lymph node dissection but not clinically apparent (If associated with greater than three positive axillary lymph nodes, the internal mammary nodes are classified as Pn3b to reflect increased tumor burden.) |
| pN2 | Metastasis in four to nine axillary lymph nodes, or in clinically apparent internal mammary lymph nodes in the absence of axillary lymph node metastasis |
| pN2a | Metastasis in four to nine axillary lymph nodes (at least one tumor deposit greater than 2 mm) |
| pN2b | Metastasis in clinically apparent internal mammary lymph nodes in the absence of axillary lymph node metastasis |
| pN3 | Metastasis in 10 or more axillary lymph nodes, or in infraclavicular lymph nodes, or in clinically apparent ipsilateral internal mammary lymph nodes in the presence of one or more positive axillary lymph nodes; or in more than three axillary lymph nodes with clinically negative microscopic metastasis in internal mammary lymph nodes or in ipsilateral supraclavicular lymph nodes |

*(continues)*

TABLE 20-1 **(continued)**

*p*N3a    Metastasis in 10 or more axillary lymph nodes (at least one tumor
         deposit greater than 2 mm), or metastasis to the infraclavicular lymph
         nodes
*p*N3b    Metastasis in clinically apparent ipsilateral internal mammary lymph
         nodes in the presence of one or more positive axillary lymph nodes; or
         in more than three axillary lymph nodes and in internal mammary lymph
         nodes with microscopic disease detected by sentinel lymph node dissec-
         tion but not clinically apparent
*p*N3c    Metastasis in ipsilateral supraclavicular lymph nodes

**Distant Metastasis (M)**
MX Distant metastasis cannot be assessed
M0 No distant metastasis
M1 Distant metastasis

**STAGE GROUPING**

| Stage | T | N | M |
|---|---|---|---|
| 0 | IS | 0 | 0 |
| 1 | 1 | 0 | 0 |
| IIA | 0 | 1 | 0 |
| | 1 | 1 | 0 |
| | 2 | 0 | 0 |
| IIB | 2 | 1 | 0 |
| | 3 | 0 | 0 |
| IIIA | 0 | 2 | 0 |
| | 1 | 2 | 0 |
| | 2 | 2 | 0 |
| | 3 | 1 | 0 |
| | 3 | 2 | 0 |
| IIIB | 4 | 0 | 0 |
| | 4 | 1 | 0 |
| | 4 | 2 | 0 |
| IIIC | Any T | 3 | 0 |
| IV | Any T | Any N | 1 |

in the mastectomy). Patients with negative sentinel nodes require no further axillary treatment. Current practice is to perform nodal dissections on sentinel node positive patients, although radiation has been shown to result in excellent regional nodal control in the clinically negative undissected axilla.

Owing to increasing public awareness of self-examination and screening mammography, the majority of patients with breast cancer in the United States present with relatively early-stage disease.[4] Depending upon a number of factors, including screening practices, the majority of breast cancer patients present with early-stage (Stage 0, I, or II) disease. In areas where screening mammography is widely utilized, women presenting with nonpalpable ductal carcinoma *in situ* represent up to 20% of newly diagnosed cases. Up to 15%–20% of breast cancer patients present

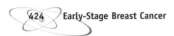

**FIGURE 20-1** Flow diagram of workup and recommendations for the patient with breast findings suspicious for early-stage breast cancer.

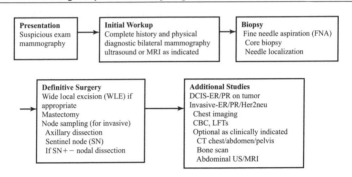

| Presentation | Initial Workup | Biopsy |
|---|---|---|
| Suspicious exam mammography | Complete history and physical diagnostic bilateral mammography ultrasound or MRI as indicated | Fine needle aspiration (FNA) Core biopsy Needle localization |

| Definitive Surgery | Additional Studies |
|---|---|
| Wide local excision (WLE) if appropriate Mastectomy Node sampling (for invasive) Axillary dissection Sentinel node (SN) If SN + − nodal dissection | DCIS-ER/PR on tumor Invasive-ER/PR/Her2neu Chest imaging CBC, LFTs Optional as clinically indicated CT chest/abdomen/pelvis Bone scan Abdominal US/MRI |

**BOX 20-2 RANDOMIZED TRIAL OF SENTINEL NODE BIOPSY VS DISSECTION**

Five hundred sixteen patients with primary breast cancers $\leq$ 2cm were randomized to sentinel node biopsy and total axillary dissection (the axillary dissection group) or to sentinel node biopsy followed by axillary dissection only if the sentinel node contained metastases (the sentinel node group). A sentinel node was positive in 32.3% of the axillary dissection group, and in 35.5% of the sentinel node group. The overall accuracy of the sentinel node status was 96.9%, the sensitivity 91.2%, and the specificity 100%. There was less morbidity in the sentinel node biopsy only group. Among the 167 patients who did not undergo axillary dissection, there were no cases of overt axillary metastasis during follow-up. The authors conclude that sentinel node biopsy is a safe and accurate method of screening the axillary nodes for metastasis in women with a small breast cancer.

Veronesi, U, et al. A randomized comparison of sentinel-node biopsy with routine axillary dissection in breast cancer. *N Engl J Med.* 2003 Aug 7;349(6):546–553.

with Stage III disease, and less than 5% present with Stage IV. Of patients presenting with early stage invasive breast cancer and a clinically negative axilla however, up to 30%–40% will have involved axillary nodes. Internal mammary nodes are involved less frequently than axillary nodes, though older studies have demonstrated internal mammary nodal involvement in over 50% of patients with positive axillary nodes and medial tumors.

## PROGNOSIS AND RISK FACTORS

While there are a wide variety of histologic subtypes of breast cancer, the vast majority of invasive cancers are of the infiltrating ductal subtype. Invasive ductal and invasive lobular tumors have a similar prognosis, while some of the other subtypes have more favorable or less favorable prognosis. Relative distribution of histological subtypes among invasive cancers and features is summarized as follows:

The majority of patients with early-stage breast cancer have a favorable prognosis with excellent overall and disease-free survival rates. As shown, overall and disease-free survival for Stage 0, I and II breast cancer are favorable, given appropriate currently available treatments with surgery,

**TABLE 20-2 Invasive Histological Subtypes**

| Histology | Frequency | Features |
|---|---|---|
| Infiltrating ductal (NOS) w/without mixed histology | 70–80% | Most common subtype of invasive cancer<br>Prognosis poorer than other common subtypes |
| Lobular | 5–10% | Often ill-defined<br>May be mammographically occult |
| Medullary | 5–8% | Favorable prognosis<br>Associated with familial breast cancers |
| Mucinous | <5% | Favorable prognosis |
| Tubular | <2% | Very favorable prognosis<br>Axillary metastasis uncommon |
| Adenocystic, Papillary, Squamous, Metaplastic, Carcinosarcoma | <1% | Rare subtypes<br>Papillary and adenocystic favorable<br>Metaplastic associated with poor prognosis |

radiation therapy, and adjuvant systemic hormonal and chemotherapy. Five-year survival rates, according to primary tumor size and nodal status for patients with invasive disease, are shown in Figure 20-2.

Numerous studies have evaluated prognostic factors in breast cancer. Nodal status and tumor size remain the most significant prognostic factors. Negative estrogen and progesterone receptor status are also poor prognostic factors, as are tumor grade and lymphvascular space invasion. Overexpression of Her2/neu has also been associated with a poorer prognosis. Young age is also associated with a poorer prognosis relating to both systemic disease and local relapse. The patient evaluation and workup should include reference to these prognostic factors. Ongoing studies include evaluation of panels of molecular markers and gene profiling studies to further refine prognosis and response to therapy for women with breast cancer.

## BREAST-CONSERVING THERAPY VERSUS MASTECTOMY

Surgical removal of the primary tumor remains the cornerstone of management for the patient with early-stage breast cancer. While traditionally this was accomplished by mastectomy with or without axillary dissection, wide local excision followed by radiation therapy to the intact breast has become the mainstay of treatment based on several randomized trials clearly demonstrating equivalent overall survival and disease-free survival to mastectomy.[5,6] While there have been numerous studies worldwide, two of the most significant studies now have follow-up of 20 years, clearly establishing the long-term safety and efficacy of breast-conserving therapy for early-stage breast cancer.

**FIGURE 20-2 Five-year survival by tumor size and nodal status.**

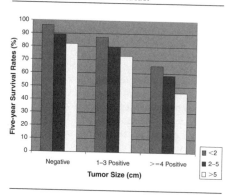

---

**BOX 20-3** RANDOMIZED STUDIES OF BREAST CONSERVATION VS. MASTECTOMY

These two landmark studies randomizing patients to breast-conserving surgery plus radiation versus mastectomy, updated with 20 year follow-up, confirm equivalent long-term disease-free and overall survival in patients treated by lumpectomy and radiation compared to mastectomy. In the NSABP trial, a third arm with lumpectomy alone was associated with a 39% risk of local relapse, compared to 14% in the lumpectomy and radiation arm, and a marginal increase in deaths due to breast cancer. In the Italian trial, rate of death from all causes was 41.7% in the conservatively managed arm and 41.2% in the mastectomy arm.

---

Fisher, et al., Twenty-year follow-up of a randomized trial comparing total mastectomy, lumpectomy, and lumpectomy plus irradiation for the treatment of invasive breast cancer. *N Engl J Med.* 2002 Oct 17;347(16):1233–1241.

Veronesi, et al. Twenty-year follow-up of a randomized study comparing breast-conserving surgery with radical mastectomy for early breast cancer. *N Engl J Med.* 2002 Oct 17;347(16):1227–1232.

## INTEGRATION OF CHEMOTHERAPY AND HORMONAL THERAPY

Based on numerous randomized trials demonstrating improvements in overall and disease-free survival, adjuvant chemotherapy is currently employed in a majority of early-stage breast cancer patients.[5,7] This is generally administered prior to radiation therapy. Although there had been some concern regarding higher local relapse rates with delayed radiation and controversy regarding the appropriate sequencing, recent studies have demonstrated acceptable local control with chemotherapy administered prior to radiation.[8,9]

---

**BOX 20-4** HARVARD CHEMO-RADIATION SEQUENCING TRIAL

In this update of the Harvard randomized trial, 244 breast cancer patients were randomized to RT first or chemo-first. With a median follow-up of 135 months there are now no differences in time to any event, distant metastasis or survival, and no significant differences in local control.

---

Bellon, J, et al. Sequencing of chemotherapy and radiation therapy in early-stage breast cancer: updated results of a prospective randomized trial. *J Clin Oncol.* 2005 Mar 20;23(9):1934–1940.

Although concurrent chemo-radiation has been employed with good results, it has generally fallen out of favor due to added toxicities, and with some exceptions, its use should be restricted to prospective controlled trials. Radiation therapy should begin between 2 and 9 weeks following the last dose of chemotherapy, in accordance with current ongoing protocol guidelines. Use of Trastuzamab (Herceptin) as adjuvant therapy has recently gained widespread acceptance.[10] While there may be some added toxicities (cardiac), Trastuzamab can be given concurrently with radiation with acceptable results.

For patients not undergoing chemotherapy, radiation treatment should begin as soon after surgery as practical. Generally, to allow for adequate wound healing, radiation should not begin prior to 3 weeks after surgery. While there are no strict guidelines regarding how long one can wait after surgery, beginning radiation within 12 weeks of surgery at the latest seems prudent and consistent with most protocols.

Based on significant improvements in overall and disease-free survival with the use of adjuvant hormonal therapy, patients with positive hormone receptors are likely to receive adjuvant hormonal therapy (Tamoxifen, Anasatrozole, Exemestane, etc.), in addition to radiation therapy and chemotherapy.[11] Although there are theoretical concerns regarding the concurrent administration of hormonal therapy and radiation, recent studies have not demonstrated any adverse effect of concurrent administration of hormonal therapy and radiation.

---

**BOX 20-5** **TAMOXIFEN-RADIATION SEQUENCING STUDIES**

These three retrospective studies were conducted independently but published together. Each study retrospectively evaluated local relapse rates as a function of whether the patients received tamoxifen during or after radiation. They all reached the similar conclusion that tamoxifen given during radiation or given following radiation had no significant impact on local control rates in the conservatively managed breast cancer patient. The Harris and Pierce study also reported no significant differences in complications with the different sequences.

Ahn, et al. Sequence of radiotherapy with tamoxifen in conservatively managed breast cancer does not affect local relapse rates. *J Clin Oncol.* 2005 Jan 1;23(1):17–23.

Harris, et al. Impact of concurrent versus sequential tamoxifen with radiation therapy in early-stage breast cancer patients undergoing breast conservation treatment. *J Clin Oncol.* 2005 Jan 1;23(1):11–16.

Pierce, et al. Sequencing of tamoxifen and radiotherapy after breast-conserving surgery in early-stage breast cancer. *J Clin Oncol.* 2005 Jan 1;23(1):24–29.

---

Radiation therapy is indicated for the majority of patients undergoing breast-conserving surgery for invasive and noninvasive breast cancer.[5,12] With few exceptions, the majority of patients are suitable candidates for breast-conserving surgery. Relative contraindications are summarized in Table 20-3. Radiation is generally not indicated for those patients with early-stage, node-negative disease who undergo mastectomy. For patients who undergo mastectomy with node-positive disease, radiation may be indicated and is discussed in the following chapter.

The widespread acceptance of breast-conserving therapy (BCS) followed by radiation therapy is based on numerous randomized trials comparing BCS with RT to mastectomy. Local relapse rates following BCS vary depending on selection factors, but generally range between 0.5% and 1% per year, with long-term local relapse rates averaging 10%–15%. A number of risk factors for local

---

**FIGURE 20-3** Current multimodality treatment of the early-stage breast cancer patient.

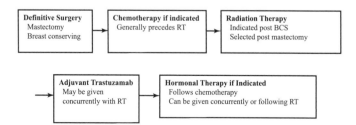

TABLE 20-3 Relative Contraindications and Controversies in Breast-Conserving Surgery/RT

| Controversy | Issue |
| --- | --- |
| Gross Multicentric Disease | Removal of all disease may result in unacceptable cosmesis |
| Persistently Positive Diffuse Margins | Though negative margins are desired, a focally involved margin may be acceptable |
| Collagen Vascular Disease | Anecdotal reports of increased complications and poor cosmesis not substantiated in several studies |
| Pregnancy | Pregnant females should not undergo radiation, but may have breast-conserving surgery (BCS) and/or chemotherapy during pregnancy, with RT following delivery |
| Prior Chest/Mantle Radiation | A relative contraindication, but there are reports of repeat irradiation in these patients with acceptable short term outcomes |

---

**BOX 20-6 COLLAGEN VASCULAR DISEASE AND BREAST CONSERVATIVE SURGERY/RT**

This case-control study of 36 patients with collagen vascular disease treated by conservative surgery and radiation and 72 matched controls similarly treated showed no significant difference in late complications, with the exception of the subgroup of patients with scleroderma. Patients with lupus, rheumatoid arthritis, and other collagen vascular diseases did not have a higher rate of G3-4 late complications compared with the controls.

Chen, et al. Breast-conserving therapy in the setting of collagen vascular disease. *Cancer J.* 2001 Nov–Dec;7(6):480–491.

---

relapse have been reported, but young age, and positive margin status are the most consistently reported risk factors for local relapse following breast-conserving therapy.[13] The use of adjuvant hormonal therapy and adjuvant chemotherapy appear to reduce the risk of local relapse significantly.[14-16]

## OMISSION OF RADIATION THERAPY FOLLOWING BREAST-CONSERVING SURGERY

Treatment by lumpectomy alone (without radiation) has been shown in numerous randomized trials to be associated with a 3-fold increase in local relapse.[17-20] Although individual trials show no compromise in survival, two recent metanalyses suggest not only a 3-fold increase in local relapse, but a small statistically significant compromise in survival by elimination of radiation.[21,22]

---

**BOX 20-7 META-ANALYSIS BCS WITH OR WITHOUT RADIATION**

This pooled metanalysis of 15 trials and over 9,000 patients randomized to conservative surgery with or without radiation confirms a 3-fold increase in local relapse with omission of radiation and an 8.6% excess mortality risk with omission of radiation following breast-conserving surgery.

Vinh-Hung, V, Verschraegen, C. Breast-conserving surgery with or without radiotherapy: pooled-analysis for risks of ipsilateral breast tumor recurrence and mortality. *J Natl Cancer Inst.* 2004 Jan 21;96(2):115–121.

*(continues)*

This metanalysis included over 7,300 patients with breast-conserving surgery (BCS) in trials of radio-therapy with 5-year local recurrence risks of 7% versus 26%, and 15-year breast cancer mortality risks 30.5% versus 35.9%; overall mortality reduction 5.3%, SE 1.8, 2p = 0.005. The authors conclude that differences in local treatment that substantially affect local recurrence rates would, in the hypothet-ical absence of any other causes of death, avoid about one breast cancer death over the next 15 years for every four local recurrences avoided, and should reduce 15-year overall mortality.

Clarke, M, Collins, R, Darby, S, et al. Effects of radiotherapy and of differences in the extent of surgery for early breast cancer on local recurrence and 15-year survival: an overview of the randomized trials. *Lancet* 2005; 366: 2087–2106.

TABLE 20-4  Randomized Trials of Breast-Conserving Therapy With or Without Radiation

| Study | n | Follow-up | Local Relapse | |
|---|---|---|---|---|
| | | | RT | No RT |
| NSABP-06 | 930 | 10 Years | 12.4% | 40.9% |
| Swedish | 381 | 10 Years | 8.5% | 24% |
| Milan | 567 | 10 Years | 5.83% | 23.5% |
| Ontario | 837 | 3 Years | 5.5% | 25.7% |
| NSABP B-21 | 1006 | 8 Years | 2.8% | 16.5% |
| German | 347 | 5.9 Years | 3.2% | 27.8% |

Collectively, the above studies clearly demonstrate the effectiveness of radiation following lumpectomy in optimizing local control; however, two recent studies suggest acceptable local con-trol rates in selected elderly women with T1 estrogen receptor positive breast cancers treated by lumpectomy and tamoxifen without radiation. Although radiation significantly lowered the risk of local-regional relapse in these patients, the risk of relapse with tamoxifen alone was felt to be acceptable, although follow-up is still relatively short.

BOX 20-8  LUMPECTOMY WITH OR WITHOUT RADIATION IN ELDERLY WOMEN

These two randomized trials compared tamoxifen with RT to tamoxifen alone in early-stage estrogen receptor positive elderly (Hughes >70 yrs, Fyles >50 yrs) women with breast cancer. Though radi-ation significantly lowered the local relapse rates, in women over the age of 70, local relapse rates were within acceptable levels, with limited follow-up of 5 years. Longer follow-up from these prospective trials is awaited.

Hughes, KS, et al. Lumpectomy plus tamoxifen with or without irradiation in women 70 years of age or older with early breast can-cer. *N Engl J Med.* 2004 Sep 2;351(10):971–977.

Fyles, AW, et al. Tamoxifen with or without breast irradiation in women 50 years of age or older with early breast cancer. *N Engl J Med.* 2004 Sep 2;351(10):963–970.

## RADIATION DELIVERY

Radiation therapy to the whole breast following lumpectomy currently remains the standard of care for the majority of early stage breast cancer patients. The patient is placed in a supine position at a slant with the arm above the head, with appropriate immobilization to ensure consistent day-to-day set-up. Recently some investigators have proposed prone positions, which may have an advantage with respect to day-to-day positioning in patients with large, pendulous breasts. The simulation set-up can be done on a conventional fluoroscopic simulator or CT-simulator. The tangential beams are angled or half beam blocked to minimize divergence into the lung, and the collimator can be rotated as needed to assure adequate coverage. Ideally, the exposed lung at the central axis of the tangential field should be kept to less than 3 centimeters. Contours or CT cuts are obtained for treatment planning. A typical tangential field setup is shown in Figure 20-4.

Wedges or other compensation methods may be employed to ensure optimal dose homogeneity within the breast. A treatment plan in Figure 20-5 demonstrates an acceptable isodose distribution with a maximum dose inhomogeneity of <10%. Current RTOG/NSABP guidelines require maximum dose to be within 15% of the prescribed dose. Although beams of 4–6 MV, with appropriate use of wedges are most commonly employed, mixed beams or beams of higher energies can be employed to optimize the treatment plan. For the majority of patients open fields with simple wedges will provide adequate coverage with acceptable homogeneity. Depending on the patient size and body habitus, other techniques including IMRT, fields within fields and "sliding window" techniques can be employed to optimize dose homogeneity within the breast.

Currently accepted practice employs daily radiation doses of 1.8–2.0 Gy to a total dose of 45–50 Gy over 5 weeks, using tangential beams directed at the whole breast.

Other fractionation schemes have been evaluated and proven acceptable, including the Canadian fractionation scheme of 42.5 Gy in 16 fractions.

**FIGURE 20-4** Tangential external beam irradiation.

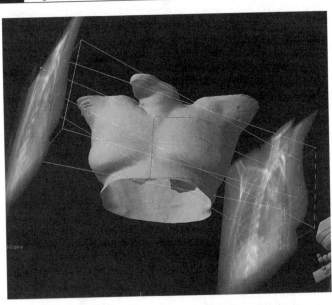

In this randomized trial of IMRT compared to standard wedges in conservatively managed breast cancer, dose distribution within the breast was significantly improved with the IMRT technique, with a reduction in the clinically significant maximum from 110% with standard wedges to 105% with IMRT, and a reduction in the relative volume of breast receiving over 105% of the prescribed dose from 16.9% with standard wedges to 7.7% with IMRT. This improvement in dosimetric performance was associated with a significant clinical gain with reduction in moist desquamation from 47.8% to 31.2%.

Pignol, et al. A multicentre randomized trial of Breast IMRT to reduce acute radiation dermatitis. *Journal of Clinical Oncology,* 2008.

Randomized trial of 1,234 women treated by lumpectomy with clear margins and negative axillary lymph nodes randomly assigned to receive whole breast irradiation of 42.5 Gy in 16 fractions over 22 days (short arm) or whole breast irradiation of 50 Gy in 25 fractions over 35 days (long arm). Five-year local recurrence-free survival was 97.2% in the short arm and 96.8% in the long arm. No difference in disease-free or overall survival rates was detected between study arms. The percentage of patients with an excellent or good global cosmetic outcome at 3 years was 76.8% in the short arm and 77% in the long arm. The authors conclude that the more convenient 22-day fractionation schedule appears to be an acceptable alternative to the 35-day schedule. This study excluded pts with a sep >25 cm.

Whelan, et al. Randomized trial of breast irradiation schedules after lumpectomy for women with lymph node-negative breast cancer. *J Natl Canc Inst* 2002: 94: 1143–1150.

This randomized trial of over 5,000 patients randomized to receive whole breast irradiation to 50 Gy with or without a 16 Gy boost, demonstrated a significant improvement in local control with the use of the 16 Gy boost (4.3% local relapse with boost compared to 7.6% without a boost, p <.001). The use of the boost was most beneficial in women under 50 years of age.

In the 2007 update, with a follow-up of 10.8 years, the local relapse rate was 10.2% in the no boost arm compared to 6.2% in the boost arm. Although the magnitude of the boost was most beneficial in younger women, the benefit was significant in all age groups. There is still no difference in overall survival with the use of the boost.

Bartelink, H, et al. Recurrence rates after treatment of breast cancer with standard radiotherapy with or without additional radiation. *N Engl J Med.* 2001 Nov 8;345(19):1378–1387.

Bartelink, H, et al. Impact of a higher radiation dose on local control and survival in breast-conserving therapy of early breast cancer: 10-year results of the randomized boost versus no boost EORTC 22881-10882 trial. *J Clin Oncol.* Aug 2007 1;25(22):3259–3265.

Use of a boost to the tumor bed following external beam whole breast irradiation is also commonly employed and has been shown in prospective randomized trials to result in slight but significantly superior local control. Although the benefit was predominantly in younger women in the original publication, a recent update demonstrated improvement in local control in all age groups.

## PARTIAL BREAST IRRADIATION

Partial breast irradiation, which can be delivered over the course of 5 days, is evolving as a potential treatment strategy for selected patients. Treatment can be administered using a variety of techniques including multiplane interstitial catheters, Mammosite balloon, or external beam

**FIGURE 20-5** Isodose plan showing improved homogeneity with the use of IMRT.

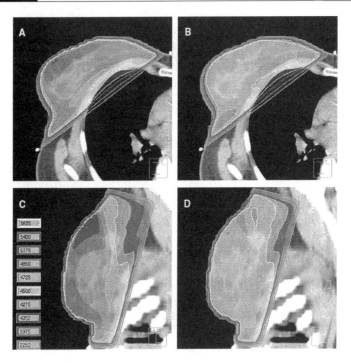

(See Color Plate 5).

conformal therapy. Single dose intra-operative techniques have also been employed.[23] A pivotal Intergroup trial is currently underway, comparing conventional whole breast irradiation to partial breast irradiation.

The eligibility and treatment schema for this trial are summarized as follows:

## Schema for Ongoing NSABP-RTOG Randomized Trial

Patient Eligibility

- All ages
- Primary lesion
  - Unicentric (if multifocal <3 cm total)
  - Stage 0, I, II breast cancer (If stage II <3 cm)
  - DCIS or invasive adenocarcinoma
  - Negative microscopic resection margin (NSABP definition)
- Axillary nodes 0–3 positive without extra capsular extension (ECE)
  - Axillary lymph node dissection (ALND) ( >6 nodes required) or negative sentinal lymph node dissection (SLN)

- Target evaluation
  - Clearly identifiable target
  - Lumpectomy cavity/whole breast volume <30% based on post-lumpectomy CT scan
- Timing
  - Randomization within 42 days of last surgery

## TREATMENT OF THE REGIONAL LYMPHATICS

Management of the regional lymphatics remains highly individualized without clearly established standards. For patients undergoing breast-conserving therapy, who are node negative by sentinel node or formal axillary sampling, treatment of the breast alone with standard tangential fields is widely employed. Patients with one to three positive nodes may be treated with tangents only, but some advocate treatment to the supraclavicular fossa with or without internal mammary radiation. For patients with node-negative disease or with less than three nodes involved, the risk of supraclavicular failure is low (<3%) and the risk of an internal mammary failure is extremely rare (<1%).[24]

Treatment of the supraclavicular nodes with or without internal mammary chain radiation is frequently considered for patients with four or more nodes. Currently, two ongoing randomized trials (NCI Canada MA20 and the EORTC) are addressing treatment of the regional lymphatics in conservatively managed breast cancer patients. In both of these trials, women at risk are randomized to whole breast irradiation alone or breast irradiation plus regional nodal irradiation. Both

---

**FIGURE 20-6** Schema of NSABP-RTOG whole breast vs. partial breast trial.

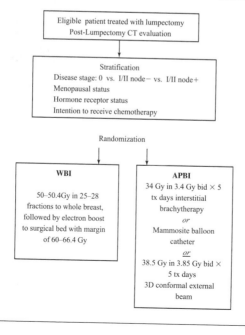

trials are open to accrual and should help to define the risks and benefits of regional irradiation in subsets of patients.

For patients who undergo axillary dissection, the risk of axillary failure is low. Treatment of the axilla remains individualized, depending on the extent of axillary dissection and involvement. For patients with a complete axillary dissection and involved nodes, our policy is to treat the supraclavicular fossa only, even in patients with multiple positive nodes. This avoids that potential morbidity of arm edema with the combination of axillary dissection and axillary radiation. However, it is reasonable to consider axillary radiation if there are multiple positive nodes with extracapsular extension, or if the axillary dissection was less than adequate.

For patients who are at risk for nodal involvement who do not undergo axillary dissection, including those patients with a sentinel node positive who do not undergo complete dissection, radiation therapy to the full axilla has been shown to provide adequate regional control with minimal morbidity. Another alternative to using a third supraclavicular field in patients who have a reasonably high risk of axillary involvement is to treat with "high tangents." With the superior field within 2 cm of the humeral head and the leading edge of the field clearing the interface of the lung/chest wall interface by 2cm, the majority of level I and level II nodes are within the tangential field has shown in Figure 20-7.

Our current institutional policy is as follows:

- Node negative by SN or dissection    Breast tangents only
- Node positive (1–3 Nodes)            Tangents $+/-$ Supraclav

**FIGURE 20-7** High tangent field demonstrating inclusion of the level I/II nodes.

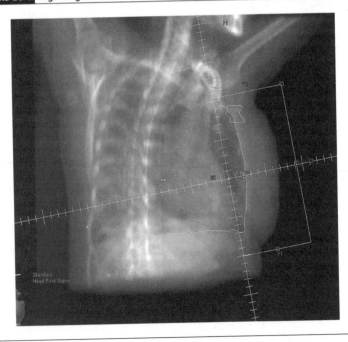

- Node positive (>=4 nodes)                          Tangents + Supraclav +/−IM
- SN+ without full dissection                        Tangents +Supraclav+Axilla
- SN+ with full dissection                           Tangents +/− Supraclav
- No dissection (risk of involvement >10%)           Tangents +Supraclav+Axilla/
                                                     Selectively consider high tangents
- No dissection (risk of involvement <10%)           Tangents only

+/− = With or without depending on clinical indications, physician preference.
*Note:* For patients with a dissected axilla, we generally do not include the axilla in the treatment. For selected patients with extensive nodal involvement, axillary treatment may be considered on an individualized basis.

Treatment of the regional lymphatics in conservatively managed breast cancer patients requires careful techniques to appropriately match the tangential breast field with the supraclavicular field and/or internal mammary field. Treatment of the internal mammary fields is reviewed in more detail in the advanced breast cancer chapter and will not be detailed here. There are several methods for matching the tangential and supraclavicular field. One method uses a single isocenter, set at the match line between the supraclavicular and tangential field and is shown in Figure 20-8. Alternatively, the supraclavicular field is half beam blocked, and the tangential fields are designed with the head of the couch rotated toward the tangent beam source to minimize divergence of the tangential beam into the supraclavicular field.

## MANAGEMENT OF DCIS

For patients with DCIS, radiation management is similar to that for patients with invasive cancer. Since the risk of nodal involvement with pure DCIS is exceedingly low, nodal treatment by dissection or irradiation is not indicated. For patients with extensive DCIS or questionable microinvasion, sentinel node sampling may be performed at the discretion of the surgeon. Patients are generally treated with tangential external beam radiation to the whole breast. I routinely employ a boost in the majority of women with DCIS; however, in patients with widely negative margins the benefit may be marginal. As with invasive cancer, several randomized trials have demonstrated

**FIGURE 20-8** Single isocenter three field breast setup.

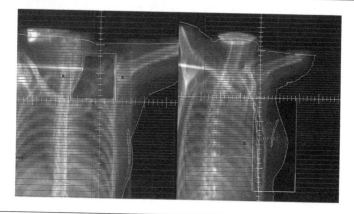

superior local control rates with radiation following lumpectomy compared to lumpectomy alone. Furthermore, improvements in local control are evident in all subgroups. The absolute benefit, however, may be small in patients with low-grade DCIS and widely negative margins.

---

### BOX 20-12 NSABP & EORTC RANDOMIZED DCIS TRIALS

Both of these landmark studies (Fisher–NSABP-17, Julien-EORTC) randomized patients with DCIS to lumpectomy alone or lumpectomy with radiation. Both studies confirm significant improvements in local control with radiation, and radiation benefited all subgroups of patients. In NSABP-17 the incidence of noninvasive relapse was reduced from 13.4% to 8.2% and the incidence of invasive relapse from 13.4% to 3.9%. In EORTC, the 4-year rate of local relapse was reduced from 16% to 9%, with similar reductions in noninvasive and invasive relapses.

Fisher, et al. Pathologic findings from the National Surgical Adjuvant Breast Project (NSABP) eight-year update of Protocol B-17: intraductal carcinoma. *Cancer.* 1999 Aug 1;86(3):429–438.

Julien, et al. Radiotherapy in breast-conserving treatment for ductal carcinoma in situ: first results of the EORTC randomised phase III trial 10853. EORTC Breast Cancer Cooperative Group and EORTC Radiotherapy Group. *Lancet.* 2000 Feb 12;355(9203):528–533.

---

The issue of offering radiation therapy to all patients remains an area of controversy and several institutions recommend observation following lumpectomy for patients with low-grade DCIS and widely negative margins, based primarily on the work from the Van Nuys group.[25] This group has proposed a classification scheme based on grade, size, margins, and age as shown in Table 20-5. For patients with low scores (<5), the risk of relapse following lumpectomy alone is low. However, in a prospective single arm trial reported by Wong et al, patients with favorable low-grade DCIS with widely negative margins were observed.[26] The trial was stopped early in accordance with preselected stopping rules because of a high local relapse rate with observation. Thirteen patients developed local recurrence at the first site of treatment failure corresponding to a 5-year rate of 12%. Nine patients (69%) experienced recurrence of DCIS and four (31%) experienced recurrence with invasive disease. Further data, including results from ongoing trials, may help to further refine selection criteria for eliminating radiation in patients with DCIS.

In patients with DCIS, there should be a discussion regarding the potential risks and benefits of tamoxifen. Although the absolute benefit is small, tamoxifen has been shown to reduce the risk of subsequent ipsilateral and contralateral events. Recent data suggest that this benefit is limited to patients with DCIS whose primary tumors are hormone receptor positive. Ongoing trials are evaluating alternative hormonal agents in DCIS.

Patients with LCIS as a component of an invasive tumor are suitable candidates for breast-conserving therapy followed by radiation. Although there are conflicting data, studies have

### TABLE 20-5 Van Nuys Prognostic Index Scoring System

| SCORE | 1 | 2 | 3 |
|---|---|---|---|
| Size | <16 mm | 16–40 mm | >=41 mm |
| Margin | >10 mm | 1–9 mm | <1 mm |
| Pathology | Not High Grade No Necrosis | Not High Grade Necrosis Present | High Grade With or Without Necrosis |
| Age | >=61 | 40–60 | <40 |

---

**BOX 20-13** | **TAMOXIFEN IN DCIS RANDOMIZED TRIAL**

In this randomized study of 1,804 women with DCIS, all treated with lumpectomy and radiation and randomized to tamoxifen (20 mg daily for 5 years) or placebo, women in the tamoxifen group had fewer breast-cancer events at 5 years than did those on placebo (8.2% vs. 13.4%, p = 0.0009). The authors conclude that the combination of lumpectomy, radiation therapy, and tamoxifen was effective in the prevention of invasive cancer in women with DCIS.

Fisher, et al. Tamoxifen in treatment of intraductal breast cancer: National Surgical Adjuvant Breast and Bowel Project B-24 randomised controlled trial. *Lancet.* 1999 Jun 12;353(9169):1993–2000.

---

demonstrated similar local relapse rates in patients with invasive cancers with or without a component of LCIS, even if the LCIS is present at or near the margins of resection. For patients with pure LCIS, bilateral mastectomy or conservative management by excision alone, without radiation is considered an acceptable alternative. There has been one retrospective study of 25 patients with LCIS treated by lumpectomy and radiation which suggests that radiation significantly lowers the expected rate of relapse and may be an acceptable treatment option.[27]

## MANAGEMENT OF THE PATIENT WITH BRCA1/BRCA2 MUTATIONS

Patients with a hereditary predisposition to breast cancer and documented germline mutation in the BRCA1 or BRCA2 gene are at high risk for breast and ovarian cancers. These patients, if diagnosed with breast cancer, have a high risk of contralateral breast cancer (up to 40%–50% by 10–15 years of follow-up), and a high risk of ovarian cancer. Genetic counseling and risk reduction strategies should be considered in such patients. Recent data suggest a relatively high rate of developing late local relapses (second primaries in the ipsilateral breast) in these patients. However, a follow-up collaborative group study has shown that prophylactic oophorectomy and/or adjuvant hormonal therapy in such patients may decrease the risk of second primary tumors. While additional data is awaited, it appears that patients electing breast conserving therapy who are BRCA1/2 mutation carriers should consider pro-active measures, such as oophorectomy and/or adjuvant hormonal therapy to decrease the risk of subsequent malignancies.

---

**BOX 20-14** | **BRCA1/2 AND BREAST CONSERVATIVE THERAPY**

These retrospective studies evaluated the risk of local ipsilateral and contralateral relapses in conservatively managed patients undergoing CS+RT. In the Haffty study, with 12-year follow-up, the risk of local relapse in BRCA carriers was approximately 40%, similar to the risk of contralateral events. None of those patients had been on tamoxifen or had prophylactic oophorectomy. In a recent large collaborative study, Pierce noted an elevated risk of ipsilateral breast events if the patients had no hormonal manipulation. However, in those BRCA patients who had undergone prophylactic oophorectomy, the risk of both ipsilateral and contralateral events was substantially reduced. These data suggest the high risk of second primary tumors in these patients may be offset by prophylactic hormonal manipulation.

Haffty, et al. Outcome of conservatively managed early-onset breast cancer by BRCA1/2 status. *Lancet.* 2002 Apr 27;359(9316): 1471–1477.

Pierce, et al. J. Clin Oncol. Ten-year multi-institutional results of breast-conserving surgery and radiotherapy in BRCA1/2-associated stage I/II breast cancer. *J Clin Oncol.* 2006 Jun 1;24(16):2437–2443.

# TOXICITIES OF RADIATION TREATMENT IN EARLY-STAGE BREAST CANCER

Conventional external beam radiation has relatively low morbidity. The most significant acute toxicity is skin reaction, with most patients experiencing some grade 1 or 2 skin reactions. Grade 3 skin reactions (moist desquamation) occurs in about 10%–20% of patients. Radiation pneumonitis and rib fractures are long term complications which occur in less than 3% of patients undergoing external beam radiation therapy. Brachial plexopathy can rarely occur in patients treated with supraclavicular radiation. There is evidence that chemotherapy given concurrently may increase the risk of acute and late toxicities. Common RTOG toxicity criteria are found in Chapter 8.

In patients undergoing radiation therapy to the intact breast, cosmesis is good to excellent in over 80%. Ten percent to 20% will have a fair cosmetic outcome and less than 5% will have a suboptimal poor cosmetic outcome.

Although, theoretically, radiation is a potent carcinogen, long term data do not demonstrate a substantial significant risk of second cancers in women undergoing radiation treatment for breast cancer using modern techniques. However, there is evidence that the risk of second malignancies is elevated from long-term follow-up of older randomized trials. Data from the Early Breast Cancer Trialists Collaborative Group demonstrated increased relative risk in each of these secondary malignancies as a function of radiation treatment for breast cancer: lung cancer-1.61($+/-$0.18, p = .007), esophagus cancer- 2.06 ($+/-$.53, p = .05), leukemia- 1.71($+/-$.36, p= .03), and sarcoma- 2.34($+/-$ .62, p = .03).[21] The total relative risk for all secondary nonbreast malignancies was 1.20 ($+/-$.06, p = .001)). The increased risk of secondary malignancies is primarily associated with trials using older techniques. Clearly, care should be taken to minimize the dose to non-target tissues to as low as is reasonably possible. However, it is evident that the benefits of radiation substantially outweigh the relatively small risks with respect to radiation-induced malignancies.

---

**BOX 20-15** **SECONDARY CONTRALATERAL BREAST CANCERS AND RADIATION**

In this large case control study of 41,109 women with breast cancer in Connecticut, 655 women who developed a second breast cancer were compared to 1,189 controls who did not. Radiation was associated with a marginally elevated risk of second malignancies. The risk was evident only in women who were treated at an age of 45 years or less. The authors conclude that radiation contributes little if any risk of second breast cancers for patients treated after the age of 45 years.

Boice, et al. Cancer in the contralateral breast after radiotherapy for breast cancer. *N Engl J Med.* 1992 Mar 19;326(12):781–785.

In this retrospective series of 1,029 early-stage patients treated with lumpectomy and radiation compared to 1,387 patients treated with mastectomy without irradiation over a 20-year span from 1970 to 1990, there was no difference in the rate of second contralateral breast cancers at 15 years. The rate of second breast cancers in the contralateral breast was 10% in both groups and the risk of any second malignancy was also nearly identical at 17.5% (CS+RT) compared to 19% (mastectomy).

Obedian, E., Fischer, D, and Haffty, B. The risk of second malignancies after treatment for early-stage breast cancer: lumpectomy and radiation versus mastectomy. *J Clin Oncol.* 2000 Jun;18(12):2406–2412.

---

# REFERENCES

1. Jemal A, Murray T, Ward E, et al. Cancer statistics, 2005. CA *Cancer J Clin* 55:10–30, 2005.
2. Ford D, Easton DF, Stratton M, et al. Genetic heterogeneity and penetrance analysis of the BRCA1 and BRCA2 genes in breast cancer families. The Breast Cancer Linkage Consortium. *Am J Hum Genet* 62:676–689, 1998.

3. Edge SB, Niland JC, Bookman MA, et al. Emergence of sentinel node biopsy in breast cancer as standard-of-care in academic comprehensive cancer centers. *J Natl Cancer Inst* 95:1514–1521, 2003.

4. Elmore JG, Armstrong K, Lehman CD, et al. Screening for breast cancer. *Jama* 293:1245–1256, 2005.

5. National Institutes of Health Consensus Development Conference Statement: Adjuvant therapy for breast cancer, November 1–3, 2000. *J Natl Cancer Inst Monogr* 2001:5–15, 2001.

6. Veronesi U, Marubini E, Mariani L, et al. Radiotherapy after breast-conserving surgery in small breast carcinoma: long-term results of a randomized trial. *Ann Oncol* 12:997–1003, 2001.

7. Fisher B, Jeong JH, Dignam J, et al. Findings from recent national surgical adjuvant breast and bowel project adjuvant studies in stage I breast cancer. *J Natl Cancer Inst Monogr*: 62–66, 2001.

8. Huang J, Barbera L, Brouwers M, et al. Does delay in starting treatment affect the outcomes of radiotherapy? a systematic review. *J Clin Oncol* 21:555–563, 2003.

9. Recht A, Come SE, Henderson IC, et al. The sequencing of chemotherapy and radiation therapy after conservative surgery for early-stage breast cancer. *N Engl J Med* 334:1356–1361, 1996.

10. Romond EH, Perez EA, Bryant J, et al. Trastuzumab plus adjuvant chemotherapy for operable HER2-positive breast cancer. *N Engl J Med* 353:1673–1684, 2005.

11. Early Breast Cancer Trialists' Collaborative Group. Tamoxifen for early breast cancer: an overview of the randomised trials. *Lancet* 351:1451–1467, 1998.

12. Early Breast Cancer Trialists' Collaborative Group. Effects of radiotherapy and surgery in early breast cancer: an overview of the randomized trials. *N Engl J Med* 333:1444–1455, 1995.

13. Freedman GM, Fowble BL. Local recurrence after mastectomy or breast-conserving surgery and radiation. *Oncology* (Williston Park) 14:1561–1581; discussion 1581–1582, 1582–1584, 2000.

14. Buchholz TA, Tucker SL, Erwin J, et al. Impact of systemic treatment on local control for patients with lymph node-negative breast cancer treated with breast-conservation therapy. *J Clin Oncol* 19:2240–2246, 2001.

15. Fisher B, Anderson S, Tan-Chiu E, et al. Tamoxifen and chemotherapy for axillary node-negative, estrogen receptor-negative breast cancer: findings from National Surgical Adjuvant Breast and Bowel Project B-23. *J Clin Oncol* 19:931–942, 2001.

16. Haffty BG, Wilmarth L, Wilson L, et al. Adjuvant systemic chemotherapy and hormonal therapy: effect on local recurrence in the conservatively treated breast cancer patient. *Cancer* 73:2543–2548, 1994.

17. Clark RM, Whelan T, Levine M, et al. Randomized clinical trial of breast irradiation following lumpectomy and axillary dissection for node-negative breast cancer: an update. Ontario Clinical Oncology Group. *J Natl Cancer Inst* 88:1659–1664, 1996.

18. Fisher B, Bryant J, Dignam JJ, et al. Tamoxifen, radiation therapy, or both for prevention of ipsilateral breast tumor recurrence after lumpectomy in women with invasive breast cancers of 1 cm or less. *J Clin Oncol* 20:4141–4149, 2002.

19. Liljegren G, Holmberg L, Adami HO, et al. Sector resection with or without postoperative radiotherapy for stage I breast cancer: five-year results of a randomized trial. Uppsala-Orebro Breast Cancer Study Group. *J Natl Cancer Inst* 86:717–722, 1994.

20. Winzer KJ, Sauer R, Sauerbrei W, et al. Radiation therapy after breast-conserving surgery: first results of a randomized clinical trial in patients with low risk of recurrence. *Eur J Cancer* 40:998–1005, 2004.

21. Clarke M, Collins R, Darby S, et al. Effects of radiotherapy and of differences in the extent of surgery for early breast cancer on local recurrence and 15-year survival: an overview of the randomized trials. *Lancet* 366:2087–2106, 2005.

22. Vinh-Hung V, Verschraegen C. Breast-conserving surgery with or without radiotherapy: pooled-analysis for risks of ipsilateral breast tumor recurrence and mortality. *J Natl Cancer Inst* 96:115–121, 2004.

23. Vicini FA, Kestin L, Chen P, et al. Limited-field radiation therapy in the management of early-stage breast cancer. *J Natl Cancer Inst* 95:1205–1210, 2003.

24. Recht A, Houlihan MJ. Axillary lymph nodes and breast cancer: a review. *Cancer* 76: 1491–1512, 1995.

25. Silverstein MJ, Lagios MD, Groshen S, et al. The influence of margin width on local control of ductal carcinoma in situ of the breast. *N Engl J Med* 340:1455–1461, 1999.

26. Wong JS, Kaelin CM, Troyan SL, et al. Prospective study of wide excision alone for ductal carcinoma in situ of the breast. *J Clin Oncol* 24:1031–1036, 2006.

27. Cutuli B, de Lafontan B, Quetin P, et al. Breast-conserving surgery and radiotherapy: a possible treatment for lobular carcinoma in situ? *Eur J Cancer* 41:380–385, 2005.

# 21

# Locally Advanced Breast Cancer

*Thomas A. Buchholz, MD*

## OVERVIEW

The prognosis for patients with locally advanced breast cancer has significantly improved over the past decade due to advances in treatment. These advances have occurred in all disciplines involved in the treatment of breast cancer, including radiation oncology. Indeed, over the past decade the role of radiation in the multidisciplinary management of breast cancer has become more clearly defined. It is now well established that all patients presenting with locally advanced breast cancer benefit from the use of radiation as a component of treatment. In this setting, the addition of radiation to surgery and systemic treatments minimizes the risk of locoregional recurrence and improves overall survival.

## EPIDEMIOLOGY AND RISK FACTORS

Although the true incidence of breast cancer continues to slowly increase, the increased use of mammography screening and heightened public education about breast cancer has led to signifi-cant decreases in the percentage of patients presenting with locally advanced disease. The data below illustrate these trends.[1]

- A 27% decrease in tumors ≥3.0 cm at diagnosis from 1980 to 1987
- A further annual 1.9% decline in ≥3.0-cm tumors from 1987 to 2000
- In 2000, only 12,000 new cases with tumors >5 cm
- In 2000, tumors >5 cm represented only 6% of total new cases

Locally advanced breast cancer represents a heterogeneous class of tumors. Some locally advanced tumors present between routine screening studies and represent disease with a rapid growth rate. This is particularly true for inflammatory breast cancer, a subcategory of locally advanced breast cancer. However, locally advanced breast cancer can also be diagnosed in patients who relate a his-tory of a slowly progressive disease that became extensive because of neglect or failure to seek medical attention.

Because of the heterogeneity of locally advanced disease, no clear risk factors have been found that are unique to patients presenting with advanced disease compared with the risk factors associated with the development of early-stage breast cancer. Established risk factors for the development of breast cancer in general have been summarized in the previous chapter.

## WORKUP AND STAGING

All cases of locally advanced breast cancer should be carefully staged to rule out the presence of distant metastases. The accepted initial workup should include the following:

- History and physical examination
- Bilateral diagnostic mammography
- Photographs of the breast
- Imaging of the liver (most commonly with diagnostic computed tomography [CT])
- Imaging of the bone (most commonly with a bone scan)
- Routine serum studies and liver function tests

As discussed later in this chapter, many patients who present with locally advanced disease will be treated with neoadjuvant chemotherapy. For such patients, it is critical that the extent of initial disease be clearly documented before treatment begins. As previously noted, medical photographs should be obtained, particularly for patients with visible breast abnormalities. In all cases, a clinical TNM (tumor–nodes–metastasis) stage should be assigned before treatment begins. For patients with locally advanced disease, this is best done with input from a multidisciplinary team that may include a surgeon, medical oncologist, and a radiation oncologist. The physical examination should include careful evaluation for evidence of skin edema ("peau d'orange") by compressing the dermis of the breast skin over the tumor and assessing skin thickening. The mobility of fixed primary tumors should be assessed with both flexion and relaxation of the pectoralis major muscle to distinguish pectoralis invasion from chest wall invasion. This is an important distinction because pectoralis muscle invasion does not affect clinical T stage, whereas chest wall invasion places primary tumors into the T4 category. During the last revision of the American Joint Committee on Cancer staging system, several changes regarding lymph node staging were implemented. Table 21-1 highlights changes in the definitions of clinical N-stage disease and pathological N-stage disease between the 1988 Fifth Edition and the 2003 Sixth Edition of the system.[2] Some of these revisions include classifying disease with infraclavicular and supraclavicular lymph node involvement as stage N3 and use of the number of positive lymph nodes in determining the pathological N-stage.

In addition to these standard tests, sonography of both the breast and the regional lymphatics (axilla, infraclavicular region, supraclavicular region, and internal mammary lymph node chain) may be of value for patients with locally advanced disease. Sonography can detect abnormalities in lymph node architecture even in small lymph nodes and thus its sensitivity for detecting metastases is higher than that of clinical examination or CT. Sonographically directed fine needle aspiration of the highest-echelon abnormal lymph node can also be done to document the extent of disease in the regional lymphatics; findings from such a study can affect the clinical N-stage in significant numbers of patients who have locally advanced disease.

Many physicians also use positron emission tomography (PET) scans or PET/CT in the initial staging of locally advanced disease, although PET remains a research tool at this time. Finally, research continues toward defining the role of breast magnetic resonance imaging (MRI) for patients with locally advanced disease.

## TREATMENT OVERVIEW

Patients who present with large primary tumors, extensive regional disease, or both, are at high risk for both distant and locoregional disease recurrence. Correspondingly, these patients benefit from both aggressive systemic therapies and locoregional treatments. The administration of these treatments requires careful coordination among all disciplines involved in oncology. Previous findings have indicated that the degree to which this coordination exists, and the experience of the treating center, can affect treatment outcome. For example, a study of breast cancer patients

**TABLE 21-1** Summary of Major Changes in the Sixth Edition of the *AJCC Cancer Staging Manual for Breast Cancer*

| | Fifth Edition | Sixth Edition |
|---|---|---|
| Size of regional lymph-node metastases | Micrometastases were defined as tumor deposits not larger than 2 mm and classified as pN1a. No quantitative distinction was made between micrometastases and isolated tumor cells. | Micrometastases are distinguished from isolated tumor cells on the basis of size. Micrometastases are defined as tumor deposits larger than 0.2 mm but not larger than 2 mm and classified as pN1mi. Isolated tumor cells are defined as tumor deposits not larger than 0.2 mm identified by either standard histology or by immunohistochemical staining. They are classified as pN0(i+). |
| Number of regional lymph-node metastases | The number of affected axillary lymph nodes was considered only in subcategories of pN1. | Major classifications of lymph-node status are defined by the number of affected axillary lymph nodes. |
| Location of regional lymph-node metastases | Metastases in infraclavicular lymph nodes (axillary level III) were considered equivalent to metastases in other axillary lymph nodes. Metastases to the internal mammary nodes were classified as N3/pN3. | Metastases in the infraclavicular lymph nodes are classified as N3, because of their assosication with extremely poor prognosis. Metastases to the internal mammary nodes are classified as N1, N2, or N3, based on the size of the lesion and the presence or absence of concurrent axillary nodal involvement. |
| The use of descriptors to indicate size and method of detection of nodal metastases | Metastases to the supraclavicular lymph nodes were classified as M1. No descritors were used. | Metastases to the supraclavicular lymph nodes are classified as N3. The descriptor (i+) is used to indicate the presence of isolated tumor cells no larger than 0.2 mm by either standard histology or by immunohistochemical staining. The descriptor (i−) means no detectable tumor cells by either histology or immuno-histochemical staining. The descriptor (sn) is used to indicate that the staging classification was based solely on sentinel lymph node dissection. The descriptor (mol+)/(mol−) is used to designate cases that are negative by standard histologic staining for regional lymph node metastasis and in which reverse transcriptase-polymerase chain reaction was used to assess the node for tumor cells. |

eprinted with permission from Singletary SE, Connolly JL. Breast Cancer Staging: Working with the Sixth Edition of the AJCC Cancer taging Manual. *CA Cancer J Clin* 56:37–47, 2006.[2]

in California found that those treated at large teaching hospitals had significantly better survival rates than those treated at small community or health maintenance organization hospitals.[3] Multidisciplinary care is of particular importance for patients with advanced disease because the optimal sequencing of various therapies is less straightforward for such patients than for those with early-stage breast cancer. Figure 21-1 illustrates a treatment approach for patients with locally advanced breast cancer. One of the first questions to address is whether a particular patient is best served by beginning the treatment process with neoadjuvant chemotherapy. Two important factors to consider in making this decision are whether the disease can be completely resected with mastectomy and whether the patient may become a candidate for breast conservation if the disease responds to neoadjuvant treatment.

## TREATMENT OUTCOME

Locally advanced breast cancer was once considered a fatal disease. Before the routine use of chemotherapy, the vast majority of patients developed distant metastases and died of the disease.[4-6] In the past, locoregional treatments such as mastectomy alone, radiation therapy alone, or combined surgery and radiation therapy were used in attempts to prevent uncontrolled locoregional disease progression. The outcomes with such strategies were poor.[4-6] Fortunately, the current outlook for patients with locally advanced breast cancer is much more optimistic. Although distant metastases remain a persistent problem, long-term disease-free survival rates have significantly improved with the use of systemic treatments.[7] This improvement in metastatic disease control has also heightened the importance of achieving locoregional control. Arguably, the

**FIGURE 21-1** Flow diagram of workup and recommendations for patients with locally advanced breast cancer. MRI, magnetic resonance imaging; CT, computer tomography.

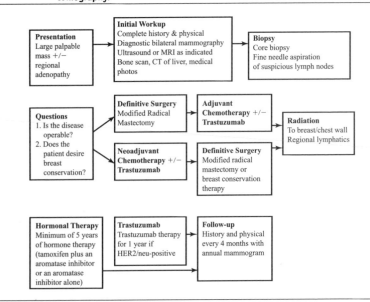

success of chemotherapy in eradicating micrometastatic disease has allowed the advances achieved in surgery and radiation therapy to also contribute to improved patient survival. Improvements in locoregional and systemic treatments have led to combined-modality therapy becoming the standard of care for all patients with Stage IIB or Stage III breast cancer.

The prognosis for patients who present with locally advanced breast cancer has improved significantly over time. Figure 21-2 shows 5-year survival data for patients with lymph node-positive breast cancer according to the size of the primary tumor and the year of treatment[8]. Overall, these data indicate an absolute 12% improvement in overall 5-year survival for patients with positive lymph nodes between the late 1970s and the late 1990s.

It is important to recognize several factors that have contributed to improvements in survival for patients with advanced disease. Clearly, advances in treatments are one of the most important reasons for the improved outcome. However, when assessing findings such as those shown in Figure 21-2, it is also important to consider the effect of "stage migration." Specifically, improvements in diagnostic imaging and other staging techniques have led to increases in the sensitivity of these modalities for detecting distant metastases at the time of diagnosis. In addition, the use of sonography in disease staging may lead to a diagnosis of N3 disease in cases that might otherwise be classified as Stage II breast cancer. Reclassification of these cases as stage III disease may lead to apparent improvements in outcome for both the Stage II and the Stage III cohorts. A similar consideration concerns sentinel lymph node surgery. The more detailed pathological assessment of sentinel lymph nodes increases the percentage of patients with lymph node-positive disease. Patients whose disease was "upstaged" by detailed pathological examination tend to have a low disease burden in the lymph nodes and therefore represent a group at the favorable prognostic end of the lymph node-positive spectrum of disease class. This upstaging simultaneously removes a less favorable cohort from the lymph node-negative group. Finally, changes in staging systems can also affect the apparent survival within a particular stage, as indicated in the study referenced in Box 21-1.

Although stage migration can bias comparisons of outcome over time, it is clear that improvements in therapy have also improved outcome for patients with advanced disease. One such improvement has been the introduction of new systemic therapies. Between 1950 and 1980, the Federal Drug Administration approved fewer than five new systemic treatments for breast cancer per decade. In contrast, six new agents were approved during the 1980s and 12 new agents were approved for breast cancer during the 1990s.[9] Moreover, these new treatments are affecting the course of the disease.

**FIGURE 21-2** Five-year survival rates for patients with positive axillary lymph nodes according to tumor size and year of diagnosis.

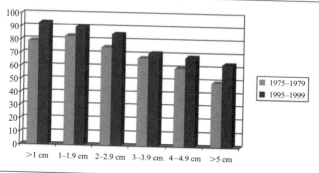

**BOX 21-1**

This interesting study showed the effect of stage migration on stage-specific survival statistics. The authors compared the stage-specific survival of 1,350 patients with breast cancer whose disease was staged according to the 1988 AJCC staging system to that of the same patients whose disease was reclassified according to the 2003 AJCC staging system. The changes in the staging system led to an increased percentage of patients being classified as having Stage III disease in the 2003 cohort. This reclassification led to apparent significant improvements in overall survival rates for both Stage II and Stage III disease within the 2003 cohort compared with the 1988 cohort.

Woodward WA, Strom EA, Tucker SL, et al. Changes in the 2003 American Joint Committee on Cancer staging for breast cancer dramatically affect stage-specific survival. *J Clin Oncol* 21:3244–3248, 2003.

Randomized clinical trials investigating adjuvant systemic treatments have found incremental improvements in the outcome of patients with lymph node-positive breast cancer (Table 21-2).

Improvements in systemic treatments have made the positive effects of locoregional therapy more important. For example, recent findings have convincingly demonstrated that patients with lymph node-positive disease derive a survival benefit from radiation therapy. The most important publication highlighting the evidence for this conclusion is from the Early Breast Cancer Trialists' Group, whose recent update of their metanalysis of radiotherapy trials in breast cancer is summarized in Box 21-2.

Advances in systemic therapy have increased the positive benefits of radiation treatment on survival. As systemic treatments continue to improve, presumably more systemic micrometastases will be eradicated by such treatments, and therefore the locoregional control benefits from radiation may have a still greater effect on overall survival for women with locally advanced disease. A second metanalysis of radiotherapy trials in breast cancer that was limited to clinical trials that included systemic treatments provides evidence for this concept and is highlighted in Box 21-3.

Finally, the benefits of radiation in both advanced and early-stage disease depend on the radiation treatment technique and dose. Treatment techniques should ensure that the areas at risk for residual microscopic disease are included in the target volume and that the risks of injury to criti-

**TABLE 21-2** Recent Incremental Improvements That Have Occurred in Adjuvant Systemic Therapy for Patients With Lymph-Node Positive Cancer

| Chemotherapy | Hormonal Therapy | Biological Therapy |
|---|---|---|
| Adjuvant chemotherapy found to offer an advantage over no chemotherapy | Adjuvant tamoxifen found to offer an advantage over no tamoxifen | Trastuzumab + chemotherapy found to offer an advantage over chemotherapy alone for tumors that overexpress HER2/neu |
| Anthracycline chemotherapy found to offer an advantage over non-anthracycline chemotherapy | Aromatase inhibitor alone or sequential tamoxifen followed by an aromatase inhibitor found to offer an advantage over tamoxifen alone | |
| Anthracycline + taxane found to offer an advantage over anthracycline only | | |
| Dose-dense scheduling of anthracycline/taxane found to offer an advantage over historical scheduling | | |

BOX 21-2

This comprehensive metanalysis of prospective radiotherapy trials is arguably one of the most important publications in breast cancer radiation oncology. The postmastectomy studies demonstrated that radiation reduced the 15-year locoregional recurrence rate from 29% to 8% for patients with lymph node–positive disease and the 10-year rate from 8% to 3% for patients with lymph node–negative disease. This benefit resulted in improved breast cancer–specific survival and overall survival for patients with positive lymph nodes but not for those with negative lymph nodes. These findings conclusively demonstrate that persistent locoregional disease can be a source of distant metastases and death and that eradication of such disease can have a significant survival benefit.

This study also demonstrated that postmastectomy radiation can lead to an increased risk of death from cardiovascular disease. This topic is further discussed later in this chapter.

Early Breast Cancer Trialists' Collaborative Group. Effects of radiotherapy and of differences in the extent of surgery for early breast cancer on local recurrence and 15-year survival: an overview of the randomized trials. *Lancet* 366:2087–2106, 2005.

cal normal structures, such as the heart, are minimized. Treatment techniques with respect to risk of normal-tissue injury will be discussed later in this chapter. Referenced in Box 21-4 is an important article concerning how the delivery of radiation affects cancer outcome.

## SEQUENCING OF TREATMENTS AND NEOADJUVANT CHEMOTHERAPY

As previously mentioned, management of locally advanced breast cancer requires multimodality therapy, which is optimally coordinated by a multidisciplinary team. One of the first therapeutic decisions concerning the management of locally advanced disease concerns the sequencing of therapy. Historically, modified radical mastectomy followed by adjuvant chemotherapy and postmastectomy radiation was the standard approach for patients with advanced but operable tumors. More recently, however, the use of neoadjuvant chemotherapy (chemotherapy given before surgery) for patients with advanced disease has significantly increased. This strategy was first adopted for patients with unresectable or marginally resectable disease, and the initial clinical findings from such patients indicated that chemotherapy led to high rates of tumor response.

The use of neoadjuvant chemotherapy affects several locoregional treatment decisions and therefore requires coordination with all disciplines involved in breast cancer care. This treatment approach has several advantages and some potential disadvantages to consider, some of which are listed in Table 21-3.

BOX 21-3

This metanalysis of prospective radiotherapy trials limited its study to only those trials that included patients with lymph node–positive disease who were also treated with systemic therapy. This analysis is important because it conclusively showed that systemic treatments do not replace the need for locoregional radiation (radiation use was associated with a 75% relative reduction in locoregional recurrence). Furthermore, radiation use was also associated with an improvement in overall survival (relative risk of death was reduced by 17%). These findings suggest that as systemic treatments reduce the risk of death from preexisting distant metastases, the benefits of radiation, both with respect to locoregional recurrence and overall survival, are increased.

Whelan TJ, Julian J, Wright J, et al. Does locoregional radiation therapy improve survival in breast cancer? A metanalysis. *J Clin Oncol* 18:1220–1222, 2000.

---

**BOX 21-4**

One of the limitations of the metanalysis conducted by the Early Breast Cancer Trialists' Collaborative Group was that it assessed the benefits of postmastectomy radiation without regard to the quality of the radiation treatments used in a particular trial. This study attempted to address this limitation by examining how radiation dose and field design affected outcome. The authors demonstrated that both locoregional control and survival benefit were much greater in the trials that had optimal radiation dose and treatment fields compared with those trials in which the dose or treatment fields were less optimal.

Gebski V, Lagleva M, Keech A, et al. Survival effects of postmastectomy adjuvant radiation therapy using biologically equivalent doses: a clinical perspective. *J Natl Cancer Inst* 98:26–38, 2006.

---

Originally, the hope was that sequencing chemotherapy before surgery might have a positive benefit in terms of eradicating systemic micrometastases and improving survival. Unfortunately the randomized trials comparing neoadjuvant chemotherapy to adjuvant chemotherapy for patients with operable breast cancer failed to show a survival difference. A positive finding of these studies, however, was that rates of breast conservation with locoregional treatments were increased. One of the most important of these studies is highlighted in Box 21-5.

## BREAST CONSERVATION AFTER NEOADJUVANT CHEMOTHERAPY

The findings from the B-18 trial suggested that a potential benefit of neoadjuvant chemotherapy for patients with locally advanced breast cancer is the ability to offer selected patients the possibility of breast-conservation therapy. The goal of breast-conservation therapy for patients with advanced disease is to achieve an aesthetically acceptable cosmetic outcome and a low risk of breast recurrence. Most patients with locally advanced breast cancer, however, will prove not to be candidates for this approach and will be best served by undergoing a mastectomy after their neoadjuvant treatment. Important selection criteria for selecting a breast-conservation approach after neoadjuvant chemotherapy include the following:

- Achievement of a partial or complete clinical response to neoadjuvant treatment
- Ability to resect the residual primary abnormality with an aesthetically acceptable outcome
- Resolution of all skin changes

---

TABLE 21-3  **Potential Advantages and Disadvantages of Neoadjuvant Chemotherapy for Patients with Operable Breast Cancer**

| Advantages | Disadvantages |
|---|---|
| May allow breast conservation or improve the aesthetic outcome of breast conservation | May make the margin status after breast conservation less certain |
| Allows assessment of response to a particular agent, so that the therapy can be modified if the disease is resistant | May increase the false-negative rate of sentinel lymph node biopsy |
| Assessment of pathological disease response allows clearer estimates of prognosis | Indications for postmastectomy radiation are less clear |
| Excellent research tool for<br>• Comparing two agents<br>• Studying the biology of chemotherapy response | |

**BOX 21-5**

The B-18 trial remains the largest and perhaps most important study to assess the value of delivering chemotherapy before surgery rather than afterward. This study randomly assigned 1,523 patients with operable breast cancer to receive four cycles of chemotherapy, given either before or after surgery. The primary endpoints of the trial were disease-free survival and overall survival, which proved to be equivalent between the two schedules. A positive finding was that neo-adjuvant chemotherapy increased the rates of breast-conservation surgery from 60% to 68%. This increase was directly due to a greater percentage of patients with T3 disease being offered breast conservation after their disease responded to the neo-adjuvant chemotherapy (22% breast conservation rate vs. 8%, respectively in the patients with T3 disease). The crude ipsilateral breast recurrence rate (first events only) was 10.7% in the patients treated with neo-adjuvant chemotherapy vs. 7.6% in those treated with adjuvant chemotherapy ($P = 0.12$).

Wolmark N, Wang J, Mamounas E, et al. Preoperative chemotherapy in patients with operable breast cancer: nine-year results from National Surgical Adjuvant Breast and Bowel Project B-18. *J Natl Cancer Inst Monogr* 30:96–102, 2001.

- Ability to achieve negative surgical margins
- Ability to resect all residual suspicious calcifications
- Noninflammatory disease

For patients with large initial primary tumors that respond favorably to neo-adjuvant chemotherapy and thus may be candidates for breast-conservative therapy, resection most often is directed at the tumor bed remaining after chemotherapy rather than the initial volume of residual disease. One concern with resecting only the post-chemotherapy volume of residual disease is that some advanced breast cancers do not respond to neoadjuvant chemotherapy by shrinking concentrically to a solitary nidus. In such cases, surgery directed at the primary core may leave a higher burden of microscopic disease around the tumor bed site, which theoretically could be associated with higher rates of breast cancer recurrence. Figure 21-3 is a diagram illustrating the ways in which breast cancers can respond to chemotherapy.[10]

A number of publications have accumulated concerning the outcome of patients treated with breast conservation after neo-adjuvant chemotherapy. Some studies have found relatively high rates of breast recurrence, and others have reported excellent outcomes. The reasons for these differences likely reflect the selection criteria used to determine candidates for breast-conservation, including the assessment of surgical margins. In addition, some studies with higher rates of recurrence used radiation without surgery for cases showing a complete clinical response to neo-adjuvant chemotherapy. A representative selection of such studies is shown in Table 21-4.[11–13]

The findings described in the table indicate that careful selection criteria and multidisciplinary coordination are key elements of success in breast-conservation therapy. One of the more successful recent large studies is further reviewed in Box 21-6.

In conclusion, these findings indicate that breast-conservation therapy is an appropriate treatment option for carefully selected patients with advanced primary tumors that respond favorably to neo-adjuvant chemotherapy. Consideration of the evidence for breast conservation in advanced disease also requires recognizing that advanced disease status also predicts locoregional recurrence after post-mastectomy radiation and distant metastases, and so removal of the breast may not necessarily enhance the likelihood of a cure.

## POSTMASTECTOMY RADIATION

As noted earlier in this chapter, most patients with locally advanced breast cancers are treated with mastectomy, and metanalyses of radiotherapy trials have indicated that the use of radiation after

**FIGURE 21-3** Three potential pathological outcomes of a primary tumor that responds to neo-adjuvant chemotherapy.

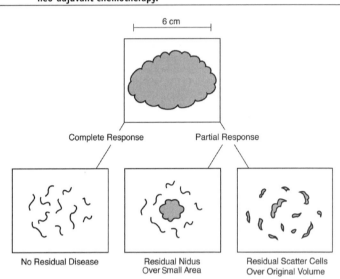

Reprinted with permission from John Wiley & Sons, Inc, Buchholz et al. *Cancer* 98:1150–1160, 2003.[10]

mastectomy can improve both locoregional control and overall survival. The three most important recent randomized trials studying the benefits of post-mastectomy radiation for patients with Stage II or Stage III breast cancer treated with mastectomy and systemic therapy are shown in Table 21-5 and in Boxes 21-7 and 21-8.[14] Collectively, these three studies indicate that selected patients are at risk of having locoregional residual disease after mastectomy and systemic therapy and that foci of residual disease can be the source of subsequent metastases and death. Correspondingly, the use of locoregional adjuvant radiation to eradicate these foci can improve survival.

The Danish Breast Cancer Cooperative Group recently updated their findings from the 82b and 82c trials.[15] After 18 years of follow-up, the rates of locoregional recurrence, with or without simultaneous distant metastases, in the combined patient data from both trials were 49% (no radiation) vs. 14% (radiation). Furthermore, the risk of developing a locoregional recurrence followed by distant metastases was 35% (no radiation) vs. 6% (radiation). These findings provide further evi

**TABLE 21-4** Local Recurrence after Breast-Conservation Therapy after Neo-adjuvant Chemotherapy in Selected Series with Mature Follow-Up Information

| Authors | Number of Patients | Follow-Up Time | Local Recurrence Rate |
|---|---|---|---|
| Wolmark et al. | 749 | 9 years | 11% |
| Mauriac et al. | 40 | 10 years | 23% |
| Rouzier et al. | 257 | 10 years | 21% |
| Bonadonna et al. | 456 | 8 years | 7% |
| Chen et al. | 340 | 10 years | 10% |

**BOX 21-6**

This report describes one of the largest single-institution studies (with 340 patients) investigating breast conservation after neo-adjuvant chemotherapy. Despite the fact that 72% of patients in the study had clinical Stage IIB or III disease, the 5- and 10-year breast cancer recurrence rates were only 5% and 10%, respectively. Four tumor-related factors were associated with breast cancer recurrence and locoregional recurrence: clinical N2 or N3 disease; lymphovascular space invasion; a multifocal pattern of residual disease; and residual disease larger than 2 cm in diameter. Interestingly, having a T3 or T4 tumor did not correlate with breast cancer recurrence overall, but those patients with T3 or T4 disease in which the primary tumor broke up and left a multifocal pattern of residual disease (similar to the right panel of Figure 23-3) had a 20% risk of local disease recurrence.

Chen AM, Meric-Bernstam F, Hunt KK, et al. Breast-conserving therapy after neoadjuvant chemotherapy: the M.D. Anderson Cancer Center experience. *J Clin Oncol* 22:2303–2312, 2004.

ence that persistent locoregional disease can be a source of subsequent distant metastases. The long-term findings from the Danish studies, like the British Columbia update, indicated that the vast majority of patients who experienced locoregional disease recurrence eventually developed distant metastases and died.

Finally, investigators in the Eastern Cooperative Oncology Group conducted a randomized study of post-mastectomy radiation for patients with advanced locoregional disease.[16] This trial also noted a reduction in locoregional recurrence but no statistically significant difference in overall survival. This trial has been criticized for the large percentage of the patients in the radiation group who either did not receive the treatment (18% of the group) or had a major treatment violation (30% of the group).[17]

## Indications for Postmastectomy Radiation

Eligibility criteria for the Danish and British Columbia postmastectomy radiation trials included any patient with lymph node-positive disease. Most of the patients enrolled in these studies had primary tumors smaller than 5 cm and one to three positive lymph nodes. Accordingly, one could

**TABLE 21-5**    **Locoregional Recurrence and Survival Rates in Randomized Trials Comparing the Use of Post-mastectomy Radiation with No Radiation for Patients Treated with Mastectomy and Systemic Therapy**

| Trial | Locoregional Recurrence Rates | Survival Rates |
|---|:---:|:---:|
| Danish 82b | | |
|    Radiation | 9% | 45% |
|    No radiation | 32% | 54% |
| | $P < 0.0001$ | $P < 0.0001$ |
| Vancouver, BC | | |
|    Radiation | 13% | 47% |
|    No radiation | 39% | 37% |
| | $P = 0.0005$ | $P = 0.03$ |
| Danish 82c | | |
|    Radiation | 8% | 45% |
|    No radiation | 35% | 36% |
| | $P < 0.0001$ | $P = 0.03$ |

---

**BOX 21-7**

The Danish 82b trial is the largest prospective randomized trial investigating the use of radiation for patients who underwent mastectomy and chemotherapy. This trial randomly assigned 1,708 pre-menopausal women to receive or not receive post-mastectomy radiation. The original results of the study found that radiation reduced the locoregional recurrence rate from 32% to 9% and improved the overall survival rate from 45% to 54% (Table 21-5). One controversy surrounding this study was the surgical component of the treatments. Specifically, the median number of lymph nodes dissected was seven, with 15% of the patients having three or fewer lymph nodes dissected. Accordingly, patients who were not treated with radiation were at risk of disease recurring from involved lymph nodes that could have been resected if a standard axillary level I/II lymph node dissection had been done.

However, an important finding that is outside of this controversy is that this trial clearly demonstrated that reducing locoregional recurrence can improve overall survival; stated another way, persistent locoregional disease can be the source of distant metastases and death.

Overgaard M, Hansen PS, Overgaard J, et al. Postoperative radiotherapy in high-risk premenopausal women with breast cancer who receive adjuvant chemotherapy. *N Engl J Med* 337:949–955, 1997.

---

conclude from the findings that postmastectomy radiation should be offered to all patients with lymph node-positive breast cancer. A caveat to this, however, is that a large percentage of patients enrolled in these trials did not undergo a standard level I/II axillary dissection. Rather, the median number of lymph nodes recovered from the axillary surgery was seven in the Danish trials (15% had zero to three lymph nodes removed) and 11 in the British Columbia study. Consequently, it is highly likely that some of the patients with one to three positive lymph nodes who were enrolled in these trials had more extensive nodal disease burden that was not completely resected. The effect of this understaging is that these patients would be at a higher risk of locoregional recurrence than would patients with this stage of disease who had undergone a standard level I/II dissection.

To provide further insight into the risk of locoregional recurrence according to the pathological extent of disease after mastectomy and chemotherapy, several groups have analyzed outcomes for patients treated in prospective clinical trials with mastectomy, chemotherapy, and no radiation. The findings from these studies, shown in Table 21-6, indicate that patients with Stage II disease with one to three positive lymph nodes have a 10-year risk of locoregional recurrence of less than 15%, which is much lower than the 30% risk reported for such patients from the Danish and British Columbia clinical trials.[18-20] In contrast, the risk for patients with four or more positive lymph nodes does approach 30% at 10 years.[18-20]

---

**BOX 21-8**

The British Columbia trial is a prospective randomized trial very similar in design to the Danish 82b trial, except that it enrolled only 318 patients. However, the 20-year results of this study also demonstrated that post-mastectomy radiation can reduce locoregional recurrence rates and improve overall survival rates for selected patients treated with mastectomy and chemotherapy (see Table 21-5). Some interesting observations from this 20-year update include the finding that 20% of patients in the no-radiation group who had a locoregional recurrence developed this recurrence after 10 years of follow-up. Furthermore, of the 39 patients who had an isolated locoregional recurrence, 37 eventually developed distant metastases and died of breast cancer.

Ragaz J, Olivotto IA, Spinelli JJ, et al. Locoregional radiation therapy in patients with high-risk breast cancer receiving adjuvant chemotherapy: 20-year results of the British Columbia randomized trial. *J Natl Cancer Inst* 97:116–126, 2005.

## Efficacy

The results of the randomized clinical trials and the metanalysis from the Early Breast Cancer Trialists' Group (Box 21-2) indicate that the addition of radiation after mastectomy and systemic treatment provides a 65%–75% proportional reduction in locoregional recurrence. Another recent study showed the same proportional reduction in a group of patients with Stage II disease and one to three positive lymph nodes even when a standard level I/II axillary dissection was performed (Box 21-9). Whether this benefit helps to improve survival remains to be seen. The metanalysis from the Early Breast Cancer Trialists' Group suggested a breast cancer survival benefit only in those trials in which the absolute improvement in locoregional recurrence with radiation exceeds 10% at 10 years.

## POSTMASTECTOMY RADIATION FOR PATIENTS TREATED WITH NEOADJUVANT CHEMOTHERAPY

In recent years, neo-adjuvant chemotherapy has become a significantly more common treatment approach for patients with Stage II breast cancer and patients with locally advanced disease. This change has led to new questions concerning the indications for post-mastectomy radiation therapy. Historically, the risk of locoregional recurrence and the corresponding indications for post-mastectomy radiation have been based on the pathological extent of disease. Neo-adjuvant chemotherapy changes the extent of pathological disease in 80%–90% of cases, and few data are

**TABLE 21-6  Locoregional Recurrence Rates in Patients Not Treated with Radiation After Mastectomy in the Danish and Canadian Randomized Clinical Trials and United States Studies (rates reflected are at 10-years)**

| Randomized Trials | Number of Patients | Locoregional Recurrence Rates |
|---|---|---|
| Danish 82b | | |
| 1–3 +LN | 516 | 30% |
| ≥4 +LN | 262 | 42% |
| Vancouver, BC | | |
| 1–3 +LN | 91 | not reported |
| ≥4 +LN | 58 | not reported |
| Overall | 149 | 37% |
| Danish 82c | | |
| 1–3 +LN | 403 | 31% |
| ≥4 +LN | 222 | 46% |
| **Patterns-of-Failure Studies** | **Number of Patients** | **Locoregional Recurrence Rates** |
| ECOG | | |
| 1–3 +LN | 400 | 13% |
| ≥4 +LN | 300 | 29% |
| M. D. Anderson | | |
| 1–3 +LN | 400 | 12% |
| ≥4 +LN | 300 | 27% |
| NSABP | | |
| 1–3 +LN | 400 | 6% to 11% |
| ≥4 +LN | 300 | 14% to 25% |

Abbreviations: +LN, positive lymph nodes; ECOG, Eastern Cooperative Oncology Group; NSABP, National Surgical Adjuvant Breast and Bowel Project

---

**BOX 21-9**

Significant controversy remains as to whether Stage II breast cancer with one to three positive lymph nodes treated with a standard modified radical mastectomy warrants postmastectomy radiation. Previously, the authors of this report found that the 10-year locoregional recurrence rate for such patients was 13%. In this study, the authors found that radiation was effective in reducing this recurrence rate to only 3% at 10 years—a similar proportional reduction in recurrence as that seen with more advanced disease. Whether an absolute reduction in locoregional recurrence of 10% can offer a slight improvement in overall survival is still unknown.

Woodward WA, Strom EA, Tucker SL, et al. Locoregional recurrence after doxorubicin-based chemotherapy and postmastectomy radiation: implications for patients with early-stage disease and predictors for recurrence after radiation. *Int J Radiat Oncol Biol Phys* 57:336–344, 2003.

---

available to help clarify how the pathological information obtained after chemotherapy treatment should guide decisions about radiation treatments. One recent study compared the pathological extent of disease with locoregional recurrence after mastectomy for patients treated either with surgery first or chemotherapy first.[21] That study showed that the locoregional recurrence rate associated with a particular pathological extent of disease was higher in patients treated with chemotherapy first than in patients treated with surgery first. These results imply that the risk of locoregional recurrence for patients treated with neo-adjuvant chemotherapy is affected by both the pretreatment clinical stage and the extent of residual disease after chemotherapy.

This same group also evaluated the efficacy of post-mastectomy radiation therapy for patients treated with neo-adjuvant chemotherapy (Box 21-10). The important message from this study was that radiation offered a similar proportional benefit in terms of reducing locoregional recurrence as was achieved for patients treated with surgery first. The investigators also found that all patients with Stage III disease, regardless of their response to chemotherapy, had a clinically relevant risk of locoregional recurrence that was significantly reduced with the addition of radiation. Finally, in this study, which consisted predominantly of patients with locally advanced breast cancer, radiation use was independently associated with an improvement in survival.

Finally, this group also investigated the risk of locoregional recurrence in 132 patients treated with neoadjuvant chemotherapy and mastectomy for clinical Stage II breast cancer. The 5-year locoregional recurrence rate for these patients, unlike that for the Stage III group, was less than 10%, except for a small subgroup of patients with clinical T3N0 disease and another small subgroup with four or more positive lymph nodes after chemotherapy.[22]

On the basis of these findings, it is reasonable to recommend post-mastectomy radiation therapy for all patients with clinical T3 or T4 tumors or clinical Stage III disease regardless of their response to the chemotherapy regimen. It is also clear that additional studies are needed to quantify the risk of locoregional recurrence for patients who present with T1 or T2 disease and have one to three positive lymph nodes after neo-adjuvant chemotherapy.

## CHEMOTHERAPY

Systemic treatments play a critically important role in the multimodality therapy of breast cancer. Over time, systemic treatments for breast cancer have shown significant incremental improvement that have positively affected patient outcome (Table 21-2). Initial randomized trials showed that the first generation of chemotherapy agents could offer a survival advantage over no systemic treatment; subsequently, anthracyclines were shown to offer an advantage over regimens that did not contain an anthracycline. More recent trials have found that the use of taxanes in addition to anthracyclines offers another incremental advantage.[23,24] The scheduling of the anthracycline,

BOX 21-10

This study compared the outcomes of 579 patients treated with neo-adjuvant chemotherapy, mastectomy, and radiation therapy with those of 136 patients treated with neo-adjuvant chemotherapy and mastectomy alone. Radiation therapy was not a randomized variable, so the groups were not equivalent in terms of T or N clinical stage; the patients treated with radiation therapy had more extensive disease. Despite this imbalance, the 10-year locoregional recurrence rates were 8% (radiation) vs. 22% (no radiation) ($P = 0.001$). More importantly, radiation therapy was associated with better overall and cause-specific survival rates in selected groups of patients with high-risk disease.

This report is important in that it describes the largest published series investigating post-mastectomy radiation for patients treated with neo-adjuvant chemotherapy. A second important finding from this study was the demonstration that patients with locally advanced clinical disease that responded to chemotherapy and were treated with mastectomy still benefited from the addition of radiation therapy. For patients with Stage III disease who achieved a pathological complete response, the locoregional recurrence rate for those treated with radiation therapy was 3% vs. 33% for those who did not receive radiation therapy ($P = 0.006$).

Huang EH, Tucker SL, Strom EA, et al. Radiation treatment improves locoregional control and cause-specific survival for selected patients with locally advanced breast cancer treated with neoadjuvant chemotherapy and mastectomy. *J Clin Oncol* 22:4691–4699, 2004.

taxane regimen in some form of an accelerated or dose-dense fashion can further improve outcome.[25] For patients with HER2/neu positive disease, recent randomized studies have shown that the addition of trastuzumab can further reduce the proportional risk of recurrence by 50% compared with chemotherapy alone.[26] This dramatic improvement is unparalleled in breast cancer history and is an advantage on top of those already achieved with standard therapies.

In addition to chemotherapy, hormonal therapy is indicated for all patients with estrogen or progesterone receptor–positive disease. For premenopausal women who continue to have ovarian function after chemotherapy, tamoxifen is the preferred therapy. For post-menopausal women, the use of an aromatase inhibitor is equally appropriate. Several options exist for post-menopausal patients, including anastrozole for 5 years, initial tamoxifen for 2 to 3 years followed by exemestane, or tamoxifen for 5 years followed by 5 years of letrozole.[27–29]

## POSTMASTECTOMY RADIATION FOR PATIENTS WITH INFLAMMATORY DISEASE

Inflammatory breast cancer is an aggressive form of locally advanced disease that typically progresses rapidly at presentation and has a high risk of early distant dissemination. Before the availability of chemotherapy, fewer than 5% of patients with inflammatory breast cancer survived more than 5 years.[30] Treatment with definitive radiotherapy, or with preoperative radiation followed by mastectomy, failed to achieve longstanding locoregional control in almost 50% of patients with inflammatory breast cancer.[31,32] However, over the past two decades, local control rates and survival for patients with inflammatory breast cancer have dramatically improved. Use of a combined-modality approach that includes chemotherapy, modified radical mastectomy, and postmastectomy radiation has significantly improved survival rates and has provided long-term local control rates of 80%–90%.[33]

The current standard of treatment sequencing for patients with inflammatory breast cancer is to begin with anthracycline- or taxane-based chemotherapy. Sequential treatment, such as weekly paclitaxel followed by FAC (5-fluouracil, doxorubicin, cyclophosphamide), or a combined regimen such as TAC (docetaxel, doxorubicin, cyclophosphamide) is appropriate. Most patients will achieve partial or complete clinical remission after such treatments and be candidates for surgery. Although breast conservation has been attempted for patients with inflammatory breast cancer that shows a complete clinical response, most findings suggest that this approach is associate with a local recurrence rate of 20% or more. Therefore, most institutions consider modified radic. mastectomy to be the current surgical standard of care. At M.D. Anderson Cancer Center, the inst tutional preference is to complete the entire anthracycline and taxane treatment course before su gery so that the total package of chemotherapy is given in the most dose-dense fashion. Howeve no data exist as yet to suggest that the outcome after this approach is superior to that after sequence strategy in which mastectomy is sandwiched in the middle of the chemotherapy cours

After the completion of chemotherapy and surgery, radiation plays a critical role in helping avoid locoregional recurrence. Treatments should be directed to the chest wall and draining lympha ics, including the undissected level III axilla, the supraclavicular fossa, and the internal mamma lymph nodes. The coverage of the chest wall should be broad in both the cranial/caudal an medial/lateral dimensions to minimize the risk of a marginal recurrence, which can develop from pe sistent disease in the lymphovascular spaces and dermal lymphatics. For patients without evidence gross disease at the time of the radiation treatments, initial fields should be treated to a minimum dos of 50 Gy in 25 fractions, with bolus doses used at appropriate intervals to ensure that a brisk skin rea tion is obtained during the later weeks of treatment. Subsequently, the regions of the chest wall an the mastectomy scar should be treated to boost doses of at least 60 Gy. Every effort should be made t avoid a treatment break, because tumor cell repopulation during treatment is a greater concern fe inflammatory breast cancer than for noninflammatory breast cancer.

M.D. Anderson has adopted an accelerated hyperfractionated approach for all patients wit inflammatory breast cancer. The initial fields are treated to 51 Gy in 1.5-Gy fractions given twice dail with a minimum of 6 hours between treatments. Subsequently, the boost fields are treated to an add tional 15 Gy in 10 1.5-Gy fractions given over 5 days. When this approach was compared with a histo ical standard, the accelerated hyperfractionated radiation appeared to improve locoregional contr and may have contributed to the improved survival noted among the most recently treated patients.

For patients with persistent inoperable disease that fails to respond to neo-adjuvant anthracy cline and taxane chemotherapy, radiation can also be used as either a preoperative treatment or a a definitive treatment. For patients who undergo preoperative radiation therapy, the dose should b limited to approximately 50 Gy to minimize the risk of postsurgical complications. For patients i whom the extent of disease precludes surgery, reduced fields should be boosted to 70–72 Gy, wit care taken to respect the tolerance of normal tissues. Unfortunately, patients with chemorefracto disease have a very poor prognosis, with high rates of both locoregional and distant recurrence.

## TREATMENT OF LOCALLY RECURRENT DISEASE

Radiation treatment is an important part of the management of locally recurrent disease. Mo patients who experience disease recurrence after breast conservation therapy have already bee treated with breast radiation, and therefore mastectomy remains the preferred approach in thes circumstances. Post-mastectomy radiation is infrequently recommended unless there are specifi extenuating circumstances concerning the extent of disease. For example, when a breast recu rence develops after lumpectomy alone, the disease can be approached in similar fashion as tha used for a primary breast cancer. For such individuals, if a second breast-conservative surgery ca achieve negative margins, radiation treatment to the breast, plus/minus lymphatics, is recom mended. If a mastectomy is performed, post-mastectomy radiation can be used selectively, wit selection criteria similar to those used for nonrecurrent disease.

The management of locally recurrent disease after mastectomy requires a comprehensive treat ment approach. Such patients represent a heterogeneous group and no clear findings from rar domized studies are available to guide decisions about treatment. A variety of poor prognosti factors have been identified, including a time to recurrence of less than 2 years, inoperable diseas at the time of recurrence, nodal vs. chest wall recurrence, inability to use radiation because of previous radiation treatments, and advanced disease at the time of original presentation.[34]

The treatment schema shown in Figure 21-4 illustrates a preferred approach for patients who develop locoregional recurrence after mastectomy and have not had previous radiation treatments. In general, the best treatment outcomes are achieved if neo-adjuvant chemotherapy and surgery can eliminate evidence of disease at the time of adjuvant radiation. For patients who present with inoperable disease, it is reasonable to begin with systemic treatments if active agents are available with which the patient has not been recently treated. If disease in such patients responds, then surgery may become a possibility. For patients with operable disease, surgery followed by radiation and possibly chemotherapy is also a reasonable approach. Although no randomized trials have been done to explore the benefits of systemic treatment, it is clear that patients who experience locoregional recurrence of locally advanced disease are at very high risk of subsequent distant failure and therefore an adjuvant systemic treatment is a reasonable approach. The optimal sequencing of adjuvant systemic treatments and radiation has not been studied and is best determined on an individual, case-by-case basis.

## RADIATION TREATMENT TECHNIQUES

The efficacy and toxicity of radiation treatments for locally advanced breast cancer depend greatly on the technique used to deliver the therapy. Treatment techniques should be evaluated with respect to both field design and radiation dosimetry. Techniques for breast-conservation therapy were reviewed in the previous chapter, so this chapter will focus on post-mastectomy radiation techniques.

**FIGURE 21-4** Flow diagram of workup and recommendations for patients who have not had previous radiation and develop locally recurrent disease after mastectomy. CT, computerd tomography; PET, positron emission tomography; ER, estrogen receptor; PR, progesterone receptor.

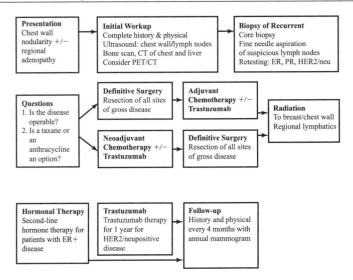

The first step in the treatment process should always be to define the target volume. The most common site of locoregional recurrence in patients treated with mastectomy is the chest wall, and inclusion of the chest wall is therefore the most important targeted region for all patients receiving post-mastectomy radiation. In general, the chest wall volume extends medially to midline, laterally to the mid-axillary line, and caudally 2 cm below the contralateral inframammary sulcus. At times, the chest wall volume needs to be further expanded to provide appropriate margins around the mastectomy scar. Patients with inflammatory breast cancer are at particular risk for recurrence at the radiation field margins, so the chest wall fields should be more generous in all dimensions.

The axillary and supraclavicular lymph nodes are a second critical target for postmastectomy radiation. Disease recurrence in the level I/II axilla is very unusual in patients who have undergone dissection of this region, so in such patients the target definition more appropriately includes the level III (superior-medial to the pectoralis minor) and supraclavicular lymph nodes. Locally advanced disease is associated with a clinically relevant risk of internal mammary lymph node involvement within the first three interspaces. Accordingly, this area is appropriate to consider as a target volume as well, although the value of internal mammary lymph node chain (IMC) irradiation is a current area of controversy.

Post-mastectomy radiation is optimally planned by using a wide-bore CT simulator. The process then proceeds according to the following steps:

- Patients are positioned supine on a 10- to 15-degree slant board, with arm abducted at approximately 110 degrees and externally rotated; radio-opaque wires are used to mark the scars and placed at the estimation of field borders.
- Patients are immobilized with a positioning cradle.
- Patients undergo CT scanning.
- The border between the supraclavicular field and the matching lower fields is set just below the head of the clavicle; the amount of exposed lung is assessed (this factor varies between individuals and may lead to adjustments).
- Field isocenters and reference marks are placed.
- Structures (internal mammary vessels in the first three interspaces, level III axilla) are contoured on axilla CT slices.
- Fields are designed to include targets while minimizing volumes of normal structures such as the heart, lung, shoulder, and spinal cord.

Several techniques can be used to safely deliver radiation doses to the target volumes. At M.D. Anderson, the most common technique is to treat the lateral chest wall with medial and lateral match photon beams. These beams have nondivergent cranial edges (couch rotation) and a nondivergent deep edge (gantry rotation). The beams are laterally positioned to include no more than 1.0–1.5 cm of lung and to avoid the heart. The medial chest wall and IMC lymph nodes are included in an electron field that matches the tangents at the skin surface. This field is angled 15–20 degrees to minimize the cold match line between this field and the tangents that occurs at a depth near the chest wall. A supraclavicular/axillary apex field with a half-beam block at the caudal border is then added.

In dosimetry planning, the weighting and wedging of the tangents field is optimized to deliver 50 Gy in 25 fractions to the chest wall. The electron energies for the IMC field are selected to ensure that the 90% isodose line covers the contoured IMC structures. The plan should be evaluated to ensure that the electron field does not deliver too much radiation to the anterior heart. If it does, this field can be split in two, with a higher energy selected for the upper field in the region of the targeted IMC and a lower energy used in the lower field to spare the heart. Similarly, the prescribed dose for the supraclavicular fossa field should ensure that the contoured level III volume receives

0%. Figure 21-5 shows examples of this technique. The chest wall/IMC can also be treated with hree matching electron fields or an electron arc.

After a 50-Gy total dose, we routinely boost the dose to the chest wall with two matched elec- ron fields an additional 10 Gy in five fractions. We also provide boost doses to sites of unresected previously involved lymph nodes in the infraclavicular, supraclavicular, and IMC.

## TOXICITY OF POST-MASTECTOMY RADIATION

Post-mastectomy radiation has important acute and late risks of normal tissue injury. Near the completion of therapy, almost all patients experience some degree of fatigue and localized skin

---

**FIGURE 21-5** Technique for postmastectomy radiation.

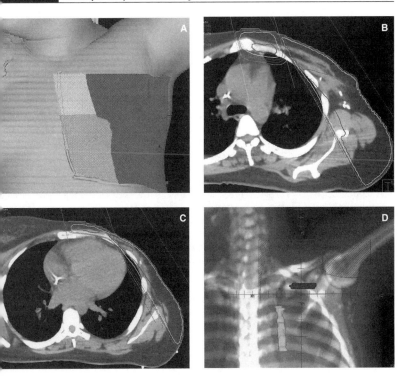

(See Color Plate 6). Radiation fields used to treat the chest wall, internal mammary lymph nodes and axillary apex/supraclavicular fossa in a patient who had undergone a left modified radical mastectomy. (A) shows a skin rendering of the radiation fields used to treat the chest wall and internal mammary lymph nodes. Two electron fields were used over the medial chest wall with a higher energy selected for the upper three inter- spaces to treat the internal mammary lymph nodes (B) axial image and a lower energy selected over the heat (C) axial image. The lateral chest wall is treated with matched tangential photon beams to nicely shape the radiation dose distribution around the heart and thoracic structures. The axillary apex/supraclavicular fields are shown in (D). The level III region of the axillary and the upper internal mammary vessels have been contoured on axial CT images and reconstructed on this image. They are used to determine depth of dose prescription.

**BOX 21-11**

In this study, the authors analyzed the Surveillance, Epidemiology, and End Results database to compare the rates of cardiac death among patients treated with radiation for a left-sided breast cancer with the rates for those treated with radiation for a right-sided breast cancer. For patients treated in the 1970s, the 15-year cardiac mortality rates were higher in the left-sided group than in the right-sided group. However, for patients treated after 1980, no difference in cardiac mortality was found between groups. These findings imply that radiation treatment delivery techniques changed after the recognition that radiation can cause heart injury and that these improved techniques have helped to minimize the risk of treatment-induced cardiac death.

Giordano SH, Kuo YF, Freeman JL, et al. Risk of cardiac death after adjuvant radiotherapy for breast cancer. *J Natl Cancer Inst* 97:419–424, 2005.

irritation, which may include areas of moist desquamation. Of more concern, however, are the late effects associated with radiation use because these often are longstanding injuries.

One of the most common late normal tissue consequences, and one that affects decisions about post-mastectomy radiation, is the detrimental effect of radiation on breast reconstruction. As a general principle, the aesthetic outcome of a breast reconstruction, immediate or delayed, is adversely affected by the use of radiation as compared with that of a skin-sparing mastectomy and immediate reconstruction without radiation. This consideration may be important when considering the risks and benefits of post-mastectomy radiation for Stage II disease. For patients with locally advanced disease, M.D. Anderson practice usually dictates a mastectomy followed by an attempted delayed reconstruction with autologous tissue.

Other sequelae of radiation include increased risks of lymphedema, radiation pneumonitis, and rarely, complications of nerves, chest wall/skin, or bone injury. Cardiovascular injuries are one of the most serious complications of post-mastectomy radiation. In the earliest trials of post-mastectomy radiation, the risk of dying from cardiovascular disease 10 years or more after treatment was higher among patients who received radiation than among patients who did not (Box 21-2). More recently, investigators from Duke University have demonstrated that irradiation of the heart can lead to perfusion changes shortly after the completion of the treatments.[35] These findings stress the importance of careful treatment planning and use of techniques that minimize the radiation dose to the heart. In the Danish randomized 82b and 82c trials, in which an electron field was used over the heart, no differences were found in cardiovascular mortality or cardiovascular hospitalizations between patients who underwent radiation therapy and those who did not.[36] In the United States, changes in techniques over time have also minimized this risk, as highlighted in Box 21-11.

## CONCLUSION

Radiation treatment has a critical role in the multidisciplinary management of breast cancer that presents at Stage II or Stage III. Emerging findings from clinical trials have indicated that for appropriately selected patients, the use of radiation after surgery and systemic treatments can reduce locoregional recurrence and improve overall survival. Further, several technological improvements in radiation oncology can help to ensure appropriate dose coverage of target volumes and to minimize the risk of injury to cardiovascular and other normal tissues.

## REFERENCES

1. American Cancer Society; *Breast Cancer Facts & Figures 2003–2004*. pp 1–25, 2003.
2. Singletary SE, Connolly JL. Breast Cancer Staging: Working with the Sixth Edition of the AJCC Cancer Staging Manual. *CA Cancer J Clin* 56:37–47, 2006.

3. Lee-Feldstein A, Anton-Culver H, Feldstein PJ. Treatment differences and other prognostic factors related to breast cancer survival. *JAMA* 271:1163–1168, 1994.

4. Haagensen CD, Stout AP. Carcinoma of the breast: criteria of inoperability. *Ann Surg* 118:859–870, 1943.

5. Fracchia AA, Evans JF, Eisenberg BC. Stage III carcinoma of the breast: a detailed analysis. *Ann Surg* 192:705–710, 1980.

6. Haagensen CD, Cooley E. Radical mastectomy for mammary carcinoma. *Ann Surg* 170:884–888, 1969.

7. Hortobagyi GN, Singletary SE, Buchholz TA. Locally advanced breast cancer. In: Singletary SE, Robb GL, GN. H, editors. *Advanced Therapy of Breast Disease,* Second Edition. Hamilton, Ontario: BC Decker, Inc.; pp. 498–508, 2004.

8. Elkin EB, Hudic C, Begg CB, et al. The effect of changes in tumor size on breast carcinoma survival in the U.S.: 1975–1999. *Cancer* 104:1149–1157, 2005.

9. Giordano SH, Buzdar AU, Smith TL, et al. Is breast cancer survival improving? *Cancer* 100: 44–52, 2004.

10. Buchholz TA, Hunt KK, Whitman G, et al. Neoadjuvant chemotherapy of breast cancer: a multidisciplinary discussion of benefits and risks. *Cancer* 98:1150–1160, 2003.

11. Mauriac L, MacGrogan G, Avril A, et al. Neoadjuvant chemotherapy for operable breast carcinoma larger than 3 cm: a unicentre randomized trial with a 124-month median follow-up. *Ann Oncol* 10:47–52, 1999.

12. Rouizer R, Extra JM, Carton M, et al. Primary chemotherapy for operable breast cancer: incidence and prognostic significance of ipsilateral breast tumor recurrence after breast-conserving surgery. *J Clin Oncol* 19:3828–3835, 2001.

13. Bonadonna G, Valagussa P, Brambilla C, et al. Primary chemotherapy in operable breast cancer: eight-year experience at the Milan Cancer Institute. *J Clin Oncol* 16(1):93–100, 1998.

14. Overgaard M, Jensen MB, Overgaard J, et al. Randomized trial evaluating postoperative radiotherapy in high-risk postmenopausal breast cancer patients given adjuvant tamoxifen: results from the DBCG 82c trial. *Lancet* 353:1641–1648, 1999.

15. Nielsen HM, Overgaard M, Grau C, Jensen AR, Overgaard J. Study of failure pattern among high-risk breast cancer patients with or without postmastectomy radiotherapy in addition to adjuvant systemic therapy: long-term results from the Danish Breast Cancer Cooperative Group DBCG82 b and c randomized studies. *J Clin Oncol* 24:1–9, 2006.

16. Olsen JE, Neuberg D, Pandya KH, et al. The role of radiotherapy in the management of operable locally advanced breast carcinoma: results of a randomized trial by the Eastern Cooperative Oncology Group. *Cancer* 79:1138–1149, 1997.

17. Fowble B. Postmastectomy radiation: a modest benefit prevails for high-risk patients. *Cancer* 79:1061–1066, discussion 1067–1068, 1997.

18. Recht A, Gray R, Davidson NE, et al. Locoregional failure 10 years after mastectomy and adjuvant chemotherapy with or without tamoxifen without irradiation: experience of the Eastern Cooperative Oncology Group. *J Clin Oncol* 17:1689–1700, 1999.

19. Katz A, Strom EA, Buchholz TA, et al. Locoregional recurrence patterns following mastectomy and doxorubicin-based chemotherapy: implications for postoperative irradiation. *J Clin Oncol* 18:2817–2827, 2000.

20. Taghian A, Jeong JH, Mamounas E, et al. Patterns of locoregional failure in patients with operable breast cancer treated by mastectomy and adjuvant chemotherapy with or without tamoxifen and without radiotherapy: results from five National Surgical Adjuvant Breast and Bowel Project randomized clinical trials. *J Clin Oncol* 22:4247–4254, 2004.

21. Buchholz TA, Katz A, Strom EA, et al. Pathologic tumor size and lymph node status predict for different rates of locoregional recurrence after mastectomy for breast cancer patients treated with neoadjuvant versus adjuvant chemotherapy. *Int J Radiat Oncol Biol Phys* 53:880–888, 2002.
22. Garg A, Strom EA, McNeese MD, et al. T3 disease at presentation or pathologic involvement of four or more lymph nodes predict for locoregional recurrence in stage II breast cancer treated with neoadjuvant chemotherapy and mastectomy without radiation. *Int J Radiat Oncol Biol Phys* 59:138–145, 2004.
23. Henderson IC, Berry DA, Demetri GD, et al. Improved outcomes from adding sequential paclitaxel but not from escalating doxorubicin dose in an adjuvant chemotherapy regimen for patients with node-positive primary breast cancer. *J Clin Oncol* 21:976–983, 2003.
24. Mamounas EP, Bryant J, Lembersky BC, et al. Paclitaxel following doxorubicin/cyclophosphamide as adjuvant chemotherapy for node-positive breast cancer: results from NSABP B-28. *Proc Annu Meet Am Soc Clin Oncol,* 22:(abst 12), 2003.
25. Citron ML, Berry DA, Cirrincione C, et al. Randomized trial of dose-dense versus conventionally scheduled and sequential versus concurrent combination chemotherapy as postoperative adjuvant treatment of node-positive primary breast cancer: first report of Intergroup Trial C9741/Cancer and Leukemia Group B Trial 9741. *J Clin Oncol* 21:1431–1439, 2003.
26. Romond EH, Perez EA, Bryant J, et al. Trastuzumab plus adjuvant chemotherapy for operable HER2-positive breast cancer. *N Engl J Med* 353:1673–1684, 2005.
27. Baum M, Buzdar AU, Cuzick J, et al. Anastrozole alone or in combination with tamoxifen versus tamoxifen alone for adjuvant treatment of postmenopausal women with early breast cancer: first results of the ATAC randomized trial. *Lancet* 359:2131–2139, 2002.
28. Coombes RC, Hall E, Gibson LJ, et al. Intergroup Exemestane Study. A randomized trial of exemestane after 2 to 3 years of tamoxifen therapy in postmenopausal women with primary breast cancer. *N Engl J Med* 350:1081–1092, 2004.
29. Goss PE, Ingle JN, Martino S, et al. A randomized trial of letrozole in postmenopausal women after 5 years of tamoxifen therapy for early-stage breast cancer. *N Engl J Med* 349:1793–1802, 2003.
30. Bozzetti F, Saccozzi R, De Lena M, Salvadori B. Inflammatory cancer of the breast: analysis of 114 cases. *J Surg Oncol* 18:355–361, 1981.
31. Barker JL, Nelson AJ, Montague ED. Inflammatory carcinoma of the breast. *Radiology* 121:173–176, 1976.
32. Zucali R, Uslenghi C, Kenda R, Bonadonna G. Natural history and survival of inoperable breast cancer treated with radiotherapy and radiotherapy followed by radical mastectomy. *Cancer* 37:1422–1431, 1976.
33. Liao Z, Strom EA, Buzdar AU, et al. Locoregional irradiation for inflammatory breast cancer: effectiveness of dose escalation in decreasing recurrence. *Int J Radiat Oncol Biol Phys* 47:1191–1200, 2000.
34. Chagpar A, Meric F, Hunt KK, et al. Chest wall recurrence after mastectomy does not always portend dismal prognosis. *Ann Surg Oncol* 10:628–634, 2003.
35. Marks LB, Yu X, Prosnitz RG, et al. The incidence and functional consequences of RT-associated cardiac perfusion defects. *Int J Radiat Oncol Biol Phys* 63:214–223, 2005.
36. Hojris I, Overgaard M, Christensen JJ, et al. Morbidity and mortality of ischaemic heart disease in high-risk breast cancer patients after adjuvant postmastectomy systemic treatment with or without radiotherapy: analysis of DBCG 82b and 82c randomized trials. *Lancet* 354:1425–1430, 1999.

# 22

# Pancreatic Cancer

*Christopher G. Willett, MD*
*Brian G. Czito, MD*
*Johanna Bendell, MD*

## OVERVIEW

Radiation therapy and 5-fluorouracil-based chemotherapy has been employed in the treatment of patients with localized pancreatic cancer in two settings: adjuvant or neoadjuvant therapy for patients with resectable disease and "definitive" therapy for patients with locally advanced and unresectable cancer. This chapter reviews the data on the role of radiation therapy in the treatment of localized pancreatic adenocarcinoma and comments on current and future areas of research.

## EPIDEMIOLOGY AND RISK FACTORS

In the year 2008, there will be an estimated 37,680 new cases of pancreatic cancer in the United States and 34,290 estimated deaths from the disease, making pancreatic cancer the fourth leading cause of cancer death in the United States.[1] At present, surgery offers the only means of cure. Unfortunately, only 5% to 25% of patients present with tumors amenable to resection. Historically, patients undergoing resection of localized pancreatic carcinoma have a long-term survival of approximately 20% and a median survival of 13–20 months.[2] Recent data suggest that the survival of patients who undergo resection of their pancreatic cancer may be improving, with contemporary 3-year survival rates around 30%.[3] Patients who present with locally advanced and unresectable pancreatic cancer have a median survival of approximately 9 to 13 months, with rare long-term survival. The highest percentage (40%–45%) of patients present with metastatic disease, which carries a shorter median survival of only 3 to 6 months.[4]

Other pertinent epidemiological facts and risk factors of pancreatic cancer include:

1. Age — Incidence increases sharply after age 45 years
2. Female: Male — 1.0:1.3
3. Race — 14.8/100,000 (black males): 8.8/100,000 (general population)
4. Risk factors — Chronic pancreatitis, smoking, diabetes mellitus, hereditary predisposition to pancreatic cancer or multiple cancers

## EVALUATION

In the recent years, significant advances have been achieved in the imaging and staging of pancreatic cancer. Currently, the principal diagnostic tools are helical CT scan, endoscopic ultrasound (EUS), and laparoscopy. These tools have facilitated the characterization of the primary tumor (resectable versus unresectable) as well as the identification of metastatic disease, so patients can be appropriately and reliably triaged to operative and non-operative therapies. With contemporary staging, the vast majority of patients with pancreatic cancer can be appropriately selected for surgery. The most commonly used diagnostic and staging examination is an abdominal computerized tomography (CT) scan. Newer generation high speed helical CT performed with contrast enhancement and thin section imaging allows high resolution, motion-free images of the pancreas and its surrounding structures to be obtained at varying phases of enhancement. Over 90% of patients deemed unresectable by CT are actually unresectable at operation. In addition, because tissue confirmation of malignancy is a necessary step prior to initiating therapy for patients with locally advanced tumors, CT can be utilized to facilitate fine needle aspiration.

Another tool for staging and diagnosis is endoscopic ultrasound (EUS). In this procedure, an endoscope with an ultrasound transducer at its tip is passed into the stomach and duodenum, where it provides high resolution images of the pancreas and surrounding vessels and facilitates needle biopsies. Frequently, endoscopic ultrasound is performed in conjunction with endoscopic retrograde cholangiopancreatography (ERCP). This combined diagnostic approach allows for staging, therapeutic stenting of the common bile duct when indicated, and retrieval of tumor cells by fine needle aspiration without exposing the peritoneum to potential tumor seeding as may occur with CT-guided biopsies.

Because current imaging techniques cannot visualize small (1–2 mm) liver and peritoneal implants, staging laparoscopy has been used preoperatively to exclude intraperitoneal metastases. This technique can detect intraperitoneal metastases in up to 37% of patients with apparent locally advanced disease by CT. If peritoneal washings or visual inspection and biopsy confirm extrapancreatic involvement, patients with locally advanced pancreatic cancer with extrapancreatic involvement or peritoneal washings at laparoscopy have the same prognosis as those with metastatic disease. These patients are more appropriately treated with systemic therapies.

## ADJUVANT THERAPY

After surgical resection of pancreatic cancer, local recurrence rates range from 50%–90% and distant recurrence rate 40%–90%, most commonly in the liver and/or peritoneum.[5–8] For this reason, adjuvant radiation therapy, chemotherapy, and combined radiation and chemotherapy have been studied in this setting in an attempt to improve patient outcomes (Table 22-1). Despite multiple trials, a definitive role for adjuvant therapy for resected pancreatic cancer has not been established.

### Prospective Trials

The Gastrointestinal Tumor Study Group (GITSG) conducted the first prospective trial of adjuvant chemoradiotherapy for patients with resected pancreatic cancer and negative surgical margins. Patients were randomized to external beam radiation therapy (ERBT) to 40 Gy delivered in split-course fashion with concurrent 5-fluorouracil (5-FU) 500 mg/m2 given as an intravenous bolus on the first 3 and last 3 days of radiation, followed by maintenance 5-FU for 2 years or until disease progression or to observation only.[9] This trial was stopped early secondary to slow accrual (43 patients over 8 years) and a positive interim analysis showing that patients treated on the chemoradiotherapy arm experienced a survival benefit. Patients receiving chemoradiotherapy had a longer median survival (21 months vs. 11 months) and improved 2-year survival (43% vs. 19%). An additional 30 patients were later enrolled to receive adjuvant chemoradiation and confirmed

**TABLE 22-1 Prospective, Randomized Trials for Adjuvant Therapy for Pancreatic Cancer**

| Series | # pts | Median survival (months) | 2-year survival | 5-year survival |
|---|---|---|---|---|
| *GITSG*[9] | | | | |
| Treatment | 21 | 21.0 | 43% | 19% |
| Observation | 22 | 10.9 | 18% | 5% |
| Treatment (expanded cohort)[10] | 30 | 18.0 | 46% | NA |
| *EORTC*[11] | | | | |
| Treatment | 60 | 17.1 | 37% | 20% |
| Observation | 54 | 12.6 | 23% | 10% |
| *ESPAC-1*[12,13] | | | | |
| Pooled data | | | | |
|   Chemotherapy | 244 | 19.7 | NA | NA |
|   No chemotherapy | 237 | 14.0 | NA | NA |
|   Chemoradiation | 178 | 15.5 | NA | NA |
|   No chemoradiation | 180 | 16.1 | NA | NA |
| 2×2 Factorial | | | | |
|   Chemotherapy | 147 | 20.1 | 40% | 21% |
|   No chemotherapy | 142 | 15.5 | 30% | 8% |
|   Chemoradiation | 145 | 15.9 | 29% | 10% |
|   No chemoradiation | 144 | 17.9 | 41% | 20% |

the survival outcomes seen in the original trial with median survival of 18 months and a 2-year survival of 46%.[10] The GITSG trial was criticized for many reasons: only 9% of patients received the 2-year maintenance chemotherapy, the radiation dose was low, the number of patients was small, accrual was slow, an unusually poor survival for the surgical control group, 25% of patients did not begin adjuvant therapy until over 10 weeks after resection, and 32% of the original treatment arm had violations of the scheduled radiation therapy. Nevertheless, this trial resulted in chemoradiation therapy being accepted as appropriate adjuvant therapy in the United States.

A second study sponsored by the European Organization for Research and Treatment of Cancer (EORTC) sought to confirm the findings of the original GITSG study. In this trial, 218 patients with resected pancreas or periampullary cancers were randomly assigned to receive 40 Gy of EBRT in a split-dose fashion with concurrent continuous infusional 5-FU or observation alone.[11] This study showed no significant improvement (p = 0.208) in median survival (24 months vs. 19 months) or 2-year survival (51% vs. 41%). Interestingly, only 114 of the patients enrolled on trial had pancreatic cancer, the remaining patients had periampullary tumors. Subset analysis of the patients with primary pancreatic tumors showed a 2-year survival of 34% for treated patients vs. 26% for the control group (p = 0.099). Criticisms of this trial include: there was no maintenance chemotherapy given in the treatment arm, patients with positive surgical margins were allowed on trial with no prospective assessment, the radiation dose was low, low numbers of patients, and 20% of patients assigned to treatment never received treatment.

The European Study Group for Pancreatic Cancer (ESPAC) then conducted the largest randomized trial evaluating adjuvant therapy for pancreatic cancer, ESPAC-1.[12,13] Treating physicians were allowed to enroll their patients onto one of three parallel randomized studies: 1) chemoradiation vs. no chemoradiation (n = 69). This consisted of 20 Gy over 2 weeks with 5-FU 500 mg/m$^2$ on days 1 through 3, then repeated after a 2-week break, 2) chemotherapy vs. no chemotherapy (n = 192). This consisted of bolus 5-FU (425 mg/m$^2$) and leucovorin (20 mg/m$^2$) given for 5 days every 28 days for 6 months, 3) a 2×2 factorial design of 289 patients enrolled on chemoradiotherapy (n = 73), chemotherapy (n = 75), chemoradiotherapy with maintenance chemotherapy (n = 72), or observation (n = 69).[12,13] The data from the treatment groups from all three parallel trials was then pooled for analysis. There was no survival difference between the 175 patients who received adjuvant chemoradiation and the 178 patients who did not receive therapy (median survival 15.5 months vs. 16.1 months, p = 0.24). There was, however, a survival benefit found for the patients who received adjuvant chemotherapy (n = 238) compared to those who did not (n = 235) (median survival 19.7 months vs. 14 months, p = 0.0005). On further follow-up, the 5-year survival rate for the patients who received chemotherapy was 21% vs. 8% for those who did not.

Like its predecessors, the ESPAC-1 trial had many criticisms: 1) Physicians and patients were allowed to choose which of the three parallel trials to enroll on, creating potential bias. 2) Patients could receive "background" chemoradiation or chemotherapy if decided by their physician. Approximately one third of the patients enrolled on the chemotherapy vs. no chemotherapy trial received "background" chemoradiation therapy or chemotherapy. 3) The radiation was given in a split-dose fashion, with the treating physician judging the final treatment dose (40 Gy vs. 60 Gy). 4) In the chemoradiation vs. no chemoradiation trial, no maintenance adjuvant chemotherapy was given, similar to the EORTC trial. Although there was no benefit seen with adjuvant chemoradiation therapy, there was a benefit to adjuvant chemotherapy.

Building from the data of benefit to adjuvant chemotherapy, investigators in Europe conducted a randomized phase III trial of adjuvant gemcitabine versus observation in patients with resected pancreatic cancer. Three hundred sixty-eight patients were enrolled to this trial and were randomized to gemcitabine 1000 mg/m$^2$ IV days 1, 8, and 15 every 4 weeks for 6 months or observation.[14] The primary endpoint was disease-free survival, and patients who were treated with gemcitabine had a statistically significantly longer disease-free survival (14.2 months vs. 7.5 months) than those who had observation only. Overall survival data are awaiting maturity.

Results from the The Radiation Therapy Oncology Group (RTOG) and GI Intergroup Trial 9704 were recently presented.[15] This is a phase III study of 538 patients with resected pancreatic cancer randomized to either: 3 weeks of continuous infusional 5-FU at 250 mg/m$^2$/day, followed by chemoradiation (50.4 Gy in 1.8 Gy daily fractions with continuous infusional 5-FU at 250 mg/m$^2$/day), then two 4-week courses of continuous infusional 5-FU at 250 mg/m$^2$/d with 2 weeks' rest between courses to begin 3 to 5 weeks after completion of chemoradiation, or three weekly doses of gemcitabine at 1000 mg/m$^2$/week followed by the same 5-FU-based chemoradiation as in the first arm, followed by 3 months of gemcitabine 1000 mg/m$^2$ given weekly 3 out of every 4 weeks. Results showed a survival advantage in patients with resected pancreatic head carcinoma receiving maintenance gemcitabine versus maintenance 5-FU.

The 3-year overall survival rate of 187 patients with resected pancreatic head carcinoma receiving maintenance gemcitabine with chemoradiation was 32%. In contrast, the 3-year overall survival rate of 194 patients receiving maintenance 5-FU with chemoradiation was 21%. Trial results of this study compared to other prospective studies are summarized in Table 22-2.

## Single Institution Experiences

Reports of single-institution experiences with adjuvant therapy for pancreatic cancer have served to provide some additional evidence to the benefit of adjuvant therapy. The largest of these series is from the Johns Hopkins Medical Institutions, where investigators reported the results of a retrospective analysis of 174 patients who had chosen either: EBRT (40 Gy to 45 Gy) with two 3-day

TABLE 22-2  Summary Results: Phase III Studies of Postop CRT for Pancreatic Head
Adenocarcinoma

| | Survival | | |
|---|---|---|---|
| Study | Median (mos) | 3-Year | 5-Year |
| GITSG[9] | | | |
| 5-FU/CRT (n = 21) | 21 | 24 | 19 |
| EORTC[11] | | | |
| 5-FU/CRT (n = 60) | 17.1 | 30 | 20 |
| RTOG 9704[15] | | | |
| 5-FU/CRT (n = 221) | 16.9 | 21 | — |
| Gem/CRT (n = 221) | 20.6 | 32 | — |

GITSG included pts with "negative" margins only
EORTC included pts with T1/2 Disease Only & ~80% had negative margins
RTOG included ~75% pts with T3/4 Disease & only ~40% had negative margins

courses of 5-FU at the beginning and end of radiation, followed by weekly bolus 5-FU (500 mg/m$^2$) for 4 months (n = 99), 2) EBRT (50.4 Gy to 57.6 Gy) to the pancreatic bed plus prophylactic hepatic irradiation (23.4 Gy to 27 Gy) given with infusional 5-FU (200 mg/m$^2$/d) plus leucovorin (5 mg/m$^2$/day) for 5 out of 7 days of the week for 4 months (n = 21), or no therapy (n = 53).[16] Patients who received adjuvant chemoradiation had a median survival of 20 months compared to 14 months for patients who were not treated. Two-year survival was 44% and 30%, respectively. There was no survival advantage to the more intensive adjuvant therapy. A follow-up report from this group of 616 patients with resected pancreatic cancer found adjuvant chemoradiation treatment as a strong predictor of outcome, with a hazard ratio of 0.5.[17]

Data with the highest seen survival after adjuvant therapy for pancreatic cancer comes from a phase II trial done at Virginia Mason University. Results from 43 of 53 enrolled patients on this study were reported in 2003. These patients were treated with EBRT to 50 Gy with concurrent chemotherapy with 5-FU 200 mg/m$^2$/day continuous infusion, cisplatin 30 mg/m$^2$ weekly, and IFN-$\alpha$ 3 million units subcutaneously every other day. After completion of chemoradiation, patients received 5-FU 200 mg/m$^2$/day continuous infusion on weeks 10 through 15 and 18 through 23.[18] The median survival, 2-year overall survival, and 5-year overall survival were 44 months, 58%, and 45%, respectively. With these encouraging data came significant toxicity, with 70% of patients experiencing grade 3 CTC toxicities, and 42% of patients requiring hospitalization. The American College of Surgeons Oncology Group (ACOSOG) has opened a larger, multicenter, phase II trial of 100 patients to further investigate this regimen, but this study has subsequently closed for poor accrual.

## NEOADJUVANT THERAPY

Even after undergoing curative resection for pancreatic cancer, 80% to 85% of patients' disease will recur. In addition, positive margins or nodal disease increases this rate of recurrence to 90%.[19,20] The use of neoadjuvant chemoradiation offers another possible way to improve upon these figures for several reasons: 1) approximately 25% of patients do not receive adjuvant therapy in a timely manner after surgery or do not receive it at all,[17 21] 2) given the high recurrence rates after surgical resection, pancreatic cancer is likely a systemic disease at the time of diagnosis in 80%–85% of patients who appear to have resectable disease,[22,23] and with neoadjuvant therapy, 20%–40% of patients will be spared the morbidity of resection because their metastatic disease becomes clinically apparent,[24] 3) preoperative therapy could theoretically be less toxic and more effective as the chemotherapy and radiation would be given without the postsurgical issues of small bowel in the radiation field and decreased oxygenation and decreased drug delivery to the remaining tumor bed,[25] and 4) patients with local and unresectable lesions may be able to be downstaged to allow for surgical resection.

At M.D. Anderson Cancer Center, multiple trials of neoadjuvant 5-FU-based chemoradiation have been performed. The first trial treated 28 patients with 5-FU 300 mg/m$^2$/day continuous infusion with concurrent EBRT to 50.4 Gy over 5.5 week.[26] Patients who underwent surgical resection also received intraoperative radiation therapy. Twenty-five percent of patients had evidence of metastatic disease on preoperative restaging. Fifteen percent had metastatic disease that was found on laparoscopy. For the patients who underwent surgery median survival was 18 months, and 41% had a pathologic partial response to therapy. However, 33% of patients treated on this study required hospitalization for gastrointestinal toxicity from therapy. For this reason, the next trials from this group focused on rapid fractionation EBRT. A prospective trial of 35 patients treated with EBRT to 30 Gy (3 Gy per fraction for 10 fractions) with concurrent 5-FU 300 mg/m$^2$/day continuous infusion found grade 3 nausea and vomiting in only 9% of patients with no grade 4 toxicitie.[27] Twenty-seven patients were taken to surgery and 20 patients underwent resection and IORT to 10 Gy to 15 Gy. Locoregional recurrence occurred in only two for the 20 resected patients. Median survival for patient who underwent surgery was 25 months with a 3-year survival of 23%.

Phase I studies have attempted to build upon the radiosensitization effects and the improved efficacy in advanced pancreatic cancer of gemcitabine in the neoadjuvant setting. Gemcitabine has also been studied in combination with other chemotherapy agents and EBRT in the neoadjuvant setting. A phase I study of 19 patients with pancreatic cancer evaluated the MTD of cisplatin when given with gemcitabine at 1,000 mg/m$^2$ weekly with EBRT to 36 Gy given in 2.4 Gy fraction.[28] Cisplatin was given on days 1 and 15 following gemcitabine. The MTD of cisplatin was 40 mg/m$^2$. Another trial from the M.D. Anderson Cancer Center evaluated a treatment schedule of gemcitabine 750 mg/m$^2$ and cisplatin 30 mg/m$^2$ given every 14 days for four treatments, followed by four weekly doses of gemcitabine at 400 mg/m$^2$ concurrent with 30 Gy of EBRT given as three Gy fractions over 2 weeks, beginning 2 days after the first dose of gemcitabin.[29] Preliminary results from 37 patients showed 67% underwent resection, with 70% of the pathologic specimens showing necrosis of >50% of the tumor. This regimen, however, had significant toxicity, with 62% of patients requiring hospitalization, most due to biliary stent occlusion.

In radiobiologic models, paclitaxel may result in enhanced radiosensitization through synchronization of tumor cells at G2/M, a relatively radiosensitive phase of cell cycle and tumor reoxygenation after apoptotic clearance of paclitaxel-damaged cells. Pisters and colleagues from M.D. Anderson Cancer Center have examined the use of paclitaxel as a radiation sensitizer in the neoadjuvant setting for pancreatic cancer.[30] In this trial, 35 patients received paclitaxel 60 mg/m$^2$ weekly with concurrent EBRT to 30 Gy. Eighty percent underwent resection with 21% percent of pathology specimens showing >50% tumor necrosis. The 3-year survival for the patients who underwent preoperative therapy and resection was 28%. Hospitalization was required in 11% of patients for toxicity, primarily nausea and vomiting. These preliminary data show an increased toxicity without a significant improvement in histological response rate or survival.

## Locally Advanced Therapy

Patients with locally advanced carcinoma of the pancreas comprise a group of patients with an intermediate prognosis between resectable and metastatic patients. These patients have pancreatic tumors which are defined as surgically unresectable, but have no evidence of distant metastases. A tumor is considered to be unresectable if it has one of the following features: 1) extensive peripancreatic lymph node involvement and/or distant metastases (typically to the liver or peritoneum), 2) encasement or occlusion of the superior mesenteric vein (SMV) or SMV/portal vein confluence, or 3) direct involvement of the superior mesenteric artery (SMA), inferior vena cava, aorta, or celiac axis. However, recent advances in surgical technique may allow for resection of selected patients with tumors involving the SMV.[31] Combined treatment with radiation and chemotherapy increases median survival for patients with locally advanced cancers to approximately 9 to 13 months, but rarely results in long-term survival. The therapeutic options of patients with locally advanced pancreatic cancer include external beam radiation therapy (EBRT) with 5-FU chemotherapy, intra-operative radiation therapy (IORT), and more recently EBRT with novel chemotherapeutic and targeted agents. In evaluating the results of these various therapies, it is useful to remember that a median survival of 3 to 6 months has been reported for this subset of patients undergoing palliative gastric or biliary bypass only.[32]

## Prospective Trials

With the exception of one trial, conventional EBRT for locally advanced pancreatic cancer has been shown to improve survival when combined with 5-fluorouracil (5-FU) compared to EBRT alone or chemotherapy alone (See Table 22-3). The Mayo Clinic undertook an early randomized trial in the 1960s in which 64 patients with locally unresectable, nonmetastatic pancreatic adenocarcinoma received 35–40 Gy of EBRT with concurrent 5-FU versus the same EBRT schedule plus placebo. A

**TABLE 22-3  Prospective Randomized Trials for Locally Advanced, Unresectable Pancreatic Cancer**

| Series | # pts | Median Survival (months) | Local Failure | 1-year Survival | 18-month Survival |
|---|---|---|---|---|---|
| *Mayo Clinic*[33] | | | | | |
| EBRT (35–40 Gy/3–4 weeks) only | 32 | 6.3 | NS | 6% | 6% |
| EBRT (35–40 Gy/3–4 weeks) + 5-Flourouracil | 32 | 10.4 | NS | 22% | 13% |
| *GITSG*[34,65] | | | | | |
| EBRT (60 Gy/10 weeks) only | 25 | 5.3 | 24% | 10% | 5% |
| EBRT (40 Gy/6 weeks) + 5-Flourouracil | 83 | 8.4 | 26% | 35% | 20% |
| EBRT (60 Gy/10 weeks) + 5-Flourouracil | 86 | 11.4 | 27% | 46% | 20% |
| *GITSG*[35] | | | | | |
| EBRT (60 Gy/10 weeks) + 5-Flourouracil | 73 | 8.5 | 58% (first site) | 33% | 15% |
| EBRT (40 Gy/4 weeks) + doxorubicin | 70 | 7.6 | 51% (first site) | 27% | 17% |
| *GITSG*[36,66] | | | | | |
| EBRT (54 Gy/6 weeks) + 5-Flourouracil and SMF | 22 | 9.7 | 45% (first site) | 41% | 18% |
| SMF only | 21 | 7.4 | 48% (first site) | 19% | 0% |
| *ECOG*[37] | | | | | |
| EBRT (40 Gy/4 weeks) + 5-Flourouracil | 47 | 8.3 | 32% | 26% | 11% |
| 5-Flourouracil only | 44 | 8.2 | 32% | 32% | 21% |

significant survival advantage was seen for patients receiving EBRT with 5-FU versus EBRT only (10.4 months vs 6.3 months).[33]

GITSG followed with a similar study comparing EBRT alone to EBRT with concurrent and maintenance 5-FU. One hundred and ninety-four eligible patients with surgically confirmed unresectable and nonmetastatic pancreatic adenocarcinoma were randomized to receive 60 Gy of split course EBRT alone, 40 Gy of split course EBRT with two to three cycles of concurrent bolus 5-FU chemotherapy or 60 Gy split course EBRT using a similar chemotherapy regimen. Patients in the latter groups received maintenance 5-FU after EBRT completion. The EBRT alone arm was closed early as a result of an inferior survival rate. The 1-year survival rate in the two combined modality therapy arms was 38% and 36%, respectively, versus 11% in the EBRT alone arm.[34]

The second GITSG trial of this series randomized 157 eligible patients with unresectable disease to 60 Gy split course EBRT with concurrent and maintenance 5-FU from the previous trial or 40 Gy continuous course radiation with weekly concurrent doxorubicin chemotherapy, followed by maintenance doxorubicin and 5-FU. A significant increase in treatment related toxicity was seen in the doxorubicin arm. However, no survival difference was observed between the two groups (median survival 37 vs. 33 weeks).[35] No clinical benefit was seen in substituting adriamycin for 5-FU.

A follow-up GITSG trial compared chemotherapy alone to chemoradiation, again in surgically confirmed unresectable tumors. Forty-three patients were randomized to receive combination streptozocin, mitomycin-C and 5-FU (SMF) chemotherapy or 54 Gy of EBRT with two cycles of concurrent bolus 5-FU chemotherapy, followed by adjuvant SMF chemotherapy. The chemoradiation arm demonstrated a significant survival advantage over the chemotherapy alone arm (1 year survival 41% vs. 19%).[36]

In contrast to the results of the prior studies, the Eastern Cooperative Oncology Group (ECOG) reported no benefit to chemoradiation versus chemotherapy only. In this study, patients with unresectable, nonmetastatic pancreatic or gastric adenocarcinoma were randomized to receive either 5-FU chemotherapy alone or 40 Gy EBRT with concurrent bolus 5-FU week 1. Patients with locally recurrent disease as well as patients undergoing surgery with residual disease were eligible for this trial. In the ninety-one analyzable pancreatic patients, no survival difference was observed between the two groups (median survival 8.2 months vs. 8.3 months).[37]

## Continuous Infusional 5-Fluorouracil

The idea that continuous infusion 5-FU allows for increased cumulative drug dose to be given without a significant increase in toxicity and for a more protracted radiosensitization effect relative to bolus 5-FU has prompted its study in locally advanced pancreatic cancer. Other trials of other gastrointestinal sites have shown an increased survival using continuous infusion 5-FU.[38] Phase I and phase II trials have been performed in pancreatic cancer, showing that the use of infusional 5-FU is without excessive treatment-related toxicity and is effective.[39-41] A phase I trial from ECOG found the maximum tolerated dose (MTD) of continuous infusion 5-FU to be 250 mg/m$^2$/day with the dose-limiting toxicity being gastrointestinal. The progression-free survival at 1 year was 40% with a median survival of 11.9 months. The 2-year survival rate for this trial was 18%. Although no randomized trials have been published, combined radiation therapy with infusional 5-FU is now commonly used, and combinations of chemotherapy with infusional 5-FU and radiation therapy for locally advanced pancreatic cancer are under investigation.

In addition, capecitabine, an oral 5-FU analog, in combination with radiation therapy for the treatment of pancreatic cancer has been reported.[42] Dosing of capecitabine has been extrapolated from combined modality trials in rectal cancer to be about 1,600 mg/m$^2$/day divided BID during radiation treatment.[43] No randomized trials have been reported with this combination. Of note, the combination of capecitabine and gemcitabine has been shown to be likely more efficacious than gemcitabine alone for patients with metastatic pancreatic cancer. A randomized trial of 533 patients with advanced pancreatic cancer were treated with either single agent gemcitabine or gemcitabine plus capecitabine.[44,45] The patients who received gemcitabine plus capecitabine had a statistically significant increase in response rate (14.2% vs. 7.1%, p = 0.008) and a statistically significant improvement in hazard ratio for overall survival (HR 0.80, 95% CI 0.65, 0.98). The confidence intervals for median survival for the two arms overlapped, however, with median survival in the gemcitabine plus capecitabine arm being 7.4 months (95% CI 6.5, 8.5) and in the gemcitabine arm 6.0 months (95% CI 5.4, 7.1 months). Further study of capecitabine in combination with radiation therapy is warranted.

In summary, with the exception of one study, conventional EBRT combined with 5-FU chemotherapy has been shown to offer a modest survival benefit for patients with locally advanced unresectable pancreatic cancer compared to radiation alone or chemotherapy alone. The median survival duration and 2-year survival rate for EBRT plus 5-FU are approximately 10 months and 2%, respectively. Because of these results, EBRT with 5-FU based chemotherapy has become a frequently employed therapy for these patients.

## Intra-operative Radiation Therapy

Because of the poor local control and results achieved with conventional EBRT and chemotherapy, specialized radiation therapy techniques that increase the radiation dose to the tumor volume have been used to improve local tumor control without increasing normal tissue morbidity. These include iodine-125 implants and intra-operative radiation therapy (IORT) as a dose escalation technique in combination with external beam irradiation and chemotherapy. A lower incidence of local failure in most series and improved median survival in some have been reported with these techniques when compared with conventional external beam irradiation, but it is uncertain whether this is due to superior treatment or case selection.[46]

A recent study from investigators of the Massachusetts General Hospital reported the results of 150 patients treated with IORT and external beam irradiation and chemotherapy.[47] Although the study spanned nearly 25 years, it is relevant because it shows for the first time that long-term survival is possible for patients with unresectable pancreatic cancer. Even though the 3- and 5-year survival rates (7%, 4%) are modest, they are not markedly different than the results reported in contemporary trials of resected pancreatic cancer patients (20%, 10%) or patients undergoing palliative pancreaticoduodenectomy (6.3%, 1.6%), especially when taking into account those patients with smaller tumors. For 25 patients treated with a small diameter applicator (5 cm or 6 cm), the 2- and 3-year actuarial survival rates were 27% and 17%, respectively. Furthermore, this study shows that postoperative and late treatment related toxicity rates were acceptable. These study results support further investigation of selected patients with small, unresectable tumors via innovative protocols employing IORT.

## Newer Chemotherapeutic Agents

Because of the high incidence of hepatic and peritoneal metastases and poor results with standard chemoradiotherapy, current and future research efforts include evaluation of EBRT with newer systemic agents (gemcitabine and paclitaxel). Interest in these agents is based on both their systemic cytotoxic effects and their radiosensitizing properties. At present, numerous investigators are pursuing phase I and II studies combining EBRT with gemcitabine. Investigators from Wake Forest University and the University of North Carolina reported the results of a phase I trial of twice-weekly gemcitabine and 50.4 Gy of concurrent upper abdominal EBRT in 19 patients with unresectable/inoperable pancreatic adenocarcinoma. In this study, the maximum tolerated dose of gemcitabine was 40 mg/m$^2$. At this dose level, gemcitabine was well tolerated. Of eight patients with a minimum follow-up of 12 months, three remain alive, and one of the three has no evidence of disease progression.[48] Following this trial, the Cancer and Leukemia Group B (CALGB) began a phase II study of this regimen for locally advanced pancreatic cancer. Data from this trial show a median overall survival for 38 patients enrolled of 8.2 months.[49] Using an alternate dosing scheme, McGinn, et al investigated weekly full dose gemcitabine combined with radiation therapy at escalating doses in a phase I trial of 37 patients with locally advanced or incompletely resected pancreatic cancer.[50] These patients received two cycles of gemcitabine at 1,000 mg/m$^2$ on days 1, 8, and 15 of a 28-day cycle with concurrent EBRT during the first 3 weeks. An optimal dose of 36 Gy in 2.4 Gy fractions was determined and recommended for a phase II trial which has completed accrual.[51]

Gemcitabine has also been studied in combination with 5-FU and radiation. ECOG performed a phase I trial of continuous infusion 5-FU at 200 mg/m$^2$, weekly gemcitabine at 50–100 mg/m$^2$, and 59.4 Gy of EBRT.[52] The patients in this trial showed a significant amount of toxicity, the five out of seven patients experiencing dose-limiting toxicities of gastric or duodenal ulcers, thrombocytopenia, or Stevens-Johnson syndrome. Because of these toxicities, the authors concluded that the combination of gemcitabine, 5-FU, and EBRT was not appropriate. However, the Massachusetts General Hospital, Dana Farber Cancer Center, and Brigham and Women's Hospital conducted a phase I/II study of continuous infusion 5-FU with weekly gemcitabine and concurrent 50.4 Gy of EBRT for locally advanced pancreatic cancer. In this study the MTD of weekly gemcitabine was 200 mg/m$^2$ when given with continuous infusion 5-FU at 200 mg/m$^2$ and concurrent EBRT. In this study, 32 patients were treated (13 at the MTD), and the severe toxicities were limited to one patient experiencing a grade 3 gastrointestinal bleed. The reason behind this is thought to be the lower dose of EBRT given, smaller treatment fields, and the continuous infusion 5-FU was given 5 days out of the week instead of 7 (Fuchs, C. preliminary data). This dosage is now being used for investigation in a phase II, multicenter trial through CALGB.

In a phase I trial at Brown University evaluating paclitaxel and 50 Gy of EBRT for patients with unresectable pancreatic and gastric cancers, the maximum tolerated dose of weekly paclitaxel with conventional irradiation was 50 mg/m$^2$.[53] The response rate was 31% among 13 evaluable pancreatic cancer patients. In the Brown University phase II study employing 50 Gy of EBRT with 50 mg/m$^2$/week of paclitaxel, six (33%) of 18 evaluable pancreatic cancer patients had a partial response; stable disease was observed in seven patients (39%); only one patient (6%) had local tumor progression after completion of treatment; and four (22%) have developed distant metastases. These data have led to an RTOG phase II study evaluating paclitaxel with EBRT for patients with unresectable pancreatic cancer.[54] The median survival of 109 patients on this study was 11.2 months (95% CI 10.1, 12.3) with estimated 1- and 2-year survivals of 43% and 13%, respectively. External irradiation plus concurrent weekly paclitaxel was well tolerated when given with large-field radiotherapy. These data provided the basis for a Radiation Therapy Oncology Group trial using paclitaxel and irradiation combined with a second radiation sensitizer, gemcitabine, and a farnesyl transferase inhibitor.

## Chemoradiation Effects on Quality-of-Life

Despite the potential survival benefits for patients with locally advanced pancreatic cancer receiving radiation therapy and chemotherapy, these gains are modest. With rare exception, all patients will ultimately succumb to their disease. In spite of this, significant palliative benefit can be achieved by chemoradiation. Pain, anorexia, fatigue, and clinical wasting are relatively common symptoms, which significantly impact on the patient's quality-of-life. Although poorly documented in many studies, reports from larger series indicate complete pain relief can be obtained in as much as 50%–80% of patients.[55] Using EBRT alone with or without chemotherapy, approximately 35%–65% of patients will experience pain resolution as well as some improvement in wasting and obstructive symptoms.[35,56,57] Definite but less dramatic improvements in performance status and anorexic symptoms may be observed as well.[56,57] Because of the high rate of morality associated with this disease, quality-of-life should be one of the important endpoints for these patients.

## Radiation Techniques

For patients undergoing laparotomy, radio-opaque clips should be placed at the superior, inferior, lateral- and medial most aspects of the tumor. Titanium clips tend to produce less artifact on CT scanning. Just prior to simulation, it may be helpful to perform an intravenous pyelogram for the purpose of better visualizing the kidneys. The patient is placed in the supine position and straightened with arms out of the field. An initial set of anteroposterior and lateral films is obtained to localize the surgical clips (if present) and renal position. Oral contrast can then be administered to better visualize the duodenal C-loop in patients who have not undergone palliative gastrojejunostomy. Generally, a four field technique consisting of anteroposterior/posteroanterior (APPA) and parallel opposed lateral fields are used to treat. For pancreatic head lesions, the primary draining lymph nodes at risk are the pancreaticoduodenal, suprapancreatic, celiac, and porta hepatic nodes, and these should be covered. The superior field border is usually placed at mid/top of T11 to allow good coverage of the celiac axis and its nodes, which are usually located at T12-mid L1. The duodenum may be invaded by pancreatic head neoplasms, and therefore the lateral and inferior borders should be set to allow adequate margin on the C-loop and pancreaticoduodenal nodes. Medially, the left side of the vertebral body should be covered with margin to allow coverage of the superior mesenteric vein and artery (whose involvement is frequently the cause of unresectability), suprapancreatic (body) nodes and any intrapancreatic extension of disease. On the lateral fields, the posterior border is at least 1.5 cm behind the anterior vertebral body to allow adequate para-aortic nodal coverage (which are at high risk with posterior extension of the tumor); anteriorly, a 2-cm margin is given on gross disease. If a biliary stent has been placed to alleviate obstruction, its course should be included to cover the common bile duct and any tumor that may have tracked superiorly. For body and tail lesions, it may be necessary to increase the superior and left borders to allow adequate coverage of the primary tumor as well as lateral suprapancreatic, splenic artery, and splenic hilar nodes; however, this also increases the volume of the left kidney in the field, and reduction in the right kidney volume being treated is accomplished by not covering the entirety of the C-loop, as duodenal involvement by tumors in these locations is uncommon. As a rule, if more than one half of one kidney is being treated on the APPA fields, more than two thirds of the other kidney should be shielded, assuming normal renal function bilaterally. Even with this reduced border, adequate coverage of the pancreaticoduodenal and porta hepatic nodes can be obtained by careful block design. The treatment by lateral fields is usually limited to 15–18 Gy secondary to the volume of kidney and liver in the field, thereby weighting treatments more heavily to the APPA fields. The total dose administered is usually 45–54 Gy, often with a field reduction after 45 Gy to minimize the amount of small bowel and stomach being treated to higher dose. These are, of course, general guidelines, and field modifications may be necessary based on the CT and other preoperative imaging, operative findings, and operative clip placement. Normal organ tolerance should always be respected, with blocks designed accordingly.

Three-dimensional conformal radiation therapy is being integrated into the treatment of a variety of malignancies, including intra-abdominal tumors. This CT-based treatment allows implementation of "unconventional" beam orientations, permitting coverage of the target volume with reductions in irradiation of nontarget tissues compared to conventional techniques. For example, an important technical consideration in the radiation treatment of pancreatic cancer is minimizing kidney irradiation, given the marked radiosensitivity of this organ. By optimizing beam orientation and weighting, significant reductions in renal irradiation have been achieved relative to standard techniques without significantly increasing the dose to other surrounding organs.[58]

**FIGURE 22-1** AP and lateral digital radiograph reconstructions of treatment fields for patient with pancreatic head cancer.

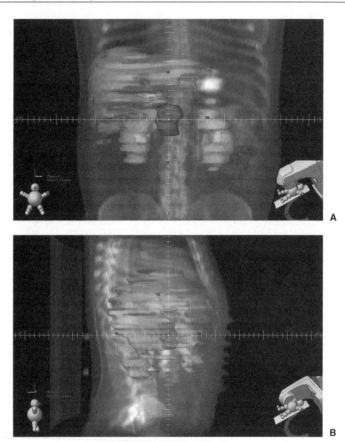

A

B

(See Color Plate 7).

Figure 22-1 demonstrates an example of a patient with an unresectable pancreatic head tumor treated using three-dimensional conformal therapy.

Further refinement of this approach is now being obtained by the use of intensity modulated radiation therapy. With this new technology, inverse treatment planning can be performed, permitting computer-based treatment optimization versus a standard "trial and error" planning approach. Secondly, a computer-controlled, nonuniform radiation treatment can be delivered to the target, permitting an even more precise and conformal dose pattern with further reductions in normal tissue irradiation. Evolution of these techniques will likely result in improved treatment tolerance and reduction of late morbidity. This is especially critical in this era of intensive chemoradiation protocols with their potential toxicity.

## Targeted Therapies/Future Directions

As the biological basis of cancer is better understood, the use of cancer specific targeted therapies are being increasingly investigated. There is preclinical evidence for either additive or synergistic effects for several of these approaches (such as antibodies against and VEGF and EGFR) with both chemotherapy and radiation therapy making these approaches especially promising. These targeted agents have been studied most extensively in the metastatic setting. Currently, the only targeted agent that has shown a statistically significant survival benefit in the metastatic setting compared to chemotherapy alone is erlotinib, an anti-EGFR tyrosine kinase inhibitor. However, the survival benefit is small, improving 1 year survival from 17% to 24%.[59] The median progression-free survival and overall survival benefits for the gemcitabine plus erlotinib arm versus the gemcitabine plus placebo arm also result in small benefits (3.75 vs. 3.55 mo p = 0.003 and 6.37 vs. 5.91 mo, p = 0.025 respectively). A phase I study of erlotinib, gemcitabine, and radiation therapy for patients with locally advanced pancreatic cancer has found an MTD of erlotinib 100 mg daily, gemcitabine 40 mg/m$^2$ biweekly, and EBRT to 50.4 Gy.[60] Of eight patients treated, seven have stable disease, and one patient was taken for R1 resection. Another phase I study has established an MTD for the combination of erlotinib, gemcitabine, paclitaxel, and radiation therapy for patients with locally advanced pancreatic cancer.[61] Another EGFR inhibitor, cetuximab, has had promising phase II results in the metastatic setting. The phase II study of the EGFR-inhibiting antibody cetuximab plus gemcitabine enrolled 41 patients with advanced pancreatic cancer. In this study, the response rate was 12%, with a median progression-free survival of 3.8 months and median overall survival of 7.1 months.[62] The phase III randomized study of gemcitabine plus cetuximab versus placebo (SWOG S0502) has recently completed accrual and results are eagerly awaited. Two small trials have reported preliminary results using cetuximab in combination with gemcitabine and radiation therapy for localized pancreatic cancer.[63,64] These studies have indicated that cetuximab can be given at full dose with chemotherapy and radiation therapy without significantly increased toxicity. Efficacy results are pending.

Preclinical data has shown that inhibition of VEGF has radiosensitizing effects. The Radiation Therapy Oncology Group is currently undertaking a phase II study combining bevacizumab, an anti-VEGF antibody with EBRT and capecitabine in the treatment of this group of patients. However, initially promising results in the metastatic setting have not shown benefit from the addition of an anti-VEGF antibody to chemotherapy. A phase II trial of the combination of gemcitabine and bevacizumab reported data from 52 treated patients with advanced pancreatic cancer. In this study, a response rate of 21% was found, with a median progression-free survival of 5.4 months and median overall survival of 8.8 months. The phase III randomized study of gemcitabine plus bevacizumab versus placebo (CALGB 80303), however, has finished accrual and was recently reported to show no benefit from the addition of bevacizumab to gemcitabine.

Pancreatic cancer remains one of the most formidable challenges in oncology. Newer imaging modalities have improved staging, thus facilitating treatment decisions. In the past 30 years, modest improvements in median survival have been attained for patients with locally advanced tumors treated by chemoradiation protocols. However, no significant impact on long-term survival has been accomplished. Local tumor control has been improved by the use of specialized radiation techniques permitting safe dose escalation. Even with these techniques, it is not clear that a survival benefit is achieved given the proclivity of metastases in this malignancy. Trials are underway testing newer systemic agents that also act as potent radiosensitizers.

Despite the recognized limitations of current therapy, palliation can be achieved for a high percentage of patients by combined modality treatment. Quality-of-life should be considered a paramount endpoint in the care and protocol design of these patients. In patients with marginal or poor performance status, gemcitabine administration alone represents a reasonable alternative to combined modality therapy. Significant improvements in long-term survival will likely be achieved through exploitation of the basic biologic anomalies of this malignancy.

## REFERENCES

1. Jemal A, Siegel R, et al. Cancer statistics, 2008. *CA Cancer J Clin* 2008:on line.
2. Geer RJ, Brennan MF. Prognostic indicators for survival after resection of pancreatic adenocarcinoma. *Am J Surg* 1993;165(1):68–72; discussion -3.
3. Lim JE, Chien MW, Earle CC. Prognostic factors following curative resection for pancreatic adenocarcinoma: a population-based, linked database analysis of 396 patients. *Ann Surg* 2003; 237(1):74–85.
4. Evans D, Abbruzzese J, Willett C. *Cancer of the Pancreas*. 6th ed. Philadephia: Lippincott, Williams, and Wilkins; 2001.
5. Tepper J, Nardi G, Sutt H. Carcinoma of the pancreas: review of MGH experience from 1963 to 1973. Analysis of surgical failure and implications for radiation therapy. *Cancer* 1976;37(3): 1519–1524.
6. Griffin JF, Smalley SR, Jewell W, et al. Patterns of failure after curative resection of pancreatic carcinoma. *Cancer* 1990;66(1):56–61.
7. Ozaki H. Improvement of pancreatic cancer treatment from the Japanese experience in the 1980s. *Int J Pancreatol* 1992;12(1):5–9.
8. Westerdahl J, Andren-Sandberg A, Ihse I. Recurrence of exocrine pancreatic cancer—local or hepatic? *Hepatogastroenterology* 1993;40(4):384–387.
9. Kalser MH, Ellenberg SS. Pancreatic cancer: adjuvant combined radiation and chemotherapy following curative resection. *Arch Surg* 1985;120(8):899–903.
10. Gastrointestinal Tumor Study Group. Further evidence of effective adjuvant combined radiation and chemotherapy following curative resection of pancreatic cancer. *Cancer* 1987;59(12): 2006–2010.
11. Klinkenbijl JH, Jeekel J, Sahmoud T, et al. Adjuvant radiotherapy and 5-fluorouracil after curative resection of cancer of the pancreas and periampullary region: phase III trial of the EORTC gastrointestinal tract cancer cooperative group. *Ann Surg* 1999;230(6):776–782; discussion 82–84.
12. Neoptolemos JP, Dunn JA, Stocken DD, et al. Adjuvant chemoradiotherapy and chemotherapy in resectable pancreatic cancer: a randomised controlled trial. *Lancet* 2001;358(9293):1576–1585.
13. Neoptolemos JP, Stocken DD, Friess H, et al. A randomized trial of chemoradiotherapy and chemotherapy after resection of pancreatic cancer. *N Engl J Med* 2004;350(12):1200–1210.
14. Neuhaus P, Oettle H, Post S, et al. A randomised, prospective, multicenter, phase III trial of adjuvant chemotherapy with gemcitabine vs. observation in patients with resected pancreatic cancer. In: *Proc Am Soc Clin Oncol* 2005.
15. Regine WF, Winter KW, RA, et al. RTOG 9704 a phase III study of adjuvant pre and post chemoradiation (CRT) 5-FU vs. gemciatbine (G) for resected pancreatic adencarcinoma. In: *Proc Am Soc Clin Oncol* 2006.
16. Yeo CJ, Abrams RA, Grochow LB, et al. Pancreaticoduodenectomy for pancreatic adenocarcinoma: postoperative adjuvant chemoradiation improves survival. A prospective, single-institution experience. *Ann Surg* 1997;225(5):621–633; discussion 33–36.
17. Sohn TA, Yeo CJ, Cameron JL, et al. Resected adenocarcinoma of the pancreas—616 patients: results, outcomes, and prognostic indicators. *J Gastrointest Surg* 2000;4(6):567–579.
18. Picozzi VJ, Kozarek RA, Traverso LW. Interferon-based adjuvant chemoradiation therapy after pancreaticoduodenectomy for pancreatic adenocarcinoma. *Am J Surg* 2003;185(5):476–480.
19. Willett CG, Lewandrowski K, Warshaw AL, Efird J, Compton CC. Resection margins in carcinoma of the head of the pancreas. Implications for radiation therapy. *Ann Surg* 1993;217(2):144–148.

0. Cameron JL, Crist DW, Sitzmann JV, et al. Factors influencing survival after pancreaticoduo-denectomy for pancreatic cancer. *Am J Surg* 1991;161(1):120–124; discussion 4-5.

1. Spitz FR, Abbruzzese JL, Lee JE, et al. Preoperative and postoperative chemoradiation strate-gies in patients treated with pancreaticoduodenectomy for adenocarcinoma of the pancreas. *J Clin Oncol* 1997;15(3):928–937.

2. Evans DB, Pisters PW, Lee JE, et al. Preoperative chemoradiation strategies for localized ade-nocarcinoma of the pancreas. *J Hepatobiliary Pancreat Surg* 1998;5(3):242–250.

3. Wayne JD, Abdalla EK, Wolff RA, Crane CH, Pisters PW, Evans DB. Localized adenocarcinoma of the pancreas: the rationale for preoperative chemoradiation. *Oncologist* 2002;7(1):34–45.

4. Raut CP, Evans DB, Crane CH, Pisters PW, Wolff RA. Neoadjuvant therapy for resectable pancre-atic cancer. *Surg Oncol Clin N Am* 2004;13(4):ix, 639–661.

5. White RR, Tyler DS. Neoadjuvant therapy for pancreatic cancer: the Duke experience. *Surg Oncol Clin N Am* 2004;13(4):ix–x, 675–684.

6. Evans DB, Rich TA, Byrd DR, et al. Preoperative chemoradiation and pancreaticoduodenectomy for adenocarcinoma of the pancreas. *Arch Surg* 1992;127(11):1335–1339.

7. Pisters PW, Abbruzzese JL, Janjan NA, et al. Rapid-fractionation preoperative chemoradiation, pancreaticoduodenectomy, and intra-operative radiation therapy for resectable pancreatic adenocarcinoma. *J Clin Oncol* 1998;16(12):3843–3850.

8. Muler JH, McGinn CJ, Normolle D, et al. Phase I trial using a time-to-event continual reassess-ment strategy for dose escalation of cisplatin combined with gemcitabine and radiation ther-apy in pancreatic cancer. *J Clin Oncol* 2004;22(2):238–243.

9. Wolff RA, Crane CH, Xiong HQ, et al. Preliminary analysis of preoperative systemic gemcitabine (GEM) and cisplatin (CIS) followed by GEM-based chemoradiation for resectable pancreatic adenocarcinoma. In: *Proc Am Soc Clin Oncol* 2004.

0. Pisters PW, Wolff RA, Janjan NA, et al. Preoperative paclitaxel and concurrent rapid-fractionation radiation for resectable pancreatic adenocarcinoma: toxicities, histologic response rates, and event-free outcome. *J Clin Oncol* 2002;20(10):2537–2544.

1. Leach SD, Lee JE, Charnsangavej C, et al. Survival following pancreaticoduodenectomy with resection of the superior mesenteric-portal vein confluence for adenocarcinoma of the pan-creatic head. *Br J Surg* 1998;85(5):611–617.

2. Gunderson LL, Haddock MG, Burch P, Nagorney D, Foo ML, Todoroki T. Future role of radio-therapy as a component of treatment in biliopancreatic cancers. *Ann Oncol* 1999;10 Suppl 4:291–295.

3. Moertel CG, Childs DS, Jr., Reitemeier RJ, Colby MY, Jr., Holbrook MA. Combined 5-fluorouracil and supervoltage radiation therapy of locally unresectable gastrointestinal cancer. *Lancet* 1969;2(7626):865–867.

4. Moertel CG, Frytak S, Hahn RG, et al. Therapy of locally unresectable pancreatic carcinoma: a randomized comparison of high-dose (6,000 rads) radiation alone, moderate dose radiation (4,000 rads + 5-fluorouracil), and high-dose radiation + 5-fluorouracil: The Gastrointestinal Tumor Study Group. *Cancer* 1981;48(8):1705–1710.

5. Gastrointestinal Tumor Study Group. Radiation therapy combined with Adriamycin™ or 5-fluorouracil for the treatment of locally unresectable pancreatic carcinoma. *Cancer* 1985;56(11):2563–2568.

6. Gastrointestinal Tumor Study Group. Treatment of locally unresectable carcinoma of the pan-creas: comparison of combined-modality therapy (chemotherapy plus radiotherapy) to chemotherapy alone. *J Natl Cancer Inst* 1988;80(10):751–755.

7. Klaassen DJ, MacIntyre JM, Catton GE, Engstrom PF, Moertel CG. Treatment of locally unre-sectable cancer of the stomach and pancreas: a randomized comparison of 5-fluorouracil alone

with radiation plus concurrent and maintenance 5-fluorouracil—an Eastern Cooperative Oncology Group study. *J Clin Oncol* 1985;3(3):373–378.

38. O'Connell MJ, Martenson JA, Wieand HS, et al. Improving adjuvant therapy for rectal cancer by combining protracted infusion fluorouracil with radiation therapy after curative surgery. *N Engl J Med* 1994;331(8):502–507.

39. Whittington R, Neuberg D, Tester WJ, Benson AB, 3rd, Haller DG. Protracted intravenous fluorouracil infusion with radiation therapy in the management of localized pancreaticobiliary carcinoma: a phase I Eastern Cooperative Oncology Group Trial. *J Clin Oncol* 1995;13(1):227–232.

40. Boz G, De Paoli A, Innocente R, et al. Radiotherapy and continuous infusion 5-fluorouracil in patients with nonresectable pancreatic carcinoma. *Int J Radiat Oncol Biol Phys* 2001; 51(3):736–40.

41. Osti MF, Costa AM, Bianciardi F, et al. Concomitant radiotherapy with protracted 5-fluorouracil infusion in locally advanced carcinoma of the pancreas: a phase II study. *Tumori* 2001; 87(6):398–401.

42. Ben-Josef E, Shields AF, Vaishampayan U, et al. Intensity-modulated radiotherapy (IMRT) and concurrent capecitabine for pancreatic cancer. *Int J Radiat Oncol Biol Phys* 2004;59(2):454–459.

43. Vaishampayan UN, Ben-Josef E, Philip PA, et al. A single-institution experience with concurrent capecitabine and radiation therapy in gastrointestinal malignancies. *Int J Radiat Oncol Biol Phys* 2002;53(3):675–679.

44. Cunningham D, Chau I, Stocken D, et al. GEM-CAP: Phase III randomised comparison of gemcitabine with gemcitabine plus capecitabine in patients with advanced pancreatic cancer. In: *ECCO* 2005.

45. Herrmann R, Bodoky G, Ruhstaller T, et al. Gemcitabine (GEM) plus capecitabine (CAP) versus GEM alone in locally advanced or metastatic pancreatic cancer. Aspects of quality-of-life in a randomized phase III study of the Swiss Group for Clinical Cancer Research (SAKK) and the Central European Coo. *European Journal of Cancer Supplements* 2005;3(2):203.

46. Roldan GE, Gunderson LL, Nagorney DM, et al. External beam versus intra-operative and external beam irradiation for locally advanced pancreatic cancer. *Cancer* 1988;61(6):1110–1116.

47. Willett CG, Del Castillo CF, Shih HA, et al. Long-term results of intra-operative electron beam irradiation (IOERT) for patients with unresectable pancreatic cancer. *Ann Surg* 2005; 241(2):295–299.

48. Blackstock AW, Bernard SA, Richards F, et al. Phase I trial of twice-weekly gemcitabine and concurrent radiation in patients with advanced pancreatic cancer. *J Clin Oncol* 1999;17(7): 2208–2212.

49. Blackstock AW, Tepper JE, Niedwiecki D, Hollis DR, Mayer RJ, Tempero MA. Cancer and leukemia group B (CALGB) 89805: phase II chemoradiation trial using gemcitabine in patients with locoregional adenocarcinoma of the pancreas. *Int J Gastrointest Cancer* 2003;34(2–3): 107–116.

50. McGinn CJ, Zalupski MM, Shureiqi I, et al. Phase I trial of radiation dose escalation with concurrent weekly full-dose gemcitabine in patients with advanced pancreatic cancer. *J Clin Oncol* 2001;19(22):4202–4208.

51. McGinn CJ, Talamonti MS, Small W, et al. A phase II trial of full-dose gemcitabine with concurrent radiation therapy in patients with resectable or unresectable nonmetastatic pancreatic cancer. In: *GI ASCO* 2004.

52. Talamonti MS, Catalano PJ, Vaughn DJ, et al. Eastern Cooperative Oncology Group Phase I trial of protracted venous infusion fluorouracil plus weekly gemcitabine with concurrent radiation therapy in patients with locally advanced pancreas cancer: a regimen with unexpected early toxicity. *J Clin Oncol* 2000;18(19):3384–3389.

53. Safran H, Akerman P, Cioffi W, et al. Paclitaxel and concurrent radiation therapy for locally advanced adenocarcinomas of the pancreas, stomach, and gastroesophageal junction. *Semin Radiat Oncol* 1999;9(2 Suppl 1):53–57.

54. Rich T, Harris J, Abrams R, et al. Phase II study of external irradiation and weekly paclitaxel for nonmetastatic, unresectable pancreatic cancer: RTOG-98-12. *Am J Clin Oncol* 2004;27(1): 51–56.

55. Termuhlen PM, Evans DB, Willett CG. *IORT in Pancreatic Cancer*. Totowa, NJ: Humana Press; 1999.

56. Haslam JB, Cavanaugh PJ, Stroup SL. Radiation therapy in the treatment of irresectable adenocarcinoma of the pancreas. *Cancer* 1973;32(6):1341–1345.

57. Dobelbower RR, Jr., Borgelt BB, Strubler KA, Kutcher GJ, Suntharalingam N. Precision radiotherapy for cancer of the pancreas: technique and results. *Int J Radiat Oncol Biol Phys* 1980; 6(9):1127–1133.

58. Steadham AM, Liu HH, Crane CH, Janjan NA, Rosen II. Optimization of beam orientations and weights for coplanar conformal beams in treating pancreatic cancer. *Med Dosim* 1999;24(4): 265–271.

59. Moore M, Goldstein D, Hamm J, et al. Erlotinib improves survival when added to gemcitabine in patients with advnaced pancreatic cancer. A phase III trial of the National Cancer Institute of Canada Clinical Trials Group [NCIC-CTG]. In: *ASCO Gastrointestinal Cancers Symposium* 2005.

60. Kortmansky J, O'Reilly E, Minsky B, et al. A phase I trial of erlotinib, gemcitabine, and radiation for patients with locally advanced, unresectable pancreatic cancer. In: *ASCO Gastrointestinal Cancers Symposium* 2005.

61. Iannitti D, Dipetrillo T, Barnett J, et al. Erlotinib and chemoradiation followed by maintenance erlotinib for locally advanced pancreatic cancer: a phase I study. In: *ASCO Gastrointestinal Cancers Symposium* 2005.

62. Xiong HQ, Rosenberg A, LoBuglio A, et al. Cetuximab, a monoclonal antibody targeting the epidermal growth factor receptor, in combination with gemcitabine for advanced pancreatic cancer: a multicenter phase II Trial. *J Clin Oncol* 2004;22(13):2610–2616.

63. Pipas JM, Zaki B, Suriawinata AA, et al. Cetuximab, intensity-modulated radiotherapy (IMRT) and twice-weekly gemcitbaine for pancreatic adenocarcinoma. In: *Proc Am Soc Clin Oncol* 2006.

64. Krempien RC, Munter MW, Timke C, et al. Phase II study evaluating trimodal therapy with cetuximab intensity-modulated radiotherapy (IMRT) and gemcitabine for patients with locally advanced pancreatic cancer (ISRCTN56652283). In: *Proc Am Soc Clin Oncol* 2006.

65. A multi-institutional comparative trial of radiation therapy alone and in combination with 5-fluorouracil for locally unresectable pancreatic carcinoma. The Gastrointestinal Tumor Study Group. *Ann Surg* 1979;189(2):205–208.

66. Phase II studies of drug combinations in advanced pancreatic carcinoma: fluorouracil plus doxorubicin plus mitomycin C and two regimens of streptozotocin plus mitomycin C plus fluorouracil. The Gastrointestinal Tumor Study Group. *J Clin Oncol* 1986;4(12):1794–1798.

# 23

# Gastric Cancer

*Sharad Goyal, MD*
*Salma K. Jabbour, MD*

## OVERVIEW

Gastric cancer, although uncommon in the United States, is a major cause of mortality worldwide. Surgical resection offers the only potential for cure in primary gastric cancer, with failures occurring both regionally and distantly. Although phase III data exist to support both preoperative chemotherapy and postoperative chemoradiotherapy, studies are ongoing to identify which therapies are most beneficial. The available literature for gastric cancer can be applied to gastroesophageal junction (GEJ) cancers; however, many centers group GEJ carcinomas into the management of esophageal cancers. As the etiology of GEJ carcinomas is commonly related to Barrett's esophagus, it is possible that a separate treatment paradigm will be defined for this subset in the future. This chapter does not specifically address GEJ carcinomas.

## INTRODUCTION

According to estimates from the American Cancer Society, approximately 21,500 cases of gastric cancer will be diagnosed in 2008 with approximately 10,880 deaths due to this disease.[1] While gastric cancer is the 15th deadliest cancer in the United States, it is the second leading cause of death worldwide, totaling almost 1 million deaths per year. Gastric cancer is most common in East Asia, and China accounts for up to 40% of the cases of gastric cancer each year. The anatomic location of gastric cancer is evolving; the incidence of proximal gastric cancers has increased by 4%–5% per year, which parallels the increase in distal esophageal cancers. Distal gastric cancers have continued to decrease in incidence, and are most commonly found in Asia.

## ANATOMY[2,3]

The stomach is a muscular organ between the gastroesophageal junction and the duodenum. The stomach can be divided into four major regions: cardia (where the contents of the esophagus empty into the proximal stomach), fundus (formed by the upper curvature of the stomach), corpus (main part of the body), and pylorus/antrum (the most distal part of the organ that facilitates emptying into the duodenum). Location is not thought to contribute to long-term outcomes because patients with comparably staged proximal and distal cancers have similar survival rates.[4]

The stomach wall consists of an inner layer compromised of epithelial and glandular cells, followed by submucosa, muscularis propria, subserosa, and the outermost serosal layer. The muscularis is composed of three layers: the innermost oblique mucosal layer, the middle circular muscle layer, and the outer longitudinal muscle layer. Due to the intimate nature of the stomach to other organs—the diaphragm and left lobe of the liver superiorly; pancreas, left adrenal gland and left kidney inferiorly; the spleen and splenic flexure laterally; the transverse colon, mesocolon, and greater omentum posteriorly; and the abdominal wall anteriorly, direct extension of cancers from the stomach to other organs can occur. For example, tumors originating from the greater curvature may directly involve the splenic hilum and tail of the pancreas, while more distal tumors may invade the transverse colon.

The gastric blood supply consists of multiple arteries that supply different portions of the organ. The right gastric artery, a branch of the common hepatic/proper hepatic artery, supplies the inferior portion of the stomach. The left gastric artery, a branch of the celiac trunk, supplies the cardia. The fundus and the upper portion of the greater curvature are supplied by the short gastric arteries, which branch from the splenic artery. The right gastroepiploic artery usually originates from the gastroduodenal artery, a branch of the common hepatic artery, and feeds the inferior portion of the stomach. The left gastroepiploic artery, which originates from the splenic artery, supplies the greater curvature. The venous supply of the stomach tends to follow the arterial supply.

The Japanese Research Society for the Study of Gastric Cancer (JRSSGC) has classified distinctive nodal groups based on their anatomic relationship to the stomach. These lymph node station designations are distinct from the AJCC staging which groups lymph nodes into N1, N2, and N3, correlating to the number of involved lymph nodes (Table 23-1).

## TABLE 23-1 JRSSGC Nodal Stations[3]

| | |
|---|---|
| N1 | Perigastric lymph nodes are located along the lesser and greater curvatures of the stomach and consist of the right pericardial, left pericardial, lesser curvature, greater curvature, suprapyloric, and infrapyloric lymph nodes |
| N2 | Lymph nodes found along the three branches of the celiac trunk: the left gastric artery, common hepatic artery, and splenic artery and include celiac and splenic hilum lymph nodes |
| N3 | Hepatoduodenal, peripancreatic, and root of the mesentery lymph nodes |
| N4 | Middle colic and para-aortic lymph nodes |

Because of the extensive nature of the nodal system, complete regional lymph node coverage with radiotherapy (RT) is challenging. When developing radiotherapy portals, knowledge of the location of the primary tumor, depth of invasion, and width of primary lesion will determine the risk of each nodal station's involvement (Table 23-2).

## TABLE 23-2 Nodal Stations at Risk[3]

| | |
|---|---|
| GE Junction or Proximal | High risk—mediastinal and pericardial<br>Low risk—gastric antrum, periduodenal, porta hepatis |
| Body | May involve any nodal sites. Usually involves nodes along the greater and lesser curvature of the stomach, closest to the primary lesion |
| Distal | May involve periduodenal, peripancreatic, porta hepatic nodes. Involvement of other nodal stations is less likely. |

Any tumor originating from the stomach has a high likelihood of spreading to nodes along the curvature of the stomach, closest to the primary lesion.

# PATHOLOGY[5,6]

Approximately 90% of gastric cancers are adenocarcinomas. Other histologies include lymphoma, sarcoma, carcinoid, small cell, squamous cell, and undifferentiated carcinoma. Gastric carcinoma can be categorized as an intestinal type or diffuse type (Table 23-3). Linitis plastica, also known as Brinton's disease, is seen in diffuse gastric cancer and has a "leather bottle" appearance. The gross pathologic description of gastric cancer, known as Borrmann's classification, is listed in Table 23-4. The discussion here will be limited to adenocarcinomas.

TABLE 23-3 Intestinal vs. Diffuse Type Gastric Cancers (Lauren Classification)

| Intestinal Type | Diffuse Type |
| --- | --- |
| Men >> women | Women >> men |
| Older population | Younger population |
| Distal | Cardia/proximal |
| Ulcerated | Infiltrative |
| Improved prognosis | Worse prognosis |
| Often preceded by precancerous lesion (intestinal metaplasia) | No association with pre-cancerous lesions |
| Dominant in epidemic areas/ environmental etiology | Endemic etiology |
| Well differentiated columnar type cells arising in areas of mucosal inflammation | Signet ring cells—poorly organized cells which are poorly differentiated and produce mucin |

TABLE 23-4 Borrmann's Classification of Gastric Cancer[3]

| | |
| --- | --- |
| Type I | Polypoid or fungating (least aggressive) |
| Type II | Ulcerating lesions surrounded by elevated borders |
| Type III | Ulcerating lesions with invasion of the gastric wall |
| Type IV | Diffusely infiltrating (linitis plastica) |
| Type V | Not classifiable (most aggressive) |

# RISK FACTORS[5,6]

- Helicobacter pylori infection
- Advanced age
- Male gender
- Cigarette smoking
- High salt intake, pickled vegetables, and smoked meats
- Diet low in fruits and vegetables
- Precursor pathologic conditions: chronic atrophic gastritis, pernicious anemia, gastric adenomatous polyps, intestinal metaplasia
- Barrett's Esophagus
- Hereditary diffuse gastric cancer—mutation in E-cadherin protein (CDH-1 gene) which causes diffuse-type gastric cancer in 25% of families with an autosomal dominance
- Previous gastric surgery with carcinoma occurring in the gastric stump
- Previous radiation therapy
- Menetrier's disease (giant hypertrophic gastritis)

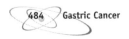

## SCREENING

Screening for gastric cancer in the United States has not yet been employed due to the low incidence of early gastric cancers which is less than 5% in most series.[7] Broad screening would not result in a decrease in mortality from gastric cancer in the U.S. population. Also there are no well defined high-risk populations where the risks of endoscopic screening (perforation, cardiopulmonary events, aspiration pneumonia, and bleeding) would outweigh the benefits of this procedure. However, in Japan, where there is a high incidence of gastric cancer, the use of screening increased the incidence of T1 lesions from 3.8% to 34.5% over a 10-year period and has significantly improved survival in these patients.[9] Confocal laser endomicroscopy (CLE) is a new endoscopic technique allowing for real-time sub-surface in vivo microscopic analysis during an endoscopy using systemically or topically administered fluorescent agents. CLE allows for targeted biopsies, potentially improving the diagnostic rate in certain diseases, including gastric cancer. More studies need to be performed to validate its utility in gastric cancer.

## PREVENTION[6]

Improvement in diet, food preservation, sanitation, cessation of smoking, and treatment of *H. pylori* will reduce the incidence of gastric cancer in certain populations. Gastric cancer has been shown to over express cyclooxygenase II (COX-2), and administration of COX-2 inhibitors has been shown to reduce the incidence of gastric cancer.[9] Future trials may incorporate COX-2 inhibitors to determine their role in chemo-prevention of gastric cancer. Early total gastrectomy is recommended in families with hereditary diffuse gastric cancer, in which a germline mutation in the E-cadherin (CDH-1) gene has been recognized.[6] Carriers of this mutation have a 70% lifetime risk of developing a gastric cancer. Pathologic analyses of prophylactic gastrectomy specimens have revealed microscopic intraepithelial neoplasia, even in patients who routinely underwent endoscopic examination with random biopsy.[10] Therefore, early total gastrectomy has been recommended for this population, and proximal and distal margins of resection must be evaluated closely since any remaining gastric mucosa can result in carcinoma.

## PRESENTATION/WORKUP[5,6]

- Symptoms—decreased appetite, abdominal discomfort, nausea, vomiting, weight loss, early satiety, hematemesis, or melena. Proximal lesions may cause dysphagia while tumors involving the pylorus may cause obstructive symptoms.
- Workup—complete history and physical exam (Table 23-5), CBC and chemistry panel with liver function tests, esophagogastroduodenoscopy with biopsy and endoscopic ultrasound, double-contrast upper GI series, colonoscopy, CT of chest, abdomen and pelvis, PET (limited role in evaluation of primary tumors, sensitive for metastatic disease), laparoscopy to rule out serosal or liver metastases if preoperative treatment is chosen.

TABLE 23-5 Classic Physical Exam Findings[3,6]

| | |
|---|---|
| Virchow's node | Nodal metastases found in the supraclavicular fossa |
| Irish's node | Nodal metastases found in the axilla |
| Sister Mary Joseph node | Nodal metastases found in the umbilical region |
| Krukenburg tumor | Palpable ovarian mass |
| Blumer's shelf | Palpable mass on rectal examination may indicate peritoneal implants to the pelvis |
| Malignant ascites | Indication of advanced disease |
| Hepatomegaly | May indicate extension of disease to the liver |

| TABLE 23-6  TNM Staging |
|---|
| T1 | Tumor invades lamina propria or submucosa |
| T2 | Tumor invades (a) muscularis propria or (b)subserosa |
| T3 | Tumor penetrates the serosa (visceral peritoneum) without invasion of adjacent structures |
| T4 | Tumor invades adjacent structures |
| N1 | Metastasis in 1–6 regional lymph nodes |
| N2 | Metastasis in 7–15 regional lymph nodes |
| N3 | Metastasis in > 15 regional lymph nodes |

| TABLE 23-7  Stage Grouping | |
|---|---|
| IA | T1 N0 M0 |
| IB | T1 N1 M0 |
|  | T2 N0 M0 |
| II | T1 N2 M0 |
|  | T2 N1 M0 |
|  | T3 N0 M0 |
| IIIA | T2 N2 M0 |
|  | T3 N1 M0 |
|  | T4 N0 M0 |
| IIIB | T3 N2 M0 |
| IV | T4 N1-3 M0 |
|  | Any N3 |
|  | Any M1 |

Used with the permission of the American Joint Committee on Cancer (AJCC), Chicago, Illinois. The original source for this material is the AJCC Cancer Staging Manual, Sixth Edition (2002) published by Springer-Verlag New York, www.springeronline.com.

## BIOLOGY[6]

The development of gastric cancer is affected by both environmental and genetic causes. Loss of tumor suppressor gene p53 predisposes cells to genetic instability and is associated with the development of malignancy. Aberrations of mismatch repair genes (hMSH3 and hMLH1) are implicated in the pathogenesis of gastric cancer; these mutations are found in hereditary nonpolyposis colorectal cancer (HNPCC) and lead to an increase in both colon and gastric cancer. Other pathways implicated in the development of gastric cancer are: 1) c-met, 2) K-sam, 3) erb-B2, 4) bcl-2, 5) telomerase activation, and 6) CD44 expression. While advances in molecular biology have enhanced our understanding of tumorgenesis, our knowledge in the realm of gastric cancer remains quite limited given the heterogeneity of its causes.

## MANAGEMENT

### Definitive Surgical Resection Alone[3]

Standard treatment for Tis, T1, or T2 N0 M0 patients is total surgical resection with a radical subtotal gastrectomy and reconstruction with gastrojejunostomy. A total gastrectomy does not provide additional locoregional control but does add significantly to morbidity and mortality. If the tumor is located in the distal stomach, a radical distal subtotal resection with removal of the first portion of the duodenum, omenta, and nodal tissue is warranted. If the tumor is proximal, attempts should be made to remove the tumor with at least 5-cm margin in an effort to preserve a portion of the stomach. If 5-cm margins are unable to be achieved, total gastrectomy should be considered.

The extent of necessary dissection is widely debated. The types of dissections can be classified based on the extent of lymph node dissection (Table 23-8). In Japan, D2 dissections are the standard of care, while in most other parts of the world, D1 dissections are employed. Two western trials randomized patients to either D1 or D2 resections, and showed no improvement in survival or locoregional control, but an increase in morbidity and mortality was apparent (Table 23-9).[11,12]

The benefit of treating Japanese patients with a D2 resection may be an effect of stage migration or tumor biology rather than surgical technique. Removal of at least 15 lymph nodes is

TABLE 23-8  **Types of Dissection[3] (see Table 23-1)**

| | |
|---|---|
| D0 dissection | No lymph node dissection |
| D1 dissection | Removal of the perigastric lymph nodes within 3 cm of the stomach |
| D2 dissection | D1 dissection contents |
| | Removal of perigastric nodes further than 3 cm of the stomach |
| | Removal of N2 lymph nodes |
| | Omentectomy |
| D3 dissection | D2 dissection |
| | Removal of N3 and N4 lymph nodes |

TABLE 23-9  **Surgical Dissection Series**

| Trial | Randomization | Complication Rate | Locoregional Recurrence Rate | 5-Year Overall Survival |
|---|---|---|---|---|
| Dutch[12] | D1 | 25% | 70% | 45% |
| | D2 | 43% | 65% | 47% |
| | | $p < 0.001$ | $p = NS$ | $p = NS$ |
| MRC[13] | D1 | — | 58% | 35% |
| | D2 | — | 45% | 33% |
| | | | $p = NS$ | $p = NS$ |

recommended by the NCCN guidelines. If the tumor is found to extend beyond the stomach, all attempts should be made to achieve negative margins.

## OVERVIEW

Five-year survival rates in patients with T1 and T2 N0 M0 tumors after complete surgical resection approach 90% and 50%–60%, respectively.[13] Patients with posterior T2 N0 M0 lesions may require adjuvant chemo-radiotherapy and should be evaluated appropriately. Patients not considered to be surgical candidates should receive combination chemo-radiotherapy consisting of 5FU concurrently with definitive external beam radiation therapy (RT) with or without maintenance chemotherapy.[14] If the patient is not able to tolerate chemotherapy, radiotherapy can be utilized as sole therapy. Patients with well-differentiated, pedunculated T1N0M0 lesions smaller than 3-cm that do not invade the submucosa may be treated with endoscopic mucosal resection (EMR). Identification of those patients who are considered to be candidates for EMR is an on-going area of research.

Patients with T3/T4 disease, node positivity, or gross residual disease after resection are at high risk of both locoregional recurrence and distant metastasis. Relapse rates in this population may be greater than 35% with the gastric bed, stump, anastomotic site, and lymph nodes at highest risk of local recurrence.[15] Furthermore, 5-year survival rates for T3 and T4 N0 M0 tumors range between 30%–50% and 5%–15%, respectively. In the node-positive population, the 5-year survival rates are 20% for N1 tumors, 10% for N2 tumors, and 0% for N3 tumors.[13] Given these findings, adjuvant therapy is recommended to improve locoregional control and survival in this patient population.

### Postoperative Therapy

There have been many studies investigating the role of adjuvant chemotherapy alone in gastric cancer but results are conflicting because of the heterogeneity of the disease, differences in surgical techniques, varying biology among distinct populations, and patient selection. Results from meta-analyses investigating the role of adjuvant chemotherapy alone after resection have been mixed, probably reflecting trial selection. One recent meta-analysis published found there to be an overall survival benefit with a reduction in relapse rate with the addition of adjuvant chemotherapy (Box 23-1).[16] Studies investigating adjuvant chemotherapy alone generally have not shown a survival benefit; however, results have differed between eastern and western trials due to a likely difference in the biology of the disease in different parts of the world.

---

**BOX 23-1   META-ANALYSIS OF ADJUVANT CHEMOTHERAPY**

This study included 23 trials with 4,919 patients (2,441 in the adjuvant chemotherapy arm and 2,478 in the observation arm) were analyzed. The survival rate for adjuvant chemotherapy was 60.6% and for observation was 53.4% with an RR of death of 0.85 (95% CI: 0.80–0.90). Of studies that reported recurrence rates, there was a reduction with adjuvant chemotherapy with an RR of 0.78 (95% CI: 0.71–0.86). They found that the number needed to treat was 14; hence, of every 14 patients treated, one would experience a survival benefit. Chemotherapy appeared to reduce the rate of metastases in the liver, peritoneum, lymph nodes, and locally.

Liu et al. An updated meta-analysis of adjuvant chemotherapy after curative resection for gastric cancer. *Eur J Surg Onc.* 2008, doi:10.1016/j.ejso.2008.02.002.

---

TABLE 23-10   **Surgery +/− Adjuvant Therapy**

| Trial | Randomization | Adjuvant Therapy | No. of Patients | 5-Year Survival (%) | Locoregional Recurrence Rate (%) |
|---|---|---|---|---|---|
| Neri et al[17] | 1) Surgery alone | — | 69 | 13 | p = NR |
| | 2) Surgery − > Chemo | Epirubicin/5-FU/ Leucovorin | 68 | 30 | |
| EORTC[18] | 1) Surgery alone | — | 159 | 36 mo | 30% local 45% distant |
| | 2) Surgery − > FAM | Modified 5-FU, Adriamycin, Mitomycin-C | 155 | 42 mo (MS) p = 0.295 | 21% local 37% distant p = NR |
| British Stomach Group[19] | 1) Surgery alone | — | 145 | 20 | 27 |
| | 2) Surgery − > FAM | 5-FU, Adriamycin, Mitomycin-C | 138 | 19 | 19 |
| | 3) Surgery − > RT | 45 Gy in 25 fractions +/− 5 Gy boost | 153 | 12 | 10 |
| Mayo Clinic[20] | 1) Surgery alone | — | 23 | 4 | 54 |
| | 2) Surgery − > RT + 5 FU | 37.5 Gy in 24 fractions + 5-FU 15mg/kg D1-3 | 39 | 23 | 39 |

One of the first prospective, randomized trials investigating combined-modality therapy in the postoperative setting was conducted at the Mayo Clinic.[20] Sixty-two patients with completely resected gastric cancer with poor prognosis were randomized to observation or RT (37.5 Gy in 24 fractions) concurrent with 5-FU (15mg/kg/d1–3 IV bolus). Patients receiving combined-modality therapy had a 5-year overall survival rate of 20% (as compared to 12% with observation, p = NS) and a reduction in locoregional recurrences (54% in observed patients vs. 39% with adjuvant treatment, p = NS). The benefit of adjuvant combined-modality therapy was then investigated in a large Intergroup trial (INT 0116).[21]

---

**BOX 23-2   INT 0116: POSTOPERATIVE CHEMO-RT VS. OBSERVATION**

Patients (n = 566) with Stage IB-IVM0 disease who underwent R0 resection of adenocarcinoma of the stomach (80%) or GEJ (20%) were randomly assigned to surgery plus postoperative chemo-RT or surgery alone. Of note, 70% of patients had T3/T4 disease and 85% were node positive. Adjuvant treatment consisted of induction 5-FU (425 mg/m$^2$ × 5 days) and leucovorin (20 mg/m$^2$/day × 5 days) followed by chemo-RT beginning 28 days after the initial cycle of chemotherapy. RT consisted of 45 Gy in 1.8 Gy per fraction concurrent with 5-FU (400 mg/m$^2$ × 5 days) and leucovorin (20mg/m$^2$/day on the first 4 days and last 3 days of RT). One month after completion of chemo-RT, two additional cycles of 5-FU and leucovorin were given one month apart, as used in the induction portion.

Overall, 54% of patients underwent a D0 resection, 36% underwent a D1 resection, and 10% of patients underwent a D2 resection. In addition, all patients underwent an R0 resection and were enrolled post-operatively; thus, the patients were selected on the basis of being fit for surgery. Also, this trial consisted of a group of mainly high-risk patients who would have benefited from additional therapy. It is also notable that radiation quality assurance was performed during the induction chemotherapy; the incidence of major/minor deviations was reduced from 35% to 6.5% before the start of RT.

Chemo-RT increased median survival to 36 months from 27 months with surgery alone (p < 0.005). Three-year relapse-free survival was improved from 31% to 48% with Chemo-RT and 3-year overall survival was improved from 41% to 50% with Chemo-RT (p < 0.001).

---

Macdonald et al. Chemo-radiotherapy after surgery compared with surgery alone for adenocarinoma of the stomach or gastroesophageal junction. N Engl J Med. 2001 Sep 6;345(10):725–730.

---

## Preoperative Therapy

Chemotherapy or RT prior to surgical resection is a paradigm that is under investigation in gastric carcinoma, and its use is extrapolated from gastrointestinal sites such as esophageal and rectal cancer. Neo-adjuvant therapy has the potential to downstage patients, possibly increasing the chances of an R0 resection. It selects patients who progress on therapy who should not receive definitive resection and delivers systemic therapy to treat micrometastatic disease earlier in the treatment course. Results using single modality RT or chemotherapy from limited trials are encouraging.

---

**BOX 23-3   PREOPERATIVE RADIOTHERAPY**

Patients (n = 370) with mostly Stage III and IV gastric adenocarcinoma were randomized to surgery alone or pre-operative RT (40Gy in 2Gy/fraction, AP-PA beams using MV beams prescribed to a partial-stomach field without regional lymph nodes) followed by surgical resection.

*(continues)*

**BOX 23-3** (CONTINUED)

Preoperative RT allowed for improved radical resection rates (80% vs. 62% with surgery alone, down-staging of disease (RT increased T2's by 8.4%, reduced T4's by 11%, and reduced nodal positivity by 20%).

The 5 and 10 year survival rates were 30% vs. 20% and 20% vs. 13% for preoperative RT vs. surgery alone (p = 0.009). Preoperative RT reduced local relapses to 39% (vs. 52% with surgery alone, p < 0.025) and distant relapses to 39% (vs. 54% with surgery alone, p < 0.005). Notably, this study is focused on a single homogenous population. Results of this study, conducted in Asia, warrants further investigation in a Western population.

Zhang et al. Randomized clinical trial on the combination of preoperative irradiation and surgery in the treatment of adenocarcinoma of gastric cardia (AGC). Report on 370 patients. *Int J Rad Onc Biol Phys.* 1998 Dec 1;42(5):929–934.

**BOX 23-4** **MAGIC TRIAL: PREOPERATIVE CHEMOTHERAPY VS. OBSERVATION**

The UK MRC conducted a phase III trial in patients with resectable Stage II-IV M0 carcinoma of the stomach (74%), GEJ (11.5%), and esophagus (14.5%). Patients (n = 503) were randomized to either surgery alone (n = 250) or chemotherapy (n = 253) consisting of three preoperative and three postoperative cycles every 3 weeks of IV epirubicin (50mg/m$^2$) and cisplatin (60mg/m$^2$) on day 1 and continuous infusion 5-FU (200 mg/m$^2$/d) for 21 days. D2 resections were performed in 40% of patients.

With a median follow-up of 4 years, there was an improvement in overall survival at 5 years (36% vs. 23%, p < 0.009) and progression-free survival with a HR of 0.66 with ECF; (95% CI: 0.53–0.81) with chemotherapy. There was no difference in rates of postoperative complications. Tumors were found to be significantly smaller and a higher proportion of downstaged tumors were found in the chemotherapy arm at the time of surgery. This study included non-gastric primaries and the pathologic complete response (pCR) rate of pCR were not reported.

Cunningham et al. Perioperative chemotherapy versus surgery alone for respectable gastroesophageal cancer. *N Engl J Med.* 2006 Jul 6;355(1):11–20.

**BOX 23-5** **PREOPERATIVE CHEMO-RT VS. OBSERVATION**

Patients (n = 113) with locally advanced adenocarcinoma of the esophagus (65%) or gastric cardia (35%) were randomized to surgery alone or neo-adjuvant chemotherapy consisting of continuous infusion 5-FU (15 mg/kg/d) on days 1–6 and cisplatin (75 mg/m$^2$) on day 7 for two cycles repeated every 6 weeks. Concurrent RT was begun on the 1st day of the 1st course of chemotherapy and consisted of 40 Gy over 15 fractions (267cGy/fraction) followed by definitive surgical resection.

There was no difference in operative morbidity or mortality with the addition of neo-adjuvant Chemo-RT. Of the patients who received neoadjuvant Chemo-RT, 25% had a pCR and a majority of the patients were downstaged. The 3-year survival rate was 37% for Chemo-RT and 7% for surgery alone (p < 0.001).

Walsh et al. A comparison of multimodality therapy and surgery for esophageal adenocarcinoma. *N Engl J Med.* 1996 Aug 15; 335(7):462–467.

Neo-adjuvant chemo-radiotherapy is another area of active clinical research. Advantages of this strategy are: 1) improved tumor oxygenation preoperatively; 2) potentially smaller RT field sizes and lower doses; 3) chemotherapy will act as a radiosensitizer and enhance locoregional control; and 4) sterilization of the tumor bed to reduce chance of intra-operative seeding.

Wydmanski et al reported a phase II study investigating various 5-FU regimens concurrent with RT prior to definitive surgical resection.[22] Radiotherapy details included treatment of the entire stomach and regional lymph nodes to 45 Gy in 25 fractions. A pathologic complete response (pCR) rate of 20% was achieved with 94% of patients undergoing an R0 resection. The RTOG has investigated neoadjuvant Chemo-RT (Box 23-6) in the phase II setting.[23]

---

**BOX 23-6  RTOG 9904: PREOPERATIVE CHEMO-RT**

Patients (n = 49) with locally advanced adenocarcinoma of the stomach or GE junction (any N+, T2–3N0 M0) were enrolled. A negative laparoscopic evaluation was required. Patients received 2 cycles of induction chemotherapy consisting of cisplatin ($20 mg/m^2/d$) on days 1–5 and continuous infusion 5-FU ($200 mg/m^2/d$) on days 1–21 every 28 days. Chemo-RT was started $\geq 28$ days after day 1 of the last induction chemotherapy cycle. Continuous infusion 5-FU ($300 mg/m^2/d$ M–F for 5 weeks) and paclitaxel ($45 mg/m^2$ on each Monday x 5 weeks) were given concurrent with 45 Gy RT. Radiotherapy portals included the entire stomach, regional lymph nodes, and margin. For lesions involving the cardia or GEJ, a 5cm margin of esophagus was included; for distal lesions near the gastroduodenal junction, a 5cm margin of duodenum was included. Patients then underwent definitive surgical resection.

Progression occurred in 17% of patients who then did not undergo surgery. Of the patients who underwent surgery, 77% of patients underwent an R0 resection, 50% had D2 dissection, 26% had a pCR. There were no treatment related deaths.

Ajani et al. Phase II trial of preoperative chemoradiation in patients with localized gastric adenocarcinoma (RTOG 9904): quality of combined-modality therapy and pathologic response. *Journal of Clinical Oncology.* 2006 Aug 20;24:3953–3958.

---

The available phase II data investigating neo-adjuvant chemo-RT demonstrate the safety and tolerability of these regimens without any additional adverse effects while achieving pathologic complete rates of 20%, a rate similar to that of other GI malignancies treated with neo-adjuvant regimens. Furthermore, neo-adjuvant chemo-radiotherapy allows patients to undergo improved surgical resection while treating micrometastatic disease earlier in their course of treatment.

### Unresectable Disease

Patients with unresectable gastric cancer are candidates for concurrent chemo-RT, which has shown to be advantageous over RT alone (Box 23-7). Nevertheless, adenocarcinoma of the stomach is fairly radioresponsive. Short-course or palliative radiotherapy (30 Gy in 10 fractions or 37.5 Gy in 15 fractions) is effective in treating symptoms such as obstruction or hematemesis.

Maintenance chemotherapy should also be utilized for unresectable disease. A randomized trial comparing supportive care and a modified FAMTx (5-FU, doxorubicin, and methotrexate) regimen was stopped early after a significant benefit in median survival (3 months vs. 10 months, p = 0.001) was found.[26] Another randomized trial comparing a FEMTx (5-FU, epirubicin, and methotrexate) regimen also found an improvement in median survival over supportive care alone (12 months vs. 3 months, p = 0.0006).[27]

**BOX 23-7  DEFINITIVE CHEMO-RT**

A study performed at the Mayo Clinic, randomized 48 patients with locally advanced, unresectable gastric cancer were to RT alone (35–37.5 Gy in 4–5 weeks) or chemotherapy (5-FU 15mg/kg D1–3) concurrent with RT. They report an improvement in median survival (13 vs. 6mo) and overall survival at 5 years (12% vs. 0%) with combined-modality therapy over radiotherapy alone.[24]

The GITSG conducted a randomized trial where patients with T4 or node positive disease with gross residual disease were randomized to:

1. Split course RT (25 Gy, 2 weeks off, 25Gy) + 5-FU followed by maintenance MeCCNU +5-FU
2. 5-FU and Methyl-CCNU (MeCCNU) alone

and found an improvement in overall survival at 4 years (18% vs. 7%, p < 0.05) with combined-modality therapy.[25]

Moertel et al. Combined 5-fluorouracil and supervoltage radiation therapy of locally unresectable gastrointestinal cancer. *Lancet.* 1969;2:865–867.

Le Chevalier et al. Chemotherapy and combined-modality therapy for locally advanced and metastatic gastric carcinoma. *Semin Oncol.* 1985;12:46–53.

## Radiotherapy Technique[6]

Prior to simulation, the pertinent medical record including pathology, preoperative and postoperative radiologic images, procedure and operative reports, and full medical history should be reviewed since this information will impact treatment volumes and field design. This information is particularly important when considering use of unconventional field arrangements or to help spare organs at risk. Precise target volumes must be delineated to avoid possible under-dosing of target volumes. Patients should be advised not to consume food or beverage for 3 hours prior to simulation to avoid falsely enlarging the stomach. This routine should be continued during the course of radiotherapy to ensure the reproducibility of organs so that the desired dose distributions may be achieved. At the time of simulation, oral and/or IV contrast should be used to help elucidate the anatomy within the thorax and abdomen. In addition, an immobilization device is recommended to ensure reproducibility of daily setup. The patient should be simulated in the supine position with their arms above their head on a wing board. CT simulation is the preferred modality of simulation to accurately determine doses to normal critical structures and target volumes. Please reference Tables 23-11, 23-12, and 23-13 for specific radiation treatment volumes based on the location of the primary tumor.

Target volumes typically include gross tumor, nodal regions at risk of involvement, and structures at risk of involvement based on the location of the primary lesion. In the postoperative setting, the inclusion of the tumor bed, anastomotic sites, the gastric stump, clips, regional lymph nodes at risk (see Tables) and residual disease is of importance. Particular attention should be given to include as much of the stomach as possible for all postoperative patients, node-positive patients, or other select patients. Any gross disease, the tumor bed, or regional nodes should be encompassed with at least a 1.5–2-cm margin to account for the clinical and planning target volume.

After an R0 resection, 45 Gy in 1.8 Gy per fraction is acceptable. In R1, R2 or unresected patients, doses of 50.4–54 Gy in 1.8 Gy per fraction may be considered if dose to critical organs is within the proper constraints; in these situations a cone-down after the initial 45 Gy should be performed to limit the additional dose to gross disease with 2-cm margin. Doses up to 54 Gy in unresected patients may be used and higher doses to smaller volumes must be used with caution since

TABLE 23-11 **Impact of Site of Primary Lesion and TN Stage on Radiotherapy Treatment Volumes: Cardia/Proximal Third of Stomach**

| Site of Primary and TN Stage | Remaining Stomach | Tumor Bed Volumes$^{\diamond\diamond}$ | Nodal Volumes |
|---|---|---|---|
| Cardia/prox third of stomach* | Preferred, but spare $^2/_3$ one kidney (usually right) | T stage dependent | N stage dependent |
| T2N0, invasion of subserosa | Variable, dependent on surgical pathologic findings$^{\diamond}$ | Medial left hemidiaphragm, adjacent body of pancreas ($\pm$ tail) | None or perigastric[◆] |
| T3 N0 | Variable, dependent on surgical pathologic findings$^{\diamond}$ | Medial left hemidiaphragm, adjacent body of pancreas ($\pm$ tail) | None or perigastric; optional: periesophageal, mediastinal, celiac[◆] |
| T4 N0 | Variable, dependent on surgical pathologic findings$^{\diamond}$ | As for T3N0 plus sites of adherence with 3–5-cm margin | Nodes related to sites of adherence $\pm$ perigastric, periesophageal, mediastinal, celiac |
| T1–2 N+ | Preferable | Not indicated for T1, as above for T2 into subserosa | Perigastric, celiac, splenic, suprapancreatic, $\pm$ periesophageal, mediastinal, pancreaticoduodenal, porta hepatis[◆◆] |
| T3–4 N+ | Preferable | As for T3N0, T4N0 | As for T1–2 N+ and T4 N0 |

*Tolerance organs or structures: kidneys, spinal cord, liver, heart, lung
$^{\diamond}$For tumors with >5-cm margins confirmed pathologically, treatment of residual stomach is not necessary, especially if this would resu[ ] in substantial increase in normal tissue morbidity.
$^{\diamond\diamond}$Use pre-operative imaging (CT, barium swallow), surgical clips, and post-operative imaging (CT, barium swallow).
[◆]Optional node inclusion for T2–3 N0 lesions if adequate surgical node dissection (D2) and at least 10–15 nodes are examined pathologica[ ]
[◆◆]Pancreaticoduodenal and porta hepatic nodes are at low risk if nodal positivity is minimal (1–2 positive nodes with 10–15 examined and this region does not need to be irradiated. Periesophageal and mediastinal nodes are at risk if there is esophageal extension.
From Gunderson LL & Tepper JE (eds): Clinical Radiation Oncology, 2nd ed. Philadelphia, Churchill Livingstone Elsevier, 2007.

they increase acute and late effects. A typical field size is $15 \times 15$cm, and postoperative fields ten[ ] to be larger than preoperative fields.

Multi-leaf collimators or physical blocks should be utilized to appropriately shield the critica[ ] organs in the field, including the spinal cord, small intestines, kidneys, liver, and heart. Eve[ ] with properly shaped fields, parts of both kidneys will receive radiation. With accurate target vol[ ] ume and field definition, doses of 45–50.4 Gy have been shown to have less than a 5% severe tox[ ] icity rate. General guidelines regarding DVH constraints for critical structures are as follows: les[ ] than 60% of the liver should receive more than 30 Gy; at least $^2/_3$ to $^3/_4$ of one kidney should b[ ] completely shielded, no more than 30% of the heart should receive more than 40 Gy; the max[ ] mum spinal cord dose is 45 Gy, maximum small bowel dose is 50 Gy. Typically, high-energy mega[ ] voltage beams are used to reduce dose to superficially located structures. AP-PA anterior[ ]

TABLE 23-12 **Impact of Site of Primary Lesion and TN Stage on Radiotherapy Treatment Volumes: Body/Middle Third of Stomach**

| Site of Primary and TN Stage | Remaining Stomach | Tumor Bed Volumes◇◇ | Nodal Volumes |
|---|---|---|---|
| Body/mid third of stomach* | Yes, but spare $2/3$ of one kidney | T stage dependent | N stage dependent, spare $2/3$ of one kidney |
| T2N0, invasion of subserosa, especially posterior wall | Yes | Body of pancreas (± tail) | None or perigastric Optional: celiac, splenic, suprapancreatic, pancreaticoduodenal, porta hepatis◆ |
| T3 N0 | Yes | Body of pancreas (± tail) | None or perigastric Optional: celiac, splenic, suprapancreatic, pancreaticoduodenal, porta hepatis◆ |
| T4 N0 | Yes | As for T3N0 plus sites of adherence with 3–5-cm margin | Nodes related to sites of adherence ± perigastric, suprapancreatic, splenic, pancreaticoduodenal, celiac, porta hepatis |
| T1–2 N+ | Yes | Not indicated for T1 | Perigastric, celiac, splenic, suprapancreatic, pancreaticoduodenal, porta hepatis |
| T3–4 N+ | Yes | As for T3N0, T4N0 | As for T1–2 N+ and T4 N0 |

*Tolerance organs or structures: kidneys, spinal cord, liver.
◇◇Use preoperative imaging (CT, barium swallow), surgical clips, and postoperative imaging (CT, barium swallow).
◆Optional node inclusion for T2–3 N0 lesions if adequate surgical node dissection (D2) and at least 10–15 nodes are examined pathologically
From Gunderson LL & Tepper JE (eds): Clinical Radiation Oncology, 2nd ed. Philadelphia, Churchill Livingstone Elsevier, 2007.

weighted (3:2) fields will reduce dose to the spinal cord. A 4-field box plan can improve dose homogeneity while reducing dose to the spinal cord and small bowel. 3D-CRT and IMRT may be warranted in certain situations. In these cases, image-guidance techniques should be used to ensure accuracy.

# MORBIDITY[5,6]

Common acute and late side effects are listed in Table 23-13:

RT should not begin until patients have fully recovered from surgery. In INT 0116, a nutritional requirement of 1500 kcal/day by oral or enterostomal alimentation was required prior to initiation of

TABLE 23-13 **Common Acute Side Effects**

Reduced blood counts
Fatigue, weight loss
Nausea, vomiting, diarrhea
Dyspepsia, gastric ulceration, abdominal cramping
Radiation dermatitis

treatment. During therapy, patients should be monitored closely for their nutritional status; weight and blood counts should be checked at least weekly. Aggressive fluid management, prophylactic anti-nausea medications, and other symptomatic management should be utilized to prevent an inpatient admission or cessation of treatment. The patients who receive pre- or postoperative chemotherapy or radiotherapy or those patients who receive definitive chemo-RT may require nutritional assistance in the form of hyperalimentation, feeding tube

**TABLE 23-14 Possible Late Side Effects**

Permanent changes in bowel habits
Small bowel obstruction
Hepatic dysfunction
Reduced renal function
Spinal cord dysfunction

**TABLE 23-15 Impact of Site of Primary Lesion and TN Stage on Radiotherapy Treatment Volumes: Antrum/Pylorus/Distal Third of Stomach**

| Site of Primary and TN Stage | Remaining Stomach | Tumor Bed Volumes$^{\diamond\diamond}$ | Nodal Volumes |
|---|---|---|---|
| Antrum/distal third of stomach* | Yes, but spare $^2/_3$ one kidney (usually left) | T stage dependent | N stage dependent |
| T2N0, invasion of subserosa | Variable, dependent on surgical pathologic findings$^{\diamond}$ | Head of pancreas ($\pm$ body), 1st and 2nd part of duodenum | None or perigastric Optional: porta hepatis, pancreaticoduodenal, celiac, suprapancreatic$^{\blacklozenge}$ |
| T3 N0 | Variable, dependent on surgical pathologic findings$^{\diamond}$ | Head of pancreas ($\pm$ body), 1st and 2nd part of duodenum | None or perigastric Optional: porta hepatis, pancreaticoduodenal, celiac, suprapancreatic$^{\blacklozenge}$ |
| T4 N0 | Preferable, dependent on surgical pathologic findings$^{\diamond}$ | As for T3N0 plus sites of adherence with 3–5-cm margin | Nodes related to sites of adherence $\pm$ perigastric, pancreaticoduodenal, porta hepatis, celiac, suprapancreatic |
| T1–2 N1+ | Preferable | Not indicated for T1 | Perigastric, celiac, pancreaticoduodenal porta hepatis, suprapancreatic |
| T3–4 N1+ | Preferable | As for T3N0, T4N0 | Optional: splenic hilum As for T1–2 N1 and T4 N0 |

*Tolerance organs or structures: kidneys, spinal cord, liver.
$^{\diamond}$For tumors with >5-cm margins confirmed pathologically, treatment of residual stomach is not necessary, especially if this would result in substantial increase in normal tissue morbidity.
$^{\diamond\diamond}$Use preoperative imaging (CT, barium swallow), surgical clips, and postoperative imaging (CT, barium swallow).
$^{\blacklozenge}$Optional node inclusion for T2–3 N0 lesions if adequate surgical node dissection (D2) and at least 10–15 nodes are examined pathologically.
From Gunderson LL & Tepper JE (eds): Clinical Radiation Oncology, 2nd ed. Philadelphia, Churchill Livingstone Elsevier, 2007.

---

**FIGURE 23-1** | AP field.

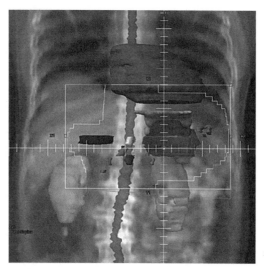

A

Postoperative radiation fields for a T3N0 poorly differentiated proximal gastric adenocarcinoma with lymphovascular invasion. The patient underwent subtotal gastrectomy, Billroth II procedure, and Roux-en-Y limb. The patient was treated adjuvantly per INT 0016. RT was delivered using a 4-field box technique prescribed to the isocenter. The AP field is shown. The field was designed to treat the Left Medial Hemidiaphragm, Surgical Clips, Porta Hepatis, Anastomotic Site, Residual Stomach, Celiac Axis (AP midline), and Superior Mesenteric Artery (AP midline). Ninety percent of the Right Kidney and 60% of the Left Kidney were able to be spared.

---

placement, or stent placement at some point during their course of treatment. Involvement of a nutritionist prior to starting treatment is optimal.

However, since the definitive treatment of gastric cancer usually involves partial or total resection of the stomach, many of these patients experience lifelong side effects from this procedure. Maintenance of adequate nutrition during and after therapy is a major problem for these patients. Patients often have early satiety and weight loss postoperatively, and management of these problems with a feeding tube should be addressed early on. Adjuvant treatment should not start until after the weight loss has stabilized. Patients also develop early dumping syndrome, reactive hypoglycemia, and nutritional deficiencies (B12, calcium, and iron) in the postoperative setting.

## FOLLOW-UP[5,6]

Patients are typically seen frequently during the acute recovery period of RT, and at 3 to 6 month intervals after completion of therapy for the first 2 to 3 years following treatment and then annually thereafter. Follow-up should consist of problem pertinent history and physical exam at each encounter. Yearly radiologic imaging and semi-annual endoscopic exams are reasonable. Blood work, including CBC and chemistries, should be performed if clinically indicated. The nutritional status of the patients should be monitored closely, including iron, calcium, and B12 levels in proximal or total gastrectomy patients. Involvement of a nutritionist is usually necessary for these patients.

## FUTURE DIRECTIONS

An Intergroup trial was activated in 2003 comparing adjuvant epirubicin, cisplatin and 5-FU (MAGIC regimen) and RT versus adjuvant 5-FU leucovorin and RT (INT 0116 regimen). This trial aims to show that an intensified chemotherapy regimen will reduce distant metastases. New approaches to therapy including targeted agents such as anti-angiogenesis inhibitors and growth factor receptor inhibitors in combination with present treatment options may also prove to be beneficial to these patients.

## REFERENCES

1. American Cancer Society: Colorectal Cancer Facts and Figures 2008. http://www.cancer.org/docroot/STT/STT_0.asp.
2. Cameron JL. *Current Surgical Therapy* (ed 8th). Philadelphia, Elsevier Mosby, 2004.
3. Yeo C. *Shackelford's Surgery of the Alimentary Tract*. Philadelphia, W.B. Saunders Company, 2007.
4. Clark GW, Smyrk TC, Burdiles P, et al. Is Barrett's metaplasia the source of adenocarcinomas of the cardia? *Arch Surg* 129:609–614, 1994.
5. Devita V, Hellman S, Rosenberg SA. *Cancer: Principles and Practice of Oncology* (ed 7th) Philadelphia, *Lippincott Williams & Wilkins,* 2005.
6. Gunderson L TJ, eds. *Clinical Radiation Oncology.* Philadelphia, Churchill Livingstone, 2007.
7. Abeloff MD, Armitage JO, Niederhuber JE, et al. *Clinical Oncology* (ed 3rd). Philadelphia, Elsevier Churchill Livingstone, 2004.
8. Prolla JC, Kobayashi S, Kirsner JB. Gastric cancer: some recent improvements in diagnosis based upon the Japanese experience. *Arch Intern Med* 124:238–246, 1969.
9. Nardone G, Rocco A. Chemoprevention of gastric cancer: role of COX-2 inhibitors and other agents. *Dig Dis* 22:320–326, 2004.
10. Chun YS, Lindor NM, Smyrk TC, et al. Germline E-cadherin gene mutations: is prophylactic total gastrectomy indicated? *Cancer* 92:181–187, 2001.
11. Bonenkamp JJ, Hermans J, Sasako M, et al. Extended lymph node dissection for gastric cancer. *N Engl J Med* 340:908–914, 1999.
12. Cuschieri A, Weeden S, Fielding J, et al. Patient survival after D1 and D2 resections for gastric cancer: long-term results of the MRC randomized surgical trial. Surgical Co-operative Group. *Br J Cancer* 79:1522–1530, 1999.
13. Noguchi Y, Imada T, Matsumoto A, et al. Radical surgery for gastric cancer: a review of the Japanese experience. *Cancer* 64:2053–2062, 1989.
14. Schein PS, Smith FP, Woolley PV, et al. Current management of advanced and locally unresectable gastric carcinoma. *Cancer* 50:2590–2596, 1982.
15. Landry J, Tepper JE, Wood WC, et al. Patterns of failure following curative resection of gastric carcinoma. *Int J Radiat Oncol Biol Phys* 19:1357–1362, 1990.
16. Liu TS, Wang Y, Chen SY, et al. An updated meta-analysis of adjuvant chemotherapy after curative resection for gastric cancer. *European Journal of Surgical Oncology,* 2008.
17. Neri B, Cini G, Andreoli F, et al. Randomised trial of adjuvant chemotherapy versus control after curative resection for gastric cancer: 5-year follow-up. *Br J Cancer* 84:878–880, 2001.
18. Lise M, Nitti D, Marchet A, et al. Final results of a phase III clinical trial of adjuvant chemotherapy with the modified fluorouracil, doxorubicin, and mitomycin regimen in resectable gastric cancer. *J Clin Oncol* 13:2757–2763, 1995.
19. Allum WH, Hallissey MT, Ward LC, et al. A controlled, prospective, randomised trial of adjuvant chemotherapy or radiotherapy in resectable gastric cancer: interim report. British Stomach Cancer Group. *Br J Cancer.* 1989 Nov; 60(5):739–744.

0. Moertel CG, Childs DS, O'Fallon JR, et al. Combined 5-fluorouracil and radiation therapy as a surgical adjuvant for poor prognosis gastric carcinoma. *J Clin Oncol* 2:1249–1254, 1984.

1. Macdonald JS, Smalley SR, Benedetti J, et al. Chemo-radiotherapy after surgery compared with surgery alone for adenocarcinoma of the stomach or gastroesophageal junction. *N Engl J Med* 345:725–730, 2001.

2. Wydmanski J, Suwinski R, Poltorak S, et al. The tolerance and efficacy of preoperative chemo-radiotherapy followed by gastrectomy in operable gastric cancer, a phase II study. *Radiother Oncol* 82:132–136, 2007.

3. Ajani JA, Winter K, Okawara GS, et al. Phase II trial of preoperative chemoradiation in patients with localized gastric adenocarcinoma (RTOG 9904): quality of combined-modality therapy and pathologic response. *J Clin Oncol* 24:3953–3958, 2006.

4. Moertel CG, Childs DS, Jr., Reitemeier RJ, et al. Combined 5-fluorouracil and supervoltage radiation therapy of locally unresectable gastrointestinal cancer. *Lancet* 2:865–867, 1969.

5. Le Chevalier T, Smith FP, Harter WK, et al. Chemotherapy and combined-modality therapy for locally advanced and metastatic gastric carcinoma. *Semin Oncol* 12:46–53, 1985.

6. Murad AM, Santiago FF, Petroianu A, et al. Modified therapy with 5-fluorouracil, doxorubicin, and methotrexate in advanced gastric cancer. *Cancer* 72:37–41, 1993.

7. Pyrhonen S, Kuitunen T, Nyandoto P, et al. Randomised comparison of fluorouracil, epidoxorubicin, and methotrexate (FEMTX) plus supportive care with supportive care alone in patients with non-resectable gastric cancer. *Br J Cancer* 71:587–591, 1995.

# 24

# Colorectal Cancer

Janet K. Horton, MD
Joel E. Tepper, MD

## OVERVIEW

Colorectal cancer is a major cause of morbidity and mortality in the United States. Advances in surgical technique, chemotherapeutics, and radiotherapy delivery have improved outcomes and are discussed in this chapter.

## INTRODUCTION

Approximately 153,760 people were diagnosed with colon and rectal cancer and approximately 52,810 died of these diseases in 2007 according to American Cancer Society (ACS) estimates. Colorectal cancer is the third most common cancer in the United States and the third leading cause of cancer death in both men and women.[1]

## ANATOMY

The colorectum consists of the cecum, ascending colon, hepatic flexure, transverse colon, splenic flexure, descending colon, sigmoid colon, and rectum. Variability in the peritoneal investment, bowel mobility, and lymph node drainage of the colon and rectum presents unique therapeutic issues.

The posterior surfaces of the ascending and descending colon are often in direct contact with the retroperitoneum while the anterior and lateral surfaces are draped with peritoneum. These posterior attachments can prevent significant mobility, increasing the difficulty of surgical resection. In contrast, the transverse colon is completely surrounded with peritoneum and supported on a long mesentery. The sigmoid colon is also completely intraperitoneal but the peritoneal covering begins to fall away as the sigmoid colon distally becomes the rectum. The rectum, approximately 12 cm in length, extends from the rectosigmoid junction to the puborectalis ring. The upper third of the rectum is draped with peritoneum anteriorly and on both sides. As the middle third of the rectum moves deeper into the pelvis, only the anterior surface is covered with peritoneum which forms the posterior border of the recto-uterine pouch or rectovesical space. The lowest third of the rectum is devoid of peritoneal covering and is in close proximity to adjacent structures including the bony pelvis. Distal rectal tumors have no serosal barrier to invasion of adjacent structures and are more difficult to resect given the close confines of the deep pelvis.[2]

Colonic nodal drainage consists of pericolic nodes and nodes in association with the vascular supply to the colon, mesenteric nodes. Because of the mobile and extensive nature of the colonic mesentery, complete regional lymph node coverage with radiotherapy (RT) is challenging but is usually well treated surgically. In contrast, the major regional groups for rectal nodal drainage can be covered within a reasonable RT field and include: perirectal, presacral, and internal iliac nodes.[2]

## PATHOLOGY

Adenocarcinomas constitute 85% of colorectal cancers (CRC). Other malignancies occurring in the colorectum include lymphoma, melanoma, carcinoid, small cell, and sarcoma.[3,4] The discussion which follows will be limited to adenocarcinomas.

## RISK FACTORS[4]

- Female:male 1:1
- Age—median seventh decade
- High-fat, low-residue diet
- Hereditary nonpolyposis colorectal cancer (HNPCC)—3%–5% of CRC, mutation in DNA mismatch repair gene with subsequent microsatellite instability
- Ulcerative colitis
- Familial adenomatous polyposis (FAP)—mutation in adenomatous polyposis coli (APC) gene, autosomal dominant

## SCREENING[3]

Because of the known progression from adenomatous polyps to frank malignancy over an extended period of time, colonoscopy is able to prevent the development of cancers by removal of polyps. Regular fecal occult blood tests have been demonstrated to decrease colorectal cancer mortality. The frequency/type of screening is determined by the risk level as follows:

- Average (70%–80% of the population)—asymptomatic, 50 years or older, no personal or familial history of colorectal, ovarian, or uterine cancer
- Moderate (15%–20%)—asymptomatic, personal history of polyps, colorectal cancer, ovarian or uterine cancer, family history (first degree relative <60 or two first degree relatives of any age) of adenomatous polyps or colorectal cancer, previous abdominal or pelvic radiation therapy
- High (5%–10%)—personal history of inflammatory bowel disease, family history of FAP or HNPCC

Based on the assigned risk group, the following tables present an adaptation of the screening approach recommended by the ACS in each of these populations.

---

TABLE 24-1 **Average Risk**[5]

At age 50, patients should initiate one of the following screening methods:

- Annual fecal occult blood test (FOBT) or fecal immunohistochemical test (FIT)
- Flexible sigmoidoscopy (FSIG) every 5 years
- Both FOBT or FIT and FSIG (combination preferred to single modality)
- Double-contrast barium enema (DCBE) every 5 years
- Colonoscopy every 10 years

### TABLE 24-2 Moderate Risk

| Risk | Initial Screening | Interval |
|------|-------------------|----------|
| Personal history of <1 cm adenomatous polyp | Colonoscopy | Repeat colonoscopy or DCBE (total colon evaluation—TCE) within 3 years, if negative follow average risk recommendations |
| Personal history of >1 cm polyp or multiple polyps | Colonoscopy | Repeat TCE within 3 years, if negative repeat every 5 years |
| Personal history of CRC treated with curative intent | TCE within 1 year of resection and perioperative TCE | If normal—TCE in 3 years, if normal at 3 years—TCE every 5 |
| Personal history of ovarian or uterine cancer | TCE within 1 year of diagnosis | TCE every 5 years |
| Family history (see risk categories) | TCE at 40 or 10 years earlier than age of earliest family diagnosis | TCE every 5 years |

### TABLE 24-3 High Risk

| Risk | Initial Screening | Interval |
|------|-------------------|----------|
| Personal history of inflammatory bowel disease | Pancolitis—8 years after initial diagnosis<br>L sided colitis—12–15 years after diagnosis—biopsy dysplasia | Repeat every 1–2 years—many believe that a patient with active colitis for >20 years should undergo colectomy |
| Family history of FAP | Puberty—endoscopic surveillance, genetic testing/counseling, specialist referral | If polyposis confirmed or testing positive consider colectomy; otherwise endoscopy every 1–2 years |
| Family history of HNPCC | At 21—colonoscopy, genetic testing/counseling | Colonoscopy every 2 years until 40 and then annually for patients not tested or + on genetic testing |

### BOX 24-1

These companion studies randomized patients to placebo versus aspirin in order to determine the effectiveness of aspirin as a chemoprevention agent.

Baron randomized 1,121 patients with a history of adenomas to placebo, 81 mg of aspirin or 325 mg of aspirin. At follow-up colonoscopy, the incidence of adenomas in the placebo group was 47%, 38% in the 81 mg aspirin group, and 45% in the 325 mg group (global $p = .04$).

*(continues)*

> **BOX 24-1** (CONTINUED)
>
> Sandler randomized 635 patients with a history of colorectal cancer to placebo versus 325 mg of daily aspirin. Subsequent colonoscopy revealed adenomas in 17% of the patients taking aspirin and 27% in the placebo group (p = .004).
>
> ---
>
> Baron JA et al. A Randomized trial of aspirin to prevent colorectal adenomas. *N Engl J Med.* 2003 Mar 6; 348(10): 891–899.
>
> Sandler RS et al. A Randomized trial of aspirin to prevent colorectal adenomas in patients with previous colorectal cancer. *N Engl J Med.* 2003 Mar 6; 348(10): 883–890.

## PREVENTION

In addition to colonoscopy, multiple agents have been explored as chemoprevention strategies. The most in-depth and successful work has been done with aspirin.

The preceding data suggest a potentially significant role for aspirin in the prevention of CRC. This simple treatment that much of the population already takes for cardiovascular prevention may also provide a significant benefit in decreasing rates of colorectal cancer. Other NSAIDs have also been shown to have a protective effect on polyp development, and to produce regression of pre-existing polyps.

Other potential prevention agents being evaluated are listed here.

---

**TABLE 24-4** Chemoprevention Agents Under Investigation

Curcumin
Folic acid
Mono- and dihydroxy vitamin $D_3$
Selenium
Ursodeoxycholic acid
Calcium

---

## PRESENTATION/WORKUP

- Symptoms—bleeding, change in bowel frequency, change in bowel character, pain, signs of blood loss, systemic symptoms
- Workup—complete history and physical, biopsy, colonoscopy, endorectal ultrasound or MR imaging to assess local extent of rectal disease, carcinoembryonic antigen (CEA)/ liver function tests, CXR or chest CT, CT abdomen/pelvis, PET—limited role in evaluation of primary tumors, sensitive for metastatic disease

## STAGING

An important change in the current American Joint Committee on Cancer (AJCC) staging system was the addition of substages to Stages II and III to reflect the differential patterns of survival and relapse within each stage. For patients with Stage III disease, invasion of the bowel wall and the extent of nodal involvement have been found to be independent prognosticators.

## BIOLOGY

Adenomatous polyps have been linked in a causal manner to the development of CRC. The presence of polyps puts an individual at increased risk for CRC, and removal of the polyps greatly reduces the risk of cancer. Multiple genetic alterations have been implicated in malignant transformation over

TABLE 24-5  **TNM Staging**

| 1 | Tumor invades submucosa |
|---|---|
| 2 | Tumor invades muscularis propria |
| 3 | Tumor invades subserosa, or nonperitonealized pericolic or perirectal tissue |
| 4 | Tumor invades other organs or structures, and/or perforates visceral peritoneum |
| 1 | 1–3 regional lymph nodes involved |
| 2 | 4 or more regional lymph nodes involved |

...ed with the permission of the American Joint Committee on Cancer (AJCC), Chicago, Illinois. The original source for this material is the *AJCC Cancer Staging Manual*, Sixth Edition (2002) published by Springer-Verlag, New York, www.springeronline.com.

...any years (United States Preventive ...ervices Task Force estimates 10–14 ...ears). There are five major pathways that ...re often implicated in the development ...f colorectal cancer and these tend to ...ccur at various stages of tumor develop-...ent, including: 1) APC/β-catenin, 2) K-...as/B-raf, 3) Smad4/TGF-βRII, 4) ...IK3CA/PTEN, and 5) p53/Bax. In addi-...on to specific mutations, the epigenetic ...nvironment has been linked to cancer ...ormation via aberrant methylation of ...umor suppressor genes. While great ...rides have been made in this area, our ...nderstanding of carcinogenesis remains quite limited.[3]

TABLE 24-6  **TNM Stage Grouping**

| I | T1-2 N0 M0 |
|---|---|
| IIA | T3 N0 M0 |
| IIB | T4 N0 M0 |
| IIIA | T1-2 N1 M0 |
| IIIB | T3-T4 N1 M0 |
| IIIC | Any T N2 M0 |
| IV | Any T Any N M1 |

Used with the permission of the American Joint Committee on Cancer (AJCC), Chicago, Illinois. The original source for this material is the *AJCC Cancer Staging Manual*, Sixth Edition (2002) published by Springer-Verlag, New York, www.springeronline.com.

Although the current staging system is based heavily on anatomic parameters, the biologic fac-...ors mentioned above are likely to play an increasing role in the way patients are grouped and subse-...uently treated. An innumerable number of predictive and prognostic factors have been and are ...urrently being evaluated.[6] Much work remains to be done before these markers can be used alone or ...n combination to assign patients to risk categories.

## MANAGEMENT

### Colon

...urgical resection is the mainstay of therapy for early-stage colon cancers. Surgery alone produces ...igh rates of 5-year survival (85%–95%) in most patients with Stage I carcinoma of the colon.[7]

BOX 24-2

Data from five randomized adjuvant rectal trials (3,791 patients) were pooled to determine the sur-vival and relapse rates according to T and N stage. The authors determined that in N0, N1, and even in N2 patients, the T stage of the tumor remained prognostically important (NT stage). Similar find-ings were noted for TN stage. These data strongly support the utility of substaging, as in the current AJCC staging system, which may ultimately guide better selection of patients for adjuvant therapy.

Gunderson LL et al. Impact of T and N stage and treatment on survival and relapse in adjuvant rectal cancer: a pooled analysis. *J Clin Oncol.* 2004 May 15; 22(10): 1785–1796.

Small tumors can be marked with India ink at the time of preoperative colonoscopy to ensure resec tion of the proper portion of bowel. The involved bowel is then taken with approximately a 10 c margin on either side, the exact margin related to the vascular supply. The associated region blood supply is resected at its origin which entails removal of a significant section of mesentery an associated nodal groups.[3]

For tumors with greater bowel wall penetration, Stage II, the 5-year survival rates with surger alone decrease to approximately 65%–70% and adjuvant therapy is sometimes indicated. Patient with Stage III tumors have only a 35%–50% cure rate with surgery alone and adjuvant chemother apy is almost always a component of definitive therapy.[7]

Adjuvant fluorouracil-based chemotherapy in colon cancer was established by Moertel et al, i the landmark trial demonstrating an absolute overall survival improvement of 16% for patient with advanced colon cancer at presentation.[8] Since that time, multiple studies using varying dru schedules established 6 months of fluorouracil (FU)/leucovorin (LV) as the standard in adjuvar treatment for high-risk colon cancer. More recently, oxaliplatin has been shown to have significar activity in metastatic colon cancer. In 2004, a randomized trial was reported that tested oxaliplati in the adjuvant setting.

---

**BOX 24-3**

Patients with Stage II or III colon cancer were eligible following complete resection. A group of 2,246 patients was randomized to adjuvant FU/LV versus FU/LV/oxaliplatin. The addition of oxali- platin was well tolerated and increased the disease-free survival rate at 3 years to 78% from 73% (p = .002) with FU/LV only.

Andre T et al. Oxaliplatin, fluorouracil, and leucovorin as adjuvant treatment for colon cancer. *N Engl J Med.* 2004 June 3; 350(23): 2343–2351.

---

These data helped to establish FU/LV/oxaliplatin as the new standard chemotherapeutic regi men in the adjuvant treatment of completely resected, high-risk colon cancer.

Radiotherapy has played a relatively limited role in colon cancer treatment given the high cu rates obtained with surgical resection alone in early-stage disease, the low risk of local failure and the benefit of adjuvant chemotherapy in advanced stages. However, several clinical scenar ios evaluated in nonrandomized institutional series may derive benefit from the addition c radiotherapy. Willett et al demonstrated favorable local control and recurrence-free survival rate in patients with locally advanced tumors (extending beyond the bowel wall into adjacent struc tures) treated with radiotherapy as compared to historical controls treated with surgical resectio alone. In addition, he noted that some patients with residual disease after resection could be sal vaged with radiotherapy.[9]

Taylor, et al, at the Mayo Clinic, demonstrated similar results in 27 patients with locally ad vanced tumors treated with postoperative radiotherapy.[10] A subsequent trial at the Massachusett General Hospital (MGH) evaluated 152 patients with T4 or residual disease treated with postopera tive radiotherapy with or without FU based chemotherapy. Seventy-nine patients treate for T4N0 or T4N+ (one lymph node positive) had a 10-year local control rate of 88% and recurrence-free survival of 58%. For the 42 patients with incomplete resections, the 10-yea recurrence-free survival was 19%.[11] These institutional data support a role for RT in those patient at high risk for local recurrence after surgical resection, and those with residual disease or invasio into surrounding structures. It is possible that this decrease in local recurrence would translat into a small survival benefit. Intergroup trial 0130 was designed to answer this question by comparing adjuvant radiation therapy in high-risk colon cancer patients to no radiation therapy.

---

**BOX 24-4**

This study evaluated the benefit of adding adjuvant radiotherapy to surgery/adjuvant chemotherapy in high-risk colon cancer patients (T4 by way of invasion/adherence to adjacent structures or T3N1-2) after complete resection. No significant differences were seen in disease-free or overall survival with the addition of radiotherapy. Although there was not even a trend toward increased survival with RT, these conclusions must be interpreted with caution given the significant methodological flaws of inadequate pathology/RT quality control.

Martenson Jr JA et al. Phase III study of adjuvant chemotherapy and radiation therapy compared with chemotherapy alone in the surgical adjuvant treatment of colon cancer: results of Intergroup protocol 0130. *J Clin Oncol.* 2004 Aug 15; 22(16): 3277–3283.

---

Unfortunately, this Intergroup trial did not definitively address the role of radiotherapy in locally advanced colon cancers. Without conclusive data, delivery of adjuvant radiotherapy should be reserved for those patients participating in clinical trials and those deemed to be at highest risk for local recurrence (residual disease or positive margins).

The role for radiotherapy in recurrent colon cancer is somewhat more clearly defined. While there are no randomized data, the group at the Mayo clinic presented a retrospective evaluation of 73 patients with recurrent colon cancer. Recurrence was local, pelvic/peritoneal, nodal, or a combination. The vast majority of patients received chemotherapy, external beam radiotherapy, surgical resection, and intra-operative radiotherapy (IORT). At 5 years, overall survival was 25%, justifying an aggressive multimodality approach for these patients.[9]

# RECTAL

## Management of Early, Favorable Lesions

As in cancers of the colon, surgical resection is a crucial component of therapy for rectal cancer. A select subgroup of patients with early rectal lesions will be candidates for conservative therapy alone.

Conservative treatment of rectal cancer may involve a limited resection or ~110 Gy in four fractions of endocavitary radiation +/− external beam pelvic irradiation. Characteristics of those tumors well suited to conservative management are listed here.

Local surgical removal of these lesions can be done via a transanal, transsphincteric, or transcoccygeal approach with local control rates in the 80%–95% range when used in conjunction with external beam radiotherapy (EBRT).[6] A phase II Cancer and Leukemia Group B (CALGB) study reported high rates of overall survival with carefully selected distal rectal tumors managed conservatively despite a failure-free survival somewhat lower than expected.

---

**TABLE 24-7 Tumors Appropriate for Conservative Surgery**

Small: < or = 3 cm
Mobile
Well or moderately differentiated
No clinical/radiographic evidence of spread beyond the bowel wall or to regional nodes
T1 or T2 disease with no ulceration

BOX 24-5

This phase II CALGB study evaluated outcomes in 177 patients with T1/T2, N0 adenocarcinomas within 10 cm of the dentate line, involving 40% or less of the rectal circumference, and 4 cm or less in diameter treated with limited, sphincter-preserving surgery. Six-year survival for the 110 patients undergoing full thickness local excision with negative margins was 85% at 48 months median follow-up. However, failure-free survival was only 78% as some of these patients required salvage therapy despite their favorable lesions.

Steele Jr GD et al. Sphincter-sparing treatment for distal rectal adenocarcinoma. *Ann Surg Oncol.* 1999: 6(5): 433–441.

Patients are at risk for failure in the untreated pelvic/perirectal nodal tissue as well as at the tumor bed after limited treatment of the primary tumor. In the CALGB series, many patients received EBRT to combat this issue. All but the most favorable tumors (T1, no lymphovascular space invasion (LVSI), negative margins, well to moderately differentiated) treated with limited local therapy should be considered for EBRT[6] which is usually combined with concurrent FU based chemotherapy.

## Surgical Management of Highly Invasive or Node-Positive Rectal Tumors

Because the anatomical constraints of the pelvis make adequate surgical resection more difficult, many patients with rectal cancer will benefit from trimodality treatment. Surgical technique in this population of patients has undergone significant change over the last 20 years. Historically, many patients with distal rectal tumors received abdominoperineal resections (APR) while those with more proximal tumors were eligible for low anterior resection (LAR). However, for both APR and LAR, conventional technique consisted of blunt dissection of the rectal fascia with local recurrence rates as high as 15%–45%.[12] Wishing to reduce the rate of APR, Heald et al explored the possibility of a more radical resection, total mesorectal excision (TME), believing that the improvements in local control gained by completely excising the mesorectum would balance the increased risk of margin reduction in distal tumors treated with LAR as opposed to APR. TME involves sharp dissection of the avascular plane surrounding the rectum and its lymphovascular mesentery, the mesorectum. In theory, excision of this entire structure will eliminate not only the primary tumor but also surrounding microscopic deposits of tumor within the perirectal soft tissue, thereby reducing the incidence of local recurrence. Heald was able to demonstrate a recurrence rate of 3.7% at 5 years despite a greater inclusion of distal tumors.[13] His work suggested that the distal margin was not the primary cause of local failure, and the previously accepted 5 cm surgical margin has since been abandoned.

The TME technique has subsequently gained widespread popularity and in 2001 a randomized trial comparing TME to preoperative radiotherapy plus TME demonstrated local failure rates <10% with surgery alone for all patients, including many with early-stage disease.

BOX 24-6

One thousand eight hundred sixty-one patients with resectable rectal tumors were randomized to short course pre-operative radiotherapy followed by TME versus TME alone. Survival was equivalent between the two groups. The addition of radiotherapy did significantly decrease the local recurrence rate to 2.4% at 2 years. Of note, however, the rate of recurrence in the surgery alone group was only 8.2%.

Kapiteijn E et al. Pre-operative radiotherapy combined with total nesorectal excision for resectable rectal cancer. *N Engl J Med.* 2001 Aug 30; 345(9): 638–646.

This study also demonstrated the necessity of adjuvant radiation therapy in patients with more advanced tumors, especially node-positive disease.

Achieving local success with TME is, in part, dependent on attaining the goals of *complete mesorectal excision*. The surgeon controls the excision, but the pathologist has a great deal of input in assessing the surgeon's success. In Nagtegaal's 2002 analysis, the role of the pathologist in quality control is illustrated.

### BOX 24-7

The pathology reports from patients participating in the nonirradiated arm of the Dutch TME trial were examined to assess a link between completeness of TME as reported by the pathologist and subsequent outcome. Of 180 cases, 24% had an incomplete mesorectal excision. These patients had a 36% rate of local and distant recurrence as compared to 20% (p = .02) in the completely resected group.

Nagtegaal ID et al. Macroscopic evaluation of rectal cancer resection specimen: clinical significance of the pathologist in quality Control. *J Clin Oncol.* 2002 April 1; 20(7): 1729–1734.

Another collaboration between surgeon and pathologist lies in the number of lymph nodes resected. The surgeon must attempt to resect an adequate number of nodes for accurate staging and the pathologist must carefully examine the pathological specimen to ensure that all nodes are evaluated. Tepper et al provides evidence to suggest the number of lymph nodes examined is crucial in determining appropriate adjuvant therapy.

### BOX 24-8

One thousand six hundred sixty-four patients with high-risk rectal cancer (T3, T4, or node-positive) treated on a national Intergroup trial with adjuvant chemotherapy/radiotherapy were assessed to determine the impact of nodal evaluation on outcome. A significant association was found between the number of nodes examined and both time to relapse and survival in node-negative patients. This relationship was not seen in node-positive patients suggesting that some patients classified as node-negative actually were node-positive patients with inadequate lymph node sampling. These patients may have benefited from adjuvant therapy. The authors conclude that 14 lymph nodes need to be examined for accurate staging.

Tepper JE et al. Impact of number of nodes retrieved on outcome in patients with rectal cancer. *J Clin Oncol.* 2001 Jan 1; 19(1): 157–163.

## Role of Combined-Modality Therapy in Invasive or Node-Positive Rectal Cancer

Table 24-8 presents the locoregional recurrence and survival data from five randomized North American trials evaluating postoperative radiotherapy after potentially curative resection of rectal cancer. Doses to the pelvis ranged from 40–48 Gy $+/-$ boost dose to 50–54 Gy. FU-based chemotherapy was used in each of the trials, either alone or in conjunction with radiotherapy.

These data suggest chemotherapy and radiotherapy work together better than either alone. Locoregional recurrence is significantly decreased with postoperative chemo-radiotherapy relative to either adjuvant single modality or surgical resection alone. It is less clear if this decrease in local recurrence translates into an overall survival benefit.

Another postoperative trial run in the late 1980s sought to clarify the delivery of chemotherapy as well as the optimal systemic regimen.

TABLE 24-8  Post-operative Radiotherapy

| Trial | Randomization | Locoregional Recurrence | Overall Survival |
|---|---|---|---|
| GITSG[14,15] | observation | 24% | 32% |
| | RT | 20% | 43% |
| | chemo | 27% | 47% |
| | chemo/RT−>chemo | 11% | 57% |
| | | | (p = .005 obs vs. chemo/RT) |
| NSABP R-01[16] | observation | 25% | 43% |
| | chemo | 21% | 53% |
| | RT | 16% | 41% |
| | | (p = .06 RT versus obs) | (p = .05 chemo versus obs) |
| NCCTG 794751[17] | RT | 25% | 48% |
| | chemo−>chemo/RT−>chemo | 14% | 58% |
| | | (p = .03) | (p = .025) |
| NSABP R-02[18] | chemo | 13% | 68% |
| | chemo−>chemo/RT−>chemo | 8% | 68% |
| | | (p = .02) | (p = NS) |
| Intergroup 0114[19] | chemo/RT−>chemo | 14% | 61–65% |
| | *various regimens | | (p = NS) |

*numbers estimated from graphs/tables when data not provided

---

**BOX 24-9**

Intergroup study 86-47-51 randomized patients to four distinct arms as follows:

1) Systemic FU/semustine plus RT with concomitant bolus FU
2) Systemic FU/semustine plus RT with concomitant protracted infusion FU
3) Systemic FU plus RT with concomitant bolus FU
4) Systemic FU plus RT with concomitant protracted infusion FU

While the addition of semustine to the systemic regimen was not associated with a benefit, the delivery of fluorouracil in a protracted manner was found to significantly increase time to relapse and overall survival relative to those receiving bolus FU. At 4 years, 60% of patients receiving bolus FU were alive as compared to 70% receiving continuous infusion FU (p = .005). These data helped to establish continuous infusion FU as the standard delivery method in the setting of concurrent chemo-radiotherapy for rectal cancer.

O'Connell MJ et al. Improving adjuvant therapy for rectal cancer by combining protracted infusion fluorouracil with radiation therapy after curative surgery. *N Engl J Med*. 1994 Aug 25; 331(8): 502–507.

As postoperative trials were ongoing, many groups were also randomizing patients to pre operative therapy. Treating patients in a preoperative setting allows the maximum number of patients to attempt preservation of bowel function. Doses ranged from 25 Gy in five fractions to 40 Gy in 20 fractions and chemotherapy was not used in conjunction with RT.

TABLE 24-9  Pre-operative Radiotherapy

| Trial | Randomization | Local Recurrence | Overall Survival |
|---|---|---|---|
| EORTC[20] | surgery alone | 30% | 59% |
| | pre-op RT | 15% | 69% |
| | | (p = .003) | (p = .08) |
| Stockholm[21] | surgery alone | 23% | 40% |
| | pre-op RT | 11% | 43% |
| | | (p < .01) | (p = NS) |
| MRC[22] | surgery alone | 46% | 19% |
| | pre-op RT | 36% | 26% |
| | | (p = .04) | (p = .10) |
| Swedish[23] | surgery alone | 27% | 48% |
| | pre-op RT | 11% | 58% |
| | | (p < .001) | (p = .004) |

(Numbers estimated from graphs/tables when data not provided.)

Even more convincing than the postoperative data, the preoperative trials demonstrated a strong, statistically significant association between adding radiotherapy and decreased local recurrence. These improvements in local control were achieved with RT alone as compared to the postoperative data where the most convincing improvements in locoregional control were obtained with concurrent chemo-radiotherapy. Extrapolating from the postoperative series, it seems likely that the addition of concurrent chemotherapy to preoperative radiotherapy would produce greater decreases in local recurrence, perhaps leading to a more obvious improvement in overall survival. In fact, even with RT alone, the preoperative data are somewhat suggestive of an overall survival trend. In an effort to clarify the impact of radiotherapy on local control and overall survival, two meta-analyses were conducted, pooling data from 14–22 randomized trials.

The data from the Colorectal Cancer Collaborative Group helped to solidify the role of radiotherapy in rectal cancer by demonstrating conclusively that pre- and postoperative RT resulted in significant reductions in rates of local recurrence. These data also supported a decrease in

## BOX 24-10

Individual patient data from 22 randomized trials were analyzed to compare outcomes of pre- (14 trials, 6,350 patients) or postoperative (8 trials, 2,157 patients) radiotherapy to no radiotherapy for rectal cancer. Preoperative treatment reduced the risk of isolated local recurrence at 10 years to 17% from 26% (p < .00001). Similarly, post-operative therapy decreased the incidence of isolated local recurrence at 5 years to 15% from 23% (p = .0002). Cause-specific mortality was decreased from 50% without radiotherapy to 46% with radiotherapy (p = .0003). In particular, preoperative regimens using biologically effective doses greater than or equal to 30 Gy demonstrated a 22% reduction in rectal cancer deaths. This benefit was negatively balanced by an increase in nonrectal cancer related deaths from 15% without RT to 19% with RT. As a result, no significant benefit was seen in overall survival at 10 years for those receiving RT.

Colorectal Cancer Collaborative Group. Adjuvant radiotherapy for rectal cancer: a systematic overview of 8,507 patients from 22 randomised trials. *Lancet.* 2001 Oct 20; 358: 1291–1303.

cancer-related deaths due to combined-modality therapy, particularly with preoperative therapy. Unfortunately, the reduction in cancer-related deaths was counterbalanced by an increase in deaths not attributable to cancer. This risk persisted throughout the first year following surgery and consisted primarily of an increase in vascular and infectious deaths. Overall, these data strongly support a role for radiotherapy in controlling local disease and suggests, particularly with preoperative radiotherapy, that this may translate into an overall survival benefit. As such, a second meta-analysis isolated those patients receiving preoperative therapy to determine if a greater impact on local control and survival was seen relative to all patients receiving RT.

---

**BOX 24-11**

Outcomes from 14 trials, 6,426 patients, evaluating pre-operative radiotherapy versus surgery alone were pooled and analyzed. Overall survival, cancer-related mortality, and local control were all significantly better in those receiving pre-operative RT. There were significantly more post-operative complications with pre-operative RT but this did not translate to increased posto-perative mortality.

The conclusions of this meta-analysis are limited by the difficulty in evaluating outcomes from heterogeneous patient populations and treatment techniques.

Camma C et al. Pre-operative radiotherapy for resectable rectal cancer: A meta-analysis. *JAMA*. 2000 Aug 23; 284(8): 1008–1015.

---

Given the controversy surrounding the optimal sequencing of chemo-radiotherapy as well as the mounting data that pre-operative therapy was superior to postoperative, the German Rectal Cancer Study Group opted to directly compare the two regimens in a randomized trial. The results from this trial were helpful in establishing the most appropriate sequencing for combined-modality therapy, particularly because conventional chemotherapy and radiotherapy fractionation schedules were incorporated into the treatment regimens.

---

**BOX 24-12**

Patients with high-risk rectal cancer (T3, T4 or N+) were randomized to conventional pre-operative radiotherapy (50.4 Gy) concurrent with continuous infusion fluorouracil versus the same post-operative chemo-radiotherapy (with the exception of the 540 cGy boost). Overall survival was not significantly different between the two groups but local recurrence was significantly decreased from 13% in the post-operative group to 6% in the pre-operative patients at 5 years (p = .006). Additionally, both acute and late toxicities were significantly less in the pre-operative group.

Sauer R et al. Pre-operative versus post-operative chemo-radiotherapy for rectal cancer. *N Engl J Med.* 2004 Oct 21; 351(17): 1731–1740.

---

Based on the accumulation of the preceding data, the current standard of care for locally advanced rectal cancer includes preoperative radiotherapy to a dose of 45–54 Gy concurrent with continuous infusion fluorouracil followed by low anterior total mesorectal resection.

After completion of preoperative radiation therapy with concurrent chemotherapy and surgical resection, patients who initially presented with T3 and/or node-positive disease generally are treated with adjuvant chemotherapy. Interestingly, the trials completed do not demonstrate a clear advantage of any chemotherapy over simple FU. However, because the data for more aggressive adjuvant chemotherapy has been so convincing in colon cancer, most medical oncologists now treat patients with regimens such as FU, leucovorin, and oxaliplatin (FOLFOX).

## Management of Locally Advanced/Unresectable Rectal Tumors

Rectal tumors deemed unresectable require aggressive, combined-modality management to effect long-term local control and survival. Nakfoor et al reported on the MGH experience using intra-operative RT in locally advanced rectal cancer. One hundred forty-five patients were treated with preoperative irradiation and ~64% also received concurrent FU. Approximately half of these patients received an IORT boost to the surgical bed. The addition of FU to preoperative radiotherapy improved both local control and disease-specific survival. The combination of complete surgical resection and IORT resulted in 89% local control and 63% disease-specific survival at 5 years. In contrast, those without complete resection receiving IORT for residual disease had rates of 65% and 32%.[24] This single institution series of patients seems to demonstrate a benefit for preoperative chemo-radiotherapy followed by maximal surgical resection with an IORT boost in patients with unresectable tumors.

Based on the preceding data, an approach to the management of rectal cancer is presented below.

---

**FIGURE 24-1**    Management of rectal cancer.

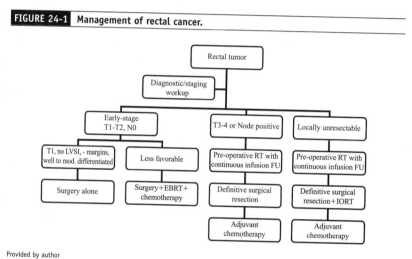

Provided by author

---

## TECHNIQUE/DOSE

Despite the fact that adjuvant radiotherapy is delivered only in a very select subset of patients with colon cancer, several general principles exist to guide the treating physician. Proper identification of the tumor bed is crucial. This may occur through registration of preoperative images, placement of surgical clips, or other suitable localization methods. The tumor bed should be encompassed with a 3–5 cm margin in all directions but the mesenteric lymph nodes are generally not covered as they are more successfully dealt with through surgical removal. The postoperative tumor bed generally receives ~45 Gy in 1.8 Gy fractions followed by a boost. The boost field and dose are limited by small bowel tolerance. For this reason, it may help to treat these patients in the left or right lateral decubitus position. The small bowel may fall away allowing the pericolic tissues to receive higher doses. Ideally, the boost region would receive 55–60 Gy, but small bowel should be completely excluded after 50 Gy.[6]

For the vast majority of patients with adenocarcinoma of the rectum, a conventional simulation procedure will suffice. The patient is typically placed in the prone position and one of the most important components of the simulation procedure is then performed, placing a marker at the anal verge. The rectum is filled with 20cc–50cc of contrast material and often additional air. In some situations it may be helpful to insert a Foley catheter into the rectum, fill the balloon with contrast, and pull it snug against the upper portion of the anal sphincter. These simple steps help to define the rectum and delineate the anal canal for better tumor coverage and normal tissue avoidance. A vaginal marker should be placed in women to possibly allow a portion of the vaginal tissue to be spared and to assure full coverage of the anterior rectal wall. Alternatively, CT planning may be performed. While an anal marker remains a critical portion of the CT setup, the remaining structures can frequently be delineated without the use of contrast. In the following example, the anal marker is difficult to visualize but is located approximately 2 cm below the inferior edge of the pubic symphysis.

The radiotherapy fields should cover the highest risk regions including the primary tumor and draining lymph nodes, which necessitates irradiating the mesorectum in its entirety and treating the areas where the surgical margins are most likely to be close or positive. In rectal cancer, this includes coverage of the rectum and perirectal tissues as well as the internal iliac, presacral, and perirectal lymph nodes. A conventional field arrangement employs AP/PA or just PA fields as well as laterals to deliver the initial 45 Gy.

Field borders are based on coverage of the at-risk volume as determined by the treating physician. The patient is treated with a full bladder to displace small bowel and buttocks taped apart. Typically the dose is delivered in fractions of 180 cGy using high-energy photons. After the initial 45 Gy, lateral fields can be used to deliver the cone down portion of the treatment, which is designed to minimize dose to the anus and small bowel. The total dose to the tumor ranges from 50.4 to 54 Gy depending on tumor extent but is generally limited to 50.4 Gy. The purpose of the boost is to increase the dose to areas that will be difficult for the surgeon to resect with an adequate margin, for example, the presacral space. In this example, the patient has a very low rectal tumor.

Radiotherapy is typically delivered in conjunction with FU-based chemotherapy. Commonly used continuous infusion regimens are 225 mg/m$^2$/day every day, or 300 mg/m$^2$/day Monday to Friday. There is an increasing use of concurrent Xeloda, which is typically given at 825 mg/m$^2$ BID,

**FIGURE 24-2** Anteroposterior views of a typical pelvic field as well as the lateral view of a boost field used in the treatment of rectal cancer.

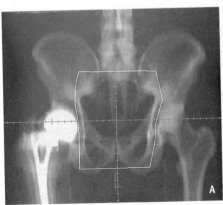
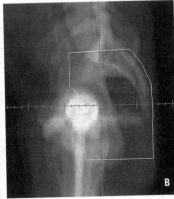

with the first dose given about 1 hour prior to radiation therapy.

## FOLLOW-UP

Patients are typically seen by the surgeon about 1 month after radiotherapy in preparation for their surgery at 4–8 weeks. Close follow-up should then continue about every 3–4 months for the first 2 to 3 years following treatment. Having the patient rotate between providers may be advantageous to the patient and the physician. The patient stays connected to each provider and benefits from the unique perspective of each discipline while the physician benefits from the input of colleagues. After the first 2–3 years, follow-up may be decreased to every 6 months until 5 years at which time the patient can return on an annual basis. Returning the patient to the primary care of his/her personal physician is at the discretion of the treating physician and the comfort level of the individual patient.

**FIGURE 24-2**  Lateral views of a typical pelvic field as well as the lateral view of a boost field used in the treatment of rectal cancer.

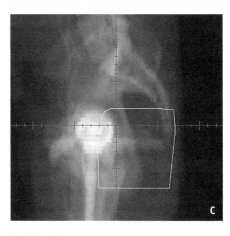

Provided by author

Follow-up should consist of problem pertinent history and physical exam at each encounter. Routine CEA levels at each visit may be helpful depending on the initial clinical scenario (if the CEA level was always normal, it may not be helpful in follow-up). CT of the abdomen and pelvis, CXR or chest CT, and colonoscopy will all be a routine part of follow-up, although the interval of use will be dictated by the initial tumor characteristics.

## MORBIDITY

Acute RT effects typically begin within a few weeks of RT initiation and persist until a few weeks after RT. Common side effects are listed here.

Fortunately, these side effects often resolve fully and quickly. The much greater risk in the use of pelvic irradiation is late bowel and anal toxicity. Late radiation injury is multifaceted and includes both fibrotic response and vascular injury. Subsequent clinical symptoms may take many years to develop but are often seen within the first 8 to 12 months after treatment. Increased rectal frequency/urgency, cramping, bleeding, and pain are all potential late effects of pelvic RT. Loss of anal function can also result from RT to the sphincter muscle. While not life-threatening, these side effects can significantly impact patient quality-of-life. The Radiation Therapy Oncology Group (RTOG) Common Toxicity Criteria can be found in chapter 8.

The most serious late complications, those requiring medical/surgical intervention, include bowel obstruction, severe bleeding, fistula formation, and intractable diarrhea. A generally accepted dose schedule to minimize late bowel complications is 50–55 Gy in fractions of 180 to 200 cGy each. In general, the addition of FU

**TABLE 24-10  Common Side Effects**

Erythema, desquamation of the perineum
diarrhea, tenesmus, rectal bleeding
dysuria, urinary urgency/frequency

chemotherapy appears to be reasonably well tolerated. While concurrent chemotherapy increases the rate and severity of acute toxicities, there does not appear to be a substantial effect on late bowel complications.[25]

Multiple treatment regimens exist to counteract the negative late effects of radiation. One of the most important, and least glamorous, methods for lessening morbidity may be simple dietary intervention. While many clinicians intuitively believe that diet and outcomes are linked, this randomized trial provides strong evidence in support of that theory and underscores the importance of aggressive dietary intervention.

---

**BOX 24-13**

One hundred eleven patients receiving radiotherapy for colorectal cancer were randomized to dietary counseling, protein supplements, or no intervention. Patients in the counseling group received guidance designed to assist them in maintaining their energy and protein requirements based on modifications of their typical diet. The second group was instructed to use protein supplements to accomplish the same goals.

Interestingly, both intervention groups enjoyed decreased symptom severity and some improvement in quality-of-life at RT completion, seemingly linked to their increased intake. At 3 months, the counseling group enjoyed persistent benefits in nutritional status and quality-of-life.

Ravasco et al. Dietary counseling improves patient outcomes: a prospective, randomized, controlled trial in colorectal cancer patients undergoing radiotherapy. *J Clin Oncol.* 2005 Mar 1; 23(7): 1431–1438.

---

Other tools in symptom management include loperamide, diphenoxylate, and cholestyramine (generally after radiation therapy to the right colon) for diarrhea. Aggressive techniques such as laser treatments or cautery can be used for bleeding bowel mucosa, bowel rest/decompression for intestinal obstruction, and surgical resection for adhesions.[25]

## FUTURE DIRECTIONS

There are two major national trials currently underway in rectal cancer. The first, conducted by the National Surgical Adjuvant Breast and Bowel Project, is evaluating the use of oral capecitabine ($825$ mg/m$^2$ BID) with pre-operative radiotherapy in locally advanced rectal adenocarcinoma as compared to conventional continuous infusion FU ($225$ mg/m$^2$/day).

The second trial is underway via the Eastern Cooperative Oncology Group. This trial evaluates the utility of adding bevacizumab to adjuvant chemotherapeutic agents FU, leucovorin, and oxaliplatin in patients with Stage II or III rectal cancer who have completed pre-operative chemoradiotherapy.

## REFERENCES

1. American Cancer Society: Colorectal Cancer Facts and Figures 2007. http://www.cancer.org/docroot/STT/stt_0_2007.asp?sitearea=STT&level=1.
2. Jessup JM, et al. Colon and Rectum. in Greene F, Page D, Fleming I, et al (eds): *AJCC Cancer Staging Handbook* (ed Sixth). New York, Springer-Verlag, 2002, pp 137–138.
3. Kelsen DP DJ, Kern SE, Levin B, and Tepper JE, eds. *Gastrointestinal Oncology Principles and Practice.* Philadelphia, Lippincott, Williams, and Wilkins, 2002.
4. Colon and Rectum, in Perez C, Brady L, Halperin E, et al (eds). *Principles and Practice of Radiation Oncology.* Philadelphia, Lippincott, Williams and Wilkins, 2004, pp 1607–1629.

5. American Cancer Society: Colorectal Cancer Risk and Screening. http://www.cancer/org/docroot/PRO/PRO_4_1_ColonMD_Risk_and_Screening.asp.

6. Horton JK, Tepper JE. Staging of colorectal cancer: past, present, and future. *Clin Colorectal Cancer* 4:302–312, 2005.

7. Gunderson L, Tepper J, eds. *Clinical Radiation Oncology*. Philadelphia, Churchill Livingstone, 2000.

8. Moertel CG, Fleming TR, Macdonald JS, et al. Levamisole and fluorouracil for adjuvant therapy of resected colon carcinoma. *N Engl J Med* 322:352–358, 1990.

9. Willett CG, Fung CY, Kaufman DS, et al. Posto-perative radiation therapy for high-risk colon carcinoma. *J Clin Oncol* 11:1112–1117, 1993.

10. Taylor WE, Donohue JH, Gunderson LL, et al. The Mayo Clinic experience with multimodality treatment of locally advanced or recurrent colon cancer. *Ann Surg Oncol* 9:177–185, 2002.

11. Willett CG, Goldberg S, Shellito PC, et al. Does postoperative irradiation play a role in the adjuvant therapy of stage T4 colon cancer? *Cancer J Sci Am* 5:242–247, 1999.

12. Kapiteijn E, Marijnen C, ID N, et al. Pre-operative radiotherapy combined with total mesorectal excision for resectable rectal cancer. *N Engl J Med* 345:638–646, 2001.

13. Heald RJ, Ryall RD. Recurrence and survival after total mesorectal excision for rectal cancer. *Lancet* 1:1479–1482, 1986.

14. Prolongation of the disease-free interval in surgically treated rectal carcinoma. Gastrointestinal Tumor Study Group. *N Engl J Med* 312:1465–1472, 1985.

15. Douglass HO, Jr., Moertel CG, Mayer RJ, et al. Survival after postoperative combination treatment of rectal cancer. *N Engl J Med* 315:1294–1295, 1986.

16. Fisher B, Wolmark N, Rockette H, et al. postoperative adjuvant chemotherapy or radiation therapy for rectal cancer: results from NSABP protocol R-01. *J Natl Cancer Inst* 80:21–29, 1988.

17. Krook JE, Moertel CG, Gunderson LL, et al. Effective surgical adjuvant therapy for high-risk rectal carcinoma. *N Engl J Med* 324:709–715, 1991.

18. Wolmark N, Wieand HS, Hyams DM, et al. Randomized trial of postoperative adjuvant chemotherapy with or without radiotherapy for carcinoma of the rectum. National Surgical Adjuvant Breast and Bowel Project Protocol R-02. *J Natl Cancer Inst* 92:388–396, 2000.

19. Tepper JE, O'Connell M, Niedzwiecki D, et al. Adjuvant therapy in rectal cancer: analysis of stage, sex, and local control—final report of Intergroup 0114. *J Clin Oncol* 20:1744–1750, 2002.

20. Gerard A, Buyse M, Nordlinger B, et al. Pre-operative radiotherapy as adjuvant treatment in rectal cancer: final results of a randomized study of the European Organization for Research and Treatment of Cancer (EORTC). *Ann Surg* 208:606–614, 1988.

21. Pre-operative short-term radiation therapy in operable rectal carcinoma. A prospective randomized trial. Stockholm Rectal Cancer Study Group. *Cancer* 66:49–55, 1990.

22. Randomized trial of surgery alone versus radiotherapy followed by surgery for potentially operable locally advanced rectal cancer. Medical Research Council Rectal Cancer Working Party. *Lancet* 348:1605–1610, 1996.

23. Improved survival with pre-operative radiotherapy in resectable rectal cancer. Swedish Rectal Cancer Trial. *N Engl J Med* 336:980–987, 1997.

24. Nakfoor BM, Willett CG, Shellito PC, et al. The impact of 5-fluorouracil and intra-operative electron beam radiation therapy on the outcome of patients with locally advanced primary rectal and rectosigmoid cancer. *Ann Surg* 228:194–200, 1998.

25. Coia LR, Myerson RJ, Tepper JE. Late effects of radiation therapy on the gastrointestinal tract. *Int J Radiat Oncol Biol Phys* 31:1213–1236, 1995.

# 25

# Anal Cancer

*Salma K. Jabbour, MD*
*Deborah Frassica, MD*

## OVERVIEW

Squamous cell carcinoma of the anal canal is rare. The incidence, however, continues to climb, likely associated with the transmission of human papillomavirus. Radiation therapy (RT) and chemotherapy are critical in the definitive management of anal cancer. Together they allow for cure via an anal sphincter preservation approach in most patients, foregoing the need for abdomino-perineal resection (APR) and permanent colostomy in those with a complete response to combined modality therapy.

## INTRODUCTION/EPIDEMIOLOGY

The incidence of anal canal carcinoma has increased notably over the last several decades, but still remains uncommon, accounting for about 1%–2% of all large bowel cancers. It is estimated that these were a total of 4,650 new cases of anal carcinoma in 2007, and 60% of these cases were diagnosed in women.[1] This represents a net increase in anal cancer incidence compared to 2002, when there were approximately 3,900 new cases.[2] An estimated 690 deaths occurred due to anal cancer in 2007.[1] Also, 67% of epidermoid carcinoma patients are women versus 42% of adenocarcinoma patients.[3] Less than 10% of patients present with distant metastases at the time of diagnosis.

## ANATOMY

The anal canal extends superiorly from the anorectal ring to the anal verge inferiorly and measures approximately 4 cm in length. The anorectal ring is palpable on digital rectal exam and is located at the level of the puborectalis sling at the apex of the anal sphincter complex.[4] The anorectal ring consists of the muscle bundle formed by the junction of the upper portion of the internal sphincter, the distal portion of the puborectalis, and the deep portion of the external sphincter. The epithelial lining at this level is characterized by columnar mucosa.[5]

The anorectal ring is 2 cm above the dentate or pectinate line (Figure 25-1). The region between them is termed the anal transitional zone and includes the anal columns of Morgagni. The columns of Morgagni are vertical mucosal folds of columnar epithelium and begin just distal to the anorectal ring and extend to the dentate line. The transitional zone lies approximately 1 cm above the

dentate line. Histologically, this 6–12 mm zone is where rectal columnar epithelium and anal squamous epithelium meet. Therefore, it consists of a mixture of rectal, transitional (urothelial) and
squamous epithelium. The dentate line is the junction between the columnar epithelium of the
proximal anal canal and the stratified squamous epithelium of the lower anal canal. The anal
glands empty through the anal valves and sinuses present here.[5]

The anal verge, or inferior margin of the anal canal, is the junction of nonkeratinized
squamous epithelium of the anal canal with hair-bearing, keratinized, perianal skin. The anal
verge is formed by the intersphincteric groove between the lower edge of the internal anal sphincter and external sphincter. At this level, the walls of the anal canal are apposed during the normal
resting state.[5]

In the past, the management of tumors of the anal margin was controversial because the definition of the proximal and distal extents of the anal canal was nonuniform. Some authorities have
defined the anal margin as beginning just below the dentate line, and the AJCC has defined
the anatomic proximal boundary to be 5–6 cm from the anal verge.[4] From a practical standpoint,
the anal verge serves as delineation between the keratinized skin (anal margin) and the nonkeratinized squamous mucosa (anal canal). Tumors originating from the skin or distal to the squamous mucocutaneous junction are anal margin tumors. Neoplasms that arise from the columnar,
transitional, or squamous mucosa of the anal canal are anal canal cancers.

## PATHOLOGY

The most common histology of anal canal carcinomas is squamous cell carcinoma, which occurs
in up to 75%–80% of cases.[3] Keratinizing squamous cell carcinomas comprise the majority and are
usually located below the dentate line. Nonkeratinizing squamous cell carcinomas (basaloid,

---

**FIGURE 25-1** Diagram of anal canal.

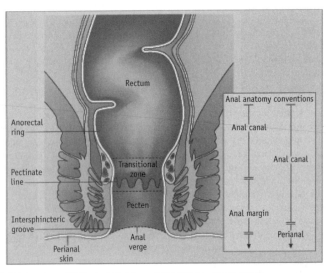

loacogenic/transitional) arise from the transitional zone above the dentate line. Traditionally, the histological subset of squamous cell carcinomas has not impacted management of anal cancer, although it is controversial whether there is truly a difference in outcome between the two subsets.[6] Adenocarcinomas can also occur in rectal type mucosa or arise from the anal glands, typically above the dentate line. Less common histologies of the anal canal malignancies include lymphoma, melanoma (2%–4%), and Kaposi sarcoma.

The WHO classification of carcinoma of the anal canal is used in AJCC staging. It includes:[4]

1. Squamous cell carcinoma (SqCCA)
2. Adenocarcinoma (including rectal type, of anal glands, and those arising within anorectal fistulas) (ACA)
3. Mucinous carcinoma
4. Small cell carcinoma
5. Undifferentiated carcinoma

The terms cloacogenic and transitional carcinoma are no longer used because both are now understood to be nonkeratinizing squamous cell carcinomas. Melanomas, sarcomas, and carcinoid tumors are excluded from the AJCC staging system for anal canal carcinomas.

Perianal skin and anal margin tumor histologies include squamous cell carcinoma, giant condyloma (verrucous carcinoma), basal cell carcinoma, Bowen's disease, and Paget's disease. These are staged as skin cancers.

## ROUTES OF SPREAD

Anal cancer can spread by direct extension, lymphatic spread, and hematogenous dissemination. Lymphatic dissemination can occur early in the disease. Conversely, distant metastatic disease tends to occur late in the course of anal cancer. There are three major pathways of lymphatic drainage from the anal canal (Table 25-1).

At presentation, involvement of perirectal lymph nodes and pelvic lymph nodes may occur in 50% and 30% of cases, respectively. Inguinal nodal metastases are detected in 15%–20% of patients at diagnosis, and an additional 10%–25% of patients later are found to have inguinal metastases.[7]

Locoregionally, tumor can extend to rectal mucosa, perianal tissues, anorectal fat, external anal sphincter, perineum, bladder, urethra, prostate, cervix, vagina, or uterus. Anal cancers most frequently metastasize to the liver and lungs.

## TABLE 25-1  Anal Cancer Lymphatic Pathways

| Location of Tumor | First Echelon Lymph Node Basin | Drainage Pathway |
|---|---|---|
| Perianal skin, Anal verge, Anal canal below dentate line | Inguinal and femoral nodes | External iliac lymphatics |
| Anal canal above dentate line | Pudendal/hypogastric/obturator<br>Inferior and middle hemorrhoidal nodes | Internal iliac lymphatics |
| Lower rectum/proximal anal canal | Perirectal nodes (anorectal, lateral sacral, perirectal)<br>Superior hemorrhoidal nodes | Inferior mesenteric lymphatics |

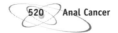

## RISK FACTORS FOR ANAL CANCER[8,9,10]

1. History of sexually transmitted disease (including HPV, genital warts, herpes, Chlamydia syphilis, and gonorrhea) (Box 25-1)
2. Anal receptive intercourse
3. History of $\geq$15 sexual partners
4. Known history of cervical, vulvar, vaginal cancer
5. Immunosuppression after solid organ transplantation
6. HIV
7. Smoking

---

**BOX 25-1 ANAL CANCER RISK FACTORS**

Telephone interviews covering possible risk factors for anal cancer were conducted in women and men diagnosed with invasive or *in situ* anal cancer. This population was compared to controls with ACA of the rectum and population controls. There was consistent and statistically significant evidence that sexual practices were associated with anal cancer including higher number of sexual partners, anal receptive intercourse, and homosexual contact in men. HPV-16 was detected in 84% of anal cancer specimens while all rectal ACA were negative for HPV. The authors concluded that anal cancer is probably sexually transmitted and is potentially preventable.

Frisch M, et al., Sexually transmitted infection as a cause of anal cancer. *N Engl J Med.* 1997 Nov 6; 337(19): 1350–1358.

---

## PRESENTATION/WORKUP

Symptoms of anal cancer can mimic benign conditions of the anus, such as *hemorrhoids*, and can cause a delay in diagnosis. Most patients with anal carcinoma present with rectal bleeding. One third of patients experience pain or anal mass. Less than 5% of patients present with gross fecal incontinence due to sphincter destruction. A tumor of the anal margin may cause pruritus, especially in the setting of Bowen's or Paget's disease. Staging workup should consist of the following

- History
  - Weight loss, tenesmus, change in stool caliber
  - Full sexual history including HIV risk factors
- Physical examination
  - Palpation of the superficial inguinal lymph nodes
  - Inspection of the perineum
  - Digital rectal examination
  - Anoscopy
    Extent of the tumor, location, size, and distance from the dentate line and anal verge
  - Women: speculum, bimanual, and rectovaginal examinations and Pap smear screening (to rule out concurrent malignancies or direct invasion from the anal tumor)
- Biopsy of any anal mass
- Fine needle aspiration of suspicious lymph nodes
- Transanal ultrasound (to assess depth of penetration and lymph node status)
- CT scan of the abdomen with IV contrast (to rule out liver metastasis)
- Pelvic CT scan or MRI (to assess for inguinal or pelvic node metastasis)
- PET scan
- Chest radiograph (to rule out lung metastasis)

- Laboratory testing
  - Complete blood cell count
  - Chemistry panel, including liver and renal function tests
  - HIV testing and CD4 count (for high risk sexual history or prior IV drug abuse)

## STAGING

Since the primary management of these tumors does not usually incorporate surgical excision, these tumors are staged clinically and less often pathologically (Table 25-2 and Table 25-3).

The location of the tumor in relation to the anorectal junction is of importance because carcinomas that overlap the anorectal junction must either be classified as rectal or anal in origin. Tumors should be staged as rectal tumors if their epicenter is located 2 cm or more from the dentate line or as anal tumors if their epicenter is less than 2 cm from the dentate line.[4] Low rectal tumors which extend distal to the dentate line are at very low risk of spread to the superficial inguinal lymph node basins.

## TREATMENT OF EARLY-STAGE ANAL CANCER

A patient with T1N0 anal cancer can be managed with wide local excision of the tumor alone if negative margins can be achieved without requiring APR. However, if APR is anticipated, then definitive chemo-radiotherapy (CRT) should be considered for primary management. In the past, RT alone for these early-stage tumors was also a reasonable treatment option.

---

**TABLE 25-2 TNM Staging Definitions[4]**

| | Definition |
|---|---|
| **Primary Tumor (T)** | |
| TX | Primary tumor cannot be assessed |
| T0 | No evidence of primary tumor |
| Tis | Carcinoma *in situ* |
| T1 | Tumor ≤2 cm in greatest dimension |
| T2 | Tumor >2 cm but ≤ 5 cm in greatest dimension |
| T3 | Tumor >5 cm in greatest dimension |
| T4 | Tumor of any size invades adjacent organ(s); vagina, urethra, bladder (involvement of sphincter muscle, rectal wall, perirectal skin, or subcutaneous tissues is not T4) |
| **Lymph Node (N)** | |
| NX | Regional lymph nodes cannot be assessed |
| N0 | No regional lymph node metastasis |
| N1 | Metastasis in perirectal lymph node(s) |
| N2 | Metastasis in unilateral internal iliac and/or inguinal lymph node(s) |
| N3 | Metastasis in perirectal and inguinal lymph nodes and/or bilateral internal iliac and/or inguinal lymph nodes |
| **Distant Metastasis (M)** | |
| MX | Distant metastasis cannot be assessed |
| M0 | No distant metastasis |
| M1 | Distant metastasis |

---

TABLE 25-3  Stage Grouping[4]

| Stage | T | N | M |
|---|---|---|---|
| Stage 0 | Tis | N0 | M0 |
| Stage I | T1 | N0 | M0 |
| Stage II | T2-T3 | N0 | M0 |
| Stage IIIA | T1-T3 | N1 | M0 |
|  | T4 | N0 | M0 |
| Stage IIIB | T4 | N1 | M0 |
|  | Any T | N2–N3 | M0 |
| Stage IV | Any T | Any N | M1 |

## TREATMENT OF LOCALIZED ANAL CANCER

Prior to the advent of combined modality CRT for anal cancer, the treatment of choice was abdomino perineal resection (APR). This extensive procedure involves removal of the sigmoid colon, rectum and anus, leaving patients with a permanent colostomy. Also, inguinal and pelvic lymph node dissec tion would be required in the setting of positive lymph nodes. The long-term survival after APR o definitive chemo-radiotherapy (CRT) is considered to be equivalent, the main benefit to CRT being anal sphincter preservation. The 5-year survival rates after APR alone range from 40%–80%.[3]

---

### BOX 25-2  THE NIGRO REGIMEN

In 1972, CRT was pioneered at Wayne State University to reduce the surgical recurrence rate in anal cancer patients after APR. The Nigro regimen, devised by Dr. Norman Nigro, was a preoperative treatment consisting of:

- Chemotherapy and RT given concurrently: 5-FU (1,000 mg/m$^2$ continuous infusion on days 1 through 4 and 29 through 32), mitomycin (15 mg/m$^2$ on day 1); Radiation therapy (30 Gy in 2 Gy per fraction)

Preliminary findings of complete pathological responses on APR specimens prompted attempts at a sphincter preservation approach. To rule out residual disease, a routine post-treatment biopsy 6 weeks after completion of CRT was started in 1975 and found to be a reasonable assessment of response, rather than proceeding directly to APR. In many cases, no recurrence of tumor was found in those patients rendered free of disease by the preoperative treatment (90%). This defined a new approach using curative CRT without requiring any surgery.

Nigro ND, et al. Combined therapy for cancer of the anal canal: a preliminary report. *Dis Colon Rectum.* 1974 May-Jun; 17 (3): 354–356.

Nigro ND, et al. Combined preoperative radiation and chemotherapy for squamous cell carcinoma of the anal canal. *Cancer.* 1983 May 15; 51910): 1826–1829.

Nigro ND, et al. Dynamic management of squamous cell carcinoma of the anal canal. *Invest New Drugs.* 1989 Apr; 7(1):83–89.

---

Subsequently, three large, randomized prospective clinical trials have helped to establish CR as the standard of care for anal cancer by showing improved local control with reduced colostom rates. Because a high local control rate can be achieved with RT alone (especially in early-stag lesions), these trials sought to evaluate the validity of the Nigro regimen and better define the role of chemotherapy in anal carcinoma.

The first trial was conducted by the United Kingdom Coordinating Committee on Cance Research (UKCCCR) (Box 25-3).

---

**BOX 25-3** UKCCCR TRIAL

This trial randomized 585 patients with all stages of anal cancer (except T1N0) to receive:

- RT alone (45 Gy in 20 or 25 fractions)
- RT with concurrent 5-FU (1,000 mg/m$^2$ over 24 hours for 4 days or 750 mg/m$^2$ by continuous infusion for 5 days during the first and last weeks of radiation therapy) and mitomycin (12 mg/m$^2$ given by IV bolus injection on day 1)

Six weeks after initial treatment, patients who had good responses (>50% response or complete remission) received boost RT (15 Gy in six fractions to a perineal field or iridium-192 implant to 25 Gy in 10 Gy per day). APR was considered in patients with <50% response.

CRT substantially reduced the chance for APR by decreasing local failures from 59% to 36% at 42 month follow-up (p > 0.0001). The mortality from anal cancer was also reduced from 39% with RT alone to 28% in the CRT arm (p = 0.02), but there was no significant improvement in overall survival (3-year survival RT = 58% vs. CRT = 65%). Increased acute morbidity occurred in the CRT arm but late morbidity occurred at similar rates. Of note, 23% of cases randomized on this study were anal margin cancers.

UKCCCR Anal Cancer Trial Working Party. Epidermoid anal cancer: results from the UKCCR randomized trial of radiotherapy alone versus radiotherapy, 5-fluorouracil, and mitomycin. *Lancet*. 1996 Oct 19; 348:1049–1054.

The second trial was led by the European Organization for the Research and Treatment of Cancer EORTC) (Box 25-4).

---

**BOX 25-4** EORTC TRIAL

One hundred ten patients with T3-T4N0-N3 or T1-2N1-3 (no T1N0 or T2N0 patients) anal cancer were randomly assigned to receive:

- RT alone (45 Gy in 1.8 Gy per fraction)
- RT with concurrent 5-FU (750 mg/m$^2$ daily on days 1 through 5 by continuous infusion and days 29 through 33) and mitomycin (single bolus injection of 15 mg/m$^2$ only on day 1)

Six weeks after completing initial treatment, patients with a complete response received a boost dose (via electrons, photons, or brachytherapy) of 15 Gy. A 20 Gy dose was prescribed for partial responders. Surgery was performed if there was an inadequate response to therapy.

This study confirmed the results of the UKCCCR trial. CRT resulted in a significant increase in the complete remission rate from 54% (RT) to 80% (CRT), which led to a benefit in local control and colostomy-free interval, both in favor of CRT (5Y LRC 68% vs. 50% (p = 0.02) and 5Y colostomy-free interval 72% vs. 40% (p = 0.002)). Event-free survival (local tumor progression, colostomy, late complications, and death) were significantly improved in the CRT arm. Similar to the UKCCR trial, no overall survival benefit was seen. Actuarial survival at 5 years for both groups was 58%.

Bartelink H, et al. Concomitant radiotherapy and chemotherapy is superior to radiotherapy alone in the treatment of locally advanced anal cancer: results of a phase III randomized trial of the European Organization for Research and Treatment of Cancer Radiotherapy and Gastrointestinal Cooperative Groups. *J Clin Oncol*. 1997 May; 15(5):2040–2049.

---

# MITOMYCIN: IS IT ESSENTIAL FOR THE TREATMENT OF ANAL CANCER?

Because of the toxicities associated with mitomycin C, including neutropenia and thrombocytopenia, the necessity for this chemotherapeutic agent was evaluated in a randomized setting through the combined Intergroup efforts of the Radiation Therapy Oncology Group (RTOG) and the Eastern

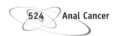 

Cooperative Oncology Group (ECOG) (RTOG protocol 87-04 and ECOG 1289). Mitomycin was found to be essential in lowering colostomy rates and improving disease-free survival (Box 25-5).

---

**BOX 25-5** **INTERGROUP TRIAL**

This study also sought to assess the role of salvage CRT in patients who had residual tumor after CRT. Three hundred and ten patients were randomized to receive:

- RT and 5-FU (1,000/mg/m2/24 hours continuous infusion on days 1 through 4, on days 1 and 28 of RT). Pelvic radiation therapy was delivered to 45 to 50.4 Gy
- RT, 5FU, and MMC (10 mg/m2 IV bolus on day 1 of each 5-FU course).

Four to 6 weeks after the completion of therapy, patients underwent a full-thickness biopsy of the primary tumor site. If the biopsy returned negative, no further treatment was given. If the post-treatment biopsy returned positive, then an additional, salvage boost of 9 Gy to the tumor with 5-FU and cisplatin was given. Post-salvage biopsy was then performed 6 weeks later, and if biopsies were positive, patients underwent APR.

Post-treatment biopsies were positive in 15% of patients in the 5-FU arm versus 7.7% in the mitomycin arm (p = 0.135). At 4 years, colostomy rates were lower (9% vs. 23%, p = 0.002), colostomy-free survival higher (71% vs. 59%, p = 0.014), and disease-free survival higher (73% vs. 51%, p = 0.0003) in the mitomycin arm. There was no improvement in survival with the use of mitomycin, and toxicity was also greater in this group. Of the patients who underwent salvage with FU and cisplatin, 50% (n = 11) were rendered disease-free at 4 years. Of note, the major benefit of mitomycin in reducing colostomy rates and improving colostomy-free survival occurred in patients whose tumors extended to skin or to adjacent organs. Therefore, in the face of greater toxicity with mitomycin, its use is justified in definitive CRT for anal cancer.

---

Flam M, et al. Role of mitomycin in combination with fluorouracil and radiotherapy, and of salvage chemoradiation in the definitive nonsurgical treatment of epidermoid carcinoma of the anal canal: results of a phase III randomized Intergroup trial. *J Clin Oncol.* 1996 Sep; 14(9): 2527–2539.

## CAN CISPLATIN REPLACE MITOMYCIN?

Cisplatin is known to be active in other squamous cell carcinomas (head and neck cancer and cervical cancer) and results from the Intergroup trial using 5-FU and cisplatin as salvage chemotherapies with RT showed efficacy in the treatment of anal canal carcinomas. In addition, cisplatin is a radiosensitizer and has resulted in a survival advantage when combined with radiotherapy in squamous cell carcinoma of the esophagus. Multiple series have addressed the role of cisplatin for the definitive management of anal canal carcinoma. Studies employing cisplatin have shown similar outcomes to standard therapy with mitomycin, 5-FU, and RT (Table 25-4).

However, preliminary results from RTOG 98-11 trial suggest that cisplatin chemotherapy should not replace mitomycin in the definitive management of anal cancer. In this study, induction and concurrent cisplatin and 5-FU were compared to standard mitomycin and 5-FU concurrent with RT (Box 25-6).

## OPTIMIZING RADIATION DOSE

Because of a 20%–30% local failure rate with CRT, dose escalation has been evaluated to attempt to increase local control and possibly survival in this disease. Despite the interest in dose escalation, the pioneering data from Nigro using a total dose of 30 Gy gave results comparable to modern day doses of 50–60 Gy (Box 25-7 and Box 25-8).

Nevertheless, due to the risk of local failure, the de facto standard radiation dose per the recently completed RTOG 9811 trial is a total of 55–59 Gy which should be delivered to the primary

**TABLE 25-4  Phase II Trials of Cisplatin in Locally Advanced Anal Carcinoma**

| Author | Number of Patients (Follow-up) | Cisplatin Dose/ Regimen | RT Dose (Gy) | Local Control/ Complete Response Rate | Colostomy-Free Survival | Overall Survival |
|---|---|---|---|---|---|---|
| Doci[11] | 35 (37 mo) | 100 mg/m$^2$ day 1 × 2–3 with 5-FU | 54–62 | 94%/94% | 86% | 94% (37 mo) |
| Gerard[12] | 95 (64 mo) | 25 mg/m$^2$/ day bolus d1-4 × 1 with 5-FU | 49–67 | 80%/90% (93% ultimate local control with salvage) | 71% (5Y) | 84% (5Y) |
| Peiffert[13] | 80 (29 mo) | Induction × 2 Concurrent × 2 with 5-FU | 60–65 | —/93% | 73% (3Y) | 86% (3Y) |
| Martenson (ECOG 4292)[14] | 19 | 75 mg/m$^2$ × 2 with 5-FU | 59.4 | —/68% | — | — |
| Hung[15] | 92 (44 mo) | 4 mg/m$^2$/ day continuous infusion 5 d/wk with 5-FU | 55 | 83%/— | 82% (5Y) | 85% (5Y) |

---

**BOX 25-6  RTOG 98-11**

This trial analyzed 598 patients with anal carcinoma who were randomly assigned to receive:

- concurrent 5-FU, mitomycin and RT or
- induction 5-FU and cisplatin followed by concurrent 5-FU, cisplatin, and RT

Preliminary 5-year estimated disease-free survival was 56% for the mitomycin arm and 48% for the cisplatin arm (p = 0.28). Also, the 5-year colostomy rate was 10% for the mitomycin arm and 20% for the cisplatin arm (p = 0.12). Grade 3 and 4 nonhematologic toxicity rates were identical, but hematologic toxicity was 20% higher in the mitomycin arm (67% vs. 27%, p = 0.0004). It was concluded that induction 5-FU/cisplatin failed to improve disease-free survival compared to standard treatment with 5-FU/mitomycin and RT.

Ajani, J A , et al. Intergroup RTOG 98-11: a phase III randomized study of 5-fluorouracil, mitomycin, and radiotherapy versus 5-fluorouracil, cisplatin, and radiotherapy in carcinoma of the anal canal. Proc ASCO 2006: Abstract 4009.

---

**BOX 25-7 | RTOG 92-08**

A single arm study conducted by the RTOG (92-08) enrolled 47 patients with tumors 2 cm or larger to assess the role of 59.6 Gy of pelvic and perineal radiotherapy delivered over 8.5 weeks with a 2-week rest period after the delivery of 36 Gy. Concurrent chemotherapy consisted of 5FU and mitomycin. The results of this trial were compared with RTOG 8704, in which identical chemotherapy was delivered, but RT was given to a lower dose of 45–50.4 Gy with only a 9 Gy boost given in the setting of a positive post-treatment biopsy.

Those treated on 92-08 had markedly lower incidences of grade 3 or higher dermal toxicity; however, they also had higher colostomy rates, a surrogate for local failure, at 1 (23% vs. 6%) and 2 years (30% vs. 7%) compared with RTOG 87-04. For 92-08, the increased toxicities included 26% with greater than grade 3 complications and 20% with hematologic side effects alone. Despite increased toxicity with higher radiotherapy doses (>50 Gy), RT must be given in a continuous fashion since it was thought that the higher local failure and colostomy rates resulted from the 2-week treatment break.

John M, et al. Dose escalation in chemoradiation for anal cancer: preliminary results of RTOG 92-08. *Cancer J Sci Am.* 1996 Jul; 2(4):205.

---

**BOX 25-8 | DOSE ESCALATION FOR ANAL CANCER**

Local control was assessed by Rich et al in 39 patients who had received low dose, continuous infusion of 5-FU with RT, which resulted in a local control rate of 50% for those receiving a total dose of < 45 Gy, 73% for those receiving 50-54 Gy, and 83% for those receiving > 60 Gy. No mitomycin C was given.

Hughes et al retrospectively assessed local control in patients who had received definitive CRT. Local control was 50% for all stages receiving 45–49 Gy, and 90% for those receiving greater than or equal to 55 Gy. These outcomes were not correlated with total 5-FU dose, although continuous infusion 5-FU was delivered without mitomycin.

Rich TA, et al. Chemoradiation for anal cancer: radiation plus continuous infusion of 5-fluorouracil with or without cisplatin. *Radiother Oncol.* 1993 Jun; 27(3): 209-215.
Hughes LL, et al. Radiotherapy for anal cancer: experience from 1979–1987. *Int J Radiat Oncol Biol Phys.* 1989 Dec; 17(6): 1153–1160.

---

tumor volume and to gross nodal metastases.[16] It has been suggested that higher doses of radiation offer improvements in local control.

## PROGNOSTIC FACTORS

Many prognostic factors have been characterized. The most important factors are size of the primary tumor and lymphatic spread of the cancer.

Positive Prognostic Factors:

1. Smaller tumor size
   Tumor size influenced the presence of residual disease after CRT. Tumors less than 5 cm achieved a 93% negative biopsy rate, as compared with 83% for patients with larger tumors (Intergroup trial).
2. Uninvolved lymph nodes (EORTC)
3. Female gender (EORTC)
4. Lack of skin ulceration (EORTC)

The overexpression of p53 has been found to be associated with a trend toward inferior locoregional control and absolute survival for patients managed with definitive CRT, as assessed from the tissue specimens of patients treated on the Intergroup Trial. Patients with p53 overexpression did have a trend toward improved outcome with the use of mitomycin with 5-FU compared to the 5-FU alone.[17]

The 5-year overall survival estimates by stage are:[3,6]

Stage I:     70%–85%
Stage II:    50%–65%
Stage III:   30%–50%
Stage IV:    15%–25%

## RADIATION TECHNIQUE AND BRACHYTHERAPY

Patients should be treated with a three-dimensional conformal plan generated with the use of a CT-simulator. Patients are simulated in a supine position. To reduce dose to small bowel, a prone position is also acceptable. The patient should fill the bladder with approximately 32 ounces of fluid prior to simulation and treatment. A radio-opaque marker should be placed over the anus or the most inferior extent of the tumor.

The initial pelvic field is treated in an identical fashion for all patients. The anus, perineum, internal and external iliac, and inguinal lymph nodes should be delineated and included in this first field. Treatment may be delivered by either an AP-PA or four-field approach. The lateral inguinal lymph nodes may be included in the AP and lateral fields, but not in the PA field.[16] Supplemental inguinal electron fields are utilized to ensure that the inguinal nodes receive full dose. Field margins are described in Table 25-5.

The final 10–14 Gy tumor boost may be designed with the patient in a supine position either with photon fields, using a PA and laterals with wedges, or a four-field approach. Alternatively, an en face field with the patient in a lithotomy position could be considered, using either photons with bolus or a direct electron field of the appropriate energy.

**TABLE 25-5 Pelvic Field Margins**

| Field | Initial | Cone-Down #1 | Cone-Down #2* |
|---|---|---|---|
| Dose | 30.6 Gy (1.8 Gy daily) | 14.4 Gy (1.8 Gy daily) | 10–14 Gy (2 Gy daily) |
| Superior Border | L5-S1 | Inferior border of the SI joints | Primary tumor volume + 2–2.5 cm |
| Inferior Border | Include anus and tumor with 2.5-cm margin | Same | Same |
| Lateral Borders | AP field Include lateral inguinal nodes with 1.5-cm margin PA field Extends 2 cm lateral to the greater sciatic notch | Same | If pelvic nodes are positive, they should be boosted if possible, depending on the dose to small bowel |
| Sum Total Dose | 30.6 Gy | 45 Gy | 55–59 Gy |

*Note:* Cone-down #2 is delivered to patients with T3, T4, N+ patients, or T2 patients with residual disease after 45 Gy.

**FIGURE 25-2** Anal cancer DRR's for an AP/PA plan.

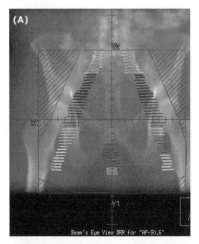

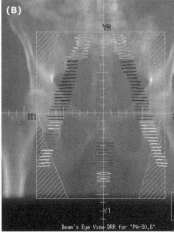

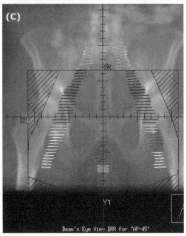

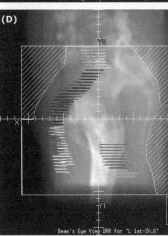

(See Color Plate 8). **(A)** AP pelvic field to 30.6 Gy. **(B)** PA pelvic field to 30.6 Gy. **(C)** AP pelvic fie
to 45 Gy. Femoral head tolerance must be calculated and should not exceed 45 Gy. **(D)** Lateral pel
field to 30.6 Gy.

With regard to the irradiation of the inguinal lymph nodes, these should be included in the A
pelvic field to 36 Gy, at a minimum of 3 cm depth from the anterior surface in all patients with an
carcinoma. It is recommended that nodal volumes be outlined on the simulation CT scan to insu
full-dose coverage. All clinically or radiographically involved lymph nodes should be treated with
2-cm margin. If patients have inguinal metastases, then the involved inguinal region is to

**FIGURE 25-2** (continued)

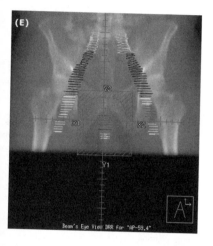

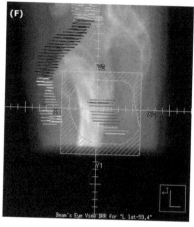

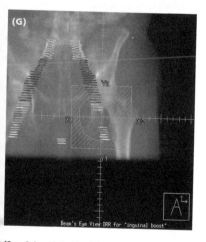

(See Color Plate 8). (E) Example of a 4-field boost to the primary anal cancer. AP field shown. (F) Boost to the primary tumor. Lateral field shown. (G) Boost to positive inguinal lymph node.

included to 45 Gy. A nodal boost dose of 10–14 Gy to the original volume of tumor plus a 2.0–2.5 cm margin would be given.[16]

The lateral inguinal lymph nodes cannot be treated with the PA photon field, so these nodes must be covered using anterior electron fields which are matched with the exit PA field. Alternatively, if electrons are not available, then an AP photon field can be used with necessary bolus to treat the lateral inguinal lymph nodes to full dose. A transmission block would be used to reduce dose through the AP pelvic portion of the field and the remaining dose to the pelvis would be delivered through the PA field. If a four-field approach is used, then the lateral inguinal nodes can be irradiated to full dose by differentially weighting the fields through the AP and laterals. Care must be taken to limit dose to the femoral heads.

In experienced hands, brachytherapy is also a reasonable option for boosting the gross tumor volume using various low dose rate interstitial methods which have had similar local control rates to EBRT and an acceptable toxicity profile.

## MORBIDITY

Combined CRT for anal cancer can result in significant acute and long-term toxicities, which are important to fully discuss with patients.

Acute toxicity is clearly increased with the addition of chemotherapy to RT compared with RT alone as was shown in the UKCCCR trial which described leukopenia ($n = 19$ vs. $n = 0$) and thrombocytopenia ($n = 14$ vs. $n = 0$) with the addition of 5-FU and mitomycin to RT compared to RT alone respectively. Skin, gastrointestinal, and genitourinary toxicity were also increased. Specifically one acute side effect that should be expected is confluent moist desquamation, which may necessitate a brief treatment break. Also, patients may experience fatigue, diarrhea, nausea, vomiting, dysuria, and urinary frequency. Rarely, hematochezia, hematuria, or vaginal bleeding may occur.

Long-term toxicities may include intermittent, chronic anorectal bleeding, fibrosis and telangactasia of the perineum, chronic diarrhea, anal stricture, vaginal stenosis, vaginal atrophy, anal ulcers, anal incontinence or fistula necessitating colostomy (2% in the Intergroup Trial), tissue necrosis, small bowel damage/obstruction, sterility, impotence, leg or genital edema, second malignancy, pelvic fracture, and osteoradionecrosis of the femoral head. Overall, the chance of a serious or life-threatening complication during or after CMT is small, but patients should be fully informed of the risks of treatment.

## FOLLOW-UP

Although the UKCCCR, EORTC, and Intergroup trials called for an initial course of treatment of 45–50 Gy followed by a 6-week break to assess tumor regression (clinically or with biopsy), most oncologists no longer adhere to this formal break from CRT. The rationale for foregoing the planned break from therapy is to improve outcome, as some series have shown that shorter treatment times of less than 40 days improve results.[18] Likewise, gaps of longer than 5 weeks may also correlate with inferior locoregional control.[19]

Patients should be re-evaluated 8 to 12 weeks after the completion of CRT with a digital rectal examination (Figure 25-3).[20]

The routine assessment of patients who have had complete remission is performed every 3 to 6 months for 5 years. At each visit, the physician should perform:

- Digital rectal examination
- Inguinal lymph node palpation
- Anoscopy
- CT scan of the abdomen and pelvis (should be done every 6 months for 5 years)

If local recurrence is discovered, APR should be performed with inguinal lymph node dissection in the setting of positive groin nodes. RT may be considered if the only evidence of local recurrence is in the inguinal lymph nodes, and these have not been previously treated. In the unfortunate scenario that distant metastases are found during follow-up, then cisplatin-based chemotherapy or a clinical trial should be offered to the patient.[20]

# ANAL MARGIN

Anal margin tumors arise from the skin at or distal to the squamous-mucocutaneous junction. There have been varied definitions for the anal canal itself, and the definition of the anal margin has also been different among authors. One commonly used definition states that the anal margin extends to a 5 cm radius around the anal verge. Anal margin cancers are more likely to spread to inguinal lymph nodes and rarely spread to pelvic nodes. The overall risk of lymph node involvement is greater with anal canal compared to anal margin cancers.

The histology of these tumors includes squamous cell carcinomas, Bowen's disease (squamous cell carcinoma *in situ*), basal cell carcinomas, verrucous carcinomas, melanomas, and Paget's disease (adenocarcinoma *in situ*). These tumors are staged as skin cancers. The initial diagnostic workup and evaluation of these cases should be approached in an identical manner to carcinomas of the anal canal.

In general, patients with squamous cell carcinoma of the anal margin have a high chance of cure with sphincter preservation with CRT or RT alone. For T1 tumors that are well differentiated, wide local excision can be chosen with adequate margins of 1 cm or more. If margins are inadequate, the lesion should be re-excised or treated with local RT- and 5-FU-based chemotherapy. Lymph nodes are only irradiated for T1 lesions if they are clinically positive. In the UKCCR trial, 23% of patients had a diagnosis of anal margin carcinoma and were managed in a similar fashion to anal canal carcinomas. Therefore, T2-T4 lesions should be managed with definitive CRT with 5-FU, mitomycin, and RT as in the paradigm for anal canal carcinoma.[20,21]

# ANAL MELANOMA

Anal melanomas originate in the mucosa of the anal canal where melanocytes are present. Anal melanomas account for 24% of mucosal melanomas but are less than 0.5% of all melanomas.[22] This disease is known to have a dismal prognosis with propensity for early dissemination to liver, lungs, and brain and 5-year survival of 20%.[22] In a Swedish series, one third of patients had either regional or distant metastases at diagnosis.[23] Patients commonly present with symptoms of rectal bleeding as with the squamous cell histology of anal cancer.

The standard of care in the past has been APR; however, local excision has been suggested as a plausible option for management of these patients, since there is no need to subject patients to an APR in light of the dismal prognosis and the lack of a known survival benefit with radical surgery. However, local excision alone is associated with higher rates of local recurrence compared with patients undergoing APR (28% (APR) vs. 58% (WLE)).[24] Most patients, however, develop distant metastases at the time of local failure, but even local failures can adversely affect a patient's remaining quality-of-life.

In the setting of anal melanoma without evidence of distant spread, it is quite sound to consider local excision followed by adjuvant RT to allow for anal sphincter preservation (Box 25-9).

**FIGURE 25-3** Evaluation after completion of CRT.

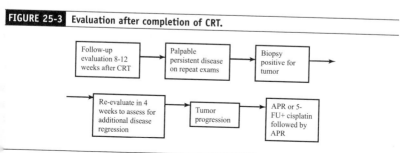

**BOX 25-9** MANAGEMENT OF ANAL MELANOMA

In this series, 23 patients with localized anal melanoma were treated with hypofractionated adjuvant RT after wide local excision (WLE). WLE was carried out to microscopically negative margins in the majority of patients and nodal dissection was performed for patients with documented regional nodal disease. If no nodal disease was suspected clinically, a sentinel lymph node dissection was performed. Five fractions of 600 cGy were delivered twice a week to a pelvic field encompassing the lateral inguinal lymph nodes. The 5-year overall survival rate was 31%, 5-year disease-free survival was 37%, and 5-year local nodal control rate was 74%. No patient had a locoregional failure as the sole site of failure, and no patient required salvage APR. Patients with nodal disease at presentation had a 5-year disease-free survival of 0%. This approach with sphincter-sparing local excision and adjuvant RT was found to be well tolerated and allowed for local control, while avoiding the morbidity of APR.

Ballo M, et al. Sphincter-sparing local excision and adjuvant radiation for anal rectal melanoma. *J Clin Oncol.* 2002 Dec 1;20(23): 4555–4558.

## ANAL ADENOCARCINOMA

Primary anal adenocarcinoma accounts for up to 20% of all anal malignancies but may also result from distal extension of a primary rectal carcinoma into the anal canal. APR has been the mainstay of therapy. These types of cancers are known to have high rates of pelvic failure and distant metastasis when compared with similarly staged patients with epidermoid histological features treated with definitive CRT. Five-year local failure and distant disease failure rates were 54% vs. 18%, 66% vs. 10% for adenocarcinomas versus epidermoid carcinomas, respectively.[25] Although there is a paucity of data regarding the optimal management of these cancers, on the basis of these failure patterns, they should probably be approached in a manner similar to rectal adenocarcinoma with primary surgery. CRT could be incorporated neoadjuvantly to maximize pelvic disease control with chemotherapy delivered postoperatively to address the problem of micrometastatic disease.[25] Other series have approached these patients with combined CRT and have acknowledged the need for aggressive management of these tumors.[26]

## HIV-POSITIVE PATIENTS

HIV-positive patients are at increased risk for HPV-related anal carcinoma due to viral immunosuppression. Anal cancer is not currently recognized as an AIDS-defining illness. Anal dysplasia, analogous to cervical dysplasia, has also been referred to as anal intra-epithelial neoplasia (AIN) or anal squamous intra-epithelial lesions (ASIL). ASIL can be divided into low- and high-grade squamous intra-epithelial lesions (LSIL or HSIL) with HSIL being considered the precursor lesion to anal cancer (Box 25-10).[27]

ASIL screening should also be performed for women with a history of cervical, vaginal, or vulvar cancer and for transplant recipients. Treatment options for ASIL include topical treatments or surgical or laser ablation.[27]

**BOX 25-10** SCREENING FOR ANAL SQUAMOUS INTRA-EPITHELIAL LESIONS

Screening of HIV-positive homosexual and bisexual men for ASIL and anal squamous cell carcinoma with anal Pap tests offers quality-adjusted life expectancy benefits at costs comparable with other accepted clinical preventative measures.

Goldie S, et al. The clinical effectiveness and cost-effectiveness of screening for anal squamous intra-epithelial lesions in homosexual and bisexual HIV-positive men. *JAMA.* 1999 May 19; 281(19): 1822–1829.

## FIGURE 25-4  Treatment overview.

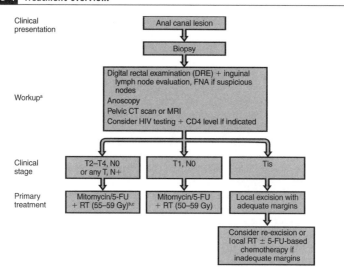

beloff et al, *Clinical Oncology*, 3rd Ed, Chapter 82: Anal Cancer, 6 1967–1980, Copyright Elsevier, 2004.

Patients who have HIV can be treated effectively and safely with CRT. Hesitancy to administer CRT in HIV-positive patients stems from concerns about lowered blood counts during treatment and a poorer ability to recover from treatment toxicity in the face of chronic immunosuppression. With the use of highly active antiretroviral therapy (HAART), CRT may be given safely at conventional doses in HIV-positive patients with comparable complete response rates to HIV-negative patients. However, for patients with CD4 counts less than or equal to 200, increased morbidity may occur requiring prolonged treatment breaks.[28] In this population with low CD4 counts, decreasing chemotherapy doses, not delivering mitomycin, or giving a lower dose treatment with 30 Gy may be considered.[29]

## FUTURE DIRECTIONS

Given the recent approval of Cetuximab in combination with radiation therapy for squamous cell carcinoma of the head and neck, biologic agents such as this one may also be given consideration for future trials. Also, the use of intensity-modulated radiation therapy (IMRT) may further permit escalation of radiotherapy doses while minimizing treatment toxicity but still requires further investigation.

## REFERENCES

1. Jemal A, Siegel R, Ward E, et al. Cancer Statistics, 2007. *CA Cancer J Clin* 57: 43–66, 2007.
2. Jemal A, Thomas A, Murray T, et al. Cancer Statistics, 2002. *CA Cancer J Clin* 52: 23–47, 2002.

3. Myerson RJ, Karnell LH, Menck HR. The National Cancer Database report on carcinoma of the anus. *Cancer* 80:805–815, 1997.
4. American Joint Committee on Cancer, Anal Canal: In Greene FL, Page DL, Fleming ID, et al, (eds) *AJCC Cancer Staging Handbook,* ed Sixth, Philadelphia: Lipincott Raven, 2002, 139–144.
5. Minsky BD, Hoffman, JP, Kelsen DP. Cancer of the Anal Region. In *Cancer Principles and Practice of Oncology* ed Sixth, (DeVita VT, Hellman S, Rosenberg SA eds), Philadelphia: Lippincott, Williams, & Wilkins, 2001, 1319–1342.
6. Klas JV, Rothenberger DA, Wong WD, et al. Malignant tumors of the anal canal: the spectrum of disease, treatment, and outcomes. *Cancer* 85:1686–1693, 1999.
7. Greenall MJ, Quan SH, Urmacher C, et al. Treatment of epidermoid carcinoma of the anal canal. *Surg Gynecol Obstet* 161:509–517, 1985.
8. Daling JR, Weiss NS, Hislop TG, et al. Sexual practices, sexually transmitted diseases, and the incidence of anal cancer. *N Eng J Med* 317:973–977, 1987.
9. Daling JR, Madeleine MM, Johnson LG, et al. Human papillomavirus, smoking, and sexual practices in the etiology of anal cancer. *Cancer* 101:270–280, 2004.
10. Ryan DR, Compton CC, Mayer RJ. Carcinoma of the anal canal. *N Eng J Med* 342: 792–800, 2000.
11. Doci R, Zucali R, La Monica G, et al. Primary chemo-radiation therapy with fluorouracil and cis-platin for cancer of the anus: results in 35 consecutive patients. *J Clin Oncol* 14: 3121–3125, 1996.
12. Gerard JP, Ayzac L, Hun D, et al. Treatment of anal canal carcinoma with high-dose radiation therapy and concomitant fluorouracil-cisplatinum. Long-term results in 95 patients. *Radiother Oncol* 46: 249–256, 1998.
13. Peiffert D, Giovannini M, Ducreux M, et al. High-dose radiation therapy and neoadjuvant plus concomitant chemotherapy with 5-fluorouracil and cisplatin in patients with locally advanced squamous cell anal canal cancer: final results of a phase II study. *Ann Oncol* 12: 397–404, 2001.
14. Martenson JA, Lipsitz SR, Wagner H, et al. Initial results of a phase II trial of high-dose radia-tion therapy, 5-fluorouracil, and cisplatin for patients with anal cancer (E4292): an Eastern Cooperative Oncology Group study. *Int J Radiat Oncol Biol Phys* 35:745–749, 1996.
15. Hung A, Crane C, Delclos M, et al. Cisplatin-based combined modality therapy for anal carci-noma: a wider therapeutic index. *Cancer* 97:1195–202, 2003.
16. Radiation Therapy Oncology Group RTOG 98-11: A phase III randomized study of 5-fluorouracil, mitomycin-C, and radiotherapy in carcinoma of the anal canal. http://www.rtog.org/members/protocols/98-11/9811.pdf.
17. Bonin SR, Pajak TF, Russell AH, et al. Overexpression of p53 protein and outcome of patients treated with chemo-radiation for carcinoma of the anal canal: a report of randomized trial RTOG 87-04. Radiation Therapy Oncology Group. *Cancer* 85:1226–1233, 1999.
18. Constantinou EC, Daly W, Fung CY, et al. Time-dose considerations in the treatment of anal can-cer. *Int J Radiat Oncol Biol Phys* 39:651–657, 1997.
19. Weber DC, Kurtz JM, Allal AS. The impact of gap duration on local control in anal canal carci-noma treated by split-course radiotherapy and concomitant chemotherapy. *Int J Radiat Oncol Biol Phys* 50: 675–680, 2001.
20. National Comprehensive Cancer Network: Practice guidelines in oncology: anal carcinoma. http://www.nccn.org/professionals/physician_gls/PDF/anal.pdf
21. Newlin HE, Zlotecki RA, Morris CG. Squamous cell carcinoma of the anal margin. *J Surg Oncol* 86: 55–62, 2004.
22. Chang AE, Karnell LH, Menck HR. The National Cancer Database report on cutaneous and non-cutaneous melanoma: a summary of 84,836 cases from the past decade. The American College

of Surgeons Commission on Cancer and the American Cancer Society. *Cancer* 83: 1664–1678, 1989.

23. Goldman S, Glimelius B, Pahlman L. Anorectal malignant melanoma in Sweden. Report of 49 patients. *Dis Colon Rectum* 33:874–877, 1990.

24. Ross M, Pezzi C, Pezzi T, et al. Patterns of failure in anorectal melanoma. A guide to surgical therapy. *Arch Surg* 125:313–316, 1990.

25. Papagikos M, Crane CH, Skibber J, et al. Chemo-radiation for adenocarcinoma of the anus. *Int J Radiat Oncol Biol Phys* 55:669–678, 2003.

26. Beal KP, Wong D, Guillem JG, et al. Primary adenocarcinoma of the anus treated with combined modality therapy. *Dis Colon Rectum* 46:1320–1324, 2003.

27. Palefsky JM, Cranston RD. Anal squamous intra-epithelial lesions (ASIL): diagnosis, screening, and treatment. www.uptodate.com.

28. Hoffman R, Welton ML, Klencke B, et al. The significance of pretreatment CD4 count on the outcome and treatment tolerance of HIV-positive patients with anal cancer. *Int J Radiat Oncol Biol Phys* 44:127–131, 1999.

29. Peddada AV, Smith DE, Rao AR, et al. Chemotherapy and low-dose radiotherapy in the treatment of HIV-infected patients with carcinoma of the anal canal. *Int J Radiat Oncol Biol Phys* 37: 1101–1105, 1997.

# 26

# Cancers of the Bladder and Kidney

*Michael G. Chang, MD, PhD*
*Michael P. Hagan, MD, PhD*

## BLADDER CANCER

### Epidemiology and Risk Factors

The American Cancer Society estimates that approximately 67,000 new cases of bladder cancer were diagnosed in the United States in 2007. Occurring more frequently in men than in women (3:1), bladder cancer is annually responsible for more than 13,000 deaths. The lifetime risk for bladder cancer is 1/28 for U.S. males.[1,2]

The two principal risk factors for bladder cancer are smoking by itself or in combination with occupational exposure to arylamines, especially benzidine and beta-naphthylamine. Arylamine-DNA adducts are enhanced by cigarette smoking and are substantially modified by the enzymes glutathione S transferase and N-acetyltransferase, which are genetically controlled. Less well established are the specific risks associated with those occupations which involve exposure to aromatic amines either in the use or production of dyes, paint, leather, rubber, plastics, organic chemicals, and textiles. Well documented increases in bladder cancer for long-haul truckers[3] and aluminum workers[4,5] are thought to be caused by exposure to the combustion products of organic materials. In all, cigarette smoking is estimated to be responsible for 50% of bladder cancers in North America and occupational exposures as much as 25%.[6,7]

Other risk factors for bladder cancer include race, age, gender, chronic inflammation, family history of bladder cancer, persistent urachal remnant, bladder extrophy, and prior exposure to ionizing radiation.

Of the factors mentioned, chronic inflammation substantially increases the risk of squamous cell cancers of the bladder. Squamous cell histology is particularly high in two populations: residents of the Nile River Valley where chronic bladder inflammation is secondary to endemic schistosomiasis and patients with spinal cord injury, where squamous cell carcinoma is associated with long-term catheter use. Squamous cell carcinomas may also present in patients who experience urinary calculi or have bladder diverticula.

## Pathology and Natural History

In North America, more than 90% of bladder cancers are of transitional cell origin. Squamous cell carcinomas account for approximately 5%, while <1% of bladder cancers are adenocarcinomas. The latter are more frequently associated (33%) with a persistent urachal remnant.[8]

Approximately 80% of bladder cancers are superficial (Tis, Ta, or T1) at the initial presentation. Of these, 60%–75% will be solitary tumors. Clinical evidence argues that there are two distinct pathways for transitional carcinoma. The most likely observed of these involves papillary growth, which is initially superficial, infrequently is of high grade or associated with CIS, and when found to be invasive is of higher curative potential. The second and more aggressive pattern is more likely to invade the muscularis propria, is commonly associated with severe dysplasia or CIS, and is at presentation more likely to be regionally spread or metastatic.[9]

Squamous cell carcinomas are frequently large and deeply invasive, even though moderate or well differentiated. Their microscopic appearance is similar to squamous cell carcinomas from other anatomy, displaying metaplasia (leukoplakia). Extravesicular spread is common, while distant metastasis occurs in only 10% at initial presentation.[10,11]

## Workup

### CBC

Chemistries: Basic metabolic profile and liver panel
CT or MRI of the abdomen and pelvis
Imaging of the upper urinary tracts: IVP, CT, or MRI-urography
Bone scan (after positive alkaline phosphatase)
Cystoscopy and examination under anesthesia include the following:
    TURBT
    Biopsies of the tumor base, suspected sites of disease, four-quadrant biopsies, biopsy of the prostatic urethral mucosa, and the prostate parenchyma if indicated
    Urine cytology

## Staging

**TABLE 26-1 TNM Staging Bladder**

| | |
|---|---|
| TX | Primary cannot be assessed |
| T0 | No evidence of primary tumor |
| Ta | Tumor limited to the mucosa |
| Tis | Carcinoma *in-situ*; flat tumor |
| T1 | Tumor invades sub-epithelial connective tissue |
| T2 | Tumor invades muscle |
| pT2a | Tumor invades superficial muscle (inner half) |
| pT2b | Tumor invades deep muscle (outer half) |
| T3 | Tumor invade perivesicular tissues |
| pT3a | Microscopic invasion |
| pT3b | Macroscopic invasion (extra-vesical mass) |
| T4 | Tumor invades any of the following: prostate, uterus, vagina, pelvic wall, abdominal wall |
| T4a | Tumor invades prostate, uterus, or vagina |
| T4b | Tumor invades pelvic wall or abdominal wall |
| | Regional lymph nodes are those within the true pelvis |
| NX | Regional lymph nodes cannot be assessed |

TABLE 26-1 (continued)

| | |
|---|---|
| N0 | Regional lymph nodes are not involved |
| N1 | Metastasis in a single lymph node, ≤2 cm in its greatest dimension |
| N2 | Metastasis in a single lymph node, >2 cm but ≤5 cm in its greatest dimension; or metastases in multiple lymph nodes, none greater than 5 cm |
| N3 | Metastasis in a lymph node greater than 5 cm |
| MX | Distant metastasis cannot be assessed |
| M0 | No evidence of distant metastasis |
| M1 | Distant metastasis |

Used with the permission of the American Joint Committee on Cancer (AJCC), Chicago, Illinois. The original source for this material is the *AJCC Cancer Staging Manual*, Sixth Edition (2002) published by Springer-Verlag New York, www.springeronline.com.

## Management

### Superficial Disease (Tis, Ta, T1)

The role for radiation therapy in the treatment of superficial transitional carcinoma, never strong, today is at best unclear. Standard treatment for Tis-T1 disease in North America begins with TURBT and fulguration. Intravesical immuno- or chemotherapy follows for high-grade, multifocal, Tis associated or recurrent disease. Unresponsive superficial tumors may require cystectomy. Recent efforts have been aimed at a tailored approach to treatment of superficial transitional cell carcinoma through stratification based upon the individual's risk for recurrence.[12]

TABLE 26-2 **TNM Stage Grouping for the Bladder**

| | |
|---|---|
| I | T1 N0 M0 |
| II | T2a N0 M0 |
| | T2b N0 M0 |
| III | T3a N0 M0 |
| | T3b N0 M0 |
| | T4a N0 M0 |
| IV | T4b Any N0 M0 |
| | Any T N1-3 M0 |
| | Any T Any N M1 |

Used with the permission of the American Joint Committee on Cancer (AJCC), Chicago, Illinois. The original source for this material is the *AJCC Cancer Staging Manual*, Sixth Edition (2002) published by Springer-Verlag New York, www.springeronline.com.

High-grade T1 tumors, however, owing to their high rate of locoregional recurrence, have been separately examined.[12–14] Given that 20%–30% of clinically-staged G3 T1 tumors are actually muscle invasive, combined chemo-irradiation may offer improved local control over intravesical therapies following TURBT. Although no randomized trial of chemo-irradiation versus intravesical therapy has been reported, the Ehrlangen group reported 5-year results for invasive progression and overall survival, 15% and 75%, respectively following chemo-irradiation (56 Gy + cisplatin or carboplatin). Table 26-3 shows that these results compare well with those from TURBT followed by intravesical treatment. Whether late recurrences are less frequent after adjuvant irradiation of G3T1 tumors remains to be established.

### Muscle-Invasive Disease (T2-T4a)

#### Radiation therapy with sensitizing chemotherapy or alone

Despite a 30% rate of pelvic nodal failures for pathologic T-stages >T2, cystectomy remains the standard therapy for nonmetastatic invasive transitional carcinoma in North America. Now that bladder conservation trials demonstrate that tri-modal therapy (TURBT followed by chemo-irradiation[15,16]) produces survival results equivalent to recent cystectomy data,[17] definitive chemo-irradiation or irradiation alone are generally reserved for patients who refuse or are medically unfit for cystectomy.

**TABLE 26-3  Radiation Therapy following TURBT for High-Grade T1 Transitional Cell Carcinoma**

| | | 5-year Results | | |
|---|---|---|---|---|
| Source | n | Progressive Recurrences (%) | Overall Survival (%) | Bladder Intact (%) |
| ChemoRT (Ehrlangen[18]) | 84 | 13 | 64 | 51 |
| RT alone (Edinburgh[19]) | 37 | 44[a] | 54 | |
| Brachy/EBRT (Netherlands[20]) | 14 | 30[a] | 75[b] | 71[b] |
| Intravesical Tx (5-series[21–25]) | 360 | 15–33 | 72[c] | 51[c] |

a. Total local recurrences.
b. 10-year results.
c. Weighted average values

**TABLE 26-4  Radiation Therapy Alone for Muscle-Invasive Bladder Cancer**

| Source | n | Stage | Overall Survival (5-yr) |
|---|---|---|---|
| Edinburgh[26] | 889 | T2-T4 | 36% |
| London Hospital[27] | 182 | T2-T3 | 40% |
| Norwegian Radium Hosp.[28] | 308 | T2-T3 | 24% |
| Princess Margaret Hosp.[29] | 121 | T2-T4 | 32% |
| Cystectomy, USC[17] | 633 | pT2-pT4 | 48% |

Data from multiple large series, shown in Table 26-4, have reported the results of radiation therapy generally performed in the 1980s. Five-year survival rates vary between ~25 and 40%. For T2-T3 tumors, local control with radiation alone is ~40%, but decreases to 20%–30% within 5 years. Both the rates of complete response and local control after 5 years are improved to approximately 60% and 45%, respectively, when irradiation is preceded by a complete TURBT.[15,16] As shown in Table 26-5, the addition of radio-sensitizing chemotherapy, most frequently via cisplatin, 5-fluorouracil, or taxol, is required to achieve overall survival results equivalent to cystectomy.

As recently shown in phase III testing reported by the National Cancer Institute of Canada, combined chemo-irradiation also significantly reduces pelvic failures.[30]

*Patient selection*

Patients considered for radical irradiation with or without sensitizing chemotherapy should have pathologically-proven TCC with evidence of invasion into or through the muscularis propria. In addition, the following should apply:

1. Workup completed as described
2. AJCC stage T2-T4a Nx-N1 and M0
3. Zubrod performance score of ≤2
4. Pretreatment TURBT completed as subsequently described within 6 weeks of the initiation of treatment
5. Workup reveals adequate renal and liver function, adequate marrow reserves, and freedom from severe comorbid disease. The latter include

**TABLE 26-5  The Importance of Tri-modal Therapy**

| Treatment 5-year Results | Local Control | Overall Survival |
|---|---|---|
| RT alone[31] | 44 | 38 |
| TURBT + RT[16] | 57 | 40 |
| TURBT + Chemo-R[15,16] | 67 | 58 |

inflammatory bowel disease, coronary artery disease associated with recent myocardial infarction or unstable angina, and class III congestive heart failure. In addition, patients who have severe symptoms of chronic obstructive pulmonary disease, diabetes mellitus, or collagen vascular diseases may not be fit for combined chemo-irradiation.

6. Evaluation by medical oncologist

---

**BOX 26-1** | **CONCURRENT CISPLATIN MAY IMPROVE PELVIC CONTROL OF LOCALLY ADVANCED BLADDER CANCER WITH PREOPERATIVE OR DEFINITIVE RADIATION**

Ninety-nine patients (T2 to T4b TCC), planned for either definitive radiotherapy or precystectomy radiotherapy, were randomized to receive cisplatin (100 mg/m$^2$) at 2-week intervals for three cycles concurrent with pelvic radiation, or radiation alone. After a median follow-up of 6.5 years, 25 of 48 control patients first recurred in the pelvis, compared with 15 of 51 cisplatin-treated patients (P = .036).

Coppin CM, Gospodarowicz MK, James K, et al. Improved local control of invasive bladder cancer by concurrent cisplatin and preoperative or definitive radiation. The National Cancer Institute of Canada Clinical Trials Group. *J Clin Oncol* (1996). 14: 2901–2907.

---

*TURBT*

Cystoscopic evaluation by a urologic surgeon will include TURBT as thorough as is safely possible and tumor mapping. Additionally, endoscopic evaluation should include biopsies of the tumor base, cold-cup biopsies of other suspicious areas, four-quadrant bladder and prostatic urethral mucosal biopsies, bimanual examination, and barbotage cytology.

*Chemotherapy*

Nonprotocol chemo-irradiation should be limited to cisplatin, paclitaxel, or 5-fluorouracil. Low-dose cisplatin (35mg/m$^2$) or paclitaxel (50mg/m$^2$) can be given as weekly outpatient treatments. Premedications typically include dexamethasone, diphenhydramine, and an H-2 blocker. Patients may require anti-emetics. Weekly, laboratory evaluations are used to monitor myelosuppression, hepatic and renal function, as well as general metabolic response. Patients are examined weekly by both the medical oncologist and radiation oncologist for treatment-related toxicities.

*Radiation*

**Patient setup.** Patient positioning for daily treatment is complicated primarily by the mobility of the bladder. In addition, during the treatment course an acute cystitis will develop, limiting the compliance of the bladder wall and temporarily reducing bladder capacity. As a result of these considerations, patients should be planned and treated in the supine position with an empty bladder. Depending on tumor morphology, the planning CT may be improved by the addition of 30–50 cc of dilute contrast. Patients are immobilized only by soft thigh/leg supports using foam wedges or an alpha cradle. During local boost irradiation, bladder distention may improve protection of the uninvolved bladder. Most patients will tolerate a comfortably full bladder for this purpose. Tumor localization with even this modest level of bladder filling should be verified via tomographic or KV-imaging daily prior to treatment.

**Dose.** Definitive irradiation with or without radio-sensitizing chemotherapy should deliver 45 Gy to small pelvic fields followed by a local boost of 20–23 Gy to the tumor. Most commonly, daily fractions of 1.8–2.0 Gy are used during both treatment phases.

**Use of altered fractionation.** A review of the available radiotherapy series supports a continuing dose response beyond the range of doses currently used for definitive treatment. Maciejewski[32] estimated the 50% tumor control dose (TCD50) for bladder to be 63.3 Gy with a decrease in tumor control from 50% to 5% when the delivery time is extended by 2 weeks. Accelerated repopulation appeared to begin after 5 to 6 weeks of therapy.[32] Since the most commonly reported dose schedules employ final dose in the range of 60–65 Gy delivered in 30–36 fractions, the potential significance of these estimates is apparent. As a result, a number of centers now routinely use both radio-sensitizing concomitant chemotherapy and accelerated fractionation for radical irradiation of the bladder. Abbreviated schedules have been developed and tested, which respect the tolerance of bowel and bladder. An optimal treatment schedule for those patients who can attend twice daily therapy would be 45 Gy delivered in 25 daily fractions to small pelvis fields combined with concomitant boost of 1.5 Gy to the tumor for the final 13 treatments. Weekly cisplatin (35 mg/m$^2$) should be used during treatment. Using this schedule, the complete response rate should be in the range of 60%–75% and associated with 45%–60% survival.[16,33]

**Target volume.** The clinical target volume (CTV) is delineated based upon pretreatment imaging (preferably MRI) and findings at cystoscopy. Regardless of the quality of this information, organ motion predominates as the most significant source of error in the planning target volume (PTV). Organ motion (a PTV consideration) and the accuracy of target delineation (a CTV consideration) also vary regionally within the bladder.[34] As a result, estimates of margin adequacy (CTV+PTV) have been as large as 4 cm for anterior lesions in the distended bladder.[35,36] More commonly, however, combined CTV+PTV margins of 1.5–2.0 cm are used for lesions limited to the trigone and bladder neck, while 2.0–2.5-cm margins are required for lesions involving bladder dome or lateral walls.[35–37] A typical four-field plan for two-phase treatment is shown in Figure 26-1(AB).

**Follow-up.** After definitive irradiation, patients are examined for recurrence quarterly in the first 2 years and thereafter at 6-month intervals. Each visit includes cystoscopy with biopsy as necessary and urine cytology. CT or MR imaging of the abdomen and pelvis should be performed at 6-month intervals, while chest films are examined at each follow-up visit. Chemistries include basic metabolic and liver panels, hemogram, and urinalysis.

Locoregional recurrences typically present with worsening frequency (65%), burning dysuria (40%), hematuria (15%), and pelvic or flank pain (more common with regional recurrences or recurrence in the upper tracts (30%). Painless gross hematuria throughout micturation is consistent with recurrence in the bladder or upper tract, while hematuria at the beginning of the stream likely reflects bleeding from the prostate or urethra. Evidence of distant metastases include weight loss, early satiety, nausea, dyspnea, fever, and bone pain.

Adenocarcinoma

One third of adenocarcinomas of the bladder arise from urachal remnants. A recent review of their CT appearance found 92% to be invasive, 88% to have a predominant extravesicular mass, and 48% presenting with evidence of distant disease. Although these tumors have been reported to be less responsive to radiation than TCC, at presentation they are frequently more advanced than TCC. Regardless, several series report long-term survivors treated only with irradiation at conventional doses. It is, therefore, likely that adenocarcinomas of the bladder do not differ substantially in their radio-sensitivity from adenocarcinomas involving other tumor sites. Their frequent involvement of the bladder dome, however, presents a highly mobile target, may extend superficially and by involving the expansile portion of the bladder, increases the morbidity of radiation treatment.

*Squamous Cell Carcinoma*

Chronic irritation increases the likelihood for the development of squamous cell carcinoma (SCC) of the bladder. Patients who require continuous catheterization due to a neurogenic bladder and those chronically infected with schistosomes experience a significantly increased risk for this

**FIGURE 26-1A** Isodose coverage for small pelvic fields.

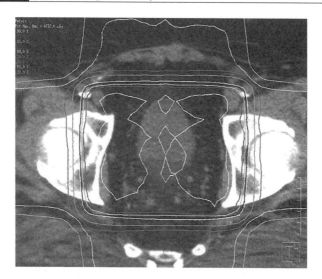

**(See Color Plate 9).** Note that the anterior coverage includes the entire bladder plus margin, but does not provide comprehensive coverage for the exteral or internal iliac nodal chains. The patient has voided prior to the simulation.

**FIGURE 26-1B** Bladder tumor boost volume.

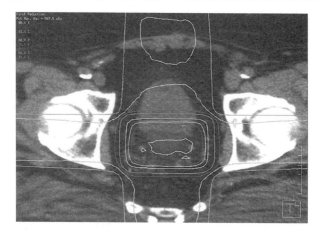

**(See Color Plate 10).** Tumor contour includes imaging evidence of involvement augmented by the urologist's tumor diagram from the pretreatment cystoscopy. Though prior to the simulation the patient has voided, still much of the anterior portion of the bladder has been excluded from the high-dose region.

disease. Though Quilty and Duncan[38] found that SCC of the bladder responds to radiation as monomodality treatment with a dose response similar to TCC, survival was poor (3-year survival of 18%). The majority of series show that the risk of pelvic failure for SCC is substantially increased and associated with low survival. For both bilharzial and nonbilharzial SCC, 75% of failures are locoregional. Trials of preoperative irradiation for SCC bladder cancers, employing various dose schedules (20–50 Gy), have shown improved local control and survival for T3/T4 tumors, tumors which are high grade, and those that are down-staged after irradiation.[39,40] For this histology, cystectomy remains the primary treatment with neo-adjuvant irradiation of the pelvis considered prior to surgery for locally advanced disease.

### Attempted bladder conservation

The prime consideration for the use of irradiation in this setting is organ-sparing with no associated reduction in overall survival. Contemporary, tri-modality treatment aimed at attempted conservation of the bladder results in ~75% of survivors, staged T2–T4a, maintaining a functional tumor-free bladder with no reduction in either overall or cause-specific survivals.

---

**BOX 26-2** **RESULTS OF SELECTIVE BLADDER PRESENTATION**

After median follow-up of 6.7 years, 5- and 10-year overall survival rates were 54% and 36%, respectively. The 5- and 10-year disease-specific survival rates were 63% and 59% (Stage T2, 74% and 66%; Stage T3-T4a, 53% and 52%), respectively. The pelvic failure rate was 8% and no patient required cystectomy due to bladder morbidity. Approximately two thirds of treated patients maintained a functional bladder. These 10-year survival rates are comparable with the results reported for radical cystectomy for patients of similar clinical and pathologic stage.

Shipley WU, Kaufman DS, Zehr E, et al. Selective bladder preservation by combined modality protocol treatment: long-term outcomes of 190 patients with invasive bladder cancer. *Urology* 60: (2002). 62–67; discussion 67–68.

---

**Tri-modal therapy.** As shown, radiation alone controls ~40% of tumors staged cT2-T4. The addition of well timed, aggressive TURBT and radio-sensitizing chemotherapy increases this value to 60%–75%. Keep in mind, however, that the rate of local control following cystectomy is ~95%. Therefore, bladder-conserving therapy must default to cystectomy without compromising either survival or the surgical approach. A flowchart for this treatment method is shown in Figure 26-2.

### Patient selection

1. Candidates for attempted bladder conservation must be medically fit for and agreeable to radical cystectomy.
2. Compatible tumor characteristics.
   a. Pathologist-confirmed invasion of the muscle propria
   b. No second focus of tumor staged ≥T1
   c. No evidence of carcinoma involving the upper tracts
   d. No lymphadenopathy (biopsy confirmed when required)
   e. No associated hydronephrosis
3. Have a functional bladder (indicated by a ≥2-hour daytime voiding interval and satisfactorily managed nocturia; patients whose *AUA symptom score* is ≥19 should be excluded)
4. Acceptable for combined chemo-irradiation
   a. Adequate renal function
   b. Acceptable hemogram

**FIGURE 26-2** Flow chart for TURBT followed by chemo-irradiation for bladder conservation.

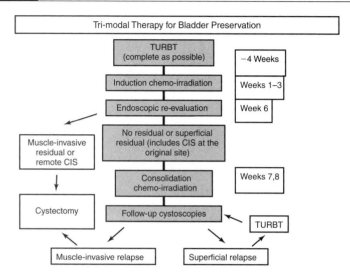

Note the delay between induction therapy and endoscopic re-evaluation presumes twice daily irradiation during induction. Although continued resorption of tumor has been reported for up to 8 weeks following 40 Gy, re-evaluation in the sixth week is planned secondary to concern for tumor repopulation.

*Organization for success*

Although bladder-conservation has become a standard treatment for muscle-invasive carcinomas of the bladders (*National Comprehensive Cancer Network, Inc. 2005/2006: NCCN v.1 2006*), the inclusion of these patients on national clinical trials will help refine treatment parameters. This is especially true of current efforts by the Radiation Therapy Oncology Group (RTOG) to examine the use of combination chemotherapy during induction.

*Transurethral Resection of Bladder Tumor (TURBT)*

1. The TURBT should accomplish the following:
   a. Maximal resection of the tumor
   b. Selective biopsies of the remaining bladder
   c. Mapping of the sites of tumor and elective biopsies
   d. Provide barbotage sample for cytology
2. Multidisciplinary evaluation of the patient should be initiated promptly following TURBT. Induction chemotherapy is more likely to be successful if initiated within 6 weeks. A re-TURBT should be considered if the delay is longer.

*Bladder-conserving treatment*

1. **Induction.** Induction treatment should deliver 40 Gy to the entire bladder and regional nodes, ensuring inclusion of the tumor plus a 2–2.5-cm margin. Irradiation is combined with Cisplatin delivered in a weekly outpatient regimen. Previously reported cisplatin dose schedules include weekly administration of 35 mg/m$^2$ × 1 day, or 20 mg/m$^2$ × 3 days.

a. **Treatment volume.** Initial treatment should include the entire bladder and a small pelvic volume. The superior border of the pelvic field is placed near the S2-S3 junction, while the inferior margin extends to the inferior aspect of the obturator foramen. Laterally, the pelvic brim is included with a 1.5–2.0-cm margin.

b. **Dose and fractionation.** The bladder tumor can be treated twice daily to provide an accelerated schedule during induction. BID treatments of the small pelvic fields at 1.5 Gy separated by 6 hours, or concomitant boost arrangements, have been well tolerated. In the concomitant boost format, the pelvis is treated at 1.8 Gy in the morning with a reduced volume receiving 1.5–1.6 Gy after a 4 to 6-hour interval. When the tumor is solitary, well defined at cystoscopy, and has not been preceded by a history of multiple superficial tumors, the boost field can be limited to the known disease plus a 2-cm margin and the dose to the whole bladder limited to 40–45 Gy. For poorly localized tumors, the entire bladder should be treated to 50–55 Gy prior to the final boost. Regardless of the acceleration and boost arrangement, the final radiation dose to the tumor should be limited to 65 Gy.

2. **Post-induction evaluation.** Patients should be scheduled for cystoscopic evaluation of the tumor response in the sixth week following the initiation of irradiation. Stopping the induction after 40 Gy results in a high incidence of regression of favorable tumors. Evaluation is delayed until the sixth week following the initiation of therapy, regardless of the dose delivery schedule. This timing represents a compromise in that continued regression has been documented beyond 8 weeks, while the treatment break allows tumor repopulation. Induction is successful when the endoscopic evaluation discloses either no residual disease or superficial disease, remote from the original site. The patient is scheduled for cystectomy when residual invasive tumor is found anywhere or Tis is found at the original tumor site.

3. **Consolidation.** When induction therapy has been successful, chemo-irradiation is continued to the following final doses:

   a. pelvic fields, 45 Gy
   b. the entire bladder, 40–55 Gy
   c. tumor, 65 Gy

4. **Adjuvant chemotherapy**. Patients who die of bladder cancer die with metastatic disease. Likewise, though contemporary multidrug therapies are associated with high response rates (*viz.*, ≥60%), few patients survive metastatic progression. Meta-analyses of the contemporary trials have identified an approximately 5% survival benefit for neo-adjuvant multidrug chemotherapy, regardless of the form of the local therapy.[41–43] A clear survival benefit has not, however, been demonstrated for chemotherapy in the adjuvant setting.[44] In general, individual trials, anticipating larger benefits, have not been powered to show this level of survival change. The exception was the combined multigroup trial of neo-adjuvant cisplatin, methotrexate, and vinblastine chemotherapy reported by the UK, Medical Research Council's (MRC) organized international collaboration of trialists.[45] The trial was initially powered to show a 10% or greater survival improvement, so the result, a 5.5% improvement in 3-year survival, displayed a wide confidence interval (95% CI: -0.5–15%).[32] Current randomized control trials are underway to test adjuvant chemotherapy combined with bladder conservation. Until there is clear outcome data to guide this decision, patients with locally advanced bladder cancer should be considered for neo-adjuvant or adjuvant multidrug therapy.

5. **Follow-up.** Bladder-conserving treatment is followed with a schedule identical to that described for definitive irradiation. The important consideration for these patients, however, is that a recommendation for prompt cystectomy will follow discovery of either an invasive recurrence or CIS remote from the original tumor. Superficial recurrences should be treated as they would be in the unirradiated bladder. Zietman and colleagues, with long-

term follow-up available for 190 patients, have observed ~25% superficial recurrences. Importantly, the response to TURBT and intravesical therapy and survival (8-year) were unchanged for these patients. Fifty percent of patients experiencing a superficial recurrence, however, eventually had cystectomy for re-recurrence or progressive disease.

## Preoperative irradiation

Four randomized trials have examined preoperative irradiation followed by immediate or delayed cystectomy. In addition to these studies, reviews by Mameghan[46] and Parsons and Million[47] have concluded that preoperative irradiation reduces by approximately one half the risk of isolated pelvic failure following cystectomy. Though small, the recent trial from NCI Canada previously detailed confirmed this finding. In this trial, patients were selected for cystectomy prior to randomization for preoperative irradiation with or without concomitant cisplatin (100 mg/m$^2$). In addition to the significant decrease in pelvic failures, survival was increased in the chemotherapy arm. Though underpowered to show statistical significance for overall survival, these data support preoperative chemo-irradiation for patients at increased risk for regional disease spread, such as T-stage $\geq$T2.

## Metastatic or Recurrent Transitional Cell Carcinoma

Although multiagent chemotherapy is the principal treatment for recurrent or metastatic transitional cell carcinoma, radiation therapy frequently provides excellent control of localized symptoms. Typically, these symptoms include pelvic pain, obstruction, hemorrhage, or extremity edema. Patients with recurrent bladder cancers, however, are likely to be elderly, severely symptomatic and may suffer from substantial comorbid disease. Therefore, palliation must be individualized. For example, though it is effective, a lengthy course such as 50 Gy in 25 fractions is generally not required, but reducing the dose to the common regimen of 30 Gy in 10 fractions Fossa and colleagues found to be sub-effective.[48] Considering patients who were elderly, medically unfit, or whose tumors were too advanced for radical treatment and were not receiving chemotherapy, the MRC examined two hypo-fractionated radiation schedules, 35 Gy in 10 daily fractions and 21 Gy in three fractions delivered in 1 week. Prescribing to the central axis and treating only the bladder, trialists found both schedules to be effective and generally well tolerated. On average, however, symptom relief lasted fewer than 4 months, while median survival for both groups was 7.5 months.[49] On average, 68% of patients experienced symptom relief from either regimen.

---

**BOX 26-3 TREATMENT OF SOLITARY BRAIN METASTASES**

Three patients with solitary lesions as the only site of metastasis received combination resection and postoperative irradiation, 40–50 Gy. Their average survival was 29 months.

Anderson RS, el-Mahdi AM, Kuban DA, Higgins EM. Brain metastases from transitional cell carcinoma of urinary bladder. *Urology* 39: (1992): 17–20.

---

Radiation relieves pain from bony metastases in ~70% of patients and should be considered following orthopedic stabilization for pending pathologic fracture or fracture.

Spinal cord compression, or cauda equina syndrome, benefits from early diagnosis and treatment. Solitary brain metastases from TCC can be treated with stereotactic irradiation or with combination surgery and postoperative irradiation.[50] Since survival following these treatments can be prolonged,[50,51] the 40% incidence of a second brain metastasis is reduced to ~20% by whole brain radiation, most commonly 30 Gy delivered in 10 fractions.

## Cancers of the Kidney, Renal Pelvis, and Ureter

### Overview

Surgery is the primary treatment modality for nonmetastatic cancers of the kidney and upper urinary tract. The role of adjuvant radiotherapy is unclear. In the setting of metastatic disease, radiotherapy continues to be an effective tool for palliation.

### Epidemiology and Risk Factors

There will be 51,000 estimated new cases of cancer of the kidney and renal pelvis and 13,000 deaths in 2007.[1] This represents 2% of adult malignancies. The male to female ratio is 1.7:1 with a median age of 55–60 years. Cancers of the ureter are uncommon with an estimated 2,100 new cases and 700 deaths in 2006.

It is estimated that up to 30% of renal carcinomas can be directly attributed to smoking. Acquired cystic disease of the kidney, obesity, and hypertension, have all been found to correlate with an increased risk of developing renal cell carcinoma (RCC). Occupational exposure to industrial solvents, asbestos, cadmium, and petroleum products have also been linked with developing RCC. The relationship between exposure to gasoline and development of renal carcinoma, though frequently studied, continues to be unclear.

Hereditary forms of renal carcinoma are associated with von Hippel-Lindau syndrome (VHL) and Birt-Hogg-Dube syndrome, and involve hereditary papillary renal carcinoma as well as hereditary renal carcinoma. Patients with VHL, associated with a proximal deletion of the short arm of chromosome 3, have been reported to have a 45% incidence of RCC, which is often bilateral. The VHL gene has also been found to be mutated in patients with nonhereditary RCC.

### Pathology and Natural History

More than 80% of primary cancers of the kidney are clear cell carcinomas, while about 5% are sarcomatoid. The sarcomatoid subtype is associated with an extremely poor prognosis. On the other hand, 80% of malignancies of the ureter and renal pelvis are transitional cell carcinomas, and 8% are SCC. SCCs are associated with a higher rate of recurrence.

For cancers of the kidney, presentation involving the classic triad of gross hematuria, flank mass, and pain is found only in 5%–10% of cases, but when present carries a worse prognosis. Separately, the symptoms of hematuria, flank mass, or pain are each present in about 50% of cases. Other common symptoms or findings at presentation include weight loss, anemia, fever, hypercalcemia, and acute varicocele.

RCC is associated with a better prognosis when discovered as an incidental finding on imaging, estimated to occur in only 7% of cases. A much larger percentage, roughly 30% of RCC patients, presents with metastatic disease. Bilateral involvement, outside of the hereditary setting, is seen in only 2% of cases. The average diameter of tumor at presentation is 7 cm.

### Workup

The diagnosis of RCC is usually made clinically and radiographically with pathologic confirmation at the time of resection. Workup typically includes history and physical, CT or MRI of the abdomen and pelvis, and may include renal ultrasound, plain films, and bone scan if indicated by elevated alkaline phosphatase. Laboratory studies should include CBC, liver and kidney function tests, and urinalysis. Metastatic workup may include CT scans of other organs when indicated.

#### Prognostic Factors

Stage at presentation is the most important prognostic factor for patients with RCC. Based on series reported in the last 10 years, the 5-year survival by stage at presentation is 95%, 85%, 65%, and

**TABLE 26-6 TNM Staging Kidney Tumors**

| | |
|---|---|
| T1 | Tumor 7 cm in greatest dimension, limited to kidney |
| T1a | Tumor 4 cm or less |
| T1b | Tumor more than 4 cm but not more than 7 cm, limited to kidney |
| T2 | Tumor more than 7 cm in greatest dimension, limited to kidney |
| T3 | Tumor extends into major veins or invades the adrenal gland or perinephric tissues but not beyond Gerota's fascia |
| T3a | Tumor invades adrenal gland or perirenal and/or renal sinus fat |
| T3b | Tumor grossly extends into the renal vein or its segmental branches or vena cava below the diaphragm |
| T3c | Tumor grossly extends into the vena cava above the diaphragm |
| T4 | Tumor invades beyond Gerota's fascia |
| N1 | Metastasis in single regional lymph node |
| N2 | Metastasis in more than one regional lymph node |
| N3 | Metastasis in lymph node >5 cm in greatest dimension |

Used with the permission of the American Joint Committee on Cancer (AJCC), Chicago, Illinois. The original source for this material is the AJCC Cancer Staging Manual, Sixth Edition (2002) published by Springer-Verlag New York, www.springeronline.com

15% for stages I, II, III, and IV, respectively. Size of the primary tumor greater than 7 cm has also been associated with a worse prognosis and has been incorporated into the current TNM staging system. The duration of survival in the presence of metastatic disease is highly variable. Patients with only one site of metastasis have been shown to have a 5-year survival as high as 25% versus 4% for patients with multiple metastases.[52]

**TABLE 26-7 TNM Stage Grouping Kidney Tumor**

| | |
|---|---|
| I | T1 N0 M0 |
| II | T2 N0 M0 |
| III | T1-3 N1 M0 |
| IV | Any T4 or any N 2-3 or any M1 |

**TABLE 26-8 TNM Staging Renal Pelvis and Ureter**

| | |
|---|---|
| Ta | Papillary noninvasive tumor |
| Tis | Carcinoma *in situ* |
| T1 | Tumor invades the sub-epithelial connective tissue |
| T2 | Tumor invades the muscularis |
| T3 | (For renal pelvis only) Tumor invades beyond the muscularis into perinephric fat or the renal parenchyma |
| T3 | (For ureter only) Tumor invades beyond the muscularis into periureteric fat |
| T4 | Tumor invades adjacent organs or through the kidney into perinephric fat |
| N1 | Metastasis in single regional lymph node >2 cm |
| N2 | Metastasis in single lymph node >2 cm but ≤5 cm or multiple lymph nodes all >5 cm |
| N3 | Metastasis in lymph node >5 cm in greatest dimension |

| TABLE 26-9 | TNM Stage Grouping Renal Pelvis and Ureter |
|---|---|
| 0a | Ta N0 M0 |
| 0is | Tis N0 M0 |
| I | T1 N0 M0 |
| II | T2 N0 M0 |
| III | T3 N0 M0 |
| IV | Any T4 or any N 1-3 or any M1 |

## Management

### Renal Cell Carcinoma

#### Surgery

The standard of care for nonmetastatic RCC is nephrectomy, nephron-sparing when indicated. While radical nephrectomy involves removing the contents within Gerota's fascia, including the tumor, kidney, adrenal gland, and perinephric fat, partial nephrectomy is now more common. Here, the adrenal gland may be left in place when the risk of its involvement is low. In the absence of evidence that lymphadenectomy improves survival, the removal of regional lymph nodes, from the diaphragm to the bifurcation of the aorta, is considered optional. Regional node dissection is still advocated as the best treatment option for those patients with micro metastases confined to the regional nodes alone. Nephron-sparing surgery is considered for patients with uni-nephric state, poor renal function, bilateral disease, or single small primaries. The approach for either surgery is usually transperitoneal, via either a thoracoabdominal, or transabdominal approach. Approximately 20% of patients undergoing radical nephrectomy have complications. The rate of perioperative mortality from large centers is about 2%.

#### Radiation Therapy

While there are no randomized controlled data that support the routine use of adjuvant radiotherapy for RCC, there are recent, more modern, retrospective series that suggest a potential benefit for radiotherapy given to patients at high risk for local recurrence. Four reported prospective randomized trials have evaluated the role of adjuvant radiotherapy. These studies, conducted largely in the pre-CT era, included a large number of patients with early-stage disease and hence a low risk of local recurrence. Two studies from the pre-CT era compared preoperative radiotherapy to the regional nodes and kidney followed by nephrectomy to nephrectomy alone. One trial from Rotterdam examined doses of 30 Gy and later 40 Gy in 2 Gy fractions, while the second trial, conducted in Sweden, delivered 33 Gy in 15 fractions.[53,54] No improvement in overall survival or local recurrence was found in either trial. The trial from Rotterdam, however, showed improved resectability following irradiation.

Two other studies have compared nephrectomy with and without adjuvant irradiation of the tumor bed and regional lymph nodes with negative results. The first trial, conducted in the United Kingdom, showed a decrement in overall survival for adjuvant radiotherapy.[55] The second trial reported no significant difference in overall survival or local relapse but a high rate of radiation-induced mortality.[56] The results of these trials could, however, be criticized for poor radiation technique and planning as well as for failure to limit treatment to patients who would most likely have benefited from radiotherapy.

Since then, more recent retrospective series have shown an improvement in local control when adjuvant radiotherapy was restricted to patients with positive margins or locally advanced disease. These patients, with a higher risk of recurrence than those treated with adjuvant radiotherapy in the previously noted trials, might be expected to have a greater potential benefit. Table 26-10 shows retrospective series in which the addition of 40–60 Gy to the regional nodes and tumor bed after radical nephrectomy improved local control by 8%–30%. One series of 184 patients showed a statistically significant improvement in local control with postoperative radiotherapy for the T3N0

---

**30X 26-4** **POSTOPERATIVE RADIOTHERAPY VS OBSERVATION**

Between 1979 and 1984, 72 Stage II and III renal cancer patients were nephrectomized and then randomized to observation versus postoperative radiotherapy of 50 Gy in 20 fractions to the operative bed and regional nodes. There was no significant difference in local control or overall survival at 5 years. Forty-four percent had significant radiotherapy-related gastrointestinal side effects and in 19% of the patients, radiation-induced complications were felt to have contributed to their death. The authors concluded that adjuvant radiotherapy was without benefit.

Kjaer M, Iversen P, Hvidt V, et al. A randomized trial of postoperative radiotherapy versus observation in Stage II and III renal adenocarcinoma. A study by the Copenhagen Renal Cancer Study Group. *Scand J Urol Nephrol* (1987): 21: 285–289.

---

ubset of patients.[57] None of these trials, however, showed an improvement in overall survival. mportantly, these trials do confirm that contemporary radiotherapy techniques and treatment lanning result in a low rate of complications.

In summary, adjuvant radiotherapy is not standard for RCC, but may be considered in the following situations:

—Preoperative radiotherapy for unresectable disease without distant metastases
—Grossly or microscopically positive disease after resection
—T3a or T3c disease

## Metastatic Disease

alliative nephrectomy is sometimes indicated for relief of pain, hematuria, or hypertension. lthough nephrectomy-induced regression of distant disease has been reported, this is a rare esponse and not an indication for surgery. Aggressive local therapy may be beneficial for patients vith solitary metastases, providing durable palliation or local control. Patients with brain metastases from RCC, similar to patients with other histologies, should be considered for radiotherapy to he whole brain or stereotactic radiotherapy. As with other histologies, excellent results have been eported with extracranial stereotactic radiotherapy for lung metastases.

## RENAL PELVIS AND URETER CARCINOMA

The standard treatment for renal pelvis and ureteral carcinoma has been radical nephroureterectomy with removal of a bladder cuff. Today, however, renal-sparing endoscopic and perutaneous treatment of TCC for selected patients has become common. Multiple centers have eported results incorporating systemic chemotherapy for locally advanced disease in the absence

---

**TABLE 26-10** **Postoperative Radiation Therapy for Renal Cell Carcinoma**

| Source | Risk Factor for Local Failure | n | RT | Local Control |
|---|---|---|---|---|
| Kao et al.[58] | Positive margins or T3 | 12 | Yes | 100% |
| | | 12 | No | 70% |
| Stein et al.[58] | T3 N0 | 37 | Yes | 90% |
| | | 30 | No | 63% |
| Makarewicz et al.[57] | T3–T4,N0–N1 | 114 | Yes | 91%* |
| | | 72 | No | 84%* |

Control rates at 5 years for T3N0 subset only.)

of metastatic spread. Owing to the relative rarity of cases, prospective trial data are not available. Therefore, the role for adjuvant radiotherapy, like that of the primary therapy itself, cannot be completely determined. Retrospective series, however, do not generally support the routine use of adjuvant radiotherapy after nephroureterectomy. Series data do suggest an improvement in local control when postoperative radiotherapy is used for Stage T3 and T4 tumors or patients with node-positive disease. In one retrospective series of 26 patients with Stage T3 and T4 tumors treated at the University of Kansas, local failure occurred in nine of 17 patients treated without radiotherapy and only one in nine patients treated with radiotherapy.[59] In general though, adjuvant radiotherapy has not been shown to improve overall survival. Metastatic disease is treated with chemotherapeutic agents that have been shown to be effective for transitional cell carcinoma of the bladder. The role of adjuvant chemotherapy for nonmetastatic disease has also not been clearly defined.

## Radiotherapy Techniques

For renal carcinoma, preoperative treatment should deliver 40–50 Gy in 1.8 to 2.0 Gy fractions. CT planning is recommended, along with conformal techniques and multiple beam angles to minimize toxicity. Fields should cover the gross tumor and regional nodes. Similar planning and field design are recommended for postoperative treatment. Doses of 45–50 Gy should be delivered to the regional nodes and tumor bed and then followed by a boost to a total of 50–56 Gy to microscopic or gross residual disease using reduced fields. Scar coverage is recommended. Organs at risk include the spinal cord, contralateral kidney, liver, and small bowel. Metastases treated to 35–40 Gy have been noted to respond about 70% of the time. Patients with small amounts of metastatic disease may benefit from higher doses, 45–50 Gy in 2.5–3.0 Gy fractions, for durable palliation.

When delivering radiotherapy preoperatively for malignancies of the renal pelvis and ureter, the target should include all gross disease plus the entire kidney, and complete course of the ureter to the bladder. Doses of 45–50 Gy using standard fractionation are recommended. Postoperatively, the tumor bed, and course of the ureter up to the bladder, are included to 45–50 Gy followed by a reduced-field boost to 50–56 Gy to microscopic or gross residual disease. Lower doses may be used if adjuvant chemotherapy is given.

## REFERENCES

1. American Cancer Society. (2007) Cancer Reference Information, http://www.cancer.org/docroot/CRI/content.
2. Jemal A, Siegel R, Ward E, et al. (2006): Cancer statistics, 2006. *CA Cancer J Clin* 56:6–130.
3. Boffetta P, Silverman DT. (2001): A meta-analysis of bladder cancer and diesel exhaust exposure. *Epidemiology* 12:125–130.
4. Gaertner RR, Theriault GP. (2002): Risk of bladder cancer in foundry workers: a meta-analysis. *Occup Environ Med* 59:655–663.
5. Tremblay C, Armstrong B, Theriault G, Brodeur J. (1995): Estimation of risk of developing bladder cancer among workers exposed to coal tar pitch volatiles in the primary aluminum industry. *Am J Ind Med* 27:335–348.
6. Silverman DT, Levin LI, Hoover RN. (1989): Occupational risks of bladder cancer in the United States: II. nonwhite men. *J Natl Cancer Inst* 81:1480–1483.
7. Silverman DT, Levin LI, Hoover RN, Hartge P. (1989): Occupational risks of bladder cancer in the United States: I. white men. *J Natl Cancer Inst* 81:1472–1480.
8. Wong-You-Cheong JJ, Woodward PJ, Manning MA, Sesterhenn IA. (2006): From the archives of the AFIP: neoplasms of the urinary bladder: radiologic-pathologic correlation. *Radiographics* 26:553–580.

9. Droller MJ. (2005): Biological considerations in the assessment of urothelial cancer: a retrospective. *Urology* 66:66–75.

0. Wong JT, Wasserman NF, Padurean AM. (2004): Bladder squamous cell carcinoma. *Radiographics* 24:855–860.

1. Shokeir AA. (2004): Squamous cell carcinoma of the bladder: pathology, diagnosis, and treatment. *BJU Int* 93:216–220.

2. Harland SJ. (2005): A second look at the pT1 G3 bladder tumour. *Clin Oncol (R Coll Radiol)* 17:498–502.

3. Rodel C, Dunst J, Grabenbauer GG, et al. (2001): Radiotherapy is an effective treatment for high-risk T1-bladder cancer. *Strahlenther Onkol* 177:82–88; discussion 89.

4. Jakse G, Algaba F, Malmstrom PU, Oosterlinck W. (2004): A second-look TUR in T1 transitional cell carcinoma: why? *Eur Urol* 45:539–546; discussion 546.

5. Shipley WU, Kaufman DS, Zehr E, et al. (2002): Selective bladder preservation by combined modality protocol treatment: long-term outcomes of 190 patients with invasive bladder cancer. *Urology* 60:62–67; discussion 67–68.

6. Rodel C, Grabenbauer GG, Kuhn R, et al. (2002): Combined-modality treatment and selective organ preservation in invasive bladder cancer: long-term results. *J Clin Oncol* 20:3061–3071.

7. Stein JP, Lieskovsky G, Cote R, et al. (2001): Radical cystectomy in the treatment of invasive bladder cancer: long-term results in 1,054 patients. *J Clin Oncol* 19:666–675.

8. Weiss C, Wolze C, Engehausen DG, et al. (2006): Radio-chemotherapy after transurethral resection for high-risk T1 bladder cancer: an alternative to intravesical therapy or early cystectomy? *J Clin Oncol* 24:2318–2324.

9. Quilty PM, Duncan W. (1986): Treatment of superficial (T1) tumours of the bladder by radical radiotherapy. *Br J Urol* 58:147–152.

0. Van der Steen-Banasik EM, Visser AG, Reinders JG, et al. (2002): Saving bladders with brachytherapy: implantation technique and results. *Int J Radiat Oncol Biol Phys* 53:622–629.

1. Kulkarni JN, Gupta R. (2002): Recurrence and progression in stage T1G3 bladder tumour with intravesical bacille Calmette-Guerin (Danish 1331 strain). *BJU Int* 90:554–557.

2. Pansadoro V, Emiliozzi P, de Paula F, Scarpone P, Pansadoro A, Sternberg CN. (2002): Long-term follow-up of G3T1 transitional cell carcinoma of the bladder treated with intravesical bacille Calmette-Guerin: 18-year experience. *Urology* 59:227–231.

3. Patard JJ, Rodriguez A, Leray E, Rioux-Leclercq N, Guille F, Lobel B. (2002): Intravesical Bacillus Calmette-Guerin treatment improves patient survival in T1G3 bladder tumours. *Eur Urol* 41:635–641; discussion 642.

4. Peyromaure M, Zerbib M. (2004): T1G3 transitional cell carcinoma of the bladder: recurrence, progression, and survival. *BJU Int* 93:60–63.

5. Shahin O, Thalmann GN, Rentsch C, Mazzucchelli L, Studer UE. (2003): A retrospective analysis of 153 patients treated with or without intravesical bacillus Calmette-Guerin for primary stage T1 grade 3 bladder cancer: recurrence, progression, and survival. *J Urol* 169:96–100; discussion 100.

6. Duncan W, Quilty PM. (1986): The results of a series of 963 patients with transitional cell carcinoma of the urinary bladder primarily treated by radical megavoltage X-ray therapy. *Radiother Oncol* 7:299–310.

7. Jenkins BJ, Caulfield MJ, Fowler CG, et al. (1988): Reappraisal of the role of radical radiotherapy and salvage cystectomy in the treatment of invasive (T2/T3) bladder cancer. *Br J Urol* 62:343–346.

8. Fossa SD, Waehre H, Aass N, Jacobsen AB, Olsen DR, Ous S. (1993): Bladder cancer definitive radiation therapy of muscle-invasive bladder cancer. A retrospective analysis of 317 patients. *Cancer* 72:3036–3043.

29. Gospodarowicz MK, Hawkins NV, Rawlings GA, et al. (1989): Radical radiotherapy for muscle-invasive transitional cell carcinoma of the bladder: failure analysis. *J Urol* 142:1448–1453; discussion 1453–1444.

30. Coppin CM, Gospodarowicz MK, James K, et al. (1996): Improved local control of invasive bladder cancer by concurrent cisplatin and preoperative or definitive radiation. The National Cancer Institute of Canada Clinical Trials Group. *J Clin Oncol* 14:2901–2907.

31. Quilty PM, Kerr GR, Duncan W. (1986): Prognostic indices for bladder cancer: an analysis of patients with transitional cell carcinoma of the bladder primarily treated by radical megavoltage X-ray therapy. *Radiother Oncol* 7:311–321.

32. Maciejewski B, Majewski S. (1991): Dose fractionation and tumour repopulation in radiotherapy for bladder cancer. *Radiother Oncol* 21:163–170.

33. Shipley WU, Kaufman DS, Tester WJ, Pilepich MV, Sandler HM. (2003): Overview of bladder cancer trials in the Radiation Therapy Oncology Group. *Cancer* 97:2115–2119.

34. Lotz HT, Pos FJ, Hulshof MC, et al. (2006): Tumor motion and deformation during external radiotherapy of bladder cancer. *Int J Radiat Oncol Biol Phys* 64:1551–1558.

35. Meijer GJ, Rasch C, Remeijer P, Lebesque JV. (2003): Three-dimensional analysis of delineation errors, setup errors, and organ motion during radiotherapy of bladder cancer. *Int J Radiat Oncol Biol Phys* 55:1277–1287.

36. Lotz HT, Remeijer P, van Herk M, et al. (2004): A model to predict bladder shapes from changes in bladder and rectal filling. *Med Phys* 31:1415–1423.

37. Turner SL, Swindell R, Bowl N, et al. (1997): Bladder movement during radiation therapy for bladder cancer: implications for treatment planning. *Int J Radiat Oncol Biol Phys* 39:355–360.

38. Quilty PM, Duncan W. (1986): Radiotherapy for squamous carcinoma of the urinary bladder. *Int J Radiat Oncol Biol Phys* 12:861–865.

39. Ghoneim MA, Ashamallah AK, Awaad HK, Whitmore WF, Jr. (1985): Randomized trial of cystectomy with or without preoperative radiotherapy for carcinoma of the bilharzial bladder. *J Urol* 134:266–268.

40. Swanson DA, Liles A, Zagars GK. (1990): Preoperative irradiation and radical cystectomy for stages T2 and T3 squamous cell carcinoma of the bladder. *J Urol* 143:37–40.

41. (2005): Neoadjuvant chemotherapy in invasive bladder cancer: update of a systematic review and meta-analysis of individual patient data advanced bladder cancer (ABC) meta-analysis collaboration. *Eur Urol* 48:202–205; discussion 205–206.

42. Winquist E, Kirchner TS, Segal R, Chin J, Lukka H. (2004): Neo-adjuvant chemotherapy for transitional cell carcinoma of the bladder: a systematic review and meta-analysis. *J Urol* 171:561–569.

43. (2003): Neo-adjuvant chemotherapy in invasive bladder cancer: a systematic review and meta-analysis. *Lancet* 361:1927–1934.

44. (2005): Adjuvant chemotherapy in invasive bladder cancer: a systematic review and meta-analysis of individual patient data. Advanced Bladder Cancer (ABC) Meta-analysis Collaboration. *Eur Urol* 48:189–199; discussion 199–201.

45. (1999): Neo-adjuvant cisplatin, methotrexate, and vinblastine chemotherapy for muscle-invasive bladder cancer: a randomized controlled trial. International collaboration of trialists. *Lancet* 354:533–540.

46. Mameghan H, Sandeman TF. (1991): The management of invasive bladder cancer: a review of selected Australasian studies in radiotherapy, chemotherapy, and cystectomy. *Aust N Z J Surg* 61:173–178.

47. Parsons JT, Million RR. (1990): The role of radiation therapy alone or as an adjunct to surgery in bladder carcinoma. *Semin Oncol* 17:566–582.

48. Fossa SD, Hosbach G. (1991): Short-term moderate-dose pelvic radiotherapy of advanced bladder carcinoma: a questionnaire-based evaluation of its symptomatic effect. *Acta Oncol* 30:735–738.
49. Duchesne GM, Bolger JJ, Griffiths GO, et al. (2000): A randomized trial of hypofractionated schedules of palliative radiotherapy in the management of bladder carcinoma: results of medical research council trial BA09. *Int J Radiat Oncol Biol Phys* 47:379–388.
50. Anderson RS, el-Mahdi AM, Kuban DA, Higgins EM. (1992): Brain metastases from transitional cell carcinoma of urinary bladder. *Urology* 39:17–20.
51. Rosenstein M, Wallner K, Scher H, Sternberg CN. (1993): Treatment of brain metastases from bladder cancer. *J Urol* 149:480–483.
52. Frank W, Stuhldreher D, Saffrin R, Shott S, Guinan P. (1994): Stage IV renal cell carcinoma. *J Urol* 152:1998–1999.
53. van der Werf-Messing B. (1973): Proceedings: carcinoma of the kidney. *Cancer* 32:1056–1061.
54. Juusela H, Malmio K, Alfthan O, Oravisto KJ. (1977): Preoperative irradiation in the treatment of renal adenocarcinoma. *Scand J Urol Nephrol* 11:277–281.
55. Finney R. (1973): The value of radiotherapy in the treatment of hypernephroma—a clinical trial. *Br J Urol* 45:258–269.
56. Kjaer M, Iversen P, Hvidt V, et al. (1987): A randomized trial of postoperative radiotherapy versus observation in stage II and III renal adenocarcinoma. A study by the Copenhagen Renal Cancer Study Group. *Scand J Urol Nephrol* 21:285–289.
57. Makarewicz R, Zarzycka M, Kulinska G, Windorbska W. (1998): The value of postoperative radiotherapy in advanced renal cell cancer. *Neoplasma* 45:380–383.
58. Kao GD, Malkowicz SB, Whittington R, D'Amico AV, Wein AJ. (1994): Locally advanced renal cell carcinoma: low complication rate and efficacy of post-nephrectomy radiation therapy planned with CT. *Radiology* 193:725–730.
59. Cozad SC, Smalley SR, Austenfeld M, Noble M, Jennings S, Raymond R. (1995): Transitional cell carcinoma of the renal pelvis or ureter: patterns of failure. *Urology* 46:796–800.

# 27

# Testicular Cancers

*Christopher R. King, MD, PhD*

## OVERVIEW

From a radiation oncologist's point of view, one must first distinguish between seminomas—where adjuvant radiotherapy is still the standard of care,[1] and non-seminomas—where the role of radiotherapy is palliative. This chapter, therefore, will focus mainly on seminomas. With cure rates approaching 100%, modern strategies are exploring chemotherapy or surveillance as possible alternative approaches in order to reduce the potential late sequelae of adjuvant radiotherapy.

## EPIDEMIOLOGY

Approximately 8,000 new cases of testicular cancer were diagnosed in the United States during 2007, with only about 300 related deaths. They represent only about 2% of all human cancers diagnosed. Interestingly, the worldwide incidence of testicular cancers has doubled in the past 40 years.[2] Although germ cell tumors can rarely occur in extra-gonadal sites, their management follows that of testicular germ cell tumors.

## RISK FACTORS

While the etiology of testicular tumors is unknown, there are several known risk factors:

- Gender: exclusively in males
- Age: predominantly in men 15 to 34 years old
- History of cryptorchidism, even after orchiopexy, by about 10- to 40-fold
- Association with dysplastic nevus syndrome and Klinefelter's syndrome
- Testicular trauma
- HIV infection
- Race: five times more frequently among white men than among black men
- Chromosomal abnormalities involving chromosomes 1 and 12

## PATHOLOGY AND SERUM TUMOR MARKERS

The majority of testicular tumors are of germ cell origin. From a therapeutic perspective, these his tologies are divided into two types, seminoma and non-seminoma germ cell tumors.

Most non-seminoma germ cell tumors are successfully managed with chemotherapy and the role of radiation therapy is limited. The majority of pure seminomas (85%) are termed "classic semi nomas." These generally enlarge the testis diffusely with a gray homogeneous appearance on cros section. While early-stage tumors generally do not penetrate the tunica albuginea, they may extend into the rete testis, epididymis, or spermatic cord. Carcinoma *in situ* precedes invasive tumors.

Germ cell tumors frequently produce proteins that can serve as tumor markers for disease burden a well as diagnosis. The two most important of these are alpha-feto protein (AFP) and the beta subunit o human chorionic gonadotropin (beta-HCG). LDH level is also used as a marker for disease burden.

It should be kept in mind, however, that these proteins are not specific to germ cell tumors. The serum half life of these tumor markers is of clinical relevance and for AFP is 4 to 6 days, and fo beta-HCG is 1 to 2 days. After five half lives, a previously elevated serum marker should return to within normal levels if all tumor cells have been eradicated. In pure seminoma, elevated beta-HCG is present about 10% of the time. By contrast, AFP is *never* present with pure seminoma.

Non-germ cell tumors are rare. In men over the age of 60, however, testicular lymphoma is the most common. Rarely, metastatic disease from the prostate, lung, kidney, and melanoma can involve the testes.

## ANATOMY AND ROUTES OF SPREAD

The lymphatic drainage from the testes originates from the testicular hilum, passes through the internal inguinal ring along with the spermatic cord, and follows the testicular veins to lymph nodes in the retroperitoneum. The right and left testes possess somewhat different lymphatic pathways of clinical relevance in designing radiation fields. The right testicular vein joins the infe rior vena cava a few cm below where the right renal vein enters the IVC. The left testicular vein, by contrast, enters the left renal vein. Hence, coverage of lymphatics in proximity to the left renal hilum is made for left-sided tumors. The lymphatics span from T11 to L4. Crossover from right to left is demonstrated by lymphangiography to be common, but is rare from left to right. After spread to this first nodal group, progression follows the lumbar retroperitoneal nodes, then supradiaphrag matic nodes in the mediastinum and supraclavicular region. Although the lymphatics from the testes do not drain into the inguinal or iliac nodes, those from the scrotum do. Distant metastatic sites include the lungs, liver, brain, and bone.

**TABLE 27-1** Histologies of Testicular Tumors

| Germ Cell Tumors (95%) | | |
|---|---|---|
| **Pure Seminoma (40%)** | | **Non-Seminoma (60%)** |
| Classic Seminoma | | Embryonal |
| Anaplastic Seminoma | | Teratoma |
| Spermatocytic Seminoma | | Choriocarcinoma |
| | | Mixed |
| Non-Germ Cell Tumors (5%) | | |
| Stromal | | |
| Lymphoma | | |

TABLE 27-2 Frequency of Serum Marker Elevation in Testicular Tumors

| Histology | AFP (%) | beta-hCG (%) |
|---|---|---|
| Seminoma | 0 | 9 |
| Teratoma | 38 | 25 |
| Embryonal | 70 | 60 |
| Choriocarcinoma | 0 | 100 |
| Yolk sac tumor | 75 | 25 |

## WORKUP AND STAGING

The classic presentation is a painless testicular mass. Among the differential diagnoses are epididymitis, orchitis, and hydrocele. Approximately 85% of patients with seminoma are Stage I at presentation, and metastatic disease at presentation occurs in about 10% of cases. Gynecomastia or breast tenderness is present in about 5% of cases resulting from increased estradiol in response to elevated HCG.

A testicular mass should be considered a tumor until proven otherwise. An ultrasound is the study of choice when presented with a testicular mass. If suspicion for a testicular tumor on the basis of history and physical examination is high, then an inguinal exploration or orchiectomy should be performed. Scrotal incisions are contraindicated because of concerns regarding the alteration of lymphatic drainage patterns. Serum markers for baseline should be obtained *prior* to surgery. Once the diagnosis of a testicular tumor has been made, the workup should include a chest X-ray or chest CT scan, an abdominopelvic CT scan, and postoperative serum markers. For patients with advanced disease a PET is useful to assess response to chemotherapy and possible further management of residual disease.

The AJCC TNM staging system is currently standard.[3]

Only stage and disease burden are of clinical prognostic significance. Neither the histologic subtype nor elevation of beta-HCG has been shown to be of prognostic value in seminoma.

## GENERAL MANAGEMENT

### Stage I (IA, IB, and IS)

The standard management for patients with Stage I seminoma includes a radical inguinal orchiectomy followed by adjuvant radiation therapy to the para-aortic and ipsilateral pelvic lymph nodes (sometimes called "dog-leg" field).[1] In instances where a scrotal approach to orchiectomy is performed, such patients are generally not considered for alternative management (such as surveillance or reduced radiation fields), and are thought to be at higher risk for scrotal recurrence. However, several studies report no increase in pelvic, abdominal, or scrotal recurrence in patients with prior scrotal surgery.[4]

For early-stage non-seminoma germ cell tumors, a retroperitoneal lymph node dissection is performed, and chemotherapy follows if there is involvement, or for a persistence of elevated serum tumor markers. With a greater propensity for hematogenous spread, adjuvant radiation therapy has been abandoned in favor of surveillance or chemotherapy and has a role in palliating residual bulky disease.

### Stage II

Stage II seminomas may also be managed with postoperative adjuvant radiation therapy provided that the retroperitoneal involvement is less than 5 cm in maximum dimension (Stage IIA and IIB).

## TABLE 27-3 TNM Staging*

### Primary Tumor

pTx Primary tumor cannot be assessed
pT0 No evidence of tumor
pTis Intratubular germ cell neoplasm (carcinoma *in situ*)
pT1 Tumor limited to the testis/epididymis (may invade tunica albuginea but not tunica vaginalis) without LVI
pT2 Limited to testis/epididymis with LVI or through tunica albuginea and involvement of tunica vaginalis
pT3 Invades spermatic cord
pT4 Invades scrotum

### Regional Lymph Nodes (clinical)

Nx Regional LN cannot be assessed
N0 No lymph node metastasis
N1 Metastasis to one or more lymph node mass, 2 cm or less
N2 Metastasis to one or more lymph node mass, greater than 2 cm but less than 5 cm
N3 Metastasis to a lymph node mass more than 5 cm

### Pathologic Lymph Nodes

pNx Cannot be assessed
pN0 No metastasis
pN1 Metastasis in one to five lymph nodes, none more than 2 cm
pN2 Metastasis in a lymph node mass greater than 2 cm but less than 5 cm, more than five nodes, none greater than 5 cm, or extranodal extension
pN3 Metastasis in a lymph node mass greater than 5 cm

### Distant Metastasis

Mx Cannot be assessed
M0 No distant metastasis
M1 Distant metastases
    M1a—non-regional lymph nodes or pulmonary metastasis
    M1b—metastases other than M1a

### Serum Tumor Markers

SX Markers not available
S0 Markers within normal limits
S1 LDH $< 1.5 \times$ normal and hCG $< 5000$ and AFP $< 1000$
S2 LDH $1.5-10 \times$ normal or hCG 5000-50,000 or AFP 1000-10,000
S3 LDH $> 10 \times$ normal or hCG $> 50,000$ or AFP $> 10,000$

### TNM Stage Grouping

| Stage 0 | pTis | N0 | M0 | S0 |
|---|---|---|---|---|
| Stage I | pT1 | N0 | M0 | S0 |
| IA | pT1-4 | N0 | M0 | SX |
| IB | pT2-4 | N0 | M0 | S0 |
| IS | any T | N0 | M0 | S1-3 |
| Stage II | any T | N1-3 | M0 | SX |
| IIA | any T | N1 | M0 | SX |
| IIB | any T | N2 | M0 | SX |
| IIC | any T | N3 | M0 | SX |
| Stage III | any T | any N | M1 | SX |

(from AJCC 6th ed.)

Recurrence after radiation therapy is directly related to initial bulk. Stage IIC patients receive chemotherapy. The role of radiation therapy for residual disease after chemotherapy is not well defined, and most of these patients are observed.

## Stage III and IV

For Stage III and IV seminomas, the current management is with platinum-based chemotherapy regimens (Platinum, Etoposide, and Bleomycin—PEB), with radiation therapy reserved for persistent or recurrent disease.

In the rare instance of a second primary early-stage seminoma after standard management for the first presentation with adjuvant radiation therapy, such patients can be considered for re-irradiation provided that lateral fields are used and that accumulated kidney doses are carefully calculated.

## Contraindications to Adjuvant Radiotherapy

Contraindications for radiotherapy include active inflammatory bowel disease, prior abdomino-pelvic radiotherapy (except as above), and a horseshoe kidney. These patients can be considered for either surveillance regimens or chemotherapy.

## RADIOTHERAPY TECHNIQUE AND DOSE

Patients are simulated supine and immobilization devices are usually not necessary. With the availability of CT simulation, an IVP to delineate the kidneys is now rarely performed. The superior border of the field is at least at the T10-11 interspace, as T11 is the highest level of lymphatic drainage. The inferior border is at the top of the obturator foramen (although bottom of foramen is acceptable). Inclusion of the inguinal orchiectomy scar within the field is not indicated. The field is usually 10–12 cm wide, although care must be taken to include the left renal hilum in left-sided tumors that may require wider fields. Standard radiotherapy field is still the "dog-leg" field that includes the para-aortic, ipsilateral iliac, and pelvic nodes.

Megavoltage photons are used in parallel opposed fields as described above, treated 5 days per week. Doses prescribed are 25 to 30 Gy, in 1.25 to 2.0 Gy fractions. There are no data to support the use of higher doses. A lower dose-per-fraction may reduce the acute sequelae. At our institution, we prescribe 25 Gy in 20 fractions.

Scattered radiation to the contralateral testis is minimized by use of a scrotal shield ("clamshell") that can reduce the dose to about 1%–2% of the

**FIGURE 27-1** AP radiotherapy field.

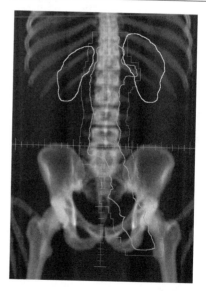

Standard AP "dog-leg" field for a Stage I testicular seminoma. Note the inclusion of nodes in proximity to the renal hilum for this left-sided tumor. Kidneys and nodes (large vessels) are drawn from CT simulation scan.

---

**BOX 27-1**

A randomized trial of 478 men with Stage I testicular seminoma compared standard dog-leg (DL) to a para-aortic (PA) field. Dose was 30 Gy in 15 fractions. Patients with disturbed lymphatic drainage were excluded. With a median follow-up of 4.5 years, nine relapses occurred in each arm. In the PA arm four of those relapses were in the pelvis. The 3-year relapse-free survival rates were similar for both arms, about 96%. One seminoma-related death occurred in the PA arm. Acute toxicity (nausea, vomiting, leukopenia) was less and sperm count higher in the PA arm. Whether this strategy provides equal cure rates or reduces second malignancies must await longer follow-up.

Fossa SD, et al. Optimal planning target volume for stage I testicular seminoma: a Medical Research Council randomized trial. *J Clin Oncol* 1999;17:1146–1154.

---

**BOX 27-2**

Some 625 patients with Stage I testicular seminoma were randomized to receive either 20 Gy in 2 weeks or 30 Gy in 3 weeks with either dog-leg (DL) or para-aortic (PA) fields. Significant lethargy was more pronounced in the 30 Gy arm at 1 month but by 3 months both arms were similar. With a median follow-up of 5 years, there were 10 and 11 relapses in the 30 Gy and 20 Gy arm, respectively. One patient died from seminoma in the 20 Gy arm. The study does not give any details of result comparisons between patients treated with DL or PA. Longer follow-up is needed to confirm the duration of efficacy of 20 Gy and any potential reduction of late toxicities including second cancers.

Jones WG, et al. Randomized trial of 30 versus 20 Gy in the adjuvant treatment of stage I testicular seminoma: a report on Medical Research Council Trial TE18, EORTC trial 30942. *J Clin Oncol* 2005;23:1200–1208.

---

prescribed dose, or 25 to 50 cGy, mostly from internal scatter. Further shielding can be achieved by extending the custom block by 5 cm below the edge of the field and adding a 10 cm lead shield supported over the scrotum.[5] Diode measurements near the contralateral testicle can be obtained to monitor the scattered radiation during treatment.

Because fewer than 10% of patients with Stage I seminoma have disease in the pelvis there is increasing interest in omitting the pelvic nodes and treating the para-aortic nodes only.

For Stage IIA, the radiation fields are the same as described above for Stage I. For Stage IIB, modification of the fields includes a margin around the bulky nodal disease as seen on CT scan. Bilateral pelvic fields are sometimes recommended as well. Doses are 25 Gy with an additional boost to the bulky nodal disease for an additional 10 Gy. There does not appear to be any benefit to prophylactic mediastinal radiation therapy[6] and it is currently not recommended.

## SEQUELAE OF RADIOTHERAPY

Acute side effects of radiation therapy are usually mild and predictable. They include nausea, vomiting and diarrhea, and a transient suppression of blood counts. The late sequelae of radiation therapy, although infrequent, are important considerations in the context of young patients and high cure rates. Among these are infertility, cardiotoxicity, gastrointestinal toxicity, second neoplasms, and immunosuppression. Second testicular tumors however are considered to stem from an underlying predisposition rather than being radiation-induced. Elective mediastinal radiation, which has been shown to be associated with an excessive number of cardiac deaths[7] has no role in Stage I or II seminoma. Less than 2% will relapse within the mediastinum with standard fields.[8] Late GI toxicity, including gastric ulceration and dyspepsia, has been observed in patients receiving higher doses (40 Gy) than are currently prescribed.

## Fertility

Infertility can be an important issue because patients are in their 20s and 30s. The contribution to infertility from surgery, radiation therapy, or a coexisting testicular abnormality is unknown. A lower testicular dose was associated with a more rapid recovery of sperm counts 1 year later.[9] Inquiry should be made regarding the patient's desire to retain fertility as many such patients already have diminished fertility and may wish to consider sperm banking prior to therapy. It would seem prudent to avoid insemination for 6 to 12 months after radiation therapy due to potentially damaged genetic material.

## Second Cancers

The incidence of second tumors attributable to radiation therapy is difficult to determine. However, data available suggest that patients with testicular cancers have higher rates of second tumors compared to an age-matched control. These included tumors of the stomach, colon, pancreas, kidney and bladder, as well as skin cancer, and leukemia.

---

**BOX 27-3**

Site-specific risks of second malignant neoplasms among 29,000 survivors of testicular cancer are reported from cancer registry databases. Second cancers were diagnosed among 5% of these patients. For seminoma patients treated with adjuvant radiotherapy the observed/expected risk was 1.5, and increased with time up to 20 years later. Significantly increased risk of stomach, pancreas, bladder, colon, kidney, and leukemias was observed. Risk was similar for seminoma as well as non-seminoma testicular tumors. Although the cause of second cancers is often attributed to carcinogenic therapies, excess second cancers are likely multi-factorial, including natural history, heightened diagnostic surveillance, environmental, and genetic determinants.

Travis LB, et al. Risk of second malignant neoplasms among long-term survivors of testicular cancer. *J Natl Cancer Inst* 1997;89:1429–1439.

---

## ADJUVANT CHEMOTHERAPY

Because seminomas are so highly sensitive to platinum chemotherapy, as well as to radiotherapy, several trials have explored the use of adjuvant platinum chemotherapy after orchiectomy for Stage I testicular seminoma, motivated in part by the desire to reduce the late sequelae of radiotherapy.

---

**BOX 27-4**

Over 1,400 patients with Stage I testicular seminoma were randomized to receive either radiotherapy (para-aortic or dog-leg field, 30 Gy) vs. one cycle of carboplatin. With a median follow-up of 4 years, relapse-free survival rates at 3 years were the same in both arms (about 95%). New primary second testicular tumors were seen in 10 patients in the RT arm and in two in the chemo arm. One seminoma-related death occurred in the RT arm. Interpreted as a non-inferiority trial, it supports continuation of chemotherapy only as part of an investigational trial and longer follow-up to confirm its durability of outcomes and late toxicities.

Oliver RT, et al. Radiotherapy versus single-dose carboplatin in adjuvant treatment of Stage I seminoma: a randomized trial. *Lancet* 2005;366:293–300.

---

Although results with a single cycle of carboplatinum are quite promising, the lack of long-term data precludes it from yet being other than investigational.

## SURVEILLANCE

In light of the high success rate of salvage chemotherapy (consisting of platinum-based regimens) the necessity of adjuvant radiation therapy after orchiectomy has been called into question. Several prospective non-randomized studies of surveillance for Stage I testicular seminoma show cause-specific survival rates approaching 100%.[10,11] These studies employed an aggressive follow-up regimen, including frequent CT scans, to detect early recurrence because most are asymptomatic and do not benefit from tumor markers.

These studies have provided important information regarding recurrence rates (hence the proportion of patients potentially benefiting from adjuvant therapies) of about 15%–20%. Median time to relapse was 12 to 18 months, with few relapses beyond 4 years. The predominant site of relapse was the para-aortic lymph nodes (in 85% of patients).

From these studies have emerged prognostic factors that should help in optimizing the selection of appropriate patients for surveillance regimens. Unfavorable factors are mainly tumor sizes larger than 4 cm (hazard ratio of 2) and rete testis invasion (hazard ratio of 1.7). Other possible factors are lymph-vascular invasion and age. The optimal surveillance schedule has not yet been determined. Beta-HCG levels above normal after orchiectomy is equivalent to a Stage II and these patients should not be considered for surveillance.

The rationale of surveillance strategies is to avoid overtreating about 85% of patients and to minimize the late sequelae of adjuvant radiotherapy or chemotherapy. However, this must be weighed against the potential harm of whole body CT scans over a 10-year surveillance period (20 scans) and the toxicities of salvage chemotherapy regimens in relapsed patients. While it may offer some advantages in well selected and compliant patients the long-term benefit has yet to be proven. It is interesting to note that in recent patterns of care surveys the option of surveillance is often not discussed.[12]

## REFERENCES

1. National Comprehensive Cancer Network (NCCN) (2006). Clinical Practice Guidelines in Oncology: Testicular Cancer. available online at nccn.org.
2. Cancer Statistics. (2005). *Cancer J Clin* 2005;55:10–30.
3. *AJCC Cancer Staging Handbook* 6E (2002). Springer-Verlag, New York.
4. Kennedy CL, Hendry F and Peckman MJ. The significance of scrotal interference in Stage I testicular cancer managed by orchiectomy and surveillance. *Br J Urol* 1986;58:705.
5. Kubo H and Shipley WU. Reduction of the scatter dose to the testicle outside the radiation treatment field. *Int J Radiat Oncol Biol Phys* 1982;8:1741.
6. Gospodarowicz M, Sturgeon JFG, and Jewitt MAS. Early-stage and advanced seminoma: role of radiation therapy, surgery, and chemotherapy. *Semin Oncol* 1998;25:160–173.
7. Hanks GE, Peters T, and Owen J. Seminoma of the testis: long-term beneficial and deleterious results of radiation. *Int J Radiat Oncol Biol Phys* 1992;24:913–919.
8. Makfoor BM, Shipley WU, and Zietman AL. Early-stage testicular seminoma: the role of radiation therapy following orchiectomy. *Front Radiat Ther Oncol* 1994;28:183–195.
9. Gordon W Jr., Siegmund K, Stanisic K, et al. A study of reproductive function in patients with seminoma treated with radiotherapy and orchidectomy (SWOG-8711): Southwest Oncology Group. *Int J Radiat Oncol Biol Phys* 1997;38:83–94.
10. Chung P, and Warde P. Surveillance in Stage I testicular seminoma. *Urol Oncol* 2006;24:75–59.
11. Daugaard G, Petersen PM, and Rorth M. Surveillance in Stage I testicular cancer. *APMIS* 2003;111:76–83.
12. Choo R, Sandler H, Warde P, et al. Survey of radiation oncologists: practice patterns of the management of Stage I seminoma of the testis in Canada and a selected group in the United States. *Can J Urol* 2002;9:1479–1485.

# 28

# Prostate Cancer

*Mark K. Buyyounouski, MD, MS*
*Eric M. Horwitz, MD*
*Alan Pollack, MD, PhD*

## OVERVIEW

There are several radiotherapy (RT) indications for men with prostate cancer. Continued progress in radiotherapy techniques and delivery have improved outcome through dose escalation, with fewer late side effects. The results of several large randomized trials are the basis for many common therapeutic decisions. Declining biochemical control rates over time, especially in the intermediate and high-risk groups, support the need for further study. Limiting the toxicity of high-dose RT and appropriate use of androgen deprivation are key to maximizing treatment success.

## EPIDEMIOLOGY AND RISK FACTORS

Prostate cancer is the most commonly diagnosed non-skin cancer in men in the United States. There will be an estimated 186,320 men with prostate cancer diagnosed during 2008.[1] Approximately 80% of these men are considered favorable or intermediate risk.[2] About 27,350 men will die of the disease this year, with African-American men more than twice as likely to die of prostate cancer as their Caucasian counterparts. The increased incidence of mortality in African-American men may be related to dietary and socioeconomic factors. However, African-American men commonly present with more aggressive and advanced disease. Pertinent epidemiological facts about prostate cancer include:

- Incidence: >186,000 (1st non-skin cancer in men)
- Deaths: >28,000 (2nd in men only to lung cancer)
- Average Age: 69

### Risk Factors for Prostate Cancer

- Age — Incidence increase with age
- Race/Ethnicity — Highest in Scandanavia
  Lowest in Asia
- Family History — Relative risk with affected father, brother or paternal relative—3.2
- Diet — High fat/caloric diets associated with increased risk

## WORKUP

Routine annual screening prostate specific antigen (PSA) and digital rectal exam (DRE) have resulted in most patients presenting early, when the risk for distant metastasis is low. An elevated PSA or suspicious DRE prompts a transrectal ultrasound (TRUS) guided biopsy of the prostate. This should be done systematically, where preferably 12 or more regions are sampled and accessioned individually. A detailed pathologic review including Gleason Score, the number of positive cores/regions, and the percentage of tumor in the cores/regions provide important information for guiding treatment. A bone scan is recommended for men with Gleason Score 8 to 10, an initial PSA >20 ng/mL or symptoms suggestive of bony disease. A CT scan to detect pelvic lymph node metastasis should be done if there is local extension outside of the prostate (T3 or T4).

The American Joint Committee for Cancer (AJCC) staging system is shown in Table 28-1. The DRE is the mainstay of prostate cancer staging. Transrectal ultrasound (TRUS) and biopsy laterality (unilateral versus bilateral) information cause stage migration.[4-8] Endorectal coil MRI, however, has proven useful to confirm or establish extra capsular extension. The utility of a two- versus three-tier T2 sub categorization system has been debated, but there is no significant difference in outcome following RT at Fox Chase Cancer Center.[7]

---

### TABLE 28-1 Clinical TNM Classification for Carcinoma of the Prostate[3]

**Primary Tumor (T)**

| | |
|---|---|
| TX | Primary tumor cannot be assessed |
| T0 | No evidence of primary tumor |
| T1 | Clinically inapparent tumor neither palpable nor visible by imaging |
| T1a | Tumor incidental histologic finding in 5% or less of resected tissue |
| T1b | Tumor incidental histologic finding in more than 5% of resected tissue |
| T1c | Tumor identified by needle biopsy (elevated PSA)* |
| T2 | Tumor confined within prostate† |
| T2a | Tumor involves one half of one lobe or less |
| T2b | Tumor involves more than one half of one lobe but not both lobes |
| T2c | Tumor involves both lobes |
| T3 | Tumor extends through the prostate capsule** |
| T3a | Extracapsular extension |
| T3b | Tumor invades seminal vesicle(s) |
| T4 | Tumor is fixed or invades adjacent structures other than seminal vesicles: bladder neck, external sphincter, rectum, levator muscles, and/or pelvic wall |

**Regional Lymph Nodes (N)**

| | |
|---|---|
| NX | Regional lymph nodes were not assessed |
| N1 | No regional lymph node metastasis |
| N2 | Metastasis in regional lymph node(s) |

**Distant Metastasis (M)**

| | |
|---|---|
| MX | Distant metastasis cannot be assessed (not evaluated by any modality) |
| M0 | No distant metastasis |
| M1 | Distant metastasis |

*Tumor that is found in one or both lobes by needle biopsy, but is not palpable or visible by imaging, is classified as T1c.
† Tumor found in one or both lobes by needle biopsy, but not palpable or reliably visible by imaging, is classified as T1c.
** Invasion into the prostatic apex or into (but not beyond) the prostatic capsule is classified not as T3 but as T2.

## Prognosis and Risk Factors

The most commonly used risk stratification schemes for clinically localized prostate cancer combine pretreatment initial PSA (iPSA), Gleason Score, and T-category (based on DRE). They are used for assigning risk of biochemical failure after external beam radiotherapy. The single factor model (modeled after D'Amico et al.)[9] classifies those with Gleason Score 8 to 10, iPSA >20 ng/mL or T3/T4 disease as high risk. An alternative three-tier system is the double factor (DF) model reported by Zelefsky et al.[10] Table 28-2 illustrates a comparison of these models. Figure 28-1 represents freedom from biochemical failure by risk group using single factor and double factor models.

A high proportion of positive biopsy cores (>50%) has been shown to correlate with lymph node metastasis, adverse pathologic features at the time of surgery (extra capsular penetration), and a higher risk of treatment failure independent of PSA and Gleason Score. Men with >50% of the biopsy cores containing Gleason Score 7 should strongly be considered for more aggressive treatment, such as the addition of androgen deprivation therapy (ADT) to radiotherapy or longer-term ADT with radiotherapy.

A PSA velocity of greater than 2 ng/mL per year prior to diagnosis has been related to an increased risk of death from prostate cancer.[12] This finding may be related to a greater risk of distant metastasis, but the best management for these patients is not established. Consideration of more aggressive treatment, such as the use of ADT, may be appropriate.

Recently, biomarker expression has been shown to be a strong predictor of outcome for men treated with RT and ADT. The Ki-67 staining index, a measure of the tumor growth fraction, was shown to be a strong predictor of distant metastasis and mortality.[13] While the optimal cut point has not been firmly established, a value greater than >7.1% appears to be the most appropriate at this time.

**TABLE 28-2** Single and Double Factor Risk Models

|  | Single Factor (NCCN) | Single Factor (Chism et al) | Double Factor (Zelefsky et al) |
|---|---|---|---|
| **Low Risk** | iPSA <10 | iPSA ≤10 | iPSA ≤10 |
|  | GS 2–6 | GS 2–6 | GS 2–6 |
|  | T1a–T2a | T1–T2c* | T1–T2c |
| **Intermediate Risk** | *Presence of 1 or more* | *Presence of 1 or more†* | *Presence of 1* |
|  | iPSA 10–20 | iPSA >10 and ≤20 | iPSA >10 |
|  | GS 7 |  | GS ≥7 |
|  | T2b–T2c |  | ≥T3 |
| **High Risk** | *Presence of 1 or more* | *Presence of 1 or more* | *Presence of 2 or 3* |
|  | iPSA >20 | iPSA >20 | iPSA >10 |
|  | GS 8–10 | GS 8–10 | GS ≥7 |
|  | T3a, T3b–T4‡ | ≥T3 | ≥T3 |

*Abbreviations:* NCCN = National Comprehensive Cancer Network

The single and double factor high-risk models are patterned after that described by NCCN Version 1.2007, D'Amico et al. and Zelefsky et al.[10]

*T2b has sometimes been considered intermediate risk and T2c has sometimes been considered intermediate or high risk. In the Fox Chase database, these patients have about the same prognosis as patients with T2a disease in univariate and multivariate analysis, and so have been grouped in a favorable category here.

† No high-risk factors present.

‡ T3b–T4 are considered locally advanced in the absence of distant metastasis.

Modified from Chism et al.,[11] with permission.

## FIGURE 28-1 Kaplan Meier freedom from biochemical failure (FFBF) by risk group.

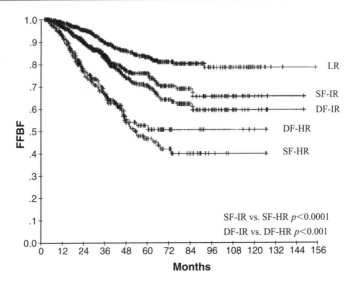

Abbreviations: LR = low risk, IR = intermediate risk, HR = high risk, SF = single factor (See Table 28-2, Chism et al), DF = double factor. Modified from Chism et al.[11], with permission from Elsevier.

### BOX 28-1

In this validation study of the Hamburg algorithm developed by Conrad et al., the risk of lymph node metastasis was determined based on the Gleason grade of systematic sextant biopsy specimens. Of the 443 men that underwent systematic sextant biopsy and staging lymphadenectomy prior to surgery, men with ≥4 of 6 regions containing any Gleason Pattern 4 disease were at highest risk for lymph node metastases (44.4%). This was in excellent agreement with the 45% rate of lymph node metastases in the original study. The risk of lymph node metastasis for men with 1 to 3 regions positive with dominant Gleason Pattern 4 disease was 20% and for all other patients was 2.5%.

Haese et al., Validation of a biopsy-based pathologic algorithm for predicting lymph node metastases in patients with clinically localized prostate carcinoma. *Cancer.* 2002 Sep 1;95(5):1016–1021.

### BOX 28-2

D'Amico et al. studied the prognostic ability of the PSA velocity to predict for prostate cancer specific survival following radiotherapy for prostate cancer. A greater than 2.0 ng/mL rise in PSA level during the year prior to diagnosis was associated with a significantly higher risk of death due to prostate cancer following RT. For all men with a PSA velocity >2 ng/mL, management similar to that for high-risk patients, RT with ADT was suggested.

D'Amico et al., Pretreatment PSA velocity and risk of death from prostate cancer following external beam radiation therapy. *JAMA.* 2005 Jul 27;294(4):440–447.

## TREATMENT OF FAVORABLE-RISK PATIENTS

Favorable-risk patients are excellent candidates for radical prostatectomy, external beam RT or a prostate brachytherapy (BT) with excellent 5-year biochemical failure-free survival. In carefully selected patients, outcomes have not been shown to differ significantly between surgery, external beam RT, and BT.

---

### BOX 28-3

Kupelian et al. compared 2,991 consecutive men with T1–T2 prostate cancer to compare biochemical relapse-free survival following external beam radiotherapy, prostate implant, radical prostatectomy, and combination external beam radiotherapy with prostate implant. The biochemical failure rates were similar among implant, high-dose (≥72 Gy) external beam RT, radical prostatectomy, and combination therapy groups. The only group with significantly lower outcome was those treated with external beam radiotherapy to doses 72 Gy.

Kupelian et al., Radical prostatectomy, external beam radiotherapy <72 Gy, external beam radiotherapy > or 572 Gy, permanent seed implantation, or combined seeds/external beam radiotherapy for stage T1-T2 prostate cancer. *Int J Radiat Oncol Biol Phys.* 2004 Jan 1;58(1):25–33.

---

Observation is also a reasonable alternative for some men. However, in the absence of serious medical comorbidities limiting their life expectancy to less than 10 years, treatment is advocated.

---

### BOX 28-4

Ten-year results from a randomized comparison between radical prostatectomy and watchful-waiting for early-stage prostate cancer (n = 695) showed that without treatment men were nearly twice as likely to die of prostate cancer. The authors concluded that while the absolute reduction in the risk of death after 10 years was small (8.6% vs. 14.4%), the reduction in metastasis (relative risk = 0.60) and local tumor progression were substantial.

Bill-Axelson et al., Radical prostatectomy versus watchful waiting in early prostate cancer. *N Engl J Med.* 2005 May 12;352(19):1977–1984.

---

Higher RT doses have not consistently benefited favorable patients in several retrospective external beam RT dose escalation studies[14–18] (see Figure 28-2). The sequential nature of these studies subjects them to inherent bias because of trends for lower Gleason Scores,[19] T-stage,[20] and PSA over time. The Proton Radiation Oncology Group (PROG) reported a randomized trial comparing 79.2 CGE (cobalt Gray equivalent) versus 70.2 CGE that demonstrated a significant improvement in biochemical control for the high-dose group. The majority of patients in the proton boost trial were favorable.

## TREATMENT OF HIGH-RISK PATIENTS

High-risk patients benefit from long-term, 2 to 3 years, ADT in randomized clinical trials comparing external beam RT with and without ADT. ADT is achieved commonly with a long-acting (3 to 4 month) luteinising hormone-releasing hormone (LHRH) agonist (leuprolide acetate or goserelin acetate).

## TREATMENT OF INTERMEDIATE-RISK PATIENTS

The intermediate-risk group appears to obtain the greatest benefit from dose escalation above 70 Gy. Level I evidence was first described in a trial from M.D. Anderson Cancer Center, with supporting evidence from the proton boost and Dutch randomized dose escalation trials.

**BOX 28-5**

In this prospective randomized PROG trial conducted between January 1996 and December 1999, 393 patients with T1b through T2b prostate cancer and iPSA <15 ng/mL were randomized to receive a combination of conformal photon and proton RT to a either 70.2 or 79.2 CGE. There was a statistically significant benefit for the high-dose group in terms of biochemical control at 5 years: 80.4% vs. 61.4% (p < 0.001). This 49% reduction in failure risk was achieved without any associated increase in Radiation Therapy Oncology Group (RTOG) grade 3 acute or late urinary or rectal morbidity.

Zietman et al., Comparison of conventional-dose vs. high-dose conformal radiation therapy in clinically localized adenocarcinoma of the prostate: a randomized controlled trial. *JAMA.* 2005 Sep 14;294(10):1233–1239.

While long-term ADT is the standard of care for high-risk patients based on the results of the trial by Bolla et al and RTOG 92-02, the addition of short-term ADT was associated with a survival benefit for intermediate- and high-risk patients in a trial from Harvard. The survival benefit was related to the addition of just 6 months of ADT. The RT dose used was below what is considered adequate today based on the current understanding of dose escalation above 70 Gy. Nonetheless, the gains from short-term ADT have been consistent and should be considered even in intermediate-risk patients treated with higher doses of radiation. The results of RTOG 92-02 indicate that for men with high-risk prostate cancer, long-term ADT is preferred over short-term ADT.

**FIGURE 28-2** PROG trial.

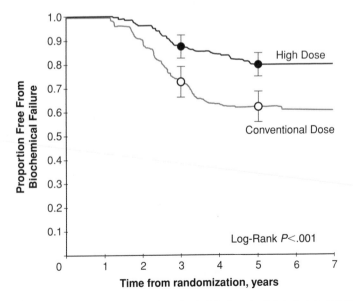

From: Zietman et al., Comparison of conventional-dose vs. high-dose conformal radiation therapy in clinically localized edenocarcinoma of the prostate: a randomized controlled trial. *JAMA.* 2005 Sep 14;294(10):1233–1239. c. 2005, American Medical Association. All right reserved.

**TABLE 28-3  Sequential 3DCRT Dose Escalation Studies of External Beam Radiotherapy**

| Author (Institution) | Year | n | Risk | 5-year Results | | p |
|---|---|---|---|---|---|---|
| | | | | %FFBF (Dose) | %FFBF (Dose) | |
| Lyons et al. | | | | | | |
| (Cleveland Clinic) | 2000 | 738 | Low | 81 (<72 Gy) | 98 (≥72 Gy) | 0.02 |
| | | | High | 41 (<72 Gy) | 75 (≥72 Gy) | 0.001 |
| Hanks et al. | | | | | | |
| (FCCC) | 2000 | 618 | Low[†] | 86 (<70 Gy) | 80 (≥70 Gy) | NS |
| | | | Int | 29 (<71.5 Gy) | 66 (≥71.5 Gy) | <0.05 |
| | | | High | 8 (<71.5 Gy) | 29 (≥71.5 Gy) | <0.05 |
| Pollack et al. | | | | | | |
| (MDACC)* | 2000 | 1213 | Low | 84 (<67 Gy) | 91 (>67–70 Gy) | NS |
| | | | Low | 91 (<67–77 Gy) | 100 (>77 Gy) | NS |
| | | | Int | 55 (<67 Gy) | 79 (>67–66 Gy) | 0.0001 |
| | | | Int | 79 (>67–77 Gy) | 89 (>77 Gy) | NS |
| | | | High | 27 (≤67 Gy) | 47 (>67–77 Gy) | 0.0001 |
| | | | High | 47 (>67–77 Gy) | 67 (>67 Gy) | 0.016 |
| Zelefsky et al. | | | | | | |
| (MSKCC) | 2001 | 1100 | Low | 77 (≤670 Gy) | 90 (>75.6 Gy) | 0.05 |
| | | | Int | 50 (≤70 Gy) | 70 (>75.6 Gy) | 0.001 |
| | | | High | 21 (≤70 Gy) | 47 (>75.6 Gy) | 0.002 |
| Pollack et al. | | | | | | |
| (FCCC) | 2004 | 839 | Low | 81 (72–76 Gy) | 78 (72–76 Gy) | NS |
| | | | Low | 78 (72–76 Gy) | 82 (>76 Gy) | NS |
| | | | Int | 24 (<72 Gy) | 65 (72–76 Gy) | 0.0051 |
| | | | Int | 65 (72–76 Gy) | 79 (>76 Gy) | 0.0096 |
| | | | High | 27 (72–76 Gy) | 34 (>76 Gy) | 0.04 |

*4-year results (published in a book chapter)

[†]based on pre-treatment PSA

*Abbreviations:* Int = intermediate; MSKCC = Memorial Sloan-Kettering Cancer Center; FCCC = Fox Chase Cancer Center; MDACC = M.D. Anderson Cancer Center; FFBF = freedom from biochemical failure; MGH = Massachusetts General Hospital.

Modified from The Prostate: In: *Radiation Oncology, Rationale, Technique, Results*, 8E. JD Cox, KK Ang (eds.), Mosby, St. Louis, MO 2003, with permission.

---

**BOX 28-6**

The EORTC randomly assigned 415 men to RT alone (70 Gy prostate, 50 Gy to the pelvic lymph nodes) or RT with immediate ADT started on the first day of irradiation and continued for 3 years. Eligible patients had high-grade T1–2 or T3–4 disease. After a median follow-up of 66 months, 5-year overall survival was 62% and 78%, respectively (p = 0.0002) and 5-year specific survival 79% and 94%. The authors concluded that immediate ADT with an LHRH analogue given during and for 3 years after RT improves disease-free and overall survival of patients with locally advanced prostate cancer.

Bolla et al., Long-term results with immediate androgen suppression and external irradiation in patients with locally advanced prostate cancer (an EORTC study): a phase III randomised trial. *Lancet.* 2002 Jul 13;360(9327):103–106.

---

**FIGURE 28-3** EORTC trial.

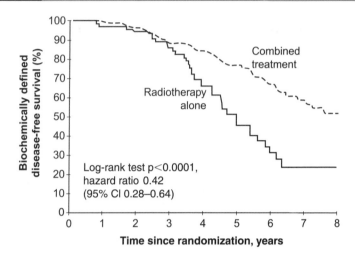

Bolla et al., Long-term results with immediate androgen suppression and external irradiation in patients with locally advanced prostate cancer (an EORTC study): a phase III randomised trial. *Lancet.* 2002 Jul 13;360(9327):103–106., with permission of Elsevier.

---

**BOX 28-7**

RTOG 92-02 randomized over 1,500 patients with T2c-T4 disease between combined RT and short-term versus long-term ADT. The RT dose was 65 Gy to 70 Gy to the prostate and 44 Gy to 50 Gy to the pelvic lymph nodes. All patients received a total of 4 months of goserelin and flutamide, 2 months before and 2 months during RT. Patients were randomly assigned to receive no additional therapy or an additional 24 months of goserelin. Overall, there was a benefit for long-term ADT in terms of biochemical control, disease-free survival, distant metastasis, local progression and cause-specific survival. In a subset of patients not part of the original study design, with men with Gleason Scores of 8 to 10, the long-term ADT+RT arm had significantly better overall survival (81.0% vs. 70.7%, p = 0.044).

Hanks et al., Phase III trial of long-term adjuvant androgen deprivation after neo-adjuvant hormonal cytoreduction and radiotherapy in locally advanced carcinoma of the prostate: the Radiation Therapy Oncology Group Protocol 92-02. *J Clin Oncol.* 2003 Nov 1; 21(21):3972–3978.

---

Combination external beam RT and interstitial brachytherapy, at low-dose or high-dose rate, have also been advocated by some for the intermediate-risk group. Toxicity from the combined treatment appears acceptable.[21,22] The RTOG is currently comparing the combination of external beam radiotherapy and brachytherapy with brachytherapy alone in men with intermediate-risk prostate cancer.

## EXTERNAL BEAM RADIOTHERAPY FOR NODE-POSITIVE DISEASE

The results of RTOG 85-13, and surgical literature[23,24] support the use of immediate ADT and pelvic RT as the standard for men with lymph node-positive (N1) disease versus RT alone.

However, these patients are sometimes not referred for RT due to physician bias regarding metastatic disease. Yet, Figure 28-4 illustrates pelvic RT results in a substantial and significant

### BOX 28-8

The M.D. Anderson trial conducted between 1993 and 1998, compared the efficacy of 70 Gy vs. 78 Gy. With a median follow-up of 8.7 years, the freedom from biochemical failure rates for the 70 Gy arm was 59% and for the 78 Gy arm 78% (p = 0.004). Dose escalation to 78 Gy preferentially benefited those with a pretreatment PSA <10 ng/mL; the biochemical control rate was 78% for the 78 Gy arm vs. 39% for those who received 70 Gy (p < 0.001). For patients with a pretreatment PSA >10 ng/mL, no significant dose response was found at 8 years (78% for 78 Gy vs 66% for 70 Gy, p = 0.237). Although no difference occurred in overall survival, the freedom from distant metastasis rate was higher for those with high-risk disease who were treated to 78 Gy (96% vs. 83%, p = 0.035). Rectal side effects were also significantly greater in the 78 Gy group. Grade 2 or higher toxicity rates at 8 years were 13% and 26% for the 70 Gy and 78 Gy arms, respectively (p = 0.013). Grade 2 or higher rectal toxicity correlated highly with the proportion of the rectum treated to >70 Gy. It was previously concluded that dose escalation techniques that limit the rectal volume that receives < 70 Gy to <25% should be used.

Kuban et al., Long term results of the M.D. Anderson randomized dose-escalation trial for prostate cancer. *Int J Radiat Oncol Biol Phys.* 2008 Jan 1;70(1):67–74.

### BOX 28-9

RTOG 8610 was the first phase III randomized trial to evaluate neoadjuvant androgen deprivation therapy in combination with external-beam RT in men with locally advanced prostate cancer. Between 1987 and 1991, 456 men with T2-4 (1998 AJCC, bulky 5 × 5 cm tumors), with or without pelvic lymph node involvement, were randomly assigned to receive goserelin (3.6 mg every 4 weeks) and flutamide (250 mg TID) for 2 months before and concurrent with RT or RT alone. Long-term follow-up results favored ADT and RT in terms of 10-year biochemical failure (65% vs. 80%, p < 0.001), distant metastasis (35% vs. 47%, = 0.006), disease free survival (11% vs. 3%, p < 0.001), and disease-specific mortality (23% vs. 36%, p = 0.01). Overall survival also favored combined treatment (10-year: 43% vs. 34%; median survival: 8.7 vs. 7.3 years) however, the difference was not statistically significant (p = 0.12). There was no impact of ADT on the risk of fatal cardiac events.

Roach M 3rd et al., Short-term neoadjuvant androgen deprivation therapy and external-beam radiotherapy for locally advanced prostate cancer: long-term results of RTOG 8610. *J Clin Oncol.* 2008 Feb 1;26(4):p.585–91.

### BOX 28-10

From December 1, 1995 to April 15, 2001, D'Amico et al. randomized 206 men with non-metastatic prostate cancer (PSA ≥10 ng/mL, a Gleason Score ≥7, or radiographic evidence of extracapsular extension) to receive 70 Gy external beam RT alone (n = 104) or in combination with 6 months of ADT (n = 102). A significantly higher survival (p = 0.04) and lower prostate cancer-specific mortality (p = 0.02) was seen after a median follow-up 4.52 years. Five-year survival rate estimates were 88% in the RT plus ADT group vs. 78% in the RT alone group. The authors concluded that the addition of 6 months of ADT to 70 Gy RT confers an overall survival benefit for patients with clinically localized prostate cancer.

D'Amico et al., 6-month androgen suppression plus radiation therapy vs. radiation therapy alone for patients with clinically localized prostate cancer: a randomized controlled trial. *JAMA.* 2004 Aug 18;292(7):821–827.

**FIGURE 28-4** M.D. Anderson trial.

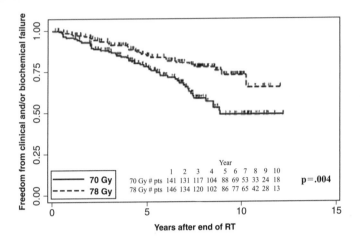

| | Year | | | | | | | | | | |
|---|---|---|---|---|---|---|---|---|---|---|---|
| | | 1 | 2 | 3 | 4 | 5 | 6 | 7 | 8 | 9 | 10 |
| 70 Gy # pts | | 141 | 131 | 117 | 104 | 88 | 69 | 53 | 33 | 24 | 18 |
| 78 Gy # pts | | 146 | 134 | 120 | 102 | 86 | 77 | 65 | 42 | 28 | 13 |

p=.004

Years after end of RT

Kuban et al., Long term results of the M.D. Anderson randomized dose-escalation trial for prostate cancer. *Int J Radiat Oncol Biol Phys.* 2008 Jan 1;70(1):67–74.

improvement in patient survival compared to age-matched expected survival as seen in a study from M.D. Anderson Cancer Center. Men with node-positive prostate cancer should not be treated with androgen deprivation alone or local therapy alone, if they have a 10-year life expectancy.

## EXTERNAL BEAM RADIOTHERAPY FOLLOWING RADICAL PROSTATECTOMY

Retrospective comparisons between adjuvant and salvage therapy are limited by selection bias. Direct comparisons between adjuvant and salvage treatment probably should not be made. The Southwest Oncology Group (SWOG) recently reported results of their randomized trial comparing immediate RT versus observation in men with pathologic T3 disease. PSA relapse and disease recurrence were significantly reduced with RT, confirming benefits seen in the large EORTC trial. In the SWOG trial, there were fewer distant metastases and a highly significant reduction in the need for

### BOX 28-11

A national prospective randomized trial of external-beam RT plus immediate ADT versus RT alone was initiated in 1985 for patients with locally advanced adenocarcinoma of the prostate. With a median follow-up of 6.5 years for all patients and 9.5 years for living patients, multivariate analysis revealed RT and immediate ADT as having a statistically significant impact on absolute survival, disease-specific failure, metastatic failure, and biochemical control with PSA less than 4 ng/mL and less than 1.5 ng/mL. The authors concluded that patients with adenocarcinoma of the prostate who have pathologically involved pelvic lymph nodes (pathologic node-positive or clinical Stage D1) should be considered for external-beam RT and immediate ADT rather ADT at the time of relapse.

Lawton et al., Androgen suppression plus radiation versus radiation alone for patients with stage D1/pathologic node-positive adenocarcinoma of the prostate: updated results based on national prospective randomized trial. Radiation Therapy Oncology Group 85-31. *J Clin Oncol.* 2005 Feb 1;23(4):800–807.

**FIGURE 28-5** RT +/− ADT for N1 disease.

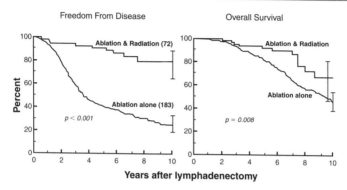

Zagars et al., Addition of radiation therapy to androgen ablation improved outcome for subclinically node-positive prostate cancer. *Urology*. 2001 Aug;58(2);233–239. Used with permission of Elsevier.

---

**BOX 28-12**

Zagars et al. retrospectively studied 255 men with lymphadenectomy-proven pelvic nodal metastases and demonstrate that early androgen ablation alone has little curative potential for node-positive prostate cancer. The study included men treated between 1984 and 1998 with either early androgen ablation alone (n = 183) or with combined ablation and radiation (n = 72). With a median follow-up of 9.4 years, the 10-year overall survival rate for those treated with early ablation alone was 46%. With a median follow-up of 6.2 years, the 10-year overall survival rate for those treated with RT and ablation was 67%. Multivariate analysis for all patients identified the addition of RT as a significant determinant of outcome for all endpoints independent of Gleason Score, T-category, and iPSA.

Zagars et al., Addition of radiation therapy to androgen ablation improves outcome for subclinically node-positive prostate cancer. *Urology*. 2001 Aug;58(2):233–239.

---

**BOX 28-13**

The SWOG randomized trial was designed to determine whether patients with pathologic T3 prostate cancer benefited from immediate adjuvant radiation therapy. From 1988 to 1995, 473 patients with pathologically determined extracapsular extension, seminal vesicle involvement, (pT3), or positive margins were randomized to radiation (60–64 Gy) versus observation. After a median follow-up of 10.6 years, biochemical free survival (PSA <0.4 ng/ml) was significantly improved with radiation, while metastatic free survival and overall survival were non-significantly improved. The benefit for radiation was seen in each of the three pathologic risk groups. There was a highly significant reduction in the need for hormonal therapy when adjuvant RT was used. When hormonal therapy was not obviated, it was delayed on average by 2.5 years. The authors concluded that pT3 patients should be given the opportunity to receive postoperative radiation.

Thompson, I. M., Jr. et al., Adjuvant radiotherapy for pathologically advanced prostate cancer: a randomized clinical trial. *JAMA*. 2006 Nov 15;296(19):2329–2335.

## BOX 28-14

The EORTC trial compared immediate external beam radiotherapy following radical prostatectomy versus prostatectomy alone for patients with positive surgical margin or pT3 prostate cancer. Over 1,000 patients were randomized to radiation (60 Gy) versus observation. After a median follow-up of 5 years, the biochemical progression-free survival was 74% in the irradiated group versus 53% in the surgery alone group (p < 0.0001). Clinical progression-free survival was also significantly improved (p = 0.0009). The cumulative rate of locoregional failure was significantly lower in the irradiated group (p < 0.0001). The authors concluded that immediate external irradiation after radical prostatectomy improves biochemical progression-free survival and local control in patients with positive surgical margins or pT3 prostate cancer who are at high risk of progression.

Bolla, M. et al., Postoperative radiotherapy after radical prostatectomy: a randomized controlled trial (EORTC trial 22911). *Lancet.* 2005 Aug 13–19;366(9485):524–525.

hormonal therapy when RT was used. However, the improvement in distant metastasis-free survival was not statistically significant. Competing factors for survival and salvage therapy in the observation group likely explain this difference.

Several factors have been associated with better salvage radiotherapy results. These include a pre-RT PSA of <1 ng/mL, Gleason Score ≤7, no seminal vesicle involvement, positive margins at prostatectomy, PSA doubling time greater than 10 months, use of androgen deprivation, and delayed rise in PSA after prostatectomy. The preliminary results from a pooled multi-institutional analysis indicate biochemical failure continues to occur between 5 and 10 years and may ultimately be as high as 80%.[25] These results provide further support for adjuvant external beam RT for men with high-risk features (especially a positive margin) at prostatectomy.

## RADIATION TECHNIQUE

### Intensity Modulated Radiotherapy (IMRT)

Intensity modulated radiotherapy (IMRT) is widely used for the treatment of prostate cancer. Advances in multileaf collimation and inverse treatment planning have resulted in dosimetric gains in terms of sharp dose fall-off and normal tissue sparing. These gains have translated to escalated doses of radiation with less toxicity, as the Memorial Sloan Kettering series has shown.

Rectal toxicity reduction is one of the most important advantages of prostate IMRT. Rectal toxicity is associated with radiation dose and rectal volume exposed to higher doses. Higher radiation dose is related to increased grade 2 or higher rectal reactions, and the volume of the rectum exposed to a specific radiation dose level is as important as the dose prescribed. High radiation doses (≥75.6 Gy) may be used when specific dose-volume criteria are applied to limit the rectal exposure.

As with any IMRT technique, the prescription dose, normal tissue constraints, and acceptability criteria are dependent upon the target and normal tissue definitions (whole rectum versus rectal wall; entire rectal length versus a smaller segment).

At Fox Chase Cancer Center, patients are simulated supine in an alpha cradle cast for immobilization with an empty rectum and partially full bladder. An empty rectum better simulates the rectal volume during treatment. A partially full bladder better enables dose sparing and visualization of the prostate when daily ultrasound localization is used. The rectum is defined from the ischial tuberosities to the sigmoid flexure, similar to the RTOG method. The femoral heads are defined to a level between the greater and lesser trochanters.

The target volume definitions used at Fox Chase Cancer Center and prescription dose for each are outlined in Table 28-4. Fused simulation CT and MRI scans are used to define the CTV. MRI is the gold standard for imaging soft tissue of the pelvis, more easily enabling identification of the prostate apex as well as the erectile structures. Alternately, a retrograde urethrogram may be used to identify the prostate apex. Detailed examples of the axial CT/MRI volumes used have been published elsewhere.[26]

Pelvic lymph node treatment remains controversial. The initial report of RTOG 94-13 showed that, overall, there was a benefit from whole pelvis RT, which substantiated the trends seen in many retrospective series. The improvement in biochemical and clinical outcome was mainly seen in the men treated with pelvic lymph node RT plus neo-adjuvant and concurrent ADT; all of the other three treatment combinations (prostate only + neoadjuvant, prostate only + adjuvant, whole pelvis + adjuvant) were worse. There may be a synergistic effect in involved lymph nodes, where tumor-stromal interactions are at a minimum as compared to the prostate and bone marrow (when involved). A recent preliminary description of an update of RTOG 94-13 no longer shows a statistical benefit for the addition of pelvic lymph node RT over prostate only RT; however, the subgroup of whole pelvis plus neo-adjuvant and concurrent ADT remained significant in most comparisons. The future of pelvic lymph RT for prostate cancer is uncertain.

The treatment plan acceptability criteria are shown in Figure 28-6. The conditions that define an acceptable plan are subdivided into dose volume histogram (DVH) criteria and spatial criteria. DVH criteria ensure that dose is delivered to the appropriate volumes without exceeding established limits. The spatial criteria require inspection of the isodose distribution on a slice-by-slice basis to ensure that the dose is distributed within the volume appropriately. For example, the rectal spatial criteria ensure that a rapid dose gradient across the rectum is achieved. Oftentimes, bladder constraints are not met. These are poorly defined and the least important.

**TABLE 28-4 Treatment Planning and Evaluation Scheme at Fox Chase Cancer Center**

| Volume | Target | Prescription |
|---|---|---|
| CTV | • Prostate<br>• Proximal seminal vesicles*<br>• Gross extracapsular extension | $D_{100\%} \geq 100\%$ prescription dose[†] |
| PTV1 | • CTV1 + 8 mm, except 5 mm posteriorly | $D_{95\%} \geq 100\%$ prescription dose[†]<br>$D_{max} < 17\%$ prescription dose[†]<br>$V_{<65Gy} < 1\%$ |
| PTV2 | • Distal seminal vesicles (CTV2) + 8 mm, except 5 mm posteriorly | $D_{95\%} \geq 100\%$ prescription dose[‡] |
| PTV3 | • Lymph nodes (CTV3) + 8 mm, except 5 mm posteriorly | $D_{95\%} \geq 100\%$ prescription dose[¶] |

Abbreviations: CTV = clinical target volume; PTV = planning target volume; $D_{XX}$ = the dose received by XX% of the volume; $V_{XX}$ = the volume receiving XX Gy; Int = intermediate.
†For T3b disease, most, if not all, of the seminal vesicles are treated to the full dose.
†Prescription dose: Low risk = 78 Gy. Int/High risk = 80 Gy.
‡Prescription dose: Low/Int risk = N/A. High risk = 56Gy§
¶Prescription dose: Low/Int risk = N/A. High risk = 56Gy§
§Delivered in 39 to 40 fractions.

## BOX 28-15

Zelefsky et al. retrospectively reviewed 772 patients with clinically localized prostate cancer and showed that acute rectal toxicity can be reduced in intensity modulated radiotherapy (IMRT). Between April 1996 and January 2001, 772 patients with clinically localized prostate cancer were treated with IMRT to 81.0 Gy (90%), and 74 patients (10%) were treated to 86.4 Gy. After a median follow-up of 24 months, 35 patients' acute grade 2 rectal toxicity (RTOG) was 4.5%, acute grade 3 or higher rectal toxicity was 0%. Acute grade 2 urinary toxicity was 28%, and one experienced urinary retention (grade 3). The 3-year actuarial likelihood of > late grade 2 rectal toxicity was 4%. The 3-year actuarial likelihood of > late grade 2 urinary toxicity was 15%. The 3-year actuarial PSA relapse-free survival rates for favorable, intermediate, and unfavorable risk group patients were 92%, 86%, and 81%, respectively. The authors concluded that acute and late rectal toxicities seem to be significantly reduced compared with what has been observed with conventional three-dimensional conformal radiotherapy techniques. Furthermore, short-term PSA control rates were at least comparable to those achieved with three-dimensional conformal radiotherapy at similar dose levels.

Zelefsky et al., High-dose intensity modulated radiation therapy for prostate cancer: early toxicity and biochemical outcome in 772 patients. *Int J Radiat Oncol Biol Phys.* 2002 Aug 1;53(5): 1111–1116.

## FIGURE 28-6 IMRT treatment planning constraints.

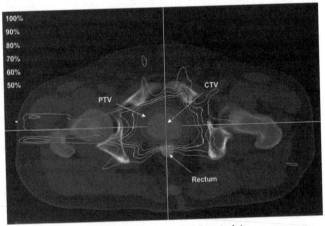

### IMRT Treatment Planning Constraints

#### DVH Criteria

1. CTV $D_{100\%}$ = 100%
2. PTV $D_{100\%}$ > 95%
3. Rectal $V_{40Gy}$ < 35%
4. Rectal $V_{65Gy}$ < 17%
5. Bladder $V_{40Gy}$ < 50%
6. Bladder $V_{65Gy}$ < 25%
7. Femoral Head $V_{50Gy}$ < 10%

#### Spatial Criteria

1. The 90% dose line encompasses no more than the half-width of the rectum on any axial cut.
2. The 50% dose line does not encompass the full-rectum width.
3. The posterior edge of the CTV to the prescription isodose line is ~3 to 8 mm.

(See Color Plate 11).

## BOX 28-16

This four arm trial tested two hypotheses: (1) Combined ADT and RT to the pelvic lymph nodes is superior to ADT and RT to prostate alone; and (2) Neo-adjuvant and concurrent ADT is superior to adjuvant ADT. Between April 1, 1995 and June 1, 1999, 1,323 patients with clinically localized prostate cancer with an estimated risk of lymph node (LN) involvement of at least 15% were randomly assigned to whole pelvis or prostate only RT. A second randomization was then performed for neo-adjuvant and concurrent ADT versus adjuvant ADT. With a median follow-up of 60 months, whole pelvis was associated with a 4-year PFS of 54% compared with 47% in patients treated with prostate only (p = 0.022). There was no difference seen between neo-adjuvant and concurrent ADT versus adjuvant ADT. When comparing all four arms, there was a progression-free difference in favor of the whole pelvis and neo-adjuvant and concurrent ADT arm (60% vs. 44% vs. 49% vs. 50%; p = 0.008).

Roach et al., Phase III trial comparing whole-pelvic versus prostate-only radiotherapy and neoadjuvant versus adjuvant combined androgen suppression: Radiation Therapy Oncology Group 9413. *J Clin Oncol.* 2003 May 15;21(10):1904–1911.

## Brachytherapy

Brachytherapy techniques vary from preplanned, preloaded needle placement to intra-operative, real-time planning with custom loaded needles. The most commonly used seeds contain either I-125 (half life, 59 days) or Pd-103 (half-life, 17 days). The difference in activity translates into different biologic effects such that the prescription dose for Iodine-125 is 145 Gy and for Pd-103 is 115-120 Gy. The American Brachytherapy Society has published guidelines for post-implant dosimetric analysis, which has helped standardize the evaluation process irrespective of the technique used.

The implant technique at Fox Chase Cancer Center utilizes transrectal ultrasound (TRUS) guidance, although CT- and MRI-guided techniques have been described. Briefly, all patients first undergo a CT/MRI volume study at least 1 week before the implant to ensure the prostate size <60 cc. Men with prostate larger in size have been shown to be at excess risk of urinary obstruction requiring a Foley catheter for days, to weeks or months.

For the actual procedure, the patient is placed in an extended dorsal lithotomy position, prepped and dressed in the usual fashion, a Foley catheter inserted, and contrast placed in the bladder. Dilute contrast material aids visualization during the procedure with portable X-rays. Two stabilization needles are placed in two central positions to limit prostate motion through the course of the implant procedure. The prostate is serially imaged from the base to apex in 0.5-cm increments.

A peripherally weighted plan is utilized with approximately 75% of the total activity placed in the periphery of the prostate. The prescription dose to the prostate is 145 Gy to 100% of the prostate volume, defined by TRUS at the time of implantation for all patients based on the AAPM TG-43 protocol. The plan is optimized such that no slice receives less than 100% of the prescribed

## BOX 28-17

Members of the American Brachytherapy Society (ABS) with expertise in prostate dosimetry evaluation performed a literature review and supplemented with their clinical experience formulated guidelines for performing and analyzing post-implant dosimetry of permanent prostate brachytherapy. This report gives recommendations regarding the technique and timing of dosimetric analyses as well as which variables are important and what criteria should be met.

Nag et al., The American Brachytherapy Society recommendations for permanent prostate brachytherapy post-implant dosimetric analysis. *Int J Radiat Oncol Biol Phys.* 2000 Jan 1;46(1):221–230.

dose and the 200% isodose lines are minimized. The urethral dose is limited to 150% at any point and the 50% isodose line should be limited to the extent of the anterior rectal wall. Two centrally located needles are introduced first to limit prostate motion. A custom loaded technique is used, and all remaining needles are placed sequentially beginning in the anterior of the prostate.

Seed placement is verified with portable plain X-ray twice during the procedure. Following insertion of all of the needles, a urologist performs a cystoscopy to ensure that there are no seeds in the bladder. CT/MRI dosimetric analysis is performed post-implant days zero and thirty. The dose received by 90% of the prostate (D90) should be at least 90% of the prescribed dose. The prostate volume receiving 100% of the prescription dose (V100) should be at least 90%. The prostate volume receiving 150% or the prescription dose should be at least 75%. The urethral dose should be limited to 150% of the prescribed dose.

Ir-192 high-dose rate after-loading brachytherapy is used by some centers as an alternative method for boosting the prostate with combination external radiotherapy. High-dose rate prostate-only brachytherapy is done infrequently outside of clinical trials.

## FOLLOW-UP

Following the completion of treatment, patients are typically seen in follow-up at 3 months, 6 months, and then annually with repeat PSA levels every 6 months. The PSA is an excellent indicator of recurrent disease and usually precedes clinical detection. Guidelines for classifying biochemical failure have been recommended by the American Society for Therapeutic Radiation and Oncology (ASTRO): three consecutive rises in PSA dated halfway between the PSA nadir and first rise. However, this definition has been found to suffer several limitations including short follow-up bias and misclassifications, especially when ADT is used. Alternatively, the PSA nadir + 2ng/mL definition has been shown to be less sensitive to length of follow-up, more predictive of continued PSA rises and eventual clinical failure, and more appropriate for comparisons between RT with and without ADT.[27] PSA nadir[28] and doubling time[29] and interval to biochemical failure[30] are other important factors that predict distant metastasis and death. Both factors should be considered when considering initiation of salvage ADT.

A CT scan of the pelvis and bone scan should be performed to exclude the presence of distant metastasis when biochemical failure is established. If these are negative, a biopsy of the prostate should be performed. Salvage cryosurgery has been shown to be safe with good results in the setting of a local recurrence.

---

**FIGURE 28-7** Peripherally loaded BT.

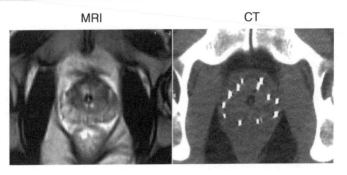

MRI    CT

For men who receive ADT, the most common additional side effects associated with ADT are weight gain, fatigue, hot flashes, osteopenia/osteoporosis, muscle loss, anemia, fluid retention, gynecomastia, and erectile dysfunction. Bone fractures may also occur, secondary to osteopenia/osteoporosis; therefore, monitoring bone density before and after treatment is suggested.

## FUTURE DIRECTIONS

Hypofractionation is a promising approach for further RT dose escalation because the alpha-beta ratio for prostate cancer is hypothesized to be low relative to the surrounding normal tissues. The dosimetric gains of IMRT have provided acceptable long-term effects with daily fractions of 250 cGy.[31] The recently completed Phase III randomized trial comparing 76 Gy in 38 fractions to 70.2 Gy in 26 fractions in intermediate- and high-risk patients at Fox Chase Cancer Center should help to further define the role of IMRT and hypofractionation for prostate cancer.[26]

## REFERENCES

1. American Cancer Society. *Cancer Facts & Figures*, 2008. [cited].
2. Miller, D.C., et al. Prostate carcinoma presentation, diagnosis, and staging: an update from the National Cancer Data Base. *Cancer*, 2003. 98(6): p. 1169–1178.
3. Prostate, in *AJCC Cancer Staging Manual*, P.D. Greene F.L., Fleming I.D., Fritz A.G., Balch C.M., Haller D.G. and Morrow M. Editor. 2002, Lippincott Raven: Philadelphia. p. 309–316.
4. Pinover, W.H., et al. Prostate carcinoma patients upstaged by imaging and treated with irradiation: an outcome-based analysis. *Cancer*, 1996. 77(7): p. 1334–1341.
5. Liebross, R.H., et al. Transrectal ultrasound for staging prostate carcinoma prior to radiation therapy: an evaluation based on disease outcome. *Cancer*, 1999. 85(7): p. 1577–1585.
6. Perrotti, M., et al. Endo-rectal coil magnetic resonance imaging in clinically localized prostate cancer: is it accurate? *J Urol*, 1996. 156(1): p. 106–109.
7. Buyyounouski, M.K., et al. Positive prostate biopsy laterality and implications for staging. *Urology*, 2003. 62(2): p. 298–303.
8. Liebross, R.H., et al. Relationship of ultrasound staging and bilateral biopsy positivity to outcome in stage T1c prostate cancer treated with radiotherapy. *Urology*, 1998. 52(4): p. 647–652.
9. D'Amico, A.V., et al. Biochemical outcome after radical prostatectomy, external beam radiation therapy, or interstitial radiation therapy for clinically localized prostate cancer. *JAMA*, 1998. 280(11): p. 969–974.
10. Zelefsky, M.J., et al. Dose escalation with three-dimensional conformal radiation therapy affects the outcome in prostate cancer. *Int J Radiat Oncol Biol Phys*, 1998. 41(3): p. 491-500.
11. Chism, D.B., et al. A comparison of the single vs. double high-risk factor stratification systems for prostate cancer treated radiotherapy without androgen deprivation. *Int J Radiat Oncol Biol Phys*, 2003. 57(2 Suppl): p. S270.
12. D'Amico, A.V., et al. Pretreatment PSA velocity and risk of death from prostate cancer following external beam radiation therapy. *JAMA*, 2005. 294(4): p. 440–447.
13. Pollack, A., et al. Ki-67 staining is a strong predictor of distant metastasis and mortality for men with prostate cancer treated with radiotherapy plus androgen deprivation: Radiation Therapy Oncology Group Trial 92-02. *J Clin Oncol*, 2004. 22(11): p. 2133–2140.
14. Lyons, J.A., et al. Importance of high radiation doses (72 Gy or greater) in the treatment of stage T1-T3 adenocarcinoma of the prostate. *Urology*, 2000. 55(1): p. 85–90.
15. Hanks, G.E., et al. Dose selection for prostate cancer patients based on dose comparison and dose response studies. *Red Journal*, 2000. 46: p. 823–832.

16. Pollack, A., L.G. Smith, and A.C. von Eschenbach. External beam radiotherapy dose response characteristics of 1,127 men with prostate cancer treated in the PSA era. *Int J Radiat Oncol Biol Phys*, 2000. 48(2): p. 507–512.

17. Zelefsky, M.J., et al. High-dose radiation delivered by intensity modulated conformal radiotherapy improves the outcome of localized prostate cancer. *J Urol*, 2001. 166(3): p. 876–881.

18. Pollack, A., et al. Prostate cancer radiotherapy dose response: an update of the Fox Chase experience. *J Urol*, 2004. 171(3): p. 1132–1136.

19. Albertsen, P.C., et al. Prostate cancer and the Will Rogers phenomenon. *J Natl Cancer Inst*, 2005. 97(17): p. 1248–1253.

20. Moul, J.W., et al. Epidemiology of radical prostatectomy for localized prostate cancer in the era of prostate-specific antigen: an overview of the Department of Defense Center for Prostate Disease Research national database. *Surgery*, 2002. 132(2): p. 213–219.

21. Lee, W.R., et al. A phase II study of external beam radiotherapy combined with permanent source brachytherapy for intermediate-risk, clinically localized adenocarcinoma of the prostate: preliminary results of RTOG P-0019. *Int J Radiat Oncol Biol Phys*, 2006. 64(3): p. 804–809.

22. Martinez, A.A., et al. Interim report of image-guided conformal high-dose rate brachytherapy for patients with unfavorable prostate cancer: the William Beaumont phase II dose-escalating trial. *Int J Radiat Oncol Biol Phys*, 2000. 47(2): p. 343–352.

23. Messing, E.M., et al. Immediate hormonal therapy compared with observation after radical prostatectomy and pelvic lymphadenectomy in men with node-positive prostate cancer. *New England Journal of Medicine*, 1999. 341: p. 1781–1788.

24. Ghavamian, R., et al. Radical retropubic prostatectomy plus orchiectomy versus orchiectomy alone for pTxN+ prostate cancer: a matched comparison. *J Urol*, 1999. 161(4): p. 1223–1237; discussion 1227–1228.

25. Pollack, A., et al. A multi-institutional analysis of adjuvant and salvage radiotherapy after radical prostatectomy. *Int J Radiat Oncol Biol Phys*, 2004. 60(Supplement 1): p. S186–S187.

26. Pollack, A., et al. Dosimetry and preliminary acute toxicity in the first 100 men treated for prostate cancer on a randomized hypofractionation dose-escalation trial. *Int J Radiat Oncol Biol Phys*, 2006. 64(2): p. 518–526.

27. Lee, N., et al. Which patients with newly diagnosed prostate cancer need a computed tomography scan of the abdomen and pelvis? An analysis based on 588 patients. *Urology*, 1999. 54(3): p. 490–494.

28. Ray, M.E., et al. PSA nadir predicts biochemical and distant failures after external beam radiotherapy for prostate cancer: a multi-institutional analysis. *Int J Radiat Oncol Biol Phys*, 2006. 64(4): p. 1140–1150.

29. D'Amico, A.V., et al. Surrogate end point for prostate cancer-specific mortality after radical prostatectomy or radiation therapy. *J Natl Cancer Inst*, 2003. 95(18): p. 1376–1383.

30. Buyyounouski, M.K. et al. Interval to biochemical failure highly prognostic for distant metastasis and prostate cancer-specific mortality after radiotherapy. *Int J Radiat Oncol Biol Phys*, 2008. 70(1): p. 59–66.

31. Kupelian, P.A., et al. Hypofractionated intensity-modulated radiotherapy (70 Gy at 2.5 Gy per fraction) for localized prostate cancer: long-term outcomes. *Int J Radiat Oncol Biol Phys*, 2005. 63(5): p. 1463–1468.

# 29

# Cervical Cancer

*Seungtaek Choi, MD*

*Patricia J. Eifel, MD*

## OVERVIEW

The overall incidence of cervical cancer and the mortality from this disease in the United States have decreased steadily over the past five decades. These decreases in incidence and mortality can be attributed to both increased use of an effective screening technique (Pap smear) and advances in diagnosis and treatment. These advances include improvements in radiation therapy planning and delivery (for both external beam radiation therapy and brachytherapy) and, for patients with locally advanced disease, the addition of chemotherapy to radiation therapy. In this chapter, we provide overviews of cervical cancer epidemiology, pathology, screening, diagnosis, and treatment and offer a detailed discussion of radiation therapy technique in the treatment of cervical cancer.

## EPIDEMIOLOGY

In the United States, cervical cancer is now the third most common gynecologic malignancy after endometrial cancer and ovarian cancer. According to the American Cancer Society, approximately 11,000 new cases of cervical cancer were diagnosed in the United States in 2007. There were approximately 3,600 deaths caused by this disease in 2005, which accounted for fewer than 2% of all cancer deaths in the United States.[1] Although these are encouraging statistics, cervical cancer continues to be a major public health problem worldwide, especially in developing countries. In 2007, cervical cancer was the second most common malignancy of women in the world, with approximately 493,000 new cases diagnosed.[2] It was also the third most common cause of cancer death in women worldwide, causing approximately 274,000 deaths, and the leading cause of cancer death in women in developing countries, where approximately 234,000 deaths from cervical cancer occurred.[2]

## ETIOLOGY AND RISK FACTORS

Invasive cervical cancer is now considered to be a sexually transmitted disease caused by the human papillomavirus (HPV).[3] The risk factors for developing cervical cancer are similar to those for developing other sexually transmitted diseases and include younger age at coitarche, multiple sexual partners, and multiparity. Although there is a suggestion that oral contraceptive use increases the risk of cervical cancer, this association is still considered to be controversial.[4] Because women who use oral contraceptives are likely to be more sexually active, oral contraceptive use may be a confounding factor rather than a true risk factor. Other factors associated with increased risk of developing cervical cancer include cigarette smoking and immunosuppression. HIV-related immunosuppression is associated with an increased risk of HPV infection and cervical intraepithelial neoplasia, but it is not clear whether HIV is associated with an increased risk of progression from cervical intraepithelial neoplasia to invasive disease.[5] Women who have been exposed to diethylstilbestrol in utero are at increased risk for developing clear cell carcinoma of the cervix and vagina, a rare subtype of adenocarcinoma.[6]

As stated earlier, HPV has been identified as the etiologic agent in the development of cervical intraepithelial neoplasia and invasive cervical cancer. Of the more than 100 strains of HPV that have been identified to date, only about 15 have been found to be associated with cervical cancer.[7] Of these, HPV-16 and HPV-18 account for approximately 70% of cervical cancers (HPV-16 alone accounts for approximately 50%). Vaccines against these two strains have been developed and have been found in clinical trials to be effective in preventing persistent infection and cytologic abnormalities[8] (See Box 29-1). The first commercial HPV vaccine was recently approved for use in the United States.[9]

---

**BOX 29-1**

A total of 1,113 patients between 15 and 25 years of age in North America and Brazil were randomized to receive either three doses of an HPV vaccine designed from the L1 virus-like particle or placebo. Among these patients, 776 patients who received all three doses of the vaccine or placebo were enrolled into the extended follow-up study. After a median follow-up of 47.7 months, the vaccine efficacy was 96.6% (95% confidence interval [CI], 81.3-99.0) against incident infection and 100% (95% CI, 33.6-100) against persistent infection with HPV-16 and HPV-18 (using a 12-month definition). There was 100% vaccine efficiency against cervical intra-epithelial neoplasia (CIN) lesions associated with HPV-16 and HPV-18. Additionally, there was protection against incident infection with HPV-45 and HPV-31 and cytohistologic abnormalities beyond those associated with HPV-16 and HPV-18. The vaccine was generally safe, well tolerated, and highly immunogenic.

Harper et al., *Lancet*, 2006, 367:1247–1255.

---

## ANATOMY

The uterus is a muscular, hollow organ located posterior to the bladder and anterior to the rectum in the pelvis.[3] The uterus is divided into the corpus and cervix by the isthmus. The uterus is attached to the surrounding pelvis by the broad and round ligaments. The broad ligaments consist of a double layer of peritoneum extending from the lateral margin of the uterus to the lateral wall of the pelvis. The broad ligaments enclose the extraperitoneal connective tissue around the uterus, including the parametrium. The round ligaments are bands of dense connective tissue and smooth muscle that contain small vessels and nerves. These ligaments extend anteriorly and laterally from their attachment in the anterolateral aspect of the uterine fundus to the lateral pelvic sidewall. The lower uterus is supported by the uterosacral ligaments, which consist of fibrous tissue with smooth muscle and extend from the uterus to the sacrum.

The cervix has an extensive network of lymphatics that can be organized into three groups.[6] The upper branches, draining the anterior and lateral cervix, follow the uterine artery. The middle branches drain into the hypogastric lymph nodes, which then drain into the external iliac lymph nodes. The lowest branches drain posteriorly to the inferior and superior gluteal, common iliac, presacral, and subaortic lymph nodes.

## PATHOLOGY

The most common histologic subtype of invasive cervical cancer is squamous cell carcinoma, which accounts for approximately 80% of all cervical cancers.[6] Adenocarcinoma accounts for approximately 15% of cervical cancers, and adenosquamous carcinoma accounts for approximately 5%. In general, adenocarcinomas and adenosquamous carcinomas of the cervix are treated similarly to squamous cell carcinomas, although several authors have reported higher risks of recurrence and death in patients with adenocarcinomas, particularly those with high-grade features.[10, 11] Other histologic subtypes, which account for less than 1% of all cervical cancers, include small cell/ neuroendocrine carcinoma, lymphoma, sarcoma, and melanoma. Small cell/neuroendocrine carcinoma is associated with a significantly worse prognosis, even when it is diagnosed at an early stage, and is associated with a high likelihood of development of metastatic disease.

## SCREENING

The Pap smear is a highly effective screening tool for cervical cancer owing to its relatively low cost, its ease of use, the long lag time for the progression of dysplasia to cancer, and the high likelihood of cure for preinvasive and early cervical cancer.[6] The Pap smear has been found to significantly reduce the incidence of and mortality from invasive cervical cancer.

Currently, the American Cancer Society recommends that women begin cervical cancer screening approximately 3 years after the onset of vaginal intercourse but no later than age 21.[12] Cervical cancer screening should be performed every year with conventional cervical cytology smears or every 2 years with liquid-based cytology techniques until age 30. After age 30, testing for HPV DNA may be added to the screening procedure. After an initial period of dual testing, women with negative results on both cytologic and HPV DNA screening do not need to be tested for another 3 years.

Women who have a negative result on cytologic screening but are positive for one of the HPV subtypes associated with cervical cancer should have repeat cytologic and HPV DNA testing in 6 to 12 months. If the result of either test is positive at that time, a colposcopy should be performed.

Women 70 years of age or older with an intact cervix who have had negative findings on at least three consecutive annual Pap smears and who have had no abnormal cytology tests within the 10-year period before age 70 may elect to cease cervical cancer screening. Women of any age with negative findings on three consecutive annual Pap smears may elect to be screened less frequently—every 2 to 3 years.

Women with a history of cervical dysplasia, cervical cancer, in utero exposure to diethylstilbestrol, or immunosuppression should undergo annual cervical cancer screening.

If a patient has abnormal findings on the speculum examination, she should undergo biopsy of the area with suspicious findings. If the patient has an abnormal Pap smear without suspicious physical findings, she should undergo colposcopy, and biopsy of abnormal areas should be performed. If biopsies show precancerous changes but not invasive cancer, the patient should undergo a cone biopsy of the cervix.

## PRESENTING SYMPTOMS

Preinvasive and microinvasive cervical cancers are usually discovered on a routine screening test or physical examination. Patients with more advanced disease usually present with abnormal vaginal bleeding.[3] Patients may also develop serosanguinous or yellowish vaginal discharge. A foul odor accompanying discharge is suggestive of a necrotic tumor. Lumbosacral or gluteal pain may indicate iliac or para-aortic lymphadenopathy with extension into the lumbosacral nerve roots. Leg edema or hydronephrosis usually indicates more advanced disease, and these symptoms are frequently associated with pelvic sidewall involvement. Urinary and rectal symptoms are worrisome as they are likely due to invasion of the cancer into the bladder or rectum.

## STAGING AND WORKUP

The most widely used staging system for cervical cancer is the International Federation of Gynecology and Obstetrics (FIGO) staging system (Table 29-1).[13] The American Joint Committee on Cancer (AJCC) has proposed its own staging system (Tables 29-2 and 29-3),[14] which is very similar to the FIGO system. However, it is important to note that the AJCC (TNM) staging system is a surgical/pathologic staging system, whereas the FIGO system is a clinical staging system. Furthermore, in contrast to the AJCC system, the FIGO system does not incorporate lymph node status. FIGO staging rules allow only palpation, inspection, endocervical curettage, hysteroscopy, cystoscopy, proctoscopy, intravenous pyelography, and plain films of the lungs and skeleton to be used for staging purposes. Computed tomography (CT) can only be used as a substitute for intravenous pyelography to evaluate for the presence of hydronephrosis. Other imaging studies, such as magnetic resonance imaging (MRI) or positron emission tomography (PET), are not allowed by FIGO staging rules. Suspected bladder involvement must be confirmed by cystoscopy with biopsy, and suspected rectal involvement must be confirmed by proctoscopy with biopsy.

The FIGO staging system has been criticized for prohibiting the use of modern imaging studies (MRI, PET scans) for staging and for not incorporating lymph node status, which is one of the most important prognostic factors for survival in patients with cervical cancer. However, it is impor-

---

**TABLE 29-1 International Federation of Gynecology and Obstetrics Staging System for Cervical Cancer**

| Stage | Description |
|---|---|
| I | Cervical carcinoma confined to the cervix |
| IA | Preclinical invasive carcinoma, diagnosed by microscopy only |
| IA1 | Tumor with an invasive component 3 mm or less in depth and 7 mm or less in horizontal spread |
| IA2 | Tumor with an invasive component more than 3 mm and not more than 5 mm in depth and 7 mm or less in horizontal spread |
| IB | Clinical lesions confined to the cervix or preclinical lesions greater than IA |
| IB1 | Clinical lesions no greater than 4 cm |
| IB2 | Clinical lesions greater than 4 cm |
| II | Cervical carcinoma invades beyond the cervix, but not to the pelvic sidewall or to the lower third of the vagina |
| IIA | Tumor without parametrial extension |
| IIB | Tumor with parametrial extension |
| III | Cervical carcinoma extends to the pelvic sidewall and/or involves the lower third of the vagina and/or causes hydronephrosis or nonfunctioning kidney |
| IIIA | Tumor involves the lower third of the vagina, with no extension to the pelvic sidewall |
| IIIB | Tumor extends to the pelvic sidewall and/or causes hydronephrosis or nonfunctioning kidney |
| IV | Cervical carcinoma invades the bladder or rectum and/or extends beyond the true pelvis and/or distant metastasis |
| IVA | Tumor invades the mucosa of the bladder or rectum and/or extends beyond the true pelvis |
| IVB | Distant metastasis |

Reproduced with permission from the International Federation of Gynecology and Obstetrics.

**ABLE 29-2** American Joint Committee on Cancer Definitions of T, N, and M Categories for Cervical Cancer

| Category | Description |
|---|---|
| | *Primary Tumor (T)* |
| x | Primary tumor cannot be assessed |
| 0 | No evidence of primary tumor |
| is | Carcinoma *in situ* |
| 1 | Cervical carcinoma confined to the cervix |
| T1a | Preclinical invasive carcinoma, diagnosed by microscopy only |
| T1a1 | Tumor with an invasive component 3 mm or less in depth and 7 mm or less in horizontal spread |
| T1a2 | Tumor with an invasive component more than 3 mm and not more than 5 mm in depth and 7 mm or less in horizontal spread |
| T1b | Clinical lesions confined to the cervix or preclinical lesions greater than IA |
| T1b1 | Clinical lesions no greater than 4 cm |
| T1b2 | Clinical lesions greater than 4 cm |
| 2 | Cervical carcinoma invades beyond the cervix, but not to the pelvic sidewall or to the lower third of the vagina |
| T2a | Tumor without parametrial extension |
| T2b | Tumor with parametrial extension |
| 3 | Cervical carcinoma extends to the pelvic sidewall and/or involves the lower third of the vagina and/or causes hydronephrosis or nonfunctioning kidney |
| T3a | Tumor involves the lower third of the vagina, with no extension to the pelvic sidewall |
| T3b | Tumor extends to the pelvic sidewall and/or causes hydronephrosis or nonfunctioning kidney |
| 4 | Tumor invades the mucosa of the bladder or rectum and/or extends beyond the true pelvis |

| | *Regional Lymph Nodes (N)* |
|---|---|
| x | Regional lymph nodes cannot be assessed |
| 0 | No regional lymph node metastasis |
| 1 | Regional lymph node metastasis |

| | *Distant Metastasis (M)* |
|---|---|
| x | Presence of distant metastasis cannot be assessed |
| 0 | No distant metastasis |
| 1 | Distant metastasis |

ant to remember that the prevalence of cervical cancer is highest in areas of the world with mited medical resources, where such imaging studies may not be readily available. The FIGO :aging system, therefore, attempts to eliminate any disparities in the staging of cervical cancer atients between different parts of the world. As for incorporating lymph node status into the taging system, this is made difficult by the lack of a standardized method of assessing lymph ode involvement.

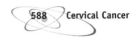

**TABLE 29-3 American Joint Committee on Cancer Stage Grouping for Cervical Cancer**

| Stage 0 | Tis | N0 | M0 |
|---|---|---|---|
| Stage I | T1 | N0 | M0 |
| Stage IA | T1a | N0 | M0 |
| Stage IA1 | T1a1 | N0 | M0 |
| Stage IA2 | T1a2 | N0 | M0 |
| Stage IB | T1b | N0 | M0 |
| Stage IB1 | T1b1 | N0 | M0 |
| Stage IB2 | T1b2 | N0 | M0 |
| Stage II | T2 | N0 | M0 |
| Stage IIA | T2a | N0 | M0 |
| Stage IIB | T2b | N0 | M0 |
| Stage III | T3 | N0 | M0 |
| Stage IIIA | T3a | N0 | M0 |
| Stage IIIB | T1 | N1 | M0 |
|  | T2 | N1 | M0 |
|  | T3a | N1 | M0 |
|  | T3b | Any N | M0 |
| Stage IVA | T4 | Any N | M0 |
| Stage IVB | Any T | Any N | M1 |

Used with the permission of the American Joint Committee on Cancer (AJCC), Chicago, Illinois. The original source for this material, *AJCC Cancer Staging Manual*, Sixth Edition (2002), published by Springer-Verlag New York, www.springeronline.com.

The current recommendations by the National Comprehensive Cancer Network for the initial workup of cervical cancer patients include history and physical examination, laboratory tests including a complete blood cell count and renal and hepatic function tests, and a chest X-ray. CT or MRI, or both, of the abdomen and pelvis are also recommended for evaluation of locoregional disease. MRI is superior to CT in the evaluation of pelvic disease and may be particularly useful in determining which patients are candidates for primary surgical resection. PET scans, although considered to be optional, have been shown to be effective in the detection of pelvic and para-aortic lymph node and distant metastases.[16] If a patient is found to have a suspicious lymph node on CT or PET, a CT-guided fine-needle aspiration of the suspicious lymph node may be indicated.

Surgical staging of pelvic and para-aortic lymph nodes in patients with cervical cancer is controversial and should be considered optional.[15] Potential benefits of surgical staging include obtaining prognostic information, identifying patients who would benefit from para-aortic radiation therapy, and debulking grossly enlarged lymph nodes. However, these procedures may delay treatment and have potential risks, including infection, bleeding, and increased risk of small bowel obstruction and lymphedema after radiation therapy. Advances in surgical technique, including the extraperitoneal approach and laparoscopic sampling of para-aortic and pelvic lymph nodes have significantly decreased the risk of side effects after surgical staging.[3]

## MANAGEMENT

### Preinvasive Disease

Preinvasive lesions are usually treated with locally ablative procedures such as cryosurgery or laser ablation, or with excisional procedures such as a cervical conization. Simple hysterectomy (removal of just the uterus and cervix) is an appropriate treatment option for women with high-grade

ervical dysplasia who no longer desire preservation of their fertility. Ablative treatment is con-
raindicated if the entire transformation zone has not been well visualized during evaluation, if there
s a marked discrepancy between the Pap smear results and colposcopy findings, or if the presence of
nvasive cancer is uncertain after colposcopy evaluation with biopsies. When there is uncertainty
egarding the presence of invasive cancer, a conization should be performed for further evaluation.

## Microinvasive Disease (FIGO Stage IA)

he standard treatment for early microinvasive disease (FIGO Stage IA1) is a simple hysterectomy
either abdominal or vaginal).[3] Because of the low risk of pelvic lymph node involvement in
atients with Stage IA1 disease (<1%), pelvic lymph node dissection is not warranted in these
atients. In patients who wish to maintain their fertility, a cone biopsy with removal of the trans-
ormation zone is an acceptable alternative as long as no dysplasia or cancer is seen at the biopsy
nargins. For patients who have significant medical comorbidities precluding surgery, FIGO Stage
A1 disease can be treated very effectively with brachytherapy alone. Treatment usually consists of
ne or two low-dose rate (LDR) intracavitary radiation treatments delivering a total dose of
,500–7,500 cGy to point A.[15] Details of intracavitary brachytherapy are covered later in this chap-
er. Ten-year local control rates, after surgery or radiation therapy, approach 100%.

The risk of lymph node involvement for FIGO Stage IA2 disease is approximately 5%. Therefore,
he standard treatment for FIGO Stage IA2 disease usually consists of a modified radical hysterec-
omy (removal of the uterus, cervix, parametria, and upper vagina) and pelvic lymph node dissec-
ion.[3] For patients who wish to maintain their fertility, a radical trachelectomy (removal of the
ervix, parametria, and upper vagina but preservation of the uterus) and pelvic lymph node dissec-
ion is an acceptable alternative.[17] Patients who are poor surgical candidates can be treated with
rimary radiation therapy using a combination of external beam radiation therapy and intracavi-
ary brachytherapy. External beam radiation therapy consists of 4,000–4,500 cGy delivered to the
elvis and to the para-aortic lymph nodes if they are involved. Intracavitary brachytherapy usually
onsists of two LDR intracavitary radiation treatments delivering an additional 3,000–3,500 cGy to
oint A (for a total dose of 7,500–8,000 cGy to point A).[15] The 5-year survival rate after either rad-
cal hysterectomy or radiation therapy is greater than 95%.

## Localized Disease (FIGO Stage IB1, Nonbulky Stage IIA)

or Stage IB1 and nonbulky Stage IIA disease (measuring 4 cm or less), treatment options include
adical hysterectomy with pelvic lymph node dissection and para-aortic lymph node sampling or a
ombination of external beam radiation therapy and intracavitary brachytherapy.[15] If there is no
linical evidence of lymph node involvement, external beam radiation therapy consists of
,000–4,500 cGy delivered to the pelvis. Intracavitary brachytherapy usually consists of two LDR
ntracavitary radiation treatments delivering an additional 4,000–4,500 cGy to point A (for a total
ose of 8,000–8,500 cGy to point A) or, in some circumstances, a radiobiologically equivalent dose
f fractionated high-dose rate (HDR) brachytherapy. The 5-year survival rate with either radical hys-
erectomy or radiation therapy is approximately 85%–90%. Concurrent chemotherapy is recom-
nended for patients with localized disease only if there is clinical evidence of lymph node metastasis.

### Adjuvant Radiation Therapy

or patients treated with radical hysterectomy who are found on pathologic examination of the
urgical specimen to have features associated with a high risk of local recurrence, the risk of local
ecurrence can be significantly reduced with adjuvant pelvic radiation therapy. Specifically,
djuvant pelvic radiation therapy is recommended for patients who have involvement of lymph
odes, parametrium, or surgical margins and may be recommended for patients who have lymph

node-negative disease and at least two of the following risk factors: (1) greater than one third stromal invasion, (2) capillary lymphatic space invasion, or (3) cervical tumor larger than 4 cm (See Box 29-2).

---

**BOX 29-2**

A total of 277 patients with Stage IB cervical cancer who underwent radical hysterectomy with at least two of three risk factors for recurrence ($>1/3$ stromal invasion, capillary lymphatic space involvement, or clinical tumor diameter of 4 cm or more) were randomized to either radiation therapy to the pelvis (RT) or no further treatment (NFT). Radiation therapy consisted of external beam radiation therapy to the pelvis (46-50.4 Gy in 1.8-2.0 Gy fractions), without any vaginal brachytherapy. In the RT arm, there was a statistically significant reduction in the risk of recurrence (hazard ratio [HR] = 0.54, p = 0.007) and a statistically significant reduction in the risk of progression or death (HR = 0.58, p = 0.009). The improvement in overall survival (HR = 0.70, 90% CI = 0.45 to 1.05, p = 0.074) with RT, although suggestive, was not statistically significant. The incidence of severe or life-threatening (Gynecologic Oncology Group grade 3 or 4) side effects was slightly higher in the RT arm (6.6% vs. 2.1%, p = 0.083).

Rotman et al. *IJROBP*, 2006, 65: 169–176.

---

Adjuvant external beam radiation therapy consists of 4,500–5000 cGy delivered to the pelvis; after hysterectomy, a four-field technique is usually used to decrease the risk of bowel complications. Some clinicians recommend additional treatment of the vaginal cuff with intracavitary brachytherapy. In these cases, the proximal third of the vagina is usually treated using HDR brachytherapy. Although a variety of fractionation schemes have been used, a typical prescription would be three treatments of 500–600 cGy each prescribed to the vaginal mucosal surface.

### Adjuvant Chemotherapy

Although the value of adjuvant chemotherapy for patients treated with radical hysterectomy who have negative lymph nodes and an increased risk of local recurrence has not been defined, Peters et al[18] (See Box 29-3) demonstrated a significant improvement in survival when patients who had positive lymph nodes, positive margins, or positive parametrial involvement received concurrent chemotherapy in addition to pelvic radiation therapy. In that trial, patients were treated with a combination of cisplatin and 5-fluorouracil during and after radiation therapy. However, many clinicians prefer to treat patients with a weekly cisplatin regimen similar to that used in trials of patients with intact cervical cancer.[19, 20]

External beam radiation therapy usually consists of 4,500–5000 cGy delivered to the pelvis (and para-aortic lymph nodes if they are involved), often followed by intracavitary vaginal brachytherapy. In patients with positive margins after surgery, a boost of 500–1,000 cGy (to a total dose of 5,500–6,000 cGy) using either three-dimensional conformal therapy or intensity-modulated radiation therapy (IMRT) to the surgical bed should be considered. However, the vaginal motion that occurs with variations in bladder and rectal filling should be carefully considered in treatment planning. If the vaginal mucosal margin is positive, then vaginal intracavitary brachytherapy should be used to increase the vaginal dose.

## Locally Advanced Disease (FIGO Stage IB2-IVA)

For most patients with locally advanced disease (FIGO Stage IB2-IVA), the standard treatment consists of concurrent chemotherapy and radiation therapy (external beam radiation therapy plus

### BOX 29-3

A total of 268 patients with clinical Stage IA2, IB, and IIA cervical cancer treated with radical hysterectomy and pelvic lymphadenectomy who had positive pelvic lymph nodes, or positive margins, or microscopic involvement of the parametrium were randomized to receive adjuvant radiation therapy (RT) or adjuvant chemoradiotherapy (RT + CT). Radiation therapy consisted of external beam radiation therapy to the pelvis (49.3 Gy in 1.7 Gy fractions), without any vaginal brachytherapy. Chemotherapy consisted of cisplatin (70 mg/m$^2$) and 5-FU (1000 mg/m$^2$/day for 4 days) given every 3 weeks for four cycles (two given during radiation therapy and two after). Progression-free survival and overall survival were both significantly improved with the addition of chemotherapy. Projected progression-free survival rates at 4 years were 63% with RT and 80% with RT + CT (hazard ratio [HR] = 2.01, p = 0.003), and projected overall survival rates at 4 years were 71% with RT and 81% with RT + CT (HR = 1.96, p = 0.007). There was increased grade 3 and 4 hematologic and gastrointestinal toxicity with the addition of chemotherapy.

Peters et al. *JCO*, 2000, 18: 1606–1613.

intracavitary brachytherapy). This recommendation is based on the results of five large randomized trials that demonstrated a significant survival benefit for the addition of cisplatin-based chemotherapy to radiation therapy (Table 29-4).[18, 19, 21–23] The most commonly used regimens are weekly cisplatin (40 mg/m2) and a combination of cisplatin and 5-fluorouracil given every 3 weeks. External beam radiation therapy consists of 4,500 cGy delivered to the pelvis and to the para-aortic lymph nodes if they are involved. Intracavitary brachytherapy usually consists of two LDR intracavitary radiation treatments delivering an additional 4,000–4,500 cGy to point A (for a total dose of 8,500–9,000 cGy to point A). Five-year survival rates of patients treated with concurrent chemotherapy and radiation therapy are 80%–85% for Stage IB2/IIA disease, 70%–80% for Stage IIB disease, 50% for Stage IIIB disease, and 15%–20% for Stage IVA disease.[3]

Some clinicians consider radical hysterectomy with pelvic lymph node dissection and para-aortic lymph node sampling as a possible treatment option for selected patients with Stage IB2 or bulky Stage IIA disease. Landoni et al compared primary radiation therapy and radical hysterectomy for patients with bulky Stage IB2 cervical cancer and found no difference between the groups in 5-year overall survival or disease-free survival[24] (Landoni, Box 29-4). However, it is important to note that 70% of the patients in the radical hysterectomy group required postoperative radiation therapy and, compared with patients treated with radiation therapy alone, patients treated with radical hysterec-

### BOX 29-4

A total of 343 patients with Stage IB and IIA cervical cancer were randomized to radical hysterectomy or radiation therapy. In women whose tumors were of surgical Stage pT2b or greater, had less than 3 mm of negative cervical stroma, a cut-through hysterectomy, or positive nodes, adjuvant radiation therapy was given. Primary radiation therapy consisted of external beam radiation therapy to the pelvis followed by one intracavitary low-dose rate brachytherapy implant. The total dose to point A ranged from 70 to 90 Gy (median 76 Gy). Chemotherapy was not given. After a median follow-up of 87 months, 5-year overall and disease-free survival rates were identical in the surgery and radiation therapy groups (83% and 74%, respectively, for both groups). Of note, 70% of patients in the surgery group required postoperative radiation therapy, which resulted in a higher rate of severe morbidity in the surgery group (28% vs. 12%, p = 0.0004).

Landoni et al. *Lancet*, 1997, 350: 535–540.

TABLE 29-4 **Summary of the Five Clinical Trials That Demonstrated a Significant Survival Benefit with the Addition of Cisplatin-Based Concurrent Chemotherapy to Radiation Therapy**

| Study | Stage | Control Group | Comparison Group | Relative Risk of Death in Comparison Group |
|---|---|---|---|---|
| Intergroup (SWOG 8797) | IB/IIA | Radiotherapy | Radiotherapy plus cisplatin and 5-FU | 0.50 |
| RTOG 90-01 | IB2-IVA | Extended-field radiotherapy | Radiotherapy plus cisplatin and 5-FU | 0.52 |
| GOG 123 | IB2 | Radiotherapy | Radiotherapy plus weekly cisplatin | 0.54 |
| GOG 120 | IIB-IVA | Radiotherapy plus hydroxyurea | Radiotherapy plus weekly cisplatin | 0.61 |
| | | | Radiotherapy plus cisplatin, 5-FU, and hydroxyurea | 0.58 |
| GOG 85 | IIB-IVA | Radiotherapy plus hydroxyurea | Radiotherapy plus cisplatin and 5-FU | 0.72 |

*Abbreviations:* 5-FU, 5-fluorouracil; GOG, Gynecologic Oncology Group; RTOG, Radiation Therapy Oncology Group; SWOG, Southwest Oncology Group. Adapted from Thomas et al.[31]

tomy and postoperative radiation had a significantly higher risk of complications after treatment. Also, patients in the primary radiation therapy group received a relatively low dose of radiation therapy (median dose to point A, 7600 cGy) and did not receive concurrent chemotherapy.

In the past, some clinicians recommended that select patients with bulky endocervical tumors be treated with a somewhat less than radical dose of radiation therapy (usually about 7500 cGy to Point A) followed 4 to 6 weeks later by extrafascial hysterectomy. However, there has never been clear evidence that patients treated with this approach have a better survival rate than those treated with radiation therapy alone. In 2003, Keys et al[21] published results of a randomized trial that showed no survival advantage for patients treated with adjuvant hysterectomy versus primary radiation therapy alone. With modern chemoradiation, local control rates are very high, further reducing the margin for improvement with the addition of adjuvant hysterectomy. Although occasional patients who have massive fibroids, poor response to radiation therapy, or involvement of the uterine fundus (which is difficult to treat adequately with brachytherapy) may benefit from adjuvant hysterectomy, the added expense and side effects of this approach probably do not justify its routine use.

## Recurrent or Metastatic Disease

Patients presenting with recurrent disease after definitive treatment for cervical cancer should be thoroughly restaged to ascertain whether they have an isolated pelvic and/or para-aortic recurrence or systemic recurrence. Recommended restaging studies are a CT scan of the chest, abdomen, and pelvis or a combined CT-PET scan, with surgical exploration as indicated.[15]

For patients initially treated with surgery alone, a localized recurrence in the pelvis or para-aortic region may be successfully treated with concurrent chemotherapy and radiation therapy. Patients who have central (vaginal) recurrences are usually treated with a combination of external beam radiation therapy and intracavitary or interstitial brachytherapy.[3] Salvage radiation therapy is particularly effective for small central recurrences limited to the vagina or paravaginal tissues. Nodal recurrences may require treatment with conformal radiation therapy techniques to permit delivery of an adequate dose of radiation to gross disease.

Most patients who have recurrence of their disease after radiation therapy are incurable. However, select patients, particularly those with isolated central recurrences, may be successfully treated with surgery; in most cases, removal of disease with adequate margins requires pelvic exenteration.[3] Candidates for this ultraradical surgery must be carefully evaluated to rule out distant or unresectable disease. In some patients who undergo pelvic exenteration, intra-operative radiation therapy may be used to treat small areas of minimal residual disease on the pelvic sidewall.

Patients with metastatic disease can be treated with either systemic chemotherapy or supportive care.[15] Cisplatin is probably the most active single agent for the treatment of cervical cancer, although ifosfamide, the taxanes (paclitaxel and docetaxel), and the camptothecins (irinotecan and topotecan) have also been found to have activity. Unfortunately, the duration of response after single-agent therapy is usually brief, ranging from 4 to 6 months, and the survival duration typically ranges from 6 to 9 months. Several combination chemotherapy regimens have been evaluated in phase II trials. Although the results of these trials show that response rates with combination chemotherapy are higher than those with single agents, no phase III trial to date has shown improved survival with combination chemotherapy regimens.[3] Table 29-5 lists the chemotherapy regimens commonly used for patients with metastatic or recurrent cervical cancer.

For patients with symptomatic metastases, radiation therapy may offer effective palliation. Common sites of metastases requiring treatment include lymph nodes, bone, and lung/

**TABLE 29-5  Chemotherapy Regimens Commonly Used for Recurrent or Metastatic Cervical Cancer**

| First-line Therapy | Possible First-line Combination Therapy | Second-line Therapy |
|---|---|---|
| Cisplatin | Cisplatin-paclitaxel | Docetaxel |
| Carboplatin | Cisplatin-topotecan | Ifosfamide |
| Paclitaxel | Cisplatin-gemcitabine | Vinorelbine |
| Topotecan | Carboplatin-paclitaxel | Irinotecan |
| | | Epirubicin |
| | | Mitomycin |
| | | 5-fluorouracil |

mediastinum. These sites are usually treated with 3,000 cGy delivered in 10 fractions, which usu
ally results in good palliation of symptoms. Radiation therapy can also be effective in the treatmen
of pelvic pain or vaginal bleeding. Various fractionation schemes can be used, including two frac
tions of 10 Gy delivered 1 month apart.

## RADIATION THERAPY TECHNIQUE

### External Beam Radiation Therapy

External beam radiation therapy is given for two primary purposes: (1) to control microscopic dis
ease in regional lymph nodes and (2) to reduce the size of the central disease to allow for optima
implant geometry and tumor dose delivery with brachytherapy. Most patients undergoing primar
radiation therapy start with external beam radiation therapy, with brachytherapy given later in
the course of treatment. Although there is some controversy among different institutions and prac
titioners regarding the optimal timing of brachytherapy in relation to external beam radiation
therapy, patients should undergo brachytherapy only after significant reduction of their disease to
allow good implant geometry and dose distribution. Although patients usually undergo their firs
brachytherapy treatment after receiving 4,000–4,500 cGy to the pelvis, they should be examined
during radiation therapy to determine their response to treatment before brachytherapy is sched
uled. Patients with good initial response may be able to undergo their first brachytherapy treat
ment before completion or during pelvic external beam radiation therapy.

#### Simulation

Simulation can be performed on either a conventional fluoroscopic simulator or a CT simulator. C
simulators are becoming more prevalent than fluoroscopic simulators and are preferred because
they allow for more accurate delineation of the target volume and normal tissues. During simula
tion, patients are usually placed in a supine position with their legs immobilized using either an
alpha or Vac-Lock cradle (MED-TEC, Orange City, IA). If there is very extensive vaginal involvement
the legs should be separated (in a frog-leg position) to reduce the dose delivered to vulvar skin
Either before or during the simulation, a radio-opaque marker is usually placed in the cervix to per
mit identification of the cervix during the planning process. Contrast material may be used to
delineate the rectum during fluoroscopic simulation but is not needed if CT simulation is per
formed. In patients with vaginal involvement, a radio-opaque seed placed at the distal edge of the
involvement may be helpful in determining the inferior border of the radiation field, and a radio
opaque marker should be placed at the anal verge so that the dose to the anus can be minimized.

#### Field Arrangements for Radiation Therapy to the Pelvis

For patients undergoing pelvic radiation therapy, the areas that need to be covered include the
cervix and the full extent of the tumor, the paracervical tissues, and the external, internal, com
mon iliac, and presacral lymph nodes. If the distal third of the vagina is involved, the inguina
lymph nodes must be covered. If the posterior vaginal wall is involved, the perirectal lymph node
must be treated as well.

Patients are usually treated with high-energy (equal to or greater than 15 MV) photons to the
pelvis using either opposed anterior and posterior (AP:PA) fields or a four-field technique (AP, PA
right lateral, left lateral). The inferior border is usually placed at the mid- or lower pubis and a
least 4 cm below the lowest extent of cervical or vaginal disease. The lateral borders of AP:PA field
are placed 1.5–2.0 cm lateral to the iliac vessels and the bony margins of the true pelvis. For
patients without pelvic lymph node involvement, the superior border is usually placed at the bifur
cation of the aorta (which is usually located at the L4–L5 interspace). For patients with pelvi

ymph node involvement, the superior border is placed approximately 4–5 cm above the superior extent of known nodal disease. However, in such cases, one must be cautious of the amount of small bowel added to the radiation field. An example of an AP field is shown in Figure 29-1.

If there is a significant amount of small bowel in the radiation field with AP:PA fields, a four-field technique may be used to spare the small bowel anterior to the iliac vessels. However, in thin patients or in patients with very bulky tumors, the four-field technique may not offer significantly improved small bowel sparing. Furthermore, it is important to remember that using the four-field technique has some disadvantages over using the AP:PA technique. Although use of the four-field technique may decrease small bowel dose, it increases the volume of irradiated bone marrow. Also, the cervix may move by as much as several centimeters within the pelvis as bladder filling changes. Therefore, great care must be taken when designing the lateral fields, as careless shielding of lateral fields (due to underestimation of organ motion and/or tumor size or involvement) may lead to undertreatment of gross tumor in patients with locally advanced disease.

The superior and inferior borders of the lateral fields are identical to those of the AP and PA fields. The anterior border is placed 1.5–2.0 cm anterior to the iliac vessels at the point where they become the femoral vessels and approximately 1.0 cm anterior to the pubic symphysis. The posterior border is usually drawn at the midline of the lumbar vertebral bodies until the L4–L5 interspace, after which point it is usually drawn at the posterior edge of the L5 vertebral body and

**FIGURE 29-1** Anteroposterior field for pelvic radiation therapy.

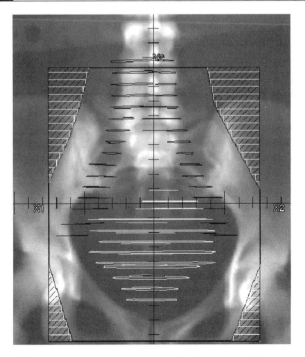

sacrum to cover the posterior motion of the cervix and the presacral lymph nodes. An example of a lateral field is shown in Figure 29-2.

### Field Arrangements for Radiation Therapy to the Para-aortic Lymph Nodes

If there is metastasis to para-aortic or common iliac lymph nodes, the para-aortic region is treated in combination with the pelvis. Several techniques have been used to treat the pelvis and para-aortic lymph nodes together in an "extended" field. Possible arrangements include large AP:PA fields for both the pelvis and para-aortic lymph nodes, AP:PA fields for the pelvis and four-field technique for the para-aortics, and four-field technique for both the pelvis and para-aortics. The first technique is seldom used because of the large amount of small bowel that would be treated in the radiation field. When the borders for the para-aortic fields are designed, the kidneys should be contoured into the treatment planning system to allow for maximal kidney sparing, especially from the lateral fields. The superior border of the para-aortic field is usually placed at the level of the renal vessels (usually located at the T11–T12 interspace). An example of a para-aortic field is shown in Figure 29-3. When AP:PA fields are used for the pelvis and four-field technique is used for the para-aortic lymph nodes, a single isocenter is used to minimize set-up error. With this beam arrangement, the lateral fields are actually half beams; the lower half of the field is completely blocked. If there is gross disease in the para-aortic lymph nodes, conformal or IMRT techniques may be required to deliver a tumoricidal dose without undue risk to adjacent normal tissues.

**FIGURE 29-2**  Right lateral field for pelvic radiation therapy.

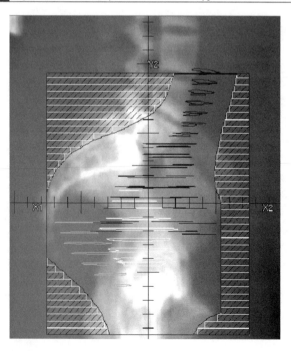

**FIGURE 29-3** Para-aortic fields.

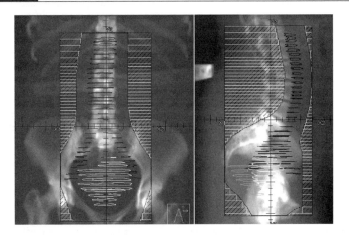

## Radiation Doses

For most patients, radiation doses between 4,500 and 5,000 cGy to the pelvis are adequate for controlling microscopic disease. However, patients found to have close or positive margins after radical hysterectomy or extracapsular extension after lymph node dissection probably require higher doses (5,500–6,000 cGy) to these areas of higher microscopic disease burden. In addition, patients with lateral paracervical or pelvic sidewall involvement and/or positive lymph nodes also require higher doses.

Patients who have persistent lateral paracervical or pelvic sidewall disease at the conclusion of pelvic radiation therapy are usually treated with AP:PA fields to the lateral pelvis to a combined total dose (from external beam radiation therapy and brachytherapy) of 6,000–6,500 cGy. The center of the pelvis should be shielded to avoid overlap with the regions treated to high dose with brachytherapy. Positive lymph nodes should be treated to a total dose of at least 6,000–6500 cGy (including the brachytherapy contribution) using AP:PA fields, three-dimensional conformal therapy, or IMRT.

## Brachytherapy

Brachytherapy is a crucial component in the treatment of intact cervical cancer. The addition of brachytherapy to external beam radiation therapy permits high doses of radiation to be delivered to the cervix and the paracervical tissues and improves pelvic disease control and survival.

It is important to remember that successful intracavitary brachytherapy requires experience, skill, and persistence (to obtain optimal positioning and packing of the implant before treatment). Therefore, it may be advisable to refer patients to centers with greater experience for their brachytherapy treatments.

### LDR Intracavitary Brachytherapy

LDR brachytherapy for cervical cancer has been used successfully for many decades. For LDR brachytherapy, a radioactive isotope, usually cesium-137, is introduced directly into the uterine cavity and vaginal fornices using special applicators. The most common applicator used in the United States is the Fletcher-Suit-Delclos system, which consists of an intrauterine tandem placed between two cylindrical vaginal colpostats ("ovoids"). The ovoids hold the radioactive sources perpendicular to the axis of the uterine tandem. The anisotropy of the sources, in addition to the anterior and posterior shielding of the ovoids, decreases the dose delivered to the bladder and rectum. An example of a tandem and ovoid implant is shown in Figure 29-4.

With LDR brachytherapy, the tandem and ovoid applicators are placed into the uterus and vagina while the patient is under general anesthesia in the operating room. Intra-operative imaging is used to verify optimal placement of the applicators before the patient is awakened from anesthesia. Once the patient has fully recovered from her anesthesia and is in a lead-shielded room, the applicators are loaded with radioactive sources. These sources can be loaded manually, or by using a remote afterloading device, which minimizes the radiation exposure to personnel. The sources are then left in place for 2 to 3 days to deliver the radiation therapy, usually at a constant dose rate of 40–60 cGy/hr. This LDR treatment allows for recovery of sublethal injury to normal tissues during the radiation exposure and permits delivery of a high dose of radiation over a relatively short period.

With computerized dosimetry, the dose rate and the total dose to a number of specific reference points in the pelvis from brachytherapy can be easily calculated. Reference points used in evaluation of brachytherapy include points A and B and the rectal and bladder points. In the classic Manchester system, point A is defined as being 2 cm above the mucous membrane of the lateral fornix in the axis of the uterus and 2 cm lateral to that axis.[25] Several alternative definitions for point A have been suggested; a commonly used alternative definition is 2 cm above the external cervical os and 2 cm lateral to the axis of the tandem. Anatomically, point A represents the lateral cervix-medial parametrium, the approximate point where the uterine artery and ureter cross. Point B is defined as being in the transverse axis of point A, 5 cm from the midline. Point B approximately represents the region of the lateral parametrium and the region of the obturator nodes. The rectal and bladder points have been defined by the International Commission on Radiation Units and Measurements (ICRU). The ICRU rectal point is defined as being 0.5 cm posterior to the posterior

**FIGURE 29-4** Tandem and ovoid implant.

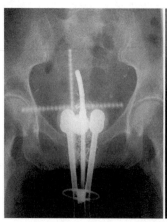
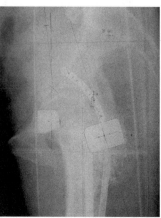

wall of the vagina, at the level of the center of the ovoids. The ICRU bladder point is determined by drawing an anterior-posterior line through the center of the Foley balloon (which is filled with 7 cc of diluted intravenous contrast) on a lateral film. The bladder point is at the intersection of the line and the posterior surface of the balloon. Although these reference points are commonly reported, they do not always accurately reflect the maximum dose to critical structures, particularly if the applicators are poorly positioned or if vaginal packing is inadequate.[25]

The dose from intracavitary brachytherapy can be reported in various ways; the most popular method involves reporting the total dose at point A. However, it is important to remember that different institutions may use slightly different definitions of point A, which can cause discrepancies in the reporting of doses and results. Many institutions also report total reference air kerma or total mgRaEq hours instead of point-A doses. For LDR brachytherapy, the dose rate at point A is typically between 40 and 60 cGy/hour. In general, a total point-A dose of 8,500–9000 cGy is recommended. However, it is crucial to note that the radiation dose that can be safely delivered depends on several factors, including patient anatomy, the size and extent of the cancer, the type of applicator, and the quality of the implant. The doses to the ICRU rectal and bladder points should usually be kept below 7,000 and 7,500 cGy, respectively. The dose to the mucosa at the vaginal apex should be kept below 12,000–14,000 cGy.

## HDR Intracavitary Brachytherapy

Over the past decade, use of HDR brachytherapy in the United States has increased significantly. With HDR brachytherapy, a single high-activity source of iridium-192 (typically 10 Ci) is stepped sequentially through various positions in the applicator to deliver a composite dose. These "dwell" positions (and times that the source is left at each position) are determined using inverse planning by the treatment planning software. Dose rates typically range between 200 and 300 cGy/min, which allow the treatment to be finished within minutes, rather than hours as with LDR. Commonly used applicators for HDR include tandem and ovoids (as for LDR) and tandem and ring.

The major advantage of HDR brachytherapy over LDR brachytherapy is that the procedure can be performed on an outpatient basis. In addition, inverse treatment planning may allow for some optimization of the radiation dose delivered by optimizing the dwell positions and times of the radiation source; however, dose optimization cannot fully make up for unfavorable anatomy or a poor-quality implant. Furthermore, when optimization is based on reference points without true three-dimensional treatment planning, major variations from standard source distributions and ratios within the tandem and vaginal applicators can lead to unforeseen overexposures of critical structures or underdosage of the tumor.

HDR brachytherapy has some disadvantages compared to LDR brachytherapy. Because the radiobiological advantages of LDR (recovery of sublethal injury to normal tissues) are absent with HDR, the dose of radiation must be divided into several fractions. Patients treated with HDR brachytherapy usually undergo five insertions, each delivering 550–600 cGy to point A. As patients are treated with these large fractions (as compared to LDR brachytherapy), great care must be taken to obtain optimal implant geometry and avoid exposing critical structures (rectum, bladder, sigmoid, and small intestine) to a large fractional dose, which can lead to higher risk of late toxicity.

The reports of the results of HDR treatment generally suggest that it is an effective method in the treatment of cervical cancer. To date, no significantly increased toxicity has been seen with HDR treatment compared to LDR treatment; however, there have been few direct comparisons of the two approaches, particularly in well controlled randomized trials.[26–29]

## Pulsed-Dose Rate Intracavitary Brachytherapy

Pulsed-dose rate (PDR) intracavitary brachytherapy represents a new paradigm in the treatment of patients with brachytherapy. In PDR brachytherapy, patients are treated with "pulses" of radiation (usually 10 to 20 minutes of radiation therapy every hour) during their implant course. PDR is usually administered using a stepping source of iridium-192 similar to that used for HDR but of lower activity. PDR brachytherapy is essentially ultrafractionated brachytherapy and has been shown to have radiobiological effects similar to those of continuous LDR brachytherapy.[30]

Applicators for PDR intracavitary brachytherapy are identical to those used for HDR brachytherapy. For gynecologic applications, patients are treated as inpatients, and the applicators are connected to a remotely afterloading source. Radiation is delivered with a single source and can be optimized using a planning computer (as with HDR brachytherapy). Therefore, PDR brachytherapy offers the flexibility of HDR in terms of treatment planning optimization with the radiobiologic advantages of LDR.

## FOLLOW-UP

Follow-up after definitive treatment of cervical cancer includes an interval history and physical examination and a speculum examination with a Pap smear every 3 months for the first year, every 4 months for the second year, every 6 months for the next 3 years, and then annually thereafter.[15] If a patient is treated with definitive radiation therapy, the first post-treatment Pap smear is usually obtained 3 to 4 months after the end of treatment; at earlier times, reactive cells may yield false-positive results. Patients should also have annual chest radiography during the first 5 years after treatment. Periodic follow-up with abdominal imaging (CT, MRI, or PET) may be indicated during the first 1 to 2 years to rule out treatable regional recurrences that may occur outside the radiation field.

## COMPLICATIONS OF RADIATION THERAPY

### Acute Side Effects

The most common side effect of external beam radiation therapy to the pelvis is diarrhea; most patients develop some diarrhea during treatment.[25] Antidiarrheal medications and dietary modification are usually effective in controlling this symptom. Less frequently, cystitis or urethritis may occur. If a urinalysis and urine culture rule out an infection, patients can be effectively treated with phenazopyridine or antispasmodics. Patients may develop very mild dermatitis during radiation treatment, including mild erythema over the treated area. In patients receiving treatment directed at the inguinal or vulvar regions, severe dermatitis may develop, including dry and moist desquamation. These patients are treated with aggressive skin care measures, including sulfasalazine cream and sitz baths. Patients who develop unexpected severe skin reactions may be infected with Candida species; in such cases, treatment with an antifungal agent may significantly improve symptoms.

Patients who are treated with concurrent chemotherapy may have additional symptoms of nausea, vomiting, and anorexia. These symptoms, particularly when combined with diarrhea, can lead to dehydration and electrolyte abnormalities. Patients should be weighed frequently, warned of the symptoms of dehydration, and given aggressive nutritional counseling to prevent serious sequelae.

### Late Side Effects

Late complications from radiation therapy usually involve the rectum, bladder, or small bowel.[25] The risk of severe hematochezia or hematuria necessitating transfusion is usually less than 3%–5%. The risk of small bowel obstruction is also less than 3%–5%, although certain risk factors significantly increase the likelihood of developing small bowel obstruction. These factors include undergoing a transperitoneal lymphadenectomy before radiation therapy, receiving a high dose of radiation to the whole pelvis (>5,000 cGy), very thin body habitus, a history of a pelvic infection, nd heavy smoking.[25] Mild to moderate apical vaginal ulceration or necrosis may occur in 5%–10% f patients.[25] In about 1% of patients, this may progress to formation of a rectovaginal or vesico-aginal fistula. Vaginal foreshortening and stenosis can occur after radiation therapy; patients ho are not sexually active are advised to use a vaginal dilator after treatment to minimize vaginal tenosis. Finally, radiation therapy to the pelvis always leads to infertility and menopause.

## 'UTURE DIRECTIONS

he wide use of Pap smear screening in the United States has significantly improved detection of oninvasive and early-stage cervical cancer. Coupled with advances in treatment (surgery, radia-ion therapy, and chemotherapy), increased use of screening has significantly decreased the inci-ence of and mortality from cervical cancer in the United States and other economically developed ations. However, cervical cancer continues to be a significant medical problem for women with oor access to medical care in this country and for women in developing countries. With results howing the efficacy of the HPV vaccine, future efforts should focus on widespread use of the accine for the prevention of cervical cancer.

In addition, the results of treatment for patients with bulky and locoregionally advanced cervi-al cancer can be improved. Several new approaches are being studied in combination with radia-ion therapy and cisplatin, including radiosensitizers, newer chemotherapy agents (such as aclitaxel and topotecan), and new molecular targeting agents (anti-epidermal growth factor eceptor and anti-angiogenesis agents).[31]

Finally, advances in the delivery of radiation therapy, including IMRT and PDR brachytherapy, lay lead to improved outcomes of cervical cancer treatment. IMRT, a method of delivering highly onformal radiation therapy, has been used with great success in the treatment of head and neck ancer and prostate cancer. However, further investigation is needed to determine the efficacy and afety of IMRT in the treatment of cervical cancer. Like IMRT, PDR will need to be investigated fur-her to determine its efficacy and safety.

## REFERENCES

1. Cancer Facts and Figures 2007. American Cancer Society, 2007.
2. Parkin DM, Bray F, Ferlay J, and Pisani P. Global Cancer Statistics, 2002. *CA Cancer J Clin*, 2005. 55(2):74–108.
3. Randall ME, Michael H, Vermorken J, and Stehman F. Uterine Cervix, in *Principles and Practice of Gynecologic Oncology, 4th Edition*, WJ Hoskins, Perez, CA Young, RC Barakat, RR Markman, M Randall, ME, Editor. 2005, Lippincott Williams & Wilkins: Philadelphia, PA.
4. Janicek MF, Averette HE. Cervical Cancer: Prevention, Diagnosis, and Therapeutics. *CA Cancer J Clin*, 2001. 51(2):92–114.
5. Palefsky, JM. Cervical human papillomavirus infection and cervical intra-epithelial neoplasia in women positive for human immunodeficiency virus in the era of highly active antiretroviral therapy. *Curr Opin Oncol*, 2003. 15(5):382–388.
6. Petereit DG, Eifel PJ, Thomas GM. Cervical Cancer, in *Clinical Radiation Oncology*, LL Gunderson, Tepper JE, Editor. 2000, Churchill Livingstone: Philadelphia, PA.
7. Munoz N, Bosch FX, de Sanjose S, Herrero R, Castellsague X, Shah KV, Snijders PJF, Meijer CJLM, and the International Agency for Research on Cancer Multicenter Cervical Cancer Study, G. Epidemiologic Classification of Human Papillomavirus Types Associated with Cervical Cancer. *N Engl J Med*, 2003. 348(6):518–527.
8. Harper DM, Franco EL, Wheeler CM, Moscicki AB, Romanowski B, Roteli-Martins CM, Jenkins D, Schuind A, Costa Clemens SA, and Dubin G. Sustained efficacy up to 4.5 years of a bivalent L1

virus-like particle vaccine against human papillomavirus types 16 and 18: follow-up from a randomised control trial. *The Lancet,* 2006. 367(9518):1247–1255.

9. FDA. FDA Licenses New Vaccine for Prevention of Cervical Cancer and Other Diseases in Females Caused by Human Papillomavirus, in *FDA News.* June 6, 2006.

10. Eifel P.J., Burke T.W., Morris M., Smith T.L. Adenocarcinoma as an independent risk factor for disease recurrence in patients with Stage IB cervical carcinoma. *Gynecologic Oncology,* 1995 59(1):38–44.

11. Rotman M, Sedlis A, Piedmonte MR, Bundy B, Lentz SS, Muderspach LI, and Zaino RJ. A phase III randomized trial of postoperative pelvic irradiation in Stage IB cervical carcinoma with poor prognostic features: follow-up of a Gynecologic Oncology Group study. *International Journal of Radiation Oncology\*Biology\*Physics,* 2006. 65(1):169.

12. *Guidelines for Early Detection of Cancer.* American Cancer Society, 2006.

13. Benedet JL, Bender H, Jones H 3rd, Ngan HY, Pecorelli S. FIGO staging classifications and clinical practice guidelines in the management of gynecologic cancers. FIGO Committee on Gynecologic Oncology. *Int J Gynaecol Obstet,* 2000. 70(2):209–262.

14. Greene FL, Page DL, Fleming, I.D., et al. *AJCC Cancer Staging Manual, Sixth Edition.* 2002 Springer-Verlag New York.

15. The NCCN Cervical Cancer Guideline, Version 1.2006, in *The Complete Library of NCCN Clinical Practice Guidelines in Oncology.* 2006.

16. Lin WC, Hung YC, Yeh LS, Kao CH, YenRF, and Shen YY. Usefulness of 18F-fluorodeoxyglucose positron emission tomography to detect para-aortic lymph nodal metastasis in advanced cervical cancer with negative computed tomography findings. *Gynecologic Oncology,* 2003 89(1):73.

17. Plante M, Renaud MC, Francois H, and Roy M. Vaginal radical trachelectomy: an oncologically safe fertility-preserving surgery, an updated series of 72 cases and review of the literature *Gynecologic Oncology,* 2004. 94(3):614.

18. Peters WA, III, Liu PY, Barrett RJ, II, Stock RJ, Monk BJ, Berek JS, Souhami L, Grigsby P, Gordon W, Jr., and Alberts DS. Concurrent chemotherapy and pelvic radiation therapy compared with pelvic radiation therapy alone as adjuvant therapy after radical surgery in high-risk early-stage cancer of the cervix. *J Clin Oncol,* 2000. 18(8):1606–1613.

19. Rose PG, Bundy BN, Watkins EB, Thigpen JT, Deppe G, Maiman MA, Clarke-Pearson DL, and Insalaco S. Concurrent cisplatin-based radiotherapy and chemotherapy for locally advanced cervical cancer. *N Engl J Med,* 1999. 340(15):1144–1153.

20. Keys HM, Bundy BN, Stehman FB, Muderspach LI, Chafe WE, Suggs CL, Walker JL, and Gersell D. Cisplatin. radiation, and adjuvant hysterectomy compared with radiation and adjuvant hysterectomy for bulky Stage IB cervical carcinoma. *N Engl J Med,* 1999. 340(15) 1154–1161.

21. Keys HM, Bundy BN, Stehman FB, Okagaki T, Gallup DG, Burnett AF, Rotman MZ, and Fowler JWC. Radiation therapy with and without extrafascial hysterectomy for bulky Stage IB cervical carcinoma: a randomized trial of the Gynecologic Oncology Group. *Gynecologic Oncology,* 2003 89(3):343.

22. Eifel PJ, Winter K, Morris M, Levenback C, Grigsby PW, Cooper J, Rotman M, Gershenson D, and Mutch DG. Pelvic irradiation with concurrent chemotherapy versus pelvic and para-aortic irradiation for high-risk cervical cancer: an update of radiation therapy oncology group trial (RTOG) 90–01. *J Clin Oncol,* 2004. 22(5):872–880.

23. Whitney CW, Sause W, Bundy BN, Malfetano JH, Hannigan EV, Fowler WC, Jr., Clarke-Pearson DL, and Liao S-Y. Randomized comparison of fluorouracil plus cisplatin versus hydroxyurea as an adjunct to radiation therapy in Stage IIB-IVA carcinoma of the cervix with negative para-

aortic lymph nodes: a gynecologic oncology group and southwest Oncology group study. *J Clin Oncol,* 1999. 17(5):1339.

24. Landoni F, Maneo A, Colombo A, Placa F, Milani R, Perego P, Favini G, Ferri L, and Mangioni C. Randomised study of radical surgery versus radiotherapy for Stage Ib-IIa cervical cancer. *The Lancet,* 1997. 350(9077):535.

25. Eifel PJ. Uterine cervix, in *Radiation Oncology: Rationale, Technique, Results, Eighth Edition,* JD Cox, Ang KK, Editor. 2002, St. Louis, MO Mosby.

26. Petereit DG, Sarkaria JN, Potter DM, and Schink JC. High-dose rate versus low-dose-rate brachytherapy in the treatment of cervical cancer: analysis of tumor recurrence—the University of Wisconsin experience. *International Journal of Radiation Oncology\*Biology\*Physics,* 1999. 45(5):1267.

27. Fu KK, Phillips TL. High-dose rate versus low-dose rate intracavitary brachytherapy for carcinoma of the cervix. *International Journal of Radiation Oncology\*Biology\*Physics,* 1990. 19(3):791–796.

28. Patel FD, Sharma SC, Negi PS, Ghoshal S, Gupta BD. Low-dose rate vs. high-dose rate brachytherapy in the treatment of carcinoma of the uterine cervix: a clinical trial. *International Journal of Radiation Oncology\*Biology\*Physics,* 1994. 28(2):335–341.

29. Eifel PJ. High-dose rate brachytherapy for carcinoma of the cervix: high tech or high risk? *International Journal of Radiation Oncology\*Biology\*Physics,* 1992. 24(2):383–386.

30. Chen C-Z, Huang Y, Hall EJ, and Brenner DJ. Pulsed brachytherapy as a substitute for continuous low-dose rate: an in vitro study with human carcinoma cells. *International Journal of Radiation Oncology\*Biology\*Physics,* 1997. 37(1):137.

31. Thomas GM. Improved treatment for cervical cancer—concurrent chemotherapy and radiotherapy. *N Engl J Med,* 1999. 340(15):1198–1200.

# 30

# Non-Cervical Gynecologic Malignancies

*Penny Anderson, MD*

*Andre Konski, MD, MBA, MA, FACR*

## ENDOMETRIAL CANCER

### Overview

Endometrial cancer is the most common cancer of the female reproductive tract. Surgery is the mainstay of treatment with radiation used in selected cases depending upon certain adverse pathologic features.

### Introduction

Approximately 41,200 new cases of endometrial cancer were diagnosed in 2006 with approximately 7,350 women dying according to American Cancer Society (ACS) statistics.[1] Uterine corpus cancer make up 6% of new cancer cases in women, the fourth most common cause of cancer in women, while constituting 3% of all cancer deaths in women, eighth most common cause of cancer deaths among women.[1]

### Anatomy

The uterus is a pear shaped organ located within the pelvis with a narrow cervix extending into the vagina and a wider body that courses superoanteriorly ending as the fundus. The uterus is a hollow organ with the lumen of the fallopian tubes, entering superiorly, in direct connection with the lumen of the uterus. The wall of the uterus consists of the peritoneum, smooth muscle or myometrium, and a glandular lining, the endometrium.

The uterus is anterior to the rectum and posterior to the bladder and can overhang the bladder anteriorly forming a right angle to the vaginal canal. The uterus has five ligaments. The broad ligament is an extension of the peritoneum from the margin of the uterus to the lateral pelvic side wall and includes the fallopian tubes, the ovarian ligament, vessels, lymphatics, and nerves. The round ligament extends laterally from the fundus between the folds of the broad ligament to the pelvic side walls and leaves the abdominal cavity through the internal ring of the inguinal canal. The two cardinal ligaments extend from the pelvic side wall to the cervix and are condensations of subserous fascia around the uterine blood vessels. The uterosacral ligaments are also condensations of subserous fascia extending from the sacrum around the rectum to the cervix. Without the uterosacral and cardinal ligaments, the uterus would prolapse through the vagina.

The uterus is supplied with arterial blood through the uterine arteries from the internal iliac artery with a venous plexus that drains into the internal iliac vein. The lymphatic drainage of the uterus ends up in numerous glands found on the rectum, anterior to the sacrum, around the iliac arteries, and high up in the abdominal cavity close to the inferior vena cava and aorta. Lymphatics are also known to course along the round ligament to reach the inguinal nodes, however, metastatic spread to these nodes is rare in the absence of spread to the lower vagina.

## Pathology

The majority of endometrial cancers are adenocarcinomas with endometrioid adenocarcinoma comprising 75%–80% of all cases. Endometrioid adenocarcinoma can be subdivided into papillary, secretory, ciliated cell, and adenocarcinoma with squamous differentiation. Other, less common histologic types include mucinous, papillary serous, clear cell, squamous cell, and undifferentiated carcinoma. Mesenchymal tumors of the endometrium comprise <5% of all uterine corpus tumors, with carcinosarcomas the most common uterine sarcoma. Papillary serous carcinoma, <10% of endometrial carcinoma, closely resembles serous carcinoma of the ovary and has a predilection for early myometrial invasion, lymphatic invasion and intra-abdominal spread. Clear cell type of endometrial carcinoma, <4% of endometrial carcinoma, usually occurs in older women exhibiting a more aggressive clinical course.

## Risk Factors

Risk factors for the development of endometrial cancer include:

- Obesity
- Nulliparity
- Early menarche and late menopause (increased number of menstrual cycles)
- Diabetes mellitus
- Hypertension
- Estrogen replacement therapy and tamoxifen
- Complex atypical hyperplasia
- A diet high in animal fat
- History of breast and/or ovarian cancer
- Family history (endometrial cancer and herditary nonpolyposis colorectal cancer [HNPCC])

## Screening

No proven tests are currently available to screen patients for endometrial cancer. The ACS has no screening recommendations for women at average risk for endometrial cancer development. Certain high-risk groups, such as patients with HNPCC or Lynch type 2 syndrome, can undergo more extensive screening evaluation including hysteroscopy and biopsy.[2]

## Prevention

The exact etiology of endometrial cancer is unknown, although excess estrogenic stimulation of the endometrium is thought to play an important role in endometrial carcinoma development. Prompt treatment of hypertension, diabetes mellitus and weight loss can lower patient's risk of developing endometrial cancer. A discussion of the potential risks and benefits of unopposed estrogen therapy can alert a patient to the potential increased risk of developing endometrial cancer with prompt interventions if symptoms, such as vaginal bleeding, develop. Patients with simple or complex atypical hyperplasia are at increased risk of developing endometrial cancer and may be treated with hysterectomy or by periodic use of progestins.

## Presentation/Workup

Endometrial cancer usually presents in the sixth and seventh decades of life with an average age of 60. The most frequent sign and symptom of endometrial cancer is irregular vaginal bleeding in up to 90% of cases. Patients can also present with a non-bloody vaginal discharge, pelvic pain, pelvic mass, pelvic pressure, and/or weight loss.

The pathology report should include the tumor type and the degree of differentiation. Workup includes a chest x-ray, full biochemistry and blood count, serum CA-125 may be helpful in advanced disease, and CT scans of the abdomen and pelvis.[2] In certain circumstances cystoscopy and/or barium enema may be helpful if extension to the bladder and rectum is suspected.

## Staging

**TABLE 30-1 Comparison of FIGO and TNM Staging of Endometrial Cancer[2,25]**

| FIGO Staging | | TNM Staging |
|---|---|---|
| | Primary tumor cannot be assessed | TX |
| | No evidence of primary tumor | T0 |
| 0 | Carcinoma *in situ* (pre-invasive carcinoma) | Tis |
| I | Tumor confined to the corpus uteri | T1 |
| IA | Tumor limited to the endometrium | T1a |
| IB | Tumor invades up to less than 50% of the myometrium | T1b |
| IC | Tumor invades up to >50% of the myometrium | T1c |
| II | Tumor invades the cervix but does not extend beyond the uterus | T2 |
| IIA | Endocervical glandular involvement only | T2a |
| IIB | Cervical stromal involvment | T2b |
| III | Local and/or regional spread as specified in IIIA, B, C | T3 and/or N1 |
| IIIA | Tumor involves serosa and/or adnexa (direct extension or metastasis) and/or cancer cells in ascites or peritoneal washings | T3a |
| IIIB | Vaginal involvement (direct extension or metastasis) | T3b |
| IIIC | Metastasis to pelvic and/or para-aortic lymph nodes | N1 |
| IVA | Tumor invades the bladder mucosa and/or bowel mucosa | T4 |
| IVB | Distant metastasis (excluding metastasis to vagina, pelvic serosa, or adnexa, including metastasis to intra-abdominal lymph nodes other than para-aortic and/or inguinal nodes) | M1 |

## Biology

Simple hyperplasia progresses to cancer 1% of the time and in 3% of patients with complex hyperplasia. Simple atypical hyperplasia progresses to cancer in 8% of patients while 29% of patients with complex atypical hyperplasia will progress to cancer.[3] More recently, links between genetic abnormalities and endometrial cancer development have been investigated. Mutations in BRAF gene, 1p deletion, and HOXB13 overexpression are but a few reports of investigations into the genetic abnormalities detected in endometrial hyperplasia and carcinoma specimens.[4-6] Further research is needed to confirm the importance of these and other biologic markers in patients with endometrial hyperplasia and carcinoma.

## Management

The primary treatment for non-metastatic endometrial cancer is surgery, often followed by radiation therapy. In 1988, the International Federation of Gynecology and Obstetrics mandated that the staging of endometrial cancer be changed from a clinical staging system to a surgical staging system because of inaccuracies in the former system. The procedures required for surgical staging include exploratory laparotomy, washings for peritoneal cytology, total abdominal hysterectomy, bilateral salpingo-oophorectomy, and an assessment of pelvic and para-aortic lymph nodes.[7] The operative procedure is performed through an abdominal incision allowing thorough intra-abdominal and retroperitoneal exploration. Upon entry into the peritoneal cavity, fluid samples are obtained for cytologic evaluation. Thorough pelvic and abdominal exploration is then performed, and biopsies or excisions of any suspicious lesions are taken. Following this, total abdominal hysterectomy and bilateral salpingo-oophorectomy are performed. After the uterus is removed, it is opened (away from the operating table), and the depth of myometrial invasion is determined by clinical observation as well as microscopic examination. In addition, the presence or absence of cervical involvement as well as tumor grade are also determined. Any suspicious pelvic or para-aortic lymph nodes should be removed for pathologic evaluation. It is recommended that pelvic and para-aortic lymph node sampling be performed if there is invasion of greater than one half of the myometrium, cervical involvement, high grade, enlarged lymph nodes, involvement of the adnexal or other extrauterine structures, or the presence of serous or clear-cell histologies. The incidence of nodal involvement in Stage I patients whose tumor is limited to the endometrium, regardless of grade, is extremely low, and therefore routine sampling of lymph nodes is not needed.

### Early-Stage Endometrial Cancer

After patients are surgically staged, the role of adjuvant radiation therapy is determined based on the prognostic factors of depth of myometrial invasion, histologic tumor grade, pathologic subtype, cervical involvement, presence of lymphovascular space invasion, and extent of disease (extrauterine involvement of serosa, adnexa, peritoneal fluid, lymph nodes, or intra-abdominal spread). Approximately 75%–80% of patients present with early-stage endometrial cancer. To date, three prospective randomized phase III trials have been conducted that have evaluated the role of postoperative pelvic RT in patients with intermediate risk early-stage endometrial cancer.

These three prospective randomized trials clearly demonstrate that adjuvant pelvic RT significantly reduces pelvic failure rates in early-stage intermediate risk patients. Evidence-based medicine suggests that these phase III trials support the role of adjuvant pelvic RT in patients with

---

### BOX 30-1

Eligible patients with clinical Stage I endometrial cancer underwent total abdominal hysterectomy, bilateral salpingo-oophorectomy without lymph node staging, and vaginal brachytherapy. These 540 patients were randomized to no further therapy versus pelvic radiation therapy (RT).

There was no difference noted in the 5-year survival between the two groups (91% no further therapy vs. 89% pelvic RT). However, pelvic RT reduced the risk of vagina/pelvic recurrence in patients with deep myometrial invasion (14.7% no further therapy vs. 6.6% pelvic RT). Pelvic RT also reduced the risk of vagina/pelvic recurrence in women with high-grade disease (14.1% no further therapy vs. 3.2% pelvic RT).

Aalders J, Abeler V, Kolstad P, et al.: Postoperative external irradiation and prognostic parameters in stage I endometrial carcinoma: clinical and histopathologic study of 540 patients. *Obstet Gynecol* 56:419–427, 1980.

**BOX 30-2**

The PORTEC (postoperative radiation therapy in endometrial cancer) trial enrolled 715 patients with Stage IB, grade 2 or 3 tumors and Stage IC, grade 1 or 2 tumors, and randomized women to receive either postoperative pelvic RT or no further therapy. All patients underwent a TAH/BSO. No surgical lymph node staging was performed. With a median follow-up of 52 months, the 5-year actuarial locoregional recurrence rate was 4% in the pelvic RT arm vs. 14% in the no further therapy arm (p < 0.001). The survival rates were similar between the two groups (81% pelvic RT arm vs. 85% in the no further therapy arm). On multivariate analysis, advanced age and not using radiation therapy were significantly associated with locoregional relapse.

Creutzberg CL, van Putten WL, Koper PC, et al.: Surgery and postoperative radiotherapy versus surgery alone for patients with Stage 1 endometrial carcinoma: multicentre randomised trial. PORTEC Study Group. Post Operative Radiation Therapy in Endometrial Carcinoma. *Lancet* 355:1404–1411, 2000.

**BOX 30-3**

Three hundred ninety-two evaluable patients with intermediate risk endometrial cancer, Stages IB, IC, and occult II underwent TAH/BSO with selective pelvic and para-aortic lymph node sampling, and were then randomized to pelvic RT vs. no further therapy. At a median follow-up of 69 months, the 2-year recurrence rate was 3% in the pelvic RT arm vs. 12% in the no further therapy arm (p < 0.01). The addition of pelvic radiation had a substantial impact on pelvic and vaginal recurrences, as 18 surgery-alone patients recurred in the pelvis/vagina compared to three in the surgery plus pelvic RT group (of which two of the three patients did not receive RT). There was a 22% pelvic recurrence rate in the no further therapy arm vs. 0% pelvic recurrence rate in the pelvic RT arm. The 4-year overall survival was 86% in the no further therapy arm vs. 92% in the pelvic RT arm which was a slight, although non-significant, difference. GOG #99 has also defined a subset population termed "high intermediate risk" (HIR) (recurrence rate >15%) which includes patients with several combinations of the major risk factors of advanced age, high-grade, deep myometrial invasion, and lymphovascular space invasion. The reported 2-year incidence of recurrence for this HIR group, comprising 132 patients (33% of the study population), was 27%. Although the majority of patients accrued to this study were low risk, this trial confirms the significant reduction of locoregional recurrence by the addition of pelvic RT.

Keys HM, Roberts JA, Brunetto VL, et al.: A phase III trial of surgery with or without adjunctive external pelvic radiation therapy in intermediate risk endometrial adenocarcinoma: a Gynecologic Oncology Group study. *Gynecol Oncol* 92:744–751, 2004.

intermediate risk features. However, recently the role of adjuvant pelvic radiation therapy has been the subject of debate, given that there has been an increase in the incidence of lymphadenectomy performed at the time of hysterectomy. There has been an interest in using vaginal brachytherapy alone in patients with pathologically negative lymph nodes. Several small retrospective series have demonstrated excellent outcomes for patients with negative lymph nodes, but without deep myometrial invasion or high-grade tumors who were treated with vaginal brachytherapy alone.

The current recommendations for adjuvant radiation treatment for early-stage endometrial cancer are illustrated in Tables 30-2 and 30-3.

In general, adjuvant pelvic radiation is recommended for patients with deep myometrial invasion, tumor grade 2 or 3, or evidence of lymphovascular invasion. Vaginal brachytherapy alone may be considered for patients with low-grade histology and superficial tumors who have had an adequate lymph node dissection.

TABLE 30-2  **Treatment Recommendations for Adjuvant Pelvic Radiation (with no lymph node sampling)**

|  | Grade | | |
|---|---|---|---|
| **Stage** | **1** | **2** | **3** |
| IA | — | — | — or VB |
| IB | — or VB | — or VB | pelvic |
| IC-IIB | pelvic | pelvic | pelvic |

— none recommended
VB vaginal brachytherapy

TABLE 30-3  **Treatment Recommendations for Adjuvant Pelvic Radiation (with lymph node sampling)**

|  | Grade | | |
|---|---|---|---|
| **Stage** | **1** | **2** | **3** |
| IA | — | — | — or VB |
| IB | — or VB | — or VB | VB |
| IC-IIB | VB | VB | VB |

— none recommended
VB vaginal brachytherapy

### *Advanced Stage Endometrial Cancer*

Patients with surgical Stages III and IV disease are at high risk of developing recurrent disease after surgery if no adjuvant therapy is administered. Approximately 10% of patients with clinically confined endometrial cancer are found postoperatively to have involvement of the serosa, adnexa, or peritoneal washings (pathological Stage IIIA); involvement of the vagina (pathological Stage IIIB); or positive pelvic or para-aortic lymph nodes (pathologic Stage IIIC).[8] The management of locally advanced endometrial cancer patients remains an evolving issue. At some institutions these patients receive adjuvant whole abdominal RT. However, with concerns over the toxicity of whole abdominal RT, increasing attention has been turned to the use of adjuvant chemotherapy. In addition, combined adjuvant chemotherapy and whole pelvic RT in these high-risk disease patients has also been investigated.

The optimal management of high-risk endometrial cancer patients remains unclear. Although the addition of chemotherapy to radiation therapy seems reasonable, the use of chemotherapy instead of radiation therapy may pose the risk of unacceptably high local recurrence rates. Mundt et al evaluated the risk of pelvic recurrence in 43 high-risk endometrial cancer patients who received adjuvant chemotherapy alone.[9] Eighty-four percent of the patients had pathologic Stage III/IV disease or unfavorable histology tumors (74%). All patients received four to six cycles of chemotherapy as adjuvant treatment (cisplatin/adriamycin). The median follow-up was 27 months. Overall, 29 (67.4%) patients relapsed. The authors reported a 39.5% pelvic recurrence rate. Thirty-seven percent (9/29 relapsed patients) developed pelvic recurrence as their only or first site of recurrence. These results support the use of locoregional RT for these high-risk endometrial patients who receive adjuvant chemotherapy.

**BOX 30-4**

Three hundred ninety-six evaluable patients with Stage III/IV endometrial carcinoma were randomized to receive whole abdominal RT (n = 202) or 194 chemotherapy consisting of doxorubicin-cisplatin (n = 194). The median follow-up was 74 months.

Of the 202 patients who received whole abdominal RT, 109 (54%) had tumor recurrence. The initial site of recurrence was limited to the pelvis in 27 (13%) patients, in the abdomen in 33 (16%) patients, and extra-abdominal disease in 45 (22%) patients. Of the 194 patients who received chemotherapy, 97 (50%) had documented tumor recurrence. The initial site of recurrence was limited to the pelvis in 34 (18%) patients, in the abdomen in 27 (14%) patients, and extra-abdominal disease in 34 (18%) patients.

At the time of final analysis, 38% of patients on the whole abdominal RT arm were predicted to be alive and disease-free compared to 50% on the chemotherapy arm. This translated into a statistically significant difference in progression-free survival between the two treatment arms (p = 0.007). In addition, there was a statistically significant difference in 5-year overall survival between the two arms of 55% for patients on the chemotherapy arm versus 42% for patients who received whole abdominal RT (p = 0.004). Of note, greater acute grade 3-4 hemotologic and gastrointestinal toxicity was observed in the chemotherapy arm compared to the RT arm. It was also noted that treatment most likely contributed to eight deaths on the chemotherapy arm versus four deaths on the RT arm.

Randall ME, Filiaci VL, Muss H, et al.: Randomized phase III trial of whole-abdominal irradiation versus doxorubicin and cisplatin chemotherapy in advanced endometrial carcinoma: a Gynecologic Oncology Group Study. *J Clin Oncol* 24:36–44, 2006.

## Technique/Dose

The standard postoperative pelvic radiation external beam dose is 45–50 Gy utilizing 1.8–2.0 Gy daily fractionation. The external beam field should extend superiorly to cover the common iliac lymph nodes and inferiorly to encompass the upper half of the vagina.

The lateral borders of the anterior/posterior treatment fields should extend 1.5 to 2.0 cm beyond the border of the bony pelvis to include the pelvic lymph nodes.

A vaginal marker is placed in the vagina to demonstrate the length of the vagina included in the radiation field. The technique for the delivery of the external beam treatment should include multiple fields treated daily, using a four-field technique, to provide a homogeneous dose distribution.

Vaginal brachytherapy is delivered utilizing either low-dose rate (LDR) or high-dose rate (HDR) technique. Excellent local control rates and low morbidity has been demonstrated using both techniques. The HDR brachytherapy treatments require multiple insertions, usually one to two per week for several weeks. Each insertion takes only several minutes and is on an outpatient basis. LDR treatments require hospitalization for several days, but are usually delivered only once.

## Follow-up

Patients are typically seen for follow-up approximately 4–6 weeks after completion of their radiation treatments. Close follow-up should then continue about every 3–4 months for the first 2–3 years following treatment. Follow-up may then be decreased to every 6 months until 5 years, at which time the patient can return for follow-up on an annual basis.

Follow-up should include a pertinent history and physical examination at each visit. Pelvic examination and cytology of the vaginal cuff should be performed at each interval visit. Interval

**FIGURE 30-1** Typical anterior field for endometrial cancer.

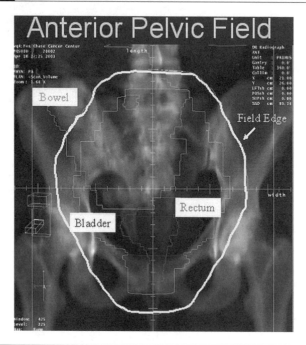

CT scans of the abdomen/pelvis, as well as a CXR or chest CT, are also part of the routine follow-up care, and the scheduling of these tests is dictated by the initial tumor stage at presentation.

## Morbidity

Acute radiation side effects of pelvic RT typically begin within a few weeks of initiation of radiation and can persist for several weeks after completion of radiation treatment. Common acute side effects include loose stools, diarrhea, cystitis, and fatigue. Late complications, seen in less than 10% of patients, include small bowel obstruction, intractable diarrhea, chronic proctitis, and chronic cystitis. Vaginal foreshortening, stenosis, and dryness can also occur and can severely alter the quality-of-life of these patients. However, these sequelae can be successfully managed or even prevented with routine use of a vaginal dilator and vaginal estrogen applications.

## Future Directions

A multicenter randomized trial is currently underway in Europe for early-stage endometrial cancer. The PORTEC-2 trial is a phase III trial comparing pelvic external beam radiation therapy to vaginal brachytherapy. The GOG recently completed a randomized phase III study of tumor volume directed pelvic radiation therapy plus or minus para-aortic radiation therapy followed by cisplatin and doxorubicin or cisplatin, doxorubicin, and paclitaxel for advanced endometrial cancer. The results are pending at the time of this publication.

**FIGURE 30-2** | Typical lateral field for endometrial cancer.

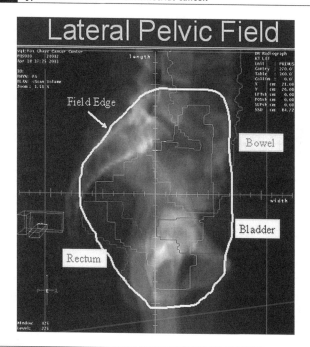

## Vaginal Cancer

### Overview

Cancers of the vagina are much less common than cancers that start elsewhere (uterus, rectum, or bladder) and spread to the vagina. The cervix or vulva cannot be involved for a cancer to be considered a vaginal cancer. Radiation is the mainstay of treatment, with surgery useful in certain situations.

### Introduction

Vaginal cancer is rare, representing 1%–3% of all cancers of the female reproductive tract. The ACS estimated there were 2,420 new cases of vaginal cancer in 2006 with 820 deaths attributable to vaginal cancer during the same time period.[1]

### Anatomy

The vagina is a canal extending from the external genitalia anterior-inferiorly to the cervix. It traverses the muscular urogenital diaphragm, the pelvic diaphragm, and passes the inferior edge of the levator ani muscle. The anterior wall is shorter than the posterior wall because the cervix extends into the anterior aspect of the superior end of the vagina. The fornices are the clefts produced by the cervix projecting into the vagina. The posterior-superior part of the vagina is covered by peritoneum, while the anterior wall does not make contact with the peritoneum.

The bladder and urethra are anterior to the vagina. The inferior end of the pelvic cavity, small intestine, rectum, and perineal body are posterior to the vagina, and the broad ligament ureters, uterine vessels, pelvic surface, or the levator ani muscle, and sphincter urethrae muscle are lateral to the vagina. The walls of the vagina are normally in contact with each other except superiorly where the cervix intervenes. The vagina is made up of smooth muscle and lined with stratified squamous epithelium.

The vagina is supplied with arterial blood from the uterine artery, from the internal iliac artery, and from the middle rectal artery. The inferior end of the vagina receives its blood flow from branches of the internal pudendal artery. The lymphatics drain to the rectum and along the iliac arteries, but lymphatics from the lower vagina may drain to the inguinal lymph nodes.

## Pathology

The majority of vaginal cancers, 85%–90%, are squamous cell carcinomas with 5%–10% of vaginal cancers being adenocarcinomas. Clear cell adenocarcinoma of the vagina occurs in young women who were exposed to diethylstilbestrol (DES) in utero. Malignant melanoma accounts for 2%–3% of vaginal cancers with an additional 2%–3% being sarcomas. Leiomyosarcoma is the most common type of sarcoma in older women while rhabdomyosarcoma occurs in children usually before the age of 3.

## Risk Factors

- Age—two thirds of occurrence in women 60 years and older
- HPV infection
- DES exposure in utero
- Cervical cancer—exposure to similar carcinogens
- Vaginal irritation
- Smoking
- Vaginal adenosis

## Screening

There are no routine screening tests for vaginal cancer. Vaginal cancers can proceed through an orderly development from precancerous areas of vaginal intra-epithelial neoplasia (VAIN) to invasive cancer, but these precancerous lesions rarely produce symptoms. VAIN and early invasive cancers can be diagnosed on routine PAP smears.

## Prevention

Other than avoidance of certain previously listed risk factors, there are currently no known interventions that can aid in the prevention of vaginal cancer.

## Presentation/Workup

Vaginal bleeding, often post-coital, is the presenting sign in 50%–75% of patients with vaginal cancer. Vaginal discharge, palpable mass, dyspaurenia, dysuria, and pelvic pain can also be presenting signs. The majority of vaginal cancers will present in the upper vagina and on the posterior vaginal wall.

Diagnostic workup includes:

- History and physical examination with bimanual pelvic examination
- Chest x-ray
- MRI of the pelvis or CT scan with contrast of the abdomen and pelvis
- Biochemistry and complete blood count
- Cystoscopy and proctosigmoidoscopy may be used to evaluate invasion into the bladder and rectum.

## Staging

**TABLE 30-4  Comparison of FIGO and TNM Staging of Vaginal Cancer[2,25]**

| FIGO | | TNM |
|---|---|---|
| | Primary tumor cannot be assessed | Tx |
| | No evidence of primary tumor | T0 |
| 0 | Carcinoma *in situ*; intra-epithelial neoplasia grade 3 | Tis |
| I | Carcinoma limited to the vaginal wall | T1 |
| II | Carcinoma has involved the subvaginal tissue but extended to the pelvic wall | T2 |
| III | Carcinoma has extended to the pelvic wall | T3 or N1 |
| IVA | Tumor invades the bladder and/or rectal mucosa and/or direct extension beyond the true pelvis (bullous edema is not sufficient evidence to classify a tumor as T4) | T4 |
| IVB | Spread to distant organs | M1 |

## Biology

Squamous cell carcinoma of the cervix can be a multi-centric disease with 5%–10% of patients with Stage 0 disease exhibiting recurrences. Overexpression of wild-type p53 in clear cell carcinoma of the vagina may result in a more favorable prognosis.[10] It has also been hypothesized that induction of genomic instability may be an important mechanism of DES-induced carcinogenesis.[11]

## Management

Due to the rarity of this disease, data regarding the treatment of vaginal carcinoma is mainly derived from small, retrospective series. Most of the literature pertaining to surgical and radiotherapeutic approaches refers to primary squamous cell carcinoma of the vagina. There is evidence that patients with highly selected early Stage I vaginal cancer, with primary lesions located in the upper vagina, can be successfully treated with surgery alone. However, surgical resection often requires a radical approach with urinary and fecal diversion in an attempt to achieve negative margins. In addition, many of these patients are elderly and unable to tolerate a radical surgical approach. Therefore, radical surgical resection has been replaced by radiation therapy in order to maximize cure and improve the quality-of-life of these patients. Radiation therapy is the most common treatment approach for vaginal cancers. Both external beam radiation therapy and brachytherapy are used as part of the treatment plan.

### Carcinoma in situ

Radiation treatment involves the use of an intracavitary vaginal cylinder to deliver radiation to the entire vaginal mucosa. Low-dose rate brachytherapy doses of 60–80 Gy have generally been used to treat the vaginal mucosa. Because vaginal cancers tend to be multicentric, the entire vaginal mucosa should be treated. In cases with discrete mucosal lesions, small portions of the mucosa may be boosted with a shielded cylinder to deliver an additional 10–20 Gy.

### Stage I

Stage I patients generally can be divided into two groups based on the depth of tumor invasion. Superficial lesions less than 0.5 cm in thickness can be treated with an intracavitary vaginal cylinder, utilizing either low-dose rate or high-dose rate brachytherapy. For Stage I patients with lesions with greater than 0.5 cm-depth of invasion, brachytherapy should be delivered using both an intracavitary and an interstitial system. The use of combined external beam radiation therapy and brachytherapy is indicated in Stage I patients with larger, more invasive, poorly differentiated disease.

### Stage II/III/IV

Radiation therapy is the primary treatment approach for Stage II disease. Surgery is used only infrequently because radical surgical procedures are often required, and these are often associated with significant morbidity and impairment of function. Radiation therapy treatment involves a combination of external beam therapy and brachytherapy. Patients with Stage III/IV advanced disease are treated with a similar approach as Stage II patients.

## Technique/Dose

### Stage I

For superficial lesions, an intracavity vaginal cylinder is commonly used. With a low-dose rate brachytherapy system, treatment is delivered in two separate applications. The first application treats the entire vaginal wall to a dose of 4,500 cGy at a depth of 0.5 cm into the vaginal mucosa. The second application treats an additional 2,500 cGy to a depth of 0.5 cm to the tumor volume. The vaginal cylinder can be custom shielded to block uninvolved mucosal areas. With the use of a high- dose rate brachytherapy system, lengthy hospital stays and bed confinement are eliminated, because high-dose rate treatments are performed on an outpatient basis. High-dose rate fractionated doses of 500 cGy to 700 cGy, prescribed to a depth of 0.5 cm into the entire vaginal mucosa, are delivered once or twice per week. The total dose delivered to the entire vaginal length is 2,100 cGy to 2500 cGy. Following this, an additional 2,100 cGy to 2,500 cGy is delivered to the tumor volume using a custom shielded vaginal cylinder. Fractionated doses of 500 cGy to 700 cGy are used, prescribing the dose to a depth of 0.5 cm. For thicker lesions, interstitial brachytherapy is used in combination with the intracavitary treatments. To deliver the interstitial implant accurately, the depth of the tumor should be delineated so as to adequately cover the tumor volume. When external beam radiation therapy is indicated, the whole pelvis is treated to 4,500 cGy in 180 cGy daily fractions. If the primary vaginal lesion involves the middle or lower third of the vagina, then the inguinal regions should also be included in the radiation fields. The external beam technique includes a parallel-opposed anterior/posterior beam arrangement that encompasses the pelvis and entire vagina inferiorly to the introitus and the inguinal regions if indicated.

### Stage II

For patients with Stage II disease, radiation treatment involves a combination of external beam radiation therapy and brachytherapy. The external beam fields include the pelvis as well as the inguinal regions, with doses of 4,500–5,040 cGy delivered in 180 cGy daily fractions. Unlike Stage I disease, Stage II lesions should be treated with an interstitial brachytherapy implant in order to cover the deep aspects of the lesion that an intracavitary implant alone would not be able to adequately cover. In this setting, interstitial brachytherapy has been shown to improve local control compared to an intracavitary implant.[12] Total tumor volume doses of 7,500–8,000 cGy from the combined external beam and brachytherapy implant are generally recommended.

### Stage III/IV

Radiation treatment for Stage III/IV disease is similar to that for Stage II disease. The external beam doses should be 4,500–5,000 cGy in combination with interstitial brachytherapy implant doses of 3,500–4,500 cGy.

## Follow-up

Patients are typically seen for follow-up approximately 4 to 6 weeks after completion of their radiation treatments. Close follow-up should continue every 3 to 4 months for the first 2 to 3 years following treatment. Follow-up may be decreased to every 6 months until 5 years, at which time the patient can return for follow-up on an annual basis.

Follow-up should include a pertinent history and physical examination at each visit. Pelvic examination and cytology of the vaginal cuff should be performed at each interval visit. Interval CT scans of the abdomen/pelvis as well as a CXR or chest CT are also part of the routine follow-up care, and the scheduling of these tests is dictated by the initial tumor stage at presentation. In addition, pelvic MRIs with particular attention to the vaginal region can be helpful as part of the routine follow-up care schedule.

## Morbidity

Common acute side effects of the external beam portion of the radiation treatment include loose stools, diarrhea, cystitis, and fatigue. Common sequelae of the combined external beam and brachytherapy treatments include vaginal stenosis, foreshortening, vaginal dryness, proctitis, and cystitis. Uncommon, yet serious, major sequelae include fistula formation, rectal ulceration, and vaginal ulceration/necrosis.

## Future Directions

Due to the rarity of this disease, there are no ongoing randomized clinical trials evaluating therapeutic approaches for the treatment of vaginal carcinoma. Quality-of-life after treatment, however, remains an important aspect in the management of this disease. Therefore, physicians treating this disease should continue to refine the skills and techniques required to accurately and safely treat these patients in order to maximize local control and minimize the potential toxic side effects that can severely alter a patient's quality-of-life after completion of treatment.

## Vulvar Cancer

### Overview

Vulva cancer is relatively rare and, in spite of its external location, many patients will present with extensive primary lesions involving the vagina, urethra, or anus. Spread to inguinal lymph nodes is common as well.

### Introduction

Vulva cancer is a relatively rare cancer, accounting for only approximately 4% of cancers in the female reproductive tract and 0.6% of all cancers in women.[1] According to ACS statistics, only 3,740 women were diagnosed with vulva cancer in the United States in 2006 with approximately 880 women dying of this cancer in 2006.

### Anatomy

The mons veneris, labia majora and minora, clitoris, and vulvar vestibule are structures that compose the vulva. The mons is a pad of fat anterior and inferior to the pubic bone. The labia majora consists of two skin folds posterior to the mons coming together anteriorly to form the anterior labial commissure and posteriorly to form the posterior labial commissure. The labia minora, medial to the labia majora, come together posteriorly to form the fourchette of the labia and anteriorly to form the frenulum of the clitoris. The clitoris is at the anterior end of the labia minora with the prepuce of the clitoris anterior to the glans of the clitoris. The clitoris, an erectile structure, consists of the glans, a body, and two crura. The vestibule of the vagina, the space between the labia minora, has two openings: the urethra and and the opening of the vagina. The greater vestibular (Bartholin's glands) and lesser vestibular glands provide lubrication of the labia minora.

The internal pudendal artery, arising from the internal iliac artery, provides the main arterial supply while the veins follow the arteries. The clitoris has an extra vein, superficial dorsal vein, and the deep dorsal vein drains directly into the pelvic cavity. Nerve supply to the vulva is provided by the pudendal nerve which divides into the perineal branch and the dorsal nerve of the clitoris. The lymphatic drainage of the vulva is important, coursing anteriorly toward the mons, turning laterally to terminate in the inguinal lymph nodes. The inguinal lymph nodes lie above the fascia lata and cribriform fascia and below Camper's fascia. The femoral lymph nodes lie below the cribriform fascia along the femoral vein. The lymph node of Cloquet or Rosenmuller, the most cephalad of the femoral lymph nodes, lies under the inguinal ligament in the femoral canal.

## Pathology

Squamous cell carcinomas make up the majority of cancers of the vulva and arise on the labia minora, clitoris, fourchette, perineal body, or medial aspect of the labia majora. A majority, approximately 60%, of the cases have vulvar intra-epithelial neoplasia (VIN) adjacent to the tumor, while lichen sclerosis can be found adjacent to the tumors in 15%–40% of the time. Malignant melanoma, verrucous carcinoma, basal cell carcinoma, Merkel cell tumors, transitional cell carcinoma, usually arising within the Bartholin's gland, adenocarcinoma, adenoid cystic carcinoma, vulvar Paget's disease, and sarcomas are other tumor types that can present in the vulvar area.

## Risk Factors

Risk factors for the development of vulvar cancer include:

- Vulvar intra-epithelial neoplasia (VIN)
- Previous human papillomavirus (HPV) infection
- Herpes simplex virus (HSV)
- Human immunodeficiency virus (HIV) infection
- Previous cervical or vaginal cancer
- Diabetes
- Smoking
- Hypertension
- Obesity
- Chronic granulomatous veneral disease and syphilis have been implicated in some countries
- Women exposed to immunosuppression therapy have also been found to be at increased risk of developing vulvar cancer

## Screening

There are no standard screening examinations for this cancer. Pelvic examinations and patient awareness of symptoms can lead to earlier diagnosis with improved chances of cure. Patients with a history of cervical or vaginal cancer should have inspection of the vulva, with or without colposcopic examination, as part of their regular follow-up.[2] Patients with VIN III or lichens sclerosis should also be kept under close surveillance.

## Prevention

Vulva cancer can be prevented by avoiding the risk factors previously listed. Regular gynecologic examinations can also lead to the discovery of precancerous lesions with subsequent removal preventing the development of invasive cancer.

## Presentation/Workup

Patients with vulva cancer can be asymptomatic, or may present with a lump in the vulva or an ulcer. The lump can be red, pink, or white with a wart-like or raw surface. It is not unusual for patients to have a long-standing history of pruritus secondary to vulvar dystrophy. Patients may also complain of pain, burning, dysuria, bleeding, or discharge. A dark pigmented lesion or a change in a mole can represent vulvar melanoma. A mass on either side of the opening of the vagina could represent a Bartholin gland carcinoma. After a full history and physical and biopsy indicating vulvar cancer, the work-up should include:

- Examination under anesthesia
- Pap smear of the cervix
- Colposcopy of the cervix and vagina because of the common association with other squamous intra-epithelial lesions
- CT of the pelvis and groins
- Routine blood count, biochemical profile, and chest x-ray
- Cystoscopy and proctoscopy as indicated by symptoms and physical examination findings

## Staging

TABLE 30-5 **Comparison of TNM and FIGO Vulvar Cancer Staging**[2,25]

| FIGO Staging | | TNM Staging |
|---|---|---|
| | Primary tumor cannot be assessed | TX |
| | No evidence of primary tumor | T0 |
| 0 | Carcinoma *in situ* (pre-invasive cancer) | Tis |
| I | Tumor confined to the vulva or vulva and perineum, $\leq$ 2cm in greatest dimension | T1 |
| IA | Tumor confined to the vulva or vulva and perineum, $\leq$ 2cm in greatest dimension and with stromal invasion $\leq$ 1.0 mm* | T1a |
| IB | Tumor confined to the vulva or vulva and perineum, $\leq$ 2cm in greatest dimension and with stromal invasion $>$ 1.0 mm* | T1b |
| II | Tumor confined to the vulva or vulva and perineum, $>$ 2 cm in greatest dimension | T2 |
| III | Tumor invades any of the following structures: lower urethra, vagina, anus, and/or unilateral regional nodal metastasis | T3 |
| IV | | T4 |
| IVA | Tumor invades any of the following: bladder, rectal or upper urethral mucosa; or is fixed to the bone and/or bilateral regional node metastasis | |
| IVB | Any distant metastasis including pelvic lymph nodes | |

*Stromal invasion is defined as the measurement of tumor from the epithelial-stromal junction of the adjacent most superficial dermal papilla, to the deepest point of invasion.

## Biology

Human papillomavirus (HPV) types 16 and 18 have been detected in vulvar tumors.[13] Vulvar cancers associated with HPV infections tend to occur in younger women and the cancers have multiple areas of vulvar intra-epithelial neoplasia (VIN). P53 gene mutation may also play an important role in undifferentiated VIN pathogenesis independent of HPV infection.[14] Herpes simplex virus (HSV) type 2 induced cytomplasmic antigens have also been identified in *in situ* squamous cell vulvar carcinomas.[15] A number of cytogenetic abnormalities have also been reported in patients with tumors of the vulva and vagina.[16]

## Management

For many years, en bloc radical vulvectomy and bilateral inguinofemoral $+/-$ pelvic lymphadenectomy using a single "butterfly" incision was the standard of care in the United States for patients with vulvar carcinoma.[17] The most common post-surgical complication was breakdown of the surgical wound in the groin. This complication was greatly reduced by changing the surgical approach to performing the vulvectomy and groin dissections through separate incisions, thereby improving primary wound healing.[18] Today, the treatment of vulvar cancer is evolving, with great emphasis on organ preservation. Radiation therapy is being increasingly used in the curative management of vulvar cancer, often concurrently with radiation-sensitizing chemotherapy.[19] Preoperative radiation therapy has reduced the indications for radical exenterative surgery in patients with locally advanced vulvar cancer. Postoperative radiation therapy directed to the pelvic and inguinal lymph nodes has been demonstrated to improve disease-free survival in vulvar cancer patients with metastatic spread to two or more inguinal lymph nodes.

---

**BOX 30-5**

One hundred fourteen patients with invasive squamous cell carcinoma of the vulva and positive groin nodes after radical vulvectomy and bilateral groin dissection were randomized to either radiation therapy or pelvic node resection. The radiation dose to the groins and to the midplane of the pelvis was 4,500–5,000 cGy in 5 to 6.5 weeks. Acute and chronic morbidity was similar between groups.

Clinically suspicious or fixed ulcerated groin nodes and two or more positive groin nodes were two major prognostic factors. A significant survival difference was found favoring patients receiving adjuvant radiation, p = 0.03. The estimated 2-year survival rates were 68% for the RT group and 54% for the pelvic node resection group. The most dramatic survival advantage for radiation therapy was in patients with either of the two major poor prognostic factors.

Homesley et al. Radiation therapy versus pelvic node resection for carcinoma of the vulva with positive groin nodes. *Obstet Gynecol* 68:733–740, 1986.

---

Radiation to the intact groin, however, was not superior to groin dissection in patients with squamous cell carcinoma of the vulva and N0-1 inguinal lymph nodes.

---

**BOX 30-6**

Fifty-eight patients with squamous cell carcinoma of the vulva and nonsuspicious (N0-1) inguinal nodes were randomized to receive either groin dissection or groin radiation (5,000 cGy to 3 cm below anterior skin surface) in conjunction with radical vulvectomy.

*(continues)*

**BOX 30-6** (CONTINUED)

The study was closed earlier after interim analysis revealed an excess number of groin relapses in patients receiving groin radiation. Eighteen percent of patients receiving groin radiation experienced a groin relapse compared to 0% in patients randomized to receive groin dissection. The groin dissection group also had a significantly better progression-free interval (p = 0.03) and survival (p = 0.04).

Stehman, F.B. et al. Groin dissection versus groin radiation in carcinoma of the vulva. A gynecologic oncology group study Int. J. Radiat. Biol. Phys. 24:389–396, 1992.

The preinvasive forms of vulvar malignancies (carcinoma *in situ* and Paget's disease) and microinvasive lesions can be treated with topical chemotherapy, cryosurgery, or surgical resection. The standard management of patients with invasive Stage I and Stage II disease includes radical vulvectomy and inguinofemoral lymphadenectomy. Adjuvant postoperative radiation therapy is given based on various prognostic factors, including clinically or pathologically positive lymph nodes, extracapsular extension in lymph nodes, surgical margin status of <8 mm in fixed tissue (corresponding to a 1-cm clinical margin), or capillary lymphatic space invasion. For locally advanced lesions that involve midline structures, such as the clitoris or encroachment of the anal sphincter or involvement of more than the distal urethra, preoperative radiation therapy in an attempt to convert the status of a patient from unresectable to resectable is a reasonable treatment approach. Definitive radiation therapy has been used to treat medically inoperable or technically unresectable vulvar cancer patients.

## Technique/Dose

The clinical and pathologic characteristics of the primary vulvar tumor and regional lymph nodes determine the radiation target volume. The target volume in patients receiving radiation therapy for pathologically positive lymph node involvement should include the bilateral groin regions and pelvic lymph nodes. In the absence of clinical or pathologic evidence of pelvic node involvement, the superior border of the external beam field should include the external iliac lymph nodes. If pelvic lymph node involvement is present, then the superior border of the radiation treatment volume should include the common iliac nodes. The lateral borders of the pelvic treatment volume are a 2-cm margin lateral to the pelvic brim. For the groins, the lateral border of the treatment volume should extend to the anterior superior iliac spine region and include the full extent of the operative dissection. For extensive groin nodal involvement, the inferior border of the treatment volume should encompass the inferior inguinal nodal chain. It has been demonstrated that the vulva and perineum should be included in the radiation treatment volume when treating the inguinal/pelvic nodes, because of the significant increased risk of local recurrence in this volume when midline shielding is used.[20] Large parallel-opposed anterior and posterior photon fields can be used, with daily fractionation of 180 cGy to deliver 4,500–5,000 cGy. Dose to involved inguinal nodes is supplemented by anterior electron fields, to deliver an additional 1,000–2,000 cGy to gross or microscopic tumor volumes. Alternatively, a large anterior photon field covering the entire target volume, a smaller posterior photon field designed to cover the perineum, pelvic nodes, medial inguinal/femoral nodes, and use of supplemental anterior electron fields to boost dose to the lateral inguinal/femoral nodes can be utilized to reduce radiation dose to the femoral heads. It is important that dose to the groin be applied at an appropriate tissue depth. The depth of the femoral arteries/groin nodes can be determined by CT scan, and depends on patient body habitus, size, enlarged lymph nodes, and whether groin dissection has been performed. Technical inadequacies in the delivery of radiation can cause significant underdosing of inguinofemoral nodes, resulting in clinical failures.[21]

The patient is usually treated in the supine "frog-leg" position, with the knees apart and the feet together, if tolerated, in order to reduce skin folds which in turn can reduce skin toxicity. An alpha cradle cast in the treatment position facilitates daily position reproducibility. During the simulation, wires should be utilized to identify surgical scars or visible or palpable lesions or lymph nodes. If there is involvement of the perineum or vagina, a radio-opaque marker should be placed to identify the lesions of the simulation radiographic films.

### Follow-up

Patients are typically seen for follow-up approximately 2 to 3 weeks after completion of their radiation treatments. Close follow-up should then continue about every 3 to 4 months for the first 2 to 3 years following treatment. Follow-up may then be decreased to every 6 months until 5 years at which time the patient can return for follow-up on an annual basis. Follow-up should include a pertinent history and physical examination at each visit. Pelvic examination should be performed at each interval visit. Interval CT scans of the abdomen/pelvis, as well as a CXR or chest CT are also part of the routine follow-up care, and the scheduling of these tests is dictated by the initial tumor stage at presentation.

### Morbidity

Acute sequelae from radiation include desquamation of the skin in the treatment field. These skin reactions can be managed with a local skin care regimen, including saline soaks, moisturizers, Nugel pads, and sitz baths. Significant chronic toxicity has been reported, including groin soft tissue necrosis. Necrosis and fracture of the femoral head/neck has been reported to occur occasionally in patients who receive doses of 5,000 cGy or higher.[22]

### Future Directions

Currently, there is a phase II GOG trial evaluating radiation therapy and weekly cisplatin chemotherapy for the treatment of locally advanced squamous cell carcinoma of the vulva. No active phase III randomized studies are enrolling patients at the present time.

## Ovarian Cancer

### Overview

The ovary is composed of germ cells, stromal cells, and epithelial cells. Benign and malignant ovarian tumors can develop from any of these cell types. Treatment will differ based upon the cell of origin. Epithelial ovarian tumors will be the focus of this chapter.

### Introduction

The incidence of ovarian cancer increases with age. Ovarian cancer is the eighth most common cancer among women, 3% of all cancers, with the ACS estimating about 20,180 new cases diagnosed in 2006.[1] Ovarian cancer ranks fifth in cancer deaths among women with approximately 15,310 deaths from ovarian cancer in 2006. The incidence of ovarian cancer has decreased 0.7% a year since 1985.

### Anatomy

The ovaries are located between the uterus and the pelvic sidewall and are suspended by the ligament of the ovary medially to the uterus and to the lateral pelvic sidewall by the suspensory ligament of the ovary. The ovaries are suspended from the posterior-superior surface of the broad ligament by a mesentery called the mesovarium. The ovaries relate to either the ileum or colon, since both structures fill the pelvic cavity. The arterial blood supply is from the ovarian arteries which arise from the aorta just inferior of the renal arteries. Like the left testicular vein, the left ovarian vein drains into the left renal vein instead of the inferior vena cava. Lymph node drainage is superior to the lumbar nodes along the inferior vena cava and aorta.

## Pathology

The majority of ovarian tumors are benign, do not spread, and do not lead to serious illness. Tumors of low malignant potential (LMP) do not grow into the supporting tissue of the ovary and usually do not grow into the lining of the abdomen. LMP of the ovary affect women at a younger age, grow slowly and are less life-threatening than most ovarian cancers, although death can occur but is uncommon. About 85%–90% of ovarian cancers are epithelial in origin. Epithelial cancers can be classified into serous, mucinous, endometriod, undifferentiated, and clear cell types.

## Risk Factors

The risk factors for ovarian cancer include:

- Age—most develop after menopause
- Obesity
- Reproductive history—early menarche, gravida 0 or low parity, first child after 30, late menopause
- Family history of ovarian, breast, or colorectal cancer
- Family history of BRCA1 or BRCA2
- Fertility drug use
- Personal history of breast cancer
- Estrogen and hormone replacement therapy
- Talcum powder use

## Screening

There is no effective screening for ovarian cancer. CA-125, ultrasonography of the pelvis, and pelvic examination have not produced satisfactory results. Patients with a strong family history should obtain genetic counseling and, if found to be at high risk, be placed on prospective screening trials.

## Prevention

Knowledge about risk factors for the development of ovarian cancer has not translated into successful prevention interventions. Using oral contraceptives can reduce the risk of women at high risk of developing ovarian cancer, especially women with BRCA1 or BRCA2 mutations. Prophylactic oophorectomy has been proposed for certain high-risk women over the age of 40, but this is controversial because it induces premature menopause. Extra-ovarian primary peritoneal carcinoma can still develop in these women.

## Presentation/Workup

Early ovarian cancer can present with vague symptoms including early satiety, abdominal discomfort or pain, nausea, dyspepsia, constipation, or obstipation. Patients may also experience vaginal bleeding, dysuria, or urinary frequency.

Workup for ovarian cancer includes:

- History and physical examination with bimanual pelvic examination
- CA125

- Transvaginal or pelvis ultrasound
- CT of the abdomen and pelvis
- Chest x-ray
- Biochemistry and complete blood count
- Barium enema or colonoscopy to rule out bowel cancer

## Staging

Ovarian cancer is surgically staged. A careful examination of all of the peritoneal surfaces, washings of the peritoneal cavity, biopsy, and/or resection of any suspicious nodules, selected lymphadenectomy of the pelvic and para-aortic nodes, TAH/BSO, and appendectomy for mucinous tumors.

## Biology

Common genetic abnormalities in ovarian cancer include abnormalities of *c-myc*, H-*ras*, K-*ras*, and the *neu* oncogenes. More recently, altered expression and loss of heterozygosity (LOH) of the LOT1

**TABLE 30-6 Comparison of FIGO and TNM Ovarian Cancer Staging[2,25]**

| FIGO | | | TNM |
|---|---|---|---|
| | | Primary tumor cannot be assesed | Tx |
| | | No evidence of primary tumor | T0 |
| 0 | | | |
| I | | Tumor confined to ovaries | T1 |
| | IA | Tumor limited to one ovary, capsule intact | |
| | | No tumor on the ovarian surface | |
| | | No malignant cells in the ascites or washings | T1a |
| | IB | Tumor limited to both ovaries, capsule intact | |
| | | No tumor on the ovarian surface | |
| | | No malignant cells in the ascites or washings | T1b |
| | IC | Tumor limited to one or both ovaries | |
| | | With any of the following: capsule ruptured, tumor on ovarian surface, positive malignant cells in the ascites or positive washings | T1c |
| II | | Tumor involves one or both ovaries with pelvic extension | T2 |
| | IIA | Extension and/or implants in uterus and/or tubes | |
| | | No malignant cells in the ascites or peritoneal washings | T2a |
| | IIB | Extension to other pelvic organs; no malignant cells in the ascites or peritoneal washings | T2b |
| | IIC | IIA/B with positive malignant cells in the ascites or positive peritoneal washings | T2c |
| III | | Tumor involves one or both ovaries with microscopically confirmed peritoneal metastasis outside the pelvis and/or regional lymph node metastasis | T3 and/or N1 |
| | IIIA | Microscopic peritoneal metastasis beyond the pelvis | T3a |
| | IIIB | Macroscopic peritoneal metastasis beyond the pelvis 2 cm or less in greatest dimension | T3b |
| | IIIC | Peritoneal metastasis beyond pelvis more than 2 cm in greatest dimension and/or regional lymph nodes metastasis | T3c and/or N1 |
| IV | | Distant metastasis beyond pelvis | M1 |

locus has been reported in the pathogenesis of ovarian cancer.[23] An association with a single nucleotide polymorphism (SNP) of matrix metalloproteinase-7 to ovarian cancer susceptibility has been reported comparing women with ovarian cancer to control women in China.[24] The importance of the BRCA1 and BRCA2 mutations in ovarian cancer development has been previously cited.

## Management

Surgical management is one of the most important components in the treatment of ovarian cancer. Comprehensive surgical staging is necessary to identify patients with Stage I and II ovarian cancer. Tumor debulking surgery plays a crucial role in the management of patients with ovarian cancer. Debulking surgery, or cytoreductive surgery, has been shown to directly affect survival independent of adjuvant therapy. Survival is directly related to the amount of residual tumor after primary cytoreductive surgery. In a woman of reproductive age with disease limited to one ovary, it may be possible to preserve the uterus, opposite ovary, and fallopian tube in order to maintain the possibility of fertility in the future.

Current management of patients with early-stage disease is dependent on the presence or absence of high-risk features. Patients with Stage IA or IB disease and well-differentiated tumors generally do not require further adjuvant therapy. High-risk features include high-grade tumors, Stage IC and II disease, and clear-cell histology. Adjuvant postoperative chemotherapy is generally recommended in early-stage tumors with high-risk features. Multiple randomized trials have demonstrated the survival benefit to the immediate use of adjuvant chemotherapy in early-stage disease. Platinum and taxane-based chemotherapy is considered the standard approach for patients with early-stage disease with high-risk features. Adjuvant chemotherapy is the standard for all patients with advanced-stage disease. Recently, the Gynecologic Oncology Group reported the results of a phase III randomized trial comparing intravenous paclitaxel followed by either intravenous cisplatin or intraperitoneal cisplatin and paclitaxel in patients with Stage III ovarian cancer.

---

**BOX 30-7**

Four hundred twenty-nine patients with Stage III ovarian carcinoma or primary peritoneal carcinoma with no residual mass greater than 1.0 cm were randomized to receive intravenous (IV) paclitaxel and cisplatin or intraperitoneal (IP) cisplatin and paclitaxel.

Grade 3 and 4 pain, fatigue, hematologic, gastrointestinal, metabolic, and neurologic toxic effects were more common in the IP group. The median duration of progression-free survival was greater in the IP chemotherapy group (23.8 months) compared to the IV chemotherapy group (18.3 months), $p = 0.05$. The median duration of overall survival in the IP group was 65.6 months compared to 49.7 months in the IV group, $p = 0.03$. Quality-of-life was worse in the IP group before cycle 4 and 3 to 6 weeks after treatment but not 1 year after treatment.

Armstrong, D.K., et al. Intraperitoneal cisplatin and paclitaxel in ovarian cancer. *N Engl J Med* 354:34–43, 2006.

---

Radiation therapy can be used in the primary management of epithelial ovarian carcinoma. Whole abdominal radiation therapy (WART) is curative in appropriately selected patients. Definitive radiation therapy should encompass all areas of potential disease recurrence, and thus the entire peritoneal cavity must be included in the radiation portal field. No prospective randomized trial has compared WART, using modern radiation techniques, with a modern chemotherapy regimen. However, there are published series demonstrating outcomes with WART that are comparable to outcomes using platinum-based chemotherapy.

## Technique/Dose

The WART treatment field must include the entire peritoneal cavity, which is at risk for dissemination of disease. The open field technique involves an open anterior and posterior portal field to treat the peritoneal cavity, including the para-aortic, pelvic, and mesenteric lymph nodes along with the entire diaphragm. The treatment fields extend from 2 cm above the domes of the diaphragm to below the obturator foramina and 2 cm laterally beyond the peritoneal reflection. The daily radiation dose is 120–150 cGy per day. The total dose to this large open field is 3,000 cGy in 20 fractions. The kidneys are shielded at 2,000 cGy and the liver is shielded at 2,500 cGy to protect these organs. The pelvic field then receives a boost for an additional 1,500–2,000 cGy using either an anterior/posterior or four-field beam arrangement. High-energy photons should be utilized to ensure minimal dose variation. Posterior kidney blocks should be used, limiting the dose to the kidneys to 1,800–2,000 cGy.

## Follow-up

Patients are typically seen for follow-up approximately 4 to 6 weeks after completion of their radiation treatments. Close follow-up should then continue about every 3 to 4 months for the first 2 to 3 years following treatment. Follow-up may then be decreased to every 6 months until 5 years, at which time the patient can return for follow-up on an annual basis. Follow-up should include a pertinent history and physical examination at each visit. Pelvic examination should be performed at each interval visit. In addition, serum marker CA-125 levels should be followed as part of the routine follow-up schedule.

## Morbidity

Common acute effects from whole abdominal radiation therapy include loose stools, diarrhea, nausea, vomiting, and fatigue. Hematologic toxicity is generally mild. Late effects include small bowel complications, including obstruction.

## Future Directions

Issues that remain unresolved and are continuing to evolve are those of the optimal administration and use of the adjuvant chemotherapy in the treatment of ovarian carcinoma. There are no current ongoing national clinical trials evaluating the role of radiation therapy in the management of ovarian carcinoma.

## REFERENCES

1. Society AC: Cancer Statistics 2006, http://www.cancer.org/downloads/stt/1.
2. Benedet J, Hacker, NF, Ngan, HYS. Staging classifications and clinical practice guidelines of gynaecologic cancers. *Int J Gyn Obstet* 70:207–312, 2000.
3. Kurman RJ, Kaminski PF, Norris HJ. The behavior of endometrial hyperplasia: a long-term study of "untreated" hyperplasia in 170 patients. *Cancer* 56:403–412, 1985.
4. Feng YZ, Shiozawa T, Miyamoto T, et al. BRAF mutation in endometrial carcinoma and hyperplasia: correlation with KRAS and p53 mutations and mismatch repair protein expression. *Clin Cancer Res* 11:6133–6138, 2005.
5. Muslumanoglu HM, Oner U, Ozalp S, et al. Genetic imbalances in endometrial hyperplasia and endometrioid carcinoma detected by comparative genomic hybridization. *Eur J Obstet Gynecol Reprod Biol* 120:107–114, 2005.
6. Zhao Y, Yamashita T, Ishikawa M. Regulation of tumor invasion by HOXB13 gene overexpressed in human endometrial cancer. *Oncol Rep* 13:721–726, 2005.

7. Barnes MN, Kilgore LC. Complete surgical staging of early endometrial adenocarcinoma: optimizing patient outcomes. *Semin Radiat Oncol* 10:3–7, 2000.

8. Grigsby PW, Perez CA, Kuske RR, et al. Results of therapy, analysis of failures, and prognostic factors for clinical and pathologic Stage III adenocarcinoma of the endometrium. *Gynecol Oncol* 27:44–57, 1987.

9. Mundt AJ, McBride R, Rotmensch J, et al. Significant pelvic recurrence in high-risk pathologic Stage I-IV endometrial carcinoma patients after adjuvant chemotherapy alone: implications for adjuvant radiation therapy. *Int J Radiat Oncol Biol Phys* 50:1145–1153, 2001.

10. Waggoner SE, Anderson SM, Luce MC, et al. p53 protein expression and gene analysis in clear cell adenocarcinoma of the vagina and cervix. *Gynecol Oncol* 60:339–344, 1996.

11. Boyd J, Takahashi H, Waggoner SE, et al. Molecular genetic analysis of clear cell adenocarcinomas of the vagina and cervix associated and unassociated with diethylstilbestrol exposure in utero. *Cancer* 77:507–513, 1996.

12. Stock RG, Mychalczak B, Armstrong JG, et al. The importance of brachytherapy technique in the management of primary carcinoma of the vagina. *Int J Radiat Oncol Biol Phys* 24:747–753, 1992.

13. Huang FY, Kwok YK, Lau ET, et al. Genetic abnormalities and HPV status in cervical and vulvar squamous cell carcinomas. *Cancer Genet Cytogenet* 157:42–48, 2005.

14. Chulvis do Val IC, Almeida Filho GL, Valiante PM, et al. Vulvar intra-epithelial neoplasia p53 expression, p53 gene mutation, and HPV in recurrent/progressive cases. *J Reprod Med* 49:868–874, 2004.

15. Kaufman RH, Dreesman GR, Burek J, et al. Herpesvirus-induced antigens in squamous-cell carcinoma *in situ* of the vulva. *N Engl J Med* 305:483–488, 1981.

16. Micci F, Teixeira MR, Scheistroen M, et al. Cytogenetic characterization of tumors of the vulva and vagina. *Genes Chromosomes Cancer* 38:137–148, 2003.

17. Byron RL, Jr., Mishell DR, Jr., Yonemoto RH. The surgical treatment of invasive carcinoma of the vulva. *Surg Gynecol Obstet* 121:1243–1251, 1965.

18. Hacker NF, Leuchter RS, Berek JS, et al. Radical vulvectomy and bilateral inguinal lymphadenectomy through separate groin incisions. *Obstet Gynecol* 58:574–579, 1981.

19. Roberts WS, Hoffman MS, Kavanagh JJ, et al. Further experience with radiation therapy and concomitant intravenous chemotherapy in advanced carcinoma of the lower female genital tract. *Gynecol Oncol* 43:233–236, 1991.

20. Dusenbery K, Carlson, JW, LaPorte, RM, Goswitz, JJ, Roback, DM, Adcock, LL, Potish, RA. Radical vulvectomy with postoperative nodal radiotherapy: a re-appraisal of the vulvar central block. *Int. J. Radiat. Oncol. Biol. Phys.* 27:199, 1993.

21. Koh WJ, Chiu M, Stelzer KJ, et al. Femoral vessel depth and the implications for groin node radiation. *Int J Radiat Oncol Biol Phys* 27:969–974, 1993.

22. Grigsby PW, Roberts HL, Perez CA. Femoral neck fracture following groin irradiation. *Int J Radiat Oncol Biol Phys* 32:63–67, 1995.

23. Cvetkovic D, Pisarcik D, Lee C, et al. Altered expression and loss of heterozygosity of the LOT1 gene in ovarian cancer. *Gynecol Oncol* 95:449–455, 2004.

24. Li Y, Jin X, Kang S, et al. Polymorphisms in the promoter regions of the matrix metalloproteinases-1, -3, -7, and -9 and the risk of epithelial ovarian cancer in China. *Gynecol Oncol* 101:92–96, 2006.

25. AJCC Cancer Staging Manual, Sixth Edition. New York: Springer, 2002.

# 31

# Soft Tissue Sarcoma

*Peter W.M. Chung, MD*

*Brian O'Sullivan, MD*

## OVERVIEW

Soft tissue sarcoma (STS) is a rare malignancy requiring multimodality management. Advances and integration of surgery, radiotherapy, and chemotherapy have improved outcomes and are discussed in this chapter.

## INTRODUCTION

Soft tissue sarcoma represents approximately 1% of adult cancers in the United States, translating into almost 9,000 new cases annually, of which 5,000 are male and 4,000 are female.[1] The disease is characterized by wide heterogeneity in anatomical site, pathologic subtype, and clinical behavior. Just over half originate in the limbs/torso with the retroperitoneum or visceral tissues representing about 35% and the head and neck about 10% of cases.

## RISK FACTORS

- Median age 50–55 years
- Prior radiation exposure
- Lymphedema (associated with lymphangiosarcoma)
- Chemical carcinogens–thorotrast, vinyl chloride and arsenic (hepatic angiosarcomas), phenoxyherbicides, chlorophenols, dioxins, phenoxyacetic acids, and certain herbicides
- Genetic conditions–Neurofibromatosis, Li-Fraumeni syndrome, retinoblastoma, Gardner's Syndrome, Carney's triad, Werner's syndrome, Gorlin's syndrome, tuberous sclerosis

## SCREENING

No population screening exists due to the low incidence and prevalence. Patients at increased risk for sarcoma should be assessed at a threshold commensurate with index of suspicion.

## PATHOLOGY

The World Health Organization (WHO) classification is the most frequently used.[2] This has largely been based on classifying tumors on the basis of their putative "tissue of origin." Gene expression profiling of STS has been used to identify a genomic-based classification scheme, and further research to enhance "classical" methods of defining subtypes of STS is ongoing. There are two main systems for grading of STS, and while both use the degree of necrosis and mitotic rate, the French system (which may be prognostically more useful)[3] relies on differentiation and the U.S. system considers location, histological subtype, cellularity, and nuclear pleomorphism. The TNM stage classification (see Table 31-1) uses a two-tiered grade classification ("low" vs. "high" grade) and a formula is used to translate three- and four-tiered grading systems.

## STAGING

The International Union Against Cancer (UICC)/American Joint Committee on Cancer (AJCC) TNM (6th edition) staging system is the most widely used. Visceral sarcoma (lack of international system), dermatofibrosarcoma protuberans (borderline malignancy), and angiosarcoma (different natural history) are excluded. In rhabdomyosarcoma, two separate classifications exist; a postoperative surgical classification developed by the North American Intergroup Rhabdomyosarcoma Study Group (IRSG) and the International Society of Pediatric Oncology (SIOP) employs a TNM presurgical staging system more in keeping with contemporary TNM staging. This system may be more appropriate as such lesions will frequently be treated with induction protocols in advance of surgery.

## MOLECULAR BIOLOGY[4]

Two major types of genetic alteration appear to play a role in the development of STS. The first type comprises specific genetic alterations that include simple karyotypes, such as fusion genes (which may account for roughly 30% of sarcomas) due to reciprocal translocations such as those found in

---

### TABLE 31-1  TNM Staging and Grouping

#### TNM Staging

| | |
|---|---|
| TX | Primary tumor cannot be assessed |
| T0 | No evidence of primary tumor |
| T1a | Superficial tumor <5 cm in greatest dimension |
| T1b | Deep tumor <5 cm in greatest dimension |
| T2a | Superficial tumor $\geq$5 cm in greatest dimension |
| T2b | Deep tumor $\geq$5 cm in greatest dimension |
| NX | Regional lymph nodes cannot be assessed |
| N0 | No regional lymph nodes involved |
| N1 | Regional lymph node(s) involved |
| MX | Distant metastasis cannot be assessed |
| M0 | No distant metastasis |
| M1 | Distant metastasis |

#### TNM Stage Grouping

| | |
|---|---|
| Stage I | G1-2 T1-2 N0 M0 |
| Stage II | G3-4 T1-T2a N0 M0 |
| Stage III | G3-4 T2b N0M0 |
| Stage IV | Any G Any T N1 M0 |
| | Any G Any T N0 M1 |

G = grade
Sobin L, Wittekind C. *TNM Classification of Malignant Tumours*, 6th ed. New York: Wiley-Liss; 2002.

the EWS family and specific point mutations such as *KIT* mutations in gastrointestinal stromal tumors. Examples of STS associated with these genetic alterations include myxoid liposarcoma, synovial sarcoma, desmoplastic small round cell sarcoma, clear cell sarcoma, and extraskeletal myxoid chondrosarcoma. The second involves complex unbalanced karyotypes and non-specific genetic alterations representing numerous genetic losses and gains. Here, the most common abnormality is the prevalence of inactivation of the p53 pathway, which may occur early in the pathogenesis, leading to progression of tumors. Tumor types that may show these changes include malignant fibrous histiocytoma, leiomyosarcoma, and fibrosarcoma.

The presence of certain genetic changes, in particular the presence of fusion genes, aids the diagnosis of the STS subtype associated with the specific genetic mutation.

Although these cytogenetic abnormalities may aid in differential diagnosis and may provide therapeutic targets, molecular prognostication and prediction of treatment response are proving more elusive. This is illustrated by the translocation t(X;18)(p11;q11), which has been used to confirm the diagnosis of synovial cell sarcoma for patients with poorly differentiated lesions. Irrespective of their histological appearance, almost all synovial sarcomas contain the t(X;18)(*SYT-SSX*) translocation involving the *SSX1* (associated with monophasic histology) *or SSX2* (associated with biphasic histology) gene, two closely related genes from chromosome Xp11, and the *SYT* gene from chromosome 18q11. The result is the formation of a chimeric gene thought to function by encoding a transcription-activating protein. It was suggested that the transcripts of these fusion genes had specific prognostic significance but results have been contradictory.

Additional biologic prognostic information has been studied and include mutations in p53 and mdm2, Ki-67 status, altered expression of the retinoblastoma gene product (pRb) in high-grade sarcomas with uncertain conclusions. Also, tissue hypoxia appears associated with the development of distant metastases independently from depth, size, and grade.

## NATURAL HISTORY

Soft tissue sarcomas spread longitudinally within the site of origin and may invade contiguous structures and envelope major neuro-vasculature. Often a "pseudocapsule" that is composed of a reactive zone of edematous tissue, neovascularization, and tumor satellites surround the main tumor mass. This sometimes encourages enucleation as it is (wrongly) interpreted as anatomic disease containment. In the extremity, barriers such as bone and major fascial planes prevent axial spread of disease beyond originating compartments. When breached, the risk of tumor contamination is significant. Similar patterns of spread occur in nonextremity lesions, and thus the fascial planes should be recognized and encompassed in surgical or radiation target volumes.

STS have a low incidence of lymph node spread except for epithelioid sarcoma, clear cell sarcoma, angiosarcoma, and rhabdomyosarcoma. Although signifying a relatively poor prognosis, isolated lymph node metastasis may not be as adverse a prognostic indicator as was once thought.

Overt metastases are present in 10% of cases at primary diagnosis. The most common site of metastatic disease is pulmonary, but osseous disease may be seen following lung metastases. Myxoid liposarcoma may develop bone metastasis as the first site of relapse and also has the curious characteristic of developing isolated soft tissue metastases. In patients with retroperitoneal sarcoma (RPS) and intra-abdominal visceral sarcomas, the liver is a more common site of first metastasis.

## SPECIFIC CLINICOPATHOLOGIC ENTITIES[4]

A full description of all of the differing clinicopathologic entities is beyond the scope of this chapter; however we have outlined several which may be encountered in the clinic.

## Malignant Fibrous Histiocytoma

This has been considered the prototypical STS and is the most frequently diagnosed in the past two decades. It now appears to be a diagnosis of exclusion and may be considered synonymous with undifferentiated pleomorphic sarcoma that may be subtyped in the majority of patients by immunohistochemical and ultrastructural means. The most common subclassifications are myxofibrosarcoma and leiomyosarcoma.

## Liposarcoma

This is the second most commonly encountered STS subtype of which myxoid liposarcoma (MLS) is a frequent variant. A translocation (t12:16) is present, resulting in the TLS-CHOP fusion; the more aggressive round cell variant also exhibits this but, generally, it is not seen in myxoid well-differentiated liposarcoma. MLS can have a multifocal presentation, which may be an unusual pattern of metastases, seen predominantly in the retroperitoneum and mediastinum; bone metastases are not uncommon. Long disease-free intervals may be enjoyed if an aggressive approach to treatment is pursued. Liposarcoma as a STS subtype also appears to have a more favorable outcome than other histological subtypes of STS. MLS is a radiosensitive tumor and may have enhanced local control with the addition of radiotherapy.

## Angiosarcoma

Superficial angiosarcoma tends to occur in the head and neck region (~50%) of older male patients, with a radial growth pattern spreading within the dermis of the scalp and facial tissues. Lesions can appear remotely from each other and exhibit a characteristic purplish maculopapular distribution. Local control is problematic due to difficulty in determining the extent of microscopic disease beyond gross tumor. This is reflected in the practical concern about the extent of surgical and radiotherapeutic margins, and hence local recurrence beyond the treatment area is frequent. Distant metastasis is common, but regional nodal disease (10%–20% rates) is also more frequent. Other sites where angiosarcoma may arise with some frequency are the breast (usually complicating previous breast cancer treatment) and the heart.

## Rhabdomyosarcoma (RMS)

This is uncommon in the adult but is the fifth most common cancer in childhood. Outcome for adults is considerably less favorable than in children. The main subtypes of RMS are embryonal (70%), alveolar (20%), and pleomorphic (10%). Most alveolar subtypes possess the t(2;13) aberration. The translocations and the gene fusion products are characteristic and the PAX3 gene family involved in the disease fingerprint may have a role in muscle development. One subtype, rarely described in adults, is the "spindle cell rhabdomyosarcoma" that in children has a relatively favorable prognosis but is aggressive in the adult. Evaluation should include bone marrow biopsy and in the case of parameningeal tumors, CSF examination. The risk of lymph node metastasis is significant and there is also an odd propensity for these tumors to metastasize to the breast in some female patients. Response rates to chemotherapy and RT are excellent in alveolar and embryonal but less so in pleomorphic subtypes, which also appear more in older patients.

## Dermatofibrosarcoma Protruberans (DFSP)

This is a superficial tumor that frequently manifests as a dermal raised purple/red lesion(s) in the lower neck, upper chest, and shoulder girdle regions with a slow but persistent growth over many years. Immunostaining for CD34 suggests evidence of neural differentiation. Histological appearance is often borderline or low grade but it has a high rate of local recurrence after simple excision even though metastases are rare. Platelet-derived growth factor beta (PDGF-B) is increased locally, resulting in autocrine or paracrine tumor growth. Although there are data supporting the use of imatinib in DFSP, most cases are treated successfully with surgery alone or supplemented with adjuvant radiotherapy.

## Synovial Sarcoma

This has a biphasic cellular pattern consisting of a stroma of fibroblast spindle-like cells and epithelial-like cells in a glandular pattern on light microscopy and immunohistochemistry. The t(x;18) translocation can almost invariably be detected with the demonstration of a fusion between the SSX1 and SYT genes. There may be calcification. These tumors are found in the para-articular areas of the tendon sheaths and joints of young adults. At least 50% of the cases are in the lower limbs (especially the knee); the remainder are mostly seen in the upper limbs but it is not limited to these areas. It is rarely encountered in regions with specific relationship to synovial structures. The risk of lymph node spread is also increased in this disease. General management is the same as for other STS but this histological subtype exhibits good response to chemotherapy and this may be included in management.[5]

## Gastrointestinal Stromal Tumors (GIST)

These tumors arise predominantly in the stomach or small intestine, but can also develop from omentum and retroperitoneum. Metastases occur predominantly within the peritoneal cavity and to the liver. GISTs harbor so-called gain-of-function mutations in the *c-kit* or *platelet-derived growth factor-receptor* (*PDGFRA*) genes in 85% and 5% of cases respectively. Through these mutations, the receptors are constitutively activated. The advent of the tyrosine kinase inhibitor imatinib (Gleevec®) was a major breakthrough in the management of advanced GIST lesions because the response rates were dramatic, and effective treatment options had not previously been available. Patients whose tumors contained exon 11 KIT mutations are more likely to respond to imatinib than those whose tumors have an exon 9 KIT mutation or those with no detectable kinase mutation.

## Clear Cell Sarcoma

This unusual tumor has also been termed malignant melanoma of soft parts or clear cell sarcoma of tendons and aponeuroses. It presents as a deep soft tissue mass and has a propensity for lymph node metastases. Clear cell sarcoma has a distinct chromosomal translocation, t(12;22)(q13;q13), involving EWS and ATF1 genes. Because of the presence of intracellular melanin and immunoreactivity for S100 and HMB45, it has been suggested that this entity is better considered a subtype of melanoma and not a soft tissue sarcoma.

### PRESENTATION

- Painless mass, pain, erythema, warmth, restriction of joint motion, or ulceration (large lesions)
- Abdominal pain, palpable mass, anorexia, subacute intestinal obstruction, weight loss (intra-abdominal sarcoma)
- Nasal obstruction, cranial nerve dysfunction, proptosis, mass effect in sensitive locations (head and neck sarcomas)

### WORKUP:

- History and clinical examination
- Prebiopsy cross-sectional imaging (CT/MRI) particularly when STS strongly suspected
- Core needle or open incisional biopsy
- CT chest (chest X-ray may be sufficient for very low grade lesions)

Evaluation of a STS patient is summarized in Figure 31-1.

**FIGURE 31-1** Evaluation of STS patient.

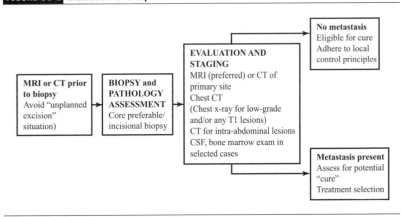

## MANAGEMENT

The overall approach to the local management of non-metastatic extremity, head and neck, and superficial trunk soft tissue sarcoma is summarized.

## EXTREMITY

The overall 5-year survival of STS patients is expected to be approximately 60% with local control of 90%.[6] The cornerstone of management is surgery, which previously was often amputation. Contemporary management of extremity STS can be traced to the landmark trial at the NCI.

**FIGURE 31-2** Management of non-metastatic extremity, head and neck, and superficial trunk soft tissue sarcoma.

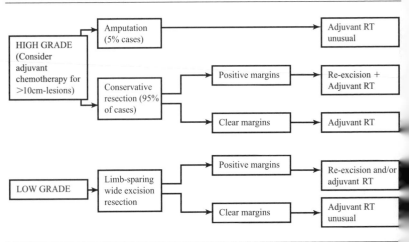

## BOX 31-1

In this study 43 patients were randomized to receive amputation vs. limb conservation and adjuvant radiotherapy in a 1:2 randomization. Local control was 100% and 85% in those amputation and conservative treatment respectively. No difference was seen in disease-free (5-year 78% vs. 71%) or overall survival (5-year 88% vs. 83%). Patients with positive margins were more likely to have local recurrence even in the presence of adjuvant radiotherapy.

The treatment of soft-tissue sarcomas of the extremities: prospective randomized evaluations of (1) limb-sparing surgery plus radiation therapy compared with amputation and (2) the role of adjuvant chemotherapy. *Ann Surg.* 1982 Sep;196(3):305–315.

Subsequently, two notable trials helped to establish the value of adjuvant radiotherapy with conservative surgery as optimal management in extremity STS.

## BOX 31-2

These two studies randomized patients to receive adjuvant radiotherapy after conservative surgery. At the NCI, patients were treated with concurrent chemotherapy depending on grade. The local control for those receiving RT was 99% compared to 70% in the control group (p = 0.0001). The results were similar for high- and low-grade tumors.

Adjuvant RT, using brachytherapy (BRT), was used at Memorial Sloan-Kettering Cancer Center with a similar effect in high-grade lesions. No improvement in local control was evident in the low-grade tumors attributed to more slowly cycling cells which are unaffected during BRT.

Yang et al. Randomized prospective study of the benefit of adjuvant radiation therapy in the treatment of soft tissue sarcomas of the extremity. *J Clin Oncol* 1998;16:197–203.

Pisters et al. Long-term results of a prospective randomized trial of adjuvant brachytherapy in soft tissue sarcoma. *J Clin Oncol* 1996;14:859–868.

Adjuvant radiotherapy allows more conservative tissue resections with less extensive operations and improves local control for STS of the extremity and also the trunk.

## BOX 31-3

This systematic overview employed data from five randomized trials, six prospective studies, 25 retrospective studies, and three additional articles involving a total of 4,579 patients. Adjuvant RT improved the local control rate in combination with conservative surgery in the treatment of STS of extremities and trunk in patients with negative, marginal, or minimal microscopic positive surgical margins. A local control rate of 90% was documented. Following intralesional surgery radiotherapy improved local control, but rates were less satisfactory. The evidence was less conclusive for STS in the retroperitoneum, head and neck, breast, and uterus.

A systematic overview of radiation therapy effects in soft tissue sarcomas. *Acta Oncol* 2003;42:516–531.

Most tumors affect either the superficial or deep compartments, unnecessary contamination of uninvolved compartments is avoided by a planned biopsy. Amputation rates have been reduced by improved surgical techniques (maintaining the principles of fascial containment) and have resulted in limb sparing for most patients. Wide excision of the lesion together with underlying fascia is required for superficial STS. When fascia is left intact, RT can be given after a negative, narrow margin of excision. If the deep compartment is involved or has been contaminated, re-excision, radiotherapy or both are required. For deep lesions, wide excision (when feasible) of the tumor and biopsy tracts is necessary, together with adjuvant RT. When margins are positive, the risk of local recurrence is almost doubled, as is the risk of distant recurrence and disease-related death.[7] However, a "planned" small positive resection margin with the intention of sparing a critical structure may have superior control when compared to an "unplanned" positive margin (local recurrence 3.6% vs. 31.6%), even with the addition of RT.[8] Simply stated, radiotherapy does not ameliorate inadequate surgery.[8,9]

There is a subgroup of patients who may be managed with conservative surgery alone and do not need RT,[10] but the challenge remains in identifying such patients. Case selection is paramount and much of the data are published from large experienced centers.[11]

In some patients, better functional outcome can be achieved with amputation.[12,13] This includes the following scenarios: (1) involvement of major neurovascular structures or multiple compartments when adequate surgical clearance is not possible; (2) major RT complication resulting from dose and volume issues; (3) below knee amputation prosthesis is functionally better than a limb damaged by extensive surgery and radiation. Occasionally, radiotherapy is required with inadequate clearance of tissues in very proximal lesions.

---

**BOX 31-4**

A series of 112 patients who underwent radiotherapy for gross disease. Local control at 5 years was 51%, 45%, and 9% for tumors less than 5 cm, 5 to 10 cm, and greater than 10 cm, respectively. Patients who received doses of less than 63 Gy had inferior outcomes, and a rise in complications was seen at doses of 68 Gy or more, providing a potential therapeutic window.

Kepka et al. Results of radiation therapy for unresected soft-tissue sarcomas. *Int J Radiat Oncol Biol Phys* 2005;63:852–859.

---

In some patients where surgery is not considered appropriate, definitive radiation may be offered as an alternative with some possibility of long term-local control.

## STRATEGIES COMBINING RADIOTHERAPY WITH OTHER AGENTS

Delaney et al have reported on preoperative chemo-radiotherapy which involved three courses of doxorubicin, ifosfamide, mesna, and dacarbazine (MAID) interdigitated with two 22 Gy courses of radiation. This was followed by surgical resection and 16 Gy boost for positive microscopic margins and three cycles of postoperative chemotherapy.[14] Patients with tumor sizes >8cm had local control rates similar to historical controls but 5-year overall survival rates seemed improved (87% vs. 58%), suggesting an effect of chemotherapy on micrometastatic disease in these high-risk patients. Febrile neutropenia occurred in 25% of patients and 29% also experienced wound complications. This regimen has been tested in a multi-institutional phase II setting by the Radiation Therapy Oncology Group (RTOG 9514).[15] Late complications included myelodysplasia.

Intra-arterial chemotherapy with doxorubicin or other agents with or without radiotherapy has been used. The total dose of radiotherapy has varied with doses of 17.5 Gy to 35 Gy preceded by a 3-day infusion of intra-arterial doxorubicin. Although an attractive concept, no benefit has been demonstrated compared to radiation alone.[16]

Isolated lymph perfusion (ILP) similar to that used in melanoma has been attempted. The combination of melphalan and tumor necrosis factor-alpha (TNF-$\alpha$) has been most popular with response rates of 76% and the limb saved in 71% of patients.[17] The selection for ILP hinges on the decision that patients would otherwise require amputation or marked functional deficit if treated conventionally. Patients who develop resectable disease usually then undergo surgery.

Higher doses of radiotherapy with concurrent dose intensified chemotherapy regimens, provide an opportunity to enhance local control. Preliminary data using a concurrent ifosfamide-based protocol exists and may help to address unresectable disease.[18] Rhomberg et al used the radiation sensitizer razoxane.[19] Among 82 patients with gross disease, RT combined with razoxane demonstrated an increased response rate compared to photon irradiation alone (74% vs. 49%) with improved local control (64% vs. 30%; p <0.05). Acute skin reactions were enhanced in the "sensitizer" arm, but late toxicity was not increased.

## SPECIFIC RADIOTHERAPY ISSUES

Currently, there are no randomized data comparing outcomes of EBRT and brachytherapy (BRT). When considering the particular strategy to be used for specific radiotherapeutic management of STS, factors that need to be taken into account include the anatomic setting and the volume of tissue irradiated, particularly if radiosensitive normal tissue is likely to limit delivery of adequate doses. In certain cases, the options may include combining brachytherapy and external beam radiotherapy, choosing preoperative external beam or using techniques such as intensity modulated radiotherapy to avoid high doses to normal tissue. Operational advantages of BRT include prompt initiation following surgery, shorter overall treatment time, and relative ease of combining with chemotherapy because there is relative skin sparing from the high RT doses. Disadvantages include lack of efficacy in low-grade tumors and poorer results when anatomy of the lesion prevents ideal implant geometry. Brachytherapy catheters can be placed intra-operatively and removed if pathological criteria are satisfactory. BRT alone is not recommended where poor CTV coverage will result from the implant, where nearby critical structures would limit the dose delivered and where there is involvement of resection margins and also the skin.[20] The combination of external beam and brachytherapy may be used in these circumstances.

The technical delivery aspects of BRT remain varied and have been defined in an empirical manner without randomized clinical trials. Various options are available that include low-dose rate (LDR) monotherapy, LDR combined with EBRT, fractionated high-dose rate (HDR), and intra-operative HDR. A summary of doses used in EBRT, brachytherapy, and combinations is shown here.

TABLE 31-2  **RT Doses**

| RT Modality | Recommended Target | Dose |
|---|---|---|
| **EBRT** | | |
| Preoperative | Phase 1: GTV plus 4cm margin for CTV | 50Gy/25/5w |
| | Phase 2: Original GTV plus 2-cm margin for CTV | 16Gy/8/1.5w if needed |
| Postoperative | Phase 1: Entire surgical field including scars and drain sites plus 4-cm margin for CTV | 50Gy/25/5w |
| | Phase 2: Original GTV and surgical scar plus 1-cm margin for CTV | 16Gy/8/1.5w |

*(continues)*

TABLE 31-2 **RT Doses** (continued)

| RT Modality | Recommended Target | Dose |
|---|---|---|
| BRT | "Surgical bed" plus 2cm | |
| LDR monotherapy | | 45–50Gy/4–6d/ ~0.45Gy/h |
| LDR with EBRT | | 15–25Gy/2–3d/ ~0.45 Gy/h |
| HDR fractionated | | 32–50Gy/4–7d/2xd, q6h |
| Fractionated HDR with EBRT | | 12–18Gy/3d/2xd, q6h |

**FIGURE 31-3A** Anterior DRR showing volume and fields for preoperative radiotherapy.

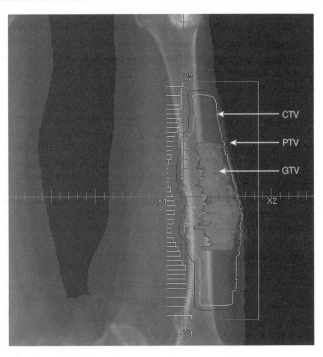

**(See Color Plate 12).** GTV—gross tumor volume, CTV—clinical target voume, PTV—planning target volume.

**FIGURE 31-3B** DRR showing postoperative field and volume outlined.

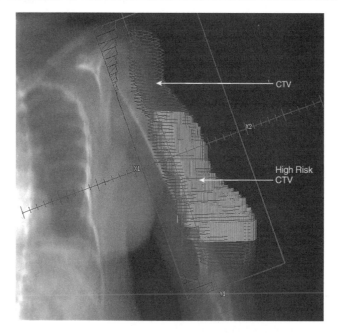

**(See Color Plate 13).** "High risk" CTV—clinical target volume in this situation includes the preoperative GTV and volume considered to be most at risk of recurrence; CTV—clinical target volume which will include the entire surgical bed and scars.

## EXTERNAL BEAM RT TARGET VOLUME

The "risk zone" around the tumor will need to be included with an appropriate margin. This may include drain sites and areas potentially contaminated by tumor through surgery. In the preoperative setting the gross tumor volume (GTV) is typically represented by the radiologically apparent tumor, but the definition of the acceptable volume margin is problematic. This margin may include soft tissues at some distance from the main tumor mass.[21,22] MRI has documented high T2-weighted signal changes surrounding soft tissue sarcomas, the so called "peritumoral edema" which may contain both edema and tumor cells. Our policy has been to use a 4-cm longitudinal CTV margin (approximating a 5-cm field margin after the PTV and penumbra are considered) beyond any imaging abnormalities, including "peritumoral edema," or areas of surgical disruption irrespective of grade or size of the tumor. Typical fields for the pre- and postoperative approaches are shown in Figures 31-3A and 31-3B.

## RT DOSE

The dose typically delivered in postoperative settings employs 60 and 66 Gy for low- and high-grade tumors respectively, often with a reduced field after 50 Gy (1.8–2 Gy per fraction). The preoperative approach may be advantageous where doses near critical structures may often be limited to 45–50 Gy to reduce risk of toxicity. The dose and scheduling of EBRT was tested in a randomized study of preoperative vs. postoperative radiotherapy.

---

**BOX 31-5**

Preoperative and postoperative external beam were tested in this Canadian randomized trial. Wound complications were twice as common with preoperative RT as with postoperative RT (35% vs. 17%), although the increased risk was almost entirely confined to patients with sarcomas of the lower extremity. With 3.3 years median follow-up, the initial report of the Canadian trial showed identical local control (in excess of 90%) between the two arms of the trial.

Preoperative versus postoperative radiotherapy in soft-tissue sarcoma of the limbs: a randomised trial. *Lancet* 2002;359:2235–2241.

---

Altered fractionation schemes using small dose per fraction (with or without chemotherapy) have been employed but gain in therapeutic ratio remains to be proven and they have not yet been widely adopted. In unresected gross disease, higher doses such as 70 Gy are needed and the therapeutic ratio may be enhanced by the addition of systemic treatments.

## LATE EFFECTS

Late radiation-induced fractures appear to be more problematic for patients treated with doses in excess of 60 Gy. Such patients have a 10% risk of fracture compared to 2% for patients treated with 50 Gy.[23] Female gender confers a higher risk of fracture, as does the addition of chemotherapy.[24,25] In addition, late fibrosis appears to be worse in those treated with higher doses to large volumes, particularly for patients treated with postoperative RT.[26]

## BRACHYTHERAPY TARGET VOLUME

The American Brachytherapy Society recommends at least 2–5-cm longitudinal margin beyond the CTV and at least 1 cm beyond the lateral edge of the CTV20.

This is based on expert panel agreement rather than robust evidence. The CTV, in general, is represented by the volume of tissue considered at risk for microscopic extension of tumor and includes the tumor bed visualized on imaging studies and under direct inspection intraoperatively.[20] The BRT protocol at MSKCC uses margins of 2 cm around the surgical bed.[27]

## BRACHYTHERAPY DOSE

The optimal adjuvant doses for postoperative brachytherapy remains undetermined.[20] In general, the dose delivered is related to the dose rate and also whether EBRT is used. The prescription point is usually at an isodose line 5–10 mm from the plane of the implant. Doses of 45–50 Gy at 0.45 Gy/h are acceptable with the skin dose not exceeding 20–25 Gy. Where LDR brachytherapy is used with external beam (45–50 Gy), doses of 15 Gy to 25 Gy are generally administered over 2 to 3 days. As a relatively new technique with limited clinical experience, fractionated HDR poses problems such as the radiobiologic issues governing serious late toxicity. When catheters are in contact with neurovascular structures, the dose per fraction should probably be reduced. Generally doses of approximately 36 Gy in 10 fractions using a 6-hour interfraction interval have been suggested, though some have used higher doses.

One novel approach for the treatment of retroperitoneal sarcoma is that of intra-operative HDR using doses of 10–15 Gy as single treatment prescribed at 5 mm to supplement EBRT doses of 45–50 Gy, depending on surgical margins.[28] The large single doses required make this a problematic approach in the vicinity of the vulnerable anatomy of the retroperitoneum.

**FIGURE 31-4**  American Brachytherapy Society guidelines on the placement of catheters.

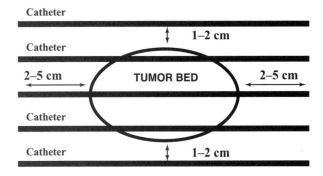

...–2 cm beyond the lateral edge of the clinical target volume (CTV) and 2–5 cm beyond the CTV in the longitudinal direction.

...ubir Nag et al, The American Brachytherapy Society recommendations for brachytherapy of soft tissue sarcomas, 11, Copyright (2001). ...*nternational Journal of Radiation Oncology/Biology/Physics, Vol. 49*, with permission from Elsevier.

## Adjuvant Chemotherapy in STS

Unlike pediatric sarcomas and certain types of chemo-sensitive sarcomas, adjuvant chemotherapy ...as not been routinely used in adult STS due to lack of proven benefit. This issue was addressed in ... large meta-analysis of randomized studies using doxorubicin-based treatment.

**BOX 31-6**

The role of doxorubicin-based adjuvant chemotherapy in STS was addressed in a landmark meta-analysis. Data from 1,568 patients in 14 randomized trials were combined, only three had a relatively large sample size. Although no difference in overall survival (p = 0.12) was seen, metastasis-free interval and overall recurrence-free survival was significantly in favor of chemotherapy. These trials included a broad spectrum of patients with various metastatic risk and thus the power of the studies to detect an effect may have been diluted.

Adjuvant chemotherapy for localized resectable soft-tissue sarcoma of adults: meta-analysis of individual data. *Lancet* 1997; 350:1647–1654.

Many low-grade patients were included in the meta-analysis and thus were at low risk of metasta-...ic disease, and this may be one reason no significant benefit was shown for adjuvant chemotherapy. ...t has been suggested that chemotherapy may benefit particular STS subtypes such as myxoid/round ...ell liposarcoma or high-grade extremity soft tissue sarcomas >10 cm, but studies designed to ...ddress this issue in patients with high-grade disease have failed to show significant benefit.[29,30]

Although adjuvant chemotherapy does not have a clear role in the management of adult STS, ...here may be an effect of chemotherapy on local control in addition to other local treatment.

Overall, adjuvant chemotherapy may have little benefit and should be delivered within the ...ontext of clinical trials. However, it may be reasonable to use in high-risk patients such as

---

**BOX 31-7**

Adjuvant chemotherapy improved local control in high-risk groups of STS, where local control has traditionally not been as satisfactory, such as head, neck, and trunk tumors. The outcome of adjuvant CYVADIC chemotherapy was compared to control in 468 patients. There was improved relapse-free survival (56% versus 43%; p = 0.007) and reduction in local recurrence (17% versus 31%; p = 0.01) but similar overall survival rates (63% versus 56%; p = 0.64).

Adjuvant CYVADIC chemotherapy for adult soft tissue sarcoma—reduced local recurrence but no improvement in survival: a study of the European Organization for Research and Treatment of Cancer Soft Tissue and Bone Sarcoma Group. *J Clin Oncol* 1994;12: 1137–1149.

---

the following: (1) those presenting with large, high-grade deep lesions, (2) younger patients with relatively chemotherapy-sensitive subtypes such as myxoid/round cell liposarcoma and synovial sarcoma, (3) patients presenting with lymph node involvement, (4) head and neck or torso sarcoma where adequate surgery and radiotherapy delivery may be compromised.

## RECURRENT AND METASTATIC DISEASE

A summary of the management of the STS patient with locally recurrent and/or metastatic disease is presented in Figures 31-5 and 31-6.

## LYMPH NODE METASTASIS

The presence of lymph node metastasis is a grave prognostic factor with outcome similar to other Stage IV disease. However, in a series of selected patients with isolated lymph node metastases who underwent radical therapy 4- and 5-year survival ranged from 24%–71%. Elective treatment of nodal region in the primary setting is unusual apart from certain high-risk histological subtypes. Radiotherapy may be added for patients where there is risk of recurrence within the surgically dissected tissues because of extracapsular nodal spread (especially when the resection margins are narrow) or when nodes are very large and/or multiple. The target volume usually includes the next nodal echelon.

## LOCALLY RECURRENT DISEASE

Salvage treatment must be individualized because some patients may enjoy long disease-free outcomes in the face of locoregional and/or pulmonary metastatic disease. Patients previously treated with surgery alone may be treated with a combined multimodality approach. Chemotherapy may be employed more often than in primary disease, and radiotherapy can be used in a similar manner as in primary disease. For patients previously irradiated, management includes wide local excision where feasible, together with brachytherapy. In cases where external beam radiotherapy is contemplated, the preoperative route is probably preferred to the postoperative route because smaller volumes and doses are required. The possibility of radiation-induced disease should also be considered as an alternate diagnosis to local recurrence.

Where local recurrence occurs with metastases, aggressive surgery is usually not indicated and local excision may delay or prevent local complications. In some situations, where there is limited systemic disease and a long disease-free interval, aggressive local management may be indicated in addition to metastasectomy.

## METASTATIC DISEASE

Metastasectomy is unlikely to be curative except in pulmonary disease. For first-time pulmonary metastasectomy, five-year survival rates range from 15%–35% and from 12%–52% for subsequent

**FIGURE 31-5** Management of locally recurrent disease.

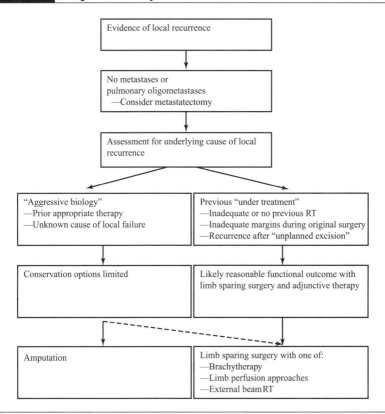

ulmonary resections.[31] The most adverse features for outcome of pulmonary metastasectomy were: 1) incomplete resection, (2) tumor doubling time exceeding 40 days, (3) more than 4 metastatic esions, and (4) disease-free interval shorter than 12 months. A retrospective study from the EORTC howed 5-year disease-free and overall survival figures of 35% and 38%.[32] The International Registry f Lung Metastases reported 2,173 bone or soft tissue sarcoma patients with pulmonary metastases esection; patients with single metastasis and long disease-free intervals had better outcomes.[33]

## PALLIATIVE TREATMENT

A multimodality approach may still be required for palliative management. Symptomatic one metastases may be treated with radiotherapy, but its use in large mass lesions may be limited, especially in the vicinity of radiosensitive structures due to dose/volume constraints. Surgery is used to relieve obstruction or for mechanical problems such as fracture. Occasionally, amputation may improve pain and ambulation in extremity tumors and debulking of relatively indolent disease may improve symptoms for a significant period of time.

**FIGURE 31-6** Management of metastatic disease.

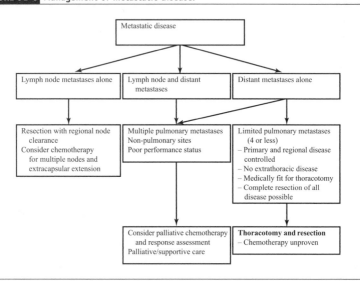

The role of chemotherapy for palliation has been well described.[5] Good performance status, young age, and absence of liver metastases had a favorable influence on both survival time and response rate following chemotherapy. Although combination chemotherapy is popular due to higher response rates, median survival with single agent doxorubicin appears to be similar.[34] Even though low-grade lesions tend to respond less well, survival is still longer; this is also true for those who have a long disease-free interval. Patients with malignant fibrous histiocytoma, which is relatively chemo-resistant, fare less well than those with liposarcoma and synovial sarcoma.

## SPECIFIC SITES

### Retroperitoneal Sarcomas (RPS)

These represent 10%–15% of all STS.[35] Liposarcoma (30%–60%) and leiomyosarcoma (20%–30%) are the most common, although all sarcoma subtypes may appear. In many cases, tumors sizes are large (>10cm) due to late onset of symptomatology. The management of a suspected RPS is summarized in Figure 31-7.

Although radiotherapy is often used as an adjuvant treatment, evidence of significant benefit remains lacking and this also applies to chemotherapy (with the exception of certain histological subtypes such as soft tissue Ewing's sarcoma and adult rhabdomyosarcoma). The treatment of RPS is often challenging and requires en-bloc excision of the tumor with involved viscera and margin of uninvolved tissue. Although complete resection rates have risen to 80%–90% in more recent reports, at best, 5-year local control rates and overall survival are 40%–60% and 50%–60%, respectively. Local relapse may continue to 10 years with mortality often related to local rather than systemic disease.

Adjuvant radiotherapy may delay rather than prevent local recurrence, and delivery of sufficient tumoricidal doses may be compromised by adjacent radiosensitive structures.[36] Thus its use remains

**FIGURE 31-7** Management of retroperitoneal sarcoma.

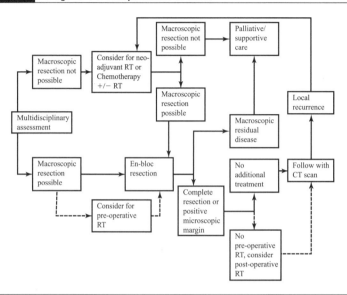

controversial. Pre-operative radiotherapy has the advantages of a well defined and undisturbed tumor acting as a tissue-expander to displace radiosensitive structures from the radiation field. Pre-operative external beam radiotherapy is well tolerated with minimal acute and late toxicity and no increase in wound healing complications.[37] This option was the subject of an American College of Surgeons Oncology Group randomized trial that, unfortunately, closed prematurely due to lack of accrual. Three-dimensional conformal radiotherapy and IMRT are particularly well suited for preoperative radiotherapy of RPS. Usually, a CTV margin of 1.5–2.0 cm around the GTV is used depending on proximity to vital radiosensitive viscera. A dose of 45–50.4 Gy in 1.8–2 Gy fractions may be given to large CTV volumes with acceptable acute and late toxicity. Intra-operative radiotherapy (IORT), with or without external beam therapy, is another alternative. Nonrandomized data has shown improved rates of local control (83%) and survival (74%).[38,39] Similarly, HDR brachytherapy with or without external beam therapy for RPS has been reported to show a 5-year actuarial local control rate of 62%. Both of these techniques have complications including bowel obstruction (18%), fistula (9%), neuropathy (6%), hydronephrosis (3%), and wound complication (3%).[28]

## Primary Gastrointestinal STS

These are uncommon and comprise approximately 0.1%–3% of all gastrointestinal neoplasms.[40] The 5-year disease specific survival of 239 patients with gastrointestinal stromal tumors (GIST) and 322 with leiomyosarcoma (LMS) was 28% and 29%, respectively. Favorable factors for overall DSS with LMS and GIST were primary presentation, tumor size <5 cm, and complete excision. Local recurrence was a component of initial recurrence in 36% of GIST and 40% of LMS; distant failure was different as pulmonary metastases were more common in leiomyosarcoma and hepatic metastases in GIST.

The role of adjunctive RT for GI sarcomas is relatively limited due to the predilection for peritoneal seeding and hematogenous metastases, but it may be considered where tumor is infiltrating pelvic or retroperitoneal wall structures and undergoes marginal resection. GIST is a distinct entity where imatinib mesylate in patients with unresectable, metastatic, or recurrent GIST has resulted in almost 90% of patients experiencing partial response or stable disease and has modest toxicity.[41] It is unknown if treatment can be curative and responding patients normally require complete resection of residual disease. Ongoing studies will elucidate the role of imatinib in the adjuvant setting.

## Head and Neck STS

These comprise about 10% of STS and in common with other sarcomas, similar issues pertain to their management. Aggressive sarcomas, such as angiosarcoma of the scalp and facial regions, and parameningeal rhabdomyosarcoma are more commonly seen in the head and neck. The overall approach to the management of head and neck soft tissue sarcoma is similar to STS elsewhere; however, clear surgical margins may be inherently more difficult due to the anatomical constraints of this region. Improvement in local control is seen with adjuvant radiotherapy, elevating the local control rate from 52% with surgery alone to 90%.[42] Data from the Princess Margaret Hospital showed that patients with clear margins treated without adjuvant RT had a control rate of 74% compared to 70% in positive-margin patients who received adjuvant radiotherapy.[12] Outcome remains linked to tumor grade and the ability to obtain a satisfactory resection, rather than tumor size because it is usual for these patients to present early due to their location. Overall, local control and survival is relatively poor (60%–70%). Although chemotherapy has thus far not improved rates of distant metastases, its role may lie in improvement in local control.

## REFERENCES

1. Jemal A, Tiwari RC, Murray T, et al. Cancer statistics, 2004. *CA Cancer J Clin* 2004;54:8–29.
2. Fletcher CDM, Unni K, Mertens K, editors. *World Health Organization Classification of Tumors: Pathology and Genetics of Tumours of Soft Tissue and Bone.* Lyon, France: IARC Press (International Agency for Research on Cancer); 2002.
3. Guillou L, Coindre JM, Bonichon F, et al. Comparative study of the National Cancer Institute and French Federation of Cancer Centers Sarcoma Group grading systems in a population of 410 adult patients with soft tissue sarcoma. *J Clin Oncol* 1997;15:350–362.
4. O'Sullivan B, Chung P, Euler C, et al. Soft Tissue Sarcoma. In: Gunderson LL, Tepper JE, editors. *Clinical Radiation Oncology*, 2nd ed. Philadelphia: Churchill Livingstone; 2007. pp. 1519–1549.
5. Van Glabbeke M, van Oosterom AT, Oosterhuis JW, et al. Prognostic factors for the outcome of chemotherapy in advanced soft tissue sarcoma: an analysis of 2,185 patients treated with anthracycline-containing first-line regimens—a European Organization for Research and Treatment of Cancer Soft Tissue and Bone Sarcoma Group Study. *J Clin Oncol* 1999;17:150–157.
6. Pollock R, Karnell L, Menck H, et al. The National Cancer Data Base report on soft tissue sarcoma. *Cancer* 1996;78:2247–2257.
7. Stojadinovic A, Leung DH, Hoos A, et al. Analysis of the prognostic significance of microscopic margins in 2,084 localized primary adult soft tissue sarcomas. *Ann Surg* 2002;235:424–434.
8. Gerrand CH, Wunder JS, Kandel RA, et al. Classification of positive margins after resection of soft tissue sarcoma of the limb predicts the risk of local recurrence. *J Bone Joint Surg* [Br] 2001;83–B:1149–1155.
9. Kepka L, Suit HD, Goldberg SI, et al. Results of radiation therapy performed after unplanned surgery (without re-excision) for soft tissue sarcomas. *J Surg Oncol* 2005;92:39–45.
10. Rydholm A, Gustafson P, Rooser B, et al. Limb-sparing surgery without radiotherapy based on anatomic location of soft tissue sarcoma. *J Clin Oncol* 1991;9:1757–1765.

11. Stotter A, Fallowfield M, Mott A, et al. Role of compartmental resection for soft tissue sarcoma of the limb and limb girdle. *Br J Surg* 1990;77:88–92.

12. Le Vay J, O'Sullivan B, Catton C, et al. Outcome and prognostic factors in soft tissue sarcoma in the adult. *Int J Radiat Oncol Biol Phys* 1993;27:1091–1099.

13. Ghert MA, Abudu A, Driver N, et al. The indications for and the prognostic significance of amputation as the primary surgical procedure for localized soft tissue sarcoma of the extremity. *Ann Surg Oncol* 2005;12:10–17.

14. DeLaney TF, Spiro IJ, Suit HD, et al. Neo-adjuvant chemotherapy and radiotherapy for large extremity soft-tissue sarcomas. *Int J Radiat Oncol Biol Phys* 2003;56:1117–1127.

15. Kraybill WG, Harris J, Spiro IJ, et al. Phase II study of neo-adjuvant chemotherapy and radiation therapy in the management of high-risk, high-grade, soft tissue sarcomas of the extremities and body wall: Radiation Therapy Oncology Group Trial 9514. *J Clin Oncol* 2006;24:619–625.

16. Eilber FR, Giuliano AE, Huth JF, et al. A randomized prospective trial using postoperative adjuvant chemotherapy (adriamycin) in high-grade extremity soft tissue sarcoma. *Am J Clin Oncol* 1988;11:39–45.

17. Eggermont AM, de Wilt JH, ten Hagen TL. Current uses of isolated limb perfusion in the clinic and a model system for new strategies. *Lancet Oncol* 2003;4:429–437.

18. Cormier JN, Patel SR, Herzog CE, et al. Concurrent ifosfamide-based chemotherapy and irradiation: analysis of treatment-related toxicity in 43 patients with sarcoma. *Cancer* 2001;92:1550–1555.

19. Rhomberg W, Hassenstein EO, Gefeller D. Radiotherapy vs. radiotherapy and razoxane in the treatment of soft tissue sarcomas: final results of a randomized study. *Int J Radiat Oncol Biol Phys* 1996;36:1077–1084.

20. Nag S, Shasha D, Janjan N, et al. The American Brachytherapy Society recommendations for brachytherapy of soft tissue sarcomas. *Int J Radiat Oncol Biol Phys* 2001;49:1033–1043.

21. Simon MA, Enneking WF. The management of soft tissue sarcomas of the extremities. *J Bone Joint Surg Am* 1976;58:317–327.

22. Enneking WF, Spanier SS, Malawer MM. The effect of the anatomic setting on the results of surgical procedures for soft parts sarcoma of the thigh. *Cancer* 1981;47:1005–1022.

23. Holt GE, Griffin AM, Pintilie M, et al. Fractures following radiotherapy and limb-salvage surgery for lower extremity soft tissue sarcomas. A comparison of high-dose and low-dose radiotherapy. *J Bone Joint Surg Am* 2005;87:315–319.

24. Lin PP, Schupak KD, Boland PJ, et al. Pathologic femoral fracture after periosteal excision and radiation for the treatment of soft tissue sarcoma. *Cancer* 1998;82:2356–2365.

25. Alektiar KM, Zelefsky MJ, Brennan MF. Morbidity of adjuvant brachytherapy in soft tissue sarcoma of the extremity and superficial trunk. *Int J Radiat Oncol Biol Phys* 2000;47:1273–1279.

26. Davis AM, O'Sullivan B, Turcotte R, et al. Late radiation morbidity following randomization to preoperative versus postoperative radiotherapy in extremity soft tissue sarcoma. *Radiother Oncol* 2005;75:48–53.

27. Alektiar KM, Leung D, Zelefsky MJ, et al. Adjuvant radiation for Stage IIB soft tissue sarcoma of the extremity. *J Clin Oncol* 2002;20:1643–1650.

28. Alektiar KM, Hu K, Anderson L, et al. High-dose rate intra-operative radiation therapy (HDR-IORT) for retroperitoneal sarcomas. *Int J Radiat Oncol Biol Phys* 2000;47:157–163.

29. Frustaci S, Gherlinzoni F, De Paoli A, et al. Adjuvant chemotherapy for adult soft tissue sarcomas of the extremities and girdles: results of the Italian randomized cooperative trial. *J Clin Oncol* 2001;19:1238–1247.

30. Cormier JN, Huang X, Xing Y, et al. Cohort analysis of patients with localized, high-risk, extremity soft tissue sarcoma treated at two cancer centers: chemotherapy-associated outcomes. *J Clin Oncol* 2004;22:4567–4574.

31. Frost DB. Pulmonary metastasectomy for soft tissue sarcomas: is it justified? *J Surg Oncol* 1995;59:110–115.
32. van Geel AN, Pastorino U, Jauch KW, et al. Surgical treatment of lung metastases: the European Organization for Research and Treatment of Cancer Soft Tissue and Bone Sarcoma group study of 255 patients. *Cancer* 1996;77:675–682.
33. Friedel G, Pastorino U, Buyse M, et al. Resection of lung metastases: long-term results and prognostic analysis based on 5,206 cases—the International Registry of Lung Metastases. *Zentralbl Chir* 1999;124:96–103.
34. Bramwell VH, Anderson D, Charette ML. Doxorubicin-based chemotherapy for the palliative treatment of adult patients with locally advanced or metastatic soft tissue sarcoma. *Cochrane Database Syst Rev* 2003:CD003293.
35. Mendenhall WM, Zlotecki RA, Hochwald SN, et al. Retroperitoneal soft tissue sarcoma. *Cancer* 2005;104:669–675.
36. Catton C, O'Sullivan B, Kotwell C, et al. Outcome and prognosis in retroperitoneal soft tissue sarcoma. *Int J Rad Oncol Biol Phys* 1994;29:1005–1010.
37. Jones JJ, Catton CN, O'Sullivan B, et al. Initial results of a trial of preoperative external-beam radiation therapy and postoperative brachytherapy for retroperitoneal sarcoma. *Ann Surg Oncol* 2002;9:346–354.
38. Gieschen HL, Spiro IJ, Suit HD, et al. Long-term results of intra-operative electron beam radiotherapy for primary and recurrent retroperitoneal soft tissue sarcoma. *Int J Radiat Oncol Biol Phys* 2001;50:127–131.
39. Petersen IA, Haddock MG, Donohue JH, et al. Use of intra-operative electron beam radiotherapy in the management of retroperitoneal soft tissue sarcomas. *Int J Radiat Oncol Biol Phys* 2002;52:469–475.
40. Clary BM, DeMatteo RP, Lewis JJ, et al. Gastrointestinal stromal tumors and leiomyosarcoma of the abdomen and retroperitoneum: a clinical comparison. *Ann Surg Oncol* 2001;8:290–299.
41. Demetri GD, von Mehren M, Blanke CD, et al. Efficacy and safety of imatinib mesylate in advanced gastrointestinal stromal tumors. *N Engl J Med* 2002;347:472–480.
42. Tran LM, Mark R, Meier R, et al. Sarcomas of the head and neck. Prognostic factors and treatment strategies. *Cancer* 1992;70:169–177.

# 3²

# Pediatrics

*Torunn I. Yock, MD, MCH*

## OVERVIEW

Childhood cancer is the fourth leading cause of death in children under 20 years of age, behind accidental injuries, homicides and suicides but the second leading cause of death in children under 15 years of age.[1] In 1998 in the United States, 12,400 children were diagnosed with malignancies and 2,500 died. Childhood cancer includes a spectrum of diseases from leukemias to solid tumors and invokes a wide array of treatments from supportive observation to the combination of surgery, chemotherapy, and radiation therapy. Advances in treatments over the last four decades have dramatically improved the mortality rates from childhood cancer.[2] Now, 70% of children with solid tumors are long-term survivors.[1] Radiotherapy plays a larger role in the control of solid tumors than in leukemia, but it is still used for cranial radiation in some higher risk leukemia patients. Although radiation therapy has played a critical role in the higher rates of cure and survivorship in the pediatric population, it is not without cost. Radiotherapy has adverse effects on growth and development of normal tissues and can, therefore, cause added morbidity above and beyond what is seen in the adult population. Furthermore, children are far more susceptible to radiation-induced second malignancies than are adults[3]; therefore, great care must be taken in designing radiotherapy treatment plans to minimize late effects and to maximize cure.

Because of the broad array of childhood malignancies, this chapter will focus on the more common tumors of childhood requiring radiation therapy. They will be broken into two groups, CNS tumors and non-CNS tumors.

## CNS TUMORS

### Introduction

Brain tumors are the most common solid tumor of childhood. In 2004, more than 2,000 patients in the United States were diagnosed with brain tumors. Approximately 70% can be cured through a variety of treatment approaches including radiation, surgery and chemotherapy.[1] Surgery usually plays an important role in the management of pediatric brain tumors, either for diagnostic purposes or as part of the definitive treatment. Many children with aggressive tumors or incomplete resection of tumors will require radiotherapy and chemotherapy. Optimal management of children with brain tumors requires a multidisciplinary team including a pediatric oncologist, neurosurgeon, radiation oncologist, and neurologist. Pediatric brain tumors and their treatment can have multiple different effects on a child's cognition, behavior, hormonal function, hearing, and vision. Therefore, it may also be important that the health care provider team include rehabilitation specialists, social work specialists, neuroendocrinologists, and neuroophthalmologists as well as child psychiatrists and psychologists.

## Presentation of Pediatric CNS Tumors

Children with brain tumors may present with a variety of symptoms that typically depend on both the age of the child and the location of the tumor within the brain. Common symptoms associated with a posterior fossa tumor include headache, morning nausea and vomiting, ataxia, and diplopia. Most of these symptoms are related to the obstruction of the flow of CSF causing hydrocephalus. On physical exam, two important signs of elevated intracranial pressure from a brain tumor include nystagmus and papilledema. In an infant, symptoms might include varying degree of failure to thrive and failure to meet developmental milestones. The signs would be a bulging fontanel and increasing head size, but due to open cranial sutures, papilledema may be absent. Supratentorial tumors are more likely to present with focal abnormalities including long track signs and seizures or inability to keep up performance in school. Tumors involving the suprasellar region/optic chiasm and hypothalamus may present with visual decline, field cuts, endocrine abnormalities or headache; however, alterations in behavior or personality are often the first symptoms of any brain tumor. Lethargy, irritability, hyperactivity, and inability to concentrate can all be manifestations of a brain tumor. Many of the presenting symptoms remit when the tumor is discovered and treated.

## Workup of Pediatric CNS Tumors

When a brain tumor is suspected, and if the child is medically stable, a gadolinium-enhanced MRI of the brain is essential to delineate the tumor margins and make a full differential diagnosis. If a child is not neurologically stable, a much quicker first step is to obtain a head CT to look for gross mass lesions and hydrocephalus. Once a lesion is identified, the subsequent workup will depend on the characteristics of the lesion found. MRI is the most sensitive imaging modality for brain tumors, but a CT scan is still superior in evaluating calcification in craniopharyngiomas and germ cell tumors. A neurosurgeon should always be consulted to discuss obtaining tissue for definitive diagnosis and if possible, surgical removal of the lesion. Children with medulloblastomas, ependymomas, PNETs (primitive neuroectodermal tumors), or germ cell tumors will also need gadolinium enhanced MRI imaging of the spine to rule out cerebral spinal fluid (CSF) spread of disease. If any of these tumors are relatively high on the differential list—such as in the case of a midline posterior fossa tumor—a spine MRI is optimally obtained prior to definitive surgery. The preoperative spine MRI helps eliminate the uncertainty of questionable leptomenigeal spread if there are blood products or an inflammatory response to the surgical procedure. Additionally, tumors that occur in the suprasellar or pineal region suspicious for germ cell tumors should have serum and CSF level of AFP and beta-HCG performed.

Once a tumor is resected, a gadolinium-enhanced MRI should be obtained, optimally in the first 48 hours after resection, to evaluate the full extent of resection. This allows evaluation of residual disease without the confounding effects of enhancement from postoperative change, which is seen for weeks after 72 hours from surgery.

Once the pathology is confirmed, the workup after the diagnosis is known depends on the tumor type. Importantly, if the tumor is a medulloblastoma or primitive neuroectodermal tumor (PNET), or other potentially seeding tumor such as an ependymoma or germ cell tumor, a CSF ample should be obtained 10 to 14 days after the surgery. If obtained more proximally to the surgery, it is possible to have a false positive cytology sample due to the previous surgical intervention and the sampling procedure will need to be repeated. Because medulloblastoma can metastasize to bone and bone marrow, a complete workup includes a bone scan and bone marrow biopsy, although many physicians would agree that this is necessary in only patients with disease dissemination within the CNS because the yield is extremely low in patients with localized disease.

## Anatomy

Nearly one half of pediatric brain tumors occur in the supratentoriam and about the same number occur in the cerebellum or brainstem. Only a small percentage of tumors occur in the spinal CNS. The supratentorial brain includes the cerebral hemispheres with the frontal, temporal, parietal and occipital lobes and the diencephalon, which includes the basal ganglia, the thalamus, the hypothalamus, the optic chiasm, and the pineal region. The infratentorial brain includes the brainstem and the cerebellum.

## Pathology

In 1993, the World Health Organization (WHO) defined a new comprehensive classification of central nervous system tumors which was modified and updated in 2000. This new system helps to standardize communication among centers around the country and world. This classification system is based on the premise that each type of tumor results from the abnormal growth of a specific cell type. The WHO tumor classification and grading (I-IV) used in many of the brain tumors informs the choice of therapy and predicts prognosis. A table modified from the WHO classification system and pared down to be most appropriate for the pediatric population of brain tumors follows.[4, 5]

## Risk Factors

Brain tumors are mostly sporadic, but there are a few recognized predisposing genetic syndromes. Neurofibromatosis I (NF1) is an autosomal dominant and a relatively common genetic disorder linked to chromosome 17q. Approximately 20% of children with NF1 will develop CNS neoplasm, usually low-grade gliomas in the visual pathway or in the diencephalon, cerebral hemispheres, or in the cerebellum. These tumors are typically less aggressive than similar gliomas in the general population and may have a waxing and waning course without treatment. Typically children identified with NF1 will be screened with MRIs for the development of these low-grade tumors, as many do not follow an indolent course and require treatment.

Children with tuberosclerosis may also develop an indolent low-grade subependymal giant cell astrocytoma which is usually treated with resection alone. Young adults and children with a p53 deletion abnormality have Li-Fraumeni syndrome which predisposes them to many different tumors commonly including breast cancer, sarcomas, and brain tumors. Radiation exposure can also result in the induction of brain tumors, with gliomas and meningiomas being the most commonly induced tumors.[6, 7] Cranial radiotherapy in combination with antimetabolite chemotherapy can dramatically increase the risk of a treatment induced brain tumor.[8]

## Technique/Dose

Because so much more morbidity from the treatment is at stake, children require extra care and attention to treatment planning. In this modern era, all children should be planned with 3-D conformal radiotherapy techniques or with intensity modulation with the goal of maximally treating the tumor while maximally sparing normal tissue. It is likely that proton radiotherapy will play an ever-increasing role in treating children with curable brain tumors because of their greater ability to spare normal tissue and the higher cost of irradiating normal tissues in pediatric patients.

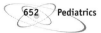

**TABLE 32-1 WHO Tumor Classification and Grading for Select Brain Tumors**

| Cell of Origin | WHO Grade |
|---|---|
| **Neuroepithelial Tissues** | |
| *Astrocytic tumors* | |
| Pilocytic Astrocytoma | I |
| Subependymal giant cell astrocytoma | I |
| Diffuse astrocytoma | II |
| (fibrillary, protoplasmic, gemistocytic) | |
| Anaplastic astrocytoma | III |
| Glioblastoma | IV |
| *Oligodendroglial tumors* | |
| Oligodendroglioma | II |
| Anaplastic oligodendroglioma | III |
| *Mixed gliomas* | |
| Oligoastrocytoma | II |
| Anaplastic oligodendroglioma | III |
| *Ependymal tumors* | |
| Myxopapillary ependymoma | I |
| Subependymoma | I |
| Ependymoma | II |
| (cellular, papillary, clear cell, tanycytic) | |
| Anaplastic ependymoma | III |
| *Choroid plexus tumors* | |
| Choroid Plexus Papilloma | I |
| Choroid Plexus Carcinoma | III |
| **Embryonal Tumors** | |
| Medulloblastoma | IV |
| (desmoplastic, large cell) | |
| Supratentorial primitive neuroectodermal tumor | IV |
| Atypical teratoid/rhabdoid tumor | IV |
| **Tumors of the Meninges** | |
| Meningioma | I |
| Atypical meningioma | II |
| Anaplastic meningioma | III |
| **Germ Cell Tumors** | |
| Germinoma | |
| Embryonal carcinoma | |
| Yolk sac tumor | |
| Choriocarcinoma | |
| Teratoma | |
| Mature | |
| Immature | |
| With malignant transformation | |
| **Tumors of the Sellar Region** | |
| Craniopharyngioma | |

Because brain tumors are usually best delineated by MRI, it is important to use the MRI in treatment planning. It is optimal, whenever possible, to anatomically register the MRI to the planning CT scan with careful review of the quality of the registration. It is ideal to use MRIs obtained expressly for this purpose. Some radiology departments will specifically protocol an MRI so that the T1 post-gadolineum, Flair, or T2 sequences can be obtained with 3 mm or better slices with no skips. This allows higher definition reformatting of the MRI to register with the CT scan and gives a better picture for target delineation. However, images of the tumor at initial presentation, at progression and preoperative and postoperative studies should be available for review and reference at the time of target delineation for radiotherapy so that the entire tumor bed at risk may be appropriately treated.

## Follow-up

Children with brain tumors need regularly scheduled visits and follow-up examinations. Generally, for the first year following treatment for an aggressive brain tumor MRI scans are required every 3 months; lower grade tumors may be followed with longer intervals. During the second year, MRI scans may be obtained every 3 to 4 months. During the third and fourth years, MRI scans may be obtained every 6 months and then yearly thereafter. An MRI should also be obtained when there is clinical suspicion of tumor progression or change in the neurological exam. Additional tests and visits to be obtained at baseline include audiological examinations if any radiation dose to the cochlea is anticipated or an ototoxic drug such as carboplatin or cisplatin will be used. Also, because radiation to the brain (specifically the pituitary and hypothalamus) and tumor near these regions has been associated with neuroendocrine abnormality, a baseline pediatric endocrine evaluation should be obtained within 3 months of diagnosis and treatment—or immediately if there are any endocrine signs or symptoms. Subsequently, semi-annual visits are likely necessary if baseline abnormalities are noted or radiation dose to the pituitary or hypothalamus is anticipated. Additionally, *all children*, regardless of whether they receive radiotherapy as part of their treatment for a brain tumor should undergo a neurocognitive evaluation by a trained psychologist. Most insurance companies will cover the expense. Many children will have baseline abnormalities as a result of the brain tumor itself.[9, 10] Individual education plans (IEPs) are devised to aid these children and their schools in getting the most out of their education.[11] Furthermore, radiotherapy can cause deficits to manifest over time that are related to the radiotherapy directly. This is more apparent in the younger patients and those who receive whole brain radiotherapy; children receiving partial brain radiotherapy have less risk of decline but are still at risk. Neurocognitive evaluations may be obtained within 3 months of radiation treatment at baseline, although optimally within 1 month of starting radiotherapy and then either yearly or every 2 years thereafter until their scores and findings stabilize. Children with tumors affecting vision or oculo-motor function should be regularly followed by an ophthalmologist because changes in this physical exam may be the first sign of tumor progression (or response to treatment).

## Morbidity

Because the majority of pediatric brain tumor patients are long-term survivors, the late effects of treatment are increasingly being recognized as a major source of morbidity and they negatively affect the survivors' quality-of-life. Major late effects of radiotherapy in brain tumor patients include neurocognitive effects, neuroendocrine effects, vascular effects, hearing effects, and second malignancies. The first two have been studied more extensively than the latter, but all are important causes of morbidity in childhood brain tumor survivors.

Neurocognitive effects have been best studied in the medulloblastoma population where whole brain radiotherapy as a part of cranial-spinal irradiation (CSI) plays a significant role in these effects. Patients under seven years of age are more greatly affected than those over seven years and the dose of CSI also plays an important role, with children under seven treated with 23.4 G losing 2.4 FSIQ points per year and those treated with 36 Gy CSI losing 3.7 points per year.[1] Dr. Merchant's team at St. Jude has done some important work modeling the effects of differen brain and cortex volumes irradiated and their effect on neurocognition. In summary, the less nor mal brain is irradiated, the better the neurocognitive outcome.[13, 14]

The endocrine effects of radiotherapy are dose related to the pituitary and the hypothalamu and direct dose to the thyroid gland and ovaries in the case of exit dose from photon CSI radiother apy. From brain radiotherapy, growth hormone, and thyroid hormone are the most likely to b reduced, with sex hormones and cortisol less commonly affected.[15, 16]

In one of the largest series from St. Jude's, second malignancies occur in 4% of all brain tumo patients by 15 years from treatment with the two most common histologies of gliomas and menin giomas, but the risk depends on age of treatment.[7] Vascular changes which may result in benig findings on MRI, or more sinister changes such as Moyamoya and stroke as a result of radiother apy, occur more often in children treated at five years of age or younger, those treated with radio therapy to the circle of Willis, and children with NF-1, but it remains a risk in all patients.[1] Ototoxicity is more of a problem in children receiving high doses of radiotherapy to the cochle (>32 Gy) and is very much exacerbated in those receiving ototoxic drugs.[18]

## Future Directions

The future of radiotherapy in the pediatric population will focus primarily on diminishin morbidity from treatment since 70% of pediatric cancer patients live to be long-term survivors The primary focus of these advances will take the form of ever-increasing conformality an decreasing the dose to non-tumor tissues. These improvements in the therapeutic profile wi capitalize on improving surgical techniques and more effective chemotherapy to either reduc dose or diminish the need for radiotherapy. However, neither of these modalities is without it toxicities as well. In radiotherapy, improved targeting through better anatomical and functiona imaging and avoidance of critical structures will play an important role in reducing morbidit from treatment.

Furthermore, proton radiotherapy will diminish the clinical side effects of radiotherapy for mor children in the future as more facilities open in the United States in the next decade. This modalit eliminates the exit dose to normal tissues and only treats normal tissues proximal to the tumo eliminating approximately 50% of unnecessary radiation to normal tissues.[19] (See Figure 32- to demonstrate dose distribution of photons compared with protons.) The long-term clinical ben efits of this approach in the pediatric population are just beginning to be reported[20] but provid the most promising form of external beam radiotherapy to date, eliminating the low-dose bat effect of multi-field 3-D conformal radiotherapy and intensity modulated radiotherapy which ma be associated with worse second malignancy rates.[21]

## Gliomas

### Anatomy

Gliomas can occur in any part of the central nervous system and are usually low grade in children Tumors occurring in the cerebellum are often completely resectable and carry an excellent progno sis. Tumors in the supratentorium can occur in the cerebral hemispheres, predominantly in th frontal and temporal lobes, or in the diencephalon. Tumors involving both thalami tend to behav more aggressively than other diencephalic tumors. Hemispheric lesions may also be resectable, bu lesions in the diencephalon are less commonly resectable without major morbidity.

**FIGURE 32-1** Photons/proton Bragg.

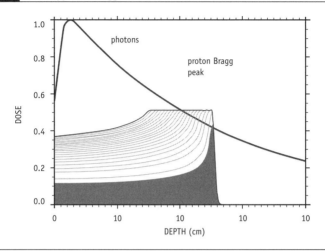

## Pathology/Biology

Most pediatric astrocytomas are low grade and either juvenile pilocytic astrocytoma (JPA, WHO grade I) or low-grade (WHO grade II) tumors. JPAs tend to behave more indolently and retain their original histology better than other low-grade tumors in the setting of recurrent disease. However, pilomyxoid astrocytomas are a more aggressive subset of JPAs and may require a more aggressive approach to treatment. Uncommonly, low-grade gliomas may present as widely infiltrating tumors involving two or more lobes of the brain that typically do not enhance on MRI and do not cause much mass effect. This entity is called gliomatosis cerebri and surgery is limited to biopsy. It responds well to radiation but can recur in less than 2 years.

High-grade gliomas (anaplastic hisologies and glioblastoma multiforme, GBM) are less common than low-grade gliomas but can occur in any part of the CNS. Children are more likely to have anaplastic lesions as apposed to GBMs and typically live longer than their adult counterparts. Lesions on MRI typically enhance and are associated with significant edema and mass effect. In contrast, the diffusely infiltrating pontine glioma may not enhance. These lesions are treated as high-grade gliomas, but studies involving biopsy have not always shown high-grade histologies. Median survival of these tumors is approximately 1 year despite multiple drug and radiotherapy trials attempting to improve it.

## Staging

There is no widely accepted staging for gliomas, but important prognostic factors include histology, grade, and extent of resection.

## Management

### Low-grade gliomas

The location of the low-grade glioma generally determines the treatment. Tumors arising in the hemispheres can often be resected unless they involve the speech cortex, the motor strip, or the dominant medial temporal lobe or other areas that make the resection too morbid. In the event of a gross total resection of a low-grade glioma, no further therapy is necessary, but regular surveillance scans are indicated. A sub-total resection may also be watched carefully with close interval MRI surveillance because many tumors are indolent for years. This approach allows for further brain development prior to the initiation of radiotherapy which may have negative consequences on further development of that part of the brain and future neurocognitive effects. Postoperative radiation therapy after a sub-total resection improves progression-free survival, but not overall survival (Pollack, 1995, NJT's book pg 80, ref 24, 14 and 61). Indications for radiation therapy include: 1) progression after resection in an area not amenable to safe second resection, 2) symptomatic disease that may be reversed by radiotherapy such as vision deficits or long-track signs in a thalamic tumor, or 3) progression by clinical manifestations or by imaging findings.

Chemotherapy can also delay the use of definitive radiation therapy and is preferentially used in the younger patients over radiation therapy. The standard first line regimen is vincristine/carboplatin or carboplatin as a single agent. Chemotherapy is rarely definitive and puts off the eventual use of definitive radiotherapy, which may be very useful in young children. Other regimens have been used with some success as well, with temazolamide as a single agent with good efficacy. However, when children progress on chemotherapy and different regimens are tried, there is a danger of permanent neurologic sequelae from the tumor in the efforts to put off the possible sequelae of radiotherapy and a balance must be struck based on the patient's neurologic status.

---

**BOX 32-1**

This study was one of the first to demonstrate that chemotherapy with carboplatin and vincristine was effective, especially in children under five years old, in controlling newly diagnosed low-grade gliomas. There were 78 children with a mean age of three years (3 months to 16 years) who were treated with carboplatin/vincristine. Median follow-up was 30 months. Fifty-six percent showed an objective response to treatment and 2- and 3-year PFS was 75% and 68%. Histologic subtype, location, maximum response, and NF-1 status did not effect PFS. However, 3 year PFS rates were better in patients $<5$ years (74% versus 39%, p $<$ 0.01).

Packer RJ et al. Carboplatin and vincristine chemotherapy for children with newly diagnosed progressive low-grade gliomas. *Journal of Neurosurgery.* 1997 May; 86(5)747–754.

---

### High-grade Gliomas

High-grade gliomas should involve a maximally safe resection and postoperative radiation therapy. Patients with anaplastic gliomas or GBMs and a gross total or near total ($>$90% resection) enjoyed 5-year PFS 44% and 26% compared with those patients with lesser resections 22% and 4%.[22] Many large academic centers treating pediatric patients are also using concurrent temozolamide with the radiotherapy or enroll the child in a pediatric cooperative group study which uses concurrent chemotherapy. The latter is the best way to evaluate the optimal role and choice of chemotherapy regimen in the pediatric population.

## Technique/Dose

Because both low- and high-grade gliomas are best delineated by MRI, it is important to use MRI in treatment planning and optimally with the most helpful images co-registered to the treatment planning CT scan.

Low-grade gliomas are usually confined to the area of abnormality seen on MRI. Therefore, using both the MRI (T1 gadolineum, Flair, or T2 sequences) and a contrast enhanced planning CT scan, the gross tumor volume should be drawn on the CT scan and a margin of 0.5 cm to 1 centimeter for clinical target volume (CTV) added with anatomically constrained barriers such as tentorium or bone. A planning target volume appropriate to the level of setup uncertainty should be added and this should not be anatomically constrained. A dose of 50.4-54 Gray at 1.8 Gy/fx is typically used for patients over three years of age and 45 -50.4 Gy for patients under three years of age. If a child has already suffered damage to a radiologically sensitive structure such as the optic chiasm or nerves, it is safer to err on the side of a lower dose in these individuals—for example 50.4 or 52.2 Gy in a patient with an optic glioma and visual deficits already.

High-grade gliomas are more infiltrative than low-grade gliomas and larger target volumes are necessary. The current COG protocol, ACNS0423 uses concurrent temozolomide with radiotherapy and adjuvant temozolomide and lomustine calls for the clinical target volume (CTV-1) to be the preoperative enhancing mass on T1 post-gadolinium MRIs plus a 2-cm margin. The current protocol calls for 54 Gy at 1.8 Gy/fx if there is a gross total resection. If there is residual disease, the boost volume (CTV-2) is the postoperative enhancing portion on gadolinium-enhanced MRI for an additional 5.4 Gy at 1.8 Gy/fx. Because studies of GBM tumors in adults have shown the area of edema seen on scans also contain tumor,[23] it is also reasonable to use the T2 or Flair abnormality on MRI to inform the margins on the enhancing portion of the tumor, rather than using a strict geometric expansion. With either approach, it is important to take into account the displaced brain that falls into the resection cavity so that more tissue is not treated than necessary.

## Follow-up

As indicated previously in the section on general follow-up of brain tumors, appropriate endocrine, neuropsychology, and other clinical referrals should be made. In addition, MRI scans should be obtained every 3 to 4 months during the first 2 years, stretching out the interval from there to annually at 5 years. Importantly, nearly half of the tumors can undergo a transient change of increased size of the lesion, increased signal intensity or enhancement, cysts or cavitations, and an increase in edema or mass effect on follow-up MRI. Most of these changes occur between 9 and 12 months after the start of conformal therapy and resolve or decrease by 15 to 21 months. Most will retain normal neurologic examinations, but a course of steroids may be needed. These changes are most often treatment-related and not a sign of progression. The transient nature of these changes, the timing and the usual lack of clinical symptoms support the diagnosis of treatment effect.[24]

## MEDULLOBLASTOMAS/PNETs/ATRT

### Staging

Medulloblastoma is broken down into two risk stratifications—standard-risk and high-risk. Standard risk patients have clinically localized disease to the posterior fossa at presentation and have had a near total or gross total resection of the primary. High-risk patients have either disease dissemination at presentation or local residual disease measuring greater than 1.5 cm in area. Of the modified Chang staging system, it is predominantly the M-stage that is used to characterize dissemination. T stage has not been shown to be as useful a prognostic factor in the modern treatment era. For supratentorial PNETs (SPNETs) and atypical teratoid rhalodoid tumors (ATRTs), both embryonal tumors as well, there is no formal staging but the same M stage is used to characterize the pattern of spread in these entities. ATRTs and SPNETs are rare and do not fare as well as medulloblastoma patients and therefore there is no risk stratification system.

### Biology (NCPO)

Medulloblastoma is the most common malignant pediatric brain tumor, accounting for 15%–20% of all pediatric brain tumors, with a median age of presentation of 6 to 7 years. It arises in the

**TABLE 32-2  Chang Staging for Medulloblastoma**

| T Stage | Description | M Stage | Description |
|---------|-------------|---------|-------------|
| T1 | Tumor <3 cm in diameter | M0 | No evidence of gross subarachnoid or hematogenous metastasis |
| T2 | Tumor ≤3 cm in diameter | M1 | Microscopic tumors cells found in CSF |
| T3a | Tumor >3 cm and with extension into aqueduct of Sylvius or foramen of Luschka | M2 | Gross nodular seeding intracranially beyond the primary site (in cerebellar/cerebral subarachnoid space or in third or lateral ventricle) |
| T3b | Tumor >3 cm and with unequivocal extension into brainstem | M3 | Gross nodular seeding in spinal subarachnoid space |
| T4 | Tumor >3 cm with extension past Aqueduct of Sylvius or down past foramen magnum | M4 | Metastasis outside cerebrospinal axis |

posterior fossa and has a tendency to spread in the CNS. ATRTs are rare tumors found most commonly in the posterior fossa and in young children.[25] Supratentorial PNETs occur either in the hemispheres, the diencephalon, or the pineal region which are called pinealblastomas. Pinealblastomas have a more favorable prognosis than SPNETs in other locations.[26]

## Management

Treatment for children older than three years with medulloblastoma requires aggressive cisplatin-based chemotherapy and radiation therapy to the entire craniospinal axis, as well as a radiotherapy boost to the posterior fossa or tumor bed. Cure rates with conventional radiotherapy and chemotherapy for patients who have standard-risk disease exceeds 80%, but for those with high-risk disease it is less.[13–15]

Currently, standard-risk children are treated with 23.4 Gy to the cranial-spinal axis (CSA), and the posterior fossa is boosted to 54 Gy. High-risk children are treated with 36 Gy to the CSA, followed by a boost to 54 Gy to the posterior fossa. Studies show that children treated with lower whole-brain doses have less neurocognitive effects.[12, 27] For this reason the current standard-risk COG protocol (ACNS 0331) randomizes patients under eight years to 18 Gy CSI with slightly increased intensity chemotherapy or 23.4 Gy CSI, which is now considered standard.

When the posterior fossa radiation boost of lateral fields is delivered with conventional photon techniques, the cochlea, temporal lobes, and other parts of the brain receive higher doses of incidental radiation because of the photon entrance and exit dose. Cisplatin chemotherapy can cause significant hearing loss, an effect compounded by radiation therapy.[28] The combined effect of radiation and cisplatin on the cochlea exacerbates the neurocognitive effects of radiation by inhibiting a child's ability to learn through hearing. Therefore, techniques to spare the cochlea from radiation using IMRT or conventional 3-D planning have been developed.[28–30] Additionally, the current phase III standard risk medulloblastoma COG study (ACNS 0331) randomizes all pediatric patients to whole posterior fossa[31, 32] or involved field (IF). Phase II studies have indicated that IF offers no increased risk of tumor relapse in the posterior fossa and can better spare the cochlea.[33] However, the resulting scatter dose to the other parts of the brain or body is higher and may have a negative effect on cognition or increased risk of second malignancy.[21, 34] Both improved cochlear sparing and no scatter dose to surrounding normal brain is achieved with proton radiotherapy which should ultimately help to diminish the neurocognitive and neuroendocrine effects. When more proton facilities are open with the capability of treating pediatric patients, a referral should be considered.

Treatment for ATRT and SPNET is less standardized. Many of the children with ATRT are under three years of age and CSI is devastating in this age group and usually avoided. However, prognosis appears to be improved for the older group getting CSI as well as tumor resection and anthracycline based chemotherapy.[25] Children with SPENTs are treated more like high-risk medulloblastoma patients if they are over three years of age with 36 Gy CSI and intensive chemotherapy[36] with a boost to the residual disease or tumor bed to 54-59.4 Gy.

# EPENDYMOMAS

Approximately 200 children per year in the United States are diagnosed with ependymomas, accounting for 8%–10% of pediatric CNS tumors. The mean age at diagnosis is between 4 and 6 years, but a significant number occur in children under three years of age.[37] A majority of these occur in the posterior fossa and both radiation and surgery play an important role in control of the disease. The lesions in the posterior fossa are often more difficult to achieve a full resection due to intimate involvement of the lower cranial nerves. The histology is divided into ependymoma and anaplastic ependymoma which is correlated with disease control in many studies.

## Management

Because a gross total resection (GTR) confers significantly better prognosis, attempts at a GTR should be made unless too much morbidity is expected. Rates of 5-year progression-free survival (PFS) and overall survival (OS), for those with a GTR or an STR (sub-total resection) include approximately 50-75% and 65-80% versus 25-50% and 0-30%. Anaplastic tumors (WHO grade III) probably fare worse than non-anaplastic tumors but the data on histology are somewhat conflicting. Post-operative radiation therapy is considered standard practice in patients with posterior fossa tumors in children over three due to high rates of local failure if radiation therapy is omitted.[38] Grade II supratentorial ependymomas may have acceptable rates of failure without postoperative radiation therapy and some may be observed. This approach is being studied in the current COG protocol. Supratentorial anaplastic ependymomas usually behave worse than ependymomas and will require radiation therapy in the postoperative setting. Until recently, it was standard practice that children under three years of age received chemotherapy in an effort to delay radiation therapy and Duffner et al showed that radiotherapy can be delayed for 1 year with intensive chemotherapy without a decrement in overall survival.[39] Other trials with chemotherapy have not enjoyed as much success and its use may result in a decrement in ultimate disease control.[40,1] Merchant et al published the St. Jude experience treating children one year and older with highly conformal involved field radiotherapy and showed that the decrement in neurocognitive function over time was minimal to not measurable (see Text Box 32-2). The results are still preliminary but encouraging and

---

**BOX 32-2**

This study established that a limited-volume of radiation can achieve a high rate of disease control and results in early stable neurocognitive outcomes even in the very young pediatric population. There were 88 pediatric patients (median age, 2.85 years) given conformal radiotherapy in which doses of 54 Gy (patients under 18 months) to 59.4 Gy were administered to the gross tumor volume and a margin of 10 mm. An age-appropriate neurocognitive battery was administered before and serially after CRT. The median length of follow-up was 38.2 months; the 3-year progression-free survival estimate was 75%. Local failure occurred in eight patients, distant failure in eight patients,

*(continues)*

and both in four patients. The cumulative incidence of local failure as a component of failure at 3 years was 15%. On univariate analysis the following were subgroups that showed significant differences in EFS: GTR 78% versus STR 43%; Differentiated 90% versus anaplasia 44%, no pre-irradiation chemotherapy 78% versus chemotherapy 60%. On multivariate analysis, anaplasia and an STR remained poor prognositic indicators. Mean scores on all neurocognitive outcomes were stable and within normal limits, with more than half the cohort tested at or beyond 24 months. However, children under three years of age were scored significantly lower at baseline than children over three years of age at diagnosis, but went on to improve after treatment. At the most recent neurocognitive follow-up all the mean scores on all neurocognitive endpoints were within ten points of the normative mean for the appropriate age group.

Merchant, T. E, et al., Preliminary results from a phase II trial of conformal radiation therapy and evaluation of radiation-related CNS effects for pediatric patients with localized ependymoma, *J. Clin Onc.,* August 1 2004, 22:3156–3162.

have formed the foundation for the current open COG phase I protocol looking at immediate postoperative radiation in children as young as one year of age and 3 months of chemotherapy with a second look surgery in those patients with an initial sub-total resection.

## Technique/Dose

All pediatric patients must be planned with 3-D conformal photon/proton or IMRT techniques and a contrast-enhanced CT scan when safely feasible. Anatomic registration of the MRIs (preoperative and postoperative) also enables more precise volume definition. At minimum, reference to the MRIs and operative report during treatment planning are critical. Although the current COG protocol prescribes doses to 59.4 Gy at 1.8 Gy/fx for children over 18 months, the standard dose off protocol is generally between 54 and 55.8. The dose in the COG protocol has been escalated due to St Jude's experience with it and local failure is a component in approximately 80% of failures. In very young patients who have been heavily treated with chemotherapy and extirpative surgery, doses as low as 50.4 Gy have been used.

The target volume has evolved smaller over the years from CSI to posterior fossa irradiation to conformal involved field radiotherapy for both ependymoma and anaplastic ependymoma. Larger fields do not offer better disease-free survival advantage.[42, 43] The gross tumor volume (GTV) includes the original tumor bed and resection cavity. Tumor that pushed normal brain aside which has collapsed back into a more normal anatomic position is not considered part of the GTV. The clinical target volume is anatomically defined and includes a 1-centimeter margin around the GTV. The PTV is not anatomically assigned and is a geometric expansion of 2-5 mm depending on the setup certainty in your institution. Care should be taken to contour and minimize dose to critical structures such as brainstem, cochlea, chiasm, pituitary, and hypothalamus.

## CRANIOPHARYNGIOMAS

### Biology

Craniopharyngiomas are benign tumors of epithelial origin arising from the remnants of Rathke's pouch in the suprasellar region. Craniopharyngiomas account for approximately 5%–9% of pediatric brain tumors in the United States. They usually present by causing visual field deficits and symptoms of raised intracranial pressure, as well as hormonal deficits. The majority of craniopharyngiomas extend retrochiasmally and become more difficult to resect with a higher risk of hypothalamic injury.

## Management

Surgical resection was the mainstay of treatment for many years, but a change in treatment patterns is occurring since the recognition that radical surgery for these lesions can be more morbid than conservative surgery followed by radiotherapy. Craniopharyngiomas have clearly defined margins and a total resection is usually curative but possible in only 50%–80% of patients. Even in patients with a gross total resection, a significant proportion will recur.[44] In those with residual disease seen on MRI after surgery, a recurrence is most likely. Additionally, about 10% of patients suffer a significant visual or neurological deficit after radical surgery. The tumor is often adherent to the optic nerves or chiasm or the major vessels around the circle of Willis. Diabetes insipidus occurs in 80%–90% of patients postoperatively and morbid hypothalamic obesity develops in 50% of patients after surgery.[45] Furthermore, a significant minority of patients lose all pituitary function after the surgery. In contrast, limited surgery consisting of debulking and immediate postoperative radiation has excellent disease control, between 83% and 96% at 10 years.[45, 46] Additionally, diabetes insipidus is only rarely caused by radiotherapy for these tumors. However, there are more common late neuroendocrinologic effects from radiation that manifest with time. In the pediatric population, growth hormone secretion is often diminished over time and thyroid hormone production is the second most likely to be affected. However, sexual development and glucocorticoid production can also be affected and may require replacement as well.[47-49] In addition, late vascular events are much more rare, but have been reported as a complication of radiotherapy.[50] There is a trade-off between the immediate side effects of surgery and the delayed side effects from radiation. However, a good neuroendocrinologist can adequately correct most of the hormonal aberrations that may arise from the surgery or radiation therapy. The complication of hypothalamic obesity rarely results from radiotherapy, but is a relatively common morbidity of radical surgery and is much more difficult to manage.

Overall survival rates of 85% at 10 to 15 years are expected, but the potential for morbidity from this tumor is great, requiring neurosurgeons and radiation oncologists to work together to optimize treatment in any given patient. The role of stereotactic radiosurgery and intracystic and intralesional radionucleotides is currently being defined but is not considered the standard of care and should be reserved for recurrence after fractionated radiotherapy.

## Technique/Dose

The gross tumor volume should include any residual solid tumor and its cyst. The clinical target volume should include any surface of the brain that was in contact with the tumor or cyst prior to surgery. A sub-total resection and cyst aspiration can dramatically decrease the volume of tissue required to be treated, but care should be taken to cover any of the surfaces that could have cyst wall or tumor attached. It is important to use the preoperative and postoperative MRIs in the treatment planning as well as the operative report to best delineate the areas at risk. The total dose required is generally 54 Gy at 1.8 Gy/fraction. If there has been chiasmal damage or visual deficits at any time during the diagnosis or treatment, it is important to consider the dose distribution of the plan and decrease the dose by a fraction or block the chiasm for the last fraction, as a previously damaged optic apparatus does not have the same tolerance to radiotherapy as one that has not suffered damage.

Many of the craniopharyngiomas have active cysts. It is very important to include the entire cyst in the treatment volume. Because cysts can continue to grow throughout treatment, it is imperative that children with cysts be scanned during the course of their radiotherapy. The speed at which a cyst is growing can often be estimated by the growth that has occurred from the postoperative MRI scan to the planning CT and MRI scans. Weekly to bi-weekly non-contrast enhanced CT scan is usually sufficient to monitor cyst growth during treatment, although serial MRIs are optimal. Often, very young children who require sedation for MRIs and radiotherapy can tolerate a

CT scan without sedation if their parent or guardian can be with them. When possible, the CT should be obtained in the treatment position and with fine cuts and no skips. Then, it should be anatomically registered to the planning CT scan and evaluated for growth. Replanning is a must if the cyst or tumor is threatening to exceed the margins of the prescription dose. In those children with growing cysts, it is wiser to put a larger CTV margin around the tumor to allow for growth during the interval between rescanning and replanning.

### Follow-up

Cysts can continue to grow for approximately 1 year after treatment and this does not denote tumor failure. Surgical drainage or aspiration may be required if the cyst causes symptoms of visual compromise, headaches, or raised intracranial pressure.

## GERM CELL TUMORS

### Biology/Presentation

Intracranial germ cell tumors occur within the diencephalic structures, usually as midline third ventricular lesions in the pineal region or the suprasellar region, but they can also uncommonly arise in the basal ganglia or thalamic nuclei. Germ cell tumors represent only 1%–3% of pediatric CNS neoplasms and germinomas are somewhat more common than non-germinoma germ cell tumors (NGGCTs). NGGCTS may be embryonal carcinomas, endodermal sinus (yolk sac) tumors, choriocarcinomas, mature teratomas, immature teratomas, or a mixture of histologies. Generally, a pathological diagnosis is best because the risks of a surgical biopsy in the pineal region are now much less than what they used to be. The primary distinction is between germinomas, NGGCTs, and mature teratomas and this distinction informs treatment. If tumor markers show a marked increase of both AFP and BHCG, then a NGGCT is the default diagnosis. Germinomas may have no elevation or only a mild elevation in b-HCG (<100 IU/ml) where as choriocarcinomas tend to have dramatic increases in b-HCG (>1000 IU/ml), but synctialtrophoblastic variants of germinoma can be intermediate.

Tumors in the pineal region may present with Parinaud's syndrome (decreased upward gaze, limited constriction to light but retained papillary response to accommodation, and limited convergence). Tumors in the suprasellar region may result in neuro-endocrine abnormalities, most classically diabetes insipidus or precocious or delayed puberty. Visual symptoms may also be apparent. If a patient with a pineal mass presents with neuroendocrine abnormalities, it must be assumed the hypothalamic and pituitary axis is also involved. Germinomas much more commonly than NGGCTs present with multiple midline lesions (approximately 5%–15% of the time).

### Management

Germinomas can be treated in multiple different ways. A GTR has not been shown to add benefit to germinoma patients but certainly helps with the pathological diagnosis. The standard of care for years which has resulted in >90% OS rates at 5 to 10 years has been CSI to approximately 25 Gy followed by an involved field boost to 45-50 Gy. However, numerous studies have shown that more limited field radiotherapy in patients well staged with CSF cytology and MRI with non-disseminated disease with whole ventricular radiotherapy (WV) or whole brain (WB) radiotherapy to 25 Gy followed by an involved field boost to 45-50.4 Gy in just as effective, or very nearly so.[51, 52] A more recent trend in pediatric oncology is to treat with chemotherapy using a platinum based regimen followed by involved field radiotherapy. It is unclear if the chemotherapy and involved field approach is as effective as a larger field radiotherapy approach. However, the neurocognitive consequences of large field radiotherapy in the pediatric population are driving this study. The proposed COG protocol for germinoma randomizes patients between radiotherapy alone with WVRT followed by IF versus induction chemotherapy followed by lower dose IF radiotherapy in the complete responders. The use of chemotherapy alone has resulted in recurrence rates in excess of 50% and was therefore judged unacceptable.

With NGGCTs, all three modalities probably play an important role both in diagnosis and in treatment. Although, it is still controversial whether a gross total resection is important in patients with NGGCTs, the disappointing best OS rates of less than 50% with postoperative radiation therapy at 5 years leads clinicians to be aggressive with this disease entity. Studies on small cohorts of patients suggest 60%–80% 5-year OS[53, 54] with trimodality therapy. However, surgery in the pineal region is challenging due to the vascular plexus surrounding it and should be performed only by a neurosurgeon who has a good experience with lesions in this region—and some will simply be unresectable.

Contemporary practice utilizes all three modalities whenever possible, with a GTR up front if not too morbid. Then, either chemotherapy with a platinum-based regimen or CSI radiotherapy to 36 Gy followed by an IF boost to 50.4–54 Gy. Currently, the COG protocol gives chemotherapy after surgery and follows it by radiotherapy in those with a CR, or second look surgery if a partial response or stable disease. If tumor markers have not normalized, the protocol calls for high dose chemotherapy followed by stem cell rescue and consolidation chemotherapy and then the radiotherapy.

## NON-CNS TUMORS

### Overview

The non-CNS tumors encompass a wide variety of tumor types. These tumors may occur in any part of the body and each of the most common ones requiring radiotherapy will be discussed below under its own subheading and will include neuroblastoma, Wilms' tumor, Ewing's sarcoma, rhabdomyosarcoma, pediatric acute lymphoblastic leukemia, Hodgkin's and non-Hodgkin's lymphoma, and retinoblastoma.

### NEUROBLASTOMA

#### Introduction

Neuroblastoma is a tumor of early childhood arising from the embryonic neural crest cells of the peripheral sympathetic nervous system, in the adrenal gland and the paraspinal sympathetic ganglia. Ninety percent of cases present before age 10, with a median age at presentation of two years. With more than 650 new cases per year, neuroblastoma is the most common extracranial solid tumor of childhood. Neuroblastoma is a unique malignancy with clinical behavior varying from spontaneous regression, spontaneous maturation, or aggressive metastatic spread.

#### Pathology/Biology

Neuroblastoma is one of the many small round blue cell tumors of childhood. There are three main subtypes in increasing order of differentiation, neuroblastoma, ganglioneuroblastoma, and ganglioneuroma. Immunohistochemistry stains are typically positive for neuro-specific enolase (NSE), synaptophysin, chromogranin A, and neuronal filaments. Several clinical and biologic factors are associated with prognosis and help to stratify patients for risk-adapted therapy. Young age (<1), low stage, stage 4s, hyperdiploidy, favorable Shimada classification, and absence of *MYCN* oncogene amplification are good prognostic factors.[55] Shimada classification is based on patient age, the presence of stroma (rich or poor) and nodularity, the mitosis-karyorrhexis index, and the degree of differentiation. Loss of heterozygosity of 1p and 11q connote a worse prognosis.[56]

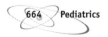

## Screening/Risk Factors

Although 90% of neuroblastomas secrete urine catecholamines (vanillyl-mandelic acid [VMA] or homovanillic acid [HVA]) in the urine which are easily quantified, screening studies have failed to show a benefit in mortality or in reduction of patients diagnosed with advanced and high-risk disease.[57, 58] There are no known proven environmental risk factors at this time. Approximately 1%–2% of patients have a family history of neuroblastoma that is inherited in an autosomal dominant pattern with incomplete penetrance.

## Presentation/WorkUp

Neuroblastomas most commonly present in the abdomen, often with an abdominal mass with fever, malaise, anorexia, weight loss, and generalized failure to thrive.[59] Other presentations depend on the site. A commonly seen presentation lesion is the dumbbell configuration where tumor extends through the neural foramina and can cause a cord compression. Metastatic disease to the bone, bone marrow, skin, or liver can be the primary cause of presenting symptoms and depends on the site of metastasis. A workup usually includes an ultrasound of the mass lesion found on physical exam (if present) and a CT and MRI scan of the primary, which helps to assess for lymph node metastasis. A classic finding for neuroblastoma is a soft tissue suprarenal mass with calcifications. Also, a chest CT, MIBG (123I-metaiodobenzyl-guanidine) scan, technetium bone scan, and bilateral bone marrow biopsies are important for assessing for distant metastatic spread.

## Management/Prognosis

For all stages of disease, children less than one year of age at diagnosis have a significantly higher overall and disease-free survival, and children have a better prognosis than adults. Patients are stratified into low, intermediate and high risk, based on prognostic variables and are assigned treatment according to risk. In general, low-risk patients are those with Stage I or II, favorable histology, favorable DNA ploidy, and lack *MYCN* amplification and these are generally managed with surgery alone. Chemotherapy is reserved for tumors that are incompletely resected or recurrent. Radiation therapy is used in the rare case of tumor recurrence following surgery and chemotherapy. Stage IVS disease with favorable histology and without *MYCN* amplification is considered low- risk disease. These patients are managed with expectant observation since there is a high rate of spontaneous regression within this group. Patients with low-risk disease have a 5-year overall survival that is greater than 95% and an event-free survival that is approximately 90%.[61] Radiation therapy in 4S disease is indicated in the setting of rapid disease

---

TABLE 32-3 **Staging: The International Neuroblastoma Staging System**

**Stage I:** Localized tumor with complete gross and microscopic excision, LN's negative (if not directly attached to the tumor).

**Stage IIA:** Localized tumor with incomplete gross excision, non-adherent LN's negative.

**Stage IIB:** Localized tumor completely or not excised with ipsilateral nonadherent LN's positive for tumor.

**Stage III:** Unresectable unilateral tumor infiltrating across the midline ($+/-$ regional LN involvement.) OR localized unilateral tumor with positive contralateral Regional LN's. OR midline tumor with bilateral extension by infiltration (unresectable) or by lymph node involvement.

**Stage IV:** Any primary tumor with spread to distant LN's, bone, bone marrow, liver, skin, etc.

**Stage IVS:** (infants <1 year of age): Localized primary tumor as defined for Stages I, IIA, or IIB, with dissemination to skin, liver, bone and/or bone marrow.

progression leading to compromise of vital organ functioning. For example, a rapidly enlarging liver causing respiratory compromise secondary to upward displacement of the diaphragm may be effectively treated with three to four fractions of 1.5 Gy/fx to quickly decrease tumor volume.[62]

Intermediate-risk disease includes children with Stage III disease who are less than one year old, children older than one with no adverse features, and infants with Stage IV disease. Intermediate-risk children have a 5-year overall survival rate greater than 90% and an event-free survival greater than 87%[63]. Treatment involves multi-drug chemotherapy to treat regional or metastatic disease followed by surgical resection of the primary tumor. Although the role of radiation therapy remains unclear, the most recent COG study of intermediate risk-disease (COG A3961) recommends radiation for progressive clinical deterioration after initial chemotherapy and surgery. Radiation therapy is also indicated for children with unfavorable histology or unfavorable biology disease who have progression after chemotherapy and surgery. Typically, 24 Gy in 1.5-1.8 Gy fractions to areas of viable gross or microscopic residual disease and involved lymph nodes after second look surgery as determined by CT, MRI and MIBG scans is delivered.

Children with high-risk disease are older than one year of age with disseminated disease or localized disease combined with unfavorable biology such as *MYCN* amplification. The prognosis for high-risk disease is considerably poorer, with 5-year overall survival of between 30%–60%.[64,65] Treatment of high-risk disease involves aggressive multimodality treatment including induction multiagent chemotherapy, surgical resection, radiation therapy, and high-dose chemotherapy with hematopoietic stem cell rescue and retinoid therapy. Radiotherapy is given to the primary tumor bed and sites of bulky disease to a total dose of 24 to 30 Gy to improve local tumor control.[66, 67]

Children presenting with cord compression can often be managed with up-front chemotherapy as the response rate is excellent and usually quick. Surgery can also play an important role to quickly decompress the spinal cord and make the diagnosis. Radiotherapy is the third viable option, but dose should be limited to 4.5-6 Gy at 1.5 Gy/fx to affect a quick response. This fractionation and regimen can also be used for peri-orbital metastasis causing visual compromise.

## WILMS' TUMOR

### Introduction/Presentation/Risk Factors

Wilms' tumor is the most common primary renal tumor in children and accounts for approximately 500 new cases diagnosed annually in the United States. A majority are under five years of age. The most common clinical presentation is a child with an asymptomatic abdominal mass. However, other relatively common presenting symptoms include fever, hematuria, abdominal pain, anemia, and hypertension from rennin secretion. Approximately 10%–25% of Wilms' tumors occur in the setting of various congenital anomalies including aniridia, hemihypertrophy, and genitourinary malformations.[68, 69]

### Pathology

Wilms' tumor can be broken into two major categories, favorable histology and unfavorable histology. Anaplasia defines the unfavorable histology and is categorized into focal and diffuse, which helps in the risk stratification for NWTS-V study. Two rare variants, rhabdoid, and clear cell are not discussed here. Genetic deletions or inactivation of WT1 (11p13) and WT2 (11p15) are associated with WAGR syndrome and Beckwith-Wiedemann syndrome.

### WorkUp

Once a Wilms' tumor is suspected based on history and physical, workup includes an abdominal ultrasound to assess if there is a renal mass and what characteristics it has, a chest X-ray, and CT of the chest, abdomen, and pelvis. If Wilms' tumor is still leading the differential, a pediatric surgeon assesses for operability. It is important to assess whether there was spillage of the tumor, either prior to or during the surgery, whether it was focal or diffuse and whether intraperitoneal seeding was noted. Also important at the time of surgery is an examination of the other kidney, an evaluation of the renal vessels for thrombus and intra-abdominal lymph nodes. From the pathologist, it is important to learn whether the histology is favorable or unfavorable, to what degree there is anaplasia, and which lymph nodes were pathologically involved.

## Staging: National Wilms' Tumor Study Group Staging

I   Tumor limited to kidney excised completely and without rupture, renal capsule intact.
II  Tumor extends beyond kidney but is completely excised, and/or vessels with tumor thrombus, local spillage confined to flank at surgery. No residual tumor.
III Residual nonhematogenous tumor confined to the abdomen (+lymph nodes, diffuse peritoneal contamination by spillage, peritoneal implants)
IV  Hematogenous metastasis (lung, liver, bone, brain)
V   Bilateral renal involvement at diagnosis

## Management

The National Wilms' Tumor Study (NWTS) and International Society of Pediatric Oncology (SIOP) have performed successive studies that evolved the treatment for Wilms' tumor over the years. Most children with Wilms' tumor (approximately 70%) do not receive radiation therapy as part of their definitive management. Patients with Stage I and II disease and favorable histology (pathologic features of Wilms' tumor without anaplastic or sarcomatous components) are generally managed with surgery and chemotherapy consisting of vincristine and actinomycin base. In the fifth National Wilms' Tumor Study (NWTS) trial, postoperative radiation in addition to three- or four-drug chemotherapy (actinomycin, vincristine, and Adriamycin; or cyclophosphamide, vincristine, Adriamycin and etoposide) is limited to children with Stage III or IV disease regardless of histology and Stage II disease with unfavorable histology. Radiation begins by postoperative day 9 because delayed radiation has been associated with increased risk of abdominal recurrence.[70, 71]

## Technique/Dose

The radiation treatment field is limited to the tumor bed, which includes the kidney and the tumor with a 1-cm margin as well as the whole vertebral body to minimize the likelihood of scoliosis. For patients with preoperative intraperitoneal rupture, diffuse peritoneal seeding, or diffuse intraoperative spillage of tumor within the abdomen, radiation therapy must encompass the entire abdomen including all peritoneal surfaces. Radiation dose is limited to the remaining kidney to 14.4 Gy and to the liver to 19.8 Gy. As the first two NWTS trials did not show an obvious dose response relationship in Wilms' Tumor, the total dose to the tumor bed is 10.8 Gy in 1.8 Gy per fraction unless there is residual disease.[71] The NWTS-5 protocol requires a 10.8 Gy boost dose to residual disease greater than 3 cm in diameter. Whole lung radiation (12 Gy) is administered to patients with chest X-ray and CT identified metastatic with areas of persistent gross disease in the lung boosted with an additional 7.5 Gy or resected. When flank irradiation and whole lung irradiation are required, they may be given together in one large field with a fractionation of 1.5 Gy/fx and an independent jaw closed on the abdomen for the last lung fraction. Figure 32-2 depicts a patient who required both flank and whole lung irradiation. The latest COG protocol investigates the omission of whole lung irradiation in the children with a rapid and complete response to chemotherapy by week six (COG AREN0533).

**FIGURE 32-2**    Anterior portals in a CT planned patient with Wilm's tumor requiring both flank and whole lung radiotherapy.

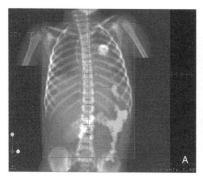 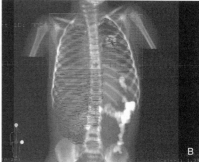

(See Color Plate 14). (A). The independent jaw was closed for the last fraction after 10.5 Gy at 1.5 Gy per fraction and was given to the larger field to bring the lung dose to 12 Gy (B).

## Morbidity

Using current treatment approaches, over 80% of children with Wilms' tumors are cured. Therefore, treatment-related late effects are of concern. The late effects from radiation may include musculoskeletal abnormalities, impaired renal function and fertility, pulmonary, and cardiac effects as well as second malignancies which are enhanced by doxorubicin.[72, 73]

## EWING'S SARCOMA

### Introduction

Ewing's sarcoma is the second most common bone tumor in childhood and represents 3% of pediatric malignancies occurring most commonly between 10 and 15 years of age, but 70% of cases present before age 20.[1, 74] Ewing's sarcoma can arise in any bone or soft tissue as extra osseous Ewing's sarcoma. The most common site of presentation is the long bones of the extremities and the bones of the pelvis. Typically, Ewing's sarcoma presents with pain and swelling with an associated soft tissue mass. There are several negative prognostic factors in Ewing's sarcoma, including the presence of metastasis, axial location, especially pelvic location, large tumor size, elevated LDH, poor histological response to induction chemotherapy at the time of surgery, and older age.[75-77] Although only 25% of Ewing's patients present with metastatic disease, most will fail with metastasis if not treated with systemic agents.

### Pathology

Ewing's tumor is another small round blue cell tumor that arises from bone. It is similar in appearance and treated the same as a PNET (peripheral primitive neuroectodermal tumor) which typically arises from soft tissue. They are believed to arise from neural crest progenitors and both have the characteristic translocation of t(11;22) about 90% of the time which is often diagnostic, although a minority may have t(21;22). PNETs and Ewing's sarcoma are similar in their marker expression, but PNET's are typically neuron-specific enolase positive and classic Ewing's is typically negative.

## WorkUp

The workup includes a complete history and physical examination focusing on the duration of symptoms, presence of pain, functional difficulties, neurologic symptomatology, and location and size of mass. After a plain film of the region which may show a bone tumor with the classical onion skin effect, a CT and MRI of the primary site are important, as are a bone scan, chest CT, bone marrow biopsy, and laboratory evaluation including an LDH and ESR. Biopsy of the primary lesion should be performed by a skilled surgeon who won't compromise the uninvolved areas, cause a hematoma, and make subsequent surgery of the lesion and the biopsy tract more extensive than it need be.

## Management

Treatment combines induction multiagent chemotherapy usually consisting of alternating cycles of vincristine, Adriamycin, cyclophosphamide (VAC), and ifosfamide/etoposide (IE) followed by local treatment (surgery, radiation, or both) at week 12 and then further chemotherapy. The choice of local treatment in Ewing's sarcoma is often made by the weighing the likelihood of achieving clear margins with a functionally and cosmetically acceptable surgery versus the side effects associated with radiation therapy including the risk of a second malignancy. Generally, when acceptable, surgery is the preferred modality due to some studies showing superior local control and the sparing of radiation associated second malignancy risk.[78,79] However, in modern series with MRI-assisted CT-based radiation planning and with ifosfamide-based chemotherapy regimens such as VAC-IE, it is not clear whether surgery alone is superior to radiotherapy.[77] Some data indicate that both modalities may be better than either modality alone.[80,81] However, these analyses of local control modality are confounded by the non-random selection of surgery and radiation therapy. Larger tumors in axial locations are more likely to be treated with radiotherapy than with surgery and these also imply a worse prognosis.

## Technique/Dose

When designing a radiotherapy plan, the pre-chemotherapy tumor volume seen on MRI and CT defines the primary tumor volume. The primary treatment volume to 45 Gy includes all bony abnormalities and soft tissue masses identified prior to chemotherapy with an anatomically restricted margin of 1.5 to 2 cm of CTV to include potential microscopic disease. The boost volume to 10.4 Gy is defined by the pre-chemotherapy *boney* tumor volume and the post-chemotherapy soft tissue volume. The total radiation dose is 55.8 Gy to gross residual disease and 50.4 Gy for microscopic disease after resection in 1.8 Gy/fraction. Radiotherapy is also used in the setting of pulmonary metastases (15-18 Gy of whole lung radiation) or other metastatic sites but dose and volume may be limited due to extent of disease.[82]

## Prognosis and Morbidity

The 5-year disease-free survival (DFS) for patients with localized Ewing's Sarcoma is 50%–75% with DFS reflecting the initial disease characteristics at diagnosis. The 5-year DFS is 20%–25% for patients with metastatic disease at diagnosis, but patients with lung-only metastasis fare better than those with multiple sites of metastasis.[83, 84] Excellent functional outcomes can be achieved with radiation therapy in most patients with appropriate treatment but depend on other normal tissues irradiated in the process.[85] It is important to use 3-D planned conformal radiation techniques to minimize complications of treatment. Post-treatment complications are related to the primary site of involvement and may include limb length discrepancy or bone fracture for extremity and pelvic primaries, wound complications for those treated pre- or postoperatively, soft tissue changes, and/or second malignancy. The risk of second malignancies is related to radiation doses and rises precipitously at doses over 60 Gy.[78, 86]

# RHABDOMYOSARCOMA

## Introduction

Rhabdomyosarcoma is a malignant tumor of mesenchymal origin that occurs in approximately 350 children per year in the United States and is the most common soft tissue sarcoma of childhood.[87] It is a curable disease in most children with localized disease who receive combined modality therapy, with more than 70% surviving 5 years after diagnosis.[88–90] While rhabdomyosarcoma most commonly presents as a mass, the presenting signs and symptoms are related to the anatomic site of the primary tumor. The most common locations of primary disease are the head and neck region, genitourinary tract, and extremities.

## Pathology

The two major histologic subtypes of rhabdomyosarcoma are alveolar and embryonal. Embryonal histology is the more common subtype and is associated with a better prognosis than alveolar rhabdomyosarcoma. Embryonal histology also encompasses two variants, botryoid, and spindle cell. Alveolar histology is associated with a characteristic translocation of t(2;13) or less commonly t(1;13).[91] Head and neck and GU rhabdomyosarcomas are most commonly of the embryonal histologic subtype whereas extremity tumors tend to present in adolescence and are frequently of alveolar histology.[92]

## WorkUp

The evaluation of a patient with a rhabdomyosarcoma includes a detailed history and physical, a CT and MRI of the primary site, a biopsy, a chest and abdomen CT, as well as a bone marrow biopsy and bone scan for metastasis evaluation, and a laboratory evaluation. If the tumor is parameningeal, then a CSF cytology and brain MRI are also necessary. Parameningeal sites include the following: nasopharynx, nasal cavity, paranasal sinuses, middle ear and mastoid region, pterygopalatine and parapharyngeal areas, and infratemporal fossa. Based on the following grouping and staging guidelines, patients are stratified into low, intermediate, and high risk discussed in the management section.

## Grouping: The IRS Grouping System

Group I:   Localized disease, completely resected
    a. Confined to muscle or organ of origin
    b. Infiltration outside the muscle or organ of origin
Group II:  Total gross resection with
    a. Microscopic residual disease
    c. Regional lymphatic spread, resected
    c. Both
Group III: Incomplete resection with gross residual disease
    a. After Bx only
    c. After major resection (>50%)
Group IV:  Distant metastatic disease present at onset

## Management

Treatment of rhabdomyosarcoma involves risk-adapted therapies that take into account tumor stage and group as well as histology. Currently, International Rhabdomyosarcoma Study (IRS) protocols are on their sixth generation of studies and have been incorporated into the COG (Children's Oncology Group) framework. Over the years, these studies have helped to stratify patients into

TABLE 32-4 TNM Pretreatment Staging Classification for IRS IV

| Stage | Sites | T (confined?) | T size | N | M | 5-yr OS |
|-------|-------|---------------|--------|---|---|---------|
| I | Orbit, H and N, GU-non bladder/prostate | Either | A or B | Any | 0 | 89 |
| II | Bladder/prostate, extremity, parameningeal (other, trunk, retroperitoneal) | Either | A (≤5 cm) | N0, Nx | 0 | 86 |
| III | Same as II but either large or node + | Either | A B | N1 N0-1 | 0 | 69 |
| IV | All | | | | 1 | 30 |

T1: confined to anatomic site of origin, T2: extension beyond anatomic site
A: ≤5 cm, B: >5 cm

three different risk groups (low, intermediate, and high). Treatment involves chemotherapy and either surgery, radiation, or both.

In general, low-risk patients have localized disease with embryonal histology at favorable sites or embryonal histology at unfavorable sites with complete resection or microscopic disease following resection. Intermediate-risk patients include embryonal histology with gross residual disease and an unfavorable site as well as patients with alveolar histology. High-risk patients include those presenting with metastatic disease.

Although it is encouraged that children treated in the United States be enrolled on the latest COG/IRS appropriate protocol, patients treated off-protocol should be treated to a radiation dose of 50.4 Gy to areas of bulky or gross residual disease and 36-41.4 Gy to areas of microscopic disease.[93]

In the IRS-V studies that have just closed, radiation therapy is determined by clinical risk group. Patients with favorable histology, low-risk disease receive no radiation for completely resected disease with negative margins, 36 Gy for residual microscopic disease and no lymph node involvement, 41.1 Gy for residual microscopic disease and lymph node involvement, 45 Gy for orbital primaries and residual gross disease, and 50.4 Gy for non-orbital primaries with gross residual disease. Patients with intermediate-risk disease and a complete resection or microscopic residual disease are given 36–41.4 Gy and 50.4 Gy for gross residual disease. Similar guidelines are followed for the high-risk patients for the primary site, but sites of metastatic disease are also irradiated.[92] Similar radiation dose and guidelines are followed for the new COG/IRS studies but the timing is somewhat different. For intermediate-risk patients, the timing of radiotherapy will be at week 4 for all patients instead of week 13 or at week 1 (day 0) for the parameningeal rhabdomyosarcomas (PM) with intracranial extension (ICE). For low-risk patients, the timing of radiotherapy in

TABLE 32-5 Risk Stratification Table Based on the Latest COG/IRS Protocols

| Risk Group | Histology | Stage | Clinical Group |
|------------|-----------|-------|----------------|
| Low | Embryonal (with variants) | I | I, II, III |
| | Embryonal (with variants) | II, III | I, II |
| Intermediate | Embryonal (with variants) | II, III | III |
| | Alveolar | I, II, III | I, II, III |
| High | Embryonal or Alveolar | IV | IV |

the newest trial will be at beginning of week 13 instead of the beginning of week 4 in the previous IRS-V study. For high-risk patients, radiotherapy begins at week 19 for the initial site and week 47 for the metastatic sites, except when the patient has a PM RMS with ICE. In the previous study, radiotherapy was delivered at week 15.

## CHILDHOOD ACUTE LYMPHOBLASTIC LEUKEMIA

Leukemia is the most common malignancy of childhood, accounting for approximately 30% of all childhood malignancies in the United States. The most common leukemia, acute lymphoblastic leukemia (ALL) is responsible for approximately 3,000 new cases each year and is the leukemia in which radiotherapy occasionally plays a role. [1, 94]ALL usually presents in children between the ages of two to five years and is found more frequently in boys than in girls. Presenting symptoms are non-specific and include fever, bleeding, bone pain, and lymphadenopathy.

Survival rates for ALL have improved significantly since the 1960s with current 5- year survival rates estimated to be better than 80%.[95] Much of the improvement is due to improved treatment of the CNS with chemotherapy and radiotherapy when necessary. Patients are again stratified into risk categories for treatment. In current protocols, CNS radiation is limited to high-risk patients which usually means they have one or more of the following: a WBC count of greater than 50,000, B-precursor disease, age over 10 years,  T-cell ALL, t(9;22) translocation (Philadelphia chromosome), or CNS involvement.[96] Children under the age of 1 are also at high risk, but radiation is not used for CNS prophylaxis in this age group. For preventive CNS therapy, the radiation therapy treatment volume includes the entire intracranial subarachnoid space and posterior aspects of the orbits. Because of neurocognitive consequences of both intensive chemotherapy, steroid treatment, and radiotherapy, the radiation dose has been reduced from 24 Gy to either 12 or 18 Gy in current protocols using 1.5 or 1.8 Gy per fraction.[97–99]

## PEDIATRIC NON-HODGKIN'S LYMPHOMA

Lymphoma is the third most common malignancy in children with over 1,700 children diagnosed each year, approximately half of which are non-Hodgkin's lymphoma (NHL) and half are Hodgkin's lymphoma.[100]

NHL in children tends to be high-grade, including Burkitt's and Burkitt's-like lymphoma, diffuse lymphoblastic lymphomas, diffuse large B cell lymphoma, and anaplastic large cell lymphoma.[100] In the modern era with more effective chemotherapy, radiotherapy plays a limited role in childhood NHL and is reserved for palliation, emergent intervention for mediastinal or spinal cord compression, adjunct therapy after an incomplete remission, and consolidation after transplant for recurrent disease.

## PEDIATRIC HODGKIN'S LYMPHOMA

### Introduction

Hodgkin's lymphoma is now highly curable, with more than 90% of children with Hodgkin's disease (HD) expecting to survive beyond 10 years.[100] Certain risk factors such as B-symptoms, (fever, drenching night sweats, >10% weight loss in the preceding 6 months), bulky mediastinal or peripheral lymph nodes, extranodal extension, hilar nodal involvement, and advanced stage are associated with a somewhat less favorable prognosis. With these high cure rates, the costs of the therapies have also come to light. The late effects of treatment, such as cardiac toxicity, secondary malignancies, and musculoskeletal growth inhibition, have led to reduction of the dose and volume of radiation fields in combination with chemotherapy as part of combined-modality therapy.[101, 102]

## Management

In general, pediatric patients are managed with chemotherapy, the intensity of which is targeted to the child's disease characteristics. Only in the most favorable patients is the involved field radiotherapy omitted, and this is done only on trial and is not currently the standard of care. To date, there have been three randomized trials evaluating chemotherapy alone, compared with combined-modality therapy in children and adolescents, and two of the three continue to show that involved field radiotherapy is beneficial to disease-free and overall survival.[103-105] Currently, radiation doses in pediatric HD are usually lower than those used in adult patients, usually between 15-25 Gy depending on the bulk of disease and the response to treatment. The definition of the involved field has varied widely by radiation oncologist, but an excellent reference article written by two Hodgkin's experts standardizes the treatment fields.[106]

## RETINOBLASTOMA

### Introduction

There are approximately 300 new cases of retinoblastoma in the United States annually and it is the most common intra-ocular tumor of childhood, occurring mostly in children under five years of age and commonly in preverbal children. Approximately one of every 15,000 to 20,000 live births is affected by retinoblastoma, which can occur in sporadic or hereditary forms. Most cases (60%–70%) are sporadic, in which both copies of the Rb tumor suppressor gene on chromosome 13 suffer a mutation in a single retinal cell causing a unilateral and unifocal tumor. However, 10%–15% of these unilateral cases arise from germinal mutations so that offspring should be screened. In the hereditary form of the disease, a predisposition to the tumor is inherited by an affected parent in whom one Rb gene is already affected. The loss of the other Rb gene results in a tumor in any given retinal cell which suffers this second loss. The hereditary form of the disease usually presents earlier, with multifocal disease and bilateral involvement. A trilateral form of the Rb occurs in 5%–10% of patients with hereditary retinoblastoma in which the pineal gland or suprasellar region can also develop a tumor (PNET). Patients with the hereditary form of the disease are predisposed to other tumors as well.[107, 108]

### Presentation/WorkUp

Infants or children with retinoblastoma may present with strabismus or poor visual acuity or, commonly, a white reflex instead of red reflex seen on a flash photograph. Workup should include a detailed history and physical with a focus on family history, an exam under anesthesia by an ophthalmologist familiar with retinoblastoma. An ultrasound of the affected eyes can help in the staging and suspicious lymph nodes should be biopsied. Laboratory examinations including blood counts, chemistries, and liver and renal function tests should also be included to be complete. An MRI of the primary site and pineal region is also required. A metastatic workup consisting of a bone marrow biopsy, CSF, Chest CT, and bone scan are necessary only if clinical symptoms or signs suggest metastatic disease or a high risk of metastatic disease. A biopsy is usually not performed because of the high risks of seeding.

### Staging

The Reese-Ellsworth staging system was designed to predict the visual outcome with external beam radiotherapy but is not as useful in this era when chemotherapy is used as a frontline modality. The International Classification System for intraocular retinoblastoma is based on the extent and location of the tumors and has been adopted by the Children's Oncology Group to risk stratify their patients for their protocol purposes. Both staging systems are given in Tables 32-6 and 32-7.

**TABLE 32-6  Reese-Ellsworth Classification of Retinoblastoma Designed to Predict an Eye's Visual Prognosis When Treated with Methods Other than Enucleation**

**Group 1: Very favorable**
1. Solitary tumor, less than 4 dd (disc diameters) in size at or behind equator.
2. Multiple tumors, none over 4 dd in size at or behind equator.

**Group 2: Favorable**
1. Solitary tumor, 4–10 dd in size at or behind equator.
2. Muliple tumors, 4–10 dd in size behind equator.

**Group 3: Doubtful**
1. Any lesion anterior to the equator.
2. Solitary tumors larger than 10 dd in size behind equator.

**Group 4: Unfavorable**
1. Multiple tumors, some larger than 10 dd.
2. Any lesion extending anterior to ora serrata (anterior termination of the retina).

**Group 5: Very unfavorable**
1. Massive tumors involving over half the retina.
2. Vitreous Seeding.

## Management/Prognosis

There is some controversy about how best to treat retinoblastoma in certain circumstances. Historically, radiotherapy and surgery were the mainstays of treatment, but platinum-based chemotherapy regimens have shown promise with very good response rates and are commonly being incorporated into the treatment of retinoblastoma for tumor reduction purposes prior to local treatment.[109] Tumors with vitreal seeds do not respond to chemotherapy as well and radiotherapy will likely need to be used.[110] Children with tumors confined to the orbit have excellent rates of survival in excess of 95%. Most agree that a local approach only for the small tumors amenable to local therapy should be used. For small intraretinal tumors distant from the fovea and optic disc, local vision sparing procedures such as cryotherapy or laser therapy may be used. For unilateral tumors that are more advanced, enucleation is considered standard, although radiotherapy is a reasonable organ-sparing alternative.[107, 108, 110]

Tumors with a positive margin after enucleation or positive lymph nodes will require adjuvant radiotherapy and chemotherapy. Tumors with a negative margin but unfavorable characteristics found on pathology after enucleation, such as choroidal invasion, concomitant choroidal and optic nerve involvement, optic nerve involvement posterior to the lamina cribrosa, scleral invasion, anterior chamber seeding, ciliary body infiltration, and iris infiltration, will generally require adjuvant chemotherapy with a carboplatin and vincristine based regimen with or without etoposide. Currently, local injections of chemotherapy (predominanantly carboplatin) are being investigated for safety and efficacy.[107, 108, 110]

Patients with bilateral retinoblastoma are at increased risk for radiation-induced second malignancy that is augmented by the use of chemotherapy.[111, 112] For this reason, external beam radiotherapy should be avoided whenever possible. However, in bilateral cases, external beam radiotherapy is often unavoidable if vision is to be preserved, due to location of the tumors and inability to treat effectively with local organ sparing measures.

## Technique/Dose

External beam radiotherapy is used when retinoblastoma is multifocal, close to macula or optic nerve, preservation of vision is desired, the tumor(s) are large, or vitreal seeds are present and

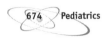 

---

TABLE 32-7  International Classification System for Intra-ocular Retinoblastoma

---

**Group A:** *Small intraretinal tumors away from foveola and disc*
  1. All tumors are 3 mm or smaller in greatest dimension, confined to the retina
  2. All tumors are located further than 3mm from the foveola and 1.5 mm from the optic disc

**Group B:** *All remaining discrete tumors confined to the retina*
  1. All other tumors confined to the retina not in Group A
  2. Tumor-associated subretinal fluid less than 3 mm from the tumor with no sub retinal seeding

**Group C:** *Discrete local disease with minimal subretinal or vitreous seeding*
  1. Tumor(s) are discrete
  2. Subretinal fluid, present or past, without seeding involving up to one fourth of the retina
  3. Local fine vitreous seeding may be present close to discrete tumor
  4. Local subretinal seeding less than 3-mm (2 disk diameters) from the tumor

**Group D:** *Diffuse disease with significant vitreous or subretinal seeding*
  1. Tumor(s) may be massive or diffuse
  2. Subretinal fluid present or past without seeding, involving up to total retinal detachment
  3. Diffuse or massive vitreous disease may include "greasy" seeds or avascular tumor masses
  4. Diffuse subretinal seeding may include subretinal plaques or tumor nodules

**Group E:** *Presence of any one or more of these poor prognosis features*
  1. Tumor touching the lens
  2. Tumor anterior to anterior vitreous face involving ciliary body or anterior segment
  3. Diffuse infiltrating retinoblastoma
  4. Neovascular glaucoma
  5. Opaque media from hemorrhage
  6. Tumor necrosis with aseptic orbital cellulites
  7. Phthisis bulbi

---

extensive. Generally, the goal is to treat the whole retina because a field defect is assumed and vitreous seeding is possible and tumor can spread via the subretinal space. All tumor should be included in the full dose range. For posteriorly located tumors, a lateral beam with a half-beam block at the bony orbit can be used which somewhat underdoses the retina anteriorly, but anterior lesions can be addressed with cryotherapy should they arise. An additional anterior field with or without a hanging two half value layer lens block weighted 1:5 anteriorly:laterally can improve the dose distribution to the anterior part of the retina. Proton radiotherapy ideally, or IMRT and SRT may also be used to get good dose to the orbit and decent dose fall off to adnexal structures. An appositional electron field with skin collimation is also a reasonable technique to provide good tumor coverage.[45, 113] Doses classically range from 35-45 Gy at 1.8 to 2 Gy per fraction depending on the use of chemotherapy, response to treatment, and the bulk of disease.

Plaque radiotherapy may be used if the tumor is less than 10 mm thick, <16 mm in its base, with minimal apical vitreal seeding, and at least 2-3 mm from the fovea and ideally at least 2 mm from the optic nerve. Referral to an institution with sufficient volume of procedures will ensure the best outcome. The guidelines given here are in accordance with the COG protocol guidelines.

Iodine-125 or Ruthenium-106 should be used to give between 30 and 45 Gy to the tumor apex at a dose rate of between 0.4 Gy/hr and 0.8 Gy/hr. The plaque should cover the tumor by 1-2 mm on every side but may be somewhat tighter if the optic nerve is close. It is placed between the sclera and the conjunctiva with gold shield to protect the other side. Plaque radiotherapy can also be used for recurrent disease.[45]

## Morbidity

Each of the three modalities, radiation, surgery, and chemotherapy carries with it risks of side effects. External beam radiotherapy is associated with impaired orbital bone growth and increased rates of second malignancy, especially in the patients with the hereditary form of the disease (see Box 32-3). However, it is also associated (albeit less commonly) with other potentially serious side effects such as retinopathy, vitreous hemorrhage, neovascular glaucoma, dry eye and keratopathy, cataracts, and photophobia—all of which can affect vision.[111,] Thus modern techniques that dramatically reduce dose to non-target tissues are of paramount importance in this group. Proton radiotherapy is rapidly gaining prominence in the United States and should be considered when external beam approaches are required. The side effects from retinal brachytherapy are similar but more localized. Unfortunately, brachytherapy cannot be used as effectively in all circumstances.

Enucleation is not without side effects either. It obviously eliminates vision in that eye and can have adverse psychological effects as well as causing chronic local effects including discharge from the orbit, contraction of the socket, and extrusion of the implant. Chemotherapy carries with it the risk of leukopenias and possible life-threatening infections. Also notably, the etoposide regimens carry a very real risk of a secondary leukemia. Carboplatin can be associated with

---

### BOX 32-3

Dr. Kleinerman and team updated their original publication delineating the risk of secondary sarcomas in a large cohort of retinoblastoma survivors treated with radiation therapy originally published in *JAMA* in 1997 by F. Wong et al.

They analyzed the risk of new cancers in 1,601 Rb survivors, diagnosed from 1914 to 1984, at two U.S. medical centers. The standardized incidence ratio (SIR) was calculated as the ratio of the observed number of cancers after hereditary and nonhereditary Rb to the expected number from the Connecticut Tumor Registry. The cumulative incidence of a new cancer after hereditary and non-hereditary Rb and radiotherapy was calculated with adjustment for competing risk of death, which differed from their previous publication. Hereditary patients continued to be at significantly increased risk for sarcomas, melanoma, and cancers of the brain and nasal cavities. The cumulative incidence for developing a new cancer at 50 years after diagnosis of Rb was 36% for hereditary and 5.7% for nonhereditary patients. Among the hereditary patients, radiotherapy increased the cumulative probability of developing a second cancer to 38.6% at 50 years, whereas the cumulative probability was 21% in the hereditary patients who did not receive radiotherapy. Furthermore, ortho-voltage radiotherapy (used prior to 1960) was associated with higher risks of second malignancy in hereditary patients compared with megavoltage techniques. Furthermore, among hereditary patients, half of the tumors diagnosed in patients older than 25 years were sarcomas, whereas only 8% of tumors diagnosed at this age were sarcomas in non-irradiated subjects. In conclusion, hereditary Rb predisposes to a variety of new cancers over time, with radiotherapy further enhancing the risk of tumors arising in the radiation field.

Kleinerman R. A. et al., Risk of new cancers after radiotherapy in long-term survivors of retinoblastoma: an extended follow-up. *J Clin Oncol.* 2005 Apr 1. 23(10):2272–2279.

ototoxicity and must be monitored. Vincristine can cause numerous neuropathies, although most are reversible. In summary, each treatment is associated with side effects, but the goals of therapy for retinoblastoma aim to minimize the side effects, preserve vision when reasonable, and maximize durable remission.[114,115]

## REFERENCES

1. Jemal, A., et al. Cancer Statistics, 2005. CA Cancer *J Clin,* 2005. 55(1): 10–30.
2. Ries, L.A.G. Childhood Cancer Mortality, in cancer incidence and survival among children and adolescents: United States SEER Program 1975–1995, Ries LAG, et al. Editors. 1999, National Cancer Institute, SEER Program. NIH Pub. No. 99-4649: Bethesda, MD. 165–169.
3. Hall, E.J. and C.S.I.H.E.J. Wuu. Radiation-induced second cancers: the impact of 3-D-CRT and IMRT. International *Journal of Radiation Oncology, Biology, Physics.,* 2003. 56(1): 83–88.
4. Kleihues, P., P.C. Burger, and B.W. Scheithauer. The new WHO classification of brain tumours. *Brain Pathol,* 1993. 3(3): 255–268.
5. Kleihues, P., et al. The WHO classification of tumors of the nervous system. *J Neuropathol Exp Neurol,* 2002. 61(3): 215–225; discussion 226–229.
6. Ron, E., et al. Tumors of the brain and nervous system after radiotherapy in childhood. *The New England Journal of Medicine,* 1988. 319(16): 1033–1039.
7. Broniscer, A., et al. Second neoplasms in pediatric patients with primary central nervous system tumors: the St. Jude Children's Research Hospital experience. *Cancer,* 2004. 100(10): 2246–2252.
8. Relling, M.V., et al. High incidence of secondary brain tumours after radiotherapy and antimetabolites. *Lancet,* 1999. 354(9172): 34–39.
9. Beebe, D.W., et al. Cognitive and adaptive outcome in low-grade pediatric cerebellar astrocytomas: evidence of diminished cognitive and adaptive functioning in National Collaborative Research Studies (CCG 9891/POG 9130). *J Clin Oncol,* 2005. 23(22): 5198–5204.
10. Carpentieri, S.C., et al. Neuropsychological functioning after surgery in children treated for brain tumor. *Neurosurgery,* 2003. 52(6): 1348–1356; discussion 1356–1357.
11. Butler, L., et al. Developing communication competency in the context of cancer: a critical interpretive analysis of provider training programs. *Psychooncology,* 2005. 14(10): 861–872; discussion 873–874.
12. Mulhern, R.K., et al. Neurocognitive consequences of risk-adapted therapy for childhood medulloblastoma. *J Clin Oncol,* 2005. 23(24): 5511–5519.
13. Merchant, T.E. Craniopharyngioma radiotherapy: endocrine and cognitive effects. *J Pediatr Endocrinol Metab,* 2006. 19 Suppl 1: 439–446.
14. Merchant, T.E., et al. Modeling radiation dosimetry to predict cognitive outcomes in pediatric patients with CNS embryonal tumors including medulloblastoma. *Int J Radiat Oncol Biol Phys,* 2006. 65(1): 210–221.
15. Hawkins, M.M. Long-term survivors of childhood cancers: what knowledge have we gained? *Nature Clinical Practice Oncology,* 2004. 1(1): 26–31.
16. Heikens, J., et al. Long-term survivors of childhood brain cancer have an increased risk for cardiovascular disease. *Cancer,* 2000. 88(9): 2116–2121.
17. Smith, E.R. and R.M. Scott. Surgical management of moyamoya syndrome. *Skull Base,* 2005. 15(1): 15–26.
18. Merchant, T.E., et al. Early neuro-otologic effects of three-dimensional irradiation in children with primary brain tumors. *International Journal of Radiation Oncology, Biology, Physics,* 2004. 58(4): 1194–1207.

19. Yock, T.I. and N. Tarbell. Technology insight: proton beam radiotherapy for treatment in pediatric brain tumors. *Nature Clinical Practice Oncology,* 2004. 1: 97–103.

20. Yock, T., et al. Proton radiotherapy for orbital rhabdomyosarcoma: clinical outcome and a dosimetric comparison with photons. *Int J Radiat Oncol Biol Phys,* 2005. 63(4): 1161–1168.

21. Miralbell, R., et al. Potential reduction of the incidence of radiation-induced second cancers by using proton beams in the treatment of pediatric tumors. *Int J Radiat Oncol Biol Phys,* 2002. 54(3): 824–829.

22. Wisoff, J.H., et al. Current neurosurgical management and the impact of the extent of resection in the treatment of malignant gliomas of childhood: a report of the Children's Cancer Group trial no. CCG-945. *J Neurosurg,* 1998. 89(1): 52–59.

23. Halperin, E.C., et al. Radiation therapy treatment planning in supratentorial glioblastoma multiforme: an analysis based on post-mortem topographic anatomy with CT correlations. *Int J Radiat Oncol Biol Phys,* 1989. 17(6): 1347–1350.

24. Bakardjiev, A.I., et al. Magnetic resonance imaging changes after stereotactic radiation therapy for childhood low-grade astrocytoma. *Cancer,* 1996. 78(4): 864–873.

25. Tekautz, T.M., et al. Atypical teratoid/rhabdoid tumors (ATRT): improved survival in children three years of age and older with radiation therapy and high-dose alkylator-based chemotherapy. *J Clin Oncol,* 2005. 23(7): 1491–1499.

26. Jakacki, R.I. Treatment strategies for high-risk medulloblastoma and supratentorial primitive neuroectodermal tumors. Review of the literature. *J Neurosurg,* 2005. 102(1 Suppl): 44–52.

27. Ris, M.D., et al. Intellectual outcome after reduced-dose radiation therapy plus adjuvant chemotherapy for medulloblastoma: a Children's Cancer Group study. *J Clin Oncol,* 2001. 19(15): 3470–3476.

28. Fukunaga-Johnson M.D., N., et al. The use of 3D conformal radiotherapy (3D CRT) to spare the cochlea in patients with medulloblastoma. *International Journal of Radiation Oncology, Biology, Physics,* 1998. 41(1): 77–82.

29. Huang, E., et al. Intensity-modulated radiation therapy for pediatric medulloblastoma: early report on the reduction of ototoxicity. *Int J Radiat Oncol Biol Phys,* 2002. 52(3): 599–605.

30. Paulino, A.C., et al. Posterior fossa boost in medulloblastoma: an analysis of dose to surrounding structures using three-dimensional (conformal) radiotherapy. *International Journal of Radiation Oncology, Biology, Physics,* 2000. 46(2): 281–286.

31. Merchant, T.E., et al. Preliminary results of conformal radiation therapy for medulloblastoma. *Neuro-Oncology,* 1999. 1(3): 177–187.

32. Wolden, S.L., et al. Patterns of failure using a conformal radiation therapy tumor bed boost for medulloblastoma. *J Clin Oncol,* 2003. 21(16): 3079–3083.

33. Mulhern, R.K., et al. Late neurocognitive sequelae in survivors of brain tumours in childhood. *Lancet Oncol,* 2004. 5(7): 399–408.

34. Hall, E.J. and C.S.I.H.E.J. Wuu. Radiation-induced second cancers: the impact of 3D-CRT and IMRT. *International Journal of Radiation Oncology, Biology, Physics,* 2003. 56(1): 83–88.

35. St Clair, W.H., et al. Advantage of protons compared to conventional X-ray or IMRT in the treatment of a pediatric patient with medulloblastoma. *International Journal of Radiation Oncology, Biology, Physics,* 2004. 58(3): 727–734.

36. Hong, T.S., et al. Patterns of failure in supratentorial primitive neuroectodermal tumors treated in Children's Cancer Group Study 921, a phase III combined modality study. *Int J Radiat Oncol Biol Phys,* 2004. 60(1): 204–213.

37. Merchant, T.E. Current management of childhood ependymoma. *Oncology (Huntington),* 2002. 16(5): 629–642, 644; discussion 645–646, 648.

38. Rogers, L., et al. Is gross-total resection sufficient treatment for posterior fossa ependymomas? *J Neurosurg*, 2005. 102(4): 629–636.
39. Duffner, P.K., et al. Postoperative chemotherapy and delayed radiation in children less than three years of age with malignant brain tumors. *New England Journal of Medicine*, 1993. 328(24): 1725–1731.
40. Merchant, T.E., et al. Preliminary results from a phase II trial of conformal radiation therapy and evaluation of radiation-related CNS effects for pediatric patients with localized ependymoma. *J Clin Oncol*, 2004. 22(15): 3156–3162.
41. Timmermann, B., et al. Role of radiotherapy in anaplastic ependymoma in children under age of three years: results of the prospective German brain tumor trials HIT-SKK 87 and 92. *Radiother Oncol*, 2005. 77(3): 278–285.
42. Paulino, A.C. The local field in infratentorial ependymoma: does the entire posterior fossa need to be treated? *Int J Radiat Oncol Biol Phys*, 2001. 49(3): 757–761.
43. Taylor, R.E. Review of radiotherapy dose and volume for intracranial ependymoma. *Pediatr Blood Cancer*, 2004. 42(5): 457–460.
44. Merchant, T.E., et al. Craniopharyngioma: the St. Jude Children's Research Hospital experience, 1984–2001. *International Journal of Radiation Oncology, Biology, Physics,* 2002. 53(3):533–542.
45. Halperin, E.C., et al. *Pediatric Radiation Oncology*, Fourth Edition 2004, Philadelphia: Lippincott, Williams & Wilkens.
46. Wisoff, J.H. Craniopharyngioma, in *Tumors of the Pediatric Central Nervous System*, R.F. Keating, J.T. Goodrich, and R.J. Packer, Editors. 2001, New York: Thieme.
47. Packer, R.J., et al. Carboplatin and vincristine chemotherapy for children with newly diagnosed progressive low-grade gliomas. *Journal of Neurosurgery,* 1997. 86(5): 747–754.
48. Pierce, S.M., et al. Definitive radiation therapy in the management of symptomatic patients with optic glioma. Survival and long-term effects. *Cancer,* 1990. 65(1): 45–52.
49. Constine, L.S., et al. Hypothalamic-pituitary dysfunction after radiation for brain tumors. *New England Journal of Medicine,* 1993. 328(2): 87–94.
50. Kortmann, R.D., et al. Current and future strategies in radiotherapy of childhood low-grade glioma of the brain. Part II: treatment-related late toxicity. *Strahlentherapie und Onkologie,* 2003. 179(9): 585–597.
51. Haas-Kogan, D.A., et al. Radiation therapy for intracranial germ cell tumors. *Int J Radiat Oncol Biol Phys*, 2003. 56(2): 511–518.
52. Zissiadis, Y., et al. Stereotactic radiotherapy for pediatric intracranial germ cell tumors. *International Journal of Radiation Oncology, Biology, Physics,* 2001. 51(1): 108–112.
53. Calaminus, G., et al. Intracranial germ cell tumors: a comprehensive update of the European data. *Neuropediatrics,* 1994. 25(1): 26–32.
54. Robertson, P.L., R.C. DaRosso, and J.C. Allen. Improved prognosis of intracranial non-germinoma germ cell tumors with multimodality therapy. *J Neurooncol,* 1997. 32(1): 71–80.
55. Weinstein, J.L., H.M. Katzenstein, and S.L. Cohn. Advances in the diagnosis and treatment of neuroblastoma. *Oncologist,* 2003. 8(3): 278–292.
56. Attiyeh, E.F., et al. Chromosome 1p and 11q deletions and outcome in neuroblastoma. *N Engl J Med,* 2005. 353(21): 2243–2253.
57. Schilling, F.H., et al. Neuroblastoma screening at one year of age. *N Engl J Med,* 2002 346(14): 1047–1053.
58. Woods, W.G., et al. Screening of infants and mortality due to neuroblastoma. *N Engl J Med,* 2002. 346(14): 1041–1046.
59. Angstman, K.B., J.S. Miser, and W.B. Franz, 3rd, Neuroblastoma. *Am Fam Physician,* 1990 41(1): 238–244.

60. Nickerson, H.J., et al. Favorable biology and outcome of stage IV-S neuroblastoma with supportive care or minimal therapy: a Children's Cancer Group study. *J Clin Oncol*, 2000. 18(3): 477–486.
61. Strother, D., et al. Event-free survival of children with biologically favourable neuroblastoma based on the degree of initial tumour resection: results from the Pediatric Oncology Group. *Eur J Cancer*, 1997. 33(12): 2121–2125.
62. Hsu, L.L., A.E. Evans, and G.J. D'Angio. Hepatomegaly in neuroblastoma stage 4s: criteria for treatment of the vulnerable neonate. *Med Pediatr Oncol*, 1996. 27(6): 521–528.
63. Matthay, K.K., Neuroblastoma: biology and therapy. *Oncology* (Williston Park), 1997. 11(12): 1857–1866; discussion 1869–1872, 1875.
64. Matthay, K.K., et al. Treatment of high-risk neuroblastoma with intensive chemotherapy, radiotherapy, autologous bone marrow transplantation, and 13-cis-retinoic acid. Children's Cancer Group. *N Engl J Med*, 1999. 341(16): 1165–1173.
65. George, R.E., et al. High-risk neuroblastoma treated with tandem autologous peripheral-blood stem cell-supported transplantation: long-term survival update. *J Clin Oncol*, 2006. 24(18): 2891–2896.
66. Marcus, K.J., et al. Primary tumor control in patients with stage three fourths unfavorable neuroblastoma treated with tandem double autologous stem cell transplants. *J Pediatr Hematol Oncol*, 2003. 25(12): 934–940.
67. Haas-Kogan, D.A., et al. Impact of radiotherapy for high-risk neuroblastoma: a Children's Cancer Group study. *Int J Radiat Oncol Biol Phys*, 2003. 56(1): 28–39.
68. Kalapurakal, J.A., et al. Management of Wilms' tumour: current practice and future goals. *Lancet Oncol*, 2004. 5(1): 37–46.
69. Morgenstern, B.Z., et al. Wilms' tumor and neuroblastoma. *Acta Paediatr Suppl*, 2004. 93(445): 78–84; discussion 84–85.
70. Kalapurakal, J.A., et al. Influence of radiation therapy delay on abdominal tumor recurrence in patients with favorable histology Wilms' tumor treated on NWTS-3 and NWTS-4: a report from the National Wilms' Tumor Study Group. *Int J Radiat Oncol Biol Phys*, 2003. 57(2): 495–499.
71. Thomas, P.R., et al. Results of two radiation therapy randomizations in the third National Wilms' Tumor Study. *Cancer*, 1991. 68(8): 1703–1707.
72. Egeler, R.M., et al. Long-term complications and post-treatment follow-up of patients with Wilms' tumor. *Semin Urol Oncol*, 1999. 17(1): 55–61.
73. Paulino, A.C., et al. Late effects in children treated with radiation therapy for Wilms' tumor. *Int J Radiat Oncol Biol Phys*, 2000. 46(5): 1239–1246.
74. Denny, C.T. Ewing's sarcoma—a clinical enigma coming into focus. *J Pediatr Hematol Oncol*, 1998. 20(5): 421–425.
75. Bacci, G., et al. Prognostic factors in nonmetastatic Ewing's sarcoma of bone treated with adjuvant chemotherapy: analysis of 359 patients at the Istituto Ortopedico Rizzoli. *J Clin Oncol*, 2000. 18(1): 4–11.
76. Cotterill, S.J., et al. Prognostic factors in Ewing's tumor of bone: analysis of 975 patients from the European Intergroup Cooperative Ewing's Sarcoma Study Group. *J Clin Oncol*, 2000. 18(17): 3108–3114.
77. Yock, T.I., et al. Local control in pelvic Ewing's sarcoma: analysis from INT-0091—a Report from the Children's Oncology Group. *Journal of Clinical Oncology*, 2006. 24(24): 3838–3843.
78. Dunst, J., et al. Second malignancies after treatment for Ewing's sarcoma: a report of the CESS-studies. *Int J Radiat Oncol Biol Phys*, 1998. 42(2): 379–384.
79. Horowitz, M.E., J.R. Neff, and L.E. Kun. Ewing's sarcoma. Radiotherapy versus surgery for local control. *Pediatr Clin North Am*, 1991. 38(2): 365–380.

80. Krasin, M.J., et al. Efficacy of combined surgery and irradiation for localized Ewing's sarcoma family of tumors. *Pediatric Blood & Cancer*, 2004. 43(3): 229–236.

81. Schuck, A., et al. Local therapy in localized Ewing tumors: results of 1058 patients treated in the CESS 81, CESS 86, and EICESS 92 trials. *International Journal of Radiation Oncology, Biology, Physics*, 2003. 55(1): 168–177.

82. Spunt, S.L., et al. Selective use of whole-lung irradiation for patients with Ewing's sarcoma family tumors and pulmonary metastases at the time of diagnosis. *J Pediatr Hematol Oncol*, 2001. 23(2): 93–98.

83. Paulussen, M., et al. Primary metastatic (stage IV) Ewing tumor: survival analysis of 171 patients from the EICESS studies. European Intergroup Cooperative Ewing Sarcoma Studies. *Ann Oncol*, 1998. 9(3): 275–281.

84. Pinkerton, C.R., et al. Treatment strategies for metastatic Ewing's sarcoma. *Eur J Cancer*, 2001. 37(11): 1338–1344.

85. Fuchs, B., et al. Complications in long-term survivors of Ewing sarcoma. *Cancer*, 2003. 98(12): 2687–2692.

86. Tucker, M.A., et al. Bone sarcomas linked to radiotherapy and chemotherapy in children. *N Engl J Med*, 1987. 317(10): 588–593.

87. Punyko, J.A., et al. Long-term survival probabilities for childhood rhabdomyosarcoma. A population-based evaluation. *Cancer*, 2005. 103(7): 1475–1483.

88. Crist, W., et al. The Third Intergroup Rhabdomyosarcoma Study. *J Clin Oncol*, 1995. 13(3): 610–630.

89. Crist, W.M., et al. Intergroup rhabdomyosarcoma study-IV: results for patients with non-metastatic disease. *J Clin Oncol*, 2001. 19(12): 3091–3102.

90. Sung, L., et al. Late events occurring 5 years or more after successful therapy for childhood rhabdomyosarcoma: a report from the Soft Tissue Sarcoma Committee of the Children's Oncology Group. *Eur J Cancer*, 2004. 40(12): 1878–1885.

91. Kelly, K.M., et al. Common and variant gene fusions predict distinct clinical phenotypes in rhabdomyosarcoma. *J Clin Oncol*, 1997. 15(5): 1831–1836.

92. Dagher, R. and L. Helman. Rhabdomyosarcoma: an overview. *Oncologist*, 1999. 4(1): 34–44.

93. Raney, R.B., et al. Rhabdomyosarcoma and undifferentiated sarcoma in the first two decades of life: a selective review of Intergroup rhabdomyosarcoma study group experience and rationale for Intergroup Rhabdomyosarcoma Study V. *J Pediatr Hematol Oncol*, 2001. 23(4): 215–220.

94. Gurney, J.G., et al. Trends in cancer incidence among children in the U.S. *Cancer*, 1996. 78(3): 532–541.

95. Pui, C.H., M.V. Relling, and J.R. Downing. Acute lymphoblastic leukemia. *N Engl J Med*, 2004. 350(15): 1535–1548.

96. Schrappe, M., et al. Improved outcome in childhood acute lymphoblastic leukemia despite reduced use of anthracyclines and cranial radiotherapy: results of trial ALL-BFM 90. German-Austrian-Swiss ALL-BFM Study Group. *Blood*, 2000. 95(11): 3310–3322.

97. Schrappe, M., et al. Long-term results of large prospective trials in childhood acute lymphoblastic leukemia. *Leukemia*, 2000. 14(12): 2193–2194.

98. Schrappe, M., et al. Long-term results of four consecutive trials in childhood ALL performed by the ALL-BFM study group from 1981 to 1995. Berlin-Frankfurt-Munster. *Leukemia*, 2000. 14(12): 2205–2222.

99. Waber, D.P., et al. Excellent therapeutic efficacy and minimal late neurotoxicity in children treated with 18 grays of cranial radiation therapy for high-risk acute lymphoblastic leukemia: a 7-year follow-up study of the Dana-Farber Cancer Institute Consortium Protocol 87-01. *Cancer*, 2001. 92(1): 15–22.

100. Percy, C.L., et al. Chapter II lymphomas and reticuloendothelial neoplasms, in Cancer Incidence and Survival among Children and Adolescents: United States SEER Program 1975–1995, L.A.G. Ries, et al. Editors. 1999, National Cancer Institute, SEER Program: Bethesda.

101. Hancock, S.L., M.A. Tucker, and R.T. Hoppe. Factors affecting late mortality from heart disease after treatment of Hodgkin's disease. *JAMA*, 1993. 270(16): 1949–1955.

102. Tucker, M.A., et al. Risk of second cancers after treatment for Hodgkin's disease. *N Engl J Med*, 1988. 318(2): 76–81.

103. Hutchinson, R.J., et al. MOPP or radiation in addition to ABVD in the treatment of pathologically staged advanced Hodgkin's disease in children: results of the Children's Cancer Group Phase III Trial. *J Clin Oncol*, 1998. 16(3): 897–906.

104. Nachman, J.B., et al. Randomized comparison of low-dose involved-field radiotherapy and no radiotherapy for children with Hodgkin's disease who achieve a complete response to chemotherapy. *J Clin Oncol*, 2002. 20(18): 3765–3771.

105. Weiner, M.A., et al. Randomized study of intensive MOPP-ABVD with or without low-dose total-nodal radiation therapy in the treatment of stages IIB, IIIA2, IIIB, and IV Hodgkin's disease in pediatric patients: a Pediatric Oncology Group study. *J Clin Oncol*, 1997. 15(8): 2769–2779.

106. Yahalom, J. and Mauch. The involved field is back: issues in delineating the radiation field in Hodgkin's disease. *Ann Oncol*, 2002. 13 Suppl 1: 79–83.

107. Abramson, D.H. and A.C. Schefler. Update on retinoblastoma. *Retina*, 2004. 24(6): 828–848.

108. Deegan, W.F., Emerging strategies for the treatment of retinoblastoma. *Curr Opin Ophthalmol*, 2003. 14(5): 291–295.

109. Friedman, D.L., et al. Chemoreduction and local ophthalmic therapy for intraocular retinoblastoma. *J Clin Oncol*, 2000. 18(1): 12–17.

110. De Potter, P. Current treatment of retinoblastoma. *Curr Opin Ophthalmol*, 2002. 13(5): 331–336.

111. Kleinerman, R.A., et al. Risk of new cancers after radiotherapy in long-term survivors of retinoblastoma: an extended follow-up. *J Clin Oncol*, 2005. 23(10): 2272–2279.

112. Wong, F.L., et al. Cancer incidence after retinoblastoma: radiation dose and sarcoma risk. *JAMA*, 1997. 278(15): 1262–1267.

113. Lee, C.T., et al. Treatment planning with protons for pediatric retinoblastoma, medulloblastoma, and pelvic sarcoma: how do protons compare with other conformal techniques? *Int J Radiat Oncol Biol Phys*, 2005. 63(2): 362–372.

114. Imhof, S.M., et al. Quantification of orbital and mid-facial growth retardation after megavoltage external beam irradiation in children with retinoblastoma. *Ophthalmology*, 1996. 103(2): 263–268.

115. Kaste, S.C., et al. Orbital development in long-term survivors of retinoblastoma. *J Clin Oncol*, 1997. 15(3): 1183–1189.

# 33

# Cutaneous Malignancies
## (including Cutaneous Lymphoma)
*Roy H. Decker, MD, PhD*
*Lynn D. Wilson, MD, MPH*

## BASAL AND SQUAMOUS CELL CARCINOMA

### Epidemiology

Skin cancer represents the most common malignancy, with more than ten million cases diagnosed annually. Basal and squamous cell carcinomas represent 80% and 20%, respectively, of non-melanoma skin cancer, but account for only a minority of skin cancer deaths.

The most important risk factor for both squamous and basal cell carcinoma is sun exposure. Childhood sun exposure is the strongest correlate with the development of basal cell carcinoma, whereas exposure in the decade preceeding diagnosis has been correlated with the development of squamous cell tumors. Other established risk factors include fair complexion, immunosuppression, chronic inflammatory states such as non-healing ulcers or burn scars (Marjolin's ulcers), or exposure to ionizing radiation or chemical agents such as arsenic or polyvinyl chloride. Genetic syndromes resulting in predisposition to skin cancers include xeroderma pigmentosum, epidermodysplasia verruciformis, and basal cell nevus syndrome.

Pre-malignant skin lesions include actinic keratoses and Bowen's disease (squamous cell carcinoma *in situ*). Erythroplasia of Queryat is an *in situ* lesion with an erythematous, plaque-like presentation on the penis or labia majora. Multiple actinic keratoses are typically located in sun-exposed areas, and may contain UV-induced loss of p53 or p16. Progression of any single actinic lesion to invasive squamous cell carcinoma occurs at a relatively low rate, usually considered to be a few percent per year.

### Pathology

The majority of basal cell carcinomas are nodular or superficial type. The former are most common, and appear as pearly, raised nodules with prominent telangiectasia. Superficial basal cell lesions are more likely to present as erythematous patches with rolled borders. Less common, but more clinically aggressive, subtypes include micronodular and morpheaform. Risk factors for local recurrence include perineural invasion, depth of invasion, and pathologic sub-type.

The clinical appearance of squamous cell carcinoma is variable, and lesions may appear as scaly plaques, nodules, or non-healing ulcers. Microscopically, atypical keratinocytes are noted to penetrate beyond the basement membrane. Poorly differentiated lesions may be non-keratinizing. Sub types of squamous cell carcinoma include adenoid, acantholytic, verrucous, adenosquamous, and spindle cell. Histopathologic risk factors for local recurrence include increased tumor thickness perineural invasion, an infiltrative border, and lack of differentiation.

## Clinical Presentation and Evaluation

The risk of lymph node or distant metastasis for basal cell carcinoma is extremely low, often quoted to be less than 0.01%. When such spread has been documented, it is primarily in the context of large, locally advanced or recurrent disease. Instead, the typical pattern of basal cell lesions is for progressive local invasion. The indolent growth pattern of basal cell carcinomas implies that deeply invasive lesions are normally limited to cases of neglect or delay in diagnosis. The exception is lesions in the area of embryologic fusion planes (the nasolabial fold), where relatively deep, occult invasion is felt to occur, although this is the subject of some controversy.

Squamous cell carcinomas, in comparison, do have a somewhat higher risk of nodal and metastatic spread, although approximately 97% of such lesions are localized at diagnosis. Characteristics of primary lesions felt to be at significant risk of nodal and/or metastatic spread include recurrent or poorly differentiated lesions, size greater than 3 cm, perineural invasion, depth of invasion greater than 4-5 mm, immunosuppressed host status, and lesions arising in burns, scars, or osteomyelitic tracts.

Both basal and squamous carcinomas have a propensity for perineural invasion, which has been correlated with local recurrence, occult nodal disease, and distant metastatic spread. Involvement of the cranial nerves may provide a route of contiguous or non-contiguous (skip lesions) spread to the central nervous system.

In all patients, a comprehensive physical examination with attention to the skin and lymphatics is appropriate. In patients with extensive local disease, imaging studies including CT or MRI may help delineate the extent of invasion.

---

**TABLE 33-1  Staging for Non-melanoma Skin Cancer, Adapted from the *AJCC* 6th Edition**

**T Stage**

| | |
|---|---|
| TX | Primary tumor not assessed |
| T0 | No evidence of primary tumor |
| Tis | Carcinoma *in situ* |
| T1 | Tumor 2 cm or less in greatest dimension |
| T2 | Tumor >2 cm and ≤5 cm in greatest dimension |
| T3 | Tumor >5 cm in greatest dimension |
| T4 | Invasion of deep tissues (cartilage, bone, skeletal muscle) |

**N Stage**

| | |
|---|---|
| NX | Nodal disease not assessed |
| N0 | No evidence of regional nodal disease |
| N1 | Regional nodal disease |

**M Stage**

| | |
|---|---|
| MX | Distant metastasis not assessed |
| M0 | No evidence of distant metastasis |
| M1 | Distant metastasis |

## Treatment with Definitive Radiotherapy

Radiation has been used as primary treatment for basal and squamous cell carcinoma with local control of 90% or greater.[1] As an alternative to wide excision or Moh's surgery, radiotherapy may offer superior cosmetic results for lesions in exposed anatomic areas such as the head and neck. There is some concern for progressive late skin atrophy and necrosis decades after radiation and for this reason surgical excision is usually felt to be a better option in younger patients (those less than 55). Local control is a function of tumor size and T stage; for small lesions, radiation is felt to offer equivalent local control to that seen with excision. Results from a large, modern series are summarized in Box 33-1.

---

**BOX 33-1**

The authors reviewed the treatment and results of 531 basal and squamous cell carcinomas of the skin treated with definitive radiation at the Mallinckrodt Institute of Radiology. Overall local control was 92% for basal cell lesions, 80% for squamous, and was significantly worse for recurrent tumors. Control was related to tumor stage as follows:

|    | Basal Cell | Squamous Cell |
|----|------------|---------------|
| T1 | 96%        | 95%           |
| T2 | 90%        | 86%           |
| T3 | 94%        | 86%           |
| T4 | 100%       | 75%           |

Cosmesis was rated good to excellent in 92% of patients and was noted to be worse following treatment of large or recurrent lesions. The authors recommend treatment in 2.5 Gy fractions 4 days per week, to total doses of 40–60 Gy depending on histology and tumor size.

This large series reports excellent local control with radiotherapy alone for epithelial skin cancer. Local control is a function of radiation dose and tumor size. Recurrent lesions are at significantly higher risk of recurrence and warrant aggressive treatment.

Locke J, Karimpour MD, Young G, et al. Radiotherapy for epithelial skin cancer. *Int J. Radiation Oncology Biol Phys*, 2001;51:748–751.

---

## Adjuvant Radiotherapy

The indications for postoperative treatment of epithelial skin cancer are based on risk factors for local recurrence after resection, established in multiple retrospective experiences. The decision to offer adjuvant radiation should include consideration of tumor factors such as size and depth of invasion, microscopic features including differentiation and perineural invasion, as well as the surgical approach and limitations of resection imposed by anatomic location.

The clearest indication for treatment is positive margins after excision or Moh's surgery. Other considerations include tumor depth greater than 4 mm and tumor size. Lesions greater than 2 cm in diameter on the trunk, or greater than 1 cm in diameter on the head and neck, carry an elevated local recurrence risk. Involvement of cartilage or bone is a strong predictor of local recurrence and consensus guidelines recommend adjuvant therapy in appropriate patients. Perineural invasion has been correlated with both local and nodal recurrence following excision,[2,3] and is a relative indication for treatment. Involvement of large, named nerves should prompt consideration of extension of the clinical target volume to include the proximal nerve tract. Other relative indications for treatment include poorly differentiated tumors, adenosquamous sub-type, and limitations imposed on excision by anatomic location. Patient factors include the presence of neurologic symptoms, implying underlying nerve involvement, and immunosuppressed host status.

The majority of data concerning local recurrence after surgical management is derived from populations who underwent simple excision. Moh's surgery has now become a more standard option, with documented lower recurrence rates. Given the meticulous inspection of the margins during the Moh's procedure, assessment of risk factors based on post-excision experiences may overestimate the actual recurrence risk.

## Nodal Irradiation

For squamous cell carcinoma, locally advanced lesions may have a significant risk of nodal metastasis. Clinically evident nodes should be surgically dissected; adjuvant radiation is recommended in the context of multiple involved nodes, a single node greater than 3 cm in size, or residual disease. In patients without clinically evident nodal disease, but with risk factors for occult disease (large tumor size, invasive > 4 mm, locally recurrent disease, perineural invasion, lymph-vascular space invasion, or immunosuppressed host status) consideration should be given to evaluation of the nodal bed with sentinel node biopsy or dissection. In patients being treated adjuvantly or definitively for locally advanced primaries with risk factors, draining lymphatics should be electively included. Primary tumors arising in the head and neck region, and draining to cervical lymph nodes, may be at increased risk of metastasis.[4] The predilection of pre-auricular tumors for metastasis to intra-parotid lymph nodes is well documented, and adjuvant radiotherapy for high risk lesions should include the parotid bed.

Basal cell carcinomas rarely metastasize, and treatment of draining lymphatics should be limited to patients with documented nodal disease.

## Radiotherapy Technique

The treatment volume should include the tumor or tumor bed, along with a 1-2-cm margin of normal tissue. Additional margin may be required by the surgical margin status or the presence of an infiltrative histologic front. Depth of coverage is dictated by known or suspected depth of the primary lesion. For lesions occurring at embryologic fusion plates, such as the area of the nasolabial folds, there is concern for deeper, occult involvement, and the treatment field should be designed appropriately.

Dose fractionation schemes represent a balance between patient convenience and the relative risk of poor cosmesis. 60-66 Gy in 2 Gy fractions is appropriate for gross disease, with higher doses indicated for lesions greater than 2–4 cm. Published experience with relatively hypofractionated treatment has shown equivalent locoregional control after 45-50 Gy in 2.5 Gy fractions, or radiobiologically equivalent doses in fraction sizes of 3 or 4 Gy.

## MALIGNANT MELANOMA

### Epidemiology

Malignant melanoma, with an annual incidence of approximately 60,000 cases per year in the United States, represents a small percentage of total skin cancer cases while accounting for the majority of skin cancer mortality. Cutaneous melanoma may arise in individuals of any age, and at any anatomic site, but is most common in middle-aged patients and in sun-exposed areas. A history of blistering sunburns in childhood, the presence of multiple dysplastic nevi, or exposure to polyvinyl chloride put a patient at increased risk. While the vast majority of melanoma are sporadic, there are familial forms, associated with mutations in p16, cdk4, and other genes, in which involved family members may have up to a 50% lifetime risk, and may develop multiple primary tumors.

# Pathology

Malignant melanoma is theorized, in many cases, to progress through distinct growth phases. During the early, radial, growth phase the cells are confined to the epidermis. During the latter, vertical, growth phase the tumor invades the dermis and deeper tissues and the risk of metastatic spread increases. The relative prevalence and chronology of progression through these phases is related to the histologic subtype.

Cytologically, melanoma may take on an epithelioid, spindle cell, or non-specific appearance. Immunohistochemical stains may be required to make the diagnosis. Common antigens which distinguish melanoma from mesenchymal tumors include S-100, HMB-45, and MART-1. The most prevalent histologic subtypes include:

- Superficial spreading melanoma represents 70% of diagnosed lesions. The primary growth pattern is radial, often for many years, before a late, vertical growth phase. The peak incidence is between ages 40 and 60. These tend to be flat, pigmented lesions with variegated color with an epithelioid microscopic appearance.
- Nodular melanoma represents approximately 20%–25% of diagnosed lesions. These are discrete and darkly pigmented or amelanotic. They may be epithelioid or spindle-shaped, and tend toward early vertical growth.
- Acral lentiginous melanoma, representing 5% of lesions, are the most common subtype diagnosed in dark skinned patients. Most common primary sites include palms, soles, and nail beds.
- Lentigo maligna is felt to be a pre-invasive lesion, most commonly identified on head and neck sites in the seventh or eighth decade. These are indolent lesions, strongly correlated with sun exposure, that often cover significant surface area over many years. They may progress to lentigo maligna melanoma.
- Desmoplastic melanoma is an uncommon subtype with peak incidence in the sixth or seventh decade. These tend to be more deeply invasive lesions, with higher local recurrence rates. There is some evidence that they tend to have a lower predilection for nodal and distant spread, and prominent neurotropism. Desmoplastic lesions are more likely to be immunohistochemically negative than other, more common, subtypes.

# Clinical Presentation and Evaluation

The evaluation of a patient with newly diagnosed malignant melanoma should include detailed history and physical with attention to family history, a complete skin survey, and biopsy of the primary lesion. Important pathologic factors include depth of invasion, measured in Clark's level or Breslow thickness (measured from the top of the granular layer of the epidermis), as well as the presence of ulceration or satellitosis. Favorable clinical factors include female gender, young age, and extremity location.

For lesions less than 1 mm in thickness, without ulceration, wide excision alone is adequate. A surgical margin of at least 1 cm of normal tissue is recommended for small lesions (those less than 2 mm thick), while 2 cm or more is recommended for more deeply invasive primaries. For lesions greater than 1 mm in depth or those with ulceration, sentinel node biopsy is recommended.

For patients with clinically or pathologically positive lymph nodes, further staging workup is appropriate with appropriate radiographic studies and basic laboratory values.

The staging system for melanoma includes evaluation of tumor thickness, ulceration, satellitosis, as well as the presence of nodal and distant metastases. Ten-year survival is correlated with stage at diagnosis: greater than 80% for Stage I, 50% for Stage II, 30%–40% for Stage III, and 10% or less for Stage IV.

**TABLE 33-2 Stage Grouping for Melanoma, Adapted from the *AJCC* 6th Edition**

| | |
|---|---|
| Stage 0 | Melanoma *in situ* |
| Stage I | ≤1 mm thick with or without ulceration, or >1 mm, and ≤2 mm thick without ulceration |
| Stage II | >1 mm thick with ulceration, or >2 mm, with or without ulceration |
| Stage III | Nodal metastasis |
| | Includes satellite lesions, in-transit metastases |
| Stage IV | Distant metastasis |

## Treatment

The role of radiotherapy in the definitive management of localized melanoma has not been conclusively established. There is evidence, however, that selected patients at increased risk of local or regional failure may benefit from adjuvant radiation.[5] In the context of metastatic disease, radiation treatment is commonly employed for palliation. For *in situ* disease (Lentigo Maligna), superficial radiation may be effective in controlling tumor growth and preventing progression.[6]

### BOX 33-2

Forty-two patients with lentigo maligna (LM) and 22 with lentigo maligna melanoma (LMM) were treated with fractionated radiation to 100 Gy in 10 daily fractions over 2 weeks. Superficial X-rays were used with the 50% isodose delivered to 1.1 mm. In LMM patients, the nodular portion of the tumor was excised prior to radiation. With a median follow-up of 15 months, there were no local recurrences in the LM patients, and only two in the LMM patients. There were pigmentation changes within the treatment field but no reported fibrosis.

High-dose superficial radiation appears to be safe and efficacious with short-term follow-up and should be considered for *in situ* lesions not amenable to excision.

Schmid-Wendtner MH, Brunner B Konz B, et al. Fractionated radiotherapy of lentigo maligna and lentigo maligna melanoma in 64 patients. *J Am Acad Dermatol* 2000;43:477–482.

## Adjuvant Therapy

Wide excision is the standard therapy for the primary tumor, with appropriate margins based on the size and thickness of the lesion. For tumors greater than 1 mm in thickness, with ulceration, or those invading the reticular dermis, sentinel node biopsy is recommended. For appropriately staged patients with localized disease at diagnosis, the most common site of failure is distant, with a risk of local failure of less than 5%.

There are risk factors which have been established in retrospective series to significantly increase the risk of local recurrence. These include tumor thickness greater than 4 mm, ulceration, satellitosis, positive surgical margins, mucosal origin, perineural invasion, and desmoplastic histology. When these risk factors are present in combination, local relapse can approach 50%.[5]

Prospective, randomized data supporting the use of adjuvant radiotherapy in the context of high risk primary lesions are lacking. Several retrospective series report the treatment of high risk melanoma with post-excision radiotherapy, with relatively low local recurrence in comparison to historical controls, suggesting a benefit. The presence of these risk factors also confers an increased risk of nodal and distant failure, and therefore improving local control may not translate into an overall survival benefit.

Overall, the role of adjuvant radiation is not yet firmly established. In high-risk lesions, treatment may be appropriate.

## Adjuvant Nodal Irradiation

In the setting of a positive sentinel node, or clinically evident nodal disease, complete dissection is indicated. While overall regional control after dissection is greater than 80%, several factors increase the risk of nodal recurrence. These include extracapsular extension, multiple (4 or more) involved nodes, $\geq$ 3 cm metastases, recurrent disease, and head and neck location.

Regional recurrence of high-risk nodal disease after dissection and adjuvant nodal irradiation has been examined in several retrospective series as well as a single-arm prospective trial. One of the largest experiences, from the M.D. Anderson Cancer Center (see Box 33-3), found that recurrence after irradiation was notably lower than reported in historical controls who did not receive radiation, although distant failure was still seen in more than 50% of patients. Late complications of radiation, including symptomatic lymphedema, were noted in a significant number of patients, and highest after irradiation of axillary or inguinal nodal regions.[7] A randomized phase III RTOG trial did not accrue and was subsequently closed.

Adjuvant radiotherapy should be considered in the setting of high-risk features following nodal dissection, although the potential benefit should be balanced against both the expected toxicity as well as the independent risk of distant failure since several features that increase the risk of nodal relapse (multiple involved nodes, extracapsular extension, recurrent disease) also portend distant metastasis. Again, whether improving regional control translates to increased survival remains questionable.

Surgical dissection following identification of a positive sentinel node provides regional control and establishes important prognostic information. While such completion dissection is standard, it may not be practical in certain clinical situations. In this setting, elective irradiation of the nodal basin should be considered.

---

### BOX 33-3

This is a retrospective study of 466 patients with node-positive melanoma managed with nodal surgery and radiation. The majority of patients had clinically evident nodal disease at diagnosis, underwent nodal dissection, and were found to have high risk disease (four or more nodes, nodes greater than 3 cm, recurrent disease, or cervical site). Radiotherapy consisted of 30 Gy in 5 fractions delivered twice weekly. The Kaplan-Meier 5-year regional control rate was 89% and 5-year disease-free survival was 42%. Treatment side effects included lymphedema in 9% of all patients, 20% in those treated to the axillary region, and 27% in those treated to inguinal nodes.

This large series of patients treated with combined modality therapy to high-risk nodal disease demonstrates excellent regional control which is superior to that seen in historical controls of node dissection alone. Treatment related side effects were significant in those treated to axillary and inguinal fields. The benefits of regional control need to be balanced against the high competing risk of metastatic failure.

Ballo MT, Ross MI, Cormier JN, et al. Combined-modality therapy for patients with regional nodal metastases from melanoma. *Int J. Radiation Oncology Biol Phys*, 2006;64:106–113.

---

## Radiotherapy Technique

Interest in hypofractionated treatment of melanoma was raised when cell culture models were found to have cell survival curves with pronounced shoulders. Several single institution retrospective series then reported improved response rates with fraction sizes of 4, 5, or 6 Gy compared to conventional fractionation.[8] The relative response rates are primarily documented in metastatic disease, and the effect most pronounced in cutaneous, rather than visceral, sites. Overall response rates reported in the literature for hypofractionation range from 30%–90%, and complete response from 24%–60%. Interestingly, a randomized multi-center trial, the RTOG 8305, failed to demonstrate a significant benefit of fraction sizes greater than 2.5 Gy delivered daily. In this study, complete response was seen in 24% of lesions treated, and the overall response rate was approximately 60%, regardless of the scheme used.

Since data suggesting a benefit to adjuvant radiation to the primary tumor or draining nodal basins derives predominantly from patients treated with hypofractionated regimens, we would recommend treatment of superficial regions with 5-6 Gy per fraction to a total dose of 30-36 Gy. For treatment of visceral sites or when toxicity is a concern, then equivalent fractionation schemes such as 40 Gy in 10 fractions or 50 Gy in 20 fractions are appropriate. Consideration should be given to radiosurgery for palliation of intracranial and extracranial metastases based on the relatively low efficacy of fractionated treatment.

## MERKEL CELL CARCINOMA

Merkel cell carcinoma, also known as neuroendocrine carcinoma or trabecular carcinoma of the skin, is an uncommon but aggressive malignancy arising from dermal sensory cells. There may be a relationship between Merkel cell carcinoma and polyomarvirus. The typical presentation is in a head and neck or extremity location, as a small and isolated violaceous nodule, in patients over 60. As many as 20% of patients will have clinically involved nodes at diagnosis, and up to 50% will have occult nodal metastases following surgical staging. Relapses following local therapy are common and typically occur within the first year. Although outcomes vary among published series, some authors report more than 50% of patients will ultimately die of this disease. Primary treatment with curative intent should address both the primary tumor site and draining lymphatics, regardless of initial tumor size.[9]

In terms of the primary tumor site, the most well established approach is wide local excision. Due to the prevalence of local microscopic infiltration and satellite lesions, margins of 3-4 cm are typically recommended. Many authors have advocated routine postoperative radiation, but a recently published modern series[10] (see Box 33-4) identifies patients at low risk of local relapse following excision alone. Large tumor size, close margins, in-transit or satellite metastases, or immunosuppressed status are all relative indications for adjuvant treatment. Additionally, when anatomic location, tumor size, or cosmesis limit excision margins, then the addition of adjuvant radiotherapy to planned conservative surgery offers comparable outcome. Locally recurrent lesions also present a higher risk of further recurrence after resection, and adjuvant radiation is indicated. Alternately, primary radiation has been used in relatively small numbers of patients with reasonable outcomes.

### BOX 33-4

This large, modern series reports the results of 251 patients with Merkel cell carcinoma treated at Memorial Sloan-Kettering Cancer Center. The majority of patients had wide local excision; many had pathologic nodal staging with sentinel node biopsy or nodal dissection. Local control after margin negative excision was 94%; there was no benefit to adjuvant radiation and no relation between recurrence and margin size.

Surgical staging of clinically negative lymph nodes was associated with improved regional control (11% vs. 44% for clinically staged patients). There was no additional benefit to nodal radiotherapy in this cohort. In clinically node positive patients regional failure was 26% after dissection, and 13% after dissection and adjuvant radiation, a result which was not statistically significant.

This is the largest surgical series to separately examine local and regional failure following operative management. In contrast to previous series in which surgery was more limited, radiotherapy was of no significant benefit. Since adjuvant radiation was administered in a small number of patients in this trial, statistical inferences concerning the value of adjuvant treatment are difficult to make. In patients with margin negative local excision and surgically staged low-risk nodal disease, routine adjuvant radiation was of no demonstrable benefit.

Allen PJ, Bowne WB, Jaques DP, et al. Merkel cell carcinoma: prognosis and treatment of patients from a single institution. *J Clin Oncology* 2005; 23:2300–2309.

Clinically node negative patients should be offered sentinel node biopsy, followed by complete dissection or nodal irradiation when nodal metastases are found. Routine postoperative radiotherapy to dissected lymph nodes appears to be of no demonstrable benefit when minimal microscopic disease is present. When multiple nodes are involved, or there is extracapsular extension, then adjuvant treatment should be considered, extrapolating from a well documented increased risk of failure after dissection alone in epithelial tumors. In patients with clinically apparent nodal disease, combined modality therapy with nodal dissection and adjuvant radiation offers the best regional control, though the relative toxicity of such treatment in certain nodal basins should be considered. In these cases, radiation alone has also been used to definitively manage undissected nodal regions with reasonable control rates.

Radiotherapy for Merkel cell carcinoma should incorporate wider margins than those used for epithelial tumors, to account for the propensity for microscopic infiltration. A 5 cm margin around primary lesions is commonly employed. If the draining nodal basin is to be treated, then the two regions should be treated in contiguity to account for in-transit disease.

In comparison to epithelial skin malignancies, Merkel cell carcinoma is a highly radiosensitive tumor. Historically, radiation doses of between 45 and 60 Gy have been used to treat both microscopic and gross tumor with excellent response rates and durable local control. Some anatomic areas, such as distal extremities, inguinal, axillary and supraclavicular fields, may not tolerate higher doses without a significant risk of late effects. In these cases, a multimodality approach of limited excision and lower dose radiation may offer the best balance of local control and limited toxicity.[11]

## Sebaceous and Eccrine Carcinoma

Sebaceous carcinomas are rare malignancies which are typically found on the upper or lower eyelid. They are thought to arise from meibomian, Zeis, or sebaceous glands in elderly individuals. Clinically they are commonly misdiagnosed as inflammatory processes (chalazion) and microscopically may be confused with basal or squamous cell carcinoma. Muir-Torre syndrome is an autosomal dominant syndrome predisposing to sebaceous carcinomas, keratocanthomas, and visceral malignancies, and may be related to hereditary non-polyposis colorectal cancer (HNPCC).

Definitive treatment is surgical, spanning local excision to orbital exenteration. Radiation therapy may be appropriate in the adjuvant setting when there is incomplete resection or in cases where resection is not felt to be practical.

Eccrine and apocrine carcinomas are rare, aggressive tumors arising in sweat glands. Apocrine tumors arise in the axilla, while eccrine lesions are most prevalent in the head and neck region. As in sebaceous lesions, surgery is the mainstay of treatment, and local and distant recurrences are common.

# KAPOSI'S SARCOMA

Kaposi's sarcoma (KS) is a previously rare malignancy whose incidence rose dramatically with the onset of AIDS, as the prevalence in such patients is 20,000 times that of the general population. Prior to the availability of effective anti-retroviral therapy, KS represented the most common malignancy seen in AIDS patients.

Clinically, KS appears as a purplish plaque or nodule. It is often multifocal at presentation, and may involve visceral and mucosal sites. There may be associated lymphadenopathy and localized lymphedema. Distinct epidemiologic subtypes are described:

- Classic KS is a low-grade tumor affecting older Mediterranean men, not associated with immune deficiency.
- Endemic KS occurs in men in equatorial Africa and is also not associated with immune deficiency.
- Epidemic KS occurs in immune suppressed patients. It is particularly prevalent in homosexual men with AIDS, likely due to coinfection with HHV-8. The latter has been strongly associated with the development of KS in AIDS patients as well as in patients who have undergone solid organ transplant.

Pathologic features of KS include spindle cells, inflammation, and neovascularization. The lesions are most commonly seen on the lower extremity and face. A minority of tumors arise in the oral mucosa or gastrointestinal tract, though autopsy series suggest under-diagnosis of such lesions in involved patients. Pulmonary involvement may also occur, especially in advanced, AIDS-related cases.

## Treatment

Treatment of KS is palliative. In AIDS patients, the initiation of highly active antiretroviral therapy (HAART) has been demonstrated to result in significant stabilization and regression of disease. Patients with widespread disease and intact immune systems may be candidates for systemic therapy with liposomal anthracyclines, paclitaxel, or other agents.

Local therapies for palliation include topical alitretinoin, intralesional chemotherapy, laser ablation, and cryotherapy. For palliation of pain, bleeding, or edema, or to preserve or improve cosmesis, radiotherapy also has an established role. Several series have reported response rates of 80%–90% or greater with excellent symptom relief. Typical palliative fractionation schemes of 30 Gy in 10 fractions, 40 Gy in 20 fractions, or the radiobiologic equivalent, may be selected based on the individual requirement of each anatomic site and patient characteristics. Superficial therapy with kilovoltage/orthovoltage photons, or electrons with modest normal tissue margin is appropriate.

Visceral lesions also have documented palliative response to radiation, although lower fraction sizes and lower total doses have been used. Systemic therapies may be appropriate and should be considered in light of the expected higher acute and late side effect profile.

# CUTANEOUS LYMPHOMA

Cutaneous T-cell and B-cell lymphomas (CTCL, CBCL) are relatively rare, constitute less than 10% of all lymphomas, usually present with either a T or B-cell phenotype, and in many cases exhibit relatively indolent behavior. Because of the variety of cell types, low incidence, various presentations, and relative lack of thoroughly documented therapeutic approaches, the cutaneous lymphomas often present diagnostic and therapeutic dilemmas for the treating physician. The pathogenesis of cutaneous lymphoma and clinical course are based on subtype, extent, and location. The staging and evaluation of patients is different than that utilized for patients with nodal lymphoma and the staging/classification systems are different for mycosis fungoides (the most common T-cell cutaneous lymphoma) compared to B-cell lymphomas. Discussion will be limited to the most common varieties of CTCL and CBCL.

## Epidemiology

Mycosis fungoides, a T-cell lymphoma, is the most common of the cutaneous lymphomas, but data from the National Cancer Institute's Surveillance, Epidemiology and End Results Program (SEER) reveal that the annual incidence has apparently reached a plateau at five cases per 1,000,000 persons in the United States (US). Of interest is that CBCL appears to have increasing incidence at a rate of approximately 3.5 per 1,000,000 (see Figure 33-1).[12]

For CBCL, lesions can involve any region of the skin surface but most commonly involve the head and neck (50%), trunk (19%), upper extremity (12%), lower extremity (12%), and multifocal location in less than 10%. CBCL is more common in men (1.4:1) and whites (2.2:1). Incidence increases with age with a peak of approximately 11 cases per 1,000,000 for those patients above the age of 80 years. The mean age is 64 years and diffuse large cell lymphoma is the most common subtype according to data gathered from SEER[12] but this is not the case based on the update from the WHO-EORTC which reveals that more indolent histologies are more common.[13]

Mycosis fungoides is most common in older patients, with a peak incidence in patients between the ages of 70 and 80. Lesions may appear on any location of the body but tend to present in "sun shielded" areas. Mycosis fungoides is more common in blacks (2.0:1) and in males (2.2:1).

Although risk factors for CTCL have been investigated, there is no clearly established relationship between infectious or exposure etiologies. For CBCL, risk factors are also not well established, but for the marginal zone subtype, *Borrelia burgdorferi* has been reported in Europe as perhaps having an etiologic relationship but not in the United States.

**FIGURE 33-1** MF-CBCL Incidence: Age-adjusted yearly incidence of primary cutaneous B-cell lymphoma (PCBCL; ▲) and mycosis fungoides (MF; ○) from 1973 to 2001. Error bars represent 95% CIs around regression lines (Joinpoint version 2.7).

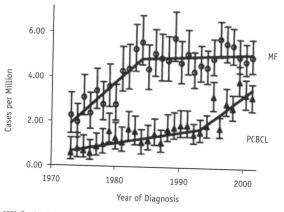

*Clin Oncol* 23:3390–3395. Reprinted with permission from the American Society of Clinical Oncology

## Pathology, Immunophenotype, and Genetics

The classification of both T-cell and B-cell cutaneous lymphomas has been challenging and recently the EORTC and WHO produced a consensus opinion in an effort to reconcile the differences inherent within these two classification systems.[13]

### Cutaneous T-cell Lymphomas

#### CTCL-Mycosis Fungoides

Mycosis fungoides typically presents with a CD4+ (helper T-cell), CD3+, CD5+(pan T-cell), CD8- (cytotoxic T-cell), CD45RO+(memory T-cell) T-cell phenotype and these cells migrate to the skin through a complicated process of molecular interactions that involve cascades of cell signaling, T-cell activation, and eventual clonal predominance in some cases. These cells are considered "epidermotropic" and the classic histologic presentation reveals what is known as a Pautrier's microabscess. Clonal T-cell receptor gene rearrangements are detectable in many cases, and chromosomal deletions at 1p, 17p, 10q have been identified. Additionally, p53 mutation has been associated with disease progression.[14]

#### CTCL-CD30+ Anaplastic Large Cell

The next most commonly encountered CTCLs after MF are the primary cutaneous CD30+ lymphoproliferative disorders which include lymphomatoid papulosis and anaplastic large cell lymphoma (ALCL). ALCL often presents without evidence of MF and histologically, cells are anaplastic or immunoblastic in appearance. These cells also generally reveal a CD4+ phenotype as seen with MF and express cutaneous lymphocyte antigen (CLA). In contrast to MF, these cells typically are not epidermotropic and are CD30+. These lesions may demonstrate clonal rearrangement of T-cell receptor (TCR genes) as in MF. In contrast to the non-cutaneous (systemic) counterpart, translocation of 2:5 is usually not seen. Overexpression of anaplasitc lymphoma kinase is not seen in anaplastic CD30+ cutaneous lymphoma.

Lymphomatoid papulosis often presents as violaceous papules and lesions may resolve spontaneously. Subtypes A, B, and C have been described with the A and C variety consisting of CD30+ T-cells and the B type may simulate classical mycosis fungoides. Lymphomatoid papulosis is considered a more clinically benign variant compared to anaplastic large cell lymphoma.

### Cutaneous B-cell Lymphomas

The most common presentations of CBCL as documented from the SEER data are diffuse large cell, follicular, and marginal zone types.[12]

#### CBCL-diffuse large B-cell

Cutaneous diffuse large B-cell lymphoma can usually be identified by centroblasts and immunoblasts with infiltrates that may extend into subcutaneous tissue. Lesions may express CD20 and CD79 and lesions from the lower extremity may express bcl-2, bcl-6 and MUM-1. It is possible for these findings to be noted in large cell lesions in other locations. These lesions may exhibit inactivation of p16 suppressor genes, additions for 18q and 7p, and loss of 6q.

#### CBCL-marginal zone

This cutaneous lymphoma is considered as part of the group of lymphomas involving mucosa associated lymphoid tissue (MALT). Marginal zone cells are identified in addition to small lymphocytes and reactive germinal centers. Cell classification reveals expression of CD20, CD79 and often bcl-2 but not bcl-6. Immunoglobulin heavy chain gene rearrangement has been identified

(IgH) and translocations of the IHG and MLT genes of chromosomes 14 and 18 respectively have been identified.

*CBCL-follicle center cell*

Histologically, these lesions often spare the epidermis and may consist of large centrocytes and reactive T-cells. A follicular pattern gives rise to the cellular designation and expression of CD20 and CD79 is usually identified. Expression of bcl-2 and MUM-1 is typically not found. In contrast to the systemic nodal counterpart, the t(14:18) translocation is atypical.

## Clinical Presentation and Evaluation[15]

When a patient is suspected of having a cutaneous lymphoma, a history and physical should be performed in conjunction with biopsy. Tissue for immunophenotyping and gene rearrangement should be obtained. It is critical that the entire skin surface be evaluated, and any suspicious areas documented and preferably photographed. Patients should be evaluated by a dermatologist, radiation oncologist, and medical oncologist. For those with MF, disease often presents in "sun shielded" regions and begins as erythema (patches and plaques) but may appear in any surface location. Typically disease presents as patches and or plaques over small areas or more extensive regions of skin surface. Such lesions may progress to tumors and lesions may ulcerate, and become infected. Some patients may develop widespread erythroderma. The Sezary Syndrome is defined as erythroderma in addition to malignant T-cell hematologic involvement. Various definitions have been used to determine blood involvement but generally one of the following five criteria should be met: 1) absolute Sezary count of > 1,000 cells/ul, 2) CD4/CD8 ratio > 10 due to an increase in CD3+ or CD4+ cells via flow cytometry, 3) aberrant expression of pan-T cell markers (CD2, CD3, CD4, CD5) by flow cytometry (deficient CD7 expression on T-cells is a tentative criterion), 4) increased lymphocyte count with a T-cell clone in the blood identified by Southern blot or polymerase chain reaction (PCR), or 5) a chromosomally abnormal T-cell clone. Nodal and visceral disease is possible but often lymph nodes are dermatopathic in nature. Any suspicious lymph nodes should be biopsied via excision.

Patients with CBCL typically have a different clinical presentation than those with CTCL. Lesions tend to be more common on the head and neck or trunk/upper extremities. Lesions typically present with a more focal papule or nodular type appearance compared to patches or plaques, although such a presentation (which is more characteristic of mycosis fungoides) is certainly possible. Generally, large areas of skin are not involved as they can be in CTCL(MF), but areas of involvement can expand locally and be noted in other anatomic locations simultaneously. Diffuse large cell type can present in any location, but in CBCL the diffuse large cell entity appears to have different clinical behavior based on location. Lesions of the lower extremity appear to behave more aggressively than lesions found on the truck or head and neck for example. Because of this more aggressive behavior, combined modality therapy is often considered despite any substantial evidence of an advantage to such an approach. The clinical evaluation of the patient with CBCL is similar to that of a patient with CTCL and includes careful documentation with photography of the lesion or lesions in question.

Bone marrow evaluation is usually not performed for patients with CTCL, but evaluation of blood via flow cytometry is recommended and an increased CD4:CD8 ratio (normal range 0.5-4.0) may be indicative of blood involvement. Bone marrow evaluation is often incorporated into the evaluation of the patient with CBCL and flow cytometry of the blood can be considered. If initial flow cytometry is negative in those with CTCL, polymerase chain reaction assay (PCR) for T-cell clonality can be considered. A complete blood count including differential with smear and chemistries should be obtained in addition to LDH. Soluble interleukin-2 receptor may be evaluated for patients with advanced CTCL. Posterior-anterior and lateral chest radiography should be performed for all patients and computed tomography (CT) is generally not recommended for CTCL patients with early-stage disease (patches and plaques, T1-T2) given the low clinical yield. Data are emerging on the use of positron emission tomography-CT (PET-CT) for patients with cutaneous lymphoma and may be helpful in staging and treatment planning for radiotherapy for those with either CTCL or CBCL. Especially in CBCL, it is critical to document that there is no visceral or nodal involvement. Should this be the case, the identification of B-cells in the skin may represent spread of nodal lymphoma and the clinical management would generally require a radically different approach.

Although a variety of classification and staging systems have been utilized for the cutaneous lymphomas, the American Joint Committee on Cancer (AJCC) utilizes a TNM based system that allows provision for lesion type and distribution, nodal status, visceral and hematologic involvement for mycosis fungoides. (Table 33-3) For CBCL, a variety of classification systems have been used based on pathologic interpretation and most recently, the WHO-EORTC system has been adopted as previously described.[13] For clinical utility in prognostication considering pathologic and clinical information together, we recommend the use of the recently developed cutaneous B-cell lymphoma prognostic index (CBCL-PI).[12] (Table 33-4)

---

### TABLE 33-3 Staging Classification for Mycosis Fungoides (TNM)

| | |
|---|---|
| $T_1$ | Patches and/or plaques involving <10% body surface area |
| $T_2$ | Patches and/or plaques involving ≥10% body surface area |
| $T_3$ | One or more cutaneous tumors |
| $T_4$ | Erythroderma |

| | |
|---|---|
| $N_0$ | Lymph nodes clinically uninvolved |
| $N_1$ | Lymph nodes clinically enlarged but not histologically involved |
| $N_2$ | Lymph nodes clinically nonpalpable but histologically involved |
| $N_3$ | Lymph nodes clinically enlarged and histologically involved |

| | |
|---|---|
| $M_0$ | No visceral disease |
| $M_1$ | Visceral disease present |

| | |
|---|---|
| $B_0$ | No circulating atypical cells <1000 (Sézary cells) |
| $B_1$ | Circulating atypical cells >1000 (Sézary cells) |

#### Stage Groupings

| | | | |
|---|---|---|---|
| IA | $T_1$ | $N_0$ | $M_0$ |
| IB | $T_2$ | $N_0$ | $M_0$ |
| IIA | $T_{1-2}$ | $N_1$ | $M_0$ |
| IIB | $T_3$ | $N_{0-1}$ | $M_0$ |
| IIIA | $T_4$ | $N_0$ | $M_0$ |
| IIIB | $T_4$ | $N_1$ | $M_0$ |
| IVA | $T_{1-4}$ | $N_{2-3}$ | $M_0$ |
| IVB | $T_{1-4}$ | $N_{0-3}$ | $M_1$ |

TABLE 33-4  Cutaneous B-cell Lymphoma Prognostic Index (CBCL-PI)

| CBCL-PI Group | Histology | Site | 5-Year Survival (%) | | Adjusted Risk of Death | | |
|---|---|---|---|---|---|---|---|
| | | | Overall | Relative | HR | 95% CI | P |
| IA | Any indolent | Any | 81 | 94 | 1.0 | | |
| IB | Diffuse large B-cell | Favorable | 72 | 86 | 1.3 | 0.99–1.7 | 0.6 |
| II | Diffuse large B-cell Immunoblastic diffuse large B-cell | Unfavorable Favorable | 8 | 60 | 2.1 | 1.6–2.7 | <.0001 |
| III | Immunoblastic diffuse large B-cell | Unfavorable | 27 | 34 | 4.5 | 2.8–7.2 | <.0001 |

Model is adjusted for age, gender, race, year of diagnosis, confirmed B-cell lineage, surveillance, epidemiology, and end results historic tage, and treatment with radiation.
Abbreviations: HR-Hazard ratio; CBCL PI-cutaneous B-cell lymphoma prognostic index.
Indolent histologies include follicular, marginal zone, small lymphocytic not otherwise specified, and lymphoplasmacytic.
Favorable skin sites include head/neck and upper extremity.
Unfavorable skin sites include trunk, lower extremity, and disseminated.
Smith BD, Smith GL, Cooper DL, Wilson LD. The cutaneous B-cell lymphoma prognostic index: a novel prognostic index derived from a population based registry. J Clin Oncol 23:3390–3395;2005.

## Therapy-CTCL

The discussion for the purpose of this chapter will focus on the use of radiotherapy, but it is important to recognize that a variety of modalities may be of use in the management of patients with cutaneous lymphomas. Generally, therapy for CTCL is divided into "skin directed therapy" versus "systemic therapy" which is generally reserved for more advanced disease. Skin directed therapy for patients with disease that is limited to the skin can be very effective with high rates of remission. For patients with localized disease, long-term survival exceeds 85% and can be achieved with any one of a variety of modalities, radiotherapy being the most effective. Skin directed therapy that is most often used in the management of mycosis fungoides includes: radiotherapy, mechlorethamine (nitrogen mustard), carmustine (BCNU), topical steroids, topical rexinoids (bexarotene gel), psoralen plus ultraviolet A light (PUVA), and ultraviolet B light (UVB). Systemic therapies generally include: interferon, retinoides, rexinoids (bexarotene), denileukin diftitox (ONTAK-recombinant fusion protein that is comprised of interleukin-2 and diptheria toxin), chemotherapy, extracorporeal photopheresis (ECP), high-dose chemotherapy with autologus or allogeneic bone marrow/stem cell transplant, new investigational agents, and combinations of the above. (Table 33-5)

TABLE 33-5  Therapeutic Modalities for Mycosis Fungoides*

**Topical**
Steroids
Radiotheapy (localized and total skin electron beam)
Bexarotene gel (Targretin)
Mechlorethamine (Nitrogen Mustard)
Carmustine (BCNU)
Psoralen + UVA light
UVB light

**Systemic**
Rexinoids (Bexarotene/Targretin)
Retinoids
Interferon
Denileukin Diftitox (Ontak)
Extracorporeal Photochemotherapy (ECP)
Chemotherapy

*Combinations are sometimes utilized together or in sequence.

It is important to keep in mind, especially in the case of topical therapy, that maintenance treatment may be necessary to offer a patient continued clearance of lesions. This is very important following the use of total skin electron beam (TSEBT) for example.

## Localized Radiotherapy

Radiotherapy for patients with CTCL can either be localized with a single field directed at the lesion or lesions on the skin, a combination of several localized fields, or the more technically challenging TSEBT. Radiotherapy is the single most effective therapy for eradication of either localized or diffuse cutaneous lymphoma. It is also an extremely effective palliative modality for patients with ulceration, tumors, nodal and visceral involvement. When localized fields are utilized for skin lesions, it may be appropriate to use electrons or superficial/orthovoltage energies. When using electrons, "bolus" material should be applied to the skin surface to ensure the appropriate dose. Often, the dosimetric plan will prescribe to the 90% isodose curve to ensure more homogeneous coverage of the lesion. Size and depth of the "bolus" material will be dependent on the energy of electrons that are suitable for the treatment of the particular lesion. Field design is straightforward and typically the field is designed with a 2-3-centimeter margin around cutaneous abnormalities. This margin will allow for adequate coverage given potential constriction of the electron beam within tissue and for appropriate coverage of any subclinical disease in the skin. Typical doses that are used range between 30-36 Gy generally in 2 Gy fractions. Local radiotherapy has been successful and well tolerated. Complete response rates are generally above 90% and there may be a dose response.[16,17] In the series by Wilson et al, the complete response rate was 97% for those patients receiving doses of > 20Gy and 5-year local control was 75%. Cotter reported no local failures in a small group of patients treated to dose greater than 30 Gy. Side effects of this treatment generally include minimal fatigue, dermatitis, erythema, and mild discomfort within the treatment field.

## Total Skin Electron Beam Therapy (TSEBT)

Total skin electron beam therapy is a technically complicated modality but has been used with great success in the management of patients with CTCL.[18] The technique should be performed in centers with significant experience, and a quality assurance program is important to ensure beam homogeneity, consistency, appropriate dose distribution, and proper clinical setup so that optimum results can be achieved. Given lack of experience at most centers and technical challenges associated with TSEBT, patients are generally offered other modalities first and TSEBT is often held in reserve for failure of more logistically straightforward modalities. TSEBT was first described by Trump and in 1960, the Stanford group published the TSEBT linear accelerator based method of delivery. Currently, the most well documented method for TSEBT delivery is a 6-field "Stanford" technique. At Yale, six fields are utilized (anterior-posterior, right posterior oblique, left posterior oblique, right anterior oblique, left anterior oblique, and a posterior anterior). The entire skin is treated over 2 treatment days which constitute a "cycle", and this cycle is performed two times per week over 4 treatment days. Boosts to the perineum (1 Gy daily to a total of 20 Gy via orthovoltage) and soles of feet (1 Gy daily to a total of 18 Gy via orthovoltage) are offered, as are ad hoc boosts to regions of tumor formation (2 Gy per day to 10-20 Gy via orthovoltage). The prescription dose is 36 Gy given over the course of 36 fractions with treatment of the AP, RPO, and LPO fields on the first day of a cycle, and the PA, LAO, and RAO are treated on the final day of the cycle. Each cycle provides a total of 2 Gy to the total skin via a 6MeV electron beam at a distance of 3.8 meters utilizing a dual gantry angle beam technique. The effective beam energy at the patient surface is 3.9 MeV.[18,19]

**FIGURE 33-2** TSEBT positions.

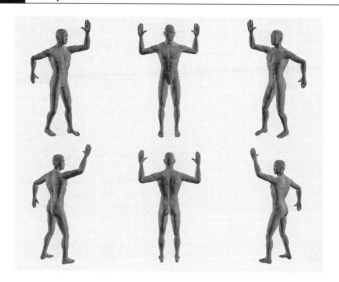

Clinical results for TSEBT are excellent for patients with T1 and T2 level disease with complete response rates in excess of 80%. Complete response rate for those with T3 disease (tumors) approaches 70% (includes supplemental boosts), and in the range of 30%–75% for those with erythroderma (Table 33-6).

**FIGURE 33-3** TSEBT depth dose curve.

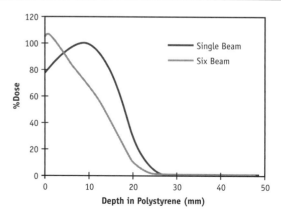

TABLE 33-6 Complete Total Skin Electron Beam Response Rates by Stage for Mycosis Fungoides Patients Who are Newly Diagnosed (CR-complete response)

| Stage | CR rate | Progression-free survival rate (2.5 yr)* |
|-------|---------|------------------------------------------|
| IA    | 95%     | 68%                                      |
| IB    | 88%     | 41%                                      |
| IIA   | 85%     | 18%                                      |
| IIB   | 75%     | 42%                                      |
| III   | 75%     |                                          |

*Data from the Hamilton Regional Cancer Center, Dr. Glenn Jones.

TSEBT can be repeated in patients who fail subsequent therapies and is safe if appropriately fractionated as described.

After patients have achieved a complete response via TSEBT, a maintenance program with either PUVA or mechlorethamine is recommended, and retrospective data from Yale and Stanford support this therapeutic philosophy in an effort to enhance disease-free survival.

There is no clear evidence to support the combination of TSEBT and other modalities with respect to overall survival benefit but this is often done. For those with T4 disease, TSEBT with ECP either during or following the TSEBT course may provide benefit with respect to progression free and cause specific survival (after adjustment for blood involvement and stage) and is extremely well tolerated.

---

**BOX 33-5**

These two studies demonstrate that repeating the course of TSEBT can be done safely and efficaciously. In the Yale study of 14 patients, the complete response rates for the second course were as good as the first course with 86% of patients achieving a complete response (93% after initial course). In the Stanford study, the second course provided a 40% complete response rate.

Patients should be considered for a second course of TSEBT when they have exhausted other modalities, have a documented excellent response to the initial course, have a long disease-free interval, and have recurred with diffuse disease.

Wilson LD, Quiros PA, Kolenik SA, et al. Additional courses of total skin electron beam therapy in the treatment of patients with recurrent cutaneous T-cell lymphoma. J Am Acad Dermatol 1999;35:69–73.

Becker M, Hoppe RT, Knox S. Multiple courses of high dose total skin electron beam therapy in the management of mycosis fungoides. Int J Radiat Oncol Biol Phys 1995;32:1445–1449.

---

**BOX 33-6**

This paper was the first to demonstrate a key advantage for maintenance therapy following TSEBT. At Yale, there has been a bias toward using PUVA as an adjuvant and the Stanford group later demonstrated that nitrogen mustard could also be used for the same purpose. Total of 39 T1 and 75 T2 patients were managed with TSEBT and 6 T1 and 8 T2 patients received adjuvant PUVA. There was no difference in overall survival for those who received PUVA following TSEBT versus those who did not, but for those who received PUVA, the disease-free survival at 5 years was 85%, and only 50% for those in the non-PUVA group (p < 0.02). For those with T2 disease, the failure rates were 25% and 55% respectively with disease-free survivals of 60 months (median not yet reached in the PUVA group) and 20 months (p < 0.03). The 5-year disease-free survival for those who were salvaged with PUVA was 50%.

Quiros PA, Jones GW, Kacinski BM, et al. Total skin electron beam therapy followed by adjuvant psoralen/ultraviolet-A light in the management of patients with T1 and T1 T-cell lymphoma (mycosis fungoides). Int J Radiat Oncol Biol Phys 1997;38:1027–1035.

## BOX 33-7

This study reconfirms the advantage of adjuvant therapy following TSEBT. A total of 55 patients with T2 disease received TSEBT with or without nitrogen mustard as an adjuvant. Following a complete response to TSEBT, those who received nitrogen mustard had a longer freedom from relapse which approached significance (p = 0.068). Additionally, both TSEBT and nitrogen mustard were effective as salvage therapies. There was no benefit in overall survival for those who received nitrogen mustard as an adjuvant following TSEBT.

Chinn DM, Chow S, Kim YH, et al. Total skin electron beam with or without adjuvant topical nitrogen mustard or nitrogen mustard alone as initial treatment of T2 and T3 mycosis fungoides. *Int J Radiat Oncol Biol Phys* 1999;43:951–958.

## BOX 33-8

Although this study has limitations of being retrospective and including relatively small numbers of patients, the addition of extracorporeal photopheresis either before, during or after TSEBT, was associated with an improvement in disease-free survival and cause-specific survival (p = 0.024 and p = 0.048 respectively) in a multivariate model with adjustment for blood involvement and stage. The combination is very well tolerated and the addition of ECP does not add any toxicity to that already associated with a standard course of TSEBT.

Wilson LD, Jones GW, Kim D, et al. Experience with total skin electron beam therapy in combination with extracorporeal photopheresis in the management of patients with erythrodermic (T4) mycosis fingoides. *J Am Acad Dermatol* 2000;43:54–60.

The sequelae of total skin electron beam are relatively well tolerated and such effects can be minimized with the fractionation and dosing as recommended in this chapter. There should be no significant bone marrow toxicity, but patients will experience a variety of skin-related effects. (Table 33-7)

### Therapy-CBCL

CBCL presents in a variety of histologic forms and clinical presentations. The more indolent forms such as marginal zone or follicle center cell tend to be associated with an excellent prognosis despite whichever therapeutic modality is selected. Treatment approaches for localized disease include observation, excision, and localized radiotherapy. The techniques for radiotherapy are similar to those for localized CTCL but doses are slightly higher in the range of 36-40 Gy in 2 Gy daily fractions. Effects of treatment are also similar to those seen in the management of CTCL. Patients with diffuse large cell histology present an interesting dilemma, as many experts believe that such patients should be managed with combined modality therapy in a similar fashion to those with diffuse large cell histology involving lymph nodes. There is no clear evidence to suggest that a combined approach will yield superior outcomes for those with diffuse large cell histology on the head and neck or trunk and if a solitary lesion, radiotherapy alone may be considered. If on the lower extremity (or if diffuse large cell lymphoma-leg type according to the WHO-EORTC), given the less favorable outcome, combined modality therapy may be utilized. If this is the

TABLE 33-7 **Common Side Effects of Total Skin Electron Beam Therapy**

Erythema of skin
Hyperpigmentation
Alopecia
Change/loss of nails
Edema of lower extremities
Hypohydrosis
Xerosis
Blisters
Atrophy

TABLE 33-8 Cutaneous B-cell Lymphoma Radiotherapy Series

|  |  | Pts | Dose | CResp | 5-yr RFS |
|---|---|---|---|---|---|
| Santucci | 1991 | 83 | 40 | 100 | <50 |
| Piccinno | 1993 | 31 | 10–40 | 100 | 41(2-yr) |
| Rijlaarsdam | 1996 | 40 | 30–40 | 100 | 85(2-yr) |
| Kirova | 1999 | 25 | 30–40 | 92 | 75 |
| Eich | 2003 | 35 | 27–54 | 100 | 50 |
| Piccinno | 2003 | 104 | 14–35 | 100 | 23 |
| Smith | 2004 | 34 | 20–48 | 100 | 55 |

CResp-complete response
Pts-number of patients

case, often systemic chemotherapy such as cyclophosphamide, adriamycin, vincristine, prednisone (CHOP) is incorporated into the treatment plan with radiotherapy following the completion of systemic therapy. Doses in the range of 30-40 Gy are recommended. The role of rituximab (Rituxan) in CBCL is unclear, but there are a variety of small series and anecdotal reports supporting its use both as a primary therapy and as part of a combined modality treatment program. Total skin electron beam has generally not been used in the management of patients with widespread CBCL or cutaneous involvement related to a nodal lymphoma given the success of systemic therapy regimens, lack of supporting data, and potential for enhanced toxicity as an adjuvant to adriamycin based chemotherapy.

The results for localized radiotherapy for CBCL are encouraging although it should be noted that most of the patients reported in the series had more indolent type histologies. The complete response rate is in excess of 90% with appropriate doses of radiotherapy and the 5-year relapse free survival is approximately 50% for those with localized disease.[20-26]

## CONCLUSION

The cutaneous lymphomas, both CTCL and CBCL present challenging clinical scenarios for the treating physician and patient. There is a relative lack of data compared to the nodal lymphomas and a paucity of phase III data. It is clear, however, that radiotherapy plays an important role in patients with CTCL and CBCL with localized disease and can afford excellent complete response rates regardless of histologic subtype with relatively few side effects. Additionally, since the clinical findings are skin-based, there are substantial psycho-social ramifications for patients with cutaneous lymphoma, and radiotherapy plays a critically essential role in palliation. For those patients with widespread mycosis fungoides or its variants, TSEBT can be an excellent definitive therapy whether provided as first line or as salvage and should be strongly considered for those patients in need of rapid palliation when they have failed other modalities.

## REFERENCES

4. Veness MJ, Palme CE, Smith M, Cakir B, Morgan GJ, Kalnins I. Cutaneous head and neck squamous cell carcinoma metastatic to cervical lymph nodes (nonparotid): a better outcome with surgery and adjuvant radiotherapy. *Laryngoscope.* 2003;113:1827-1833.

5. Ballo MT, Ang KK. Radiotherapy for cutaneous malignant melanoma: rationale and indications. *Oncology (Williston Park).* 2004;18:99-107.

6. Schmid-Wendtner MH, Brunner B, Konz B et al. Fractionated radiotherapy of lentigo maligna and lentigo maligna melanoma in 64 patients. *J Am Acad Dermatol.* 2000;43:477-482.

7. Ballo MT, Ross MI, Cormier JN et al. Combined-modality therapy for patients with regional nodal metastases from melanoma. *Int J Radiat Oncol Biol Phys.* 2006;64:106-113.

8. Habermalz HJ, Fischer JJ. Radiation therapy of malignant melanoma: experience with high individual treatment doses. *Cancer.* 1976;38:2258-2262.

9. Poulsen M. Merkel-cell carcinoma of the skin. *Lancet Oncol.* 2004;5:593-599.

10. Allen PJ, Bowne WB, Jaques DP, Brennan MF, Busam K, Coit DG. Merkel cell carcinoma: prognosis and treatment of patients from a single institution. *J Clin Oncol.* 2005;23:2300-2309.

11. Decker RH, Wilson LD. Role of radiotherapy in the management of merkel cell carcinoma of the skin. *J Natl Compr Canc Netw.* 2006;4:713-718.

12 Smith BD, Smith GL, Cooper DL, Wilson LD. The cutaneous B-cell lymphoma prognostic index: a novel prognostic index derived from a population-based registry. *J Clin Oncol.* 2005;23: 3390-3395.

13. Willemze R, Jaffe ES, Burg G et al. WHO-EORTC classification for cutaneous lymphomas. *Blood.* 2005;105:3768-3785.

14. Girardi M, Heald PW, Wilson LD. The pathogenesis of mycosis fungoides. *N Engl J Med.* 2004;350:1978-1988.

15. Foss FM, Edelson RL, Wilson LD. Cutaneous Lymphoma. In: Devita VT, Lawrence TS, Rosenberg SA, eds. *Principles and Practice of Oncology.* Philadelphia: Lippincott; 2008.

16. Cotter GW, Baglan RJ, Wasserman TH, Mill W. Palliative radiation treatment of cutaneous mycosis fungoides—a dose response. *Int J Radiat Oncol Biol Phys.* 1983;9:1477-1480.

17. Wilson LD, Kacinski BM, Jones GW. Local superficial radiotherapy in the management of minimal stage IA cutaneous T-cell lymphoma (mycosis fungoides). *Int J Radiat Oncol Biol Phys.* 1998;40:109-115.

18. Chen Z, Agostinelli AG, Wilson LD, Nath R. Matching the dosimetry characteristics of a dual-field Stanford technique to a customized single-field Stanford technique for total skin electron therapy. *Int J Radiat Oncol Biol Phys.* 2004;59:872-885.

19. Jones GW, Kacinski BM, Wilson LD et al. Total skin electron radiation in the management of mycosis fungoides: consensus of the European Organization for Research and Treatment of Cancer (EORTC) Cutaneous Lymphoma Project Group. *J Am Acad Dermatol.* 2002;47:364-370.

20. Santucci M, Pimpinelli N, Arganini L. Primary cutaneous B-cell lymphoma: a unique type of low-grade lymphoma. Clinicopathologic and immunologic study of 83 cases. *Cancer.* 1991;67: 2311-2326.

21. Piccinno R, Caccialanza M, Berti E, Baldini L. Radiotherapy of cutaneous B cell lymphomas: our experience in 31 cases. *Int J Radiat Oncol Biol Phys.* 1993;27:385-389.

22. Rijlaarsdam JU, Toonstra J, Meijer OW, Noordijk EM, Willemze R. Treatment of primary cutaneous B-cell lymphomas of follicle center cell origin: a clinical follow-up study of 55 patients treated with radiotherapy or polychemotherapy. *J Clin Oncol.* 1996;14:549-555.

23. Kirova YM, Piedbois Y, Le Bourgeois JP. Radiotherapy in the management of cutaneous B-cell lymphoma. Our experience in 25 cases. *Radiother Oncol.* 1999;52:15-18.

24. Piccinno R, Caccialanza M, Berti E. Dermatologic radiotherapy of primary cutaneous follicle center cell lymphoma. *Eur J Dermatol.* 2003;13:49-52.

25. Eich HT, Eich D, Micke O et al. Long-term efficacy, curative potential, and prognostic factors of radiotherapy in primary cutaneous B-cell lymphoma. *Int J Radiat Oncol Biol Phys.* 2003;55:899-906.
26. Smith BD, Glusac EJ, McNiff JM et al. Primary cutaneous B-cell lymphoma treated with radiotherapy: a comparison of the European Organization for Research and Treatment of Cancer and the WHO classification systems. *J Clin Oncol.* 2004;22:634-639.

# 34

# Hodgkin Lymphoma

*Joachim Yahalom, MD*

## Epidemiology and Risk Factors

In the year 2007, approximately 8,000 new cases of Hodgkin Lymphoma (HL) will be diagnosed in the United States. Over the past four decades, advances in radiation therapy and the advent of combination chemotherapy have tripled the cure rate of patients with HL. In 2008, more than 80% of all newly diagnosed patients can expect a normal, disease-free life span.

Pertinent epidemiological facts about HL include:

- **Gender**—Male-to-female ratio of HL is 1.3:1.0.
- **Age**—The age-specific incidence of the disease is bimodal, with the greatest peak in the third decade of life and a second, smaller peak after the age of 50 years.
- **Race**—Lower in African-Americans (2.3 cases per 100,000 persons) than in Caucasians (3.0 per 100,000 persons).
- **Geography**—The age-specific incidence of HL differs markedly in various countries. In Japan, the overall incidence is low and the early peak is absent. In some developing countries, there is a downward shift of the first peak into childhood.

## Etiology and risk factors

The cause of HL remains unknown, and there are no well-defined risk factors.

- **Familial factors**—Have a role, but its magnitude is unknown. The monozygotic twin sibling of a patient with HL has a 99 times higher risk of developing HL than a dizygotic twin sibling of a patient with HL and same-sex siblings of patients with HL have a 10 times higher risk for the disease. Patient-child combinations are more common than spouse pairings.
- **Socio-economic**—More common with higher socio-economic background. Higher risk for HL is associated with few siblings, single-family houses, early birth order, and fewer playmates; all of which decrease exposure to infectious agents at an early age.
- **Viruses**—The Epstein-Barr virus (EBV) has been implicated in the etiology of HL by both epidemiologic and serologic studies, as well as by the detection of the EBV genome in 20%–80% of tumor specimens. There have been no conclusive studies regarding the possible increased frequency of HL in patients with human immunodeficiency virus (HIV) infection. However,

HL in HIV-positive patients is associated more commonly with an advanced-stage and less favorable therapeutic outcome.

## DIAGNOSIS

- **Biopsy**—The initial diagnosis of HL can only be made by biopsy. Incisional or core biopsy is required and needle aspiration is inadequate because the architecture and adequate immunostaining of the lymph node is important for diagnosis and histological sub classification.
- **The Reed-Sternberg (R-S) cell**—The diagnostic tumor cell that must be identified within the appropriate cellular milieu of lymphocytes, eosinophils, and histiocytes. The R-S cell is characterized by its large size and classic binucleated structure with large eosinophilic nucleoli. Two antigenic markers are thought to provide diagnostic information: CD30 and CD15. These markers are present on R-S cells in "classical" HL, but not in the less common type of HL called lymphocyte predominance HL LPHL.

## CLASSIC HL SUBTYPES (95% OF CASES)

- **Nodular sclerosis**—The most common subtype. It is typically seen in young adults (more commonly in females) who have early-stage supradiaphragmatic presentations.
- **Mixed Cellularity**—Is the second most common histology. It is more often diagnosed in males, who usually present with generalized lymphadenopathy or extra nodal disease and with associated systemic symptoms.
- **Lymphocyte Rich Classical Hodgkin Lymphoma**—Relatively uncommon (4%) with features of classical HL and lymphocyte predominant HL and an excellent prognosis.
- **Lymphocyte Depletion**—Rarely seen in current practice.

## LYMPHOCYTE-PREDOMINANT HL (5% OF CASES)

- **Histology**—This is an infrequent form of HL in which few R-S cells or their variants may be identified. The cellular background consists primarily of lymphocytes in a nodular or sometimes diffuse pattern. The R-S variants express a B-cell phenotype (CD20-positive, CD15-negative).
- **Clinical features**—Lymphocyte-predominant HL is often localized, involves peripheral lymph nodes and not the mediastinum. Bulky disease and B symptoms are rare. It is usually treated effectively with radiation alone, and may relapse late (a clinical feature reminiscent of low-grade lymphoma). The 15-year disease-specific survival is excellent (> 90%).

## STAGING

The staging system is detailed in Table 34-1.

### FAVORABLE OR UNFAVORABLE EARLY-STAGE HL

Most recent studies in Stage I/II disease distinguish between favorable and unfavorable early-stage disease, according to the European Organization for Research and Treatment of Cancer (EORTC) definitions outlined in table 34-2.

### CLINICAL EVALUATION AND WORKUP

- **Commonly involved lymph nodes**
  More than 80% of patients with HL present with lymphadenopathy above the diaphragm, often involving the anterior mediastinum; the spleen may be involved in about 30% of patients. Less than 10%–20% of patients present with lymphadenopathy limited to regions below the diaphragm. The commonly involved peripheral lymph nodes are located in the

---

**TABLE 34-1 The Cotswold's Staging Classification for Hodgkin Lymphoma**

**Stage Description**
- **Stage I**
    Involvement of a single lymph node region or lymphoid structure
- **Stage II**
    Involvement of two or more lymph node regions on the same side of the diaphragm (the mediastinum is a single site, hilar lymph nodes are lateralized). The number of anatomic sites should be indicated by a subscript (II2).
- **Stage III**
    Involvement of lymph node regions or structures on both sides of the diaphragm
- **Stage IV**
    Involvement of extra nodal site(s) beyond that designated E

**Designations applicable to any disease stage**
A—   No symptoms
B—   Fever, drenching sweats, weight loss
X—   Bulky disease
    $>1/3$ the width of the mediastinum
    $>10$ cm maximal dimension of nodal mass
E—   Involvement of a single extra nodal site, contiguous, or proximal to a known nodal site
CS—  Clinical stage
PS—  Pathologic stage

---

cervical, supraclavicular, and axillary areas; para-aortic pelvic and inguinal areas are involved less frequently.
- **Extra nodal involvement**
HL may affect extra nodal tissues by direct invasion (contiguity; the so-called E lesion) or by hematogenous dissemination (Stage IV disease). The most commonly involved extra nodal site is the lung. Liver, bone marrow, and bone may also be involved.
- **B symptoms**
About one third of patients will have B symptoms. In each anatomic stage, the presence of B symptoms is an adverse prognostic indicator and may affect treatment choices. B symptoms are carefully defined in the staging system. Unexplained fever should be $> 38°C$ (100°F) and recurrent during the previous month, night sweats should be drenching and recurrent and unexplained weight loss should be significant only if $> 10\%$ of body weight has been lost within the preceding 6 months. Pruritus and, less commonly, pain in involved regions after ingestion of alcohol are not considered B symptoms.

---

**TABLE 34-2 EORTC Prognostic Definition of Early-stage Disease**

- **Favorable** CS I and II (maximum 3 involved areas) and $< 50$ years *and* ESR $< 50$ mm/h (no B symptoms) *or* ESR $< 30$ mm/h (B symptoms present) *and* MT ratio $< 0.33$
- **Unfavorable** CS II $\geq 4$ nodal areas involved *or* age $\geq 50$ years *or* ESR $\geq 50$ mm/h (no B symptoms) *or* ESR $\geq 30$ mm/h (B symptoms present) *or* MT ratio $\geq 0.33$

CS = Cotswold's staging; EORTC = European Organization for Research and Treatment of Cancer; ESR = erythrocyte sedimentation rate; MT = mediastinal/thoracic

- **Laboratory studies**

  Studies should include a CBC with WBC differential and platelet count, erythrocyte sedimentation rate (ESR), tests for liver and renal function, and assays for serum alkaline phosphatase and lactate dehydrogenase (LDH). A moderate to marked leukemoid reaction and thrombocytosis are common, particularly in symptomatic patients, and usually disappear with treatment. The ESR may provide helpful prognostic information. At some centers, treatment programs for patients with early-stage disease are influenced by the degree of ESR elevation. In addition, changes in the ESR following therapy may correlate with response and relapse.

  Abnormalities of liver function studies should prompt further evaluation of that organ, with imaging and possible biopsy. An elevated alkaline phosphatase level may be a nonspecific marker, but it may also indicate bone involvement that should be appropriately evaluated by a radionuclide bone scan and directed skeletal radiographs.

- **Imaging studies**

  Imaging studies should include a chest X-ray and CT scan of the chest, abdomen, and pelvis with IV contrast. FDG PET scan will provide important information on the extent of disease, serves as a baseline for evaluation of response to treatment, and is highly recommended. Radionuclide bone scan, MRI of the chest or abdomen, and CT scan of the neck are contributory only under special circumstances.

  The thoracic CT scan details the status of intrathoracic lymph node groups, the lung parenchyma, pericardium, pleura, and chest wall. Since the chest CT scan may remain abnormal for a long time after the completion of therapy, the evaluation of pretreatment involvement and response to therapy is assisted by the use of an FDG-PET scan.[1]

- **Bone marrow biopsy**

  Bone marrow involvement is relatively uncommon, but because of the impact of a positive biopsy on further staging and treatment, unilateral bone marrow biopsy should be part of the staging process of patients with Stage IIB disease or higher.

## Treatment

HL is sensitive to radiation and many chemotherapeutic drugs, and, in most stages, there is more than one effective treatment option. Disease stage is the most important determinant of treatment options and outcome. All patients, regardless of stage, can and should be treated with curative intent.

## TREATMENT OF EARLY-STAGE (STAGES I–II) HL

- **The preferred treatment—combined modality[2]**

  The treatment of choice for favorable and unfavorable early-stage classic HL is brief chemotherapy followed by involved-field radiotherapy (IFRT).[3] Most of the experience that yielded excellent treatment results with low toxicity was with ABVD (Adriamycin [doxorubicin], bleomycin, vinblastine, and dacarbazine) for four cycles and IFRT of 30 to 36 Gy. Table 34-3 summarizes data from randomized studies that reported on the combination of short chemotherapy (four or even only two cycles) followed by IFRT. The three top randomized studies have also indicated that adding extended-field radiotherapy to chemotherapy is not necessary and the small involved field is adequate. The most recent (and as yet not fully mature) excellent results are with shortening the duration of chemotherapy to only two cycles of ABVD in favorable patients and reducing the IFRT dose to 20 Gy (GHSG HD10). If the excellent results obtained by the German Hodgkin's Study Group prevail with additional follow-up, brief ABVD and low-dose IFRT will become the standard of care for favorable early-stage HL.[4]

**TABLE 34-3** Studies Comparing Involved Field Radiation with Extended Radiation in Combined Modality Programs for Favorable and Unfavorable Early-Stage HL

| Study (Years) | Treatment Regimens | FFTF or RFS | | OS |
|---|---|---|---|---|
| Milan[5] | ABVD (4) + STLI | 97% | | 93% (5) |
| (133 pts) | ABVD (4) + IFRT | 94% | | 94% |
| | | NS | | NS |
| GHSG HD[6] | COPP/ABVD (4) + EFRT | | 86% | 91% (5) |
| (1064 pts) | COPP/ABVD (4) + IFRT | | 84% | 92% |
| | | NS | | NS |
| EORTC/GELA H8U[7] | MOPP/ABV (6) + IFRT | 94% | | 90% (4) |
| (995 pts) | MOPP/ABV (4) + IFRT | 95% | | 95% |
| | MOPP/ABV (4) + STLI | 96% | | 93% |
| | | NS | | NS |

Abbreviations: EFRT—extended-field radiotherapy; IFRT—involved-field radiotherapy; STLI—subtotal lymphoid irradiation; The numbers in parenthesis represent the years of disease-free survival results.

**TABLE 34-4** Chemotherapeutic Regimens Used for the Treatment of Hodgkin Lymphoma

| Regimen | Dosage and Schedule | Frequency |
|---|---|---|
| **MOPP** | | |
| Mechlorethamine | 6 mg/m$^2$ IV on day 1 | |
| Oncovin | 1.4 mg/m$^2$ IV on day 1 and day 8 (maximum dose, 2.0 mg) | |
| Procarbazine | 100 mg/m$^2$ PO on days 1-7 | Repeat cycle every 28 days |
| Prednisone[a] | 40 mg/m$^2$ PO ON DAYS 1-14 | |
| **ABVD** | | |
| Adriamycin | 25 mg/m$^2$ IV on days 1 and 15 | |
| Bleomycin | 10 mg/m$^2$ IV on days 1 and 15 | |
| Vinblastine | 6 mg/m$^2$ IV on days 1 and 15 | Repeat cycle every 28 days |
| Dacarbazine | 375 mg/m$^2$ IV on days 1 and 15 | |
| **BEACOPP** | | |
| Bleomycin | 10 mg/m$^2$ IV on day 8 | |
| Etoposide | 100 mg/m$^2$ (200 mg/m$^2$)d IV on days 1–3 | |
| Adriamycin | 25 mg/m$^2$ (35 mg/m$^2$)[d] IV on day 1 | |
| Cyclophosphamide | 650 mg/m$^2$ (1,200 mg/m$^2$)[d] IV on day 1 | |
| Oncovin | 1.4 mg/m$^{2e}$ IV on day 8 | |
| Procarbazine | 100 mg/m$^2$ PO on days 1–7 | |
| Prednisone | 40 mg/m$^2$ PO on days 1–4 | Repeat cycle every 21 days |
| G-CSF from day 8 | | |

*(continues)*

**TABLE 34-4 (continued)**

| Regimen | Dosage and Schedule | Frequency |
|---|---|---|
| **Stanford V** | | |
| Doxorubicin | 25 mg/m$^2$ IV on days 1 and 15 | Repeat cycle every |
| Vinblastine[b] | 6 mg/m$^2$ IV on days 1 and 15 | 28 days for a |
| Mechlorethamine | 6 mg/m$^2$ IV on day 1 | total of 3 cycles |
| Vincristine[b] | 1.4 mg/m$^2$ IVc on days 8 and 22 | Radiotherapy to |
| Bleomycine | 5 U/m$^2$ IV on days 8 and 22 | initial sites $\geq$ 5 cm |
| Etoposide | 60 mg/m$^2$ IV on days 15 and 16 | (dose: 36 Gy) |
| Prednisone | 40 mg/m$^2$ PO every other day (maximum dose, 2.0 mg) | |

[a] In the original report, prednisone was given only in cycles 1 and 4.
[b] Vinblastine dose decreased to 4 mg/m$^2$ and vincristine dose to 1 mg/m$^2$ during cycle 3 for patients $\geq$50 years of age.
[c] Tapered by 10 mg every other day starting at week 10.
[d] Increased dose for BEACOPP.
[e] Maximal dose of 2 mg.
G-CSF = granulocyte colony-stimulating factor.

## SUBTOTAL LYMPHOID IRRADIATION (STLI)

Irradiation of the mantle and para-aortic fields, termed STLI, was the standard treatment in the past and remains an adequate alternative treatment of clinically or pathologically staged favorable (non-bulky and without B symptoms) early-stage HL (stage I/II). Yet, STLI is no longer the treatment of choice due to the risk of second tumors and (to a lesser degree) coronary artery disease in long-term survivors of extensive radiotherapy alone as practiced in the past. In classic (non–lymphocyte predominant) HL, subtotal lymphoid irradiation is adequate for patients who are not candidates for a chemotherapy-containing strategy.

## CHEMOTHERAPY ALONE

Some claim that chemotherapy alone is a reasonable option for patients with favorable early-stage HL.[8] Several groups have already tested the hypothesis that chemotherapy alone could provide equivalent disease control to that achieved with combined-modality therapy. The studies targeted mostly early-stage favorable and unfavorable patients and were conducted in adults, children and adolescents, or in both. In some, the randomization was upfront; in others, it was limited to patients who achieved a clear complete response (CR) with chemotherapy. The results are summarized in Table 34-5.

All studies (with the exception of the small MSKCC study) showed a significantly superior EFS or freedom-from-progression when radiation was added to chemotherapy. Only in the study with the longest follow-up (8 years), superior initial disease control has translated into a significantly better overall survival. In HL, most randomized studies have not been able to document a significant survival advantage for the superior disease control arm, even when one arm was clearly more effective (CALGB study of MOPP vs. ABVD vs. MOPP/ABVD or the stem cell salvage trials) and thus was accepted as the standard treatment. There are many reasons for this phenomenon: good salvage for failures, long survival with disease, and (but not only) possibly more toxic events in the more effective arm. To make a conclusion based on survival in HL, follow-up that is longer and more complete than most study groups currently provide is necessary.

**TABLE 34-5 Randomized Studies Comparing Combined Modality to Chemotherapy Alone**

| | Stage | Treatment Program | EFS or FFP (%) | P | OS P | Comments |
|---|---|---|---|---|---|---|
| CCG 5942[9] (501 pts) | I-IV (I-II 68%) | COPP/ABV × 4-6 Same + IF 21Gy | 85* 93* | .02* | NS 3 yrs | No-RT arm closed early (many relapses) |
| Mumbay[10] (251 pts) | I-IV (I-II 55%) | ABVD × 6 ABVD × 6 + IF 30Gy | 76 88 | .01 | 0.02 8 yrs | |
| EORTC/GELA H9F[11] (489 pts) | I-II Favorable | EBVP × 6 EBVP × 6 + IF 20Gy EBVP × 6 + IF 36Gy | 69 84 87 | .001 | NA 4 yrs | No-RT arm closed early (many relapses) |
| NCIC/ECOG HD6[12] (276 pts) | I-II Unfavorable, but no B, or bulky | ABVD × 4–6 ABVD × 2 + STLI | 88 95 | .004 | NS 5 yrs | Designed for OS evaluation @12 yrs |
| MSKCC[13] (152 pts) | I-III A/B Non-bulky | ABVD × 6 ABVDx6 + EF/IF | 81 86 | NS | 0.08 5 yrs | Not powered to detect differences <20% |

CCG, Children's Cancer Group; EFS, Event-free Survival; FFP, Freedom-from Progression; NA, not available; EBVP' epirubicin, bleomycin, vinblatine, and prednisone; NCIC, National Institute of Canada; ECOG, Eastern Cooperative Oncology Group; NS, not significant; MSKCC, Memorial Sloan-Kettering Cancer Center; EF, extended-field; IF, involved-field
*Analyzed as treated

The inferior results with chemotherapy alone, the need to increase the number of chemotherapy courses in order to substitute for radiotherapy and the excellent results with short chemotherapy and mini-radiotherapy make chemotherapy alone less desirable and at this point is not accepted as the standard of care.[14]

**BOX 34-1**

The most important recent study of patients with favorable early-stage HL is the HD 10 study of the GHSG. It was designed to test how far the treatment may be reduced. One thousand three hundred and seventy patients with favorable early-stage HL were randomized upfront into four arms: ABVD × 4 or ABVD × 2, and each chemotherapy group was further randomized for treatment to be followed by IFRT of either 30 Gy or 20 Gy. At a median follow-up of 5 years, FFTF was similar in all groups—92%, and overall survival was 96%. Reducing chemotherapy appeared safe, and, at this point, there was no difference between the excellent results of the two different RT doses (30 Gy vs. 20 Gy). The current GHSG study for favorable patients (HD 13) is testing the exclusion of bleomycin and dacarbazine from the shorter chemotherapy regimen, while maintaining IFRT at 30 Gy.

Behringer K, Diehl V: Twenty-five years clinical trials of the German Hodgkin Study Group (GHSG). *Eur J Haematol Suppl*:21–25, 2005.

## TREATMENT OF PATIENTS WITH *UNFAVORABLE* EARLY-STAGE HL

Most patients in this common category will have disease Stage I–II disease with either bulky mediastinum and/or B symptoms (see Table 34-2 for all other factors). The standard treatment consists of chemotherapy followed by involved field radiotherapy. Different chemotherapy regimens are considered effective and there are no reported significant differences between them. Most commonly used in the United States are ABVD ×4–6 and Stanford V (See details in Table 34-4). In Europe BEACOPP is often used. Radiation therapy is limited to the involved field. Stanford V regimen includes radiotherapy to all sites that were initially ≥ 5cm. Many who use ABVD limit IFRT to the bulky site(s). The dose is 30–36 Gy.

---

**BOX 34-2**

The HD11 study of the GHSG targeted patients with unfavorable early-stage and randomized them to either ABVD × 4 or bleomycin, etoposide, doxorubicin, cyclophosphamide, vincristine, procarbazine and predisone (BEACOPP) × 4, either program was followed by either 20 Gy or 30 Gy to the involved field. The interim analysis at 2 years has not shown a difference between the arms with FTTF of 90%. At this point, it appears that BEACOPP has no advantage over ABVD, is more toxic, confers no advantage over ABVD. It is too early to reduce the IFRT dose below 30 Gy in bulky disease patients.

Behringer K, Diehl V: Twenty-five years clinical trials of the German Hodgkin Study Group (GHSG). *Eur J Haematol Suppl*:21–25, 2005.

---

## Lymphocyte-Predominant Hodgkin Lymphoma (LPHL)

Most (>75%) patients with LPHL present at an early stage; the disease is commonly limited to one peripheral site (neck, axilla, or groin) and involvement of the mediastinum is extremely rare.[15] The treatment recommendations for LPHL differ markedly from those for classic HL. In both North America and Europe the guidelines recommend *involved-field radiation alone* as the treatment of choice for early-stage LPHL.[2] It should be emphasized that even if regional radiation fields are selected, the uninvolved mediastinum should not be irradiated, thus avoiding the site most prone for radiation-related short- and long-term side effects. Although there has not been a study that compared extended-field RT (commonly used in the past) with involved field RT, retrospective data suggest that involved-field is adequate. The radiation dose recommended is between 30 to 36 Gy with an optional additional boost of 4 Gy to a (rare) bulky site. Patients with advanced-stage and/or B symptoms (rare) are treated with combined modality therapy.

## Advanced-Stage HL

In this category, patients with Stage III and IV are included. The commonly used prognostic factors for this group are described in Table 34-6.

Patients with 0–3 poor prognostic factors had a 5-year freedom from progression (FFP) of 70% and an overall survival of 83%, while patients with >4 prognostic factors had 47% and 59%, respectively.[16] The most commonly used effective regimens for advanced-stage patients are ABVD X6, Stanford V and standard and escalated BEACOPP (see Table 34-4).

**TABLE 34-6  International Prognostic Factors (1998) Used for Advanced-stage HL**

- Age ≥ 45
- Male sex
- Stage IV
- Hemoglobin < 10.5 g/dlL
- Serum Albumin < 4.0 g/dL
- Leukocytosis ≥ 15 × 10$^9$/L
- Lymphocytopenia < 0.6 × 10$^9$/L or 8% of the WBC

## Role of Radiation in Advanced-Stage HL

Although the role of consolidation radiotherapy after induction chemotherapy remains controversial, irradiation is often added in patients with advanced stage HL who present with bulky disease or remain in uncertain complete remission after chemotherapy. Retrospective studies have demonstrated that adding low-dose radiotherapy to all initial disease sites after chemotherapy induced complete response, decreases in the relapse rate by ~25%, and significantly improved overall survival. Interpretation of the impact of radiation in prospective studies has been controversial. However, a Southwest Oncology Group (SWOG) randomized study of 278 patients with Stage III or IV Hodgkin's disease suggested that the addition of low-dose irradiation to all sites of initial disease after a complete response to MOP-BAP (mechlorethamine, Oncovin [vincristine], prednisone, bleomycin, Adriamycin [doxorubicin], and procarbazine) chemotherapy improves remission duration in patients with advanced-stage disease. An intention-to-treat analysis showed that the advantage of combined-modality therapy was limited to patients with nodular sclerosis.[17] No survival differences were observed. A meta-analysis of several randomized studies demonstrated that the addition of radiotherapy to chemotherapy reduces the rate of relapse but did not show survival benefit for combined-modality compared to chemotherapy alone.[18]

More recently, EORTC reported the results of a randomized study that evaluated the role of IFRT in patients with Stage III/IV Hodgkin's disease who obtained a CR after MOPP/ABV.[19] Patients received six or eight cycles of MOPP/ABV chemotherapy (number of cycles depended upon the response). Patients who did not receive a CR (only 40% of patients) were not randomized to receive chemotherapy and received IFRT. Of the 418 patients who reached a CR, 85 patients were not randomized to receive treatment for various reasons. A total of 161 patients were randomized to receive no RT and 172 patients were randomized to receive IFRT. The authors concluded that IFRT does not improve the treatment results in patients with Stage III/IV Hodgkin's disease who reached a CR after six to eight courses of MOPP/ABV chemotherapy. The 5-year overall survival rates were 91% and 85%, respectively ($P=0.07$). The data indicated that in comparison with chemotherapy alone, there were more cases of leukemia second tumors on the CR combined modality, but surprisingly not on the PR combined-modality arm. In partial responders after six cycles of MOPP/ABV, the addition of IFRT yielded overall survival and event-free survival rates that were similar to those obtained in CR to chemotherapy patients. Among the 250 patients in partial remission after chemotherapy, the 5-year event-free and overall survival rates were 79% and 87%, respectively. The EORTC study has several limitations that detract from its applicability to many advanced-stage patients. First, a relatively small fraction of patients were determined to be in CR and thus eligible for randomization on the study. The regimen of MOPP/ABV $\times$ 6–8 is quite toxic and this regimen is no longer used in North America. Second, only few patients with bulky disease were randomized on the EORTC study. Lastly, the claim that added RT caused more secondary malignancies on the combined modality has not been evident in patients with PR receiving even higher doses of RT to multiple areas after MOPP/ABV.

The only randomized study questioning the role of consolidation RT after CR to ABVD $\times$ 6 (the most common regimen currently used for advance-stage HL) was performed at Tata medical center in India. The study included patients of all stages, but almost half were Stage III and IV. A subgroup analysis of the advanced-stage patients showed a statistically significant improvement of both 8-year event-free survival and 8-year overall survival with added RT compared to ABVD alone (EFS 78% vs. 59%; p<0.03 and OS 100% vs. 80%; p<0.006).

When advanced-stage HL is treated with the new highly effective and less toxic treatment program of Stanford V, it is imperative to follow the brief chemotherapy program with involved field radiotherapy to sites originally larger than 5 cm or to a clinically involved spleen. When radiotherapy was fully of partially omitted on this program the results were inferior.

In summary, patients in CR after full dose chemotherapy program like MOPP/ABV may not need RT consolidation. Yet, patients with bulky disease, or with incomplete or uncertain CRp or patients treated on brief chemotherapy programs will benefit from involved field RT to originally bulky or residual disease.

## SAVAGE PROGRAMS FOR REFRACTORY AND RELAPSED HL

High-dose therapy supported by autologous stem cell transplantation (ASCT) has become a standard salvage treatment for patients who relapsed or remained refractory to chemotherapy or to combined-modality therapy. Many of the patients who enter these programs have not received prior radiotherapy or have relapsed at sites outside the original radiation field. These patients could benefit from integrating radiotherapy into the salvage regimen.

Poen and colleagues from Stanford analyzed the efficacy and toxicity of adding cytoreductive (pre-transplant; n=18) or consolidative (post-transplant; n=6) RT to 24 of 100 patients receiving high-dose therapy. This study showed that most (69%) relapses after ASCT occurred in sites known to be involved immediately before transplantation.[21] When these sites were irradiated prior to transplantation, no in-field failures occurred. While only a trend in favor of IF-RT could be shown for the entire group of transplanted patients, for patients with Stages I–III, freedom from relapse was significantly improved. Limiting the analysis to patients who received no prior RT also resulted in a significant advantage to IF-RT. Fatal toxicity in this series was not influenced significantly by IF-RT.

At MSKCC, we developed a program that integrated RT into the high-dose regimen for salvage of HD.[22] We scheduled accelerated hyperfractionated irradiation (b.i.d. fractions of 1.8 Gy each) to start after the completion of re-induction chemotherapy and stem cell collection and prior to the high-dose chemotherapy and stem cell transplantation. Patients who had not been previously irradiated received involved field RT (18 Gy in 5 days) to sites of initially bulky (>5cm) disease and/or residual clinical abnormalities followed by total lymphoid irradiation (TLI) of 18 Gy (1.8 Gy per fraction, b.i.d.) within an additional 5 days. Patients who had prior RT received only involved-field RT (when feasible) to a maximal dose of 36 Gy. This treatment strategy has been in place since 1985 with more than 350 patients treated thus far. The first generation program demonstrated the feasibility and efficacy of the high-dose combined modality regimen resulting in an event-free survival of 47% for the patients receiving TLI followed by cyclophosphamide-etoposide chemotherapy. The recent report of the second generation two-step high-dose chemoradiotherapy program indicated that after a median follow-up of 34 months, the intent-to-treat event-free survival and overall survival were 58% and 88%, respectively. For patients who underwent transplantation, the event-free survival was 68%. Treatment-related mortality was 3% with no treatment-related mortality over the last 8 years. The results of this treatment program in refractory patients were similar to those of relapsed patients. Both groups showed favorable event-free survival and overall survival compared to most recently reported series. Most failures in this salvage program occurred in either unirradiated extranodal sites or in nodal sites that could not be further irradiated. The pattern of failure may suggest that the extensive use of nodal irradiation in our program contributed to its overall success. A recently reported study from Chicago comparing TLI-containing salvage regimen to a chemotherapy only regimen demonstrated a significantly improved outcome in the TLI/chemotherapy treated group.[23]

## RADIATION FIELDS: PRINCIPLES AND DESIGN

In the past, radiation-fields design attempted to include multiple involved and uninvolved lymph node sites. The large fields known as "mantle," "inverted Y," and "total lymphoid irradiation (TLI)" were synonymous with the radiation treatment of HL. These fields should rarely be used nowadays. The involved-field, or its slightly larger version—the regional field—encompasses a significantly smaller, but adequate volume when radiotherapy is used as consolidation after chemotherapy in HL. Even when radiation is used as the only treatment (early-stage follicular, marginal zone and lymphocyte predominant HL), the field should be limited to the involved site or to the involved sites and immediately adjacent lymph node groups. Further, even more limited radiation fields restricted to the originally involved lymph node, are currently under study by several European groups.

The many terminologies given to radiation field variations in HL caused significant confusion and difficulties in comparing treatment programs. While the final determination of the field may vary from patient to patient and depends on many clinical, anatomic and normal tissue tolerance considerations, general definitions and guidelines are available and should be followed.[24]

The following are definitions of types of radiation fields used in HL:

## Involved Field

This field is limited the site of the clinically involved lymph node group (Figure 34-1). For extra-nodal sites—the field includes the organ alone (if no evidence for lymph node involvement). The "grouping" of lymph nodes is not clearly defined, and involved field borders for common presentation of HL will be discussed below.

## Regional Field

This field includes the involved lymph node group field plus at least one adjacent clinically uninvolved group (Figure 34-1). For extranodal disease, it includes the involved organ plus the clinically uninvolved lymph nodes region.

---

**FIGURE 34-1** Radiation fields used in Hodgkin lymphoma.

### Involved Field

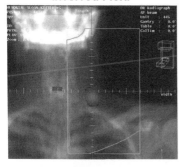

### Mantle

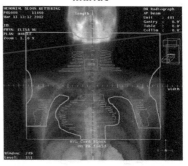

### Regional Field

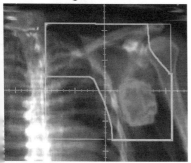

### Inverted Y

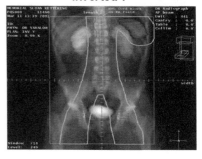

## Extended Field

This field includes multiple involved and uninvolved lymph node groups. If the multiple sites are limited to one side of the diaphragm, the upper field is called the *mantle* field (Figure 34-1). The extended field that includes all lymph nodes sites below the diaphragm (with or without the spleen) is called after its shape—*inverted Y* (Figure 34-1).

When radiation treatment includes all lymph nodes on both sides of the diaphragm, these large areas are combined, the resulting field is called *total lymphoid irradiation (TLI)* or *total nodal irradiation (TNI)*, if the pelvic lymph nodes are excluded the field is called *sub-total lymphoid irradiation (STLI)*.

## Involved Lymph Node(s) Field [25]

This is the most limited radiation field that has just recently been introduced. The clinical treated volume (CTV) includes only the originally involved lymph node(s) volume (pre-chemotherapy) with the addition of 1-cm margin to create planned treatment volume (PTV) (Figure 34-2).

## Suggested Guidelines for Delineating the Involved Field to Nodal Sites[24]

1. IFRT is treatment of a region, not of an individual lymph node.
2. The main involved field nodal regions are: neck (unilateral), mediastinum (including the hilar regions bilaterally), axilla (including the supraclavicular and infraclavicular lymph nodes), spleen, para-aortic lymph nodes, inguinal (including the femoral and iliac nodes).
3. In general, the field includes the involved pre-chemotherapy sites and volume, with an important exception that involves the transverse diameter of the mediastinal and para-

---

**FIGURE 34-2** Involved lymph node radiotherapy. An example of patients with involvement of lymph node in the left neck and the determination of the filed extent based on the pre-chemotherapy lymph node size.

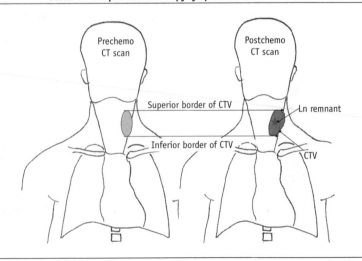

aortic lymph nodes. For the field width of these sites, it is recommended to use the reduced post-chemotherapy diameter. In these areas, the regression of the lymph nodes is easily depicted by CT imaging and the critical normal tissue is saved by reducing the irradiated volume.

4. The supraclavicular lymph nodes are considered part of the cervical region and, if involved alone or with other cervical nodes, the whole neck is unilaterally treated. Only if the supraclavicular involvement is an extension of mediastinal disease and the other neck areas are not involved (based on CT imaging with contrast and gallium/PET imaging, when appropriate) the upper neck (above the larynx) is spared. This is to save on irradiating the salivary glands when the risk for the area is low.

5. All borders should be easy to outline (most are bony landmarks) and plan on with a 2-D standard simulation unit. CT data are required for outlining the mediastinal and para-aortic region and will also help in designing the axillary field.

6. Pre-chemotherapy and post-chemotherapy information (both CT and PET) regarding lymph node localization and size is critical and should be available at the time of planning the field.

## Involved Field Guidelines for Common Nodal Sites

### I. Unilateral Cervical/Supraclavicular Region

Involvement at any cervical level with or without involvement of the supraclavicular (SCL) nodes.

Arm position: akimbo or at sides. *Upper Border:* 1–2 cm above the lower tip of the mastoid process and midpoint through the chin. *Lower Border:* 2 cm below the bottom of the clavicle. *Lateral Border:* To include the medial two thirds of the clavicle. *Medial Border:* a) If the supraclavicular nodes are not involved, the border is placed at the ipsilateral transverse processes except when medial nodes close to the vertebral bodies are seen on the initial staging neck CT scan. For medial nodes, the entire vertebral body is included. b) When the supraclavicular nodes are involved, the border should be placed at the contra-lateral traverse processes. For Stage I patients, the larynx and vertebral bodies above the larynx can be blocked (assuming no medial cervical nodes). *Blocks:* A posterior cervical cord block is required only if cord dose exceeds 40 Gy. Mid-neck calculations should be performed to determine the maximum cord dose, especially when the central axis is in the mediastinum. A laryngeal block should be used unless lymph nodes were present in that location. In that case the block should be added at 20 Gy (Figure 34-1).

### II. Bilateral Cervical/Supraclavicular Region

Both cervical and supraclavicular regions should be treated as described above regardless of the extent of disease on each side. Posterior cervical cord and larynx blocks should be used as described above. Use a posterior mouth block if treating the patient supine (preferably with an extended travel couch at greater than 100 cm FSD) to block the upper field divergence through the mouth (Figure 34-1).

### III. Mediastinum

Involvement of the mediastinum and/or the hilar nodes: In HL, this field includes also the medial SCL nodes even if not clinically involved. In NHL, the volume is limited to the mediastinum.

Arm position: akimbo or at sides. The arms up position is optional if the axillary nodes are involved. *Upper Border:* C5–C6 interspace. If supraclavicular nodes were also involved, the upper border should be placed at the top of the larynx and the lateral border should be adjusted as described in the section on treating neck nodes. *Lower Border:* The lower of: a) 5 cm below the carina or b) 2 cm below the *pre-chemotherapy* inferior border. *Lateral Border:* The *post-chemotherapy* volume with 1.5-cm margin. *Hilar Area:* To be included with 1-cm margin unless initially involved where as the margin should be 1.5 cm.

### IV. Mediastinum with Involvement of the Cervical Nodes

When both cervical regions are involved, the field is a mantle without the axilla, using the guidelines described above. If only one cervical chain is involved in the vertebral bodies, contralateral upper neck and larynx can be blocked as previously described. Because of the increased dose to the neck (the isocenter is in the upper mediastinum), the neck above the lower border of the larynx should be shielded at 30.6 Gy. If paracardiac nodes are involved, the whole heart should be treated to 14.4 Gy, and the initially involved nodes should be treated to 30.6 Gy (Figure 34-1).

### V. Axillary Region

The ipsilateral axillary, infraclavicular, and supraclavicular areas are treated when the axilla is involved. Whenver possible, use CT-based planning for this region. Arms akimbo or arms up. *Upper Border:* C5–C6 interspace. *Lower Border:* The lower of the two of: a) the tip of the scapula or b) 2 cm below the lowest axillary node. *Medial Border:* Ipsilateral cervical transverse process. Include the vertebral bodies only if the SCL are involved. *Lateral Border:* Flash axilla.

### VI. Spleen

The spleen is treated only if abnormal imaging was suggestive of involvement. The *post-chemotherapy* volume is treated with 1.5-cm margins.

### VII. Abdomen (Paraaortic Nodes)

*Upper Border:* Top of T11 and at least 2 cm above pre-chemotherapy volume. *Lower Border:* Bottom of L4 and at least 2 cm below pre-chemotherapy volume. *Lateral Borders:* The edge of the transverse processes and at least 2 cm from the post-chemotherapy volume.

### VIII. Inguinal/Femoral/External Iliac Region

These ipsilateral lymph node groups are treated together if any of the nodes are involved.

*Upper Border:* Middle of the sacro-iliac joint. *Lower Border:* 5 cm below the lesser trochanter *Lateral Border:* The greater trochanter and 2 cm lateral to initially involved nodes. *Medial Border:* Medial border of the obturator foramen with at least 2 cm medial to involved nodes. If common iliac nodes are involved, the field should extend to the L4–L5 interspace and at least 2 cm above the initially involved nodal border.

## SIDE EFFECTS AND SUPPORTIVE CARE

Side effects of radiotherapy depend on the irradiated volume, dose administered, and technique employed. They are also influenced by the extent and type of prior chemotherapy, if any, and by the patient's age. Today, most of the information that we use to estimate risk of radiotherapy is derived from strategies that used radiation alone. The field size and configuration, doses and technology have all changed drastically over the last decade; thus it is probably misleading to judge current radiotherapy for HL and inform patients solely on the basis this of different past practice of using radiotherapy in treating HL.

## Acute Effects

Radiation, in general, may cause fatigue and areas of the irradiated skin may develop mild sun-exposure-like dermatitis. The acute side effects of irradiating the full neck include mouth, dryness change in taste, and pharyngitis. These side effects are usually mild and transient. The main potentia side effects of subdiaphragmatic irradiation are loss of appetite, nausea, and increased bowel movements. These reactions are usually mild and can be minimized with standard antiemetic medications.

Irradiation of more than one field, particularly after chemotherapy, can cause myelosuppression, which may necessitate short treatment interruption and very rarely administration of G-CSF, erythropoietin type drugs or platelet transfusion.

## Early Side Effects

### Lhermitte's sign

Fewer than 5% of patients may note an electric shock sensation radiating down the backs of both legs when the head is flexed (Lhermitte's sign) 6 weeks to 3 months after mantle-field radiotherapy. Possibly secondary to transient demyelinization of the spinal cord, Lhermitte's sign resolves spontaneously after a few months and is not associated with late or permanent spinal cord damage.

### Pneumonitis and pericarditis

During the same period, radiation pneumonitis and/or acute pericarditis may occur in < 5% of patients; these side effects occur more often in those who have extensive mediastinal disease. Both inflammatory processes have become rare with modern radiation techniques.

## Supportive Care During Treatment

It is important to prepare the patient for the potential side effects, and many organizations and cancer centers also provide written patient information regarding radiotherapy of lymphomas. Since some level of mouth dryness is often associated with radiotherapy that involves the upper neck and/or lower mandible and mouth, attention to dental care is advised. If dryness is a concern, it is advised to arrange for an expert dental appointment for overall dental evaluation and consideration of mouth guards (from scatter) and/or supplemental fluoride treatment during and after radiotherapy.

Soreness of the throat and mild to moderate difficulty of swallowing solid and dry food may also occur during neck irradiation at a dose of approximately 20 Gy. These side effects are almost always mild, self-limited, and subside shortly after completion of radiotherapy. Skin care with use of sun screen is advised for all patients undergoing radiotherapy. Temporary hair loss is expected in irradiated areas and recovery is observed after several months.

We normally recommend a first post-RT follow-up visit 6 weeks after the end of treatment and obtain post-RT baseline blood count, standard biochemistry test, as well as TSH levels and lipid profile (if applicable) at that visit. Follow-up imaging studies normally commence 3 months after completion of treatment. Other follow-up studies are included in the NCCN guidelines for HL.

## Late Side Effects

### Subclinical Hypothyroidism

Irradiation of the neck and/or upper mediastinum can induce subclinical hypothyroidism in about one third of patients. This condition is detected by elevation of thyroid-stimulating hormone (TSH). Thyroid replacement with levothyroxine (T4) is recommended, even in asymptomatic patients, to prevent overt hypothyroidism and decrease the risk of benign thyroid nodules.

### Infertility

Only irradiation of the pelvic field may have deleterious effects on fertility. In most patients, this problem can be avoided by appropriate gonadal shielding. In females, the ovaries can be moved into a shielded area laterally or inferomedially near the uterine cervix. Irradiation outside of the pelvis does not increase the risk of sterility.

### Secondary Malignancies

Hodgkin's disease patients who were cured with radiotherapy and/or chemotherapy have an increased risk of secondary solid tumors (most commonly, lung, breast, and stomach cancers, as well as melanoma), and NHL 10 or more years after treatment. Unlike MOPP and similar chemotherapy combinations or etoposide, radiotherapy for Hodgkin's disease is not leukemogenic.

#### Lung cancer

Patients who are smokers should be strongly encouraged to quit the habit because the increase in lung cancer that occurs after irradiation or chemotherapy has been detected mostly in smokers.

#### Breast cancer

For women whose HD was successfully treated at a young age, the main long-term concern is the increased risk of breast cancer.[26] During the last decade, multiple studies have documented and characterized the risk of breast cancer after HD and have established that the increase in breast cancer risk is undoubtedly associated with the use of radiation.[27–29] The magnitude of risk is not completely clear and different methods of risk reporting and data are found in the literature with relative risk ratios from 2 to 450.[26,30] Unfortunately, RR, absolute risk and actuarial risks are often cited without detailing specifics that could have influenced the findings (length of follow-up for the group and for the individuals; age group, age-incidence and actuarial risk of the malignancy in an untreated population; and quality of follow-up, which may result in event overestimation).[28] The largest long-term follow-up study of second neoplasms in survivors of HD, which included data from 16 cancer registries of more than 35,000 patients, revealed that the RR for breast cancer in women was 2 and the absolute excess risk (AER) was 10.5.[26]

The increase in breast cancer risk is inversely related to the patient's age at Hodgkin's disease treatment; no increased risk has been found in women irradiated after 30 years of age. It is also inversely related to the radiation dose to the breast and the volume of breast tissue exposed.[27,28] In a recent study, Travis and colleagues from 13 centers in 7 countries reported a large case-control study that included 105 women who developed breast cancer within a cohort of more than 3,800 1-year female survivors of HD diagnosed at age 30 or less.[28] Unique to this study is the use of patients who received a very low radiation dose (less than 4 Gy) or no radiation to the breast area where breast cancer developed. This approach allowed isolating treatment factors and analyzing the radiation dose and chemotherapy dose-risk relationships. For all patients who received RT alone ($\geq$4 Gy) the relative risk (RR) of breast cancer is 3.2 and increases to 8 in the highest radiation dose group. The results reported by Travis et al clearly demonstrate the influence of radiation dose on the risk of breast cancer. Within the range of doses to which the breast was exposed in past years, more radiation translates into a higher risk of developing breast cancer. This information, as well as data from earlier publications showing a significantly lower risk of second tumors when radiation was reduced from 40 Gy to 20 Gy, support the notion that "lower is better" as long as the radiation dose used augments HD cure rate.

Radiotherapy alone had been the standard treatment and primary curative modality for HD through the 1970s and early 1980s. Irradiating all lymph node regions, regardless of clinical involvement with HD, has been standard practice, and relatively high doses (over 40 Gy) have been used. Consequently, a substantial amount of breast tissue has been exposed to either the full prescribed dose or to an attenuated dose (at field margins or under the lung shields) in almost all women irradiated for HD. Most breast exposure in the "mantle" era, resulted from the radiation of the axillae (65% of tumors in this study developed in the outer part of the breast), and to a lesser extent from wide mediastinal and hilar irradiation. Approximately two thirds of women with early-stage HD do not require radiation of the axillae, and additional protection to the upper and medial aspects of the breast could be provided by further reducing field size using careful CT-based planning that usually allows for smaller mediastinal volumes, especially post-chemotherapy. During the last decade, reduction in field size has been the most important change in radiation therapy of HD. Reduction in the volume of exposed breast tissue together with dose reduction (from over 40 Gy to a dose in the range of 20–30 Gy) is likely to dramatically change the long-term risk profile of young male and female patients cured of HD. Emerging data from trials using smaller fields and lower doses support the expectation that the modern application of "mini-radiotherapy" will be associated with a significantly lower risk of breast cancer as well as other solid tumors and cardiac sequela.[6,32–34] Yet, longer follow-up of studies that employ smaller fields and lower doses is necessary.

Breast cancer is curable in its early stages, and early detection has a significant impact on survival. Breast examination should be part of the routine follow-up for women cured of Hodgkin's disease, and routine mammography should begin about 8 years after treatment.

### Coronary Artery Disease

An increased risk of coronary artery disease among patients who have received mediastinal irradiation has recently been reported. To reduce this hazard, patients should be monitored and advised about other established coronary disease risk factors, such as smoking, hyperlipidemia, hypertension, and poor dietary and exercise habits. There are data supporting the notion that reduced fields and lower doses to the mediastinum have reduced the risk of heart disease in irradiated patients.[33,35]

### Effects on Bone and Muscle Growth

In children, high-dose irradiation will affect bone and muscle growth and may result in deformities. Current treatment programs for pediatric Hodgkin's disease are chemotherapy-based; radiotherapy is limited to low doses.

## REFERENCES

1. Hutchings M, Loft A, Hansen M, et al. FDG-PET after two cycles of chemotherapy predicts treatment failure and progression-free survival in Hodgkin lymphoma. *Blood* 107:52–59, 2006.
2. Hoppe RT, al. NCCN physician guidelines: Hodgkin Disease 2006 v.1, www.nccn.org, 2006.
3. Yahalom J. Favorable early-stage Hodgkin lymphoma. *J Natl Compr Canc Netw* 4:233–240, 2006.
4. Behringer K, Diehl V. Twenty-five year clinical trials of the German Hodgkin Study Group (GHSG). *Eur J Haematol* Suppl:21–25, 2005.
5. Bonadonna G, Bonfante V, Viviani S, et al. ABVD plus subtotal nodal versus involved-field radiotherapy in early-stage Hodgkin's disease: long-term results. *J Clin Oncol* 22:2835–2841, 2004.
6. Engert A, Schiller P, Josting A, et al. Involved-field radiotherapy is equally effective and less toxic compared with extended-field radiotherapy after four cycles of chemotherapy in patients with early-stage unfavorable Hodgkin lymphoma: results of the HD8 trial of the German Hodgkin Lymphoma Study Group. *J Clin Oncol* 21:3601–3608, 2003.
7. Ferme C, Eghbali H, Hagenbeek A, et al. MOPP/ABV hybrid and irradiation in unfavorable supradiaphragmatic clinical stages I-II Hodgkin's disease: comparison of three treatment modalities. Preliminary results of the EORTC-GELA H8-U randomized trial in 995 patients. *Blood* 96:A576, 2000.

8. Canellos GP. Chemotherapy alone for early Hodgkin lymphoma: an emerging option. *J Clin Oncol* 23:4574–4576, 2005.

9. Nachman JB, Sposto R, Herzog P, et al. Randomized comparison of low-dose involved-field radiotherapy and no radiotherapy for children with Hodgkin's disease who achieve a complete response to chemotherapy. *J Clin Oncol* 20:3765–3771, 2002.

10. Laskar S, Gupta T, Vimal S, et al. Consolidation radiation after complete remission in Hodgkin's disease following six cycles of doxorubicin, bleomycin, vinblastine, and dacarbazine chemotherapy: is there a need? *J Clin Oncol* 22:62–68, 2004.

11. Noordijk E, Thomas J, Ferme C, et al. First results of the EORTC-GELA H9 randomized trials: the H9-F trial (comparing 3 radiation dose levels) and H9-U trial (comparing 3 chemotherapy schemes) in patients with favorable or unfavorable early-stage Hodgkin lymphoma (HL). *J Clin Oncol* 21 (supp 1):Abstract # 6506, 2005.

12. Meyer RM, Gospodarowicz MK, Connors JM, et al. Randomized comparison of ABVD chemotherapy with a strategy that includes radiation therapy in patients with limited-stage Hodgkin lymphoma: National Cancer Institute of Canada Clinical Trials Group and the Eastern Cooperative Oncology Group. *J Clin Oncol* 23:4634–4642, 2005.

13. Straus DJ, Portlock CS, Qin J, et al. Results of a prospective randomized clinical trial of doxorubicin, bleomycin, vinblastine, and dacarbazine (ABVD) followed by radiation therapy (RT) versus ABVD alone for stages I, II, and IIIA nonbulky Hodgkin disease. *Blood* 104:3483–3489, 2004.

14. Yahalom J. Don't throw out the baby with the bathwater: on optimizing cure and reducing toxicity in Hodgkin lymphoma. *J Clin Oncol* 24:544–548, 2006.

15. Diehl V, Sextro M, Franklin J, et al. Clinical presentation, course, and prognostic factors in lymphocyte-predominant Hodgkin's disease and lymphocyte-rich classical Hodgkin's disease: report from the European Task Force on Lymphoma Project on Lymphocyte-Predominant Hodgkin's Disease. *J Clin Oncol* 17:776–783, 1999.

16. Hasenclever D, Diehl V. A prognostic score for advanced Hodgkin's disease. International Prognostic Factors Project on Advanced Hodgkin's Disease. *New England Journal of Medicine* 339:1506–1514, 1998.

17. Fabian C, Mansfield C, Dahlberg S, et al. Low-dose involved field radiation after chemotherapy in advanced Hodgkin's disease. *Ann Intern Med* 120:903–912, 1994.

18. Loeffler M, Brosteanu O, Hasenclever D, et al. Meta-analysis of chemotherapy versus combined modality treatment trials in Hodgkin's disease. International Database on Hodgkin's Disease Overview Study Group. *Journal of Clinical Oncology* 16:818–829, 1998.

19. Aleman BM, Raemaekers JM, Tirelli U, et al. Involved-field radiotherapy for advanced Hodgkin lymphoma. *N Engl J Med* 348:2396–2406, 2003.

20. Aleman BM, Raemaekers JM, Tomisic R, et al. Involved-field radiotherapy for patients in partial remission after chemotherapy for advanced Hodgkin lymphoma. *Int J Radiat Oncol Biol Phys* 67:19–30, 2007.

21. Poen JC, Hoppe RT, Horning SJ. High-dose therapy and autologous bone marrow transplantation for relapsed/refractory Hodgkin's disease: the impact of involved field radiotherapy on patterns of failure and survival. *International Journal of Radiation Oncology, Biology, Physics* 36:3–12, 1996.

22. Yahalom J, Gulati SC, Toia M, et al. Accelerated hyperfractionated total-lymphoid irradiation, high-dose chemotherapy, and autologous bone marrow transplantation for refractory and relapsing patients with Hodgkin's disease. *J Clin Oncol* 11:1062–1070, 1993.

23. Evens A, Altman J, Mittal B, et al. Phase I/II trial of total lymphoid irradiation and high-dose chemotherapy with autologous stem-cell transplantation for relapsed and refractory Hodgkin lymphoma. *Ann Oncol*, 2007.

24. Yahalom J, Mauch P. The involved field is back: issues in delineating the radiation field in Hodgkin's disease. *Ann Oncol 13 Suppl* 1:79–83, 2002.

25. Girinsky T, van der Maazen R, Specht L, et al. Involved-node radiotherapy (INRT) in patients with early Hodgkin lymphoma: concepts and guidelines. *Radiother Oncol* 79:270–277, 2006.

26. Dores GM, Metayer C, Curtis RE, et al. Second malignant neoplasms among long-term survivors of Hodgkin's disease: a population-based evaluation over 25 years. *J Clin Oncol* 20:3484–3494, 2002.

27. van Leeuwen FE, Klokman WJ, Stovall M, et al. Roles of radiation dose, chemotherapy, and hormonal factors in breast cancer following Hodgkin's disease. *J Natl Cancer Inst* 95:971–980, 2003.

28. Travis LB, Hill D, Dores GM, et al. Breast cancer following radiotherapy and chemotherapy among young women with Hodgkin's disease. *JAMA* 289, 2003.

29. Yahalom J. Breast cancer after Hodgkin disease: hope for a safer cure. *Jama* 290:529–531, 2003.

30. Bhatia S, Robison LL, Oberlin O, et al. Breast cancer and other second neoplasms after childhood Hodgkin's disease. *New England Journal of Medicine* 334:745–751, 1996.

31. Doria R, Holford T, Farber LR, et al. Second solid malignancies after combined modality therapy for Hodgkin's disease. *J Clin Oncol* 13:2016–2022, 1995.

32. Salloum E, Doria R, Schubert W, et al. Second solid tumors in patients with Hodgkin's disease cured after radiation or chemotherapy plus adjuvant low-dose radiation. *Journal of Clinical Oncology* 14:2435–2443, 1996.

33. Salloum E, Tanoue LT, Wackers FJ, et al. Assessment of cardiac and pulmonary function in adult patients with Hodgkin's disease treated with ABVD or MOPP/ABVD plus adjuvant low-dose mediastinal irradiation. *Cancer Invest* 17:171–180, 1999.

34. Chronowski GM, Wilder RB, Tucker SL, et al. Analysis of in-field control and late toxicity for adults with early-stage Hodgkin's disease treated with chemotherapy followed by radiotherapy. *Int J Radiat Oncol Biol Phys* 55:36–43, 2003.

35. Hancock SL, Tucker MA, Hoppe RT. Factors affecting late mortality from heart disease after treatment of Hodgkin's disease. *JAMA* 270:1949–1955, 1993.

# 35

# Non-Hodgkin Lymphomas

*Joachim Yahalom, MD*

## EPIDEMIOLOGY AND RISK FACTORS

In 2007, approximately 63,000 new cases of non-Hodgkin Lymphomas (NHL) were diagnosed in the United States and almost 24,000 people died from it.[1] The incidence of NHL has increased by 150% since 1950. An increase of 50% was documented between 1973 and 1988 (3%–4% increase each year). This is one of the largest increases reported for any cancer over the last two decades. The increase was more common in the elderly and in spite of improved therapies the death from this disease has also increased.

It is important to remember that NHL is a group of more than 30 lympho-proliferative malignancies with different epidemiology, natural history, treatment approaches, and outcome, and the those most relevant to the radiation oncologists will be discussed separately. Yet, some general features of the whole group are outlined below.

Pertinent epidemiological facts about NHL include:

**Gender:** Male-to-female ratio of HL is 1.5:1.0.

**Age:** NHL incidence rises exponentially with age. In persons older than 65 the incidence is 68/100,000. Burkitt's lymphoma and lymphoblastic lymphma are more common in children and young adults.

**Race:** Caucasians have a higher incidence than blacks.

**Geography:** NHL is more common in developed countries; the highest rate is in the United States, the lowest in China. Endemic geographic factors influence the risk of NHL in specific areas.

## Etiology

Human HTLV-1-associated adult T-cell lymphoma/leukemia (ATLL) occurs in areas endemic with HTLV-1 in southern Japan and the Caribbean.

Burkitt's lymphoma in Africa is associated with malaria and EBV infection. Carriers of HIV have a higher risk of developing aggressive types of NHL, particularly primary central nervous system lymphoma. The cumulative incidence of NHL among the HIV-infected population is now 5% to 10% over a decade. Molecular genetics studies indicate that more than one pathogenic mechanism is operative in HIV-associated NHL.

The presence of the bacteria *Helicobacter pylori* has been closely associated with the development of mucosa-associated lymphoid tissue (MALT), lymphoma of the stomach, and even in some cases, eradication of *H. pylori* by antibiotic treatment may result in lymphoma regression.

Several epidemiologic studies have shown that agricultural workers have a high incidence of the disease. Some researchers have attributed this to pesticide exposure. There is also suggestive evidence that hair dyes may play a role in the etiology of lymphoma. Ionizing radiation alone has little or no effect on risk of NHL, but patients with HD treated with radiation therapy and chemotherapy have an increased risk of developing secondary large-cell lymphoma.

## CYTOGENETICS AND MOLECULAR BIOLOGY

Several lymphomas are associated with non-random chromosomal abnormalities. These abnormalities often correlate with the histologic type, immunophenotype, and clinical behavior. For example, translocation t(14:18) (q32;q21) occurs commonly in follicular lymphoma. It results in the transposition of the *bcl-2* oncogene of chromosome 18 to become adjacent to the heavy chain immunoglobulin gene on chromosome 14. The *bcl-2* oncogene is essential for apoptosis or programmed cell death. The t(14:18) translocation interferes with the normal senescence and death of the follicular center cell and is possibly engaged in its malignant transformation. Most patients with Burkitt's lymphoma have translocation t(8:14) or one of its variants and *c-myc* is the relevant translocated oncogene. The *c-myc* product is an important transcription factor, and its dysregulation is probably involved in the proliferative process. Translocation t(11:14) involving *bcl-1* is characteristic of recognition of mantle cell lymphoma. The gene product of *bcl-1*, cyclin D, is directly involved in the regulation of cell division. Rearrangement of *bcl-6* has been reported in one third of patients with diffuse large-cell lymphoma. t(11:18) has been detected in 25%–40% of patients with MALT lymphoma and indicates an unlikely response of MALT lymphoma of the stomach to antibiotic therapy of an associated *H. pylori* infection.

## PATHOLOGIC CLASSIFICATION

In consideration of the clinical and histologic diversity of the lymphoid malignancies that are grouped under the generic title non-Hodgkin's lymphoma, it is crucial to obtain clear and detailed pathologic information about the biopsy specimen. An adequately processed pathologic specimen should be analyzed by a hemato-pathologist who is well versed in interpreting modern immuno-histopathologic and molecular genetics techniques required for modern diagnosis and classification of NHL.

The current classification of lymphomas is the WHO classification.[2] In Table 35-1 the more common histologies are listed by the WHO classification and are grouped as low-grade (indolent), intermediate-grade (aggressive), or high-grade (highly aggressive), a terminology that is still in clinical use.

## STAGING AND PROGNOSTIC FACTORS

Although histology is the predominant determinant of prognosis in this diverse group of lymphoid malignancies, stage remains important for selection of treatment strategy and predicting the prognosis in each histologic category. The Ann Arbor Staging Classification system, developed originally for HD, has been used also for NHL. The staging system is described in the chapter on Hodgkin Lymphoma.

This system reflects the number of sites of involvement and their relation to the diaphragm, the existence of B symptoms, and the presence of extranodal disease. Patients can be assigned a clinical stage or a pathologic stage. In NHL, most patients are staged clinically based on physical examination, imaging studies, and bone marrow biopsy. Staging laparotomy and splenectomy are rarely performed in the evaluation of patients with NHL, and a distinction between clinical stage and pathologic stage is not commonly used in NHL. The Ann Arbor staging system is considered by

TABLE 35-1 **Abridged Version of the WHO Lymphoma Classification Organized by Clinical Groups**

### Low-Grade (Indolent)

Follicular lymphoma (FL) (grades I–II)
Small lymphocytic lymphoma (SLL)
Marginal zone lymphoma (MZL): Extranodal (MALT lymphoma)
    Nodal
    Splenic
Mycosis fungoides (T-Cell lymphoma of skin)

### Intermediate-Grade (Aggressive)

Diffuse large B-cell (including immunoblastic and mediastinal B cell) lymphoma (DLBCL)
Follicular lymphoma (grade III)
Mantle cell lymphoma (MCL)
T-cell lymphomas: Peripheral T-cell lymphoma (PTCL)
    Angiocentric
    Angioimmunoblastic
    NK lymphoma
Anaplastic large cell lymphoma (ALCL)

### High-Grade (Highly Aggressive)

Lymphoblastic lymphoma
Burkitt's lymphoma
High-grade B-cell, Burkitt's-like

many to be inadequate for NHL. Furthermore, the modification of the Ann Arbor staging system (Cotswolds modification) addressed issues mostly relevant for HD but not for NHL.

## THE INTERNATIONAL PROGNOSTIC INDEX

In addition to stage, important other prognostic factors have been identified in patients with NHL.[3] These prognostic factors frequently include patient parameters such as age (less or over 60 years) and performance status as well as tumor burden indicators such as bulk (smaller or larger than 10 cm), number of involved sites (mostly extranodal), and lactate dehydrogenase (LDH) level.

An international team developed a prognostic model to predict outcome of patients with aggressive NHL (Table 35-2).

The international index (IPI) identified five significant risk factors prognostic of overall survival: age (<60 vs. <60), serum LDH (normal vs. elevated), performance status (0 or 1 vs. 2–4), stage (I or II vs. III or IV), and extranodal site involvement (0 or 1 vs. 2–4). These features were incorporated into a model that identified four groups of patients with significantly different outcome following treatment. These were determined by adding the number of adverse risk factors, thus creating low-risk (0–1 factor), low-intermediate (2 factors), high-intermediate (3 factors), and high-risk (4–5 factors) groups. The predicted 5-year survival rates for these groups were 73%, 51%, 43%, and 26%, respectively. When only patients under 60 years old were evaluated, stage, performance status, and LDH levels remained significant for poor prognosis (age-adjusted IPI). After validation by several centers, the major cooperative groups have accepted this index for the design of new protocols. The model is simple to apply, is reproducible, and predicts outcome even

**TABLE 35-2 International Prognostic Index for Aggressive NHL**

*All Patients*
- Age > 60
- Serum LDH above normal
- ECOG performance status > 2
- Ann Arbor clinical Stage III or IV
- Number of involved extranodal sites > 1

|  | IPI Score | 5-Year Survival (%) |
|---|---|---|
| Low-risk | 0–1 | 73 |
| Low-intermediate | 2 | 51 |
| High-intermediate | 3 | 43 |
| High-risk | 4–5 | 26 |

*Patients < = 60 years*
- Serum LDH above normal
- ECOG performance > 2
- Ann Arbor Stage III or IV

|  | Age-Adjusted IPI Score | 5-Year Survival (%) |
|---|---|---|
| Low-risk | 0 | 83 |
| Low-intermediate | 1 | 69 |
| High-intermediate | 2 | 46 |
| High-risk | 3 | 32 |

*Patients with Early-Stage (I–II) Disease*
- Age > 60
- Serum LDH above normal
- Stage II disease
- ECOG performance status ≥ 2

| Modified IPI Score | 10-Year Survival (%) |
|---|---|
| 0 | 90 |
| 1–2 | 56 |
| 3 | 48 |

after patients have achieved complete response. Although originally designed for aggressive lymphomas, it has been shown to be of predictive in relapsing patients undergoing salvage therapy with or without high-dose therapy and stem-cell support.

For follicular lymphoma, the follicular lymphoma international prognostic index (FLIPI) has been shown to be a valuable prognostic tool.[4] It is depicted in Table 35-3.

## ESSENTIAL WORKUP STUDIES FOR STAGING AND IPI

Table 35-4 details the essential workup of patients with NHL.
Essential and useful workup studies:

- Physical examination: attention to node-bearing areas, including Waldeyer's ring, and to size of liver and spleen
- Performance status
- B symptoms
- CBC, differential, platelets

**TABLE 35-3  The International Prognostic Index for Follicular Lymphoma**

| | | |
|---|---|---|
| | Age | ≥60 y |
| | Ann Arbor stage | III–IV |
| | Hemoglobin level | < 12 g/dL |
| | Serum LDH level | > ULN (upper limit of normal) |
| | Number of nodal sites[d] | ≥ 5 |
| **Risk group according to FLIPI chart** | | |
| | | Number of factors |
| | Low | 0–1 |
| | Intermediate | 2 |
| | High | ≥3 |

**TABLE 35-4  Radiotherapy Alone for Stage I and II Indolent Lymphomas**

| Reference | Patients, n | Stage | Relapse-free Survival, % (yr) | Overall Survival, % (yr) |
|---|---|---|---|---|
| Vaughn et al[8] | 208 | I | 47 (10) | 64 (10) |
| Suttcliffe et al[9] | 190 | I–II | 53 (12) | 58 (12) |
| MacManus[5] | 177 | I–II | 44 (15) | 40 (15) |

- LDH
- Comprehensive metabolic panel
- Uric acid
- Chest X ray, PA, and lateral
- CT of chest, abdomen, pelvis
- Unilateral or bilateral bone marrow biopsy
- FDG-PET scan

*In selected cases:*
   Neck CT
   - Head CT or MRI
   - HIV testing
   - Determination of ejection fraction: MUGA scan or echocardiogram
   - Lumbar puncture, if: paranasal sinus, testicular, parameningeal, periorbital, CNS, paravertebral, bone marrow involvement or HIV positive
   - Discussion of fertility issues and sperm banking

## THE MORE COMMON LYMPHOMAS AND THE ROLE OF RADIATION THERAPY

The types of lymphomas that are more likely to require radiation oncology attention will be discussed. Table 35-5 displays the types of HL and NHL most likely to benefit from radiation therapy.

## LOW-GRADE LYMPHOMAS

### Follicular Lymphomas

Follicular lymphomas (FL) are the most common types of lymphoma in the United States. These closely related entities constitute together as much as 35% of adult NHL; the incidence is apparently lower in other parts of the world. This is a disease of adults with a median age of 59 years

**TABLE 35-5 Indications for Radiotherapy in the Treatment of Lymphomas**

*Radiation Alone—Potentially Curative*
- Hodgkin lymphoma—Lymphocyte Predominance Stage I–II
- Hodgkin lymphoma—Classical* Stage IA–IIA (non-bulky)
  - ° Combined modality is treatment of choice
- Follicular lymphoma Stage I–II Stage III (rarely used)
- Extranodal marginal zone (MALT) lymphoma Stage IE-IIE
- Nodal marginal zone lymphoma Stage I–II
- Mycosis fungoides Stage IA, IB, IIA
- Anaplastic large cell lymphoma of skin Stage IE

*Radiation is Part of a Potentially Curable Combined Modality Program*
- Hodgkin lymphoma—Classical Stage I–II (favorable and unfavorable)
- Hodgkin lymphoma Advanced Stage

- For bulky sites, incomplete response, and as part of brief chemotherapy program (Stanford V)
- Diffuse large B-cell lymphoma Stage I–II
- Primary mediastinal lymphoma Stage I–II
- Peripheral T-cell lymphoma Stage I–II
- Extranodal NK/ T-cell lymphoma-nasal type
- Primary CNS lymphoma
- In high-dose therapy programs for Hodgkin lymphoma, diffuse large B-Cell lymphoma, follicular lymphoma, and mantle cell lymphoma

*Radiation is Effective for Palliation and Local Control*
Highly Sensitive
- Follicular lymphoma
- Mantle cell lymphoma
- Small lymphocytic lymphoma/ CLL
- Marginal zone lymphoma
- Mycosis fungoides
Moderately Sensitive
- Diffuse large cell lymphoma

and male to female ratio of 1:1.7. Follicular lymphomas, particularly of grade I, constitute a very favorable prognostic subtype of lymphoma with a median survival of 8 to 10 years reported in selected populations. Reproducible distinction between grade I and grade II is difficult and of questionable significance.

The disease involves predominantly lymph nodes; bone marrow is involved in approximately 40% of the patients. Of particular interest to the radiation oncologist is the fact that one third of the patients present with localized (Stage I and Stage II) disease. This group of localized disease patients is largely curable with radiation therapy.[5] Although patients with advanced-stage disease may have an indolent course, there is no curative treatment and there is an inexorable relapse rate of 15% to 20% per year. In many patients, follicular lymphomas[6] eventually evolve into aggressive and unresponsive disorders manifested by histologic transformation to diffuse pattern and large cell morphology, clinical progression, and abnormal cytogenetic findings in addition to t(14; 18). Diffuse large-cell lymphomas that evolve from follicular lymphomas lack the curability of diffuse large-cell lymphomas. A recent study disclosed a transformation risk of 28% in 10 years.[7] The median survival after transformation was only 1.2 years.

Most FL patients present with in an advanced-stage (III-IV). Their treatment is primarily with systemic chemotherapy and/or immunotherapy (rituximab, an anti CD-20 antibody) and patients with low-burden disease are frequently being managed with expectant observation.

Approximately 20% of patients with low-grade follicular lymphomas present in localized stages (I–II). The standard treatment for these patients is regional or involved-field radiotherapy. Results from large series of patients with Stage I and II indolent lymphomas who were treated with radiotherapy alone are summarized in Table 35-6. It should be noted that in past series no clear distinction was made between early stages of follicular lymphomas and the less frequent currently recognized low-grade histologies of marginal zone and small lymphocytic lymphoma (SLL). The report of patients with Stage I and II low-grade follicular lymphoma from Stanford with long-term follow-up indicated that a substantial number of patients in this category have, indeed, been "cured" by radiotherapy.[5] The median follow-up was 7.7 years and observation has maintained for up to 31 years. The median survival after radiotherapy was 14 years. The actuarial survival rates at 5, 10, 15, and 20 years were 82%, 64%, 44%, and 35%, respectively. Freedom from relapse (FFR) at 5, 10, 15, and 20 years was 55%, 44%, 40%, and 37%, respectively. Only 5 of 47 patients who reached 10 years without a relapse developed a late recurrence. There was no significant FFR difference between Stage I and Stage II or between nodal or extranodal disease. The survival of patients irradiated after the age of 60 years was significantly shorter than the survival of younger patients, but the decrease of survival in this age group was strongly affected by death from other causes.

Most relapses in early-stage patients occur in unirradiated sites during the first 5 to 6 years following therapy.[9] In the Stanford series, administration of radiotherapy to nodal sites on both sides of the diaphragm was associated with a significantly better FFR compared with more localized treatment but did not translate into a clear survival benefit.[5] Similar experience was reported from MD Anderson.[10] In the absence of a clear survival benefit for total lymphoid irradiation in this setting, the common involvement of mesenteric nodes that may require whole abdominal irradiation, and in consideration of the fact that almost half of the patients will eventually require chemotherapy for relapse, a limited field is preferred. Involved or regional field irradiation for these patients is currently the standard of care.

The optimal radiation dose for indolent lymphoma has not been determined in a prospective study. However, most current radiotherapy series for Stage I and II indolent lymphomas usually employ 30–40 Gy, and in-field recurrences have been uncommon. Data from the Princess Margaret Hospital showed in-field disease control in 78% of patients treated with doses of less than 25 Gy and 91% control with doses greater than 25 Gy.[11] At MD Anderson excellent local control was achieved with 30 Gy to lesions smaller than 3 cm.[10] A recent (yet unpublished) prospectively randomized British study showed that 24 Gy provide similar response and local control rates to those obtained with 40-45 Gy.[12] At MSKCC, a dose of 24 to 36 Gy to involved sites (36 Gy, if bulky) is the standard of care.

Several prospective randomized trials failed to demonstrate that the use of radiation followed by chemotherapy was superior to radiation alone in early-stage indolent lymphoma.

The rare histology of nodal marginal zone lymphoma in early stage is treated like FL with IFRT alone.[6]

TABLE 35-6　Role of Radiotherapy in Stage I–II Aggressive Lymphomas: Randomized Studies

| Reference | Patients, n | Progression/Failure-Free Survival, % | | P value |
|---|---|---|---|---|
| | | CHOP % | CHOP-RT | |
| Horning et al[34] | 345 | 39 | 54 | 0.06 |
| Miller et al[35] | 401 | 66 | 77 | 0.01 |

## Extra Nodal Marginal Zone Lymphomas (MZL) or MALT Lymphomas

Marginal zone lymphomas constitute 7% to 8% of all B-cell lymphomas. When marginal zone lymphomas involve the nodes, they are called monocytoid B-cell lymphomas; when they involve extranodal sites, they are called MALT lymphomas.[2] These are tumors of adults, most in the sixth to eighth decade of life with a 1.5:1 male predominance.

Marginal zone lymphomas are characterized by cellular heterogeneity, including marginal zone (centrocyte-like) cells, monocytoid B cells, small lymphocytes, and plasma cells. In epithelial tissue, the marginal zone cells typically infiltrate the epithelium, forming lymphoepithelial lesions. The immunophenotype of marginal zone lymphomas helps to distinguish them from other neoplastic proliferations of small lymphoid cells. Although positive for pan-B-cell antigens and express surface immunoglobulin, they are negative for both CD5 (unlike small lymphocytic and mantle cells) and CD10 (unlike follicle center cells).

The MALT lymphomas have been identified in many extranodal sites; most commonly in the stomach, but also in the salivary glands, Waldeyer's ring, large and small intestine, thyroid, eye (orbit and conjunctiva), lung, breast, and skin. Some of these sites do not have mucous membranes but contain columnar epithelium, which may be the common feature. Most of these lymphomas are limited to the involved site at diagnosis with occasional involvement of adjacent lymph nodes. The clinical course is indolent in even advanced-stage patients.

There is considerable evidence to suggest that MALT lymphoma develops as a result of prolonged antigenic stimulation and in some situations may depend on continuous stimulation. MALT lymphoma may develop in the thyroid gland of patients with Hashimoto's thyroiditis and in salivary glands of patients with Sjögren's syndrome. Most *Helicobacter pylori* infection of the stomach has been shown to be the etiological factor in many patients with MALT lymphoma of the stomach and lymphoma regression has been documented following eradication of *H. pylori* with antibiotics. For patents with MALT lymphoma of the stomach and evidence for active *H. pylori* presence in the stomach, omeprazole with antibiotics is the first line of lymphoma eradication treatment.

Yet, approximately 30% to 50% of patients with *H. pylori*-positive gastric MALT lymphoma (GML) will show persistent or progressing lymphoma even after eradication of *H. pylori* with antibiotic therapy and even in complete responders, almost 15% will relapse within 3 years, suggesting that about half of patients with GML will eventually be considered for additional therapies.[13] Most of those will still have disease limited to the stomach. In these patients and in those who present with no evidence of *H. pylori* infection, involved-field radiation therapy with relatively low radiation dose is the treatment of choice.[6,14]

Several institutions reported excellent results using involved-field radiotherapy of the stomach in *H. pylori*-independent GML patients who either failed antibiotic therapy or had no evidence for *H. pylori* infection.[15-18] The recent update of the Memorial Sloan-Kettering Cancer Center experience included 51 patients with GML (Stage I-39; Stage II-10; Stage IV-2) who were either *H. pylori* negative (30) or remained with persistent lymphoma after antibiotic therapies and adequate observation (21).[19] All patients were treated with radiation to the stomach and peri-gastric nodes; the median total dose was 30 Gy in 4 weeks. All patients had regular follow-up endoscopic evaluations and biopsies. Ninety-six percent (49/51) patients obtained a biopsy-proven complete response. Of three patients who relapsed, two were salvaged. Three patients died of other malignancies, all second tumors developed outside the radiation field. At a median follow-up of 4 years, freedom from treatment failure, overall survival, and cause-specific survival were 89%, 83% and 100%, respectively. Treatment was well tolerated, with no significant acute or chronic side effects. The experience from Toronto and Boston using the same radiation approach was equally successful,[20-22] supporting the approach that modest dose involved-field radiotherapy is the treatment of choice for patients with persistent GML who have exhausted the antibiotic therapy approach or are unlikely to respond to it (*H. pylori*-negative patients).[23,24] The treatment techniques for treatment of gastric lymphoma have been recently published.[25]

MALT lymphomas have also been described in various non-gastric sites, such as salivary glands, skin, orbit, conjunctiva, lung, thyroid, larynx, breast, kidney, liver, bladder, prostate, urethra, small intestine, rectum, pancreas, and even in the intracranial dura.[24]

The optimal management of non-gastric MALT lymphomas has not yet been clearly established. Retrospective series included patients treated with surgery, radiotherapy, and chemotherapy, alone or in combination. Marginal-zone lymphomas (ML) are exquisitely sensitive to relatively low doses of radiation. Specifically, ML in sites such as salivary glands, ocular, conjunctiva, thyroid, breast, bladder, have been successfully eradicated with involved-field RT encompassing the involved organ alone with a dose of 24 Gy to 36 Gy.[20,22] Even unusual sites (such as larynx, base of skull, urethra, prostate) not easily amenable to surgery have been well controlled by involved-field RT.

### *Radiation Therapy for Relapsed and Refractory Low-Grade Lymphomas*

While chemotherapy and antibody therapy are the primary treatments of advanced-stage low-grade lymphomas, the very high sensitivity of these lymphomas to radiation should not be ignored. Even extremely low doses of radiation can provide longstanding local control and effective palliation. Several European groups showed that patients with low-grade lymphoma and persistent or relapsed disease following several regimens of chemotherapy, responded to only two treatments of 2 Gy each (a total of 4 Gy). Using this schedule, a Dutch group reported on 109 patients (304 symptomatic sites) mostly with FL, with an overall response rate of 92% and a complete response rate of 61%.[26,27] The 2-year actuarial freedom from local progression (FFLP) rate was 56%. Similarly, a French team reported an objective response of 81% of the sites, with 57% attaining a complete remission. The 2-year actuarial freedom from local progression (FFLP) rate was 56%.[28]

## THE INTERMEDIATE-GRADE (AGGRESSIVE) LYMPHOMAS

### Mantle Cell Lymphoma

While mantle cell lymphoma (MCL) presents as Stage IV in most patients and is treated primarily with chemotherapy, its exquisite sensitivity to radiation should be appreciated. A British Columbia Cancer Center study indicated that patients with MCL Stages I–II, benefited significantly from localized RT alone or combined with chemotherapy. The 5-year progression-free survival (PFS) was 68% for those receiving RT compared to 11% in patients not receiving RT (p = 0.002), 6-year overall survival was 71% and 25%, for RT versus no RT (p = 0.13).[29] At MSKCC, we used low-dose RT for local control and palliation of 38 sites in 21 patients previously treated with chemotherapy. Local control with radiation was obtained in all sites and a complete response was achieved in 64% of the sites.[30] Ninety-four percent of symptomatic patients obtained pain control with RT. Local progression occurred in 34% of patients at a median time to progression of 10 months. Since only low-dose radiation is required (15–30 Gy) in MCL, large nodal sites may be treated with only minor side effects and without jeopardizing other future therapeutic options.

### Diffuse Large B-Cell Lymphoma

Diffuse large cell lymphoma (DLBCL) is the most common aggressive lymphoma and constitutes approximately 30% of all NHLs. Its incidence has been increasing over the past few decades. The median age of patients is in the seventh decade, but the range is broad and includes children. Male/female ratio is equal. The immunophenotype is characterized by pan-B-cell markers (CD19, CD20, CD22) and clonal surface immunoglobulin (usually IgM) in about 75% of patients and CD10 in about 25% of patients. The *bcl-2* rearrangement and t(14;18) are found in about 30% of patients and probably represent transformation of CD10 follicular follicle center lymphomas. Recently, *bcl-6* rearrangements were identified in a significant subset of patients characterized by primary involvement of extranodal tissues, lack of bone marrow involvement, and favorable prognosis.

Patients with DLBCL typically present with a rapidly enlarging, often symptomatic mass at a single nodal or extranodal site. Forty percent are at least initially confined to extranodal sites. Although DLBCL is an aggressive disease that, without treatment, has a rapidly lethal course with a median survival of 8 months, it is potentially curable in all stages. About 40% of patients in advanced-stage and approximately 80% to 90% of patients with Stages I to II disease are curable with chemotherapy or with combined-modality therapy, respectively. Almost half of the patients present with localized disease. Radiation therapy, as part of a combined modality approach, has an important role in their treatment.

An important subset of patients with DLBCL present with predominant mediastinal disease. Patients with mediastinal B-cell lymphoma are usually young (fourth decade) and female gender predominates. This lymphoma is locally invasive and may cause airway compromise and superior vena cava syndrome. The treatment approach is similar to that of other localized aggressive lymphomas: combination chemotherapy followed by involved field radiotherapy.

### Early-Stage DLBCL

In the past, radiation alone was considered an appropriate treatment for patients with localized (Stage I–II) diffuse large B-cell lymphoma (DLBCL). Young patients with low-bulk Stage I DLBCL obtained 10 years survival of 87%, but other patients have relapsed in a rate higher than 50%. Most of the relapses in patients treated with radiotherapy alone were extranodal or occurred outside the irradiated field.

The advent of effective chemotherapy made radiotherapy alone obsolete for most patients with early-stage aggressive lymphoma. Several randomized studies indicated that adjuvant chemotherapy following involved (IFRT) or extended field radiotherapy results in significantly better relapse-free survival and overall survival rates than treatment with radiation alone in early-stage aggressive lymphoma. Over the last two decades, the treatment of early-stage diffuse large B-cell lymphoma with three to six courses cyclophosphamide, doxorubicin, vincristine, and prednisone (CHOP) followed by IFRT has become the standard of care. More recently, several randomized studies showed that adding Rituximab (anti CD-20) to the chemotherapy improves outcome. R-CHOP followed by IFRT is currently the preferred treatment for early-stage DLBCL.

The question of whether the addition of radiotherapy improves the relapse-free survival rate and overall survival rate in patients with early-stage aggressive lymphoma who attained a complete response with chemotherapy is frequently an issue of controversy.[31,32]

Adjuvant radiation therapy has become standard of care in early-stage aggressive NHL following the analysis of two large randomized studies by the Eastern Cooperative Oncology Group (ECOG) and the Southwest Oncology Group (SWOG).[33] These studies are summarized in Table 35-5. The ECOG study involved patients with bulky or extranodal Stage I and Stage II intermediate-grade NHL.[34] All patients received eight cycles of CHOP chemotherapy. Patients who attained only a partial response following chemotherapy received involved field radiotherapy to 40 Gy, and 28% converted to complete-response status. Patients in complete response (61%) following chemotherapy alone were randomly assigned either to receive radiotherapy of 30 Gy to site pretreatment involvement or to observation alone. The recent 15-year update showed a statistically significant advantage to the adjuvant radiotherapy arm. The patients who received adjuvant radiotherapy attained a better failure-free survival rate than those receiving CHOP alone (54% vs. 39%; $P = 0.06$).[34] Overall survival that included all courses of death in this aging population was better in the irradiated group (60% vs. 44%), but the difference was not statistically significant. Cause-specific survival was not reported.

The SWOG study enrolled patients with Stage I and non-bulky Stage II aggressive NHL. The patients were randomly assigned to receive either eight cycles of CHOP chemotherapy alone or three cycles of CHOP followed by an involved field of 40 Gy (with an optional boost of up to 55 Gy). At a median follow-up of 4 years, the progression-free survival rate was significantly greater for the short-course CHOP plus radiotherapy group: 77% compared with 66% in the group receiving eight cycles of CHOP with no radiotherapy. The combined-modality treatment also resulted in a superior overall survival rate (87% vs. 75%; $P = 0.01$). Additionally, reversible toxicity occurring during therapy also favored the combined modality arm.[35] Recent analysis is of the SWOG data suggested that patients with early-stage modified high IPI had inferior survival and may require more than three cycles of chemotherapy.[36]

The results of both randomized studies confirm the importance of adjuvant radiation therapy to the involved field in patients who attained a complete response following short (three cycles) or long (eight cycles) chemotherapy. A relatively low dose of 30 Gy was adequate for patients who attained a complete response in the ECOG study (using eight cycles of CHOP), while a higher dose (40–55 Gy) was used in the short chemotherapy arm of the SWOG study. At MSKCC the standard consolidation dose is 30 to 36 Gy for patients who attained an unquestionable complete response following three to six cycles of chemotherapy. This is based on our and others' excellent local control data with this dose range. A recent randomized study from England confirmed the adequacy of 30 Gy as well.[12] At MSKCC a higher dose (40–50 Gy) is still advised for uncertain complete responses or for patients who failed chemotherapy but are still potentially curable. For evaluating response, it is now recommended to obtain a PET-CT scan prior to and following chemotherapy, since a positive PET scan following chemotherapy may indicate an incomplete response that mandates a more aggressive approach.

### Advanced-Stage DLBCL

The standard treatment for patients with advanced-stage (III or IV) aggressive lymphoma is combination chemotherapy, and R-CHOP is the most commonly used combination.[36] In North America, radiation therapy as consolidation to even bulky sites or incomplete responders is rarely being considered, although supported by retrospective studies.[37] Surprisingly, the data regarding the irrelevance of radiotherapy in these situations are scanty and/or indirect, at best.[38]

Unfortunately, while the superiority of combined modality over chemotherapy alone has been established for early stages, the concept and the feasibility have not been tested in trials for advanced-stage NHL in the United States. It is of interest that recent randomized studies from other countries suggest that radiotherapy, particularly if administered to areas of originally bulky disease, may significantly improve the relapse-free survival and overall survival of patients who attained a CR with chemotherapy.[39-42]

Investigators from Mexico City conducted two consecutive randomized studies with a similar design. In the first study, 218 patients with Stage IV diffuse large cell lymphoma were included. Following chemotherapy, 155 patients (71%) achieved a complete response. Of the complete responders, 88 patients (56%) originally presented with bulky disease (>10 cm) and therefore were prospectively randomized to observation or to receive involved-field radiotherapy to a dose of 40-50 Gy. At 5 years, 72% of 43 patients randomized to receive radiotherapy were alive and disease-free as compared with only 35% of the 45 patients who were not irradiated (P < 0.01). Most of the relapses occurred in the original site. Overall survival was also improved for the irradiated patients (81% vs. 55%; P < 0.01).[39] In the more recent study, 341 patients with aggressive DLCL and presence of nodal bulky disease (tumor mass <10 cm) in pathological proven complete response after intensive chemotherapy were randomized to receive either radiotherapy (involved fields, 40 Gy) or not. The 5-year EFS and OS in radiated patients were 82% and 87%, respectively, which were superior to the control group: EFS- 55%

(P < 0.001) and OS- 66% (P < 0.01) respectively. Radiotherapy was considered "well tolerated," acute toxicity was "mild."[42]

In Milan, 97 patients with Stages III–IV diffuse, large cell lymphoma that were in CR after chemotherapy were either observed or received consolidation radiotherapy. At 5 years, patients with bulky disease (<10 cm) who received radiotherapy had a significantly longer time to relapse and a better overall survival (P = 0.05) compared with patients who were not irradiated. A multivariate analysis showed that the use of radiotherapy was an independent favorable prognostic factor for relapse (P = 0.001) and survival (P = 0.05).[40]

In Paris, patients with NHL who underwent high-dose chemotherapy with stem-cell transplantation as up-front treatment or treatment for relapse and received post-transplantation radiotherapy had a better event-free survival compared with patients who had not received radiotherapy (P = 0.02 in multivariate analysis). Other studies have also supported the use of consolidation radiotherapy after high-dose chemotherapy and bone marrow transplantation.[41]

These data support the notion that although intermediate-grade NHL is a systemic disease, all stages should primarily be treated with chemotherapy. Yet, radiotherapy to bulky or residual disease may improve the outcome of the treatment program. While more studies should address the potential benefit of radiation therapy in advanced-stage disease, the above data provide an adequate basis to justify the combined-modality approach in selected cases.

### Primary Mediastinal Lymphoma

In most patients the disease is bulky and limited to the mediastinum. Consolidation with involved field radiotherapy of the mediastinum after a complete, uncertain, or partial response with chemotherapy is a standard approach in most centers.[43,44] Several large retrospective studies indicated the superiority of a combined-modality approach in primary mediastinal lymphoma over chemotherapy alone.[45] Yet, prospective randomized studies evaluating the contribution of RT in mediastinal lymphoma have not been reported.

## RADIATION FIELDS

This section is covered in detail in the chapter on Hodgkin lymphoma. In almost all clinical scenarios radiotherapy is given as an involved field to either the involved organ or to the involved lymph node group. This IFRT approach is recommended for either treatment with RT alone or when radiotherapy is used for consolidation or palliation.

## ACUTE AND LONG-TERM SIDE EFFECTS

Side effects and complications are site-specific and in general are covered in the chapter on Hodgkin lymphoma. In general, the decrease in radiation dose used for lymphoma in recent years has made the treatment simpler and safer.

## REFERENCES

1. Jemal A, Siegel R, Ward E, et al. Cancer statistics, 2007. *CA Cancer J Clin* 57:43–66, 2007.
2. Harris NL, Jaffe ES, Diebold J, et al. Lymphoma classification—from controversy to consensus: the R.E.A.L. and WHO Classification of lymphoid neoplasms. *Ann Oncol* 11 Suppl 1:3–10, 2000.
3. Shipp MA. Prognostic factors in aggressive non-Hodgkin lymphoma: who has "high-risk" disease? *Blood* 83:1165–1173, 1994.
4. Solal-Celigny P, Roy P, Colombat P, et al. Follicular lymphoma international prognostic index. *Blood* 104:1258–1265, 2004.

5. MacManus MP, Hoppe RT. Is radiotherapy curative for stage I and II low-grade follicular lymphoma? Results of a long-term follow-up study of patients treated at Stanford University. *J Clin Oncol* 14:1282–1290, 1996.

6. Zelenetz AD. NCCN physician guidelines: non-Hodgkin lymphoma 2007 v.1. www.nccn.org, 2007.

7. Montoto S, Davies AJ, Matthews J, et al. Risk and clinical implications of transformation of follicular lymphoma to diffuse large B-cell lymphoma. *J Clin Oncol,* 2007.

8. Vaughan Hudson B, Vaughan Hudson G, MacLennan KA, et al. Clinical stage 1 non-Hodgkin lymphoma: long-term follow-up of patients treated by the British National Lymphoma Investigation with radiotherapy alone as initial therapy. *Br J Cancer* 69:1088–1093, 1994.

9. Sutcliffe SB, Gospodarowicz MK, Bush RS, et al. Role of radiation therapy in localized non-Hodgkin lymphoma. *Radiother Oncol* 4:211–223, 1985.

10. Wilder RB, Jones D, Tucker SL, et al. Long-term results with radiotherapy for stage I-II follicular lymphomas. *Int J Radiat Oncol Biol Phys* 51:1219–1227, 2001.

11. Bush RS, Gospodarowicz M, Sturgeon J, et al. Radiation therapy of localized non-Hodgkin lymphoma. *Cancer Treat Rep* 61:1129–1136, 1977.

12. Hoskin P. Radiation dose in non-Hodgkin lymphoma: preliminary results of UK NCRN randomized trial. *Ann Oncol* 16, 2005.

13. Bertoni F, Conconi A, Capella C, et al. Molecular follow-up in gastric mucosa-associated lymphoid tissue lymphomas: early analysis of the LY03 cooperative trial. *Blood* 99:2541–2544, 2002.

14. Zelenetz AD. NCCN physician guidelines: non-Hodgkin lymphoma 2004 v.1. www.nccn.org, 2004.

15. Fisher RI, Dahlberg S, Nathwani BN, et al. A clinical analysis of two indolent lymphoma entities: mantle cell lymphoma and marginal zone lymphoma (including the mucosa-associated lymphoid tissue and monocytoid B-cell subcategories): a Southwest Oncology Group study. *Blood* 85:1075–1082, 1995.

16. Coiffier B, Salles G. Does surgery belong to medical history for gastric lymphomas? *Ann Oncol* 8:419–421, 1997.

17. Wotherspoon AC, Doglioni C, Isaacson PG. Low-grade gastric B-cell lymphoma of mucosa-associated lymphoid tissue (MALT): a multifocal disease. *Histopathology* 20:29–34, 1992.

18. Schechter NR, Portlock CS, Yahalom J: Treatment of mucosa-associated lymphoid tissue lymphoma of the stomach with radiation alone. *J Clin Oncol* 16:1916–1921, 1998.

19. Yahalom J, CS. P, Gonzales M, et al. H. Pylori-independent MALT lymphoma of the stomach: excellent outcome with radiation alone. *Blood* 100:160a, 2002.

20. Tsang RW, Gospodarowicz MK, Pintilie M, et al. Stage I and II MALT lymphoma: results of treatment with radiotherapy. Int J Radiat *Oncol Biol Phys* 50:1258–1264, 2001.

21. Fung CY, Grossbard ML, Linggood RM, et al. Mucosa-associated lymphoid tissue lymphoma of the stomach: long-term outcome after local treatment. *Cancer* 85:9–17, 1999.

22. Hitchcock S, Ng AK, Fisher DC, et al. Treatment outcome of mucosa-associated lymphoid tissue/marginal zone non-Hodgkin lymphoma. *Int J Radiat Oncol Biol Phys* 52:1058–1066, 2002.

23. Gospodarowicz MK, Pintilie M, Tsang R, et al. Primary gastric lymphoma: brief overview of the recent Princess Margaret Hospital experience. *Recent Results Cancer Res* 156:108–115, 2000.

24. Yahalom J. MALT lymphomas: a radiation oncology viewpoint. *Ann Hematol* 80:B100-105, 2001.

25. Dell Bianca C, Hunt M, Furhang E, et al. Radiation treatment planning techniques for lymphoma of the stomach. *International Journal of Radiation Oncology, Biology, Physics,* 2005.

26. Haas RL, Poortmans P, de Jong D, et al. High response rates and lasting remissions after low-dose involved field radiotherapy in indolent lymphomas. *J Clin Oncol* 21:2474–2480, 2003.

27. Haas RL, Girinsky T. HOVON 47/EORTC 20013: chlorambucil vs 2x2 Gy involved field radiotherapy in stage III/IV previously untreated follicular lymphoma patients. *Ann Hematol* 82:458–462, 2003.

28. Girinsky T, Guillot-Vals D, Koscielny S, et al. A high and sustained response rate in refractory or relapsing low-grade lymphoma masses after low-dose radiation: analysis of predictive parameters of response to treatment. *Int J Radiat Oncol Biol Phys* 51:148–155, 2001.

29. Leitch HA, Gascoyne RD, Chhanabhai M, et al. Limited-stage mantle cell lymphoma. *Ann Oncol* 14:1555–1561, 2003.

30. Rosenbluth BD, Yahalom J. Highly effective local control and palliation of mantle cell lymphoma with involved field radiation therapy (IFRT). *Int J Radiat Oncol Biol Phys* 65:1185–1191, 2006.

31. Ng AK, Mauch PM. Role of radiation therapy in localized aggressive lymphoma. *J Clin Oncol* 25:757–759, 2007.

32. Longo DL. Combined-modality therapy for localized aggressive lymphoma: enough or too much? *J Clin Oncol* 7:1179–1181, 1989.

33. Miller TP. The limits of limited-stage lymphoma. *J Clin Oncol* 22:2982–2984, 2004.

34. Horning SJ, Weller E, Kim K, et al. Chemotherapy with or without radiotherapy in limited-stage diffuse aggressive non-Hodgkin lymphoma: Eastern Cooperative Oncology Group study 1484. *J Clin Oncol* 22:3032–3038, 2004.

35. Miller TP, Dahlberg S, Cassady JR, et al. Chemotherapy alone compared with chemotherapy plus radiotherapy for localized intermediate- and high-grade non-Hodgkin lymphoma. *N Engl J Med* 339:21–26, 1998.

36. Fisher RI, Miller TP, O'Connor OA. Diffuse aggressive lymphoma. *Hematology (Am Soc Hematol Educ Program)*:221–236, 2004.

37. Schlembach PJ, Wilder RB, Tucker SL, et al. Impact of involved field radiotherapy after CHOP-based chemotherapy on stage III-IV, intermediate-grade and large-cell immunoblastic lymphomas. *Int J Radiat Oncol Biol Phys* 48:1107–1110, 2000.

38. Shipp MA, Klatt MM, Yeap B, et al. Patterns of relapse in large-cell lymphoma patients with bulk disease: implications for the use of adjuvant radiation therapy. *J Clin Oncol* 7:613–618, 1989.

39. Aviles A, Delgado S, Nambo MJ, et al. Adjuvant radiotherapy to sites of previous bulky disease in patients with stage IV diffuse large cell lymphoma. *Int J Radiat Oncol Biol Phys* 30:799–803, 1994.

40. Ferreri AJ, Dell'Oro S, Reni M, et al. Consolidation radiotherapy to bulky or semibulky lesions in the management of stage III-IV diffuse large B-cell lymphomas. *Oncology* 58:219–226, 2000.

41. Fouillard L, Laporte JP, Labopin M, et al. Autologous stem-cell transplantation for non-Hodgkin lymphomas: the role of graft purging and radiotherapy post-transplantation—results of a retrospective analysis on 120 patients autografted in a single institution. *J Clin Oncol* 16:2803–2816, 1998.

42. Aviles A, Fernandezb R, Perez F, et al. Adjuvant radiotherapy in stage IV diffuse large cell lymphoma improves outcome. *Leuk Lymphoma* 45:1385–1389, 2004.

43. Aviles A, Garcia EL, Fernandez R, et al. Combined therapy in the treatment of primary mediastinal B-cell lymphoma: conventional versus escalated chemotherapy. *Ann Hematol* 81:368–373, 2002.

44. Zinzani PL, Martelli M, Bertini M, et al. Induction chemotherapy strategies for primary mediastinal large B-cell lymphoma with sclerosis: a retrospective multinational study on 426 previously untreated patients. *Haematologica* 87:1258–1264, 2002.

45. Todeschini G, Secchi S, Morra E, et al. Primary mediastinal large B-cell lymphoma (PMLBCL): long-term results from a retrospective multicentre Italian experience in 138 patients treated with CHOP or MACOP-B/VACOP-B. *Br J Cancer* 90:372–376, 2004.

# 36
# Leukemias and Plasma Cell Disorders

*Bouthaina Dabaja, MD*

*Chul Soo Ha, MD*

## LEUKEMIAS

### Overview

Leukemias are uncontrolled neoplastic proliferation of the hematopoietic system. Eventually the neoplastic proliferation will replace the function of the normal marrow cells causing the signs and symptoms seen in leukemias.

Leukemias are divided into acute and chronic types. The main difference is that acute leukemias are derived from primitive immature progenitor cells in contrast to chronic leukemias that are derived from more mature cells. However, chronic leukemias can transform into acute leukemias during the course of the disease.

Leukemias are either of myeloid origin like acute myelogenous leukemia (AML), chronic myelogenous leukemia (CML), chronic myelomonocytic leukemia, chronic eosinophilic leukemia, myelofibrosis or of lymphoid origin like acute lymphoblastic leukemia (ALL), chronic lymphoid leukemia (CLL), T and B cell prolymphocytic leukemia.

Myelodysplastic disorders, known as oligoblastic leukemia, range from clonally derived refractory anemia to refractory anemia with excess blasts but not enough to be called AML.

Some lymphomas, like lymphoblastic lymphomas and Burkitt's lymphoma, are derived from immature cells, and they have the outcome and behavior of leukemias.

### Epidemiology

The incidence in the United States:[1]

2.5 per 100,000 Persons for AML
1.3 per 100,000 persons for ALL.
2 per 100,000 men and 1.1 per 100,000 females for CML
3.9 per 100,000 men and 2 per 100,000 females for CLL.

The median age of occurrence:[1,2]

66 years for AML
11 years for ALL

66 years for CML
65 years for CLL

## Risk Factors

### Acute Leukemias[3–5]

- Atomic bomb survivors/radiation exposure
- Smoking
- Occupational exposure to benzene
- No definite evidence that relates viruses to leukemias

### Chronic Leukemias

- Atomic bomb survivors and patients treated for ankylosing spondylitis with radiation therapy are at risk of developing CML[3,4]
- No risk factor is confirmed in patients with CLL

## Classification of Leukemias

The French-American-British (FAB) classification is falling out of favor because it depends mainly on morphologic and cytochemistry typing of acute leukemias. Currently more physicians favor the World Health Organization classification that incorporates morphologic, immunophenotyping and genotypic data into the classification.[6]

## Clinical Presentation

### Acute Leukemias

Acute leukemia occurs when one mutant hematopoietic cell gains a growth and survival advantage compared to normal pool of stem cells. The result of this proliferation is inhibition of normal hematopoiesis, resulting in depression of normal neutrophil count, red blood cell count, and platelet count. Patients develop signs and symptoms of anemia, infections, and spontaneous hemorrhage. Lymphoblasts in ALL have the ability to accumulate in the meninges, gonads, thymus, liver, spleen, and lymph nodes.

### Chronic Leukemias

Patients with CML are commonly asymptomatic and diagnosis is often made on routine blood tests. The most common presenting symptoms are those related to anemia and splenomegaly.

Although patients with CLL can be asymptomatic, they can also present with fatigue, lymphadenopathy, and recurrent infections. Splenomegaly or hepatomegaly can occur in advanced stage. Autoimmune disorders occur in up to 20% of cases of CLL.[7]

## Prognostic Factors for Poor Outcome

1. AML[8]
   a. Age > 60
   b. Cytogenetics abnormalities
      i. −5, del (5q), −7, del (9q), +11, +13, trisomy 8 are associated with a worse prognosis.
      ii. t(15;17), inversion 16, and t(8;21) are associated with a better prognosis.
   c. Failure to achieve remission to chemotherapy
   d. Antecedent hematological disorder/secondary AML

2. ALL[9,10]
   a. Older age
   b. High white blood cell count
   c. Mature B cell type
   d. Presence of Philadelphia chromosome t(9;22)
   e. Longer time to achieve complete remission
3. CML[11]
   a. Age > 20 years for transplant candidates and > 40 years for others
   b. Duration of chronic phase < 12 months
   c. > 5% marrow blasts
   d. Splenomegaly
   e. > 15% total basophil + eosinophil count in peripheral blood
   f. Platelets count > $700 \times 10^9$
   g. Marrow fibrosis
4. CLL[12,13]
   a. Age > 65 years
   b. Advanced stage
   c. Doubling time < 6 months
   d. Elevated $\beta_2$ microglobulin
   e. Expression of CD 38
   f. Trisomy 12
   g. Diffuse replacement of the marrow with clonal lymphocytes

# Diagnosis

## Acute Leukemias

The following tests are usually used to determine if the leukemia is myeloid or lymphoid:

   a. Morphology inspection identifies leukemia blast cells in the peripheral blood and marrow. This can be further specified to B-cell or T-cell lymphocyte progenitor in ALL, or erythroblastic, megakaryocytic, myelocytic progenitors in AML.
   b. Identification of myeloperoxidase activity is specific for AML blast cells.
   c. Identification of cluster of differentiation (CD) antigens includes
      i. CD13, 33 in AML
      ii. CD 2, 5, 7 in T cell ALL
      iii. CD10, 19, 22 in B cell ALL
   d. Cytogenetics typing is essential for diagnosis, outcome, and treatment and this includes
      i. t (9;22), t (4;11) in ALL
      ii. t(15;17), t (8;21), inversion 16, trisomy 8, –5, del (5q), -7, del (9q), +11, +13 in AML

## Chronic Leukemias

The diagnosis of CML includes

   a. Peripheral blood with full spectrum of myeloid cells from blasts to neutrophils including basophilia and eosinophilia with occasional thrombocytosis
   b. Low or undetectable blood level of leukocyte alkaline phosphatase
   c. Bone marrow markedly hypercellular, with predominance of myeloid cells in full maturation
   d. Identification of Philadelphia chromosome t(9;22) a translocation involving ABL and BCR genes usually present in > 90% of cases

The diagnosis of CLL includes

a. Lymphocytosis $> 5 \times 10^9$/L with monoclonal cells and marrow infiltration with lymphocytes $> 30\%$
b. Identification of CD antigens
   i. CD 5 aberrantly co-expressed with B cell markers such as CD 19, CD 20, CD 21, CD 23, and CD 24
c. Cytogenetic typing
   i. 13q deletion found in 55% and 11q deletion in 18%[14]

## TREATMENT OUTCOME OF LEUKEMIAS

### Acute Leukemias

Chemotherapy is the main treatment for both AML and ALL. The purpose of treatment is eradication of leukemic clones present in the bone marrow, hoping for restoration of normal lineage when patients recover from the pancytopenia caused by chemotherapy.

#### Treatment of Acute Myelogenous Leukemia

*Chemotherapy*

Treatment consists of induction chemotherapy to achieve remission, followed by post-remission chemotherapy or consolidation chemotherapy. The patient will develop severe pancytopenia after each chemotherapy. In patients with AML, anthracycline and cytarabine based chemotherapy, achieves complete remission (CR) in 30%–50% of patients over 60 years of age and 50%–80% of younger patients.[15]

One exception to standard of care is the treatment of acute promyelocytic leukemia (APL), characterized clinically by coagulopathy with risk for lethal hemorrhage and cytogenetically by t(15;17). APL is treated with all transretinoic acid (ATRA) and anthracyclines. About 90%–95% of patients with newly diagnosed APL are expected to achieve CR with this regimen.[16]

*Allogeneic and Autologous Bone Marrow Transplantation*

Eventually the majority of patients with AML relapse, and this leads investigators to consider high dose therapy after first CR. Allogeneic bone marrow transplantation (Allo BMT) using an HLA-compatible donor for patients in first CR results in a 5-year disease-free survival of 45%–50%. Although the relapse rate after Allo BMT is only 10%–20%, this does not translate into prolonged survival because many patients will succumb to transplant-related complications.[17]

On the other hand, using autologous bone marrow transplant is associated with higher relapse rate because of undetectable residual leukemias in the patient's bone marrow.[18]

*Role of Radiation*

Radiation can be used as part of a conditioning regimen for transplant.

Also, radiation can be palliative for patients who develop chloroma, a cluster of leukemia cells forming a mass that can occur anywhere in the body. Typically, chloroma is sensitive to radiation; however, a wide range of doses are used depending on the institutions. To achieve a local control, the dose of radiation should be $> 1100$ cGy.[19]

*Outcome of Patients with AML*

Survival of patients with AML depends on age at diagnosis.[20] The 5-year survival rate is 45% for patients <45 years, 26% for patients 45 to 54 years, and it drops to 6% for patients older than 65 years.

## Treatment of Acute Lymphocytic Leukemia

### Chemotherapy

The treatment consists of induction, consolidation, maintenance, and central nervous system (CNS) prophylaxis.

Induction therapy consists of "four-drug" (vincristine, prednisone, anthracycline, and cyclophosphamide or asparaginase) or "five-drug" (vincristine, prednisone, anthracycline, cyclophosphamide, and asparaginase) regimens.

Consolidation therapy consists of cytosine arabinoside containing regimens.

Maintenance therapy usually lasts for 2 years to 3 years with various chemotherapy, including methotrexate, vincristine, cyclophosphamide, and mercaptopurine.

Testicles, eyes, and CNS are considered sanctuary sites with risk of involvement on presentation of 5%–10%. Since CNS is the most common sanctuary site, prophylaxis is typically achieved with high-dose IV methotrexate along with intrathecal methotrexate. This regimen replaced the cranial irradiation that was used in the 1970s.[21] Cranial irradiation is still being used in some pediatric protocols when patients present with T cell ALL and high white blood cell count. The typical dose ranges from 1200 cGy to 1800 cGy.[22] The field of radiation should cover the entire intracranial meninges, including the cribriform plate, and the posterior aspect of the retina and orbits.

### Role of Radiation Therapy

Radiation therapy is indicated in the treatment of lymphoblastic lymphoma (LBL). LBL is treated like ALL, but the role of local radiation therapy to the mediastinum after completion of chemotherapy is controversial. In a retrospective study, patients treated with mediastinal radiation had a significant decrease in the rate of mediastinal recurrence compared to those who were not treated.[23]

### Outcome of Treatment

CR can be achieved in 65%–90% but eventually only 30% of adults with ALL are cured.[24,25]

## Chronic Leukemias

### Treatment of Chronic Myelogenous Leukemia

There are three phases of the disease: chronic, accelerated, and blastic phase.

For patients in chronic phase, Allo BMT is regarded as the best curative modality, but a matched donor is not always available. Other treatment modalities include hydroxyurea, interferon, and cytosine arabinoside. Imatinib mesylate, a tyrosine kinase inhibitor, is now used as the initial therapy for patients who are not getting transplant.[26] When compared to interferon and cytosine arabinoside regimen, imatinib mesylate achieved better hematological and cytogenetic response, and lower risk of transformation into accelerated and blastic phase.[27]

Total body irradiation (TBI) is sometimes used as part of the conditioning regimen prior to Allo BMT. A commonly used TBI regimen is 1200 cGy fractionated over 6 days.[28,29,30]

Total lymphoid irradiation is recently introduced in non-myeloablative regimens. Non-myeloablative regimens have the advantage of decreasing the intensity of conditioning regimens. These regimens rely more on donor immunity against the residual leukemia rather than on myeloablation.[31]

### Outcome of treatment

The outcome and survival of patients with CML improved over time with the introduction of Allo BMT and imatinib mesylate. The median survival reported with busulfan and hydroxyurea ranged from 39 to 47.[32,33] The 5-years survival rate improved with addition of interferon from 42% to 57% compared to chemotherapy.[34] The reported 4-year survival rates with imatinib mesylate are 49% for poor risk group and up to 96% for good risk group.[35]

## Treatment of Chronic Lymphoid Leukemia

CLL is an indolent disease, and the decision to start treatment depends on the presence of many factors, including:

1. Constitutional symptoms
2. Progressive marrow failure
3. Progressive splenomegaly or lymphadenopathy
4. Immune disorders, such as autoimmune thrombocytopenia
5. Doubling time of lymphocytosis < 6 months

Alkylating agents with or without prednisone have been the mainstay of treatment. It has been shown recently that a purine analogue, fludarabine, achieves a higher overall response rate compared to alkylating agents. However, it does not appear to impact overall survival.[36]

Rituximab, chimeric monoclonal antibody targeted against the CD20 antigen, has been also used in combination with fludarabine in recent studies.

### Role of radiation

Radiation therapy is useful in treating bulky lymph nodes causing pain, nerve impingement, or vital organ compromise. Radiation therapy can also be used for splenomegaly-causing symptoms or adverse blood counts. Multiple regimens have been used for this purpose. Usually these regimens used up to a few hundred cGy in fractionated doses at 25 to 100 cGy per fraction.[37,38]

### Outcome of treatment

There is no established cure for CLL. The survival of patients with CLL depends on the age and stage at presentation. The median survival for low risk (Rai stage 0) can be > 12 years, compared to 19 months for high risk (Rai Stage III and IV).

## MYELOMA

### Overview

Plasma cell neoplasms are a spectrum of diseases characterized by clonal proliferation and accumulation of terminally differentiated B cells. The spectrum includes clinically benign conditions such as monoclonal gammopathy of unknown significance (MGUS) as well as rare disorders such as Castleman's disease, indolent conditions such as Waldenström's macroglobulinemia (WM), solitary plasmacytoma, the more common malignant entity plasma cell myeloma, a disseminated B-cell malignancy, and a more aggressive form, plasma cell leukemia with circulating malignant plasma cells in the blood. Our discussion in this section will be limited to solitary plasmacytoma and multiple myeloma.

### Epidemiology

Multiple Myeloma (MM) is an uncommon malignancy in the United States, representing 1% of all malignancies in whites and 2% in African Americans. Among hematologic malignancies, it constitutes 10%, and is the second most frequently occurring hematologic cancer in the United States after non-Hodgkin's lymphoma.[39]

- Prevalence    50,000 patients
- Incidence    15,000 patients a year
- Deaths    10,900 patients a year
- Female/Male    4.7/3.2 per 100,000 persons in whites and 10/7 in blacks
- Average Age    71 years

# Etiology

## Risk Factors

Exposure to ionizing radiation is the strongest single factor linked to an increased risk of MM. This has been documented in atomic bomb survivors with a five times greater incidence than the control group.[40]

Other factors[41,42] include exposure to:

- Metals: nickel
- Agriculture chemicals
- Benzene and petroleum product
- Aromatic hydrocarbons
- Silicon
- Mineral oil used as laxative

Myeloma can occur among siblings, although direct genetic lineage has not been established.[43,44]

## Cytogenetic Abnormality

The most important being partial or complete deletion of chromosome arm 13q that confers poor prognosis even after high-dose therapy.[45,46] There are other translocations found in MM and these are believed to promote MM cell proliferation.

- t(11;14)(q13;q32) and the involved gene is Cyclin D1[47]
- t(4;14) and t(14;16)
- Abnormalities in p16 and p15 are reported in up to 75% of cases of myeloma, suggesting a defect in Rb regulatory pathway.[48]

## Role of Cytokines

- Interleukin 6 (IL-6) and insulin-like growth factor-1 (IGF-1) play an important role in survival of myeloma cells preventing apoptosis of malignant plasma cells.[49]
- Vascular endothelial growth factor (VEGF) promotes cell migration and angiogenesis.[50]
- Tumor necrosis factor-a (TNF-a) induces secretion of IL-6 and NFB which leads to binding of myeloma cells to bone marrow with the subsequent cell adhesion-mediated drug resistance.[51]
- Interleukin 21 (IL-21) induces proliferation and inhibits apoptosis.[52]
- Stromal cell-derived factor-1 (SDF-1) plays a role in mediating migration of myeloma cells.[51]

## Clinical Manifestations

The clinical presentation of plasmacytoma is related to the mass effect and the location of the mass. As for MM, patients can be asymptomatic and diagnosed on routine blood testing, they can present with bone-related problems, infections, various organ dysfunctions, neurologic complaints, or bleeding tendencies. These symptoms and signs result from direct involvement of bone marrow, or the effect of the protein produced by the tumor cells deposited in various organs.

Specific clinical manifestations in multiple myeloma include:

- Normochromic normocytic anemia secondary to marrow infiltration and inadequate erythropoietin responsiveness.
- Renal failure: multifactorial in origin including
  - Development of light-chain tubular casts leading to interstitial nephritis (myeloma kidney).
  - Hypercalcemia and hypercalciuria.
  - Light-chain deposition disease causing amyloidosis.

- Bone disease: bony changes are due to an increase in osteoclast-activating factors produced predominantly by the bone marrow microenvironment, but also by myeloma cells.
- Infection: bacterial infections due to deficiencies in both humoral and cellular immunity.
- Neurologic symptoms: caused by mass effect, hypercalcemia or hyperviscosity.
  - Amyloid deposition might lead to polyneuropathy, which is part of POEMS syndrome (polyneuropathy, organomegaly, endocrinopathy, monoclonal gammopathy, and skin changes).
- Hyperviscosity: occurs when the serum Ig levels exceed certain level. The incidence is highest with IgM, followed by IgA myeloma, and is least common in IgG myeloma.
- Coagulopathy
  - Related to high level of paraprotein.
  - Due to specific antibody activity that leads to a clinical syndrome similar to acquired deficiency of factor VIII.
  - Due to protein C and S deficiency.

## Diagnosis of Plasma Cell Disorders

### Diagnosis of Multiple Myeloma

Diagnosis of MM needs specific criteria that include major criteria, minor criteria, or a combination of both. Table 34-1 illustrates the details of diagnosis.

The initial evaluation for MM includes:

- Hemogram, chemistry profile (creatinine, calcium, total protein, albunin, lactate dehydrogenase)
- Complete skeletal radiographic survey
  - Demineralization of bone (osteoporosis) is one of the common manifestations of myeloma, measurement of bone mineral density (BMD) by dual-energy x-ray absorptiometry is an important evaluation at diagnosis. Other manifestations on radiographs can be well-demarcated lytic lesions.
  - Magnetic resonance imaging (MRI) of bone marrow provides a better assessment of tumor burden and is essential in the workup of patients with solitary plasmacytomas of bone. More than 95% of myeloma patients have abnormalities on MRI.

---

TABLE 34-1 **Criteria Used for MM Diagnosis According to Durie-Salmon**

Major Criteria

1. Plasmacytoma on tissue biopsy
2. Bone marrow plasmacytosis with >30% plasma cells
3. Monoclonal globulin spike on serum electrophoresis; IgG > 35 g/l, IgA > 20 g/l, light-chain excretion on urine electrophoresis ≥ 1g/24 hours in the absence of amyloidosis.

Minor Criteria

a. Bone marrow plasmacytosis with 10%–30% plasma cells
b. Monoclonal globulin spike present, but lower levels than defined above
c. Lytic bone lesions
d. IgM > 500 mg/l, IgA > 1 g/l, or IgG > 6 g/l

The diagnosis of MM requires a minimum of one major and one minor criterion or three minor criteria that must include (a) + (b).

- o Positron emission tomography has also been evaluated in a small number of studies and may provide a better functional definition of lesions observed on MRI or computed tomography (CT), as well as allowing selection of lesions for biopsy.
- Serum and urine protein electrophoresis and immunofixation, quantitative Ig levels, urinary protein excretion in 24 hours. Among patients with myeloma, 70% have IgG subtype, whereas 20% have IgA subtype, with an additional 5% to 10% having production of monoclonal light chains only. Less than 1% produce monoclonal IgD, IgE, or IgM or have nonsecretory myeloma.
- Bone marrow aspiration and biopsy. Various degrees of bone marrow infiltration with clonal proliferation of CD 38 expressing malignant plasma cells are observed in myeloma starting at 5% or more.
- Cytogenetics analysis to determine any chromosomal abnormalities

## Staging and Prognostic Factors of MM

The most accepted and used staging system is the Durie-Salmon system. (Table 34-2.) Besides staging, serum (2 microglobulin $> 2.5$ mg/L) and low albumin level are both powerful prognostic indicators.[53]

Other prognostic factors for poorer outcome include:

- Elevated serum IL-6
- Elevated C-reactive protein (CRP) levels
- Number of lytic lesions

---

### TABLE 34-2  Myeloma Staging System

**Stage I (low tumor burden)**

All of the following:

- Hemoglobin $> 10$ g/dl
- Normal serum calcium ($<12$ mg/dl)
- Normal skeletal survey or solitary bone plasmacytoma
- Low paraprotein production rates
  - o IgG value $< 5$ g/dl
  - o IgA value $< 3$ g/dl
  - o Urine light-chain M component on electrophoresis $> 4$ g/24 hours

**Stage II (intermediate tumor burden)**

Laboratory and radiological parameters intermediate between Stages I and III

**Stage III (high tumor burden)**

At least one of the following criteria must be satisfied:

- Hemoglobin $< 8.5$ g/dl
- Serum calcium $> 12$ g/dl
- Skeletal survey: advanced lytic lesions
- High paraprotein production rates:
  - o IgG $> 7$ g/dl
  - o IgA $> 5$ g/dl
  - o Urine light chain $> 12$ g/24 hours
    - (A) Serum creatinine $< 2$ mg/dl
    - (B) Serum creatinine $\geq 2$ mg/dl

---

- Percent of monoclonal plasma cells in peripheral blood > 4%.
- Poor performance status
- Cytogenetic abnormalities: deletion of chromosome 13

### Diagnosis of Plasmacytoma

Plasmacytoma can present as either extramedullary plasmacytoma (EMP) or solitary bone plasmacytoma (SBP). They account for around 5%–8% of plasma cell disorders.

EMP typically presents as a well-localized submucosal mass or swelling. It occurs in the upper aerodigestive system in more than 80% of patients; most often in the nasal cavity, paranasal sinuses, nasopharynx, tonsils, and larynx.[48,54]

SBP typically presents with pain related to a lytic lesion. The most common sites are the vertebral bodies or pelvic bones.

Diagnosis of solitary plasmacytoma of bone or soft tissue requires intense investigation to rule out systemic disease. Bone marrow examination in a true solitary lesion should be normal. MRI evaluation for myelomatous involvement of the bone marrow helps detect early lesions before their detection by radiographic examination. Detection of such lesions and cytologic confirmation through CT or MRI-guided fine-needle aspiration biopsy may help confirm solitary plasmacytoma. Limited elevation of serum or urine myeloma protein can be found in patients with solitary plasmacytoma.[55]

## Treatment and Outcome of Plasma Cell Disorders

### Multiple Myeloma

An objective response to treatment is defined by the reduction of at least 75% of the calculated serum paraprotein level or at least 90% of urinary light chains. The overall response ranges from 50%–60% with melphalan-prednisone to 84% with vincristine-adriamycin-dexamethasone (VAD) regimen. A meta-analysis of 6,633 patients from randomized trials showed that the median survival with the currently used regimens of chemotherapy is 3 to 4 years.[56]

#### Chemotherapy

- Treatment with melphalan-prednisone was introduced more than three decades ago. Other types of chemotherapy include various combinations of vincristine, cyclophosphamide, carmustine, doxorubicin, and prednisone. A recent meta-analysis of 18 published studies showed no difference between melphalan-prednisonse and other combinations.[57]
- High-dose dexamethasone given alone or with VAD regimen has shown high response rate and improved survival.[58]

#### Novel Biologically-Based Agents

- Thalidomide: an antiangiogenic agent used in newly diagnosed patients with MM alone or in combination with Dexamethasone[59]
- Bortezomib: a prototype proteasome inhibitor that acts directly on myeloma cells to induce apoptosis[60]
- Arsenic Trioxide: known to induce apoptosis in vitro, currently being tested in phase I and II trials[51]
- Bisphosphonates pamidronate and zoledronate: reduce skeletal complications and bone pain by down-regulating the osteoclast activity and decreasing IL-6 production

## High-dose Chemotherapy with Peripheral Blood Stem Cell Support

- The benefit in overall survival of using high-dose chemotherapy with stem cell rescue has been shown in several randomized trials. Attal et al reported a 5-year overall survival of 52% for high dose, versus 12% for conventional chemotherapy.[61-63]
- Double transplant is indicated in partial responders to the first transplant. In a randomized trial comparing single versus double transplant, single transplant had an overall survival rate of 11% compared to 42% for double transplant at 7 years of follow-up. This benefit was limited to partial responders to the first transplant.[62,64]

## Radiation Therapy

1-The indication for radiation therapy in multiple myeloma is palliation.

  a. Impending pathologic fracture
  b. Spinal cord compression
  c. Bone pain or symptomatic soft tissue masses

  The dose of palliative radiation therapy range from 1,500 to 2,500 cGy at conventional fractionation.[65,66] With this dose only around 6% of patients will be re-treated to the same area at a later date. A generous local field is sufficient, and it is unnecessary to treat the entire bone.[56]

  Radiation oncologists should be cautious while treating a large bone marrow-containing area such as the pelvis if there is an anticipated need for stem cell collection.

  The use of total body radiation as a part of high-dose therapy protocols is controversial. A phase III study conducted by the Intergroupe Francophone du Myelome (IFM 90) compared melphalan 140 mg/m2, plus total body radiation 8 Gy in four daily fractions to melphalan 200 mg/m2. The study showed no difference in event-free survival, but there were more toxicities (mucositis, pancytopenia, and toxic death) in the total body radiation arm.[67] Certain toxicity, such as fatal radiation pneumonitis, has led some investigations to abandon this approach. However other institutions continue to use it for specific indications.[46,68]

## Solitary Plasmacytoma

The standard treatment for solitary plasmacytoma is radiation therapy, and the recommended dose ranges from 3,000 to 5,000 cGy. Mendenhall et al[69] reported a minimum required dose of 4,000 cGy in their retrospective dose response analysis. Tsang et al reported that a median dose of 3,500 cGy (fraction 175–400) was enough, especially for tumor size <5 cm. Liebross et al recommend higher doses of 4,500 to 5,000 cGy at 2 Gy per fraction.[55,68]

The reported local control ranges from 80%–96% according to published series.[70,71]

## Development of multiple myeloma

There is a direct correlation between the subsequent development of MM and the persistence of abnormal myeloma protein following radiation therapy. The persistence of myeloma protein carries a risk of over 50% of developing MM. The 10-year rate of progression to MM according to the published literature varies from 32% to 86%[53,71-73] for SBP and from 8%–44% for EMP.[54,73,74]

The median time of progression is usually 2 to 3 years, but it can be as long as 12 years.[72]

One needs to keep in mind that the risk of developing MM also depends on the thoroughness of the initial workup to rule out MM. For example, patients who had involvement of the vertebral bodies by MM ruled out by MRI would have a lower chance of developing MM compared to those who had only plain films of the vertebral bodies.[72]

The reported 10-year overall survival for SBP is around 50% with a wide reported range (33%–65%). However, the 10-year overall survival for EMP appears higher with a reported range of 43% to 80%.[73,75]

## REFERENCES

1. Jemal A, Murray T, Samuels A, et al. Cancer statistics, 2003. *CA Cancer J Clin* 53:5–26, 2003.
2. Redaelli A, Bell C, Casagrande J, et al. Clinical and epidemiologic burden of chronic myelogenous leukemia. *Expert Rev Anticancer Ther* 4:85–96, 2004.
3. Brown WM, Doll R. Mortality from cancer and other causes after radiotherapy for ankylosing spondylitis. *Br Med J* 5474:1327–1332, 1965.
4. Preston DL, Kusumi S, Tomonaga M, et al. Cancer incidence in atomic bomb survivors: part III. Leukemia, lymphoma and multiple myeloma, 1950–1987. *Radiat Res* 137:S68–S97, 1994.
5. Sandler DP, Shore DL, Anderson JR, et al. Cigarette smoking and risk of acute leukemia: associations with morphology and cytogenetic abnormalities in bone marrow. *J Natl Cancer Inst* 85:1994–2003, 1993.
6. Harris NL, Jaffe ES, Diebold J, et al. World Health Organization classification of neoplastic diseases of the hematopoietic and lymphoid tissues: report of the Clinical Advisory Committee meeting-Airlie House, Virginia, November 1997. *J Clin Oncol* 17:3835–3849, 1999.
7. Diehl LF, Ketchum LH. Autoimmune disease and chronic lymphocytic leukemia: autoimmune hemolytic anemia, pure red cell aplasia, and autoimmune thrombocytopenia. *Semin Oncol* 25:80–97, 1998.
8. Mrozek K, Heinonen K, de la Chapelle A, et al. Clinical significance of cytogenetics in acute myeloid leukemia. *Semin Oncol* 24:17–31, 1997.
9. Hoelzer D, Thiel E, Loffler H, et al. Prognostic factors in a multicenter study for treatment of acute lymphoblastic leukemia in adults. *Blood* 71:123–131, 1988.
10. Gaynor J, Chapman D, Little C, et al. A cause-specific hazard rate analysis of prognostic factors among 199 adults with acute lymphoblastic leukemia: the Memorial Hospital experience since 1969. *J Clin Oncol* 6:1014–1030, 1988.
11. Sokal JE, Cox EB, Baccarani M, et al. Prognostic discrimination in "good-risk" chronic granulocytic leukemia. *Blood* 63:789–799, 1984.
12. Binet JL, Auquier A, Dighiero G, et al. A new prognostic classification of chronic lymphocytic leukemia derived from a multivariate survival analysis. *Cancer* 48:198–206, 1981.
13. Lee JS, Dixon DO, Kantarjian HM, et al. Prognosis of chronic lymphocytic leukemia: a multivariate regression analysis of 325 untreated patients. *Blood* 69:929–936, 1987.
14. Dohner H, Stilgenbauer S, Dohner K, et al. Chromosome aberrations in B-cell chronic lymphocytic leukemia: reassessment based on molecular cytogenetic analysis. *J Mol Med* 77:266–281, 1999.
15. Rai KR, Holland JF, Glidewell OJ, et al. Treatment of acute myelocytic leukemia: a study by cancer and leukemia group B. *Blood* 58:1203–1212, 1981.
16. Huang ME, Ye YC, Chen SR, et al. Use of all-trans retinoic acid in the treatment of acute promyelocytic leukemia. *Blood* 72:567–572, 1988.
17. Stockerl-Goldstein K BK (ed). Allogeneic hematopoietic cell transplantation for adult patients with acute myeloid leukemia. Malden, MA: Blackwell Science, 1999.
18. Brenner MK, Rill DR, Moen RC, et al. Gene-marking to trace origin of relapse after autologous bone-marrow transplantation. *Lancet* 341:85–86, 1993.
19. Chak LY, Sapozink MD, Cox RS. Extramedullary lesions in non-lymphocytic leukemia: results of radiation therapy. *Int J Radiat Oncol Biol Phys* 9:1173–1176, 1983.

20. Lichtman MA, Rowe JM. The relationship of patient age to the pathobiology of the clonal myeloid diseases. *Semin Oncol* 31:185–197, 2004.

21. Conter V, Schrappe M, Arico M, et al. Role of cranial radiotherapy for childhood T-cell acute lymphoblastic leukemia with high WBC count and good response to prednisone. Associazione Italiana Ematologia Oncologia Pediatrica and the Berlin-Frankfurt-Munster groups. *J Clin Oncol* 15:2786–2791, 1997.

22. Schrappe M, Reiter A, Ludwig WD, et al. Improved outcome in childhood acute lymphoblastic leukemia despite reduced use of anthracyclines and cranial radiotherapy: results of trial ALL-BFM 90. German-Austrian-Swiss ALL-BFM Study Group. *Blood* 95:3310–3322, 2000.

23. Dabaja BS, Ha CS, Thomas DA, et al. The role of local radiation therapy for mediastinal disease in adults with T-cell lymphoblastic lymphoma. *Cancer* 94:2738–2744, 2002.

24. Kantarjian HM, Walters RS, Keating MJ, et al. Results of the vincristine, doxorubicin, and dexamethasone regimen in adults with standard- and high-risk acute lymphocytic leukemia. *J Clin Oncol* 8:994–1004, 1990.

25. Kantarjian HM, O'Brien S, Smith TL, et al. Results of treatment with hyper-CVAD, a dose-intensive regimen, in adult acute lymphocytic leukemia. *J Clin Oncol* 18:547–561, 2000.

26. Peggs K, Mackinnon S. Imatinib mesylate—the new gold standard for treatment of chronic myeloid leukemia. *N Engl J Med* 348:1048–1050, 2003.

27. O'Brien SG, Guilhot F, Larson RA, et al. Imatinib compared with interferon and low-dose cytarabine for newly diagnosed chronic-phase chronic myeloid leukemia. *N Engl J Med* 348:994–1004, 2003.

28. Clift RA, Buckner CD, Thomas ED, et al. Marrow transplantation for chronic myeloid leukemia: a randomized study comparing cyclophosphamide and total body irradiation with busulfan and cyclophosphamide. *Blood* 84:2036–2043, 1994.

29. Deeg HJ, Flournoy N, Sullivan KM, et al. Cataracts after total body irradiation and marrow transplantation: a sparing effect of dose fractionation. *Int J Radiat Oncol Biol Phys* 10:957–964, 1984.

30. Socie G, Clift RA, Blaise D, et al. Busulfan plus cyclophosphamide compared with total-body irradiation plus cyclophosphamide before marrow transplantation for myeloid leukemia: long-term follow-up of four randomized studies. *Blood* 98:3569–3574, 2001.

31. Attal M, Harousseau JL, Facon T, et al. Single versus double autologous stem-cell transplantation for multiple myeloma. *N Engl J Med* 349:2495–2502, 2003.

32. Cervantes F, Rozman C. A multivariate analysis of prognostic factors in chronic myeloid leukemia. *Blood* 60:1298–1304, 1982.

33. Sokal JE, Baccarani M, Russo D, et al. Staging and prognosis in chronic myelogenous leukemia. *Semin Hematol* 25:49–61, 1988.

34. Interferon alfa versus chemotherapy for chronic myeloid leukemia: a meta-analysis of seven randomized trials: Chronic Myeloid Leukemia Trialists' Collaborative Group. *J Natl Cancer Inst* 89:1616–1620, 1997.

35. Kantarjian HM, Cortes JE, O'Brien S, et al. Long-term survival benefit and improved complete cytogenetic and molecular response rates with imatinib mesylate in Philadelphia chromosome-positive chronic-phase chronic myeloid leukemia after failure of interferon-alpha. *Blood* 104:1979–1988, 2004.

36. Rai KR, Peterson BL, Appelbaum FR, et al. Fludarabine compared with chlorambucil as primary therapy for chronic lymphocytic leukemia. *N Engl J Med* 343:1750–1757, 2000.

37. Chisesi T, Capnist G, Dal Fior S. Splenic irradiation in chronic lymphocytic leukemia. *Eur J Haematol* 46:202–204, 1991.

38. Guiney MJ, Liew KH, Quong GG, et al. A study of splenic irradiation in chronic lymphocytic leukemia. *Int J Radiat Oncol Biol Phys* 16:225–229, 1989.

39. Cohen HJ, Crawford J, Rao MK, et al. Racial differences in the prevalence of monoclonal gammopathy in a community-based sample of the elderly. *Am J Med* 104:439–444, 1998.
40. Ichimaru M, Ishimaru T, Mikami M, et al. Multiple myeloma among atomic bomb survivors in Hiroshima and Nagasaki, 1950–76: relationship to radiation dose absorbed by marrow. *J Natl Cancer Inst* 69:323–328, 1982.
41. Bergsagel DE, Wong O, Bergsagel PL, et al. Benzene and multiple myeloma: appraisal of the scientific evidence. *Blood* 94:1174–1182, 1999.
42. Lundberg I, Milatou-Smith R. Mortality and cancer incidence among Swedish paint industry workers with long-term exposure to organic solvents. *Scand J Work Environ Health* 24: 270–275, 1998.
43. Brown LM, Linet MS, Greenberg RS, et al. Multiple myeloma and family history of cancer among blacks and whites in the *U.S. Cancer* 85:2385–2390, 1999.
44. Grosbois B, Jego P, Attal M, et al. Familial multiple myeloma: report of fifteen families. *Br J Haematol* 105:768–770, 1999.
45. Sawyer JR, Waldron JA, Jagannath S, et al. Cytogenetic findings in 200 patients with multiple myeloma. *Cancer Genet Cytogenet* 82:41–49, 1995.
46. Barlogie B, Jagannath S, Desikan KR, et al. Total therapy with tandem transplants for newly diagnosed multiple myeloma. *Blood* 93:55–65, 1999.
47. Zhan F, Hardin J, Kordsmeier B, et al. Global gene expression profiling of multiple myeloma, monoclonal gammopathy of undetermined significance, and normal bone marrow plasma cells. *Blood* 99:1745–1757, 2002.
48. Alexiou C, Kau RJ, Dietzfelbinger H, et al. Extramedullary plasmacytoma: tumor occurrence and therapeutic concepts. *Cancer* 85:2305–2314, 1999.
49. Chauhan D, Uchiyama H, Urashima M, et al. Regulation of interleukin 6 in multiple myeloma and bone marrow stromal cells. *Stem Cells* 13 Suppl 2:35–39, 1995.
50. Dankbar B, Padro T, Leo R, et al. Vascular endothelial growth factor and interleukin-6 in paracrine tumor-stromal cell interactions in multiple myeloma. *Blood* 95:2630–2636, 2000.
51. Hideshima T, Chauhan D, Hayashi T, et al. The biological sequelae of stromal cell-derived factor-1alpha in multiple myeloma. *Mol Cancer Ther* 1:539–544, 2002.
52. Brenne AT, Ro TB, Waage A, et al. Interleukin-21 is a growth and survival factor for human myeloma cells. *Blood* 99:3756–3762, 2002.
53. Bataille R, Durie BG, Grenier J, et al. Prognostic factors and staging in multiple myeloma: a reappraisal. *J Clin Oncol* 4:80–87, 1986.
54. Liebross RH, Ha CS, Cox JD, et al. Clinical course of solitary extramedullary plasmacytoma. *Radiother Oncol* 52:245–249, 1999.
55. Liebross RH, Ha CS, Cox JD, et al. Solitary bone plasmacytoma: outcome and prognostic factors following radiotherapy. *Int J Radiat Oncol Biol Phys* 41:1063–1067, 1998.
56. Catell D, Kogen Z, Donahue B, et al. Multiple myeloma of an extremity: must the entire bone be treated? *Int J Radiat Oncol Biol Phys* 40:117–119, 1998.
57. Gregory WM, Richards MA, Malpas JS. Combination chemotherapy versus melphalan and prednisolone in the treatment of multiple myeloma: an overview of published trials. *J Clin Oncol* 10:334–342, 1992.
58. Alexanian R, Barlogie B, Dixon D. High-dose glucocorticoid treatment of resistant myeloma. *Ann Intern Med* 105:8–11, 1986.
59. Weber D, Rankin K, Gavino M, et al. Thalidomide alone or with dexamethasone for previously untreated multiple myeloma. *J Clin Oncol* 21:16–19, 2003.
60. Richardson PG, Barlogie B, Berenson J, et al. A phase II study of bortezomib in relapsed, refractory myeloma. *N Engl J Med* 348:2609–2617, 2003.

51. Child JA, Morgan GJ, Davies FE, et al. High-dose chemotherapy with hematopoietic stem-cell rescue for multiple myeloma. *N Engl J Med* 348:1875–1883, 2003.
52. Barlogie B, Jagannath S, Vesole DH, et al. Superiority of tandem autologous transplantation over standard therapy for previously untreated multiple myeloma. *Blood* 89:789–793, 1997.
53. Attal M, Harousseau JL, Stoppa AM, et al. A prospective, randomized trial of autologous bone marrow transplantation and chemotherapy in multiple myeloma. Intergroupe Francais du Myelome. *N Engl J Med* 335:91–97, 1996.
54. Attal M, Harousseau JL, Facon T, et al. Single versus double autologous stem-cell transplantation for multiple myeloma. *N Engl J Med* 349:2495–2502, 2003.
55. Leigh BR, Kurtts TA, Mack CF, et al. Radiation therapy for the palliation of multiple myeloma. *Int J Radiat Oncol Biol Phys* 25:801–804, 1993.
56. Mill WB, Griffith R. The role of radiation therapy in the management of plasma cell tumors. *Cancer* 45:647–652, 1980.
57. Moreau P, Facon T, Attal M, et al. Comparison of 200 mg/m(2) melphalan and 8 Gy total body irradiation plus 140 mg/m(2) melphalan as conditioning regimens for peripheral blood stem-cell transplantation in patients with newly diagnosed multiple myeloma: final analysis of the Intergroupe Francophone du Myelome 9502 randomized trial. *Blood* 99:731–735, 2002.
58. Hu K, Yahalom J. Radiotherapy in the management of plasma cell tumors. *Oncology* (Williston Park) 14:101–108, 111; discussion 111–112, 115, 2000.
59. Mendenhall CM, Thar TL, Million RR. Solitary plasmacytoma of bone and soft tissue. *Int J Radiat Oncol Biol Phys* 6:1497–1501, 1980.
60. Ozsahin M, Tsang RW, Poortmans P, et al. Outcomes and patterns of failure in solitary plasmacytoma: a multicenter Rare Cancer Network study of 258 patients. *Int J Radiat Oncol Biol Phys* 64:210–217, 2006.
61. Tsang RW, Gospodarowicz MK, Pintilie M, et al. Solitary plasmacytoma treated with radiotherapy: impact of tumor size on outcome. *Int J Radiat Oncol Biol Phys* 50:113–120, 2001.
62. Wilder RB, Ha CS, Cox JD, et al. Persistence of myeloma protein for more than one year after radiotherapy is an adverse prognostic factor in solitary plasmacytoma of bone. *Cancer* 94:1532–1537, 2002.
63. Knowling MA, Harwood AR, Bergsagel DE. Comparison of extramedullary plasmacytomas with solitary and multiple plasma cell tumors of bone. *J Clin Oncol* 1:255–262, 1983.
64. Susnerwala SS, Shanks JH, Banerjee SS, et al. Extramedullary plasmacytoma of the head and neck region: clinicopathological correlation in 25 cases. *Br J Cancer* 75:921–927, 1997.
65. Bolek TW, Marcus RB, Mendenhall NP. Solitary plasmacytoma of bone and soft tissue. *Int J Radiat Oncol Biol Phys* 36:329–333, 1996.

# 37
# Benign Diseases
*Prabhakar Tripuraneni, MD*

## OVERVIEW

Although the use of radiation therapy in benign diseases has declined, it is useful in carefully selected situations.

## INTRODUCTION

The exact use of radiation therapy in benign diseases is unknown in the United States. It appears to vary significantly in different parts of the country and throughout the world. Until recently, the practice of vascular brachytherapy (VBT) was the most dominant use of radiotherapy in benign diseases beginning in the early 2000s.[1] The need for VBT has dropped significantly due to the advent of drug eluting stents (DES).

## ANATOMY

All organs and systems of the body may be involved.

## PATHOLOGY

These conditions range from chronic inflammatory conditions to hyperproliferative disorders to benign non-malignant disorders.

## RISK FACTORS

There are no known universal risk factors for benign diseases treated with radiotherapy.

## PRESENTATION/WORKUP

It is common practice that patients with benign conditions are referred for radiotherapy after the usual treatment schema are exhausted or there exists a high risk of recurrence of that benign condition. Certain groups of patients with high risk of heterotopic ossification (HO) are evaluated, and those with high-risk factors such as ankylosing spondylitis (AS), diffuse idiopathic skeletal hyperostosis (DISH), or exuberant osteoarthritis, are given consideration for pre or postoperative radiotherapy for the prevention of HO.

## INFORMED CONSENT

The informed consent must be written in clear, unambiguous language understandable to a lay person. The patient must be made aware of the benign nature of the condition, the multiple treatment options available and tried, the rationale for proposing radiotherapy with available alternatives including the pros and cons for each of them, along with the potential long range effects of radiation, especially carcinogenesis.

Guidelines for offering radiation therapy for benign conditions:[2]

1. Determine the consequence of no treatment and the natural history of the disease.
2. Determine the alternative methods of treatment and the risk benefit ratio regarding radiation therapy and other treatments.
3. Consider radiation therapy if the conventional treatment has not succeeded in alleviating the condition. If the risk of other therapies is greater than the risk of radiation therapy and the potential consequence of no further treatment is unacceptable, then radiation therapy may be considered.
4. Determine the potential long-term risk of radiation therapy, taking into consideration the type of radiation, dose, fractionation schema, underlying organs at risk, underlying disease, and age of the patient.
5. Informed consent must include the potential long-range risks along with the usual components of informed consent.

## BIOLOGY

The most common examples of radiotherapy in benign diseases are vascular brachytherapy for in-stent restenosis, radiotherapy for the prevention of heterotopic ossification, and radiotherapy for the prevention of keloid formation. These three conditions are unique in the sense that they are considered hyperproliferative disorders, usually triggered by the injury of stenting or further surgery. Usually, the condition recurs within 6–18 months of the procedure. With relatively modest doses of radiation therapy applied immediately prior to or immediately after the procedure, they are highly preventable.

## MANAGEMENT

This category covers a wide range of conditions. The common conditions in which radiotherapy is implemented will be reviewed. For uncommon conditions, the reader is referred to the book on radiation therapy in benign diseases or the exhaustive chapter in the text book on radiation oncology.[1,2]

### Coronary In-Stent Restenosis

During the last decade, brachytherapy was extensively tested in decreasing in-stent restenosis in rigorously controlled double blind randomized trials enrolling more than 2,000 patients over a span of 5 years.[3,4,5] With vascular brachytherapy, repeat in-stent restenosis was decreased from about 40% to 10% in several trials. In fact, all of the trials testing various systems with different isotopes testing the efficacy of brachytherapy in reducing in-stent restenosis were all positive with significant decrease in target lesion revascularization. Based on the above trials, the FDA has given its approval for the use of vascular brachytherapy in coronary in-stent restenosis for three different systems. Neointimal hyperplasia was thought to be a cause of in-stent restenosis. The radiation therapy is applied immediately after the repeat angioplasty during the same procedure in the cardiac catheterization lab. During the peak use of vascular brachytherapy, it is estimated that 60,000 procedures were done in the United States to decrease repeat in-stent restenosis. In the early

2000s, drug eluting stents that have proven to significantly decrease the incidence of in-stent restenosis were introduced into the market, thereby significantly reducing, if not eliminating the need for vascular brachytherapy. This is an excellent example of a new innovation in medicine eliminating categories of standards of practice.

The Beta-Cath system is the only system currently manufactured for in-stent restenosis. $^{90}$Sr is a pure β emitter with a 28.5-year half life and 546-KeV maximum β energy. The Beta-Cath system contains sources that are 0.6 mm in diameter and 2.5 mm in length. Source trains of 12 seeds (30 mm), 16 seeds (40 mm), and 24 seeds (60 mm) are commercially available. A nonradioactive marker seed is located both proximally and distally to the radioactive sources. This helps with fluoroscopic verification of the position of the radioactive seeds and allows verification of the return of the sources to the delivery device. For lesions longer than 60 mm, a "pullback technique" is used where the most distal portion of the lesion is treated first, then the catheter is carefully pulled back to treat the more proximal lesion.

The Beta-Cath system consists of four main components: the source train, transfer device, delivery catheter, and accessories. The sources are stored in a hand-held transfer device and are advanced by a closed-loop hydraulic system that uses sterile water to advance (and then retract) the sources. The advantage of the Beta-Cath system is the relatively short treatment times (3 to 5 minutes) and the absence of radiation exposure to catheterization laboratory staff. The long half life of the isotope permits the sources to be exchanged once every 6 months, with no need to change the treatment times during that 6-month period. A potential disadvantage of this system is the inferior depth–dose gradient compared with the γ source, attenuation by calcifications or stents, and the lack of utility in larger vessels.

A dose of 18.4 Gy is prescribed at 2-mm radius at the center of the source axis for vessels with a reference diameter between 2.7 mm–3.3 mm. For reference diameters between 3.4 mm–4 mm, a dose of 23 Gy is prescribed.[4] The gross target volume is the stenotic area itself. The clinical target volume is the dilated part of the vessel. The planning target includes at least 5 mm proximal and distal to the clinical target volume.

With the widespread use of drug eluting stents and longer follow-ups, a few drug resistant in-stent restenosis occurrences are seen. They are initially treated with the alternating drug-coated stent such as Rapamycin- or Paclitaxel-coated stents. After the second failure, patients are considered for vascular brachytherapy after repeat recanalization of the coronary vessel. With multiple failures prior to vascular brachytherapy, this group of patients is probably at a higher risk for sub-acute thrombosis and may need to be on prolonged periods of platelet inhibitors such as Plavix. The vascular brachytherapy in DES resistant in-stent restenosis appears to be effective in scattered individual studies and prospective collection of the longitudinal data in progress.

The TAXUS V study and the SISR randomized trials demonstrate that DES may be superior to VBT in treating coronary in-stent restenosis.[5] Nevertheless, there may be circumstances where VBT continues to play a role, such as in drug-resistant in-stent restenosis, bifurcation lesions, small-diameter vessels, and for treatment of recurrent, multi-DES resistant restenosis.[6,7]

## Peripheral Vessel Stenosis and In-Stent Restenosis

Peripheral vascular disease (PVD) involves more organs than CAD, hence there are more diverse clinical situations, manifestations, and end points. Unlike coronary vessels, most peripheral vessels have a diameter greater than 3 mm, and, in fact, generally range from approximately 7 to 10 mm. Peripheral vascular lesions tend to be much longer and are more likely to be multifocal. Compared with trials in CAD, peripheral vascular disease clinical trials testing the efficacy of VBT in reducing restenosis are in their early stages. VBT has now been tried in numerous sites outside of the coronary arteries including vein grafts, renal artery in-stent restenosis, femoropopliteal

**FIGURE 37-1** BetaCath system.

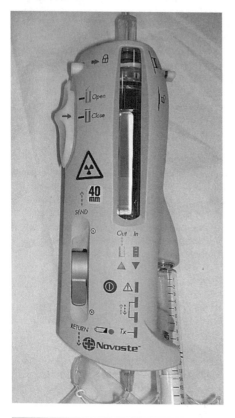

arteries, and even the carotid arteries.[8] The Vienna II and III trials, single-institution randomized trials, supported its efficacy in PVD. However, other trials have shown mixed results, particularly in high-risk patients. The multinational PARIS trial testing the efficacy of vascular brachytherapy in reducing femoral popliteal stenosis was a negative trial. Currently, there are no clinical trials nor any approved systems available in the United States to treat peripheral vascular disease with radiation therapy.

## HETEROTOPIC OSSIFICATION

HO is most common around periacetabular regions, occurring in those patients with exuberant osteoarthritis, following trauma, or previous hip replacements. The risk of forming HO is significantly higher in patients with Ankylosing spondylitis, DISH, etc. Approximately one third of patients with HO have limited hip movement and associated pain. Corticosteroids and nonsteroidal anti-inflammatory drugs were used with limited success in patients with minimal HO. Prophylactic radiation therapy, delivered either immediately before or after usual hip replacement surgery is very effective in preventing HO. Traditional doses of a single fraction of 7–8 Gy or fractionated 10–20 Gy in the immediate perioperative period was found to be effective.[9] Randomized trials comparing preoperative radiation therapy within 4 hours before surgery and postoperative radiotherapy appear to be equally effective. A single dose of 7 Gy delivered preoperatively appears to be as effective as postoperative fractionated radiotherapy delivered within 72 hours from surgery.[10] The dose response has been established indicating that 7 Gy single fraction is more effective than a single fraction of 5.5 Gy. In general, with the above data, the common practice is to deliver a single fraction of 7 Gy preoperatively within 4 hours of surgery, as it is less traumatic for the patient and easier to deliver. In cases where preoperative radiotherapy is not feasible, postoperative radiotherapy within 72 hours of surgery either at a single fraction of 7–8 Gy or fractionated radiotherapy are also effective.

## KELOIDS

Keloids form after skin trauma with excessive production of fibrous tissue that extends beyond the wound, becomes hyalinized and does not regress spontaneously. In susceptible individuals, keloids can occur after infection, burns, and more commonly after surgical wounds. Scars on the

**FIGURE 37-2** Field for preoperative radiotherapy for heterotopic ossification.

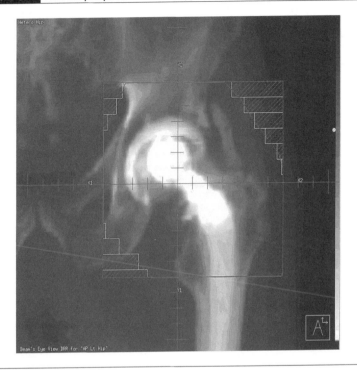

sternal region, shoulders, and back are more likely to spread, as are lobular masses after ear piercing. The usual treatment is excision along with local injection of steroids and/or immediate postoperative radiation therapy. The fields are usually tailored to the surgical excision bed with custom cutouts and low energy electrons with appropriate bolus. The doses are 10–15 Gy delivered in 2–5 fractions starting within 24 hours of surgery.[11] With immediate postoperative radiation therapy, the local controls are in the range of 70%–90%. Studies have confirmed the dose response rates with local control of 40% with less than 9 Gy, and 77% with more than 9 Gy. There appears to be a trend for slightly better local control at doses of 15 Gy.[12]

## DESMOID TUMORS/AGGRESSIVE FIBROMATOSIS

These are low-grade-locally invasive, nonmetastasizing tumors of connective tissue origin, probably related to other fibromatoses such as keloids. Aggressive surgical resection with wide margins is the treatment of choice and the reported recurrence rates after surgery are in the 30% range. Recurrences are usually salvaged with repeat resection with or without postoperative radiation therapy. If the lesion is inoperable or requires mutilating surgery, then radiation therapy alone is an effective option. The recommended doses for either gross disease or microscopic disease are the same and are in the range of 50–60 Gy in 6 to 7 weeks. The irradiation portals should be generous with wide margins. The local control rates are in the range of 70% to 85%.[13]

## PTERYGIUM

After surgical excision of pterygium, the recurrence rate is approximately 20%–30%. Several studies have confirmed the benefit of immediate postoperative radiation therapy delivered within 8 hours or so in decreasing the recurrences. The typical application of radiotherapy is with beta irradiation using a dose of 20 Gy as a single fraction to multiple fraction regimens such as three weekly fractions of 8 Gy each, starting in the immediate postoperative period.[14,15] Recurrent pterygia can also be treated with immediate postoperative radiotherapy with three weekly fractions of 10 Gy with good local control.

## EXOPHTHALMOS

The pathogenesis of Grave's Exophthalmos is thought to be due to activated T lymphocytes invading orbit and stimulating glycosaminoglycan production in fibroblasts, resulting in edema and enlargement of extraocular muscles. The usual presentation consists of bilateral exophthalmos, extraocular muscle dysfunction, diplopia, blurred vision, chemosis, lid lag, eye lid and periorbital edema, and compressive optic neuropathy. Radiation therapy is most effective in the soft tissue symptoms such as redness, chemosis, edema, etc. The response rates of various symptoms range from 40% to 80%. In more than 75% of patients, the steroids can usually be discontinued after radiation therapy. A randomized study of prednisone and radiation therapy in moderately severe Grave's Exophthalmos confirmed almost equally successful outcomes of about 50%. Side effects during prednisone administration were more common and severe than those observed with radiation therapy.[16,17] Small opposed lateral fields with a split beam or five-degree posterior angulation to avoid dose to lens with megavoltage are used. Immobilization, CT-based treatment planning, and beam shaping are used to minimize radiation beyond the retro-orbital region. A dose of 20 Gy at midplane in 10 fractions is effective. Higher doses do not seem to improve the outcome.

## GYNECOMASTIA

Gynecomastia is a common side effect of estrogen or Casodex® administration. A study was done on patients starting estrogen therapy whereby one breast was irradiated while the other breast was not irradiated, but kept as a control. Gynecomastia occurred in 90% of nonirradiated breasts and in only 17% of irradiated breasts. Radiation therapy of breast tissue to prevent gynecomastia involves treating with 9–12 MeV electrons with 6–10-cm diameter circular cutouts or tangential photon fields to a dose of 12–15 Gy in 3 fractions.[18] It is reasonable to start hormone therapy a few days after the completion of radiation therapy. For those patients who have developed painful gynecomastia, radiation therapy to a dose of 20 Gy in 5 fractions would be a consideration and offer good symptomatic relief.[19]

## OVARIAN CASTRATION

Ovarian castration has been used in patients with breast cancer. Pelvic irradiation to a dose of 14 Gy in 4 fractions is quite effective in ovarian ablation in premenopausal women of 40 years or older. For women younger than 40, higher doses are needed to ablate. The recommended dose is 20 Gy in 10 fractions with anterior and posterior fields with adequate coverage to include the variation of ovarian position.[20]

## FUTURE DIRECTIONS

The use of radiotherapy in benign conditions should be applied very judiciously and will most likely continue to remain at very low usage levels, as it should be. The development of vascular brachytherapy in a short span of 5 years in the context of randomized clinical trials is a shining example of an introduction to new applications of radiation therapy and serves as an excellent model for any potential future applications of radiotherapy.

# REFERENCES

1. Perez, CA, Brady LW, Halperin EC et al (eds). *Principles and Practice of Radiation Oncology.* Philidelphia: Lippincott, Williams, & Wilkins, 2004; pp 2332–2351.

2. Order SE, Donaldson SS (eds) in *Radiation Therapy of Benign Diseases,* Springer Verlag, 1998.

3. Tripuraneni P. Coronary artery radiation therapy for the prevention of restenosis after percutaneous coronary angioplasty, II: outcomes of clinical trials. *Semin Radiat Oncol* 2002; 12: 17–30.

4. Suntharalingam M, Laskey W, Lansky W, et al. Analysis of clinical outcomes from the START and START 40 trials: the efficacy of Sr-90 radiation in the treatment of long lesion in-stent restenosis. *Int J Radiat Oncol Biol Phys* 2001; 51[Suppl 3]: 142.

5. Popma JJ, Suntharanlingam M, Lansky AJ, et al. Randomized trial of 90Sr/90Y b radiation versus placebo control for treatment of in-stent restenosis. *Circulation* 2002; 106: 1090–1096.

6. Stone GW, Ellis SC, O'Shaughnessy CD, et al. Paclitaxel-eluting stents versus vascular brachytherapy for in-stent restenosis within bare metal stents: the TAXUS V ISR randomized trial. *JAMA* 2006; 295:1253–1263.

7. Tripuraneni P. The future of CART in the era of drug-eluting stents: it's not over until it's over. Counterpoint. *Brachytherapy* 2003; 2:74–76.

8. Tripuraneni P, Giap H, Jani S. Endovascular brachytherapy for peripheral vascular disease. *Semin Radiat Oncol* 1999; 9:190–212.

9. Lo Tc, Healy WL, Covall DJ et al. Heterotopic bone formation after hip surgery: prevention with single-dose postoperative irradiation. *Radiology* 1988; 168:851.

10. Seegenschmiedt MH, Martus P, Goldmann AR et al. Preoperative versus postoperative radiotherapy for prevention of heterotopic ossification: first results of a randomized trial in high risk patients. *Int J Radiat Oncol Biol Phys.* 1994; 30:63.

11. Dornobos DB, Stoffel TJ, Hass AC et al. The role of kilovoltage irradiation in the treatment of keloids. *Int J Radiat Oncol Biol Phy* 1990; 18:833.

12. Kovalic JJ, Perez CA. Radition therapy following keloidectomy. A 20-year experience. *Int J Radiat Oncol Biol Phy* 1989; 17:77.

13. Leibel SA, Wara WM, Hill DR, et al. Desmoid tumors: local control and patterns of relapse following radiation therapy. *Int J Radiat Oncol Biol Phys* 1983; 9:1167.

14. Paryani SB, Scott WP, Well JW et al. Management of pterygium with surgery and radiation therapy. *Int J Radiat Oncol Biol Phy* 1994; 28:101.

15. Cooper JS. postoperative irradiation of pterygia. Ten more years of experience. *Radiology* 1978; 128:753.

16. Petersen IA, Kriss JP, McDougall IR et al. Prognostic factors in the treatment of Grave's ophthalmopathy. *Int J Radiat Oncol Biol Phy* 1990; 19:259.

17. Prummel MF, Mourits MP, Blank L et al. Randomized double blind trial of prednisone versus radiotherapy in Grave's ophthalmopathy. *Lancet* 1993; 343:949.

18. Alftahn O, Holsti LR. Prevention of gynecomastia by local roentgen irradiation in estrogen treated prostate carcinomas. *Scand J Urol Nephrol* 1969; 3:183.

19. Chou JL, Easley JD, Feldmeier JJ et al. Effective radiotherapy in palliation mammalgia associated with gynecomastia after DES therapy. *Int J Radiat Oncol Biol Phys* 1988; 15:749.

20. Leung SF, Tsao SY, Teo PM et al. Ovarian ablation failures by radiationp: a comparison of two dose schedules. *Br J Rdiol* 1991; 64:537.

# Index

**Note:** page numbers followed by f, t, or b denote figures, tables, or boxes respectively

# H

## O

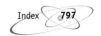

# Color Plates

| **Tonsil cancer: unilateral neck treatment.**

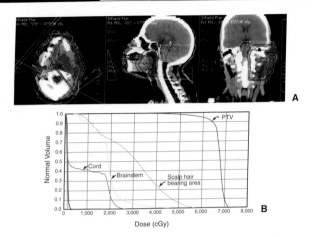

**(A)** Tonsil cancer. Unilateral neck treatment technique. The patient is a 50-year-old female who had a T2N0 left tonsil cancer and was treated unilaterally. She was treated with a three-field plan to minimize dose to the contralateral parotid.

**(B)** Dose-volume histogram of this plan showing good coverage of the target volume and adequate protection of the surrounding normal structures.

| **Intensity modulated radiation therapy for oropharynx cancer.**

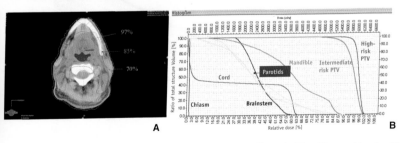

**(A)** Intensity modulated radiation therapy for oropharynx cancer. The patient is a 62-year-old male with a T2N2bM0 squamous cell carcinoma of the left base of tongue who received chemoradiation with IMRT to a dose of 60 Gy to the primary and involved nodes and 54 Gy elective treatment to the contralateral neck and three cycles of concurrent cisplatin. Subsequently, he underwent planned neck dissection and brachytherapy implant boost to 20 Gy.

**(B)** Dose volume histogram shows that 95% of the PTV's received the intended dose, respecting the dose tolerance of the parotids and normal critical structures.

**COLOR PLATE 3: FIGURE 13-1**

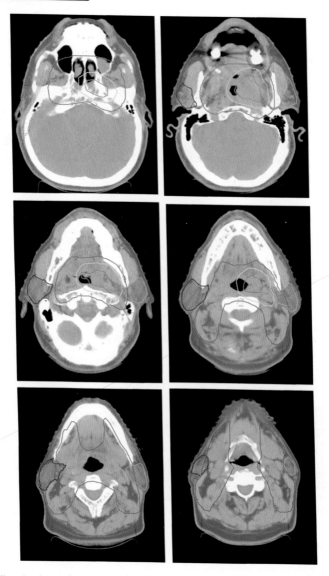

Target delineation for a T2bN0M0 nasopharyngeal carcinoma receiving definitive IMRT. GTV, light blue; PTV70, yellow; PTV59.4, red; right parotid gland, dark blue; left parotid gland, orange.

From Bortfeld T, Schmidt-Ulrich, De Neve W, Wazer D: Image-Guided IMRT. Springer Berlin Heidelberg 2006: 324.

**COLOR PLATE 4: FIGURE 19-2** | IMRT distribution on axial perspective and DVH.

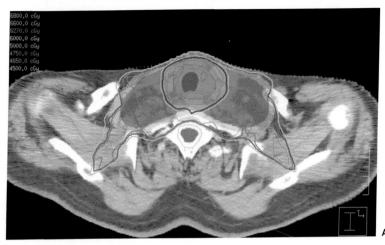

**A**

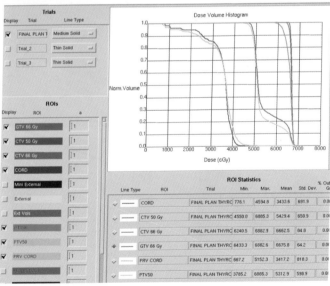

**B**

A 58-year-old man with 5 cm papillary thyroid carcinoma, invading into the trachea (pT4N1aM0), treated with total thyroidectomy, shave excision of disease from trachea, and RAI (150 mCi). External beam IMRT plan, for 50 Gy to thyroid bed and adjacent lymph nodes, with boost 16 Gy to area of tracheal invasion. Seven fields of 6 MV at the following gantry angles: 0, 40, 120, 160, 200, 240, and 320. **(A)** Axial Isodose Distribution (CTV$_{50Gy}$ is shaded blue, and CTV$_{66Gy}$ is shaded orange). **(B)** Dose Volume Histograms for the Clinical Target Volumes, and Spinal Cord.

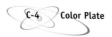

**COLOR PLATE 5: FIGURE 20-5** | Isodose plan showing improved homogeneity with the use of IMRT.

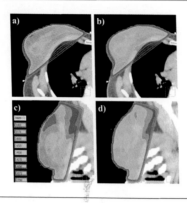

**COLOR PLATE 6: FIGURE 21-5** | Technique for postmastectomy radiation.

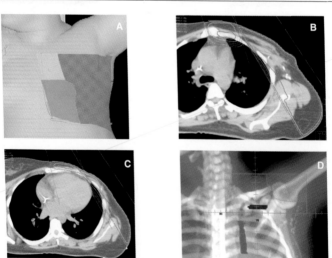

Radiation fields used to treat the chest wall, internal mammary lymph nodes and axillary apex/supraclavicular fossa in a patient who had undergone a left modified radical mastectomy. **(A)** shows a skin rendering of the radiation fields used to treat the chest wall and internal mammary lymph nodes. Two electron fields were used over the medial chest wall with a higher energy selected for the upper three interspaces to treat the internal mammary lymph nodes **(B)** axial image and a lower energy selected over the heat **(C)** axial image. The lateral chest wall is treated with matched tangential photon beams to nicely shape the radiation dose distribution around the heart and thoracic structures. The axillary apex/supraclavicular fields are shown in **(D)**. The level III region of the axillary and the upper internal mammary vessels have been contoured on axial CT images and reconstructed on this image. They are used to determine depth of dose prescription.

**COLOR PLATE 7: FIGURE 22-1** AP and lateral digital radiograph reconstructions of treatment fields for patient with pancreatic head cancer.

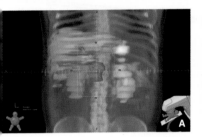
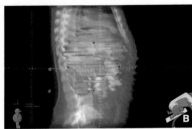

**COLOR PLATE 8: FIGURE 25-2** Anal cancer DRR's for an AP/PA plan.

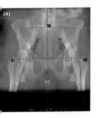
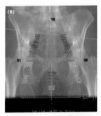
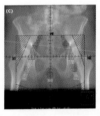
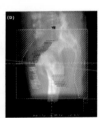

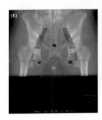
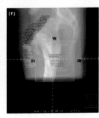
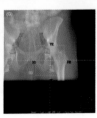

(A) AP pelvic field to 30.6 Gy. (B) PA pelvic field to 30.6 Gy. (C) AP pelvic field to 45 Gy. Femoral head tolerance must be calculated and should not exceed 45 Gy. (D) Lateral pelvic field to 30.6 Gy. (E) Example of a 4-field boost to the primary anal cancer. AP field shown. (F) Boost to the primary tumor. Lateral field shown. (G) Boost to positive inguinal lymph node..

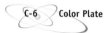

**COLOR PLATE 9: FIGURE 26-1A** Isodose coverage for small pelvic fields.

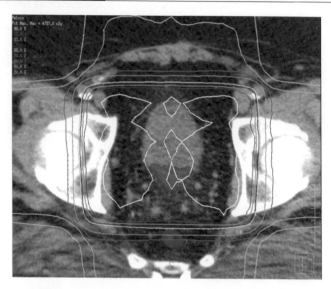

Note that the anterior coverage includes the entire bladder plus margin, but does ot provide comprehensive coverage for the exteral or internal iliac nodal chains. The patient has voided prior to the simulation.

**COLOR PLATE 10: FIGURE 26-1B** Bladder tumor boost volume.

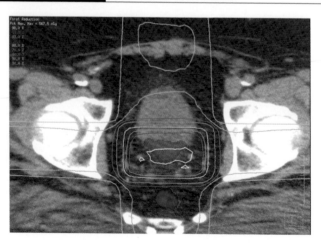

Tumor contour includes imaging evidence of involvement augmented by the urologist's tumor diagram from the pre-treatment cystoscopy. Though prior to the simulation the patient has voided, still much of the anterior portion of the bladder h as been excluded from the high-dose region.

**COLOR PLATE 11: FIGURE 28-6**   IMRT treatment planning constraints.

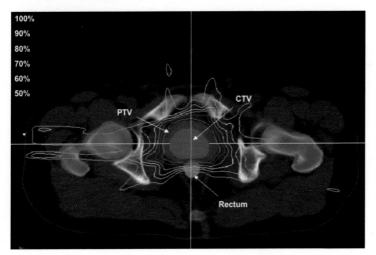

## IMRT Treatment Planning Constraints

### DVH Criteria

1. CTV $D_{100\%}$ = 100%
2. PTV $D_{100\%}$ > 95%
3. Rectal $V_{40Gy}$ < 35%
4. Rectal $V_{65Gy}$ < 17%
5. Bladder $V_{40Gy}$ < 50%
6. Bladder $V_{65Gy}$ < 25%
7. Femoral Head $V_{50Gy}$ < 10%

### Spatial Criteria

1. The 90% dose line encompasses no more than the half-width of the rectum on any axial cut.
2. The 50% dose line does not encompass the full-rectum width.
3. The posterior edge of the CTV to the prescription isodose line is ~3 to 8 mm.

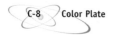

## COLOR PLATE 12: FIGURE 31-3A

Anterior DRR showing volume and fields for preoperative radiotherapy.

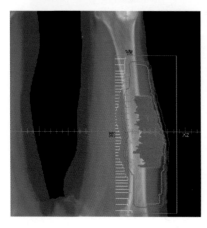

GTV—gross tumor volume (red), CTV—clinical target voume (green), PTV—planning target volume (blue).

## COLOR PLATE 13: FIGURE 31-3B

DRR showing postoperative field and volume outlined.

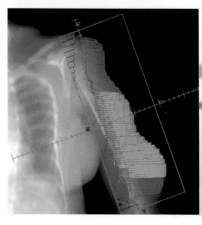

"High risk" CTV—clinical target voume (orange) in this situation includes the pre-operative GTV and volume considered to be most at risk of recurrence; CTV—clinical target volume (purple) which will include the entire surgical bed and scars.

## COLOR PLATE 14: FIGURE 32-2    Anterior portals in a CT planned patient with Wilm's tumor requiring both flank and whole lung radiotherapy.

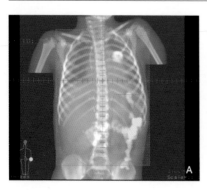

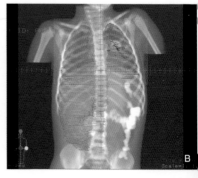

**(A)** The independent jaw was closed for the last fraction after 10.5 Gy at 1.5 Gy per fraction was given to the larger field to bring the lung dose to 12 Gy **(B)**.